Treatments of Psychiatric Disorders

Third Edition

Treatments of Psychiatric Disorders

Third Edition

VOLUME 1

Glen O. Gabbard, M.D.
Editor-in-Chief

American Psychiatric Publishing, Inc.

Washington, DC
London, England

Note: The authors have worked to ensure that all information in this book concerning drug dosages, schedules, and routes of administration is accurate as of the time of publication and consistent with standards set by the U.S. Food and Drug Administration and the general medical community. As medical research and practice advance, however, therapeutic standards may change. For this reason and because human and mechanical errors sometimes occur, we recommend that readers follow the advice of a physician who is directly involved in their care or the care of a member of their family. A product's current package insert should be consulted for full prescribing and safety information.

Manufactured in the United States of America on acid-free paper

04 03 02 01 4 3 2 1
Third Edition

American Psychiatric Press, Inc.
1400 K Street, N.W.
Washington, DC 20005
www.appi.org

Library of Congress Cataloging-in-Publication Data
Treatments of psychiatric disorders / Glen O. Gabbard, editor-in-chief.—3rd ed.
p. ; cm.
Includes bibliographical references and index.
ISBN 0-88048-910-3 (v. 1 : alk. paper) — ISBN 0-88048-911-1 (v. 2 : alk. paper)
1. Mental illness—Treatment. I Gabbard, Glen O.
[DNLM: 1. Mental Disorders—therapy. WM 400 T7866 2001]
RC480.T69 2001
616.89'1—dc21

00-050815

British Library Cataloguing in Publication Data
A CIP record is available from the British Library.

The correct citation for this book is *Treatments of Psychiatric Disorders*, 3rd Edition, Volumes 1 & 2. Gabbard GO, Editor-in-Chief. Washington, DC, American Psychiatric Press, 2001.

Contents

VOLUME 1

Section 1

General Considerations in Psychiatric Treatment

Section Editor: Glen O. Gabbard, M.D.

Section 2

Disorders Usually First Diagnosed in Infancy, Childhood, or Adolescence

Section Editors: John F. McDermott Jr., M.D., and Elizabeth B. Weller, M.D.

Section 4

Substance-Related Disorders

Section Editors: Herbert D. Kleber, M.D., and Marc Galanter, M.D.

Section 5

Schizophrenia and Other Psychotic Disorders

Section Editors: Richard L. Munich, M.D., and Carol A. Tamminga, M.D.

The complete index can be found at the end of each volume.

VOLUME 2

Section 6

Mood Disorders

Section Editor: A. John Rush, M.D.

Section 7

Anxiety Disorders, Dissociative Disorders, and Adjustment Disorders

Section Editors: David Spiegel, M.D., Lisa Mellman, M.D., and Franklin R. Schneier, M.D.

Section 8

Somatoform and Factitious Disorders

Section Editor: Charles V. Ford, M.D.

Section 9

Sexual and Gender Identity Disorders

Section Editors: R. Taylor Segraves, M.D., Ph.D., and Stephen B. Levine, M.D.

Section 10

Eating Disorders

Section Editors: Katherine A. Halmi, M.D., and Paul E. Garfinkel, M.D., F.R.C.P.C.

Section 11

Personality Disorders

Section Editors: John G. Gunderson, M.D., and Glen O. Gabbard, M.D.

Section 12

Sleep Disorders

Section 13

Disorders of Impulse Control

The complete index can be found at the end of each volume.

Contributors

Gene G. Abel, M.D.
Director, Behavioral Medicine Institute of Atlanta, and Professor of Clinical Psychiatry, Emory University School of Medicine and Morehouse School of Medicine, Atlanta, Georgia

W. Stewart Agras, M.D., F.R.C.P.C.
Department of Psychiatry and Behavioral Sciences, Stanford University School of Medicine, Stanford, California

Thomas F. Anders, M.D.
Professor, Department of Psychiatry, and Executive Associate Dean, University of California–Davis School of Medicine, Sacramento, California

David B. Arciniegas, M.D.
Assistant Professor, Departments of Psychiatry and Neurology, University of Colorado Health Sciences Center, and Research Associate Physician, Denver Veterans Affairs Medical Center, Denver, Colorado

Lesley M. Arnold, M.D.
Associate Professor of Psychiatry and Director, Division of Women's Health Research, Department of Psychiatry, University of Cincinnati College of Medicine, Cincinnati, Ohio

Joan Rosenbaum Asarnow, Ph.D.
Professor of Psychiatry and Biobehavioral Sciences, University of California–Los Angeles, Neuropsychiatric Institute, Los Angeles, California

Adam Keller Ashton, M.D.
Clinical Associate Professor of Psychiatry, Department of Psychiatry, State University of New York at Buffalo, School of Medicine, Buffalo, New York

Richard Balon, M.D.
Professor of Psychiatry, Department of Psychiatry and Behavioral Neurosciences, Wayne State University School of Medicine, Detroit, Michigan

Kimberly Barrett, Ed.D.
Senior Lecturer, Department of Psychology, University of Washington, Seattle, Washington

Douglas Beer, M.D.
Assistant Professor, Department of Psychiatry and Human Behavior, Brown University School of Medicine, Butler Hospital, Providence, Rhode Island

Joseph H. Beitchman, M.D.
Professor and Head, Division of Child Psychiatry, University of Toronto, Toronto, Ontario, Canada

Tami Benton, M.D.
Director of Clinical Services, Department of Child and Adolescent Psychiatry, The Children's Hospital of Philadelphia, and Department of Psychiatry, University of Pennsylvania, Philadelphia, Pennsylvania

Joseph Biederman, M.D.
Chief, Joint Program in Pediatric Psychopharmacology, Massachusetts General Hospital and McLean Hospital, Harvard Medical School, and Professor of Psychiatry, Department of Psychiatry, Harvard Medical School, Boston, Massachusetts

Daryl L. Bohac, Ph.D.
Assistant Professor of Psychiatry, Department of Psychiatry, University of Nebraska Medical Center, Omaha, Nebraska

Lisa Borg, M.D.
Senior Research Associate, Laboratory on the Biology of Addictive Diseases, The Rockefeller University, and Clinical Assistant Professor of Psychiatry in Medicine, Weill Medical College of Cornell University, New York, New York

Thomas D. Borkovec, Ph.D.
Distinguished Professor of Psychology, Department of Psychology, Penn State University, University Park, Pennsylvania

Kathleen T. Brady, M.D., Ph.D.
Professor of Psychiatry, Department of Psychiatry and Behavioral Sciences, Center for Drug and Alcohol Programs, Medical University of South Carolina, Charleston, South Carolina

George R. Brown, M.D.
Chief of Psychiatry and Director of Psychiatric Research, Department of Psychiatry, Mountain Home Veterans Affairs Medical Center; Professor of Psychiatry, Department of Psychiatry, and Associate Chairman, East Tennessee State University, Johnson City, Tennessee

Thomas M. Brown, M.D.
Chief, Investigational Psychopharmacology, Alamo Mental Health Group, Christus Primary CareNet of Texas, San Antonio, Texas

William J. Burke, M.D.
Professor of Psychiatry, Department of Psychiatry, University of Nebraska Medical Center, Omaha, Nebraska

John W. Burruss, M.D.
Assistant Professor of Psychiatry, Department of Psychiatry, and Deputy Chief of Psychiatry, Ben Taub General Hospital, Baylor College of Medicine, Houston, Texas

Daniel J. Buysse, M.D.
Associate Professor of Psychiatry, Department of Psychiatry, University of Pittsburgh School of Medicine, Pittsburgh, Pennsylvania

Gabrielle A. Carlson, M.D.
Professor of Psychiatry and Pediatrics, Department of Psychiatry and Behavioral Sciences, State University of New York at Stony Brook, Stony Brook, New York

Gabrielle M. Cerda, M.D.
Assistant Professor, Department of Psychiatry, University of California San Diego, San Diego, California

Greg L. Clary, M.D.
Clinical Associate Professor, Departments of Internal Medicine and Psychiatry, Duke University Medical Center, Durham, North Carolina

Catherine Classen, Ph.D.
Senior Research Scholar, Department of Psychiatry and Behavioral Sciences, Stanford University School of Medicine, Stanford, California

Donald J. Cohen, M.D.
Irving B. Harris Professor of Psychiatry, Psychology, and Pediatrics, Yale Child Study Center, New Haven, Connecticut

Stephen A. Cole, M.D., A.M.
Staff Psychiatrist, Health Care and Rehabilitation Service of Southeastern Vermont, Bellows Falls, Vermont, and Adjunct Assistant Professor, Department of Psychiatry, Dartmouth Medical College, Hanover, New Hampshire

Arnold M. Cooper, M.D.
Stephen Tobin and Dr. Arnold M. Cooper Professor Emeritus in Consultation-Liaison Psychiatry, Weill Medical College of Cornell University, New York, New York

Paul Crits-Christoph, Ph.D.
Professor of Psychology, Department of Psychiatry, University of Pennsylvania Health Systems, Philadelphia, Pennsylvania

Scott J. Crow, M.D.
Associate Professor, Department of Psychiatry, University of Minnesota School of Medicine, Minneapolis, Minnesota

Jeffrey L. Cummings, M.D.
Augustus S. Rose Professor of Neurology and Professor of Neurology and Psychiatry and Biobehavioral Science, UCLA School of Medicine, and Chief, Behavioral Neuroscience Section, Psychiatry Service, West Los Angeles Veterans Affairs Medical Center, Los Angeles, California

Christopher Dare, M.D.
Reader and Head, Section in Psychotherapy, Department of Psychiatry, Institute of Psychiatry, London, England

George De Leon, Ph.D.
Director, Center for Therapeutic Community Research, and Clinical Professor, Department of Psychiatry, New York University Medical School, New York, New York

Pedro L. Delgado, M.D.
Douglas Danford Bond Professor and Chairman, Department of Psychiatry, Case Western Reserve University and University Hospitals of Cleveland, Cleveland, Ohio

Steven L. Dubovsky, M.D.
Professor, Department of Psychiatry, University of Colorado Health Sciences Center, Denver, Colorado

Robert L. DuPont, M.D.
President, Institute for Behavior and Health, Inc., Rockville, Maryland, and Clinical Professor of Psychiatry, Georgetown University School of Medicine, Washington, D.C.

Stuart J. Eisendrath, M.D.
Director, Ambulatory Services, Department of Psychiatry, Langley Porter Psychiatric Hospital and Clinics, University of California–San Francisco, San Francisco, California

Chad D. Emrick, Ph.D.
Assistant Clinical Professor, Department of Clinical Psychology in Psychiatry, University of Colorado Health Sciences Center, Denver, Colorado, and Staff Psychologist, Substance Abuse Treatment Program, Denver Veterans Affairs Medical Center, Denver, Colorado

Brigette A. Erwin, M.A.
Doctoral student in clinical psychology, Temple University, Philadelphia, Pennsylvania

Maurizio Fava, M.D.
Director, Depression Clinical and Research Program, Massachusetts General Hospital, and Associate Professor of Psychiatry, Harvard Medical School, Boston, Massachusetts

Jan Fawcett, M.D.
Stanley G. Harris Sr. Professor and Chairman, Department of Psychiatry, Rush–Presbyterian–St. Luke's Medical Center, Chicago, Illinois

Wayne S. Fenton, M.D.
Deputy Director, Clinical Affairs, Division of Mental Disorders, Behavioral Research and AIDS, National Institute of Mental Health, Bethesda, Maryland, and Associate Clinical Professor of Psychiatry and Behavioral Sciences, George Washington University School of Medicine, Washington, D.C.

Edna B. Foa, Ph.D.
Professor and Director, Center for the Treatment and Study of Anxiety, Department of Psychiatry, Medical College of Pennsylvania, Philadelphia, Pennsylvania

Charles V. Ford, M.D.
Professor, Department of Psychiatry and Behavioral Neurobiology, and Director, University of Alabama Neuropsychiatry Clinic, University of Alabama School of Medicine, Birmingham, Alabama

Richard J. Frances, M.D.
President, CEO, and Medical Director, Silver Hill Hospital, New Canaan, Connecticut, and Clinical Professor, Department of Psychiatry, Division of Alcoholism and Drug Abuse, New York University School of Medicine, New York, New York

John E. Franklin, M.D.
Associate Professor and Director of Addiction Psychiatry, Northwestern University Medical School, Chicago, Illinois

Jennifer B. Freeman, Ph.D.
Postdoctoral Fellow, Brown University School of Medicine, Rhode Island Hospital, Providence, Rhode Island

Kimberly Frost-Pineda, M.P.H.
Research Coordinator, Department of Psychiatry, University of Florida Brain Institute, Gainesville, Florida

Glen O. Gabbard, M.D.
Callaway Distinguished Professor of Psychoanalysis and Education, Karl Menninger School of Psychiatry, The Menninger Clinic, Topeka, and Clinical Professor of Psychiatry, University of Kansas School of Medicine, Wichita, Kansas

Marc Galanter, M.D.
Professor of Psychiatry and Director, Division of Alcoholism and Drug Abuse, New York University School of Medicine, New York, New York, and Research Scientist, World Health Organization Collaborating Center, Nathan Kline Institute, Orangeburg, New York

Don Gallant, M.D.
Professor Emeritus, Department of Psychiatry and Neurology, Tulane Medical School, New Orleans, Louisiana

Paul E. Garfinkel, M.D., F.R.C.P.C.
President and CEO, Centre for Addiction and Mental Health, and Professor of Psychiatry, University of Toronto, Toronto, Ontario, Canada

Alan J. Gelenberg, M.D.
Professor and Head, Department of Psychiatry, University of Arizona College of Medicine, Tucson, Arizona

Mark S. Gold, M.D.
Professor, Departments of Psychiatry, Neuroscience, and Community Health and Family Medicine, University of Florida Brain Institute, Gainesville, Florida

Sarah J. Golden, Ph.D.
Clinical psychologist, Tucson, Arizona

Carlos A. González, M.D.
Assistant Clinical Professor of Psychiatry, Yale University School of Medicine, New Haven, Connecticut, and Attending Psychiatrist and Chief, Crisis Intervention Service, Griffin Hospital, Derby, Connecticut

Ross Greene, Ph.D.
Staff, Pediatric Psychopharmacology Clinic, Massachusetts General Hospital, and Assistant Professor of Psychiatry, Department of Psychiatry, Harvard Medical School, Boston, Massachusetts

John H. Greist, M.D.
Distinguished Senior Scientist, Madison Institute of Medicine, and Clinical Professor of Psychiatry, Department of Psychiatry, University of Wisconsin Medical School, Madison, Wisconsin

Ezra E. H. Griffith, M.D.
Deputy Chair for Clinical Affairs, and Professor of Psychiatry and of African-American Studies, Department of Psychiatry, Yale University School of Medicine, New Haven, Connecticut

Leonard C. Groopman, M.D.
Assistant Professor of Clinical Psychiatry, Weill Medical College of Cornell University, New York, New York

John G. Gunderson, M.D.
Director, Personality and Psychosocial Research, McLean Hospital, Belmont, and Professor, Department of Psychiatry, Harvard Medical School, Boston, Massachusetts

Robert E. Hales, M.D.
Professor and Chair, Department of Psychiatry, University of California–Davis School of Medicine, Sacramento, California

Katherine A. Halmi, M.D.
Professor, Department of Psychiatry, Weill Medical College of Cornell University, White Plains, New York

James C. Harris, M.D.
Director, Developmental Neuropsychiatry, and Professor of Psychiatry and Behavioral Sciences, Pediatrics, and Mental Hygiene, Johns Hopkins University School of Medicine, Baltimore, Maryland

Catherine Hayer, M.S.
Pervasive Developmental Disorders Clinic and Autism Research Program, Langley Porter Psychiatric Institute, University of California–San Francisco, San Francisco, California

Richard G. Heimberg, Ph.D.
Professor of Psychology, Temple University, Philadelphia, Pennsylvania

Donald M. Hilty, M.D.
Assistant Professor, Department of Psychiatry, University of California Davis Medical Center, Sacramento, California

Rudolf Hoehn-Saric, M.D.
Professor Emeritus of Psychiatry, Department of Psychiatry and Behavioral Science, Johns Hopkins University School of Medicine, Baltimore, Maryland

Steven D. Hollon, Ph.D.
Professor of Psychology, Department of Psychology, Vanderbilt University, Nashville, Tennessee

Mardi J. Horowitz, M.D.
Professor, Department of Psychiatry, University of California–San Francisco, San Francisco, California

Michael Y. Hwang, M.D.
Staff Physician and Director of Schizophrenia Research, Department of Psychiatry, East Orange Veterans Affairs Medical Center, East Orange, New Jersey, and Associate Professor of Psychiatry, UMDNJ–Robert Wood Johnson Medical School, Piscataway, New Jersey

James W. Jefferson, M.D.
Distinguished Senior Scientist, Madison Institute of Medicine, and Clinical Professor of Psychiatry, Department of Psychiatry, University of Wisconsin Medical School, Madison, Wisconsin

Martin P. Kafka, M.D.
Clinical Assistant Professor, Department of Psychiatry, Harvard Medical School, Boston, Massachusetts, and Senior Attending Psychiatrist, Department of Psychiatry, McLean Hospital, Belmont, Massachusetts

John M. Kane, M.D.
Chairman, Department of Psychiatry, Hillside Hospital, Division of Long Island Jewish Medical Center, Glen Oaks, and Professor of Psychiatry, Albert Einstein College of Medicine, Bronx, New York

Allan S. Kaplan, M.Sc., M.D., F.R.C.P.C.
Head, Program for Eating Disorders, Department of Psychiatry, Toronto General Hospital, University Health Network; Director, Postgraduate Education, and Associate Professor, Department of Psychiatry, University of Toronto, Toronto, Ontario, Canada

Anwarul Karim, M.D.
Research Associate, Department of Psychiatry, Mount Sinai School of Medicine, New York, New York

Edward F. Kaufman, M.D.
Clinical Professor, Department of Psychiatry and Human Behavior, University of California–Irvine, Irvine, California

Edward J. Khantzian, M.D.
Clinical Professor of Psychiatry, Harvard Medical School at The Cambridge Hospital, Cambridge, and Associate Chief of Psychiatry, Tewksbury Hospital, Tewksbury, Massachusetts

Herbert D. Kleber, M.D.
Professor of Psychiatry and Director, Division on Substance Abuse, Department of Psychiatry, Columbia University College of Physicians and Surgeons and New York State Psychiatric Institute, New York, New York

Richard P. Kluft, M.D.
Director, Dissociative Disorders Program, The Institute of Pennsylvania Hospital, and private practice, Bala Cynwyd, Pennsylvania

Alex Kopelowicz, M.D.
Assistant Professor of Psychiatry, Department of Psychiatry and Biobehavioral Sciences, UCLA School of Medicine, and Medical Director, San Fernando Mental Health Center, Los Angeles, California

Thomas R. Kosten, M.D.
Professor, Department of Psychiatry, Yale University School of Medicine, VA Connecticut Healthcare System, West Haven, Connecticut

K. Ranga Rama Krishnan, M.D.
Professor and Chair, Department of Psychiatry, Duke University Medical Center, Durham, North Carolina

Andrew D. Krystal, M.D.
Associate Professor, Department of Psychiatry and Behavioral Sciences, Duke University Medical Center, Durham, North Carolina

David J. Kupfer, M.D., Ph.D.
Thomas Detre Professor and Chairman, Department of Psychiatry, University of Pittsburgh School of Medicine, Western Psychiatric Institute and Clinic, Pittsburgh, Pennsylvania

Pantelis G. Lazaridis, M.D.
Rector, University of Thessaly, Volos, Greece

James F. Leckman, M.D.
Neison Harris Professor of Child Psychiatry and Pediatrics, Yale Child Study Center, New Haven, Connecticut

Sandra Risa Leiblum, Ph.D.
Professor of Psychiatry, Department of Psychiatry, and Professor of Clinical Obstetrics and Gynecology, Department of Obstetrics and Gynecology, University of Medicine and Dentistry of New Jersey–Robert Wood Johnson Medical School, Piscataway, New Jersey

Henrietta L. Leonard, M.D.
Director of Training, Division of Child and Adolescent Psychiatry, and Professor, Department of Psychiatry and Human Behavior, Brown University School of Medicine, Rhode Island Hospital, Providence, Rhode Island

Stephen B. Levine, M.D.
Clinical Professor of Psychiatry, Department of Psychiatry, Case Western Reserve University School of Medicine, Cleveland Ohio, and Co-Director, Center for Marital and Sexual Health, Beachwood, Ohio

Robert Paul Liberman, M.D.
Professor of Psychiatry, Department of Psychiatry and Biobehavioral Sciences, and Director, Psychiatric Rehabilitation Program, UCLA School of Medicine, Los Angeles, California

Jacob Lindy, M.D.
Training and Supervising Analyst, Cincinnati Psychoanalytic Institute, and Associate Clinical Professor of Psychiatry, University of Cincinnati, Cincinnati, Ohio

Paul S. Links, M.D., F.R.C.P.C.
Clinical Program Director, Mental Health Service, The Wellesley/St. Michael's Hospital, and Professor of Psychiatry, University of Toronto, Toronto, Ontario, Canada

Don R. Lipsitt, M.D.
Clinical Professor, Department of Psychiatry, Harvard Medical School, Boston, Massachusetts; Medical Director, Institute for Behavioral Science in Health Care, and Chairman Emeritus, Department of Psychiatry, Mount Auburn Hospital, Cambridge, Massachusetts

Richard J. Loewenstein, M.D.
Medical Director, Trauma Disorders, Sheppard Pratt Health Systems, and Associate Clinical Professor, Department of Psychiatry and Behavioral Sciences, University of Maryland School of Medicine, Baltimore, Maryland

Joseph LoPiccolo, Ph.D.
Professor of Psychology, Department of Psychology, University of Missouri, Columbia, Missouri

R. Bruce Lydiard, M.D., Ph.D.
Professor of Psychiatry and Behavioral Sciences, and Director, Mood and Anxiety Program, Medical University of South Carolina, Charleston, South Carolina

Avram H. Mack, M.D.
Resident Psychiatrist, Brigham and Women's Hospital, and Clinical Fellow in Psychiatry, Harvard Medical School, Boston, Massachusetts

Robert J. Malcolm, M.D.
Professor of Psychiatry, Department of Psychiatry and Behavioral Sciences, and Medical Director, Center for Drug and Alcohol Problems, Medical University of South Carolina, Charleston, South Carolina

Anil K. Malhotra, M.D.
Chief, Unit of Molecular Psychiatry, Hillside Hospital, Long Island Jewish Medical Center, Glen Oaks, New York

John T. Maltsberger, M.D.
Senior Consultant, Psychotherapy Consultation Services, McLean Hospital, Belmont, and Lecturer in Psychiatry, Harvard Medical School, Boston, Massachusetts

John March, M.D., M.P.H.
Director, Programs in Child and Adolescent Anxiety Disorders, Child Psychiatry, Duke University Medical Center, Durham, North Carolina

G. Alan Marlatt, Ph.D.
Professor of Psychology, Department of Psychology, and Director, Addictive Behaviors Research Center, University of Washington, Seattle, Washington

Randall D. Marshall, M.D.
Assistant Professor of Clinical Psychiatry, Columbia University College of Physicians and Surgeons, New York, New York

Donna L. Masterman, M.D., M.S.
Assistant Clinical Professor, Department of Neurology, UCLA School of Medicine, Los Angeles, California

Kathryn May, M.Sc.
Senior Lecturer in Psychosexual Therapy, Lancashire Postgraduate School of Medicine and Health, University of Central Lancashire, Preston, United Kingdom

William E. McAuliffe, Ph.D.
Associate Professor of Sociology and Director, Substance Abuse Research, Harvard Medical School at The Cambridge Hospital, Cambridge, Massachusetts

Marita P. McCabe, Ph.D., F.A.P.S.
Professor of Psychology, School of Psychology, Deakin University, Burwood, Victoria, Australia

Philip K. McCullough, M.D.
Assistant Professor of Clinical Psychiatry, Department of Psychiatry and Behavioral Sciences, Northwestern University Medical School, Chicago, Illinois

John F. McDermott Jr., M.D.
Chair, Department of Psychiatry, University of Hawaii, John A. Burns School of Medicine, Honolulu, Hawaii

David M. McDowell, M.D.
Medical Director, Substance Treatment and Research Service (STARS), and Assistant Clinical Professor of Psychiatry, Columbia University College of Physicians and Surgeons, Division on Substance Abuse, New York Psychiatric Institute, New York, New York

Susan L. McElroy, M.D.
Professor of Psychiatry and Director, Biological Psychiatry Program, Department of Psychiatry, University of Cincinnati College of Medicine, Cincinnati, Ohio

Traci McFarlane, Ph.D., C.Psych.
Staff Psychologist, Department of Psychiatry, Toronto General Hospital, University Health Network, Toronto, Ontario, Canada

W. W. Meissner, S.J., M.D.
University Professor of Psychoanalysis, Boston College, Chestnut Hill, and Training and Supervising Analyst, Boston Psychoanalytic Institute, Boston, Massachusetts

Lisa Mellman, M.D.
Associate Clinical Professor of Psychiatry, Columbia University College of Physicians and Surgeons, New York, New York

J. Reid Meloy, Ph.D.
Associate Clinical Professor, Department of Psychiatry, University of California–San Diego School of Medicine, and Adjunct Professor, University of San Diego School of Law, San Diego, California

Delinda E. Mercer, Ph.D.
Counseling Psychologist, Department of Psychiatry, University of Pennsylvania, Philadelphia, Pennsylvania

Barbara Milrod, M.D.
Assistant Professor of Psychiatry, Weill Medical College of Cornell University, New York, New York

James E. Mitchell, M.D.
Professor and Chair, Department of Neuroscience, University of North Dakota School of Medicine and Health Sciences, Fargo, North Dakota

Lynda Molleken, M.D., F.R.C.P.C.
Staff Psychiatrist, Department of Psychiatry, Toronto General Hospital, University Health Network, Toronto, Ontario, Canada

Charles M. Morin, Ph.D.
Associate Professor of Psychology and Psychiatry, École de Psychologie, Université Laval, Ste-Foy, Quebec, Canada

Richard L. Munich, M.D.
Medical Director and Chief of Staff, The Menninger Clinic, Topeka, Kansas

Carol C. Nadelson, M.D.
Clinical Professor of Psychiatry, Harvard Medical School, Boston, Massachusetts, and Editor-in-Chief, American Psychiatric Press, Inc., Washington, D.C.

Andrew A. Nierenberg, M.D.
Associate Director, Depression Clinical and Research Program, and Medical Director, Bipolar Programs, Massachusetts General Hospital, and Associate Professor of Psychiatry, Harvard Medical School, Boston, Massachusetts

Malkah T. Notman, M.D.
Clinical Professor of Psychiatry, Harvard Medical School, Boston, and President, Boston Psychoanalytic Society, Boston, Massachusetts

Edward V. Nunes, M.D.
Research Psychiatrist and Assistant Professor, New York State Psychiatric Institute, Columbia University College of Physicians and Surgeons, New York, New York

Charles P. O'Brien, M.D., Ph.D.
Chief of Psychiatry, Philadelphia Department of Veterans Affairs Medical Center, and Professor and Vice Chairman, Department of Psychiatry, University of Pennsylvania, Philadelphia, Pennsylvania

Judith K. Ockene, Ph.D.
Professor of Medicine and Director, Department of Medicine, Division of Preventive and Behavioral Medicine, University of Massachusetts Medical School, Worcester, Massachusetts

Marion P. Olmsted, Ph.D., C.Psych.
Director of Ambulatory Care for Eating Disorders and Staff Psychologist, Department of Psychiatry, Toronto General Hospital, University Health Network, and Associate Professor in Psychiatry, University of Toronto, Toronto, Ontario, Canada

Dan A. Oren, M.D.
Research Associate, U.S. Department of Veterans Affairs, West Haven, Connecticut, and Associate Professor of Psychiatry, Yale University, New Haven, Connecticut

Candice Osborn, M.A.
Director of Sex Offender Services, Behavioral Medicine Institute of Atlanta, Atlanta, Georgia

Michael W. Otto, Ph.D.
Director, Cognitive-Behavior Therapy Program, Massachusetts General Hospital, Boston, Massachusetts, and Associate Professor of Psychology in Psychiatry, Harvard Medical School, Boston, Massachusetts

Michael V. Pantalon, Ph.D.
Assistant Professor of Psychiatry (in Psychology), Department of Psychiatry, Substance Abuse Center, Yale University School of Medicine, New Haven, Connecticut

Lori Pbert, Ph.D.
Assistant Professor of Medicine, Department of Medicine, Division of Preventive and Behavioral Medicine, University of Massachusetts Medical School, Worcester, Massachusetts

Robert N. Pechnick, Ph.D.
Associate Director of Research, Department of Psychiatry, Cedars–Sinai Medical Center, Los Angeles, California

J. Christopher Perry, M.P.H., M.D.
Director of Research, Institute of Community and Family Psychiatry, Sir Mortimer B. Davis–Jewish General Hospital, and Professor of Psychiatry, McGill University, Montreal, Quebec, Canada, and Visiting Professor, Department of Psychiatry, Harvard Medical School at the Austen Riggs Center, Stockbridge, Massachusetts

Alexandra M. Phipps, Ph.D.
Behavioral Medicine Institute of Atlanta, Atlanta, Georgia

Sarah Reiff-Hekking, Ph.D.
Instructor of Medicine, Department of Medicine, Division of Preventive and Behavioral Medicine, University of Massachusetts Medical School, Worcester, Massachusetts

Charles F. Reynolds III, M.D.
Professor of Psychiatry, Department of Psychiatry, University of Pittsburgh School of Medicine, Pittsburgh, Pennsylvania

Alan Riley, M.Sc., M.B., B.S., M.R.C.S., F.F.P.M.
Professor of Sexual Medicine, Lancashire Postgraduate School of Medicine and Health, University of Central Lancashire, Preston, United Kingdom

Jonathan I. Ritvo, M.D.
Clinical Professor of Psychiatry and Training Director, Addiction Psychiatry Program, Denver Health Medical Center, University of Colorado Health Sciences Center, Denver, Colorado

Robert G. Robinson, M.D.
Professor and Head, Department of Psychiatry, University of Iowa College of Medicine, Iowa City, Iowa

Angela Cartagena Rochas, M.A.
Research Assistant, Department of Psychiatry, Mount Sinai School of Medicine, New York, New York

Jerrold F. Rosenbaum, M.D.
Chief of Psychiatry (Interim), Massachusetts General Hospital, and Professor of Psychiatry, Harvard Medical School, Boston, Massachusetts

Norman E. Rosenthal, M.D.
Clinical Professor of Psychiatry, Georgetown University, Washington, D.C.

Barbara Olasov Rothbaum, Ph.D.
Associate Professor in Psychiatry, Emory University School of Medicine, Atlanta, Georgia

Pedro Ruiz, M.D.
Professor and Vice Chair for Clinical Affairs, Department of Psychiatry, University of Texas Medical School at Houston, Houston, Texas

A. John Rush, M.D.
Betty Jo Hay Distinguished Chair in Mental Health and Professor, Department of Psychiatry, University of Texas Southwestern Medical Center, Dallas, Texas

Andrew T. Russell, M.D.
Professor of Clinical Psychiatry, Department of Psychiatry and Biobehavioral Sciences, University of California–Los Angeles, Neuropsychiatric Institute, Los Angeles, California

Gary S. Sachs, M.D.
Director, Harvard Bipolar Research Program, Massachusetts General Hospital, and Associate Professor of Psychiatry, Harvard Medical School, Boston, Massachusetts

Laura E. Sanchez, M.D.
Assistant Professor of Child Psychiatry, University of Pennsylvania, and Director, Child and Adolescent Psychopharmacology Research Clinic, Philadelphia Child Guidance Clinic, Philadelphia, Pennsylvania

Franklin R. Schneier, M.D.
Associate Professor of Clinical Psychiatry, Columbia University College of Physicians and Surgeons, and Associate Director, Anxiety Disorders Clinic, New York State Psychiatric Institute, New York, New York

Sidney H. Schnoll, M.D., Ph.D.
Professor, Departments of Internal Medicine and Psychiatry, Division of Addiction Medicine, Medical College of Virginia, Virginia Commonwealth University, Richmond, Virginia

Richard S. Schottenfeld, M.D.
Professor of Psychiatry, Yale University School of Medicine, New Haven, Connecticut

Marc A. Schuckit, M.D.
Professor of Psychiatry, University of California–San Diego Medical School and San Diego Veterans Hospital, San Diego, California

R. Taylor Segraves, M.D., Ph.D.
Professor, Department of Psychiatry, Case Western Reserve University, and Chair, Department of Psychiatry, MetroHealth Medical Center, Cleveland, Ohio

Edward C. Senay, M.D.
Professor Emeritus of Psychiatry, The University of Chicago, Chicago, Illinois

David Shaffer, M.B., B.S., F.R.C.P., F.R.C.Psych.
Irving Philips Professor of Child Psychiatry, Columbia University College of Physicians and Surgeons, New York, New York

James H. Shore, M.D.
Chancellor, University of Colorado Health Sciences Center, Denver, Colorado

Bryna Siegel, Ph.D.
Director, Pervasive Developmental Disorders Clinic and Autism Research Program, Langley Porter Psychiatric Institute, University of California–San Francisco, San Francisco, California

Amrita K. Singha, Ph.D.
Research Fellow, Yale University School of Medicine, VA Connecticut Healthcare System, Department of Psychiatry, West Haven, Connecticut

William H. Sledge, M.D.
Professor of Psychiatry, Department of Psychiatry, Yale University School of Medicine; Medical Director, Yale–New Haven Psychiatric Hospital, and Master, Calhoun College, New Haven, Connecticut

David E. Smith, M.D.
Founder and Medical Director, Haight Ashbury Free Clinics, San Francisco, California, and Professor, University of California, San Francisco

G. Richard Smith Jr., M.D.
Professor and Vice Chairman of Psychiatry and Director, Centers for Mental Health Research, University of Arkansas for Medical Sciences, Little Rock, Arkansas

Thomas Spencer, M.D.
Assistant Director, Pediatric Psychopharmacology Clinic, Massachusetts General Hospital, and Associate Professor of Psychiatry, Department of Psychiatry, Harvard Medical School, Boston, Massachusetts

David Spiegel, M.D.
Professor and Associate Chair, Department of Psychiatry and Behavioral Sciences, and Director, Psychosocial Treatment Laboratory, Stanford University School of Medicine, Stanford, California

Marlene Steinberg, M.D.
Associate Professor of Psychiatry, Department of Psychiatry, University of Massachusetts School of Medicine, Worcester, Massachusetts

Peter Steinglass, M.D.
Executive Director, Ackerman Institute for the Family, and Clinical Professor of Psychiatry, Cornell University Medical College, New York, New York

Michael H. Stone, M.D.
Professor of Clinical Psychiatry, Columbia University College of Physicians and Surgeons, New York, New York

James J. Strain, M.D.
Professor of Psychiatry and Director, Division of Behavioral Medicine and Consultation, Department of Psychiatry, Mount Sinai School of Medicine, New York, New York

Mark D. Sullivan, M.D., Ph.D.
Associate Professor, Department of Psychiatry and Behavioral Sciences, University of Washington at Seattle, Seattle, Washington

Suzanne M. Sutherland, M.D.
Assistant Consulting Professor, Department of Psychiatry, Duke University Medical Center, Durham, North Carolina

Susan E. Swedo, M.D.
Chief, Pediatrics and Developmental Neuropsychiatry Branch, National Institute of Mental Health, Bethesda, Maryland

Carol A. Tamminga, M.D.
Deputy Director, Maryland Psychiatric Research Center, University of Maryland School of Medicine, Baltimore, Maryland

Peter E. Tanguay, M.D.
Ackerly Professor of Child and Adolescent Psychiatry, Bingham Child Guidance Center, Department of Psychiatry and Behavioral Sciences, School of Medicine, University of Louisville, Louisville, Kentucky

Lenore Terr, M.D.
Clinical Professor of Psychiatry, University of California–San Francisco, San Francisco, California

Gunvant K. Thaker, M.D.
Director, Schizophrenia Related Disorders Program, Maryland Psychiatric Research Center, University of Maryland School of Medicine, Baltimore, Maryland

Michael E. Thase, M.D.
Director, Division of Mood, Anxiety, and Related Disorders, Western Psychiatric Institute and Clinic, and Associate Professor of Psychiatry, University of Pittsburgh School of Medicine, Pittsburgh, Pennsylvania

Kenneth E. Towbin, M.D.
Chief, Clinical Child and Adolescent Psychiatry, National Institute of Mental Health; and Professor of Psychiatry and Behavioral Sciences, George Washington University School of Medicine, Washington, D.C.

Javier I. Travella, M.D.
Former Fellow, Department of Psychiatry, University of Iowa College of Medicine, Iowa City, Iowa; and Staff, San Lucas Institute, Rosario, Argentina

Michelle Tullis, Ph.D. candidate
Research Associate, Department of Counselor Education, University of Florida College of Education, Gainesville, Florida

J. Thomas Ungerleider, M.D.
Professor Emeritus, Department of Psychiatry, UCLA Medical Center, Los Angeles, California

Walter Vandereycken, M.D., Ph.D.
Professor of Psychiatry, Catholic University of Leuven, Leuven, Belgium

Charles J. Wallace, Ph.D.
Professor of Psychiatry, Department of Psychiatry and Biobehavioral Sciences, UCLA School of Medicine, Los Angeles, California

Heather J. Walter, M.D., M.P.H.
Medical Director, Outpatient Services, Department of Psychiatry, Children's Memorial Hospital, and Associate Professor of Psychiatry and Behavioral Sciences, Northwestern University Medical School, Chicago, Illinois

Michael F. Weaver, M.D.
Assistant Professor, Departments of Internal Medicine and Psychiatry, Division of Addiction Medicine, Medical College of Virginia, Virginia Commonwealth University, Richmond, Virginia

Richard D. Weiner, M.D., Ph.D.
Professor, Department of Psychiatry and Behavioral Sciences, Duke University Medical Center, and Chief, Mental Health Service Line, Department of Veterans Affairs Medical Center, Durham, North Carolina

Roger D. Weiss, M.D.
Clinical Director, Alcohol and Drug Abuse Program, McLean Hospital, Belmont, and Associate Professor of Psychiatry, Harvard Medical School, Boston, Massachusetts

Elizabeth B. Weller, M.D.
Professor, Departments of Psychiatry and Pediatrics, University of Pennsylvania, and Frederick H. Allen Chair, Department of Child and Adolescent Psychiatry, Children's Hospital of Philadelphia, Philadelphia, Pennsylvania

Donald R. Wesson, M.D.
Vice President, Clinical Development, DrugAbuse Sciences, Inc., Los Altos, California

Timothy Wilens, M.D.
Staff, Pediatric Psychopharmacology Clinic, Massachusetts General Hospital, and Associate Professor of Psychiatry, Department of Psychiatry, Harvard Medical School, Boston, Massachusetts

G. Terence Wilson, Ph.D.
Oscar K. Buros Professor of Psychology, Graduate School of Applied and Professional Psychology, Rutgers, The State University of New Jersey, Piscataway, New Jersey

Michael G. Wise, M.D.
Clinical Professor, Department of Psychiatry, University of California Davis Medical Center, Sacramento, California, and Adjunct Professor, Department of Psychiatry, Uniformed Services University of the Health Sciences, Bethesda, Maryland

George E. Woody, M.D.
Professor, Department of Psychiatry, Veterans Affairs Medical Center, University of Pennsylvania School of Medicine, Philadelphia, Pennsylvania

Daniel Yaeger, B.A.
Administrator, Psychiatric Rehabilitation Program, UCLA School of Medicine, Los Angeles, California

Alayne Yates, M.D.
Professor, Department of Psychiatry, University of Hawaii, John A. Burns School of Medicine, Honolulu, Hawaii

Arlene R. Young, Ph.D.
Psychologist and Clinic Co-Head, Children's Developmental Neuropsychiatry Clinic, Child Psychiatry Programme, Centre for Addiction and Mental Health, Clarke Division, Toronto, Ontario, Canada

Carolyn M. Young, M.D.
Assistant Clinical Instructor, Department of Psychiatry, State University of New York at Buffalo, School of Medicine, Buffalo, New York

Stuart C. Yudofsky, M.D.
D. C. and Irene Ellwood Professor and Chairman, Department of Psychiatry and Behavioral Sciences, Baylor College of Medicine, Houston, Texas

Sheldon Zimberg, M.D., M.S.
Clinical Professor of Psychiatry, Columbia University College of Physicians and Surgeons, and Senior Attending, Department of Psychiatry, St. Luke's–Roosevelt Hospital Center, New York, New York

Kenneth J. Zucker, Ph.D.
Head, Child and Adolescent Gender Identity Clinic, Child Psychiatry Program, Centre for Addiction and Mental Health—Clarke Division, University of Toronto School of Medicine, Toronto, Ontario, Canada

Introduction

This third edition of *Treatments of Psychiatric Disorders* appears nearly 20 years after the idea for this project was first conceived. In 1982 Daniel X. Freedman, M.D., in his capacity as president of the American Psychiatric Association, appointed a Task Force on Treatment of Psychiatric Disorders. The charge to the task force was to produce a comprehensive statement describing current thinking on the optimal treatment of psychiatric disorders. Experts in the treatment of the major psychiatric disorders were collected together in groups of panels that exhaustively reviewed the treatment literature in the service of reaching consensus on the various psychiatric disorders. Outside consultants were contacted for additional opinions.

After an extensive review process, the first edition of *Treatments of Psychiatric Disorders* was published in 1989 as a task force report of the American Psychiatric Association. Encompassing four volumes, it was encyclopedic in scope and rapidly became the leading reference on treatment in American psychiatry. As chairperson of the task force and editor of the first edition, T. Byram Karasu, M.D., modestly acknowledged in his introduction to the text that psychiatry has an evolving knowledge base and that treatments outlined in the book should not be regarded as rigid guidelines but simply as useful approaches to the major psychiatric disorders designed to assist clinicians in treatment planning.

When it came time to respond to that evolving knowledge base with a second edition, the American Psychiatric Association Board of Trustees gave the task to American Psychiatric Press. Dr. Karasu declined to continue as editor-in-chief, and Dr. Carol Nadelson approached me with an invitation to become the new editor-in-chief.

With help from a distinguished group of section editors, we produced *Treatments of Psychiatric Disorders, Second Edition* in 1995. By decreasing the number of sections and limiting chapter length, we managed to reduce the second edition to only two volumes instead of four. We also insisted that the authors confine their contributions to treatment, with the assumption that readers can familiarize themselves with diagnostic issues by reading other textbooks.

The second edition was a highly successful compendium, but as the century neared its close, we recognized that some of the material in it was becoming dated. Therefore we set out to create a third edition that would update our rapidly expanding knowledge on the various treatments available to psychiatrists and other mental health professionals. In the tradition of the second edition, this book is deliberately pluralistic in its approach to psychiatric treatment. Knowing that a cornerstone of the art and science of clinical psychiatry is adjusting the treatment to the needs of a particular patient, chapter authors were told to include all major modalities applicable to the disorder for which they were responsible. A major emphasis in the text is on the results of randomized controlled trials, when available. However, because of concerns about whether the data emerging from controlled trials are generalizable to the naturalistic settings in which frontline clinicians practice, we have not limited the material in each chapter to results from such trials. We have also included data from uncontrolled studies as well as accumulated clinical wisdom when there is little empirical research from which to draw. Some authors have also provided highly sophisticated integrative models of treatment to help the clinician select among the available modalities and combine them in a rational conceptual framework designed to maximize the effectiveness of the overall treatment plan.

I collected a group of outstanding section editors, all chosen because they were recognized experts in the disorders for which they were responsible. They include John F. McDermott Jr., M.D., and Elizabeth B. Weller, M.D., for disorders usually first diagnosed in infancy, childhood, or adolescents; Stuart C. Yudofsky, M.D., and Robert E. Hales, M.D., for delirium, dementia, and amnestic and other cognitive disorders; Herbert D. Kleber, M.D., and Marc Galanter, M.D., for substance-related disorders; Richard L. Munich, M.D., and Carol Tamminga, M.D., for schizophrenia and other psychotic disorders; A. John Rush, M.D., for mood disorders; Franklin Schneier, M.D., Lisa Mellman, M.D., and David Spiegel, M.D., for anxiety disorders, dissociative disorders, and adjustment disorders; Charles B. Ford, M.D., for somatoform and factitious disorders; R. Taylor Segraves, M.D., and Stephen Levine, M.D., for sexual and gender identity disorders; Katherine A. Halmi, M.D., and Paul E. Garfinkel, M.D., F.R.C.P.C., for eating disorders; and John G. Gunderson, M.D. (in collaboration with yours truly), for personality disorders. Two sections, sleep disorders and disorders of impulse control, were small enough that they did not require section editors.

In working with the section editors, we faced a key decision: Should all sections be uniform in their organization, or should section editors be given more or less free rein to organize the chapter contributions in a manner that was most "reader friendly"? By overwhelming consensus, we agreed that the latter option would serve us better. In other words, a rigid uniformity might undermine the ease with which the text could be used as a reference book by the reader. For example, in the section on anxiety disorders, dissociative disorders, and adjustment disorders, it seemed eminently sensible to organize the chapters along the lines of diagnostic entities, because a myriad of different disorders are represented in the section and various treatments are applicable to each disorder. In contrast, in the section on mood disorders, which comprises fewer conditions, it was more rational to organize the section according to treatment modalities.

All chapter authors were instructed to update their chapters with references from 1995 up to the moment of submission for publication so as to make the third edition as current as possible. Also, in the interest of avoiding any dramatic expansion in the length of the text, we asked the chapter authors to delete older information from the second edition version of their chapters in an amount that was proportional to the new material added. We recognize the existence of additional conditions potentially in need of clinical attention that do not appear in this volume. For example, clinicians commonly treat the sequelae of physical or sexual abuse in childhood, relational problems, bereavement, and phase-of-life problems. The fact that such conditions are not covered in this text should not be taken to imply that they do not require careful and thoughtful psychiatric evaluation and treatment. Nor does absence of mention or coverage of a disorder imply that it is rare.

The treatments described for some disorders in this text are surrounded by controversy, and we anticipate that some readers may disagree with the approaches endorsed by chapter authors. We certainly recognize that the clinical judgment of the clinician must always be brought to bear in tailoring final treatment decisions to a particular patient. This compendium does not represent official policy of the American Psychiatric Association or any other body; furthermore, it must not be construed as a rigid standard for psychiatric care that the profession must follow. Rather, the book should be viewed as a collection of expert opinions intended to aid clinicians who are faced with the complexity of treatment planning.

A large textbook is a team effort. The section editors and the chapter authors deserve a lion's share of the credit. I am deeply grateful to them for their diligent efforts. I also wish to express appreciation to the many consultants who carefully read drafts of the chapters and offered thoughtful advice about possible revisions.

Many individuals at American Psychiatric Press also deserve acknowledgment. Carol Nadelson, M.D., editor-in-chief of American Psychiatric Press, and a longtime friend and mentor, was instrumental in the overall planning of this book. Claire Reinburg, Stacy Jobb, Pam Harley, Rebecca Richters, and other members of the editorial staff were meticulous in their preparation of the text.

Faye Schoenfeld, my editorial assistant, kept track of an extraordinary number of communications and chapter drafts for almost 2 years and was pivotal in keeping the entire project on track. I especially want to express my gratitude for her help.

Glen O. Gabbard, M.D.

SECTION 1

General Considerations in Psychiatric Treatment

Section Editor

Glen O. Gabbard, M.D.

1

Mind and Brain in Psychiatric Treatment

Glen O. Gabbard, M.D.

Although Engel (1982) proposed the biopsychosocial model as appropriate for all of medicine, his vision has the greatest potential for achievement in psychiatry. Psychiatrists are unique among medical specialists in that inherent in the specialty is the notion that psychosocial and biological factors must be integrated both in diagnostic understanding and in treatment planning. However, as we contemplate psychiatry in the 21st century, we must acknowledge that one of the greatest risks we face is reductionism. This issue has specific historical antecedents. In the 1950s and 1960s, the psychiatric enterprise tended to be construed as narrowly psychoanalytic. Today, with the extraordinary advances in neuroscience research, the specialty is at risk of being reductionistic in a biological direction. Subjective experience, interpersonal processes, and self-awareness are aspects of psychiatric study that must not be overlooked in the excitement about neurotransmitters and molecular genetics. Indeed, another aspect of psychiatry as a specialty is its interest in defining the unique features of the individual person (Cawley 1993).

The extraordinary breadth of psychiatry, however, creates some formidable challenges for the clinician. The effort to bring together diverse disciplines requires a highly synthetic and integrative capacity. The conceptual dilemma for the psychiatrist, as succinctly summarized by Slavney (1993), is that the "mind and brain can neither be fully integrated nor separated" (p. 59). Just as the physicist must simultaneously think in terms of particles and waves, the psychiatrist must speak of motives, wishes, and meanings in the same breath as genes, neurochemistry, and pharmacokinetics.

In this discussion of mind and brain in psychiatric treatment, three broad areas will be considered systematically. First, the mind-body problem, which has preoccupied philosophers for centuries, lies at the heart of the conceptual underpinnings of psychiatry. Second, any discussion of treatment cannot avoid causes and mechanisms, so a detailed examination of etiology and pathogenesis must precede an effort to integrate therapeutic modalities. Finally, the primary task of clinicians is to use their conceptual and theoretical knowledge to inform their choice of interventions in the crucible of clinical practice with complex human beings who come for help.

The Mind-Body Problem

While we know that mind and brain are ultimately inseparable, our literature and our practice do not always reflect that integrative view. The mind-body problem has vexed philosophers for centuries, and most scholars would agree that it is ultimately insoluble. A discussion of modern thinking about the mind-body problem must begin with Descartes, who in the 17th century described the notion of substance dualism. In short, his idea was that the world consisted of *res cogitans* (thinking things) and *res extensa* (extended things). The former category involved things that do not actually exist in space and time and therefore cannot be externally observed. The latter category consisted of directly observable physical entities. Descartes, who encountered just as much difficulty in integrating the two entities as have all subsequent scientists and philosophers, postulated that these two separate realms communicated through the pineal gland.

Dualism has long since fallen out of favor. The fundamental error in dualistic thinking, according to Damasio (1994), is conceptualizing the operations of the mind as somehow separate from the biology of the brain. Moreover, how can one observe the laws of conservation of energy and mass and at the same time postulate that a material phenomenon is caused by something nonmaterial, and vice versa (Edelson 1988)? William James (1890/1950) was instrumental in leading the way out of dualism when he noted that consciousness should be regarded as a process rather than as substance. He paved the way for a series of attempts to reframe the problem in terms of materialism. Theories of materialism generally reduce the mental to the physical. Materialism, however, varies widely in the degree to which the importance of mental activity is recognized. In its most extreme form, eliminative materialism, a psychology of the mind, is irrelevant and is regarded as entirely replaceable by constructs of neuroscience (Edelson 1988). A brief and selective survey of contemporary thought about the mind-body problem will illustrate the diversity of approaches to the complexities of a materialistic model.

Neural Darwinism is essentially a materialistic theory of the mind advanced by Edelman (1992) that attempts to account for psychology and is therefore useful to the clinical psychiatrist. Based on neuronal group selection and mapping, Edelman's theory is grounded in a process of selection acting on the primary neuronal units. He believes that only the fundamental motor and sensory operations, such as reflexes, are programmed from birth. The infant is otherwise free to construct a world of personal meanings and references that reflect environmental experiences as well as the infant's internal perception. This point of view is compatible with the ideas of Stern (1985), whose infant observation studies focused on the emergence of the sense of self. The infant actively correlates, categorizes, and connects experiences in the context of a self-other experience with a mothering or caregiving figure. Modell (1993) has elaborated on Edelman's work by pointing out that the neuronal mappings are symbolic systems of meaning that reflect how the self is created and re-created through the internalization of experience.

In an examination of the scientific status of psychoanalysis, Edelson (1988) argued that the mind-body problem is at heart a metaphysical question about the ultimate nature of being and can therefore never be solved by the presentation of empirical data. He suggested that the issue was most usefully reconceptualized as an issue involving the relationship between two disciplines or two theories (i.e., a theory of neuroscience and a theory of the mind). Within this context he suggested that because psychoanalysis is a theory of mental states involving symbolic representations of the self and others, it cannot be reduced to neuroscientific explanations. Moreover, Edelson asserted that this point of view is nevertheless compatible with materialism because all mental states are embodied and a physical state coexists with every mental state. In Edelson's view, reduction from the mental to the physical is not possible.

Materialism, then, can accommodate wide-ranging views on the relevance of psychology and a theory of mind. Although most contemporary commentators would agree that what we call "mind" can be understood as the activity of the brain (Andreasen 1997), not everyone agrees that such a conclusion leads to a reductive materialism. Searle (1992, 1998), for example, opines that we should not even raise the questions of dualism and materialism. Dismissing any dichotomy between the physical and mental, Searle stresses the irreducible subjectivity of the mental. In his view, which he terms *biological naturalism*, consciousness is a higher-order feature of the brain, but it can never be reduced to a "third-person phenomenon" that can be studied by neuroscientists. Searle emphasizes that consciousness involves subjective states and processes that can only be experienced by a conscious subject and are therefore in the domain of "first-person phenomena."

McGinn (1999) takes a "mysterian" position regarding the mind-body problem. He also rejects both materialism and dualism. We can never solve the mind-body problem, he asserts, because we are unable to see the mind. Consciousness is introspection-based, whereas the brain is perception-based. We can study the brain and examine physical correlates of a conscious state with a positron-emission tomography (PET) scan, but this is quite different from perceiving the individual's state of consciousness itself. Consciousness is rooted in some unknowable and mysterious natural property of the brain and is not explainable by processes studied by neuroscientists.

What we can say with certainty is that mental experience affects the brain. Using PET, Pardo and colleagues (1993) compared cerebral blood flow in seven healthy subjects at rest and in the same subjects when they imagined or recalled a situation that made them sad. The investigators detected significant differences in regional cerebral blood flow, primarily in the inferior and orbitofrontal cortices. Indeed, we now know that the brain is constructed of an elaborate interplay of genes and the environment, and that the organism's experience of the environment creates patterns of neural networks.

An extension of this observation is that psychotherapeutic interventions may result in permanent alterations in brain functioning. Kandel (1979, 1983, 1989, 1993, 1998) has elegantly demonstrated in a series of experiments with the marine snail *Aplysia* that synaptic connections can be strengthened and permanently altered through the regulation of gene expression connected with learning from the environment. Kandel (1979) concluded that "it is only insofar as our words produce changes in each other's brains that psychotherapeutic intervention produces changes in patients' minds. From this perspective the biological and psychological approaches are joined" (p. 1037). Kandel's work with *Aplysia* suggests an intriguing model for how this might happen. Given that the brain itself is a plastic and dynamic structure, representations of self and object may change through psychotherapeutic experiences. Kandel stresses that the sequence of the gene, or its *template* function, will not be affected by experiences with the environment. However, the *transcriptional* function of the gene—that is, the ability of a particular gene to direct the manufacture of specific proteins—is quite responsive to environmental factors.

Kandel's work with *Aplysia* has provocative correlates in studies with mammalian species. Preliminary research with rats has also demonstrated plasticity of the brain in response to environmental input. Rats raised in a social environment that requires complex learning for survival have significantly greater numbers of synapses per neurons compared with rats raised in isolation (Greenough et al. 1987).

Etiology and Pathogenesis of Psychiatric Disorders

The foregoing discussion of the influence of the environment on the brain leads directly into a consideration of the complex interplay between genes and environment in the etiology and pathogenesis of psychiatric disorders. To say to a patient that his or her condition is "a chemical imbalance" or "a psychological disturbance" is likely to be a partial explanation. The fact that biochemical processes are altered does not automatically mean that they are the causal agents (Lipowski 1989). An event in the environment, and particularly the subjective meaning of that event, may be the direct cause of a neurochemical change that then becomes the mediating mechanism of the illness (Gabbard 1992a).

Intensive study of the genetic contributions to psychiatric disorders has led geneticists to conclude that Mendelian patterns of heritability do not apply to psychiatric disorders. Incomplete penetrance and variable expressivity are typical of the major disorders, suggesting that developmental and environmental factors must interact with genes to produce mental illness. The study of brain plasticity has shown that once genes are activated by cellular developmental processes, the rate at which those genes are expressed is highly regulated by environmental signals throughout life (Hyman 1999).

The impact of environmental factors on gene expression explains why there are phenotypic differences between identical twins and discordance for such illnesses as schizophrenia. Heritable characteristics of children influence the kind of parenting they receive, so that two children in the same household may experience a profoundly different environment. Reiss et al. (1995) investigated the relative contributions of family environment and genetic factors to adolescent psychopathology. They studied 708 families with a variety of different constellations of same-sex siblings: 99 families with dizygotic twins, 93 families with monozygotic twins, 95 with ordinary siblings, 110 with full siblings in stepfamilies, 181 with full siblings brought from a previous marriage into the current marriage by the mother, and 130 families with genetically unrelated siblings in stepfamilies. Negative and conflictual parental behavior focused specifically at one adolescent accounted for almost 60% of the variance in adolescent antisocial behavior and 37% of the variance in depressive symptoms. The study suggested that the construct of the nonshared family environment, which has become a key factor in differentiating genetic versus environmental contributions to the pathogenesis of psychiatric disorders, often refers to parenting behavior that is directed specifically at one child. In other words, children in the same family may have different experiences with the parents that result in different outcomes.

These investigators also concluded that an individual's genetic endowment influences the type of parenting that he or she receives. The input from parents and other caregivers may in turn influence genetic expression. Reiss et al. (1995) noted that aggressiveness in parents interacted with a tendency to yield to the child's coercion, which then resulted in inconsistent parenting. Obviously, the brain is not a tabula rasa, so the impact of the environment is constrained by the particular genetic endowment of the individual. On the other hand, we now know that environmentally derived activity appears to drive the development of dendrites so that they can form the cognitive schemes related to the construction of internal representations. Neural connections between the cortex, the limbic system, and the autonomic nervous system become linked together into circuits in accordance with specific experiences of the developing organism. Memory and emotions are linked together because of consistent patterns of connection due to stimuli from the environment. This developmental pattern has been summarized as follows: "Cells that fire together wire together" (Schatz 1992, p. 64).

Schore (1997) has noted that the orbitofrontal region in the right prefrontal cortex may be particularly relevant to the "wiring" of internal representations. This area receives multimodal input from all sensory portions of the posterior cortex and also relays information to motor areas in the anterior cortex. In addition, the orbitofrontal region of the brain projects extensive pathways to other limbic structures in the temporal pole and amygdala, to subcortical drive centers in the hypothalamus, to arousal and award centers in the midbrain, and to vagal nuclei and autonomic centers in the medulla. Because the cortically processed visual information from the posterior cortex can be integrated in this area with the subcortically processed information regarding one's internal visceral state, the orbitofrontal region has the operational capacity to generate internal representations of self and other and an affective state linking the two. The orbital prefrontal region is also instrumental to empathic perception of emotional states in others. It is noteworthy, in this regard, that the orbital prefrontal area is especially expanded in the right cortex, which is dominant for the expression, regulation, and processing of emotional information. Schore (1997) noted that this area of the brain undergoes a critical period of growth at the end of the first year and into the second year of infancy. Developmental experiences with a mother or primary caregiver who is affectively misattuned can create a deficit in the maturing corticolimbic system.

There is growing evidence from research on lower species that an organism's experience of the environment profoundly affects the brain. Investigators identified a neuron in crayfish whose response to the neurotransmitter serotonin differs greatly depending on the animal's social status (Yeh et al. 1996). This particular neuron controls the tail-flip reflex in crayfish, which is relevant to the fight-flight response. In a dominant animal, serotonin makes the neuron more likely to fire. However, the same neurotransmitter suppresses firing in subordinate animals. The response to serotonin is not permanently encoded. If the animal's social status changes, the effect of serotonin on the neuron also changes. For example, when two subordinate crayfish were placed together, one would eventually become dominant. When the newly dominant animal was later tested, the neuron's response to serotonin was consistent with that seen in dominant animals (i.e., serotonin stimulated the tail-flip reflex rather than suppressing it). If we take a speculative leap, these findings suggest that one's perception of one's place in a relationship may influence the activity of neurotransmitters and their effect on the brain.

Changes in relationships have also been shown to produce enduring biochemical changes in rhesus monkeys (Suomi 1991). When separated from their mothers, infant monkeys developed a variety of behavioral abnormalities, which could be reversed when they were matched with "therapist" monkeys (i.e., socially competent infant partners). However, these isolated monkeys still manifested abnormal behavior when encountering stressful or novel situations. In infants reared by peers, separations at 6 months of age were associated with higher levels of plasma cortisol and adrenocorticotropic hormone (ACTH) than were found in those infants that were reared by their own mothers. In addition, the peer-raised group manifested lower cerebrospinal fluid (CSF) levels of norepinephrine and higher CSF levels of 3-methoxy-4-hydroxyphenylglycol (MHPG). These observations confirmed the theories of Bowlby (1969, 1973) regarding the importance of attachment objects early in life. The "therapist" monkeys simply were not as effective as the actual mothers in serving as a secure base from which the infants could explore new situations or in being able to comfort the infant monkeys and reduce their fear.

Suomi's (1991) research provides persuasive evidence that the nature of early attachment relationships is essential to psychological health. In addition, his research supports the notion that genetic-constitutional vulnerability must be taken into account. Approximately 20% of infant monkeys reared by their mothers reacted to brief social separations with increased cortisol and ACTH, depressive reactions, and exaggerated norepinephrine turnover. This inborn vulnerability, however, could be overcome when infants in this group were reared by unusually nurturant mothers. In fact, when raised by these outstanding mothers, infant monkeys showed accelerated development and even achieved dominant social status. One interpretation of these findings is that the unusually nurturant mothers help the young monkeys develop their innate sensitivity in an adaptive manner that allowed them to be more attuned to social cues and to respond to those cues in a way that was advantageous to them.

Mild trauma has also been studied in primates and appears to produce specific biochemical and behavioral changes. Rosenblum and Andrews (1994) randomly assigned infant monkeys either to normal mothers or to mothers temporarily made anxious by an unpredictable feeding schedule. The offspring of anxious mothers showed diminished capacity for normal social interaction and were socially subordinate. However, the changes did not manifest themselves until adolescence, confirming a basic psychoanalytic notion that disturbances in early phases of development can produce psychopathological effects in later developmental periods. These behavioral changes were also associated with serotonergic and noradrenergic alterations. Because genetic influences were controlled by random assignment, the findings suggest that distraction and anxiety in the mother were central to the identified changes.

Research data of this kind suggest that there are windows in time during which a gene is dependent on a certain type of developmental influence to determine its expression. Recent investigators have been finding similar windows in human development for periods of major structural change in brain formation: early childhood (15 months to 4 years), late childhood (6–10 years), puberty, and mid-adolescence (Ornitz 1996). Several research teams have postulated interactions between childhood trauma and structural brain maturation. Pynoos et al. (1997) have suggested that trauma induces changes in neuromodulation and physiological reactivity manifested in anxiety associated with traumatic expectations and increased attentiveness to external stimuli to detect danger. Perry et al. (1995) argued that early childhood trauma can alter midbrain, limbic, and brain-stem structures through use-dependent modifications secondary to extended alarm reactions. They also noted that cortical development may be retarded by experiences of neglect and deprivation early in life, thus reducing cortical modulation of limbic, brain-stem, and midbrain responses to fear and danger.

Bremner et al. (1997) has shown that adults with posttraumatic stress disorder who had experienced childhood physical and sexual abuse had dramatically reduced left hippocampal volume when compared with matched controls. It may well be that traumatic experiences during unstable periods of brain development can produce a form of regression to an earlier stage of neural function and structure (Pynoos et al. 1997). Preliminary data by Putnam and Trickett (1997) from a longitudinal study comparing sexually abused girls with nonabused controls indicate that those girls who were abused appeared to have altered regulatory dynamics of the neuroendocrine system, different neuroendocrine responses to stressors, and hypersecretion of corticotropin-releasing hormone (CRH) that induced an adaptive downregulation of CRH receptors in the anterior pituitary.

The Diathesis-Stress Model

Extensive data support the notion that many psychiatric disorders are caused by a combination of genetic-constitutional vulnerability and environmental or psychosocial stressors that activate that inborn vulnerability. As Suomi's data indicate (see previous section), inborn diatheses may be compensated for by extraordinary responses from the environment. Therefore, just as we should be skeptical of either/or reductionism in the biological and psychological polarities of etiology, we should also be suspicious of thinking in either/or terms about genetics and environment.

Social phobia is one disorder that beautifully illustrates this interaction between constitution and environment (Gabbard 1992b, 2000). Kagan and colleagues (1988) studied cohorts of children using a longitudinal design that compared consistently inhibited with consistently uninhibited children. Those children who were behaviorally inhibited clearly belonged to a qualitatively distinct category of infants apparently born with a lower threshold for limbic-hypothalamic arousal in response to unexpected changes in the environment or novel events that cannot be easily assimilated. Kagan et al. (1988) regarded this temperamental disposition as *behavioral inhibition to the unfamiliar.* In addition, these authors noted that some form of chronic environmental stress was necessary to activate the original temperamental disposition and thereby lead to an end result of shy, quiet, and timid behavior at 2 years of age. They suggested that stressors such as humiliation and criticism from an older sibling, death or separation from a parent, or parental arguments might be significant in this regard.

Rosenbaum et al. (1992) extended this work by systematically evaluating parents of behaviorally inhibited children from a nonclinical cohort studied by Kagan. Parents of these children were clearly at greater risk for anxiety disorders, primarily social phobia. Also, parents of those children with both behavioral inhibition and anxiety had significantly higher rates of two or more anxiety disorders compared with two different sets of parents in control groups. One tentative interpretation of these authors' findings was that those children with behavioral inhibition who go on to develop anxiety disorders may have been exposed to parents with greater anxiety, who in turn conveyed to their children that the world is a dangerous place.

Shear et al. (1993) have suggested that interactions of temperament and environment are involved in the etiology and pathogenesis of panic disorder. These authors propose that the same temperament described by Kagan et al. (1988) may predispose to early fearfulness. When these vulnerable children are then exposed to behaviors by their parents that confirm that the world is a fearful place, they develop characteristic patterns of object relations as well as persistent conflicts involving dependency that ultimately evolve into fears of being suffocated, unable to escape, and unable to get help. Frustration and resentment are stressors that frequently precede the onset of discrete panic attacks in adults.

Another possible underlying pathogenetic mechanism for panic disorder is that early parental loss may trigger inherited neurophysiological vulnerability (Gabbard 2000). Kendler et al. (1992) studied the relationship between parental loss prior to age 17 years and adult psychopathology in 1,018 pairs of female twins. These authors observed that panic disorder was significantly and strongly associated with both parental death and separation. Moreover, maternal separation early in life was much more likely to result in panic disorder than was paternal separation. Indeed, contrary to conventional wisdom, the impact of parental loss was three times greater for panic disorder than it was for major depression.

One of the most sophisticated efforts to tease out the relative contributions of genetics, environmental trauma, and psychological vulnerability derives from the Kendler et al. (1993) prediction study of major depression in women. Multiple assessments over time of 680 female-female twin pairs of known zygosity were used to construct an integrated etiological model for the prediction of major depressive episodes. Kendler et al. found that genetic factors play a "substantial but not overwhelming" etiological role (1993, p. 1144). The single most influential predictor and risk factor for major depression was recent stressful events. Neuroticism as derived from the Eysenck Personality Questionnaire (Eysenck and Eysenck 1975) was also a powerful predictor of future episodes of major depression, in part because it served to reduce the level of social support. Interpersonal relations, as measured by parental warmth, social support, and recent difficulties, also played an important role in predicting major depression.

In a further communication from the study, Kendler et al. (1995) reported on 2,164 members of female-female twin pairs, whom they followed for an average of 17 months. Recent stressful events were once again the most powerful risk factor for an episode of major depression. Those with the lowest genetic risk had only a 0.5% probability of depression onset per month if they were unexposed to a stressful life event. If a severe life stressor occurred, their probability of a depressive episode increased to 6.2%.

Those with the highest genetic risk had only a 1.1% probability in the absence of a stressor, but the risk escalated to 14.6% if a stressor was present. Genetic factors appeared to alter the sensitivity of individuals to the depression-inducing effect of stressful life events. Hence, the investigators concluded that gene expression was not static but rather was highly responsive to environmental stressors.

In some cases, a person with a temperament that predisposes to the development of depression may alienate others, and this may lead to chronic difficulty in maintaining social support, which in turn further predisposes to the development of depression. In a subsequent analysis of the twin study, Kendler et al. (1999) found that about one-third of the association between stressful life events and onset of depression was noncausal, because those individuals predisposed to major depression selected themselves into high-risk environments.

The Role of Meaning

If the diathesis-stress model is limited simply to environmental trauma in interaction with genetic vulnerability, there is a risk of neglecting the importance of the personal meanings of stressors (Robbins 1993). Why does one person respond to a stressor with a severe psychiatric disorder while another person does not? Obviously, genetic vulnerability is one answer. Another possibility, not mutually exclusive from the first, is that the same stressor has different meanings for different individuals. Hammen (1995) noted that "the field has reached considerable consensus that it is not the mere occurrence of a negative life event but rather the person's interpretation of the meaning of the event and its significance in the context of its occurrence" (p. 98). In a longitudinal study of the link between depressive reactions and stressors, she and her colleagues found that those stressors whose content matched the patient's area of self-definition were particularly likely to precipitate depressive episodes (Hammen et al. 1985). In other words, in someone whose sense of self is partly defined by social connectedness, loss of significant interpersonal context may precipitate a major depression.

When considering the psychodynamic aspects of illness, the clinician must make a distinction between causes and meanings. Certain behaviors that have clearly biological underpinnings may nevertheless have conscious and unconscious meanings to the individual. One study of 50 hallucinating psychiatric inpatients (Miller et al. 1993), for example, found that many of the patients regarded their hallucinations in a positive way and had attributed adaptive meanings to them. Similarly, the compulsive rituals and obsessional thoughts of a patient with obsessive-compulsive disorder (OCD) may be biological in origin but may have highly idiosyncratic meanings to the patient. Often preexisting psychodynamic conflicts attach themselves to the biologically driven compulsions and obsessions, and the symptoms then function as a vehicle for the expression of the conflicts (Gabbard 1992a). Symptoms of depression, for example, may be mediated by neurochemical changes but may be regarded by the patient as well-deserved punishment for unforgivable transgressions (Gabbard 2000).

A case vignette will illustrate how meaning can be derived from psychotic symptoms:

> Ms. A, a 24-year-old single woman with schizoaffective disorder, had been in treatment with me for approximately 6 months when she had to deal with my upcoming 3-week summer vacation. I was treating her with both medication and psychotherapy, and her psychotic episodes had been well controlled. My attempts to explore the impact of my absence were met with indifference. She steadfastly maintained that my departure would have no impact on her.
>
> When I returned from vacation, the colleague covering my patients informed me that Ms. A had become psychotic and had had to be hospitalized. I went to see her in the hospital and found her actively hallucinating. She explained to me that she was having a conversation with her brother Tom, and she asked me not to interrupt. I complied with her request and listened as she laughed and joked with her hallucinated companion. As I sat patiently, I found myself feeling strangely excluded, as though I was of no importance to Ms. A. I also noted a growing sense of irritation that I was unable to reconnect with her despite several efforts to inquire gently about what had happened while I was away. Each time I asked, she would turn to me and say, "Shush!"
>
> Eventually it dawned on me that Ms. A had turned the tables on me. I was now feeling excluded and angry in the same way she had felt during my holiday. I offered the following observation: "I wonder if you're wanting me to feel excluded in the same way you felt while I was on vacation." Ms. A broke away from her absorbing conversation with her hallucinated brother and retorted emphatically, "I don't need you! I have my own family! Why don't you go back on vacation with your family?!"
>
> The meaning of the hallucinated brother had become clear: he was a source of comfort, a bulwark against feelings of loss to Ms. A, and a vehicle to make me feel excluded in a way that allowed her to actively master a passively experienced trauma. She was able to projectively disavow her anger and hurt at being excluded by inducing similar feelings in me. While I adjusted her medication to deal with the biochemical underpinnings of the psycho-

sis, I also examined the transference-countertransference dimensions of the relationship to understand the specific meaning of the symptoms to Ms. A. As the treatment went on, I came to realize that she had attached herself to her older brother Tom in childhood because of her perception that her parents had emotionally abandoned her.

Treatment Considerations

Comprehensive treatment planning must take into account the biological forces within the patient, the social and cultural environmental stressors, and intrapsychic factors such as self-esteem, unconscious meaning and conflict, and internal representations of self and others. There was a time in psychiatry when psychotherapy was regarded as the treatment of choice for so-called psychological disturbances and pharmacotherapy was reviewed as the treatment of choice for so-called biological disturbances. Such distinctions are no longer clear-cut. In an editorial on treatment of depression, Freedman (1989) made the following observation:

> Effective treatments (e.g., digitalis) do not directly comment on etiology—or even about cherished theories of etiopathology. If psychotherapy is elected, the well-established observations of striking responsivity to one or another of the various old and new antidepressants should caution against an exclusion of pharmacotherapies based solely on ideology or limited professional competencies. The observation that psychological supports as well as particular therapies can aid should signal to all physicians that the management of proved pharmacotherapies can be assisted by prudent supportive approaches. (p. 983)

Recent investigations have demonstrated that psychosocial and psychopharmacological interventions may have similar effects on brain functioning. For example, Baxter et al. (1992) used PET to investigate local cerebral metabolic rates for glucose in patients with OCD before and after treatment with either behavior therapy or fluoxetine. Both treatments produced similar decreases in cerebral metabolic rates in the head of the right caudate nucleus.

Psychodynamic therapy may have a significant impact on serotonin metabolism (Viinamäki et al. 1998). At the beginning of a 1-year psychotherapy process, single photon emission computed tomography (SPECT) imaging was undertaken with a 25-year-old man suffering from borderline personality disorder and depression. Another man with similar problems also underwent imaging but did not receive psychotherapy or any other treatment. Initial SPECT imaging showed that both patients had markedly reduced serotonin uptake in the medial prefrontal area and the thalamus compared with 10 healthy control subjects. After 1 year of psychodynamic therapy, repeat SPECT imaging showed that the patient who received the psychotherapy had normal serotonin uptake, while the control patient who did not receive psychotherapy continued to have markedly reduced serotonin uptake. Because the patient who received psychotherapy did not take medication in conjunction with the therapy, the findings suggest that the dynamic therapy itself may have normalized the serotonin metabolism. Clearly, further research is needed to confirm this preliminary finding.

Cognitive-behavior therapy appears to make biological changes in patients with panic disorder. Panic attacks can be triggered by lactate infusion in those with panic disorder. However, a study by Shear et al. (1991) has demonstrated that lactate induction of panic can be effectively reversed with successful cognitive therapy. In other words, panic disorder patients who had attacks precipitated by injection of lactate prior to therapy no longer responded in that manner after therapy.

Cognitive therapy also appears to influence thyroid hormone levels in patients with major depression. In a study by Joffe et al. (1996), patients who responded to cognitive-behavior therapy showed striking decreases in their levels of thyroxine (T_4). The nonresponders to the therapy showed increases in T_4. Another study of depressed patients found that the biological changes in sleep architecture produced by cognitive therapy were identical to those produced by antidepressant medication (Thase et al. 1998).

Psychotherapeutic interventions may have a significant impact on the rest of the body through their effect on the brain. In one study, breast cancer patients who underwent supportive-expressive group therapy lived an average of 18 months longer than did a randomly assigned control sample who received standard treatment but no therapy (Spiegel et al. 1989). Forty-eight months after the onset of the study, all of the control patients had died, whereas one-third of the patients in the psychotherapy treatment sample were still living. Similarly, Fawzy et al. (1993) reported that malignant melanoma patients who had been randomly assigned to their support group protocol had more favorable mortality rates and more lengthy remissions than did the control group patients. Richardson et al. (1990) found that lymphoma and leukemia patients who were offered a combination of home visits and counseling lived longer than control patients, even when differences in cooperation with medical treatment were controlled.

These promising data suggest that psychotherapy has far-ranging influences on a variety of physiological systems. The mechanisms underlying that influence are not entirely clear. Effects on the endocrine and immune systems are highly likely. Fawzy et al. (1993) found that in their study the support group patients had greater activity of natural killer cells.

There are also fascinating implications from our growing understanding about the manner in which genetic biological factors interact with the environment. Family therapy has the potential to alter how parents respond to the heritable characteristics of their children in a way that positively influences genetic expression. Two examples of this modality are functional family therapy (Alexander and Parsons 1982), which has demonstrated significant improvement in conduct disorder and prevention of first episodes of the disorder in siblings, and family therapy of depressed parents (Beardslee et al. 1993) to prevent serious psychopathology of the children.

The observation that psychotherapeutic interventions may affect the brain certainly does not preclude the notion that medication may act independently of psychotherapy and alter different biological substrates in some cases. Although recent surveys of practice (Pincus et al. 1999) suggest that the majority of psychiatric patients receive combined medication and psychotherapy, this combination is not nearly as well studied as either treatment alone. Nor is it systematically taught in most psychiatric residency programs. Indeed, teaching how to choose a single or combined treatment for a particular patient can be a formidable challenge. We have little data to guide us in these choices.

With a common disorder such as major depression, we know that both psychotherapy and medication are useful, but we do not always know when to use either modality alone versus a combination. We have some data suggesting that antidepressant medication tends to have greater impact on symptoms such as insomnia, appetite disturbance, and hopelessness, whereas psychotherapy appears to be more efficacious in improving work function and interpersonal relationships (DiMascio et al. 1979; Hollon et al. 1991; Weissman et al.

1974). In addition, analysis of the data from the National Institute of Mental Health (NIMH) Treatment of Depression Collaborative Research Program (Sotsky et al. 1991) has provided investigators with some tentative guidelines as to predictors of differential treatment outcome. For example, relatively mild impairment in cognitive dysfunction predicted superior response to cognitive-behavior therapy and to imipramine. Similarly, relatively limited social dysfunction predicted superior response to interpersonal therapy. Significant vocational impairment predicted superior response to imipramine. High depression severity and impairment predicted superior response to imipramine and to interpersonal therapy.

Combining medication and psychotherapy may be particularly useful in the more severe depressions. Medication may work more rapidly than psychotherapy and may provide more reliable relief from acute distress, while the psychotherapeutic modalities appear to enhance social functioning and to extend the relapse-free period. A 1997 "mega-analysis" (Thase et al. 1997) examined a number of studies to compare outcomes of unipolar depressed patients treated with psychotherapy alone with those of patients who received combined medication and psychotherapeutic treatment. The investigators found that there was a striking advantage of the combination in more severe depressions that are recurrent.

A randomized controlled trial involving the combination of medication and psychotherapy in the maintenance phase of major depressive disorder with 107 elderly patients also found some advantage for combined treatment (Reynolds et al. 1999). In this group of patients, the recurrence rates over a 3-year period were only 20% when nortriptyline and interpersonal therapy were combined. Nortriptyline and medication clinic visits alone led to a 43% relapse recurrence rate, while interpersonal therapy and placebo resulted in a 64% recurrence rate.

There is much less literature to guide us on most other disorders, with the possible exception of schizophrenia. The addition of psychoeducational family therapy to an antipsychotic regimen has been shown to reduce the relapse rate of patients with schizophrenia by half (Hogarty et al. 1991). In addition, an innovative form of individual therapy, termed *personal therapy*, was tested in a 3-year controlled trial using random assignment (Hogarty et al. 1997). The combination of personal therapy and antipsychotic medication administered intramuscularly was more effective than supportive and family therapies in preventing psychotic and affective relapse as well as noncompliance. It is notable, however, that this difference was demonstrated only for those schizophrenia patients who were living with their families.

Preliminary data suggest that combined treatments may also have an advantage in some anxiety disorders (Mavissakalian 1993), some cases of opiate dependence (McLellan et al. 1993), and bulimia nervosa (Walsh et al. 1997).

Although data are sparse, much creative work is being done to understand the optimal integration of medication and psychotherapy. Cloninger et al. (1993) have constructed a psychobiological model of temperament and character that consists of four dimensions of temperament and three dimensions of character. Based on extensive genetic research, these investigators have determined that the four dimensions of temperament—novelty seeking, harm avoidance, reward dependence, and persistence—are 50%–60% heritable (independently of one another), manifest themselves early in life, and involve preconceptual biases in perceptional memory and habit formation. The other 50% of personality is determined by character variables, including self-directedness, cooperativeness, and self-transcendence. These dimensions of character are shaped by family and environmental influences.

This research team has found that character variables distinguish whether or not a personality disorder is present. Temperament variables tend to be influential in determining the subtype of a personality disorder as well as susceptibility to those diagnostic entities on Axis I. Making the distinction between character and temperament can be helpful for planning treatment for a particular patient. Medications such as the selective serotonin reuptake inhibitors (SSRIs) target temperament constructs, such as impulsivity and affective lability, while psychotherapeutic interventions may deal directly with character variables, such as cooperativeness and self-directedness.

Psychiatrists who undertake combined pharmacotherapy and psychotherapy must develop what Docherty et al. (1977) have described as "bimodal relatedness." The psychiatrist must regard the patient as a distressed person with both subjective symptoms and a dysfunctional brain. The clinician must shift back and forth between an objective medical model approach and an empathic intersubjective approach.

Even if the clinician selects an exclusively psychopharmacological approach, he or she must pay attention to the patient's subjective experience of the medication and monitor the therapeutic relationship. The American Psychiatric Association's (1993) "Practice Guideline for Major Depressive Disorder in Adults" points out that "psychotherapeutic management" is an essential component of every pharmacotherapeutic treatment plan. Psychodynamic principles, such as transference, resistance, and countertransference, apply as much to pharmacotherapy as to psychotherapy (Gabbard 2000). Similarly, a pharmacotherapeutic alliance is essential to the pharmacotherapist in the same way that a psychotherapeutic alliance is to the psychotherapist (Gutheil 1982).

The role of the therapeutic alliance was studied in an analysis of the outcomes of 225 depressed outpatients enrolled in the Treatment of Depression Collaborative Study sponsored by NIMH (Krupnick et al. 1996). The patients were given one of four treatments: 1) 16 weeks of interpersonal therapy, 2) 16 weeks of cognitive-behavior therapy, 3) 16 weeks of imipramine plus clinical management, or 4) 16 weeks of placebo plus clinical management. Trained raters scored the therapeutic alliance for all patients in the project with the assistance of videotapes and an instrument designed to measure therapist and patient behaviors. Outcome was also assessed by using standard depression-rating measures. The researchers discovered that the therapeutic alliance was just as important for pharmacotherapy as for psychotherapy. In fact, the quality of the therapeutic alliance accounted for more of the variance in treatment outcome (21%) than did the treatment method itself (1%). The patient's contribution to the alliance, rather than the therapist's, seemed to be the significant factor related to outcome.

Conclusions

In the absence of the kind of data for all disorders that is available for major depression, clinicians must rely on their own clinical judgment regarding the optimal therapeutic approach. To an increasing extent, the structure and economics of the mental health delivery system are dictating the treatment and removing the clinician's autonomy and the patient's choice in the clinical decision-making process. Unfortunately, the most appropriate treatment for a given patient is not necessarily the most cost-effective. We practice in an era of constraint, and often clinicians must present a convincing argument to do what is best for the patient.

Another dimension to the ultimate choice of the treatment approach is the patient's interests and capacities. Many patients do not have the psychological mindedness, motivation, or commitment for dynamic psychotherapy. Other patients do not have the desire or perseverance to complete a regimen of behavior therapy. Still others resent the idea of medication because they view their symptoms as arising from a psychological matrix that requires understanding. We also live in an era of consumer orientation, and we must be attuned to the wishes of the patient in addition to the demands of those who pay the bills, as well as to the literature on efficacy and outcome.

The complexity of the mind-body problem may become obscured by the vicissitudes of the marketplace in day-to-day practice, but we must never lose track of the need to address both the person and the illness. We continue to walk a tightrope between the twin pitfalls of biological and psychological reductionism. The balancing act requires unswerving attention and concentration, but the satisfactions derived from practicing on the cutting edge of the mind-brain interface more than make up for the occasional loss of footing and the struggle to regain a safe and sensible position on the high wire.

References

Alexander JF, Parsons BV: Functional Family Therapy: Principles and Procedures. Monterey, CA, Brooks/Cole, 1982

American Psychiatric Association: Practice guideline for major depressive disorder in adults. Am J Psychiatry 150 (suppl):1–26, 1993

Andreasen ND: Linking mind and brain in the study of mental illness: a project for a scientific psychopathology. Science 275:1586–1593, 1997

Baxter LR Jr, Schwartz JM, Bergman KS, et al: Caudate glucose metabolic rate changes with both drug and behavior therapy for obsessive-compulsive disorder. Arch Gen Psychiatry 49:681–689, 1992

Beardslee WR, Salt P, Porterfield K, et al: Comparison of preventive interventions for families with parental affective disorder. J Am Acad Child Adolesc Psychiatry 32:254–263, 1993

Bowlby J: Attachment and Loss, Vol 1: Attachment. New York, Basic Books, 1969

Bowlby J: Attachment and Loss, Vol 2: Separation: Anxiety and Anger. New York, Basic Books, 1973

Bremner JD, Randall P, Vermetten E, et al: Magnetic resonance imaging–based measurement of hippocampal volume in posttraumatic stress disorder related to childhood physical and sexual abuse: a preliminary report. Biol Psychiatry 41:23–32, 1997

Cawley RH: Psychiatry is more than a science. Br J Psychiatry 162:154–160, 1993

Cloninger CR, Svrakic DM, Pryzbeck TR: A psychobiological model of temperament and character. Arch Gen Psychiatry 50:975–990, 1993

Damasio AR: Descartes' Error. New York, Grosset/Putnam, 1994

DiMascio A, Weissman MM, Prusoff BA, et al: Differential symptom reduction by drugs and psychotherapy in acute depression. Arch Gen Psychiatry 36:1450–1456, 1979

Docherty JP, Marder SR, van Kammen DP, et al: Psychotherapy and pharmacotherapy: conceptual issues. Am J Psychiatry 134:529–533, 1977

Edelman GM: Bright Air, Brilliant Fire: On the Matter of the Mind. New York, Basic Books, 1992

Edelson M: Psychoanalysis: A Theory in Crisis. Chicago, IL, University of Chicago Press, 1988

Engel GL: The biopsychosocial model and medical education: who are to be the teachers? N Engl J Med 306:802–805, 1982

Eysenck HJ, Eysenck SBG: Eysenck Personality Questionnaire Manual. San Diego, CA, Educational and Industrial Testing Service, 1975

Fawzy FI, Fawzy NW, Hyun CS, et al: Malignant melanoma: effects of an early structured psychiatric intervention, coping, and affective state on recurrence and survival 6 years later. Arch Gen Psychiatry 50:681–689, 1993

Freedman DX: Editorial note (especially for the media). Arch Gen Psychiatry 46:983, 1989

Gabbard GO: Psychodynamic psychiatry in the "Decade of the Brain." Am J Psychiatry 149:991–998, 1992a

Gabbard GO: Psychodynamics of panic disorder and social phobia. Bull Menninger Clin 56 (No 2, Suppl A):A3–A13, 1992b

Gabbard GO: Psychodynamic Psychiatry in Clinical Practice, 3rd Edition. Washington, DC, American Psychiatric Press, 2000

Greenough WT, Black JE, Wallace CS: Experience and brain development. Child Dev 58:539–559, 1987

Gutheil TG: The psychology of psychopharmacology. Bull Menninger Clin 46:321–330, 1982

Hammen CL: Stress and the course of unipolar and bipolar disorders, in Does Stress Cause Psychiatric Illness? Edited by Mazure CM. Washington, DC, American Psychiatric Press, 1995, pp 87–110

Hammen C, Marks T, Mayol A, et al: Depressive self-schemas, life stress, and vulnerability to depression. J Abnorm Psychol 94:308–319, 1985

Hogarty GE, Anderson CM, Reiss DJ, et al: Family psychoeducation, social skills training, and maintenance chemotherapy in the aftercare treatment of schizophrenia, II: two-year effects of a controlled study on relapse and adjustment. Arch Gen Psychiatry 48:340–347, 1991

Hogarty GE, Greenwald D, Ulrich RF, et al: Three-year trials of personal therapy among schizophrenic patients living with or independent of family, II: effects on adjustment of patients. Am J Psychiatry 154:1514–1524, 1997

Hollon SD, Shelton RC, Loosen PT: Research considerations in evaluating combined treatment, in Integrating Pharmacotherapy and Psychotherapy. Edited by Beitman BD, Klerman GL. Washington, DC, American Psychiatric Press, 1991, pp 353–375

Hyman SE: Look into the future: the role of genetics and molecular biology in research on mental illness, in Psychiatry in the New Millennium. Edited by Weissman S, Sabshin M, Eist H. Washington DC, American Psychiatric Press, 1999, pp 97–117

James W: The Principles of Psychology (1890). New York, Dover, 1950

Joffe, R, Segal Z, Singer W: Change in thyroid hormone levels following response to cognitive therapy for depression. Am J Psychiatry 153:411–413, 1996

Kagan J, Reznick JS, Snidman N: Biological bases of childhood shyness. Science 240:167–171, 1988

Kandel ER: Psychotherapy and the single synapse: the impact of psychiatric thought on neurobiological research. N Engl J Med 301:1028–1037, 1979

Kandel ER: From metapsychology to molecular biology: explorations into the nature of anxiety. Am J Psychiatry 140:1277–1293, 1983

Kandel ER: Genes, nerve cells, and the remembrance of things past. J Neuropsychiatry Clin Neurosci 1:103–125, 1989

Kandel ER: Genes, synapses and declarative forms of memory. Lecture given at the 146th annual meeting of the American Psychiatric Association, San Francisco, CA, May 1993

Kandel ER: A new intellectual framework for psychiatry. Am J Psychiatry 155:457–469, 1998

Kendler KS, Neale MC, Kessler RC, et al: Childhood parental loss and adult psychopathology in women: a twin study perspective. Arch Gen Psychiatry 49:109–116, 1992

Kendler KS, Kessler RC, Neale MC, et al: The prediction of major depression in women: toward an integrated etiologic model. Am J Psychiatry 150:1139–1148, 1993

Kendler KS, Kessler RC, Walters EE, et al: Stressful life events, genetic liability, and onset of an episode of major depression in women. Am J Psychiatry 152:833–842, 1995

Kendler KS, Karkowski LM, Prescott CA: Causal relationship between stressful life events and the onset of major depression. Am J Psychiatry 156:837–848, 1999

Krupnick JL, Sotsky SM, Simmens S, et al: The role of therapeutic alliance in psychotherapy and pharmacotherapy outcome: findings in the National Institute of Mental Health Treatment of Depression Collaborative Research Program. J Consult Clin Psychol 64:532–539, 1996

Lipowski ZJ: Psychiatry: mindless or brainless, both or neither? Can J Psychiatry 34:249–254, 1989

Mavissakalian MR: Combined behavioral and pharmacological treatment of anxiety disorders, in Review of Psychiatry, Vol 12. Edited by Oldham JM, Riba NB, Tasman A. Washington, DC, American Psychiatric Press, 1993, pp 565–586

McGinn C: The Mysterious Flame: Conscious Minds in the Material World. New York, Basic Books, 1999

McLellan AT, Arndt IO, Metzger DS, et al: The effects of psychosocial services in substance abuse treatment. JAMA 269:1953–1959, 1993

Miller LJ, O'Connor E, DiPasquale T: Patients' attitudes toward hallucinations. Am J Psychiatry 150:584–588, 1993

Modell AH: The Private Self. Cambridge, MA, Harvard University Press, 1993

Ornitz EM: Developmental aspects of physiology, in Child and Adolescent Psychiatry: A Comprehensive Textbook, 2nd Edition. Edited by Lewis M. Baltimore, MD, Williams & Wilkins, 1996, pp 39–51

Pardo JV, Pardo, PJ, Raichle ME: Neural correlates of self-induced dysphoria. Am J Psychiatry 150:713–719, 1993

Perry BD, Pollard RA, Blakley TL, et al: Childhood trauma, the neurobiology of adaptation and "use-dependent" development of the brain: how "states" become "traits." Infant Mental Health Journal 16:271–291, 1995

Pincus HA, Zarin DA, Tanielian TL, et al: Psychiatric patients and treatments in 1997: findings from the American Psychiatric Practice Research Network. Arch Gen Psychiatry 56:441–449, 1999

Putnam FW, Trickett, PK: Psychobiological effects of sexual abuse: a longitudinal study, in Psychobiology of Posttraumatic Stress Disorder. Edited by Yehuda R, McFarlane AC. New York, New York Academy of Sciences, 1997, pp 150–159

Pynoos RA, Steinberg AM, Ornitz EM, et al: Issues in the developmental neurobiology of traumatic stress, in Psychobiology of Posttraumatic Stress Disorder. Edited by Yehuda R, McFarlane AC. New York, New York Academy of Sciences, 1997, pp 176–193

Reiss D, Hetherington EM, Plomin R, et al: Genetic questions for environmental studies: differential parenting and psychopathology in adolescence. Arch Gen Psychiatry 52:925–936, 1995

Reynolds CF, Frank E, Perel JM, et al: Nortriptyline and interpersonal psychotherapy as maintenance therapies for recurrent major depression: a randomized controlled trial in patients older than 59 years. JAMA 281:39–45, 1999

Richardson JL, Shelton DR, Krailo M, et al: The effect of compliance with treatment on survival among patients with hematologic malignancies. J Clin Oncol 8:356–364, 1990

Robbins M: Experiences of Schizophrenia: An Integration of Personal, Scientific, and Therapeutic. New York, Guilford, 1993

Rosenbaum JF, Biederman J, Bolduc EA, et al: Comorbidity of parental anxiety disorders as risk for childhood-onset anxiety in inhibited children. Am J Psychiatry 149:475–481, 1992

Rosenblum LA, Andrews MW: Influences of environmental demand on maternal behavior and infant development. Acta Paediatrica Supplement 397:57–63, 1994

Schatz CJ: The developing brain. Sci Am 267:60–67, 1992

Schore AN: A century after Freud's project: is a rapprochement between psychoanalysis and neurobiology at hand? J Am Psychoanal Assoc 45:807–840, 1997

Searle JR: The Rediscovery of the Mind. Cambridge, MIT Press, 1992

Searle JR: Mind, Language, and Society: Philosophy in the Real World. New York, Basic Books, 1998

Shear MK, Fyer AJ, Ball G, et al: Vulnerability to sodium lactate in panic disorder patients given cognitive-behavioral therapy. Am J Psychiatry 148:795–797, 1991

Shear MK, Cooper AM, Klerman GL, et al: A psychodynamic model of panic disorder. Am J Psychiatry 150:859–866, 1993

Slavney PR: The mind-brain problem, epistemology, and psychiatric education. Academic Psychiatry 17:59–66, 1993

Sotsky SM, Glass DR, Shea MT, et al: Patient predictors of response to psychotherapy and pharmacotherapy: findings in the NIMH Treatment of Depression Collaborative Research Program. Am J Psychiatry 148:997–1008, 1991

Spiegel D, Bloom J, Kraemer HC, et al: Effect of psychosocial treatment on survival of patients with metastatic breast cancer. Lancet 2:888–891, 1989

Stern DN: The Interpersonal World of the Infant: A View From Psychoanalysis and Developmental Psychology. New York, Basic Books, 1985

Suomi SJ: Early stress and adult emotional reactivity in rhesus monkeys, in Childhood Environment and Adult Disease (Symposium No 156, CIBA Foundation Symposium Staff). Chichester, UK, Wiley, 1991, pp 171–188

Thase ME, Greenhouse JB, Frank E, et al: Treatment of major depression with psychotherapy or psychotherapy-pharmacotherapy combinations. Arch Gen Psychiatry 54:1009–1015, 1997

Thase ME, Fasiczka AL, Berman SR, et al: Electroencephalographic sleep profiles before and after cognitive behavior therapy of depression. Arch Gen Psychiatry 55:138–144, 1998

Viinamäki H, Kuikka J, Tiihonen J, et al: Change in monoamine transporter density related to clinical recovery: a case-control study. Nordic Journal of Psychiatry 52:39–44, 1998

Walsh BT, Wilson GT, Loeb KL, et al: Medication and psychotherapy in the treatment of bulimia nervosa. Am J Psychiatry 154:523–531, 1997

Weissman MM, Klerman GL, Paykel ES, et al: Treatment effects on the social adjustment of depressed patients. Arch Gen Psychiatry 30:771–778, 1974

Yeh SR, Fricke RA, Edwards DH: The effect of social experience on serotonergic modulation of the escape circuit of crayfish. Science 271:366–369, 1996

2

Gender Issues in Psychiatric Treatment

Carol C. Nadelson, M.D.
Malkah T. Notman, M.D.

As in all areas of health care, gender is an important variable in the treatment of a variety of psychiatric symptoms and disorders. Gender affects and is affected by psychosocial factors. There are also physiological or metabolic differences between men and women. Gender can influence a patient's choice of caregiver, the "fit" between caregiver and patient, and the sequence and content of the clinical material presented. It also affects diagnosis, treatment duration, and even treatment outcome, from psychosocial and biological perspectives.

In this chapter we focus on the relationship between gender and treatment and consider psychosocial and biological variables. We examine biological influences, developmental and life experiences, gender differences in personality styles, and the effects of stereotypes and values.

Introduction

Despite heroic efforts to reconceptualize existing paradigms, the dichotomization of "brain disease" and "mind disease" continues to be prevalent. There is growing support, however, for an interactional construct that unifies brain and mind, biological and psychosocial, based on increasingly sophisticated and complex scientific data and conceptualizations. As

Eisenberg (1995) has stated, "Nature and nurture stand in reciprocity, not opposition. All children inherit, along with their parents' genes, their parents, their peers, and the places they inhabit" (p. 1568). This idea about reciprocity and interaction of nature and nurture applies to gender differences.

Evidence of gender differences in the nervous system beginning in fetal life suggests that, from birth, boys and girls may not perceive and experience the world in the same way (Pilgrim and Riesert 1992). Gender differences in neural maturity and organization influence behavior and reactions in infants, which in turn can affect caretakers' responses, further reinforcing male-female differences. Because experience can modify the structure and function of neurons and neuronal networks and can even change gene expression, these differences in reactions serve to further alter the growth and development of neuronal pathways (Kandel 1999).

Another area in which the integration of biological and psychosocial phenomena has relevance is research on the consequences of early abuse. Early childhood physical and sexual abuse is associated with limbic system brain dysfunction. Teicher et al. (1993) concluded that their findings were "consistent with a complex biopsychosocial hypothesis: namely, that sociological factors leading to early abuse may result in biological alterations in the development of the central nervous system, with these alterations manifesting as persistent behavioral disturbances that are in turn associated with long-term psychiatric sequelae and a proclivity for the intergenerational transfer of abusive and aggressive behavior" (p. 305).

Studies also demonstrate that brain metabolism and function are affected by psychotherapy. These findings reinforce our understanding of the plasticity of the brain and how it is affected by behavior and experience, so that it can functionally organize and reorganize (Baxter et al. 1992; Schwartz et al. 1996; Thase et al. 1996).

These data underscore that the distinction between the biological and the psychosocial is both artificial and misleading. Brain differences between men and women could not explain the plethora of manifestations and meanings of gender differences for each individual. These complex relationships between biological and psychosocial have direct implications for treatment.

Values and Treatment

Personal and societal values affect standards of normality and influence the perception, diagnosis, and treatment of mental disorders and emotional problems (Nadelson and Notman 1977, 1982b; Person 1983). Labeling a behavior as deviant or psychopathological reflects a judgment about normality and affects the way a symptom is understood and whether and how it is treated.

Although there have been changes in how normality, mental illness, and deviancy are conceptualized, evidence suggests that there continue to be differences in what is considered normal for men and women. Broverman et al. (1970), in their classic study, found that when male and female psychotherapists were asked to describe a mentally healthy person, psychological health was more closely associated with descriptions of "healthy, mature, socially competent" men than with concepts of maturity or mental health in women. In both male and female therapists, standards of what was mentally healthy more closely approximated stereotypical conceptions of the normal male than those of the normal female ("normal" was thus equated with "like a man"). A 1990 report (Kaplan et al. 1990) concluded that attitudes toward gender roles have changed to some extent. Male and female psychiatrists' beliefs regarding gender-appropriate behavior have become more similar and less stereotyped. However, using ratings derived from the Bem scale (Bem 1974), the authors found that female psychiatrists were still more likely to choose masculine traits as optimal for women, whereas male psychiatrists were more likely to choose an undifferentiated pattern as optimal.

In the past, the attitudes of physicians toward patients were paternalistic, with authority residing in the doctor. This also has changed in the last few decades. However, the psychological forces that create the expectation that the physician be powerful and helpful remain. The gender makeup of the physician-patient dyad affects the nature of the relationship and also physician and patient behaviors. For example, compared with men, women visit physicians more often, see physicians earlier in the course of an illness, make more return visits, obtain more preventive care (especially if they see a woman physician), and take a more interactive role in their care. More interpersonal interchange occurs between doctor and patient when the doctor is female and the patient female than when the doctor is male and the patient female, and less paternalism and more support are reported. In addition, female patients volunteer more information to female doctors. On average, women physicians spend more time with individual patients than do men physicians (Bedakis 1998).

Differences persist in the ways that men and women patients are treated. Women's symptoms, for example, have more often been pejoratively labeled "psychogenic," implying that their complaints are not to be taken seriously (Lennane and Lennane 1973). Although women are more ready to report symptoms, their symptoms, in fact, may be regarded as unimportant. This tendency to discount women's symptoms may, in part, explain some of the gender differences in the diagnosis and treatment of some diseases. For example, women are diagnosed later and have different treatments prescribed, even for cardiac disease, which is often recognized at a later stage in women (Wenger and Speroff 1993). There is evidence suggesting that women are more likely to have certain preventive screening tests, such as Pap smears and mammograms, if they see female rather than male physicians (Lurie et al. 1993).

Although concepts and standards of what is considered "normal" masculine and feminine behavior have shifted, these changes in expressed values and attitudes are not necessarily integrated into a cohesive view of normality for either men or women. Even if treaters consciously adopt gender-neutral attitudes, their unconscious views about what is "normal" may remain unchanged. Those behaviors and attitudes of the patient that are markedly different from the therapist's may be judged as pathological, and such judgments can affect treatment (Nadelson and Notman 1977).

In all areas of health, values are communicated to patients in both overt and subtle ways in the process of evaluation and referral as well as during treatment (Nadelson and Notman 1977; Person 1983). In psychotherapy, therapists communicate values by their selection of material to question or to comment on, by the timing of their interpretations, and by their affective reaction to the content of what is said by the patient. Because it is the therapist's task to help the patient define priorities as well as to express and understand what is said, this subtle communication conveys the therapist's judgment. For example, the therapist may emphasize or ignore the patient's references to menstruation, to taking drugs, or to engaging in risky sexual behavior. On the basis of values, a therapist may respond more to the relationship-related problems of women patients and to the work-related concerns of men. By responding this way, the therapist in effect expresses a judgment of what is important and to whom and consequently may misinterpret the importance of these issues for the patient.

Values and attitudes are also meaningful in other areas of treatment. If a patient perceives that a psychopharmacologist is primarily interested in specific medication effects and side effects, the patient may respond to those specific questions and leave out other relevant data that he or she sees as unimportant to the doctor. Similarly, the psychopharmacologist may not ask psychosocial questions that are pertinent to an understanding of the symptom picture. For example, a history of sexual abuse may be important in the differential diagnosis between depression and posttraumatic stress disorder (PTSD), because aspects of treatment are different. Thus, both patient and clinician can inadvertently collude in the incompleteness of the history. The history given by the patient can be influenced by the cues the clinician gives as well as by the patient's expectations.

Gender also affects treatment priorities and approaches. It has been suggested, for example, that concern about some more characteristically male behavior, such as violence related to alcohol abuse, may lead to the development of treatment methods that are more suitable for men. Although these methods may also be used with women, there is evidence that they are less effective (Reed 1991; Weisner 1991). More attention may be paid to treating an adolescent male with schizophrenia or substance abuse, because of the threat of violence, than to treating a seriously handicapped but less threatening female with PTSD or depression.

Pharmacological treatment has accorded little attention to the different presentations and resource needs of men and women. For example, because of their smaller body size and higher body fat content, women show higher blood alcohol concentrations than do men after consuming the same amount of alcohol. Furthermore, in women, the gastric mucosa elaborates less alcohol dehydrogenase than it does in men (Frezza et al. 1990; Merkatz et al. 1993). Women also show greater susceptibility to the hepatotoxic effects of alcohol than do men; cirrhosis of the liver is twice as common in women as it is in men. From a clinical perspective, men tolerate more alcohol without symptoms than do women; stated another way, women may appear to be more drunk than men after ingesting less alcohol.

Less is known about the epidemiology and treatment of alcoholism and substance abuse in women than in men. The relative paucity of data on women with these disorders has led to the assumption that illness patterns and effective treatments are similar for men and women. Most treatment approaches have been male oriented and do not account for the psychological and behavioral factors affecting women (Kauffman et al. 1995). For example, many treatment programs attempt to dissociate abusers from their drug-using peers, a strategy that places women abusers at a disadvantage, since they are more likely to live with partners who also abuse substances and who discourage or prevent them from seeking help, often by means of threats or actual physical and/or sexual abuse. In contrast, male substance abuse patients are less likely to have substance-abusing partners. Most treatment programs also expect total abstinence as part of the treatment plan. This is impossible for most female abusers, who usually continue to live in drug- and alcohol-abusing environments. In addition, the confrontational approach used by many of the 12-Step programs to elicit complete disclosure often makes women uncomfortable. Many groups employ aggressive and punitive methods, including shouting and verbal assaults. Women respond better to relationally based treatment programs. They find women's groups more helpful, and they frequently do not attend mixed-gender groups or do not participate if they do attend. Because women's substance use more frequently occurs at home and is less public than men's use, their abuse is often not known by family and friends, so they are not encouraged to seek treatment. In addition, because women are more likely than men to be primary caregivers to dependent children, they are less likely to come to treatment if they lack child care.

One report of a group therapy program with chemical dependency patients indicated that women attended sessions less often than did men because the groups were less attractive to them. The authors hypothesized, as have other researchers, that women may experience groups with men as more confrontational or uncomfortable (Comtois and Ries 1995).

Gender and Choice of Therapist

Patients give many reasons for their choice of therapist. These reasons are often based on stereotyped views, such as that men tend to perpetuate patriarchal values or that women are more nurturant.

For a woman, the choice to be treated by a woman can also represent a wish to restore the relationship with her mother or to have a better mother. A desire to see only a male can be based on the desire to avoid this maternal kind of relationship or the anxiety that these feelings arouse, or it may reflect anxiety about the intense attachment that may be evoked by a woman (Nadelson and Notman 1991).

The search for a role model has also been an important determinant of choice of therapist (Person 1983). Women frequently feel that a woman therapist would be more responsive to their wishes for achievement, success, and self-actualization, or that because she has faced similar conflicts, she could empathize with them more easily. Although this idea may facilitate the development of an alliance, it does not, by itself, resolve the patient's difficulties (Notman et al. 1978). Men may search for a role model in a therapist for different reasons, such as a wish to learn how to be a good father, because most men have had many role models for achieving professional success but few role models for being a good family member or father.

Women may also request to see a woman because they want permission to succeed in certain goals, particularly those involving their work. Permission, explicit or implicit, can result in improvement and can enable the patient to compete and succeed, even if the issues are not taken up specifically and explicitly (Person 1983).

Identification with a therapist is also important. Although the reasons for the choice may be based on stereotypes, without regard for the characteristics of the specific therapist, the patient's feeling of greater comfort or empathy can facilitate the initial development of a positive therapeutic alliance.

More recently, concerns about sexualization and sexual relationships in treatment have become important factors in requests based on gender. For those patients who have actually been abused in a previous treatment, trust can be severely damaged. It may be particularly difficult for such patients to see anyone who serves as a reminder of the previous experience.

Women therapists are often asked to see women patients who have had sexual involvements with male therapists (Person 1983). Although it does occur, women are less likely to become sexually involved with their patients, either male or female, than are men (Gabbard 1989; Gartrell et al. 1986; Holroyd and Brodsky 1977).

Sexual orientation has also become a consideration. Many gay individuals request treatment from gays, who they feel not only will better understand and empathize with them but will also be less likely to judge their sexual object choice as pathological (Krajeski 1984). Although there has been controversy about the appropriateness of this disclosure, some therapists have indicated that disclosure of their sexual orientation to patients may be beneficial in therapy (Gartrell 1984; Isay 1989).

The patient's gender-based choice and expectations can also derive from idealized fantasies about the characteristics and capacities of the clinician and of what he or she can do for the patient. For example, if the clinician is prominent in the media or in the community, expectations based on this status can affect the therapeutic relationship (Nadelson and Notman 1991). This is true for both men and women, as treaters and as patients. Quasi-omnipotent qualities can be conferred on the therapist.

If the patient makes a choice because of the particular political views, sexual orientation, or cultural heritage of the therapist, treatment may begin with positive feelings, only to have these reversed if, in the course of treatment, the patient is disappointed. The recognition that the therapist is not omnipotent repeats past life experience. If there is a negative outcome, it may be blamed on the therapist's gender. If the therapist is a woman who is not the fantasied omnipotent mother who can transform the patient, devalued ideas about women can be confirmed.

Choosing a therapist of a particular gender with the expectation that this will resolve the patient's problems can also be a resistance to therapy. A woman may want to see a female therapist for treatment because she feels unlovable and unattractive to men and can, in this way, avoid the experience of confronting her feelings (Thompson 1938). A woman may seek a woman therapist initially because she wants support, and later devalue the therapist or find herself in an angry, competitive interaction, which can be a repetition of her relationship with her mother (Notman et al. 1978). She may be unaware of the origins of her feelings or the reasons for her choice of therapist. Although there are conscious reasons for choices, unconscious factors or needs such as fear of anger or a search for mothering may be important and should be considered in the initial encounter with a patient.

Specific gender-based recommendations in the choice of a therapist have also been made. It has been suggested that because some women victims of sexual abuse find it difficult to work with men, they choose to be treated by women. Some clinicians believe that adolescents should be treated by someone of the same sex because sexual issues are so pressing, embarrassing, and intrusive at this life stage that they can interfere with therapeutic progress. Many support the view that women should be treated by women in order to avoid being misunderstood or treated from a male-oriented perspective. However, this view oversimplifies the effects of gender and minimizes the necessary working through of ambivalence and conflict in the therapeutic relationship.

Stereotypes and expectations about women affect male patients as well. A man may seek treatment from a woman in order to avoid a competitive or authoritarian relationship with a man, to avoid homosexual feelings, or to work on relationship issues with a woman because he has had poor relationships with women in the past. His expectations may be that a woman will provide the cure for his problems with intimacy.

In an effort to avoid being labeled as sexist, a male therapist may not focus on or confront certain problems. Some have described feeling intimidated by the successful women who are their patients. They may not feel free to raise questions about the motivation or specific behavior of such a patient, fearing accusations about being sexist or unsympathetic. Some women avoid female therapists who they fear might confront them more directly about this behavior.

The Therapeutic Process

Understanding the concept of transference can clarify aspects of the doctor-patient relationship that may otherwise be difficult to comprehend. The attitudes and feelings brought to a relationship from past experiences with important figures, such as parents, are important components of future interactions. The need to please or to gain love by acquiescent or seductive behavior can be brought into the doctor-patient relationship. This behavior may appear to be a genuine reaction to the physician rather than a pattern of response to anyone in authority carried over from past relationships.

The classical conceptualization of transference assumed that both maternal and paternal transference could be developed toward both male and female therapists. Thus, the therapist's gender was not a particularly salient consideration. Freud (1931/1961) came to believe that transference responses to a male analyst differed from those to a female analyst. Subsequently, however, Horney (1967) emphasized the importance of the competitive transference with the same-sex analyst, and Greenacre (1959) stated that strong wishes about the choice of analyst with regard to gender should be respected but also carefully analyzed, because prior wishes, expectations, and fantasies could affect not only the choice of analyst but also the course of the analytic process. Zetzel (1966/1970) observed that the content of the transference neuroses in the psychoanalysis of adult patients was influenced by the gender of the analyst or therapist. She indicated that transference repeats both the patient's actual identification with the same-sex parent and the patient's wish for love from the opposite-sex parent. The current view is that the person of the therapist is important and that therapy is affected by real characteristics of both the therapist and the patient.

Age, race, and other variables can affect the initial relationship and the early and evolving transference, as well as the sequence in which therapeutic issues emerge and the pace at which therapy progresses. For example, working with a woman therapist can evoke maternal transference material earlier in the treatment (Turkel 1976).

Therapists often do not attend sufficiently to the transference issues that encourage or inhibit discussion of particular material. This insufficient attention may be based on a number of factors, including gender. It can be seen at any phase in a therapeutic interaction and can occur with any patient or in any treatment modality. For example, a black patient may not tell a white therapist something that the patient sees as potentially reinforcing a stereotype about black people that he or she believes the therapist shares with other whites. For women patients who are also members of minority ethnic or social groups, there are additional issues in being what has been described as "double minorities" (Nadelson and Zimmerman 1992). As expressed by sociologist Deborah King (1987; quoted in Collins 1989), they are members of both groups and yet stand apart and are outside. This double position promotes the development of what King termed "multiple consciousness"—a sometimes inescapable sense both of belonging and of not quite being present.

As we suggested earlier, patients also may fail to reveal details of sexual abuse or other sexual experiences to a male or female therapist depending on the patient's view of how the therapist might hear or react to this information. This lack of disclosure may be related to the patient's stereotypic ideas as well as to the particular characteristics of both patient and therapist or the nature of the transference.

Many women feel that it is more difficult for a man to empathize with some issues that are gender specific; this may also be true for women who must empathize with male issues. Women report that they do not tell male therapists details of menstrual-related symptoms or even discuss concerns about hysterectomy or past histories of abortion or miscarriage. These "censorships" create the potential for inappropriate treatment.

The persistence of conventional sex-stereotyped attitudes and behaviors can be seen in some clinical examples. The concerns of a woman who decides to have children late in life or is ambivalent about childbearing, or those of the man who wants custody of his young children, are still often not appreciated. Therapists treating women may see themselves as advocates and may not fully acknowledge their patients' conflicts, such as that of balancing career and family. The woman executive who wants to have a baby but has recently undertaken a very demanding job may need to explore why she chose to make that commitment at the time she did, just as a woman of 40 with an established career who suddenly decides to have a baby and feels she must give up her career would do well to understand this behavior. Both women may be acting defensively as well as making positive choices. Countertransference issues are evoked by these situations (Nadelson and Notman 1991).

Changing Therapists

Change or reassignment of a therapist on the basis of gender has been widely discussed and is often recommended. Some have suggested that a change of therapist might mobilize a stalemated situation. Transfers on the basis of the therapist's gender have also been made when there is a therapeutic impasse or failure.

Unless there has been a sexual interaction, however, it is rare that gender per se is the significant variable in the majority of cases that are not successful. A transfer based on gender may be a way of avoiding responsibility for failure or dealing with the embarrassment of negative outcome. Person (1983) suggested that women therapists are often referred particularly difficult patients as second treatments. Because gender affects trust, and even compliance, in other modes of treatment, as well as in psychotherapy, change in the treater based on gender might be helpful in some situations.

Choice of Therapist Gender in Couples and Family Therapy

So far we have focused primarily on individual therapy. As with all forms of therapy, however, gender is a consideration in the choice of a therapist for couples or families. In general, as with individual therapy, issues related to gender choice should be clarified and addressed. A couple with marital difficulties may request a female therapist because it is the wife who has made the call and it is her preference, perhaps because she feels intimidated by men or because she fears that she could be left out of the male dyad if the therapist were male. On the other hand, the husband may choose a woman or comply with his wife's choice of a female therapist because he is more comfortable and less threatened by women, because he does not take the therapy seriously, or because he has negative feelings about women. The choice of a male therapist for some couples may re-create, in the transference, a paternal or authoritarian relationship or even the fantasy of possible sexual abuse. This can be a special problem if abuse has actually occurred.

During the course of therapy, attention must be paid to bias regardless of whether the therapist is male or female. Transference issues in couples and family therapy are multiple and more complex because there are more people directly involved in the therapy. For example, each partner, and the couple as a unit, will have different transference reactions to the therapist and to each other. If there are additional family members involved, they too will add to the transference complexity.

Changes in family patterns have also presented an increasing array of challenging issues for therapy. For example, the stress and demands of dual-career or commuting families, especially those with two achievement-oriented partners, can create enormous tension. This may be a greater source of conflict if the wife is earning more money, or if there is a job offer for either partner in another city. Because the husband's work has traditionally been the motivating factor in a relocation, a wife's job offer can create tensions, especially involving competition. A wife who achieves success later in life can be on a different timetable than her husband, who may wish to retire earlier.

The demands of parenting or of caring for elderly relatives can also stress a delicate marital balance. At times, the solution chosen to a particular problem at a particular time is a compromise between old expectations and new realities; for example, a wife will temporarily put her career on hold while her husband builds his, which does not take into account the decreased income that may result or the long-term effect on the wife's career. The husband who defers to his wife's work faces additional problems, because this has traditionally been the less accepted choice and he may feel isolated, demeaned, or "unmasculine."

Life-cycle issues have also increasingly become a concern of couples and families. Career paths take many turns, and career directions may change throughout the life cycle. There are unexpected opportunities and disappointments that stress families at different times. For example, if a husband's career plateaus by his 40s and his wife is just emerging from a period of lowered career activity because of child rearing, their interests and activities may diverge.

The increasing divorce and remarriage rates have also brought a larger number of so-called reconstituted or recombined families. The members of these families often experience divided and conflicted loyalties between their family of origin and their new family. There are also unexpected pressures related to childbearing at different phases of the life cycle with many of these relationships. For example, a childless woman in her late 30s may marry a man in his 50s with grown children, and the couple may be in conflict about having additional children. Although they may have previously agreed that children were not an option, often the wife, who is younger, changes her mind, and marital problems ensue.

As men gain permission to express their dependent needs and wishes for nurturance, they experience conflicts that are not dissimilar to those that women have traditionally encountered. A man caught in an unsatisfying and even destructive marriage may find himself torn between pursuing a new and gratifying relationship and potentially losing the intimacy and experience of his children's growth if he leaves his family. The alternatives are to remain in the marriage, leave and attempt to gain custody, or work out joint arrangements. The therapist can be influenced by his or her attitudes and values about divorce, marriage, and custody.

Feminist critiques of family therapy express concerns about the structural/hierarchical dominant role of males in the family, mother blaming, assumptions about sharing power and responsibility embedded in systemic concepts, and assumptions about therapist neutrality (Nutt 1992; Stabb et al. 1997). Family therapy has recently been criticized for biased treatment of men—for example, for reinforcing the socialized limitations of male roles (Stabb et al. 1997).

Group Therapy

As with couples and family therapy, there are gender issues in group therapy. When group therapy is sought or recommended, the gender of the group therapist is not frequently considered, although the gender composition of the group often becomes an important factor. There are some data suggesting that group behavior both between group members and with the leader is affected by gender (A. Bass 1990; Mayes 1979).

Women often seek women's groups because in groups of men or even in mixed groups they feel powerless, intimidated, and uncomfortable about speaking up. One need only look at classrooms, professional meetings, and business groups to recognize that women speak less often than men, and when they do speak, their comments are more often ignored or attributed to others. Women report the same experiences, regardless of professional status or income (Nadelson 1987). They may feel supported and less anxious in same-sex groups, although mixed groups may be helpful in confronting these issues.

Most often single-sex groups have been used for support and consciousness-raising. Both male and female self-help groups often form around a specific focus (e.g., substance abuse, divorce, family violence) and use problem-solving approaches.

It has also been suggested that issues deriving from early developmental experiences surface more frequently in single-sex groups, whereas in mixed groups these issues may be overlooked or avoided because heterosexual interpersonal issues receive more attention. An argument can be made for mixed-sex groups when there are problems of professional development, because colleagueship between men and women continues to be problematic.

McNab (1990) reported that men set themselves apart to a greater extent than do women at the start of group therapy and become integrated into the group later.

Therapy groups with both male and female leaders permit men and women to deal with transference issues, both as peers and as leaders. It is important, however, that the leaders' relationships with each other, just as with male and female therapists in family therapy, be a facilitating rather than inhibitory factor. Mistrust, competition, and anger that are not addressed in either leaders or group members can be unproductive and inhibitory to group process.

The Role of Life Experiences

The patient's life experiences can be viewed differently by male and female therapists, particularly if these experiences are gender specific. Reproductive events, decisions, and choices, for example, can have different significance for men and women, and the treatment process can be affected. Because reproductive issues are more likely to be addressed for female patients, male patients may find that their reproductively related concerns are not dealt with. Therapists often share patients' reluctance to explore these issues. This avoidance may result from the general belief that reproduction is a women's issue or from the conscious or unconscious conviction that exploration of a man's infertility or sexual dysfunction would constitute too great a threat to the patient's view of his "masculinity."

Person (1983) suggested that certain kinds of material are not so much consciously withheld as "overlooked." Menstrual symptoms, for example, may not be discussed by a female patient because she thinks they are irrelevant, and male therapists, especially younger males, are less likely to ask about such symptoms. Supervisors report that trainees may ignore certain material or interpret behavior as "regressed" or "primitive" because they fail to understand the critical importance of a particular event that may have to do with gender. For example, one senior resident, in presenting a couples therapy case to a supervisor, discussed the difficulty the husband was having with his wife's "regressive" behavior. The resident described the wife as "borderline." It was only at the end of the supervisory session that the resident casually reported that the wife was scheduled for a hysterectomy the next day. This particular example raises many questions, such as the following: Would an anxious male patient have communicated his anxiety in a way that was more likely to be recognized by a male therapist? If a male patient were to have a similar response to a prostatectomy, would it have been judged to be "regressed"? Would a male resident have failed to mention a male patient's surgery in a similar supervisory circumstance?

Gender Influences and Differences in Early Development

Early influences and endowments, both biological and psychosocial, are important in the shaping of personality. In childhood, the presence or absence of continued stable care, styles of child rearing, the responsiveness and nurturance of people in the environment, physical health and illness, loss, and trauma, as well as biological endowment, are all determinants of the ultimate configuration of personality.

Complex integrative functioning, such as conceptualization and learning of language and social skills, derives from both biological and psychosocial influences. These may differ between males and females. The effects of particular cultural practices, including gender differences in child rearing, are also manifested very early in life and affect development. Gender differences in parental behavior, especially related to male and female roles, are powerful developmental forces.

Ideas about the determinants of gender identity have changed from the early view that the major determinants of gender development were anatomic genital differences to a view that there are differing developmental experiences and paths. Complex processes take place beginning in the prenatal period. These different experiences include the hormonal environment, the structure of the family, the presence and roles of other siblings, the mother's past pregnancies, and many aspects of the child's relationships with others.

Gender identity development starts early, with prenatal expectations of parents and others about the child's gender and its meaning. By the second and third year of life, developmental goals include the growth of a sense of independence and the capacity to explore the world and, at the same time, to have a consistent, predictable, and close relationship with parents and others and to evolve a stable self-image. Important aspects of this developmental phase are the presence of an internalized image of the parent that remains, even when the parent is physically absent, and the ability to sustain a sense of closeness in the face of other conflicting feelings. If there is a disruption, such as a serious illness, a major loss, trauma, or family dysfunction, there may be greater vulnerability to psychopathology, particularly depression and some personality disorders (G. Adler 1985; Zanarini et al. 1989).

The connection between early trauma and the development of personality disorders, especially borderline personality disorder, has been widely discussed in the literature (Gunderson and Sabo 1993; Herman 1992; Herman et al. 1989; Johnson et al. 1999; Perry and Herman 1993; Zanarini 1997). Some characteristics of borderline personality disorder, which is more commonly diagnosed in women than in men, are consistent with the hypothesis that developmental disruptions occur when an individual is traumatized early in life. Some women's difficulty tolerating being alone and their intense fear of abandonment may be affected by early traumatic experiences (Clarkin and Kernberg 1993; Gunderson 1984). It is not clear why some people appear to withstand early trauma with greater resilience than do others (Gunderson and Sabo 1993).

Gender Identity and Gender Role

The concepts of gender identity and gender role have become important in treatment (Person and Ovesey 1983; Stoller 1976). Gender identity is the internalized sense of maleness or femaleness, and the knowledge of one's biological sex, including the associated psychological attributes. It begins to evolve in early childhood and appears to be firmly established by the age of about 18 months. It derives from many influences, including identifications with parents and their attitudes, expectations, and behaviors, as well as biological and cultural factors (Hines and Green 1991; Kleeman 1976; Money and Ehrhardt 1972).

Gender role is a cultural construct referring to the expectations, attitudes, and behaviors that are considered to be appropriate for each gender in that particular culture. There are enormous differences in the roles and expectations of men and women in different societies. Some societies dictate more rigid and fixed roles than others, and not all value the same traits or see traits as gender specific in the same ways.

The range of roles assigned to men and women in different cultures varies considerably. For example, despite their smaller size and lesser physical strength, women in some cultures are assigned the heavy work. However, the role consistently assumed by women across cultures is child rearing (LeVine 1991). In all cultures, the mother remains the child's primary caregiver during early development. For both boys and girls, the earliest bond is more likely to be made with the mother, who becomes the primary identification figure in early childhood. Thus, for girls, the first identification is with the parent of the same sex. For boys, the first identification is with the parent of the opposite sex.

As a girl grows up, this same-sex identification does not have to change in order for her feminine gender identity to consolidate. That is, she learns, consciously and unconsciously, about being female via her identification with her mother. In order for the boy to consolidate his masculine identity, however, he must shift his primary identification away from his mother and develop an identification with a male figure. In this process he moves away from his early attachment.

Many of these developmental differences have been thought to be important determinants of the personality differences that have been observed between men and women (Chodorow 1978). For men, the pull toward an early attachment to their mother can feel regressive and create a wish for distance and separation from these early ties. Closeness and intimacy can seem threatening, as if leading inevitably to regression. Clinically, we often see qualitative differences in intimacy, dependency, and attachment between men and women. The complex process of establishing a male identity and the separation from early attachments that seems necessary to the process of the development of a masculine identity may be factors accounting for the higher incidence of gender identity disorders in males (American Psychiatric Association 1987).

Although girls usually function better as students in the primary grades than do boys, and they present fewer behavior problems and less overt psychopathology, these characteristics also represent conformity to social stereotypes. Girls are often expected to be more compliant and conforming, and the later repercussions appear to be that the activity and ambition that lead to a sense of competence and self-esteem can be inhibited (Wellesley College Center for Research on Women 1992).

For girls, the continuity of attachment to their mothers, or primary caregivers, and the fear of loss of love if they manifest open aggression may make it more difficult to establish autonomy and independence while holding on to important relationships. Aggression, competitiveness, and anger may be difficult to manage, because expression of these feelings can threaten relationships. Women may be caught between the need to express themselves freely, especially when they experience anger and aggression, and the need to preserve relationships. This dilemma may be seen later in life in a woman's conflict about aggression, manifested in her difficulty in being appropriately assertive and in her inhibited risk-taking behavior (Nadelson et al. 1982). Cultural values such as independence, initiative, and competitiveness have traditionally been considered to be positive characteristics for males, but not for females.

Because of the primacy of relational ties, women also may be more vulnerable to loss throughout their lives. One of the syndromes that has been seen as related to the conflict about autonomy and independence, and the sense of vulnerability to loss, is agoraphobia, which is more commonly diagnosed in women than in men (Bourdon et al. 1988; Symonds 1971). Although this syndrome likely has biological determinants as well, it may represent anxiety about moving out into the world and feeling alone. Depression is more frequently diagnosed in women than in men (Weissman 1991). In contrast, disturbances involving violent, aggressive behavior and problems with impulsiveness are more often diagnosed in men (Weissman 1991). Conflicts around intimacy and socialization toward aggression and action are consistent with this picture in men. These findings raise questions about the factors affecting the process of diagnosis itself, particularly, although not exclusively, with Axis II disorders. Because these disorders more generally reflect clusters of observed personality characteristics rather than specific symptoms, the incidence figures may reflect biases and sex-role stereotypes (D. A. Adler et al. 1990; Sprock et al. 1990). It is interesting to note, in this regard, that approximately 75% of those diagnosed with borderline personality disorder are women (Gunderson et al. 1991). Male patients who have the characteristics of borderline personality disorder are more often diagnosed as having narcissistic or antisocial personality disorder (Gabbard 2000).

At times, women may also fail to act in their own best interests because of their desire to preserve relationships, even if these are abusive. For some women, this can result in behavior that may continue to put them at risk for victimization. The threat of loss, then, may motivate behavior that can be interpreted as masochistic. For women, the conflict experienced around aggression can result in turning aggression on themselves, such as occurs in the form of excessive self-criticism, with diminished self-esteem. Culturally supported passivity, and consequent feelings of helplessness, can be risk factors for depression.

For girls, problems in the development of self-esteem appear to be intensified in adolescence (Gilligan 1987). Gilligan (1987) found that there are gender differences in self-concept and identity in adolescence. Males generally define themselves in terms of individual achievement and work, and females more often in relational terms. Gilligan found that in mid-adolescence, girls experienced a crisis of connection involving conflicts between selfish or individual solutions to relational problems and selflessness and self-sacrifice. This period is also one in which girls become more vulnerable to depression compared with boys; it is a time when they begin to assume adult feminine identities and roles. The coalescence of biological and psychosocial factors makes it necessary to integrate rather than polarize our conceptualization of development.

Body Image and Reproduction

As puberty approaches, girls and boys experience their reproductive identities in different ways. For girls, menarche signals a capacity for pregnancy. This change also brings a potential vulnerability for girls that is not in boys' experience. Menarche is both a positive experience and a source of risk and anxiety. A girl also develops a new "organ," breasts, that transform her body. This has no parallel in boys (Notman et al. 1991). Menarche, for a girl, is an organizer of her sense of sexual identity. It is also an undeniable physical experience, and it can be a source both of pride and of conflict about growing up and being female. The adolescent girl in Western cultures is bombarded with media images of women who are loved because of their physical appearance. A specific model of physical attractiveness continues to be more important for women than for men, for whom strength and performance are more valued. For both, however, self-esteem and self-confidence rest heavily on physical attributes and body image, especially during adolescence.

Conflicts around self-image and body image become more prominent during adolescence and can be expressed differently for boys and girls. Discomfort with body image, and fear and ambivalence about mastery, independence, separation from family, and adulthood, including sexuality, are difficult issues that are thought to contribute to the dramatic incidence of eating disorders in adolescent girls, some of whom may literally attempt to starve themselves back into childhood.

Gender Differences in Life-Cycle Events

Women's life cycles are closely connected to their reproductive potential in a way that differs from men's life cycles. A woman's reproductive capacity is an important component of her sense of identity and femininity, regardless of whether or not she actually bears children. The knowledge that there is a finite time period for reproduction also influences her concept of time and her own life cycle. She must make decisions about career and family in a way that men are not compelled to do (Nadelson and Notman 1982a, 1982b; Notman and Lester 1988; Notman et al. 1991). This difference can obviously affect her emotional state and her decision to seek treatment if she feels the pressure of time passing and is concerned or unhappy about how her life is going, as well as the issues that will be raised in the course of treatment (Nadelson 1989). It is rare, for example, for a man in his 30s to seek treatment to resolve a problem about having children, whereas it is not uncommon for a woman to do so.

Pregnancy as a life event marks a transition to motherhood and raises many issues for a woman, including her relationship and identification with her own mother. This transition may parallel a man's experience of fatherhood, but the life event is not the same. A woman's vulnerability to specific psychiatric disorders can manifest during pregnancy, particularly in the postpartum period.

Infertility is also a different experience for men and women, and there are different issues to consider in treatment. Historically as well as in some cultures today, women have been "blamed" for infertility. A woman's pregnancy has also been viewed as a confirmation of a man's masculinity and potency. Infertility can be as threatening and distressing a problem for a man as it is for a woman, but in different ways. Social norms have supported men's resistance to be involved in infertility workups and treatment. Thus, a feeling of failure ensues when couples attempt to conceive and there has been inadequate evaluation or treatment because of resistance on the part of one of the partners.

Menopause is a marker of a woman's life cycle that has no equivalent in men. Stereotypical expectations about women's life cycles and the attribution of any symptoms that occur during this time to menopause have resulted in confusion of the experiences of this time of life, such as concerns about aging, family changes, shifts in expectations, and retirement, with the effects of the physiological event of cessation of menses. Menopause has been linked with depression and feelings of loss, but there is no evidence supporting an inevitable connection. Women who become depressed in midlife are generally those who have had depressions at other times in their lives.

In fact, the peak incidence of depression in women is in early adulthood (Weissman 1991). Estrogen replacement therapy does not address psychiatric problems, and many women have been referred to menopause clinics for treatment of depression or other symptoms that are not related to menopause. Responses to menopause are also strongly influenced by cultural expectations; in many cultures, women regard the cessation of menses and childbearing with relief.

Hysterectomy has been considered to be a procedure that produces a high risk for depression. Here, too, depression is not linked to the actual procedure. Most of the data supporting the link have not taken into account the woman's age, the diagnosis (e.g., cancer), the type of procedure performed (e.g., whether it is accompanied by oophorectomy and thus precipitates an abrupt menopause), or other circumstances, such as other events in a woman's life (McKinlay and McKinlay 1989).

Sexual Abuse

For those who have experienced early trauma, especially sexual abuse, which, as previously noted, is more common in women, the impact of the trauma and the betrayal by parental or other authority figures can result in psychopathology that emerges later. Sexual abuse can be understood as an etiological factor in the increased likelihood that survivors of childhood abuse will be victimized as adults (Herman 1992). Studies also report profoundly self-destructive behaviors emerging after victimization (Lystad 1986). The aftermath of abuse, particularly repeated abuse, is often a residual sense of helplessness and loss of autonomy (Nadelson and Notman 1979; Notman and Nadelson 1976) that may intensify conflicts about dependency and stimulate self-criticism, shame, and guilt in many areas of life. Difficulty handling anger and aggression and persistent feelings of vulnerability are also common repercussions.

Long-term consequences of early abuse appear to be different for women and men. There are some data suggesting that abused men tend to identify with the aggressor and are more likely later to victimize others, whereas women are more likely to establish relationships with abusive men in which the women and their children are victimized (Carmen et al. 1984; Jaffe et al. 1986; van der Kolk 1989). These findings are consistent with what we have seen are differences in the meaning of relationships for men and women, and the importance of relationships for the development and maintenance of self-esteem, as well as differences between men and women in the perception and expression of aggression and dependency (Chodorow 1978; Gilligan 1982; Miller et al. 1981).

In those who have been abused, the ability to form a trusting therapeutic alliance may be impaired, and, as we suggested earlier, this may lead to requests for a therapist of a particular gender. Although there is little in the literature suggesting profound differences in therapy outcome by therapist gender, this is an example of a situation in which patients may not seek or continue therapy if they are not comfortable with the therapist, and in this way gender may be an important variable.

Some of the responses and behaviors of those who have been victimized evoke profound countertransference reactions in treaters. There have been reports of gender differences in how physicians interact with abused women (Saunders and Kindy 1993). It may be difficult for some therapists to work with battered and abused women, who often evoke frustration and anger because of their tendency to displace anger, their passivity and failure to follow through on suggestions, and the frequency with which they return to the abusive situation. Some therapists overidentify with abused patients and may also project their own feelings, fantasies, or experiences onto their patients. These projections may include judgments about the appropriateness of the patient's earlier responses. Rescue fantasies may occur in both male and female therapists when they treat abuse victims. The therapist may attempt to become the loving, nonabusive parent that he or she thinks the patient should have had (Gabbard and Wilkinson 1994). These countertransference problems can compromise the therapeutic relationship.

Treatment Outcome

There are abundant data indicating that women have a greater incidence of some mental disorders and men of others. A 1991 report published by the Institute of Medicine cited gender differences in lifetime rates of mental and addictive disorders that have been replicated by other researchers (Weissmann et al. 1994) (Table 2–1).

There are also gender differences (Thase et al. 1994) in symptom reporting (Silverstein and Perlick 1991), treatment seeking (Angst and Dobler-Mikola 1985; Warren 1983), coping styles (Nolen-Hoeksema 1987), and a number of neurobiological variables. One study involving a community-based sample reported that depressed women had longer episodes of depression and a lower rate of spontaneous remission than men (Sargeant et al. 1990).

Evidence also indicates that men and women respond differently pharmacologically. For example, women may respond less favorably to tricyclic antidepressants than to monoamine oxidase inhibitors (Davidson and Pelton 1986; Yonkers et al. 1992), whereas men show a better response to tricyclics (Davidson and Pelton 1986) or to a combination of tricyclic antidepressants and psychotherapy (Frank et al. 1988).

As noted earlier, there are pharmacokinetic (i.e., potential differences in drug absorption, distribution, metabolism, and elimination) and pharmacodynamic (the basic mechanism of action of a drug at the cellular or receptor level) factors that can influence drug dosage requirements. Age, hormonal status (puberty, pregnancy, lactation, menopause), interaction with other drugs being taken, illnesses, and genetics affect drug action (Merkatz et al. 1993).

It may be useful to summarize the sex differences relevant to pharmacological treatment. Compared with men, women have

- lower body weight and thus attain higher concentrations of most medications when administered the same dose.

TABLE 2–1. Mental and addictive disorders in women and men

Disorder	Male lifetime rate/100	Female lifetime rate/100	Odds ratio[a]
Somatization	0.0002	0.4	7.34
Major depression	2.7	5.7	2.41
Panic disorder	0.8	1.8	2.31
Dysthymia	1.9	3.9	2.06
Phobias	9.5	18.3	1.98
Schizophrenia	1.0	1.6	1.48
Obsessive-compulsive disorder	1.8	2.4	1.33
Bipolar disorder	0.6	0.8	1.29
Drug abuse	6.2	3.7	0.64
Antisocial personality	3.7	0.8	0.18
Alcohol abuse	21.2	4.3	0.15

[a]Odds ratios are adjusted for age and socioeconomic status.
Source. Reprinted from Weissman MM: "Gender Differences in the Rates of Mental Disorders," in *Assessing Future Research Needs: Mental and Addictive Disorders in Women.* Washington, DC, Institute of Medicine, 1991, pp. 8–13. Copyright © 1991. Used with permission.

- a higher proportion of body fat in which psychotropic medications concentrate, which increases the necessary doses of some agents.
- slower gastric emptying time, in part related to estrogen and progesterone secretion, which may lower the effective amount of a medication that reaches the brain, thus requiring an increase in the required dose.
- 40% less gastric acid, which means that some medications (e.g., tricyclics, benzodiazepines, some antipsychotics) may not be neutralized by gastric acid before they are absorbed. Required dosages of these medications are thus lower for women.
- hormonal fluctuations and the potential for drug interaction with hormones during the menstrual cycle as well as during menopause, which can alter the effects of drugs such as antidepressants, lithium, and antianxiety agents (M. Bass and Howes 1991).
- hormonal changes during pregnancy, which may lower the capacity of some serum proteins to bind drugs, thus leaving more medication free to reach the brain.
- other changes that occur during pregnancy that may decrease the amount of medication present at the end organ. For example, cardiac pumping activity is greater during pregnancy; thus, drugs are metabolized and cleared more rapidly from liver and kidneys, which means that for some drugs, women may need higher dosages (however, these might be dangerous to the fetus).
- variations in drug effects as a result of interaction with contraceptives and estrogen replacement therapy (an increase in ovarian hormones may slow drug absorption, thus increasing the dosage required). In addition, the required dosage for some drugs (tricyclics, some benzodiazepines, propranolol, clomipramine, some antipsychotics) is lower because liver metabolism is inhibited.

There are gender influences on both the biological and the psychosocial variables that affect drug dosage, including side effects, compliance, and treatment outcome. Research findings on gender and substance abuse, noted above, illustrate this point.

Most of the early research on treatment outcome did not consider gender as a salient variable. This is beginning to change, particularly in the biological areas of psychiatry. In the psychotherapy literature, while there is increasing emphasis on outcome, gender has not been well studied. The analysis and interpretation of outcome data considering gender and psychotherapy, as with any outcome data, require consideration of a number of variables, including therapist/patient selection mechanisms and match, type of treatment, treatment goals, therapeutic process, length of treatment, measured and perceived therapeutic outcome, and patient satisfaction.

Most of the data on gender and therapeutic outcome have come from short-term types of treatment. Investigators in these studies have attempted to use easily controllable treatment techniques and protocols and to include patients with specific diagnoses, and they have assessed specific outcomes that are often behavioral (e.g., a decrease in alcohol intake or impulsive behavior) or measurable with specific objective criteria (e.g., depression or anxiety scales). Because affective and intrapsychic processes have been less amenable to the kinds of measures traditionally employed, there are many fewer studies of long-term psychotherapy and psychoanalysis.

Cavenar and Werman (1983), in their early critique of studies of psychotherapy outcome, emphasized the importance of specifying the treatment approach. They indicated that the gender of the therapist may be more relevant in modalities such as supportive psychotherapy, in which identification with the therapist and restoration of defenses are more critical. With insight-oriented psychotherapy, the goal of self-understanding and the difference in process may change the way interpretations are made and perceptions evolve (Cavenar and Werman 1983).

Mogul (1982) summarized views about gender and therapy, suggesting that therapist sex matters least in traditional psychoanalysis; however, this is not as true for face-to-face psychotherapies, which are less intensive, involve more partial transference reactions, and are more oriented to symptom alleviation, and for patients with developmental defects involving impaired ego functions or object relations. The issue, however, may have more to do with the alliance and the transference than the modality or the diagnosis. Person (1983) suggested that gender effects are more subtle in psychoanalysis than in psychotherapy but may be just as pervasive.

Popular belief is that women patients do better in therapy with women therapists because women therapists are more relational and empathic and are less likely to disempower women patients. Although there is empirical evidence supporting both sides of the efficacy argument for a gender effect in treatment, most studies conclude that no such effect exists (Zlotnick et al. 1998). However, no data are available from naturalistic studies.

One controlled study (Zlotnick et al. 1996) of the effect of gender on short-term treatment of depressed patients found no effect on patients' level of depression at termination, attrition rates, or patients' perceptions of the therapist's degree of empathy early in treatment and at termination. Likewise, patients' beliefs that a male or female therapist would be more helpful, and their match or mismatch in the study protocol, were not significantly associated with the results of the measures of treatment process or measures of outcome employed. Gender did not interact with therapist level of experience in these studies. It is possible that a patient's perception of a specific therapist is influenced not by gender stereotypes but rather by the patient's experience with the specific person.

Other controlled studies of short-term psychotherapy have reported that female therapists formed a more effective therapeutic alliance than did male therapists (Jones and Zoppel 1982) and that patients treated by female therapists experienced more symptomatic improvement (Jones et al. 1987). However, these results may be attributable to differences in methodologies and outcome measures. Some studies used self-reports; others used manualized treatment (Zlotnick et al. 1998). Given the rigid training and protocols used in these studies, naturalistic responses or differences in attitudes and behaviors might not emerge. In the study reporting a difference in symptom improvement by therapist gender (Jones et al. 1987), male therapists saw recently bereaved women who had lost a husband or father. Thus, the reported effects may have been related to the specific circumstances in which the symptoms originated or to the effect of seeing a male therapist as a possible replacement for the lost husband or father.

With regard to choice of therapeutic modality, much of the literature derives from methodologically problematic studies that are now dated. More current work continues to suggest, however, that males are more likely to be referred to a male therapist and that female therapists receive fewer referrals of male patients (Mayer and de Marneffe 1992). This finding implies that gender stereotypes continue to operate.

Studies conducted in the 1970s reported little outcome difference by gender of patient or therapist for short-term psychotherapy (Abramowitz et al. 1976; Blase 1979; Goldenholz 1979; Gurri 1977; Malloy 1979; Orlinsky and Howard 1976). Kirshner et al. (1978) studied a large number of therapist-patient matches in short-term individual psychotherapy and found that female patients showed greater responsiveness to psychotherapy and that greater patient satisfaction and self-rated improvement occurred with female therapists. More improvement was seen in attitudes toward careers, academic motivation, academic performance, and family relations. At the same time, however, these researchers also reported that the female patients of female therapists were less likely to describe their therapists as competent than were the patients of other gender dyads. When therapist experience and gender were considered, more experienced therapists seemed to have had better therapeutic results and showed fewer gender effects than did less experienced therapists, regardless of sex (Kirshner et al. 1978).

Other studies of gender differences focus on additional variables. For example, one study (Thase et al. 1994) reported that patients with higher pretreatment levels of depressive symptoms, especially women, had poorer outcomes. Another investigation (Frank et al. 1988) reported that among patients with recurrent depression, men demonstrated a more rapid response to treatment than did women. Still other research indicates that posttreatment outcomes are similar for men and women, that male and female patients suffering from major depression have generally similar outcomes over time-limited courses of cognitive-behavioral therapy (Sotsky et al. 1991; Thase et al. 1996), and that men and women have similar responses to different treatment modalities. Samstag and colleagues (1998) reported that the women in their sample were more likely either to have good overall outcome or to drop out of therapy, whereas the men were more likely to remain regardless of outcome. They pointed out that this result is consistent with reports in the literature indicating that women attend more to relational cues (Gilligan 1982; Gilligan et al. 1991). Samstag et al. (1998) suggested that the women in their study might have been more sensitive in assessing the quality of the interpersonal match in therapy and less likely to remain when they expected a poor outcome, whereas the men were more likely to see the therapy through to completion, regardless of the quality of the relationship. A further analysis of their data indicated that the subjective meaning of the alliance seemed to be the most critical factor. These data certainly suggest that more study is needed on gender effects.

Studies of psychotherapy efficacy have mostly been conducted with female patients and, as noted above, frequently do not consider other salient variables (e.g., age, race). There are also differences of opinion about the importance of therapist experience, with some studies showing that experience is an important variable and that it interacts with gender. Thus, the gender of a less experienced therapist may have a more negative impact on outcome than the gender of a more experienced therapist. There are data suggesting that less experienced female therapists do better with female patients than do less experienced male therapists. The theoretical orientation of a therapist may also be important. For example, some data indicate that the therapists who are most effective tend to have a psychological rather than a biological orientation, but that therapy (especially for depression) is longer with psychologically oriented therapists (Blatt et al. 1996). Some studies reveal that men and women prefer therapists of their own gender (Simons and Helms 1976).

In conclusion, it is apparent that gender is an important treatment variable and that attention to gender effects, together with better understanding of the complex interaction of gender and other variables, will shed light on the therapeutic process and contribute to greater therapeutic effectiveness.

References

Abramowitz SI, Roback HB, Schwartz JM, et al: Sex bias in psychotherapy: a failure to confirm. Am J Psychiatry 133:706–709, 1976

Adler DA, Drake RE, Teague GB: Clinicians' practices in personality assessment: does gender influence the use of DSM-III Axis II? Compr Psychiatry 31:125–133, 1990

Adler G: Borderline Psychopathology and Its Treatment. New York, Jason Aronson, 1985

American Psychiatric Association: Diagnostic and Statistical Manual of Mental Disorders, 3rd Edition, Revised. Washington, DC, American Psychiatric Association, 1987

Angst J, Dobler-Mikola A: The Zurich Study: a prospective epidemiological study of depressive, neurotic, and psychosomatic symptoms, IV: recurrent and nonrecurrent depression. Eur Arch Psychiatry Neurol Sci 234:408–416, 1985

Bass A: Studies find workplace still a man's world. Boston Globe, March 12, 1990, p 39

Bass M, Howes J: Towards a Women's Health Research Agenda: Findings of the Scientific Advisory Meeting. Washington, DC, Society for the Advancement of Women's Health Research, 1991

Baxter LR Jr, Schwartz JM, Bergman KS, et al: Caudate glucose metabolic rate changes with both drug and behavior therapy for obsessive-compulsive disorder. Arch Gen Psychiatry 49:681–689, 1992

Bedakis KD: Physician gender and physician-patient interaction, in Behavioral Medicine and Women: A Comprehensive Handbook. Edited by Blechman EA, Brownell KD. New York, Guilford, 1998, pp 849–853

Bem SL: The measurement of psychological androgyny. J Consult Clin Psychol 42:155–162, 1974

Blase J: A study on the effects of sex of the client and sex of the therapist on client's satisfaction with psychotherapy. Dissertation Abstracts International 49:6107–6107B, 1979

Blatt SJ, Sanislow CA III, Zuroff DC, et al: Characteristics of effective therapists: further analyses of data from the National Institute of Mental Health Treatment of Depression Collaborative Research Program. J Consult Clin Psychol 64:1276–1284, 1996

Bourdon K, Bloyd J, Rae D, et al: Gender differences in phobias: results of the ECA community survey. J Anxiety Disord 2:227–241, 1988

Broverman IK, Broverman DM, Clarkson FE, et al: Sex-role stereotypes and clinical judgments of mental health. J Consult Clin Psychol 34:1–7, 1970

Carmen E[H], Rieker PP, Mills T: Victims of violence and psychiatric illness. Am J Psychiatry 141:378–383, 1984

Cavenar JO Jr, Werman DS: The sex of the psychotherapist. Am J Psychiatry 140:85–87, 1983

Chodorow N: The Reproduction of Mothering: Psychoanalysis and the Sociology of Gender. Berkeley, University of California Press, 1978

Clarkin JF, Kernberg OF: Developmental factors in borderline personality disorder and borderline personality organization, in Borderline Personality Disorder: Etiology and Treatment. Edited by Paris J. Washington, DC, American Psychiatric Press, 1993, pp 161–184

Collins TH: The social construction of black feminist thought. Signs 14:745–773, 1989

Comtois KA, Ries RK: Sex differences in dually diagnosed severely mentally ill clients in dual diagnosis outpatient treatment. Am J Addict 4:245–253, 1995

Davidson J, Pelton S: Forms of atypical depression and their response to antidepressant drugs. Psychiatry Res 17:87–95, 1986

Eisenberg L: The social construction of the human brain. Am J Psychiatry 152:1563–1575, 1995

Frank E, Carpenter LL, Kupfer DJ: Sex differences in recurrent depression: are there any that are significant? Am J Psychiatry 145:41–45, 1988

Freud S: Female sexuality (1931), in Standard Edition of the Complete Psychological Works of Sigmund Freud, Vol 21. Translated and edited by Strachey J. London, Hogarth, 1961, pp 221–243

Frezza M, diPadove C, Pozzato G, et al: High blood alcohol levels in women: the role of decreased gastric alcoholic dehydrogenase activity and first-pass metabolism. N Engl J Med 322:95–99, 1990

Gabbard GO: Sexual Exploitation in Professional Relationships. Washington, DC, American Psychiatric Press, 1989

Gabbard GO: Psychodynamic Psychiatry in Clinical Practice, 3rd Edition. Washington, DC, American Psychiatric Press, 2000

Gabbard GO, Wilkinson SM: Management of Countertransference With Borderline Patients. Washington, DC, American Psychiatric Press, 1994

Gartrell N: Issues in psychotherapy with lesbian women, in Work in Progress, 83–04. Wellesley, MA, Stone Center for Developmental Services and Studies, Wellesley College, 1984

Gartrell N, Herman J, Olarte S, et al: Psychiatrist-patient sexual contact: results of a national survey, I: prevalence. Am J Psychiatry 143:1126–1131, 1986

Gilligan C: In a Different Voice: Psychological Theory and Women's Development. Cambridge, MA, Harvard University Press, 1982

Gilligan C: Adolescent development reconsidered, in Adolescent Social Behavior and Health (New Directions for Child Development No 37). Edited by Irwin C. San Francisco, CA, Jossey-Bass, 1987, pp 63–92

Gilligan C, Rogers AG, Tolman DL: Women, Girls and Psychotherapy: Reframing Resistance. New York, Harrington Park Press, 1991

Goldenholz N: The effect of the sex of therapist-client dyad upon outcome of psychotherapy (abstract). Dissertation Abstracts International 40:492B, 1979

Greenacre P: Certain technical problems in the transference relationship. J Am Psychoanal Assoc 7:484–502, 1959

Gunderson JG: Borderline Personality Disorder. Washington, DC, American Psychiatric Press, 1984

Gunderson JG, Sabo AN: The phenomenological and conceptual interface between borderline personality disorder and PTSD. Am J Psychiatry 150:19–27, 1993

Gunderson J, Zanarini M, Kisiel C: Borderline personality disorder: a review of data on DSM-III-R descriptions. J Personal Disord 5:340–352, 1991

Gurri I: The influence of therapist sex, client sex, and client sex bias on therapy outcome (abstract). Dissertation Abstracts International 38:898–899B, 1977

Herman JL: Trauma and Recovery. New York, Basic Books, 1992

Herman JL, Perry JC, van der Kolk BA: Childhood trauma in borderline personality disorder. Am J Psychiatry 146:490–495, 1989

Hines M, Green R: Human hormonal and neural correlates of sex-typed behaviors, in American Psychiatric Press Review of Psychiatry, Vol 10. Edited by Tasman A, Goldfinger SM. Washington, DC, American Psychiatric Press, 1991, pp 536–555

Holroyd JC, Brodsky AM: Psychologists' attitudes and practices regarding erotic and nonerotic physical contact with patients. Am Psychol 32:843–849, 1977

Horney K: Feminine Psychology. Edited by Kelman H. New York, WW Norton, 1967

Isay RA: Being Homosexual: Gay Men and Their Development. New York, Farrar, Straus & Giroux, 1989

Jaffe P, Wolfe D, Wilson SK, et al: Family violence and child adjustment: a comparative analysis of girls' and boys' behavioral symptoms. Am J Psychiatry 143:74–77, 1986

Johnson JG, Cohen P, Brown J, et al: Childhood maltreatment increases risk for personality disorders during early adulthood. Arch Gen Psychiatry 56:600–606, 1999

Jones EE, Zoppel C: Impact of client and therapist gender on psychotherapy process and outcome. J Consult Clin Psychol 50:259–272, 1982

Jones EE, Krupnick JL, Kerig PK: Some gender effects in a brief psychotherapy. Psychotherapy 24:336–352, 1987

Kandel ER: Biology and the future of psychoanalysis: a new intellectual framework for psychiatry revisited. Am J Psychiatry 156:505–524, 1999

Kaplan MJ, Winget C, Free N: Psychiatrists' beliefs about gender-appropriate behavior. Am J Psychiatry 147:910–912, 1990

Kauffman E, Dore MM, Nelson-Zlupko L: The role of women's therapy groups in the treatment of chemical dependence. Am J Orthopsychiatry 65:355–363, 1995

King D: Race, class and gender salience in black women's womanist consciousness. Dartmouth College, Department of Sociology, Hanover, NH, 1987 typescript

Kirshner L, Genack A, Hauser S: Effects of gender on short-term psychotherapy. Psychotherapy: Theory, Research & Practice 15:158–167, 1978

Kleeman JA: Freud's views on early female sexuality in the light of direct child observation. J Am Psychoanal Assoc 24 (no 5, suppl):3–27, 1976

Krajeski JP: Psychotherapy with gay and lesbian patients, in Innovations in Psychotherapy With Homosexuals. Edited by Hetrick ES, Stein TS. Washington, DC, American Psychiatric Press, 1984, pp 75–88

Lennane JK, Lennane JR: Alleged psychogenic disorders in women—a possible manifestation of sexual prejudice. N Engl J Med 288:288–292, 1973

LeVine RA: Gender differences: interpreting anthropological data, in Women and Men: New Perspectives on Gender Differences. Edited by Notman MT, Nadelson CC. Washington, DC, American Psychiatric Press, 1991, pp 1–8

Lurie N, Slater J, McGovern P, et al: Preventive care for women: does the sex of the physician matter? N Engl J Med 329:478–482, 1993

Lystad MH (ed): Violence in the Home: Interdisciplinary Perspectives. New York, Brunner/Mazel, 1986

Malloy T: The relationship between therapist-client interpersonal compatibility, sex of therapist, and psychotherapeutic outcome (abstract). Dissertation Abstracts International 40:456B, 1979

Mayer EL, de Marneffe D: When theory and practice diverge: gender-related patterns of referral to psychoanalysts. J Am Psychoanal Assoc 40:551–585, 1992

Mayes S: Women in positions of authority: a case study of changing sex roles. Signs 4:556–568, 1979

McKinlay SM, McKinlay JB: The impact of menopause and social factors on health, in Menopause: Evaluation, Treatment and Health Concerns. Edited by Hammond B, Hazeltine F, Schiff I. New York, AR Liss, 1989, pp 137–161

McNab T: What do men want? Male rituals of initiation in group psychotherapy. International Journal of Group Psychotherapy 40:139–154, 1990

Merkatz RB, Temple R, Subel S, et al: Women in clinical trials of new drugs: a change in Food and Drug Administration policy. The Working Group on Women in Clinical Trials. N Engl J Med 329:292–296, 1993

Miller JB, Nadelson CC, Notman MT, et al: Aggression in women: a reexamination, in Changing Concepts in Psychoanalysis. Edited by Klebanow S. New York, Gardner, 1981, pp 157–167

Mogul KM: Overview: the sex of the therapist. Am J Psychiatry 139:1–11, 1982

Money J, Ehrhardt AA: Man and Woman, Boy and Girl: The Differentiation and Dimorphism of Gender Identity From Concept to Maturity. Baltimore, MD, Johns Hopkins University Press, 1972

Nadelson CC: Women in leadership roles: development and challenges. Adolesc Psychiatry 14:28–41, 1987

Nadelson CC. Issues in the analysis of single women in their thirties and forties, in The Middle Years. Edited by Liebert R, Oldham J. New Haven, CT, Yale University Press, 1989, pp 105–122

Nadelson C, Notman M: Psychotherapy supervision: the problem of conflicting values. Am J Psychother 31:275–283, 1977

Nadelson CC, Notman MT: Psychoanalytic considerations of the response to rape. International Review of Psycho-Analysis 6:97–103, 1979

Nadelson C[C], Notman M[T]: To marry or not to marry, in The Woman Patient, Vol 2: Concepts of Femininity and the Life Cycle. Edited by Nadelson CC, Notman MT. New York, Plenum, 1982a, pp 111–120

Nadelson CC, Notman MT: Social change and psychotherapeutic implications, in The Woman Patient, Vol 3: Aggression, Adaptations, and Psychotherapy. Edited by Notman MT, Nadelson CC. New York, Plenum, 1982b, pp 3–16

Nadelson CC, Notman MT: The impact of the new psychology of men and women on psychotherapy, in American Psychiatric Press Review of Psychiatry, Vol 10. Edited by Tasman A, Goldfinger SM. Washington, DC, American Psychiatric Press, 1991, pp 608–626

Nadelson CC, Zimmerman V: Culture and psychiatric care of women, in Culture, Ethnicity, and Mental Illness. Edited by Gaw A. Washington, DC, American Psychiatric Press, 1992, pp 501–515

Nadelson CC, Notman MT, Miller JB, et al: Aggression in women: conceptual issues and clinical implications, in The Woman Patient, Vol 3: Aggression, Adaptations, and Psychotherapy. Edited by Notman MT, Nadelson CC. New York, Plenum, 1982, pp 17–28

Nolen-Hoeksema S: Sex differences in unipolar depression: evidence and theory. Psychol Bull 101:259–282, 1987

Notman MT, Lester EP: Pregnancy: theoretical considerations. Psychoanalytic Inquiry 8:139–159, 1988

Notman MT, Nadelson CC: The rape victim: psychodynamic considerations. Am J Psychiatry 133:408–413, 1976

Notman MT, Nadelson CC, Bennett M: Achievement conflict in women: psychotherapeutic considerations. Psychother Psychosom 29:203–213, 1978

Notman MT, Klein R, Jordan JV, et al: Women's unique developmental issues across the life cycle, in American Psychiatric Press Review of Psychiatry, Vol 10. Edited by Tasman A, Goldfinger SM. Washington, DC, American Psychiatric Press, 1991, pp 556–577

Nutt RL: Feminist family therapy: a review of the literature. Topics in Family Psychological Counseling 1:13–23, 1992

Orlinsky D, Howard K: The effects of sex of therapist on the therapeutic experiences of women. Psychotherapy: Theory, Research & Practice 13:82–88, 1976

Perry JC, Herman JL: Trauma and defense in the etiology of borderline personality disorder, in Borderline Personality Disorder: Etiology and Treatment. Edited by Paris J. Washington, DC, American Psychiatric Press, 1993, pp 123–139

Person ES: The influence of values in psychoanalysis: the case of female psychology, in Psychiatry Update: The American Psychiatric Association Annual Review, Vol 2. Edited by Grinspoon L. Washington, DC, American Psychiatric Press, 1983, pp 36–50

Person ES, Ovesey L: Psychoanalytic theories of gender identity. J Am Acad Psychoanal 11:203–226, 1983

Pilgrim C, Riesert I: Differences between male and female brains—developmental mechanisms and implications. Horm Metab Res 24:353–359, 1992

Reed BG, Linkages: battering, sexual assault, incest, child sexual abuse, teen pregnancy, dropping out of school and the alcohol and drug connection, in Alcohol and Drugs Are Women's Issues, Vol 1. Edited by Roth P. Metuchen, NJ, Scarecrow, 1991, pp 130–149

Samstag LW, Batchelder ST, Muran JC, et al: Early identification of treatment failures in short-term psychotherapy: an assessment of therapeutic alliance and interpersonal behavior. J Psychother Pract Res 7:126–139, 1998

Saunders DG, Kindy PJ: Predictors of physicians' responses to woman abuse. J Gen Intern Med 8:606–609, 1993

Sargeant JK, Bruce ML, Florio LP, et al: Factors associated with 1-year outcome of major depression in the community. Arch Gen Psychiatry 47:519–526, 1990

Schwartz JM, Stoessel PW, Baxter LR, et al: Systematic changes in cerebral glucose metabolic rate after successful behavior modification treatment of obsessive-compulsive disorder. Arch Gen Psychiatry 53:109–113, 1996

Silverstein B, Perlick D: Gender differences in depression: historical changes. Acta Psychiatr Scand 84:327–331, 1991

Simons JA, Helms JE: Influence of counselor's marital status, sex and age on college and noncollege women's preference. Journal of Counseling Psychology 23:380–386, 1976

Sotsky SM, Glass DR, Shea MT, et al: Patient predictors of response to psychotherapy and pharmacotherapy: findings in the NIMH Treatment of Depression Collaborative Research Program. Am J Psychiatry 148:997–1008, 1991

Sprock J, Blashfield RK, Smith B: Gender weighting of DSM-III-R personality disorder criteria. Am J Psychiatry 147:586–590, 1990

Stabb SD, Cox DL, Harber JL: Gender-related therapist attributions in couples therapy: a preliminary multiple case study investigation. J Marital Fam Ther 23:335–346, 1997

Stoller RJ: Primary femininity. J Am Psychoanal Assoc 24 (no 5, suppl):59–78, 1976

Symonds A: Phobias after marriage: women's declaration of dependence. Am J Psychoanal 31:144–152, 1971

Teicher MH, Glod CA, Surrey J, et al: Early childhood abuse and limbic system ratings in adult psychiatric outpatients. J Neuropsychiatry Clin Neurosci 5:301–306, 1993

Thase ME, Reynolds CF III, Frank E, et al: Do depressed men and women respond similarly to cognitive behavior therapy? Am J Psychiatry 151:500–505, 1994

Thase ME, Simons AD, Reynolds CF III: Abnormal electroencephalographic sleep profiles in major depression: association with response to cognitive behavior therapy. Arch Gen Psychiatry 53:99–108, 1996

Thompson C: Notes on the psychoanalytic significance of the choice of analyst. Psychiatry 1:205–216, 1938

Turkel AR: The impact of feminism on the practice of a woman analyst. Am J Psychoanal 36:119–126, 1976 van der Kolk BA: The compulsion to repeat the trauma: reenactment, revictimization, and masochism. Psychiatr Clin North Am 12:389–411, 1989

Warren LW: Male intolerance of depression: a review with implications for psychotherapy. Clin Psychol Rev 3:147–156, 1983

Weisner C: Treatment services research and alcohol problems: treatment entry, access, and effectiveness, in Assessing Future Research Needs: Mental and Addictive Disorders in Women. Washington, DC, Institute of Medicine, 1991, pp 85–90

Weissman MM: Gender differences in the rates of mental disorders, in Assessing Future Research Needs: Mental and Addictive Disorders in Women. Washington, DC, Institute of Medicine, 1991, pp 8–13

Weissman M, Kessler RC, McGonagle KA, Zhao S, et al: Lifetime and 12-month prevalence of DSM-III-R psychiatric disorders in the United States. Arch Gen Psychiatry 51:8–19, 1994

Wellesley College Center for Research on Women: How Schools Shortchange Girls. Washington, DC, American Association of University Women, 1992

Wenger NK, Speroff LPB: Cardiovascular health and disease in women. N Engl J Med 329:247–256, 1993

Yonkers KA, Kando JC, Cole JO, et al: Gender differences in pharmacokinetics and pharmacodynamics of psychotropic medication. Am J Psychiatry 149:587–595, 1992

Zanarini MC: Role of Sexual Abuse in the Etiology of Borderline Personality Disorder. Washington, DC, American Psychiatric Press, 1997

Zanarini MC, Gunderson JG, Marino MF, et al: Childhood experiences of borderline patients. Compr Psychiatry 30:18–25, 1989

Zetzel ER: The doctor-patient relationship in psychiatry (1966), in The Capacity for Emotional Growth. New York, International Universities Press, 1970, pp 139–155

Zlotnick C, Shea T, Pilkonis P, et al: Gender, type of treatment, dysfunctional attitudes, social support, life events, and depressive symptoms over naturalistic follow-up. Am J Psychiatry 153:10–17, 1996

Zlotnick C, Elkin I, Shea T: Does the gender of a patient or the gender of a therapist affect the treatment of patients with major depression? J Consult Clin Psychol 66:655–659, 1998

3

Cross-Cultural Issues in Psychiatric Treatment

Carlos A. González, M.D.
Ezra E. H. Griffith, M.D.
Pedro Ruiz, M.D.

The study of cultural, ethnic, and racial differences between groups of people has long been one of the endeavors of the social sciences. The discipline of psychiatry, however, accorded this area of work relatively little systematic attention during the discipline's formative years. The early work of psychiatry focused mainly on exploring intrapsychic processes and less on assessing the influence of the external world on intrapsychic development and identity formation. Over the past few decades, however, the field of psychiatry and allied professions have moved to expand their conceptual framework to include a more comprehensive view of development, function, and psychopathology. This is, in part, a consequence of the growing acceptance of cross-cultural psychiatry throughout the world and the resultant increase in the number of psychiatrists and mental health professionals whose own cultures and ethnicities differ greatly from the ethnocultural milieu in which psychoanalytic thinking originated.

The fourth edition of the American Psychiatric Association's *Diagnostic and Statistical Manual of Mental Disorders* (DSM-IV; American Psychiatric Association 1994) reflects a growing skepticism about the applicability of theories and assumptions originating in one culture to the diagnosis of an individual from a different racial or ethnic background. If the process of diagnosis needs reexamination with regard to its cross-cultural applicability, then the process of psychiatric treatment must be similarly reevaluated. As Thomas and Sillen (1972) noted, "A growing body of evidence has demonstrated that there is a dynamic interaction between the human organism and its culture, and that it is impossible to abstract an individual's lifestyle from the culture that helps to mold it and through which it is expressed" (p. 59).

In this chapter we explore the influence of culture on development, symptom expression, and diagnosis, and the impact of race, ethnicity, and culture on psychotherapy and pharmacotherapy.

Definitions

Certain terms deserve clarification and emphasis because we shall return to them at several points throughout our discussion.

Culture may be defined as a set of meanings, behavioral norms, and values utilized by members of a particular society as they construct their unique view of the world. These values or reference points may include social relationships, language, nonverbal expression of thoughts and emotions, religious beliefs, moral thought, technology, and financial philosophy. Furthermore, culture is not a static notion but one that changes as it is taught by one generation to the next.

Ethnicity refers to a subjective sense of belonging to a group of people with a common origin and with shared social and cultural beliefs and practices. Although its importance varies with each individual, ethnicity is a component of everyone's sense of identity, and, as such, it needs to be examined as a source of data regarding an individual's self-image and intrapsychic life.

Race, while it is often used in reference to physical, biological, and genetic characteristics, is also commonly employed as a psychosocial concept under which humans have chosen to group themselves, based primarily on general physiognomy. Although the validity of this concept is highly questionable (Lock 1993), its impact on the individual and on groups has been critical and remains undeniably strong throughout the world.

Psychosomatic and behavioral medicine have reemphasized the traditional value given to patients' own accounts of their troubles during the diagnostic process. Additionally, because psychiatrists do not routinely have at their disposal instruments, procedures, and sophisticated imaging techniques, a psychiatrist's principal diagnostic (and, often, therapeutic) instrument is the actual encounter with the patient. During this encounter, the patient's complaints must be put into an accurate clinical context as a prerequisite to arriving at an effective treatment. Several authors (Blue and González 1992; Comas-Díaz and Jacobsen 1991; Wohl 1989) have stressed that the therapeutic encounter does not occur without significant input from each participant's culture and ethnicity, and that ethnocultural differences between the patient and the clinician can lead to interesting and unforeseen outcomes, both positive and negative, depending on the flexibility and cultural sensitivity of the psychiatrist.

In the most general terms, the psychotherapeutic process is intended to improve the interpersonal functioning and the subjective comfort of the patient. The roots of modern psychotherapy lie in turn-of-the-century Western Europe, so it is not surprising that the discipline's cross-cultural validity has been called into question by those who point out that its theories

- espouse a predominantly psychological view of subjective experience, at times seeing somatic expressions of distress as more primitive.
- endorse independence and autonomous function at the expense of interdependence and belonging to a larger social unit.
- fail to see the individual's position in his or her family, society, and culture as an important determinant of the clinical presentation.
- often fail to recognize the importance to the individual of the religious or spiritual meaning of symptoms and suffering.

It is necessary to keep such "charges" in mind when trying to improve the scope of psychotherapy and psychiatry. Psychiatry can indeed be seen as a culture itself or as having its own cultural milieu. Yet, this must not be taken to imply that the culture of psychiatry cannot change—it has been changing for decades, much as any society's culture changes to accommodate science and learning. It is therefore not our aim in writing this chapter to "free" psychiatry from culture, but rather to incorporate a comprehensive working view of cultural difference into the culture of psychiatric practice.

Cultural psychiatry concerns itself with the relationship between mental illness and the matrix created by the interplay of society, culture, and environment (Griffith and González 1999). Initially, the thrust of cultural psychiatry was along the lines of viewing phenomena occurring in other cultural settings and finding a way to compare these with phenomena occurring in "our" culture. More recently, cultural psychiatrists have endeavored to expand the scope of psychiatry in general to allow for a more accurate view of the world through the eyes of the individual, rather than a view of the individual through the eyes of psychiatry (Kleinman 1988; Littlewood 1991; Wohl 1989).

General Considerations

A number of key issues affect the practice of psychiatry in cross-cultural settings. Although the names given most of these subjects may seem unusually arbitrary, we think it essential for the reader to understand that these concepts are fundamental to an understanding of the influence of culture on psychiatric treatment.

Biology and Environment

Culture needs to be regarded as an important determinant of an individual's mental state. For example, cultural milieu determines whether an individual's behavior or emotional state is regarded as "normal" or "abnormal." It is within an individual's culture that stressors originate whose impact leads the person to coping methods that themselves are culturally influenced. Culture also influences development and character formation, which in turn have an impact on an individual's sense of fitting in to his or her environment. Moreover, an individual's conceptualization of illness varies with culture, as do the available ways for coping or overcoming such illness (Marsella 1988).

The recent upsurge of neuroscientific, or "biological," research in psychiatry has focused almost exclusively on how biological mechanisms affect an individual's relationship to his or her environment. However, there is an equally compelling body of evidence suggesting that the environment has an important impact on neurobiological development and adult learning. The role of the environment was an important theme in the seminal work of René Spitz, who used the term *hospitalism* to describe the severe maturational disabilities incurred by children brought up without proper environmental stimulation (Spitz 1945). More recent workers have confirmed the need for environmental stimulation for appropriate structural development of the mammalian brain (Greenough and Schwark 1984; Greenough et al. 1987). Learning in adults has also been associated with acquired changes in synaptic connectivity (Greenough et al. 1987), leading to a modern view of neurobiology and environment as complementary influences on behavior and emotion.

In view of the above, Marsella (1988) stated that the cultural variability of a mental disorder will vary inversely with the degree of biological determination of such a disorder. A neurological event, such as a hemorrhagic infarct of the brain, will have relatively little cross-cultural variability, whereas a dissociative disorder is usually etiologically related to environmental trauma, and its manifestation will be influenced both by the nature of the traumatic event and by the culturally compatible coping strategies available to the patient.

Emic Versus Etic

As used in cross-cultural psychiatry, the term *emic* refers to the conceptually narrow view by people in a given culture of a phenomenon occurring within that culture. In some cultures, for example, an emic explanation of a severe stomachache may suggest that the cause of the abdominal discomfort is derived from the mixing of foods of different temperatures in the stomach. The term *etic* refers to a presumed universal approach to the viewing of such problems. Westermeyer (1985) warned against thinking that a diagnosable phenomenon is explainable in completely emic or etic terms, but rather formulates the issue as the extent to which a given diagnostic entity is emic versus the extent to which it is etic. When observers from culture A impose their cultural perspectives on their observations about culture B, the result is a "pseudoetic" or "imposed etic" view that may include a number of distortions about culture B. Berry (1975) argued that this imposed etic view needs to be tempered with emic considerations acquired through observation, in order to eventually achieve a "derived etic" view of the specific psychiatric issue.

Autonomy and Interdependence

Various experts have commented on the fact that equating mental well-being with autonomy or self-actualization is not a global outlook, but rather a "Western" (i.e., North American and Western European) one. For instance, Neki (1976) noted that even within the confines of Western psychotherapy, the question of how much dependence is normal or pathological remains a point of discussion. The degree of tolerance for dependence as part of mature behavior is determined by the culture and is highly variable cross-culturally. Kleinman (1997) referred to an institutional culture in Western clinical settings that idealizes individual autonomy and that, in doing so, may alienate patients whose culture emphasizes social obligation. This potential conflict between the culture of the therapist and that of the patient may be most crucial when family therapy is undertaken and thus requires the utmost attention to avoid alienating the family (Kaslow et al. 1995).

Tsui and Schultz (1985), in discussing the failure of therapeutic engagement with Asian patients, remarked that relatively unacculturated Asians will expect the therapist to be an authoritative, active giver of structure and advice, rather than a silent, questioning, unapproachable figure. Other investigators (Gilligan 1982; Kobayashi 1989) have criticized the extant high regard for the ideal of autonomy not only as being the product of the

Western world, but also as being biased in favor of the masculine point of view. Kobayashi (1989) pointed out striking similarities between North American "Self-in-Relation" theory and the interdependency ideal that is the cultural norm in Japan, where growth is viewed not as a process resulting in separation and independence, but rather as a deepening of the individual's relational competence and empathy.

Internal and External Loci of Control

A corollary of the "autonomy versus interdependence" dilemma is the individual's perception of the so-called locus of control, defined as "the extent to which a person believes that reinforcements in life are contingent upon his own efforts (internal control) or determined by outside forces such as luck, chance, fate, or powerful others (external control)" (Kuo et al. 1979, p. 177). In this context, Asian culture has been said to promote the perception of an external locus of control, viewing the individual as subject to situational forces usually beyond his or her control. Similarly, Ruiz and Langrod (1982) have described the trait of "fatalism" as a culturally derived outlook endorsed by peoples of Hispanic origin. Fatalism, also, refers to a sense that fate cannot be changed and that what is meant to happen will take place regardless of human intervention. It is important to realize that immigrants to the United States often face a dominant culture that they see as rigid, authoritarian, and generally oppressive to those of low socioeconomic status. Thus, a culturally derived perception of an external locus of control can actually be reinforced by the traumatizing experience of migration to a milieu that one perceives as oppressive and harsh.

Somatic and Psychological Experience and Expression of Distress

The view that stress leads to an emotional state that in turn may result in somatic discomfort or pain is historically quite recent, despite being rooted in outdated theories of mind-body duality. It is not a view that the rest of the world shares with the "psychologically minded" Western European and North American cultures (Patel and Winston 1994). Many have commented on the fact that the overwhelming majority of Asian, African, and Central and South American peoples not only express subjective distress in somatic terms but actually experience this distress somatically, such that psychological interpretations of suffering may not be of much use cross-culturally (Escobar et al. 1987; Kleinman 1982; Tsui and Schultz 1985; White 1982). This is not to say that psychotherapeutic principles do not apply cross-culturally, but rather that an astute psychotherapist must be mindful not to use culture-bound constructs in such situations. A brief case vignette may best illustrate this point:

> A 62-year-old Puerto Rican woman was referred for evaluation of incapacitating abdominal pain for the previous 9 months, as a medical diagnostic evaluation of this pain was negative. The pain had begun approximately 1 month after her substance-abusing son had been jailed for killing his lover, whom the patient "loved like a daughter." The patient expected that the psychiatrist would prescribe medication that would take her pain away, and she was initially distressed to learn that she was expected to talk about her life. While not ruling out the use of medication, the therapist explained to her that her pain might be related to the wrenching emotional ordeal of the past year. The therapist made it a point to validate her pain and took great care not to imply that the pain was "merely" the expression of unacknowledged emotion. In particular, he told her that he understood her pain to be very real

and that he did not expect her pain to be gone overnight. This approach allowed the patient to engage in a course of brief psychotherapy during which her conflicted feelings about her substance-abusing offspring were examined, though these feelings were never specifically identified as the cause of her pain. Eventually the patient felt strong enough to make drastic changes in her role as enabler of her children, at which point she reported that her pain was much improved.

White (1982) studied the differences between North American and Hong Kong Chinese students in Hawaii with regard to the explanations the students used to explain particular behaviors or somatic complaints. An important finding was that when attempting to interpret "somatic" or "affective-somatic" complaints, both groups arrived at similarly sophisticated precipitating factors. Yet, the North Americans referred more often to psychological constructs, whereas the Chinese students made use of explanations based on situational stressors, dwelling less on any emotional intermediate between a stressor and a symptom or behavior. White cautioned that this could be construed as a surplus step in reasoning by the North Americans ("psychologization") rather than a deficit in the causal reasoning by the Chinese.

Ethnocentricity and Decentering

When there are obvious differences between any two ethnic or racial groups, it is the unfortunate human reaction of those individuals who see themselves as belonging to one group to fear those who are different and to attempt to compensate for this fear with animosity toward nonmembers. When one of these groups is overwhelmingly dominant with regard to the other, this "us versus them" mentality breeds discrimination and promotes racism as a system (Group for the Advancement of Psychiatry 1987). Such forces will have an impact on any human relationship, and the therapeutic relationship is not an exception.

Piaget believed that a childhood task for the individual was to learn how to "de-center"—that is, to progress from a stage of reasoning that allows no other point of view but one's own toward a cognitive stage that is marked by the ability to see the world through the eyes of another and to understand another's position in life. Aboud (1993) expanded on this concept to explain why children's high levels of prejudice at ages 3–7 years are lower a few years later, when the children's development allows them to surpass an egocentric stance and achieve a cognitive stage that includes acceptance of another's reality and perspective. It is indeed unfortunate that cognitive development is not the only driving force behind adult individual and group behavior. It would seem that a decentered approach is still to be achieved by most societies when it comes to overcoming racial and ethnic bias.

Mental Illness and Stigma

Beyond the universality of stigma associated with mental disorder, many have remarked that this stigma is much more marked in non-Western societies. Chinese and Chinese-American patients are said to view mental disorder as a "sign of social and even supernatural disharmony leading to a 'loss of face' for individual and family alike" (White 1982, p. 1520). There is an equally strong cultural bias against mental illness in many Hispanic and Hispanic-American cultures, particularly for men, because having emotional problems is equated with weakness of character. Because of this bias, many individuals are reluctant to approach a mental health professional with any complaint, but rather take their concerns to a general practitioner, expecting an examination and some straightforward counseling on how to be rid of the problem. This factor may act as a barrier to utilization of mental health services, as well as resistance to treatment once an individual is engaged. It also makes sense to expect that if mental health services are seen as the last resort, a person of Asian or Hispanic descent may request treatment at a more advanced stage of his or her illness and may thus exhibit marked symptoms upon presentation.

Cultural Variability Within Groups

There is considerable variability within ethnic and racial groups living in the United States. This variability results in part from the common confusion of race and ethnicity as well as from the loose categorization of ethnic and racial groups. Such groupings of people are often arbitrary and convenient and are based on a single supposedly binding commonality, rather than on systematic contrasts or likenesses. Lock (1993) traced back the development of the concept of race to 18th-century scientists' rudimentary attempts at taxonomy, which were eventually found to be without scientific basis. Despite this lack of foundation, the concept was apparently solidified by political forces in the 19th century, and its continued present use and acceptance as a "biological" entity are a testimony to the durability of a convenient myth.

In addition, the category *black* has been used in many studies, with the accompanying fallacious assumption that "blacks," despite coming from places as diverse as Jamaica, the United States, Great Britain, and Haiti, all share the same cultural values. Similarly, "Hispanics," "Hispanic Americans," or "Latinos" are so labeled regardless of their country of origin and cultural background, thereby leading to research categories that are virtually meaningless, because such things as social outlook, belief systems, and traditional healing practices vary greatly among the many Hispanic groups. The use of the term "Asian" to describe all Chinese, Japanese, Korean, Vietnamese, and Filipino peoples is similarly problematic.

It should also be understood that immigrants to the United States who hail from the same geographic area may acculturate differently to the social environment encountered on their arrival in this country. Indeed, even members of the same family adapt differently to this cultural transplantation. The phenomenon of acculturation is influenced by many factors, such as age, gender, race, socioeconomic status, education, religious beliefs, and political orientation.

It is therefore important to note that the use of ethnic and racial categories may in some cases be a matter of mere convention and may, in any event, unduly evoke stereotyped expectations in the psychiatric treatment context.

Culture and Development

Culture influences the amount of time and the nature and intensity of the interaction between mother and child. Culture also is a factor in determining who else within the family will interact with a child, to what degree, and in what type of relationship. Stoller and Herdt (1982) described the way in which boys were raised by the Sambia of New Guinea with the aim of promoting maleness and warriorhood. A very strong bond is initially fostered between mother and male child, only to be broken in elaborately ritual fashion, the usual result being a strongly heterosexual male.

Kobayashi (1989) contrasted the North American ideal of autonomy with the Asian view that children be raised to consider themselves first and foremost as part of a social unit rather than as individuals. She commented on the closeness of the mother-child relationship in the Asian culture and on the culturally determined expectation that such closeness will last for as long as mother and child live. Kobayashi and others have noted that the concept of "codependence," developed by North American chemical dependence treaters, has limited cross-cultural use, given the marked differences in upbringing and family values across cultures, especially in Hispanic and Asian societies (Inclán and Hernández 1992).

In a number of traditional Hispanic and Hispanic-American cultures, *machismo* is the norm in the interpersonal relations of men. Men are expected to be dominant, to be personally and sexually assertive, and to exhibit little in the way of tender emotions, which are regarded as a sign of femaleness or weakness. As a result, mothers are more indulgent and accommodating to male children, whereas they are more strict and careful with girls, who are expected to mature into submissive, unassertive mates (Gómez et al. 1983; Torres 1998).

The African-American experience of slavery, of subsequent overt racism and oppression, and, more recently, of covert bias in social arenas has been postulated by some to lead to personality traits that reflect mistrust of the Caucasian majority. It is not uncommon to discover that an African-American individual, regardless of level of function, may possess a certain amount of reality-based paranoia, an aversion for sharing emotions, and a manner of coping with stressors by bargaining rather than by overtly attempting to control the sources of stress (Thomas and Sillen 1972). The generally obvious physical differences between African Americans and Caucasians heighten the contrast between the two races and promote racial bias, which continues to exist to date. Zimmerman and colleagues (1995) compared the perceptions of African-American, non-Hispanic white, and Hispanic teachers regarding students of all three backgrounds. Non-Hispanic white and Hispanic teachers viewed African-American children as having significantly more problems than did African-American teachers questioned about the same children. In addition, the children viewed as problematic by these teachers also perceived the teacher as behaving in a derogatory manner toward them. Zimmerman and colleagues (1995) commented on the need for increasing mutual understanding of teachers' and students' expectations as a way to begin to alleviate these differences.

Besides the more traditional cultural influences, it is unfortunately true that poverty and oppression contribute to the formation of a particular brand of cultural milieu, which in turn has an influence on development. Growing up in such a culture of poverty may demand adaptive behaviors and attitudes in a child that in a different cultural setting may be regarded as antisocial (Reid 1985). Family instability and parental inconsistency are bound to occur more frequently in a fatherless family headed by an undersupported, relatively inexperienced young woman, and these dynamics have been linked to later psychopathology in children, including conduct disorder, a known harbinger of antisocial personality disorder (Cohen and Brook 1987).

Culture not only influences personality development but also acts as a factor in the manner that an individual's personality style is interpreted by others. In most cultures, males and females are raised with different parental and societal expectations, and it is likely that this difference acts in complementary fashion with biological factors to determine intersex differences in attitudes, behavior, and manner of relating. The case has been made that the predominantly male viewpoint of early and not-so-early theorists may have led to attempts to classify, diagnose, and treat females by standards that were inappropriate or inaccurate because this viewpoint did not acknowledge these culturally based differences between men and women (Gilligan 1982; Kobayashi 1989).

Culture, Symptom Expression, and Diagnosis

Culture and Symptom Expression

The International Pilot Study of Schizophrenia (IPSS), in its endeavor to investigate psychopathology in cross-cultural settings, experimented with the use of structured rating scales to assess symptoms and signs of psychiatric illness. With regard to cross-cultural diagnosis, the investigators concluded that interrater reliability was best for the assessment of symptoms, because these are reported by the patient, but noted that reliability declined in the assessment of signs, which are gathered by observation. The worst reliability was reported in the area of historical information, which is necessarily a function of the relationship formed between interviewer and subject during the accumulation of data (Strauss et al. 1976).

The Epidemiologic Catchment Area (ECA) study was another large-scale effort to obtain information on the symptomatology and prevalence of mental illness in various settings throughout the United States. A particular finding from this study serves to illustrate a problem with the use of diagnostic schema constructed in one cultural setting to diagnose people from a different cultural group. The ECA study revealed that Puerto Ricans assessed with the Diagnostic Interview Schedule (DIS) reported a higher number of somatization symptoms than other populations. In many instances, however, this proclivity toward somatic symptoms did not lead to a diagnosis recognized by the classification in use at that time (DSM-III; American Psychiatric Association 1980), so it was essentially an invisible finding. Guarnaccia et al. (1989), however, approached the phenomenon from the side of the native culture and created a measure to detect the symptoms of an *ataque de nervios*, a culturally determined, somatically based syndrome used to express great personal distress. These authors reported an association between the excess somatic symptoms found by the ECA project and the presence of *ataques de nervios* in this population. Because the DIS was not created in a cultural setting where such a pattern of symptoms had a particular meaning, its structured format did not allow for the detection of *ataques* as an entity, despite the syndrome's unquestionable clinical significance.

Language is an important component of culture, and its contribution to cross-cultural differences cannot be underestimated, especially in a discipline such as psychiatry, in which language is one of the principal diagnostic and therapeutic media available to the practitioner. In any encounter between two people from different cultures, language is a primary consideration. Even regional and generational differences within the same general cultural setting can impair understanding and mask meaning. For example, one need only note the different meanings within the United States attached to such words as "radical," "bad," "fresh," "awesome," "outrageous," "nasty," "funky," and even "gay," from generation to generation and from region to region.

Marcos (1979, 1988) took a thorough look at the role of language in the interaction between patient and clinician, at one point by audiotaping emergency evaluations of Asian and Hispanic psychiatric patients conducted through an interpreter. Marcos pointed out the numerous distortions that take place in even the simplest exchanges. He showed that there is an inherent inclination on the part of any interpreter to "make sense" of the patient's words. Consequently, the interpreter may organize a patient's answers to the point at which even a floridly psychotic patient can be made to sound quite sane (Marcos 1979). Furthermore, Marcos argued that even when an interview is conducted in English and the patient appears to be able to answer questions, the tone and phrasing of English spoken as a second language may be misinterpreted as reflecting guardedness, negative transference, or a personality trait.

Many people who learn English as their second language do so on their own, through repeated attempts to communicate with English-speaking friends and co-workers. It is likely that the novice English speaker will often learn stock phrases and clichés first as a way of establishing some rapport with others (Blue and González 1992), and this may contribute to the use of what Marcos (1988, p. 40) calls "sterile language" when such a person is stressed by probing questions. Finally, it is important to realize that many bilingual people possess a certain amount of independence between their two languages, resulting in not only different vocabularies but also different affects and connections associated with the language they may be employing at a particular time. Consequently, a nonbilingual clinician is receiving not only a verbally incomplete account of a patient's internal world but also an impoverished sense of the patient's emotional and cognitive experience.

If the alternative of using an interpreter is available, this interpreter should be well acquainted with clinical mental health practice, should not be part of the patient's family, and should be trained in translating everything said in verbatim fashion. Another practice suggested by Marcos (1979) is that of having the interviewing clinician and the translator meet together both before and after the interview. A meeting before the interview will serve to plan any strategies for eliciting symptoms and observing signs, and a meeting after the interview will help in the immediate processing of any nonverbal cues that might have been picked up by the interpreter but might not have been obvious to the interviewer.

Suicide as a Symptom

Suicide is one of the most salient and telling nonverbal communications, and its cross-cultural variability reflects the impact of culture on the existence of an individual. The Committee on Cultural Psychiatry of the Group for the Advancement of Psychiatry (1989) reviewed the available data on suicide among four major ethnic groups in the United States (African Americans, Asian Americans, Hispanic Americans, and Native Americans). The work revealed interesting similarities and differences between the suicide rates for these groups and the rate for whites. Suicide in the adolescent and young adult populations showed similar increases in African Americans, Hispanic Americans, and Native Americans, and this similarity was partially attributed to the impact of acculturative stress on identity formation, as people in this age range are often the ones who feel most strongly the brunt of negotiating with the dominant culture while still in contact with their culture of origin. Another finding was relatively low suicide rates for elderly African Americans, Hispanic Americans, and Native Americans, and it was suggested that this finding was due to their more supported and protected position within the extended family, as well as their experience of prolonged contact with the dominant culture.

Culture and Diagnosis

There is no doubt that culture has a sizable impact on the creation of diagnostic classifications, due in part to culture's effect on the experience of distress and the expression of symptoms. In addition, culture supplies the background against which illness behavior is viewed, and this results in further possible cross-cultural variability in ideas of normalcy.

In an effort to explore the cross-cultural aspects of psychiatric diagnosis, the National

Institute of Mental Health convened an international group of experts to make recommendations to the American Psychiatric Association's DSM-IV Task Force with the aim of improving the manual's applicability to cultures other than those of North America and Western Europe. This Group on Culture and Diagnosis made important contributions to the manual, including

- the addition, within the Introduction of the manual, of a section titled "Ethnic and Cultural Considerations," which emphasizes the need for clinicians to become familiar with a patient's cultural frame of reference in order to make an accurate diagnosis.
- the addition of a set of "cultural considerations" for each major category of disorders to assist clinicians in recognizing the impact of culture and ethnicity on the expression of symptoms.
- the development of a Cultural Formulation, outlined in Appendix I, as a method for including culture as an important consideration in the clinical practice of psychiatric assessment. Appendix I also contains a Glossary of Culture-Bound Syndromes that provides descriptions of emic syndromes that may not correlate with existing diagnostic categories but that nevertheless serve to legitimize the phenomenology of some "non-Western" clinical entities.

In addition to these changes, the research and efforts of the Group on Culture and Diagnosis led to at least two important publications: *Culture and Psychiatric Diagnosis: A DSM-IV Perspective* (Mezzich et al. 1996) and the third volume of *The DSM-IV Sourcebook* (Widiger et al. 1997), each containing many of the original recommendations and supporting work of the Task Force.

Race and Diagnosis

Although the concept of race does not appear to delimit groups as solidly as once was thought, it has been useful to highlight some differences between groups. It is not clear, however, whether these differences are intrinsically valid or merely stem from observer bias or inaccurately calibrated psychometric assessments.

Adebimpe (1981; Adebimpe et al. 1982) suggested that race was a factor in the frequent misdiagnosis of mood disorders in African-American patients as schizophrenic disorders. Cultural differences, rather than biological or genetic ones, have been endorsed by workers in this field as accounting for such misdiagnosis. In addition, simplistic racial stereotypes held by treaters, cultural differences in symptom expression, and patients' racially based suspicion of non–African-American treaters have all been implicated as contributing factors.

Many psychometric instruments are currently in use that have not been appropriately validated using norms obtained by the testing of African Americans. Greene (1987) made this point about the Minnesota Multiphasic Personality Inventory (MMPI), and others have added that the MMPI's utility in the African-American population is limited by its neglect of social, economic, and political factors (Dana and Whatley 1991). With regard to intelligence testing, the controversy has been marked. Whereas some workers have maintained that testing is valid, even if only as an index of an African-American person's adaptation to white norms, others have remarked that the test's standardization using white subjects makes for poor predictive power with regard to African Americans (Williams 1987).

Traditional Spiritual Healing

Religion and Psychiatric Healing

Lukoff and colleagues (1992) have argued quite forcefully that psychiatry has often been insensitive to the religious and spiritual issues that patients bring into treatment. Such insensitivity has resulted in a "religiosity gap" between clinicians and patients that the authors thought might at least be partially closed by their recommendations for improved training for therapists about religious and spiritual issues in treatment. The authors' recommendations led to the inclusion of the diagnosis of Religious or Spiritual Problem in DSM-IV, for use when the focus of treatment or diagnosis is a psychoreligious or psychospiritual problem that is not attributable to a mental disorder (American Psychiatric Association 1994, p. 685). Lukoff and his colleagues felt that the inclusion of such a category would require differentiation among three types of problems: "a) purely religious or spiritual problems; b) mental disorders with religious or spiritual content; and c) psychoreligious or psychospiritual problems not attributable to a mental disorder" (p. 677). The authors further explained that religious problems concern conflicts generated by questions of faith and doctrine, such as a woman's struggle with family planning alternatives. Mental disorders with religious content could be seen in patients suffering from obsessive-compulsive disorder who use religious ritual as a symbol for expressing compulsiveness. Psychoreligious problems not attributable to a mental disorder could be manifested through a patient's struggle with his or her loss of faith that led to a depressive syndrome.

A review by Giglio (1993) emphasized the fact that the culture of psychodynamic psychotherapy initially regarded religious beliefs as part of an individual's system of defenses rather than as part of the individual's sense of self and a part of his or her culture, thereby neglecting to consider the role of religion in development. However, a more current and culturally informed view would consider it important for a mental health practitioner to be aware of countertransferential reactions when discussing a patient's religious life and to retain as pragmatic a view of religion as possible, cognizant of the fact that a thorough discussion of a patient's religious views may at times serve to define further that patient's view of the world. Griffith and colleagues (1984), in analyzing the therapeutic elements of a service held on Wednesday nights in an American black church, pointed out how there was considerable comparability between the church members' thoughts about the service and the six curative factors that Yalom (1975) identified as present in groups considered therapeutic: instillation of hope, group cohesiveness, altruism, universality, catharsis, and existential factors. The work by Griffith and his collaborators made it clear that certain cultural groups use religious faith and church ritual as important factors in their life, both as elements of celebration and as mechanisms for coping with difficulty in their daily lives.

Other Traditional Healing Practices

In Puerto Rico and other Hispanic Caribbean settings, *Espiritismo* has long been a culturally sanctioned religious practice and/or philosophy that attempts to explain existence and helps its adherents find workable solutions to human suffering. *Espiritismo* is based on the belief that many of life's misfortunes and conflicts can be helped by contact with the world of spirits that is said to surround the material world (Comas-Díaz 1981; Ruiz 1976, 1979). An *espiritista,* or spiritual healer, is consulted by a person in crisis and determines whether the client's suffering is caused by his or her spirit's need for "evolution." This spiritual evolution takes place with the help of the healer and the healer's contacts with the spirit world, which may direct the sufferer to atone for a presumed misdeed in order to relieve the suffering (Ruiz 1979).

Santería is a belief system native to Cuba that has been born of a syncretism between the religion of African slaves and the Catholic beliefs of their Spanish masters. A number of Yoruba gods have been imbued with some of the qualities of particular Catholic figures, out of similarities perceived by the slaves and their descendants, and perhaps out of the need on the part of slaves to disguise beliefs that would have been regarded as pagan by their masters (Sandoval 1979). These saints/gods are utilized by the movement's healers, called *santeros,* for the purpose of counseling, managing crises, and, in general, securing an improved lot in life for those who need it. Sacrifices and offerings can be made as attempts to improve one's prosperity, to reduce outbursts of anger, to enhance one's sexual ability, and to remove illnesses that may have been occasioned by ill will. *Santería* is characterized by some as more "real and efficient" than either the Catholic saints or the spirits of *Espiritismo* (Sandoval 1979).

In Brazil, similar syncretism has occurred between the African Yoruba beliefs and the Catholic credo, which has led to the formation of cults called *Umbanda* and *Candomblé,* and the addition of the European theories of Allen Kardec has resulted in *Kardecismo* (Pressel 1973). Although the healing practices of these systems vary, all three are united by beliefs in the duality of spirit and body, the ability of spirits to contact the material world, and the assumption that spirits can be used in healing (Krippner 1987).

Castillo (1997) described folk healing, or "symbolic healing" (Castillo 1997, p. 82), as a process during which an individual's illness is viewed by the treating clinician in a manner that is congruent with the individual's cultural outlook. The clinician's intent is to arrive with the patient at a joint definition of reality, or an explanation for the illness that makes sense for both the patient and the clinician. What follows is a process during which the clinician uses symbols taken from this schema of reality to change the patient's cognitive appraisal of his or her ailment. For example, a folk healer and an ailing person may both agree that the person's suffering is caused by possession by spirits. The healer will then use his or her knowledge of the cultural matrix to propose a symbolic task or ritual that will serve to reshape the patient's view of the problem and allow for healing to take place. A traditional ceremony, during which the possessing spirit is cajoled or forced into leaving, perhaps allows the patient to voice in a culturally recognized forum the emotional content associated with the illness behavior, which then leads to healing.

This process of symbolic healing is exemplified in the practices of the *Zar* cult of the Northern Sudan, described as a healing movement practiced by women for the benefit of women (Constantinides 1977, 1985; Kahana 1985; Littlewood and Lipsedge 1987). In that society, women wield very little official power, the culture dictating that men conduct business and make political decisions among themselves, while women are relegated to domestic chores. Furthermore, infibulation—the practice of female circumcision (including clitoridectomy)—is still practiced at puberty, leaving the infibulated woman severely limited in her ability to enjoy sex other than as a way of producing children. In that society, when a Muslim woman feels ill and the illness does not fit any known pattern of medical dysfunction or religious explanation, she may consider herself possessed by a *Zar* spirit and seek help from a native healer, usually female, well versed in the workings of the *Zar* spirits. A *Zar* ceremony is then planned and attended solely by women. Such a ceremony may last several days and will include a number of meals, ritualized music and dances, and occasional trance states during which the sufferer is possessed by the *Zar* spirit, which speaks through her and is eventually appeased by the ceremony. At the end of the ritual, the sufferer is returned to her husband in a state in which she can again function within the family. Constantinides (1985) contrasted the woman-run, woman-promoted, and woman-healing aspect of this powerful ritual with the lack of power otherwise associated with being female and Muslim in Northern Sudan. She hypothesized that one of the purposes of such a ritual is that of allowing otherwise oppressed women to emphasize the importance of their role in society as procreators.

The aforementioned examples of religious ritual and doctrine do not at all exhaust the large number of culturally different groups to be found in the United States. But these practices all highlight the central point made by Lukoff and his co-workers (1992): that clinicians must make an effort to understand the nature of the connection between their patients and religious or spiritual faith and practice, as such an understanding may facilitate healing.

Migration and Mental Health

A component of cross-cultural psychiatry particularly important in the United States is the effect of migration and acculturation on the mental health of the individual. Berry and Kim (1988) have postulated four possible outcomes of the acculturative process, depending on how the acculturating individual answers the following questions:

1. Is one's own culture of value and worth retaining?
2. Is the culture of the dominant society of value, and is it therefore worthwhile to associate and establish positive relations with the dominant society?

It has been postulated that an individual who answers both questions in the affirmative has developed a stance of *integration* with regard to the dominant culture without losing touch with his or her own culture of origin. Such persons are considered to adopt a stance of "biculturalism" and are hypothesized to experience the least amount of acculturative stress. A person who answers both questions in the negative, on the other hand, neither feels strongly tied to his or her culture of origin nor is disposed to obtain support from the dominant culture. This person adopts a stance of *marginalization* and may be subject to the greatest amount of acculturative stress, as it is thought that this person would have no system of support available to mediate acculturation. The stance of *separation* is adopted by those persons who feel tied to and supported by their culture of origin, to the point of not seeing any benefit in taking in the majority culture or in associating with members of the dominant society. This stance is exemplified by some Native American groups and various fundamentalist sects within the United States, and was evident in the Black Panther movement of the 1960s and 1970s. Although constant friction with the dominant culture seems to be an inevitable consequence of this strategy, group members may also derive a good sense of support from such a tightly knit organization. The stance of *assimilation* was said to be the outcome of those persons who decide to embrace the dominant culture while partially or completely discounting the importance of their own culture of origin. It is hypothesized that these persons, although seemingly successful in their attempts, may experience unhealthy levels of stress arising from their need to identify with a culture that is not their own and a neglect of the part of their sense of identity that is tied to their culture of origin.

Berry and Kim's (1988) theory is supported by recent work by Kvernmo and Heyerdahl (1998), who compared the rate of behavioral problems among children belonging to the indigenous minority Sami ethnicity with that among children belonging to the Norwegian majority in northern Norway. Using the above model, they found that those Sami children who were monoethnic and lived in a setting that was not supportive of their ethnicity exhibited the most problems. The authors commented on the particular problem of forced assimilation of indigenous populations, which can lead to marginalization and high levels of acculturative stress. It is therefore important for clinicians to be acutely aware of the acculturative status of patients, as such information can provide important insights that can deepen the level of understanding between clinician and patient.

Culture and Psychotherapy

The practice of any form of psychotherapy is predicated on the general theory that change in a patient can occur as a consequence of that person's controlled social interaction with another individual, whether such relationship occurs in a group or family setting, individually or with a significant other, and regardless of the particular theoretical bent of the psychotherapist. The traditional healing practices described above share a number of qualities with the more modern psychotherapies, as outlined by Frank (1961), who postulated six elements that characterize healing of this type:

1. Emotional stirring of the individual
2. Existence of a healer on whom the individual depends for help and who holds out hope of relief
3. Arousal of the individual's expectations by the healer's personal attributes
4. Evocation of hope
5. Bolstering of self-esteem
6. Strengthening of the individual's ties with a supportive group

Any therapy of this kind requires that an intense bond be created between therapist and patient and that this bond be one of the principal tools available to the therapist in effecting positive change. Ethnocultural difference will have an impact on all phases of the therapeutic process, including engagement, development of a therapeutic alliance, development of transference and countertransference, and ability of the therapist to communicate effectively through interpretations.

The engagement of a person in a therapeutic relationship and the development of an alliance may be markedly more complicated when the two participants come from different ethnic and/or racial backgrounds. Many authors have mentioned the "healthy cultural paranoia" held by African Americans (Brantley 1983; Jones and Gray 1986; Ridley 1984) about Caucasians in general, stating that this frequently leads to an initial presentation remarkable for a decreased affective range, limited spontaneous verbalization, and some veiled hostility toward a Caucasian therapist. Such a presentation can "confirm" countertransferential feelings of guilt, fear, and hatred in an inexperienced Caucasian therapist, and the consequent disruption of the therapeutic alliance can lead to patient dropout.

In the case of Asians and Asian-American patients, not only are racial physical differences visible, but these can be compounded by patient expectations of treatment that are quite divergent from what many non-Asian psychotherapists are prepared to offer. For example, it is not uncommon for Chinese patients, regardless of educational achievement or cognitive capacity, to expect that a psychiatrist should be able to point things out for them to improve in their everyday lives, and that this will be sufficient to improve their mental health (Blue and González 1992).

Marsella (1993) offered a number of general recommendations specifically aimed at promoting (or at least not disrupting) a working therapeutic relationship with a patient of Japanese extraction. He stated that formality should prevail in a therapeutic relationship and that an informal style may lead to the patient's sense of embarrassment for the therapist. Marsella mentioned the culturally derived inclination within the Japanese culture to express emotions quite indirectly and subtly and added that the therapist must be acutely aware of nonverbal or process-oriented modes of communication. Yamamoto and Acosta (1982) also advocated that a therapist project a much more authoritative, confident persona when seeing a traditionally oriented Chinese or Japanese patient, as this stance may be more compatible with the culturally derived expectations of such patients.

It is possible for either an Asian or a Hispanic patient to present with multiple somatic complaints and to be characterized as being hysterical or as having a limited capacity for insight by a clinician who is poorly informed about cross-cultural trends. Furthermore, the overrepresentation of Hispanic Americans and African Americans in the lower socioeconomic levels of this country can lead to an initial presentation of a patient who is in great immediate distress, resulting from very real stressors, including finances, crime, bias, and family strife. Such a patient may choose to request help in resolving these pressing issues, rather than focus on relational or characterological problems.

Transference can be defined as the development of conscious and unconscious responses to the therapist that derive from the patient's early experiences with significant figures. Such early experiences always occur within a specific social and cultural matrix, thus accounting for the ever-present influence of culture on the development of the transference. The therapist also brings his or her own culturally determined experiences to the relationship, thereby ensuring that countertransference will also have cultural determinants, whether such countertransference be derived primarily from the therapist's own conflicts or facilitated by the actual behavior of the patient (Gorkin 1986).

Psychodynamic psychotherapy with members of racial or ethnic minority groups necessitates consideration of interesting variations in the area of transference and countertransference. Comas-Díaz and Jacobsen (1991) commented on the various possibilities for transference relationships in interethnic therapeutic dyads. Mistrust and suspicion can be the predominant emotions when the therapist comes from the dominant group and the patient is from a chronically oppressed group. Alternatively, an overly compliant transference can develop in a patient who is attempting to break the perceived stereotype of being a difficult patient. Intraethnic transference can provide its own type of distortions, sometimes resulting in the idealization of the therapist as someone exceptionally able to understand the patient, while in other instances the therapist may be viewed as someone who has abandoned his or her culture of origin. The phenomenon of internalized racism can also lead a patient, consciously or unconsciously, to devalue a therapist from the patient's own ethnic or racial group.

Gorkin (1986) discussed the special situation of Jewish therapists working with Arab patients, in which the therapist's sense of guilt and discomfort can lead to disregard of obvious and significant differences, or even to excessive curiosity about differences at the expense of focusing on the patient's complaints. Various workers have advocated the addressing of ethnocultural differences with patients not only as a way of avoiding colluding with the patient in ignoring the difference, but also because discussion of such differences can often lead to quite fruitful elucidation of the patient's core conflict (Blue and González 1992; Brantley 1983; Comas-Díaz and Jacobsen 1991; Gorkin 1986; Varghese 1983).

In psychotherapeutic work with Chinese and Japanese patients, Tung (1991) contended that intense transference in non-Asian patients may be due to the fact that Western culture requires that an individual separate from his or her family of origin, thus resulting in the patient's internalization of unresolved and intensely conflicted relationships with parents. This leads to a similarly intense and conflictual transference in a therapeutic situation. Tung believed that Asians, who do not actually ever leave their families of origin, develop less intense transference, because their "core conflict is worked out directly with the original cast of characters" (Tung 1991, p. 192). Tamura and Lau (1992) have reminded us that the very idea of health as self-actualization clashes with the Japanese view of health as balance and harmony within the family and societal unit. The authors give numerous clinical examples in the setting of family therapy in which treatments devised by Western psychiatrists focus on promoting individuation, whereas an Asian psychiatrist is much more likely to frame problems in terms of failure of family integration and arrive at recommendations that are aimed at improving the family relationships.

The special case in which the therapist belongs to an ethnic minority group and the patient comes from the dominant group was discussed by Blue and González (1992). They described the special situation of a minority therapist, existing in a theoretical space that borders on his or her culture of origin, the dominant culture, and the culture of psychotherapy. The therapist's increased knowledge and expertise have expanded his or her horizons and prevented reimmersion in his or her culture of origin. The therapist has also become acutely aware of ethnocultural differences and therefore is less likely to desire assimilation into the dominant culture. Finally, he or she is aware that the culture of psychodynamic psychotherapy has a certain amount of ethnocentric bias and is therefore not to be espoused without constant careful scrutiny.

Race/Ethnicity and Pharmacotherapy

Research has highlighted some differences among racial groups in their response to psychopharmacological intervention. In their review of psychopharmacological treatment and the Asian population, Lin and associates (1991) mentioned various clinically important differences. Polymorphisms of aldehyde dehydrogenase and alcohol dehydrogenase are more common in Asians than in Caucasians or African Americans, and these result, respectively, in the "flushing response" to ethanol observed in Asians and in their lower tolerance to ethanol. In comparison with Caucasians and African Americans, a much larger percentage of Asians are said to be "fast acetylators," and this may have an impact on the metabolism of drugs such as clonazepam, caffeine, and phenelzine. The higher incidence of dyskinesia in Asian patients with Parkinson's disease has been associated with racial differences in the activity of catechol-*O*-methyltransferase.

A more recent review by Lin and associates (1995) discussed enzyme polymorphism as the cause of significant differences in drug metabolism across ethnic groups. The cytochrome P450 2D6 isoenzyme is active in the metabolism of tricyclic antidepressants (TCAs), selective serotonin reuptake inhibitors (SSRIs), and traditional and "atypical" antipsychotics, including clozapine and risperidone. This enzyme is significantly less active in Asians and African Americans than in Caucasians, which partly explains the higher blood haloperidol levels achieved in Asian individuals when comparable doses are given to Asian and Caucasian groups. A preliminary study by Ruiz et al. (1999) revealed that Hispanic-American patients suffering from schizophrenia respond to lower doses of traditional antipsychotics than those required to treat African Americans and non-Hispanic whites, suggesting differences in drug metabolism that are yet undefined.

The cytochrome P450 2C19 isoenzyme exhibits similar ethnic variability, in that a higher percentage of African Americans and Asians are poor metabolizers, and this is a likely factor in the slower metabolism of diazepam and the slower demethylation of TCAs noted in these populations (Lin et al. 1995; Strickland et al. 1991).

Although the metabolism of lithium appears to exhibit little interethnic difference, it has been well documented that Asians respond to lower blood levels of the drug than those necessary to treat Caucasians. Similarly, African Americans seem to have a less active mechanism for the countertransport of sodium and lithium and thus are more susceptible to side effects from the drug (Strickland et al. 1995).

Conclusions

No other discipline attempts to understand a person in as many ways or as comprehensively as psychiatry does. Perhaps this is based on the belief that understanding leads to the best attempts at a cure. Our ever-expanding outlook now includes biological and molecular dimensions that were not present a generation ago and that no doubt will grow even faster in the next generation. It is important that in exploring this inner frontier we remain focused on the individual as a person and as the product of the unavoidable interplay between biological and environmental forces. The viewpoint of psychiatry is invaluable because it is indeed comprehensive, and efforts must continue to expand the frontiers of psychiatry toward seeing the individual as existing within a social context, within a familial context, and within the pervasive and influential context of culture.

References

Aboud FE: The developmental psychology of racial prejudice. Transcultural Psychiatric Research Review 3:229–242, 1993

Adebimpe VR: Overview: white norms and psychiatric diagnosis of black patients. Am J Psychiatry 138:279–285, 1981

Adebimpe VR, Chu C, Klein HE, et al: Racial and geographic differences in the psychopathology of schizophrenia. Am J Psychiatry 139:888–891, 1982

American Psychiatric Association: Diagnostic and Statistical Manual of Mental Disorders, 3rd Edition. Washington, DC, American Psychiatric Association, 1980

American Psychiatric Association: Diagnostic and Statistical Manual of Mental Disorders, 4th Edition. Washington, DC, American Psychiatric Association, 1994

Berry JW: Ecology, cultural adaptation and psychological differentiation: traditional patterning and acculturative stress, in Cross-Cultural Perspectives on Learning. Edited by Brislin R, Bochner S, Lonner W. New York, Wiley, 1975, pp 207–231

Berry JW, Kim U: Acculturation and mental health, in Health and Cross-Cultural Psychology: Toward Applications. Edited by Dasen P, Berry JW, Sartorius N. Newbury Park, CA, Sage, 1988, pp 207–236

Blue HC, González CA: The meaning of ethnocultural difference: its impact on and use in the psychotherapeutic process, in New Directions for Mental Health Services No 55, Treating Diverse Disorders With Psychotherapy. Edited by Greenfeld D. San Francisco, CA, Jossey-Bass, 1992, pp 73–84

Brantley T: Racism and its impact on psychotherapy. Am J Psychiatry 140:1605–1608, 1983

Castillo RJ: Culture and Mental Illness: A Client-Centered Approach. Pacific Grove, Brooks/Cole, 1997

Cohen P, Brook J: Family factors related to the persistence of psychopathology in childhood and adolescence. Psychiatry 50:332–345, 1987

Comas-Díaz L: Puerto Rican espiritismo and psychotherapy. Am J Orthopsychiatry 51:636–645, 1981

Comas-Díaz L, Jacobsen FM: Ethnocultural transference and countertransference in the therapeutic dyad. Am J Orthopsychiatry 61:392–402, 1991

Constantinides PM: Ill at ease and sick at heart: symbolic behaviour in a Sudanese healing cult, in Symbols and Sentiments: Cross Cultural Studies in Symbolism. Edited by Lewis I. London, Academic Press, 1977, pp 61–84

Constantinides P: Women heal women: spirit possession and sexual segregation in a Muslim society. Soc Sci Med 21:685–692, 1985

Dana RH, Whatley PR: When does a difference make a difference? MMPI scores and African-Americans. J Clin Psychol 47(3):400–406, 1991

Escobar JI, Burnam MA, Karno M, et al.: Somatization in the community. Arch Gen Psychiatry 44:713–718, 1987

Frank JD: Persuasion and Healing: A Comparative Study of Psychotherapy. Baltimore, MD, Johns Hopkins University Press, 1961

Giglio J: The impact of patients' and therapists' religious values on psychotherapy. Hospital and Community Psychiatry 44:768–771, 1993

Gilligan C: In a Different Voice: Psychological Theory and Women's Development. Cambridge, MA, Harvard University Press, 1982

Gómez E, Gómez EA, Ruiz P: Mental health care of Hispanic-Americans in the US: a cultural and clinical perspective. World Journal of Psychosynthesis 15(1):19–23, 1983

Gorkin M: Countertransference in cross-cultural psychotherapy: the example of Jewish therapist and Arab patient. Psychiatry 49:69–79, 1986

Greene RL: Ethnicity and MMPI performance: a review. J Consult Clin Psychol 55:497–512, 1987

Greenough WT, Schwark HD: Age-related aspects of experience: effects upon brain structure, in Continuities and Discontinuities in Development. Edited by Emde RN, Harmon RJ. New York, Plenum, 1984, pp 69–91

Greenough WT, Black JE, Wallace CS: Experience and brain development. Child Dev 58:539–559, 1987

Griffith EEH, González CA: The basics of cultural psychiatry, in The American Psychiatric Press Textbook of Psychiatry, 3rd Edition. Edited by Hales RE, Yudofsky SC, Talbott JA. Washington, DC, American Psychiatric Press, 1999, pp 1463–1492

Griffith EEH, Young JL, Smith DL: An analysis of the therapeutic elements in a black church service. Hospital and Community Psychiatry 35:464–469, 1984

Group for the Advancement of Psychiatry, Committee on Cultural Psychiatry: Suicide and Ethnicity in the United States. New York, Brunner/Mazel, 1989

Group for the Advancement of Psychiatry, Committee on International Relations: Us and Them: The Psychology of Ethnonationalism. New York, Brunner/Mazel, 1987

Guarnaccia PJ, Rubio-Stipec M, Canino G: Ataques de nervios in the Puerto Rican Diagnostic Interview Schedule: the impact of cultural categories on psychiatric epidemiology. Cult Med Psychiatry 13:275–295, 1989

Inclán J, Hernández M: Cross-cultural perspectives and codependence: the case of poor Hispanics. Am J Orthopsychiatry 62:245–255, 1992

Jones BE, Gray BA: Problems in diagnosing schizophrenia and affective disorders among blacks. Hospital and Community Psychiatry 37:61–65, 1986

Kahana Y: The Zar spirits, a category of magic in the system of mental health care in Ethiopia. Int J Soc Psychiatry 31:125–143, 1985

Kaslow NJ, Celano M, Dreelin ED: A cultural perspective on family theory and therapy. Psychiatr Clin North Am 18:621–633, 1995

Kleinman AM: Neurasthenia and depression: a study of somatization and culture in China. Cult Med Psych 6(2):117–189, 1982

Kleinman AM: Rethinking Psychiatry: From Cultural Category to Personal Experience. New York, Free Press, 1988

Kleinman A: Triumph or pyrrhic victory: the inclusion of culture in DSM-IV. Harv Rev Psychiatry 4:343–344, 1997

Kobayashi JS: Depathologizing dependency: two perspectives. Psychiatric Annals 19:653–658, 1989

Krippner S: Cross-cultural approaches to multiple personality disorder: practices in Brazilian spiritism. Ethos 15(3):273–295, 1987

Kuo WH, Gray R, Lin N: Locus of control and symptoms of psychological distress among Chinese-Americans. Int J Soc Psychiatry 25:176–187, 1979

Kvernmo S, Heyerdahl S: Influence of ethnic factors on behavior problems in indigenous Sami and majority Norwegian adolescents. J Am Acad Child Adolesc Psychiatry 37:743–751, 1998

Lin KM, Poland RE, Smith MW, Strickland TL, et al: Pharmacokinetic and other related factors affecting psychotropic responses in Asians. Psychopharmacol Bull 27:427–439, 1991

Lin KM, Anderson D, Poland RE: Ethnicity and psychopharmacology: bridging the gap. Psychiatr Clin North Am 18:635–647, 1995

Littlewood R: Against pathology: the new psychiatry and its critics. Br J Psychiatry 159:696–702, 1991

Littlewood R, Lipsedge M: The butterfly and the serpent: culture, psychopathology and biomedicine. Cult Med Psychiatry 11:289–335, 1987

Lock M: The concept of race: an ideological construct. Transcultural Psychiatric Research Review 3:203–227, 1993

Lukoff D, Lu F, Turner R: Toward a more culturally sensitive DSM-IV: psychoreligious and psychospiritual problems. J Nerv Ment Dis 180:673–682, 1992

Marcos LR: Effects of interpreters on the evaluation of psychopathology in non-English-speaking patients. Am J Psychiatry 136:171–174, 1979

Marcos LR: Understanding ethnicity in psychotherapy with Hispanic patients. Am J Psychoanal 48:35–42, 1988

Marsella AJ: Cross-cultural research on severe mental disorders: issues and findings. Acta Psychiatr Scand 78:7–22, 1988

Marsella AJ: Counseling and psychotherapy with Japanese Americans: cross-cultural considerations. Am J Orthopsychiatry 63:200–208, 1993

Mezzich JE, Kleinman A, Fabrega H, et al: Culture and Psychiatric Diagnosis. Washington, DC, American Psychiatric Press, 1996

Neki JS: An examination of the cultural relativism of dependence as a dynamic of social and therapeutic relationships. Br J Med Psychol 49:11–22, 1976

Patel V, Winston M: "Universality of mental illness" revisited: assumptions, artefacts and new directions. Br J Psychiatry 165:437–440, 1994

Pressel E: Umbanda in Sao Paulo: religious innovation in a developing society, in Religion, Altered States of Consciousness, and Social Change. Edited by Bourguignon E. Columbus, Ohio State University Press, 1973, pp 264–318

Reid WH: The antisocial personality: a review. Hospital and Community Psychiatry 36:831–837, 1985

Ridley CR: Clinical treatment of the nondisclosing black client. Am Psychol 39:1234–1244, 1984

Ruiz P: Folk healers as associate therapists, in Current Psychiatric Therapies. Edited by Masserman JH. New York, Grune & Stratton, 1976, pp 269–275

Ruiz P: Spiritism, mental health, and the Puerto Ricans: an overview. Transcultural Psychiatric Research Review XVI (April): 28–43, 1979

Ruiz P, Langrod J: Cultural issues in the mental health of Hispanics in the United States. Am J Soc Psychiatry 2(2):35–38, 1982

Ruiz P, Varner RV, Small DR, et al: Ethnic differences in the neuroleptic treatment of schizophrenia. Psychiatric Q 70:163–172, 1999

Sandoval MC: Santería as a mental health care system: an historical overview. Soc Sci Med 13B:137–151, 1979

Spitz RA: Hospitalism: an inquiry into the genesis of psychiatric conditions in early childhood. Psychoanalytic Study of the Child 1:53–74, 1945

Stoller RJ, Herdt GH: The development of masculinity: a cross-cultural contribution. J Am Psychoanal Assoc 30:29–59, 1982

Strauss JS, Carpenter WT Jr, Bartko JJ: A review of some findings from the international pilot study of schizophrenia, in Annual Review of Schizophrenic Syndrome, Vol 4. Edited by Cancro R. New York, Brunner/Mazel, 1976, pp 74–88

Strickland TL, Ranganath V, Lin KM, et al: Psychopharmacologic considerations in the treatment of Black American populations. Psychopharmacol Bull 27:441–448, 1991

Strickland TL, Lin KM, Fu P, et al: Comparison of lithium ratio variation between African-American and Caucasian bipolar patients. Biol Psychiatry 37:325–330, 1995

Tamura T, Lau A: Connectedness versus separateness: applicability of family therapy to Japanese families. Fam Proc 31:319–340, 1992

Thomas A, Sillen S: Racism and Psychiatry. Secaucus, NJ, Citadel Press, 1972

Torres JB: Masculinity and gender roles among Puerto Rican men: machismo on the US mainland. Am J Orthopsychiatry 68:16–26, 1998

Tsui P, Schultz GL: Failure of rapport: why psychotherapeutic engagement fails in the treatment of Asian clients. Am J Orthopsychiatry 55:561–569, 1985

Tung M: Insight-oriented psychotherapy and the Chinese patient. Am J Orthopsychiatry 61:186–194, 1991

Varghese FTN: The racially different psychiatrist—implications for psychotherapy. Aust N Z J Psychiatry 17:329–333, 1983

Westermeyer J: Psychiatric diagnosis across cultural boundaries. Am J Psychiatry 142:798–805, 1985

White GM: The role of cultural explanations in "somatization" and "psychologization." Soc Sci Med 16:1519–1530, 1982

Widiger TA, Frances AJ, Pincus HA, et al. (eds): The DSM-IV Sourcebook, Vol 3. Washington, DC, American Psychiatric Press, 1997

Williams CL: Issues surrounding psychological testing of minority patients. Hospital and Community Psychiatry 38:184–189, 1987

Wohl J: Integration of cultural awareness into psychotherapy. Am J Psychother 43:343–355, 1989

Yalom ID: The Theory and Practice of Group Psychotherapy, 2nd Edition. New York, Basic Books, 1975

Yamamoto J, Acosta FX: Treatment of Asian Americans and Hispanic Americans: similarities and differences. J Am Acad Psychoanal 10:585–607, 1982

Zimmerman RS, Khoury EL, Vega WA, et al: Teacher and parent perceptions of behavior problems among a sample of African American, Hispanic, and non-Hispanic white students. Am J Community Psychol 23:181–197, 1995

SECTION 2

Disorders Usually First Diagnosed in Infancy, Childhood, or Adolescence

Section Editors

John F. McDermott Jr., M.D.,

Elizabeth B. Weller, M.D.

Introduction

The treatment of psychiatric disorders in infancy, childhood, and adolescence reflects incremental advances in the development of evidence-based, diagnosis-specific psychosocial and psychopharmacological interventions since the second edition of *Treatments of Psychiatric Disorders*. In the following chapters, our experts summarize the natural history and clinical features of each DSM-IV condition and then focus on the scientific knowledge base for its treatment, emphasizing practical applications for clinical practice (i.e., which treatment is best tailored to the needs of each child and the family).

First, in Chapter 4, James Harris outlines the treatment of psychiatric disorders in persons with mental retardation, with both cognitive level and social adaptive functioning, in the context of the most recent understanding from the neurosciences.

Next, in Chapter 5, Arlene Young and Joseph Beitchman present the latest understanding of learning disorders and their subtypes in this rapidly changing field. Emphasizing a multimodal, multidisciplinary approach to treatment, they address both the core deficit in each type of learning disorder and the need to develop coping strategies to compensate for that deficit.

Bryna Siegel, Catherine Hayer, and Peter Tanguay present, in Chapter 6, major behavioral and pharmacological interventions for autism that are supported by empirical research. They offer a model to the clinician for formulating which interventions may be most suitable for which individual with pervasive developmental disorder.

The disruptive behavior disorders are separated into two chapters. In Chapter 7, Joseph Biederman, Thomas Spencer, Timothy Wilens, and Ross Greene summarize the vast research literature on the treatment of attention-deficit/hyperactivity disorder (ADHD). In their authoritative consideration of drug dosages, side effects, indications, and contraindications, they offer special consideration of treatment-refractory patients, complicating comorbidity, and clinical guidelines for psychosocial and pharmacological treatment, including the differential use of first- through fourth-line medications for ADHD. In Chapter 8, Alayne Yates approaches the other disruptive behavior disorder—conduct disorder, one notoriously resistant to interventions—by considering the pros and cons of each treatment in turn, including promising new medications.

The treatment of tic disorders is reviewed in Chapter 9 by a group of researchers who have studied them most intensively. Kenneth Towbin, Donald Cohen, and James Leckman describe behavioral intervention programs for home and school, as well as indications and guidelines for psychotherapy and family therapy. In reviewing the range of psychopharmacological interventions, the authors consider special medication issues (e.g., related disorders that may be alternative expressions of the same underlying genetic etiology) and address the controversy about whether stimulants exacerbate tics.

In Chapter 10, Donald Shaffer presents an assessment protocol for elimination disorders that is both scientific and practical. Indeed, the author found that simply doing a baseline assessment of bed-wetting reduces the symptoms in a significant number of patients. The most effective treatment for enuresis, the night alarm, is described and evaluated, as is drug therapy. In the treatment of encopresis, the choice between behavioral and medical management gives way to the treatment of choice: multimodality therapy that combines behavioral approaches with laxative therapy.

In Chapter 11, Tami Benton and Laura Sanchez consider the wide range of symptoms presenting in children with anxiety disorders in developing a formulation that includes specific individual goals. Their thorough review of empirically researched pharmacological agents is followed by a comprehensive consideration of the various psychotherapies (e.g., cognitive and other behavioral techniques, psychoanalysis, psychodynamic therapies, and family therapy).

In Chapter 12, Gabrielle Carlson and Joan Rosenbaum Asarnow review the research base in the use of antidepressant medication for mood disorders, cover procedures for the administration of medication, and examine the discrepancies between research and practice. The interim status of pharmacological research is contrasted with the real advances in our knowledge base for psychosocial treatments, and the authors conclude with a short but comprehensive discussion of the management of suicidal behaviors.

Next, in a most practical consideration of the management of posttraumatic stress disorder, Lenore Terr details the elements of trauma-focused psychotherapy, combining cognitive-behavioral with psychodynamic principles. She reviews the early stages of evidence-based treatments, including medications, group therapy, and large-scale interventions, as well as the controversial and unproven eye movement desensitization and restructuring.

The dramatic changes in our understanding of obsessive-compulsive disorder are described by Jennifer Freeman, Henrietta Leonard, Douglas Beer, John March, and Susan Swedo in Chapter 14. The current role of psychotherapy, modified to meet the new neurobiological understanding of the disorder, is presented. Several of the best-researched cognitive-behavioral therapy approaches are outlined; pharmacotherapeutic treatments, including clomipramine, selective serotonin reuptake inhibitors, and investigational agents, are also considered.

Next, in Chapter 15, Heather Walter offers a unique developmental approach to substance abuse, relating stages in its development to interventions. Individual and group therapy techniques in inpatient and outpatient settings are emphasized, with analysis of comparative effectiveness and outcomes.

Childhood-onset schizophrenia is a rare condition, with the scientific knowledge base for this disorder in its early stages of development. Andrew Russell, in Chapter 16, discusses both standard and atypical antipsychotic drugs, the latter rapidly becoming the drugs of choice, despite very limited research data in their use with children and adolescents. Psychosocial interventions, special education, family approaches, and social skills training are also described.

Finally, in Chapter 17, Thomas Anders offers a comprehensive approach to difficulties falling asleep or maintaining sleep and disruptions of and intrusions into sleep. The author compares the pros and cons of hypnotics and the more effective behavioral strategies. The section on circadian rhythm dyssomnias in adolescence will be especially welcomed by clinicians.

In summary, we believe the authors of these chapters have assembled the most current and comprehensive set of evidence-based treatment approaches for the disorders of childhood and adolescence available in the field today.

4

Psychiatric Disorders in Mentally Retarded Persons

James C. Harris, M.D.

Psychiatric involvement with mentally retarded persons has a long history, one that begins in the 19th century; neuropsychiatrists were frequently superintendents of the early institutions for mentally retarded persons. Interest in mental retardation among psychiatrists subsequently waned for several reasons: 1) insight-oriented therapy became the primary form of treatment, and persons with mental retardation were generally considered to be poor candidates; 2) an emphasis on normalization emerged that emphasized educational approaches and behavior modification techniques that tended to minimize the diagnosis of psychiatric disorder; and 3) psychotropic medications were used excessively in state facilities for behavior reduction without adequate attention being given to comprehensive treatment programs, leading to increasing involvement of nonmedical professionals in the treatment of mental retardation. However, with the emergence of improved assessment (State et al. 1997; Szymanski and King 1999), a biopsychosocial approach to treatment, and the acknowledgment that school and community placements most commonly fail because of disruptive behavior, there has been a renewed focus on psychiatric treatment and on better understanding how mental disorders present in mentally retarded persons.

Adapted in part from Harris J: *Assessment, Diagnosis, and Treatment of Developmental Disorders.* New York, Oxford University Press, 1998.

Advances in the neurosciences, developmental psychology, developmental psychopathology, phenomenology and classification, family therapy, behavior therapy, and drug treatments have led to a new perspective in psychiatry and a renewed commitment to diagnosis and treatment of mentally retarded individuals with mental illness. Recognition of the interface and of the role of experience in brain development and a better understanding of the natural history of specific mental retardation syndromes have led to participation of psychiatrists with other professionals in the habilitation of mentally retarded persons with psychiatric disorders.

The prevalence of associated mental disorders is three to four times greater in mentally retarded persons than in the general population; moreover, the full range of mental disorders may be diagnosed. In addition, mentally retarded individuals are at greater risk for exploitation and physical or sexual abuse than are nonretarded persons, which further increases their risk for mental disorders. Because adaptive behavior is, by definition, impaired in mental retardation, social stressors are particularly problematic. Yet, in protective social environments where adequate support is available, social impairments, particularly in mildly retarded persons, may not be obvious. Considerable advances have been made in understanding the cognitive and emotional processes involved in the development of persons with mental retardation, in identifying factors that contribute to disturbed behavior, and in clarifying which treatments for emotional, behavioral, and interpersonal problems are effective.

Both cognitive level and social adaptive functioning must be carefully evaluated in developing a treatment program for persons with mental retardation. Mildly cognitively impaired individuals experience the same range of mental disorders as do nonretarded persons. The same diagnoses and modalities of treatment that are used with non–mentally retarded persons are implemented for persons with mental retardation; however, some modifications in technique are needed for psychotherapeutic interventions. For severely and profoundly mentally retarded persons, the emphasis must shift to greater involvement with those family members and community caregivers who can function as co-therapists. Psychiatric diagnosis in mentally retarded persons is more difficult and may require substantial input from other informants. Although behavior management techniques and drug treatments are used in the treatment of these individuals, family and interpersonal therapies are essential. Therefore, application of functional communication approaches and attachment theory are important elements in developing a treatment program. Behavior management techniques are frequently used in conjunction with functional communication therapies in developing care plans. Aggressive and self-injurious behaviors are common complaints for severely and profoundly mentally retarded persons and in some instances may be components of an unrecognized major mental disorder.

In this chapter, I provide background information on the definitions of mental retardation and review approaches to treatment of mental disorders in mentally retarded persons. Throughout this chapter, the terms *persons with mental retardation* and *mentally retarded persons* are used to emphasize their individuality because humane treatment has often been lacking and stigmatization is a continuing concern. To highlight the need for humane treatment, in 1972 the General Assembly of the United Nations passed a "Declaration on the Rights of Mentally Retarded Persons," which stated that "the mentally retarded person has, to the maximum degree of feasibility, the same rights as other human beings."

The prevalence of mental retardation is about 1% of the general population; approximately 85% of those affected test in the mild range of mental retardation. Genetic causes are identified in about 35%; fewer than 10% have a malformation syndrome of unknown etiology. Prenatal, perinatal, postnatal, or other external factors, including infection, trauma, toxins, complicated birth, and prematurity, account for one-third of cases. Currently unidentified causes account for the remainder of cases.

Because mental retardation describes such a heterogeneous group of disorders, treatment must be individualized. Community surveys have documented the prevalence of psychiatric disorders with mental retardation in the community (Bouras and Drummond 1992; Gillberg et al. 1986; Griffin et al. 1987; Lund 1985; Reiss 1990; Rutter 1970; Wing and Gould 1979). Treatment approaches include individual, family, behavioral, and pharmacological interventions. Prevention of those forms of mental retardation secondary to gestational substance abuse involves the psychiatrist whenever alcohol or other substances are abused by women of childbearing age.

Definition

Mental retardation is the currently accepted designation for an intellectual and adaptive behavioral disability that begins in the early developmental period. Although *mental retardation* is the term included in both ICD-10 (see World Health Organization 1992) and DSM-IV (American Psychiatric Association 1994), the terms *mental deficiency* and *mental handicap* also have been used in the past. Such variations in terminology derive from longstanding concern about the stigma of a diagnosis of mental retardation. Although the term *mental retardation* is currently used in the major classification systems, the term *intellectual disability* is increasingly being used internationally. Because of the onset in the developmental period, the terms *developmental intellectual disability* and *developmental cognitive disability* also have been proposed. Reflecting these changes, the International Association for the Scientific Study of Mental Deficiency (IASSMD) is now designated the International Association for the Scientific Study of Intellectual Disability (IASSID).

In defining mental retardation, both cognitive capacity and the ability to adapt and master tasks in the real world are assessed. The advantage of using intellectual capacity in the definition is that physical, educational, and behavioral impairment can then be judged independently. In addition to cognitive tests, scales of adaptive functioning need to be completed by interviewing parents or care providers who are familiar with the individual's performance of daily activities required for personal and social sufficiency. If intellectual level and social adaptation are not both considered, then the assessment is simply a provisional estimate. Tests of adaptive behavior that are used together with intelligence tests include the American Association on Mental Retardation (AAMR) Adaptive Behavior Scale (Kazuo et al. 1993; Lambert et al. 1993) and the Vineland Adaptive Behavioral Scales (Sparrow et al. 1984). With the development of these adaptive behavioral instruments, guidelines are being established to determine what constitutes a significant impairment in adaptive functioning. The following domains are considered: communication, daily living skills/self-help, socialization/social functioning/interpersonal skills, and motor skills.

Although a sociocultural etiology (Zigler 1967) has been suggested to account for the milder forms of mental retardation, recent medical advances, such as the recognition of the increased prevalence of fragile X syndrome and evidence for mild mental retardation in this disorder, suggest that a neurobiologically based cognitive deficit may underlie the majority of cases. Yet, despite the cognitive defect, mental retardation is not a static disorder but a dynamic condition that has multiple etiologies that must be considered in treatment planning. Mental retardation is not a disease or an illness in itself (Clarke et al. 1985) but instead constitutes a heterogeneous group of conditions ranging from genetic and metabolic disorders to functional changes that follow trauma to the nervous system at birth or later during the developmental period. Because of this heterogeneity, each case must be considered independently according to whether an associated syndrome (e.g., fragile X syndrome or Down syndrome) or an associated etiology (e.g., head trauma) is present. Consequently, there is no single cause, mechanism, clinical course, or prognosis for mental retardation. Thinking is not characteristically disordered and perception is not distorted unless a concurrent mental disorder exists.

Diagnosis and Classification

The American Psychiatric Association (1987, 1994) in DSM-III-R and DSM-IV, the World Health Organization (1992) in ICD-10, and the AAMR (American Association on Mental Retardation 1992) have formally defined mental retardation (see Table 4–1). Although all of the definitions include IQ and adaptive functioning, each provides a different emphasis, so it is important to be familiar with each of them. In applying the definitions, it should be kept in mind that specific adaptive abilities often coexist with strengths in other adaptive skills or personal capabilities; therefore, adaptive strengths must be carefully considered.

TABLE 4–1. DSM-IV diagnostic criteria for mental retardation

A. Significantly subaverage intellectual functioning: an IQ of approximately 70 or below on an individually administered IQ test (for infants, a clinical judgment of significantly subaverage intellectual functioning).

B. Concurrent deficits or impairments in present adaptive functioning (i.e., the person's effectiveness in meeting the standards expected for his or her age by his or her cultural group) in at least two of the following areas: communication, self-care, home living, social/interpersonal skills, use of community resources, self-direction, functional academic skills, work, leisure, health, and safety.

C. The onset is before age 18 years.

Code based on degree of severity reflecting level of intellectual impairment:

317 **Mild mental retardation:** IQ level 50–55 to approximately 70

318.0 **Moderate mental retardation:** IQ level 35–40 to 50–55

318.1 **Severe mental retardation:** IQ level 20–25 to 35–40

318.2 **Profound mental retardation:** IQ level below 20 or 25

319 **Mental retardation, severity unspecified:** when there is strong presumption of mental retardation but the person's intelligence is untestable by standard tests

In DSM-IV, mental retardation is divided into four levels of severity indicating the degree of intellectual impairment: mild, moderate, severe, or profound (Table 4–1). These levels are described in detail in DSM-IV-TR (American Psychiatric Association 2000, pp. 43–44). The diagnosis of dementia can be made but "may not be appropriate until the child is between ages 4 and 6 years" (American Psychiatric Association 2000, p. 47). Clarification of a diagnosis of dementia is important because mental retardation is a developmental disability.

In ICD-10, mental retardation is defined as a disorder of psychological development and takes a somewhat different approach than that used by DSM-IV. ICD-10 notes that intelligence is not a "unitary characteristic but is assessed on the basis of a large number of different, more or less specific skills" (World Health Organization 1992, p. 226). Such skills ordinarily will develop to a similar degree in a nonretarded person; however, because mental retardation is a heterogeneous disorder, one may see large discrepancies among these skills. There may be severe impairments in one area (e.g., language); in other instances, there may be an area of higher skill level that is maintained, often referred to as a "splinter skill" (e.g., better visuospatial abilities in a severely retarded person). This variance in abilities presents difficulties when the clinician is determining what subgroup of mental retardation best represents the patient's condition.

ICD-10 specifies that IQ levels are provided as a guide only and should not be applied rigidly because they are divisions of a complex continuum that cannot be defined with absolute preciseness. The appropriate test must be selected based on the individual's level of functioning and the presence of any associated disabling conditions, such as expressive language difficulties, physical handicaps, and hearing or visual problems.

The AAMR (American Association on Mental Retardation 1992) includes the same three basic criteria in its definition of mental retardation (i.e., significantly subaverage intellectual functioning, limitations in adaptive skills, and onset before age 18) as does DSM-IV (Table 4–1). However, in its revision, the AAMR has proposed an extension of this definition that focuses more on the individual's needs and what can be done to improve functioning. This revision represents a major change in the way persons with mental retardation are described for purposes of classification. The AAMR definition of mental retardation emphasizes a functional orientation to the mentally retarded person and does not include specific levels of mental retardation. Instead, it specifies "profile and intensities of psychosocial supports needed" (i.e., intermittent, limited, extensive, and pervasive) that are not directly comparable to the levels specified in DSM-IV (American Association on Mental Retardation 1992, pp. 32–33). The AAMR definition emphasizes the risks of a unidimensional approach that focuses only on disability.

The AAMR description considers the congruence of intellectual and adaptive abilities along with stressors that affect adaptive functioning. Assessment of adaptive functioning is essential because IQ tests alone are not an accurate measure of a mentally retarded person's ability, although adaptive skills are closely related to intellectual limitations. Deficits in adaptive ability have been defined as "significant limitations in an individual's effectiveness in meeting the standards of maturation, learning, personal independence, and/or social responsibility that are expected of his [or her] age level and cultural group" (Grossman 1983, p. 11). Areas of ability include social/interpersonal skills and responsibility, communication, self-care, home living, use of community resources, self-direction, functional academic skills, work, leisure, health, and safety. As in DSM-IV, at least two of these areas must be involved before a generalized limitation can be diagnosed. Because these skills will vary with chronological age, the assessment must take age into account.

The major elements of the AAMR assessment approach are 1) instrumental competence (cognition and learning) and social competence (practical and social intelligence) that result in adaptive skills; 2) overall functioning (i.e., the ability to cope with ordinary challenges of everyday living in the community); and 3) environments where an individual lives, works, and learns. Mental retardation is not viewed as a static condition; the treatment goal is to establish a "best-fit match" of the person with environmental supports to maximize his or her adaptive ability.

The AAMR definition takes into account cultural issues, communication, and behavioral differences. The expectation is that with appropriate supports that continue over a sustained period, the life functioning of the person with mental retardation will generally improve because each person has unique strengths as well as limitations. Although deficits in adaptive functioning in mental retardation may not be lifelong, supports may be needed for an extended period and, in some instances, throughout life. Improvement in functioning is expected for the majority, but for some persons, supports will be needed to maintain a basic level of functioning or to slow the regression process.

Multiaxial Classification/Multidimensional Approaches

One of the major advances in DSM-III (American Psychiatric Association 1980) was the establishment of the multiaxial classification system to deal with the multiple areas that require care. Unlike a multiple category system, the multiaxial system provides for specific axes and specifies rules for their use and, if all axes (five in the case of DSM-III) are used, constitutes a far more comprehensive perspective than does a single diagnostic axis.

In DSM-IV, the multiaxial system is continued; however, it was not introduced into the ICD-10 classification. In DSM-IV, the diagnosis of mental retardation remains on Axis II, thus highlighting the importance of considering cognitive level in developing a treatment plan. Psychiatric diagnoses for mentally retarded persons are placed on Axis I to emphasize the importance of listing specific diagnoses for mentally retarded persons rather than simply focusing on associated behaviors. If known, a particular mental retardation syndrome is coded on Axis III (i.e., general medical disorders). In addition, the Axis IV and Axis V categories are domains that should be included for all mentally retarded persons. Axis IV refers to specific stressors (i.e., psychosocial and environmental problems), and Axis V is the Global Assessment of Functioning (GAF) Scale, which provides a means to categorize overall adaptive ability. The complexity of a clinical situation can be demonstrated by describing comorbidity to highlight the heterogeneity of persons with a similar or the same diagnosis. The multiaxial system is of particular value in evaluating long-term prognosis, because diagnoses on the various axes contribute to outcome risks.

In ICD-10, a different approach is taken. Provision is made for a fourth character to be added to the standard diagnostic code to specify the degree of behavioral impairment, if another ICD-10 mental disorder diagnosis is not appropriate. For example, mental retardation with a fourth character "0" indicates no or minimal behavioral impairment. The digit "1" indicates specific behavioral impairment requiring attention or treatment.

The AAMR classification provides its own multidimensional support systems approach (Table 4–2). Four dimensions are used to provide a more comprehensive picture of the individual: intellectual functioning and adaptive skills, psychological and emotional considerations, general health and physical considerations, and environmental considerations. Detailed information on how to apply the multidimensional system is provided in the AAMR manual *Mental Retardation: Definition, Classification, and Systems of Support* (American Association on Mental Retardation 1992).

Developmental Issues/Normalization

Although mental retardation is a chronic condition and is not curable, the extent of habilitation that can be accomplished can be substantial. A developmental model of mental retardation emphasizes the capacity for growth and stresses independent living. This model

TABLE 4–2. AAMR multidimensional classification system

Dimension	Classification
Dimension I: intellectual functioning and adaptive skills	Cognitive Adaptive Developmental
Dimension II: psychological/emotional considerations	DSM-IV
Dimension III: physical/health/etiology considerations	ICD-10 Etiology
Dimension IV: environmental considerations	Ecological analysis

Source. American Association on Mental Retardation 1992.

specifically emphasizes that adaptive behavior may improve with habilitation. The developmental model constitutes an important aspect of normalization. Normalization refers to a mentally retarded individual's entitlement to services that are as culturally normative as possible to help him or her establish and maintain appropriate personal behavior (Wolfensberger 1972). Normalization means that mentally retarded persons should live in community settings, attend classes in regular schools, and be encouraged to seek competitive employment. They should be responsible for their behavior, and it should not be assumed that their mental retardation precludes their being able to take on such responsibility. In addition, their behavior should be monitored and skills should be taught to assist them in reaching the standards for nonretarded persons of a comparable developmental age.

Personality Development

Studies of mentally retarded persons have focused primarily on intellectual and cognitive functioning and have often neglected social and personality development. Problems associated with cognitive functioning have often overshadowed a needed focus on adaptive and maladaptive personality features (Reiss et al. 1982), although personality variables and personal motivation are essential for predicting social and vocational adjustment. It is mentally retarded persons' behavior and social deficits that most commonly lead them to psychiatric referral.

Investigations of personality dysfunction in mentally retarded persons suggest characteristics such as overdependency, low ideal self-image, limited levels of aspiration, and an outer-directed approach to problem solving (Zigler and Burack 1989). These personality characteristics may have their origin in negative psychosocial experiences, such as repeated failure and disapproval, leading to self-doubts about the capability to be successful. Experiences of rejection and the lack of consistent social support may lead to excessive reliance on others for guidance. Out of a need for recognition by others, persons with mental retardation may suppress the desire to become more independent, or they may assume a "cloak of competence." *Cloak of competence* is a term introduced by Edgerton (1993) to describe how mentally retarded persons cope with the stigma of mental retardation and their own low self-esteem.

During adolescence, parental restrictiveness and overprotection, peer rejection, and continuing low self-confidence often limit mastery of developmental tasks involved in establishing self-concept, sexual awareness, and identity. Mentally retarded adolescents may view their lives as being less fulfilling than those of their peers. They commonly experience dissatisfaction with their physical appearance and become frustrated when they find it hard to control their impulses, emotions, and behavior. Such experiences may lead to social isolation, loneliness, and dysphoric mood. Operant behavior modification programs tend not to address interpersonal needs. Such programs do not focus on making choices, but rather emphasize contingency management. As a result, the transition to vocational programs after completion of schooling may be difficult.

The failure to master developmental tasks may lead to maladaptive personality styles in adulthood. As many as one-half of the adults with mental retardation may have dysfunctional behavioral styles. Although the use of the diagnosis of personality disorder in persons with mental retardation has been questioned, several personality disorder diagnostic inventories that show adequate interrater and test-retest reliability have identified dysfunctional personality traits and personality disorders in adolescents and adults with mental retardation. The types of maladaptive personality characteristics most often found on these inventories include affective instability, explosive and disruptive behaviors, and introverted personality patterns (Dana 1993; Reid and Ballinger 1987). Menolascino (1988) studied 543 admissions for psychiatric care over a 5-year period. He found that 13% of those age 16 and older had received a diagnosis of personality disorder; passive-aggressive and antisocial types were the most common. The presence of a seizure disorder, especially one involving the temporal lobes, may increase the risk for a personality disorder among mentally retarded persons. Moss et al. (1997) reviewed personality disorder and other behavioral presentations.

Sexuality and Mental Retardation

Several stereotypes regarding sexual behavior are suggested for persons with mental retardation. These include their being sexually uninhibited, being sexually immature (sexual interests corresponding to their mental rather than their chronological age), or lacking sexual interests altogether. However, indiscriminate sexual behavior is not a characteristic feature in mentally retarded persons (Bregman and Harris 1995). Yet, based on stereotypes about uninhibited or indiscriminate sexual behavior, sterilization was routinely practiced in the past. Intermarriage has been prohibited in the past as a means of reducing the incidence of mental retardation. Because of these attitudes, a mentally retarded person may have limited opportunities to socialize or develop an intimate relationship with someone of the opposite sex.

Sexual interest is usually associated with the onset of puberty; therefore, mental retardation syndromes associated with delays in puberty will influence sexual interest. However, the most severely and profoundly retarded persons often show little interest in sexual activity with others regardless of the age at pubertal onset. Still, mildly retarded and many moderately retarded persons may have normal pubertal development, express sexual interests, and establish sexual identities. When the expression of sexual interest is prohibited or prevented in this group, inappropriate sexual activity may occur as a response. Moreover, sexual behavior may be used as a way to demonstrate self-importance. During adolescence, sexual behavior can be part of an attempt to gain acceptance from others in a peer group, as is the case in peer groups of nonretarded persons. Encouragement of relationships with others and the teaching of appropriate social skills are prerequisites to facilitate the development of normal sexual identification. A focus on interpersonal relationships should be emphasized along with specific instruction about sexual activity.

Mildly and moderately retarded adolescents frequently lack a basic understanding of sexual anatomy, venereal disease, and contraceptive issues and are at risk for sexual exploitation. Knowledge of sexuality may not be well established because the usual sources of information are not available or are limited. These sources normally include sex education in the schools, intimate peer discussions, and printed reading material. In addition, family members may be reluctant to review or discuss sexual matters with their mentally retarded children or young adult family members. For nonretarded persons, knowledge of sexuality is based on life experience and sexual opportunity and not on systematic education.

Assessment

The psychiatric evaluation of persons with mild and moderate mental retardation covers the same areas that are addressed with nonretarded individuals, with some slight modifications. The etiology of mental retardation should be established when possible because it may clarify the prognosis, provide information on the natural history in regard to medical and behavioral complications, and suggest treatment. A comprehensive assessment includes a diagnosis of mental retardation; a review of present concerns and symptoms; past and present developmental, genetic, medical, social, psychiatric, and family history; individual patient interview; review of past cognitive testing; physical examination; diagnostic formulation; treatment plan; an informing conference; and follow-through (Szymanski and King 1999). Caregivers who know the patient well are used as informants, and data from interdisciplinary team assessments are relied on. Disorders of interpersonal functioning, communication, emotion, and behavior should be included in the assessment.

The interview procedure must consider the patient's cognitive and adaptive limitations. Interviews are more structured, more directive, and shorter than those conducted with nonretarded individuals. After establishing rapport, the interviewer should provide overt support and establish the context of the interview so that the patient does not consider the interview a test he or she might fail. Particular care must be taken to allow adequate time and avoid leading questions. Communication devices may be required for those with language disorders and sensory handicaps (e.g., blindness and deafness). Finally, interpretations about emotional and behavioral functioning should be offered within the context of the individual's overall communication skills, life experiences, and developmental level.

Standardized assessment instruments and procedures have been developed to improve the reliability and validity of psychiatric evaluation for mentally retarded persons. However, because of variability in cognitive functioning and the use of multiple informants (e.g., physicians, psychologists, educators, direct care providers), it is more difficult to show reliability and validity for these instruments. Nevertheless, several behavior checklists and semistructured interview schedules have been designed for use with mentally retarded persons and caregivers who are informants. Some of these instruments focus on making a specific diagnosis, whereas others are used to assess the range and severity of affective and behavioral symptoms.

Aman (1991a, 1991b) evaluated instruments for assessing emotional and behavioral disorders in individuals with mental retardation. The following items were most commonly found among the instruments for adults that he reviewed with factor-analytic methodology:

1) aggressive or antisocial behavior; 2) withdrawal; 3) stereotypic behavior; 4) hyperactivity; 5) repetitive verbalization; 6) anxious, tense, and fearful behavior; and 7) self-injurious behavior. Rating scales for children are in the process of being validated. The most commonly used instruments are the Aberrant Behavior Checklist (Aman 1991a; Aman and Singh 1988), the Psychopathology Instrument for Mentally Retarded Adults (PIMRA; Matson 1988), and the Reiss Screen for Maladaptive Behavior (Reiss 1988). No one screening instrument can be recommended for preschool children; however, the Reiss Scales for Children's Dual Diagnosis (Reiss and Valenti-Hein 1990, 1994) should be considered for school-age children and adolescents. For the assessment of broad behavioral dimensions, the Aberrant Behavior Checklist and the Developmentally Delayed Child Behavior Checklist (DDCBCL; S. L. Einfeld, B. J. Tonge: "Development of an Instrument to Measure Psychopathology in Mentally Retarded Children and Adolescents," unpublished manuscript, University of Sydney, Sydney, Australia, 1990) should be considered. Moss et al. (1993) developed a semistructured clinical interview—the Psychiatric Assessment Schedule for Adults With Developmental Disability (PAS-ADD)—that includes parallel interviewing of patient and informant, a three-tier structure to provide a flexible interview that can be targeted to the patient's intellectual level, the use of a memorable "anchor event" in the patient's life to enhance time focus, and simplified wording and organization.

Spectrum of Psychiatric Disorders

The number of studies of psychopathology manifested by children, adolescents, and adults with mental retardation is growing. Systematic investigations show that the full spectrum of recognized psychiatric disorders can be identified among individuals with mental retardation. Chart reviews of clinical diagnoses, however, indicate that psychotic disturbances are overdiagnosed and that anxiety, mood, and personality disorders are underrecognized (Bregman 1991).

Children and adults with mild to moderate mental retardation present with psychiatric symptoms and disorders similar to those found in the nonretarded population. Clinicians have used standardized methods of assessment to report attention-deficit/hyperactivity disorder (ADHD), pervasive developmental disorder, conduct disorders, eating disorder, anxiety disorders (phobias, obsessive-compulsive disorder, generalized anxiety), mood disorders, personality disorders, posttraumatic stress disorder, and schizophrenia and other psychotic disorders. Mental disorders due to a general medical condition, such as hypothyroidism with depression in Down syndrome, also must be considered. Some psychiatric symptoms and behaviors occur with particular frequency among community residents, including feelings of social inadequacy, dependency, and sensitivity to criticism (affecting 25%–50%); anxiety (affecting approximately 33%); and aggressive behavior (affecting 20%–25%) (Bregman and Harris 1995).

The prevalence of ADHD in persons with mental retardation is similar to that in the general population, with estimates of between 4% and 11% (Feinstein and Reiss 1996). Because many of the criteria are based on observable behavior, the diagnosis may be made in nonverbal children. Although some criteria are written to suggest that symptoms be considered based on developmental level, it has been proposed that chronological age be used instead (Pearson and Aman 1994). The differential diagnosis must consider situation-specific hyperactivity that may be elicited when demands are too great for cognitive mastery, hyperactivity associated with neurogenetic disorders (Harris 1998) (e.g., fragile X syndrome, phenylketonuria, tuberous sclerosis), neurodevelopmental disorders (e.g., fetal alcohol syndrome), and side effects of certain medications (e.g., akathisia from antipsychotics) (Harris et al. 1981).

Disruptive behavior disorders (e.g., oppositional defiant disorder and conduct disorder) are frequently diagnosed in mentally retarded persons; S. A. Richardson et al. (1985) reported a prevalence of conduct disorder of 33% in children and adolescents with mild mental retardation. There is a risk for overdiagnosis of disruptive behavior disorders because "noncompliance" is a common reason for referral; therefore, the context of the behavior, the individual's capacity to appreciate the meaning of social rules, and recent stressors must be considered in the assessment process.

Mood disorders (e.g., major depression, bipolar disorder, dysthymia) are often underdiagnosed in mentally retarded persons. Moreover, those referred for disruptive behavior may have an underlying mood disorder. It is now recognized that the prevalence of mood disorder in mentally retarded persons is equal to or greater than that in the general population (Reiss 1994; Sovner and Pary 1993). Depressed mood may be more frequent in some mental retardation syndromes such as Down syndrome (Harris 1988). Directed informant ratings, loss of interest in usual activities, self-report of distress, and tearfulness may be better guides to diagnosis than self-reports of sadness on formal mental status examinations. However, Masi et al. (1999) successfully used the Kiddie–Schedule for Affective Disorders and Schizophrenia (K-SADS) in a group of mildly mentally retarded adolescents to reliably diagnose depressed mood, irritability, guilt, and low self-image. The authors found high rates of comorbid generalized anxiety.

Suicidal threats and behavior are of concern in children, adolescents, and adults with mental retardation (Benson and Lamar 1988; Sturmey 1994; Walters et al. 1995). Rapid-cycling affective disorder and mixed affective states are more common in those with mental retardation, but hypothyroidism and temporal lobe epilepsy must be ruled out (Glue 1989; Jan et al. 1994; Santosh and Baird 1999). Anxiety disorders (e.g., generalized anxiety disorders, panic attack, phobias, posttraumatic stress disorder, and obsessive-compulsive disorder) have been reported with a prevalence of 25% in an outpatient sample (Feinstein and Reiss 1996).

Schizophrenia and other psychotic disorders have been reported to occur in mentally retarded persons at a rate two to three times higher than that reported in the general population (Reid 1982, 1989). However, more recent reports suggest that the prevalence is similar with and without mental retardation (Reiss 1994). Because the presence of symptoms such as hallucinations, delusions, and thought disorder requires a certain level of verbal competence, it is difficult to make these diagnoses in subjects with an IQ lower than 45. Moreover, symptoms are generally expressed more concretely and with less elaboration than in the general population. Comparisons of mentally retarded and nonretarded schizophrenic patients show that the former group has an earlier age at onset and a less favorable premorbid history.

Those with severe and profound mental retardation have a different profile of psychopathology. Certain symptoms such as delusions, hallucinations, ideas of reference, obsessions, and guilty ruminations are generally not reported, probably because of limitations in cognitive and symbolic processes. Other symptoms such as stereotyped behaviors occur more frequently. Finger flicking and hand flapping are present in 15%–50% of these individuals, and self-injurious behaviors, such as eye gouging and head banging, are present in 10%–20%, depending on the setting (Harris 1992). Several psychiatric disorders are more common among children and adults with severe to profound mental retardation. These include autistic disorder and related pervasive developmental disorders and stereotypic movement disorder. As many as 4%–8% of mentally retarded children meet the criteria for autistic disorder, which is approximately 10 times the prevalence of this disorder in the general population. Conversely, approximately 75% of autistic children and adults test in the mentally retarded range. Although severely and profoundly mentally retarded individuals may have poor verbal language and self-stimulatory behaviors, a pervasive developmental disorder is diagnosed only if, after considering developmental level, significant impairment in social understanding and skills is found. For adult subjects, a detailed early developmental history may be needed to make the diagnosis. The category stereotypic movement disorder is used to classify the stereotypical self-stimulatory, nonfunctional movement disorders that are often associated with severe mental retardation. This category is commonly used with the specifier "with self-injurious behavior" for those referred for psychiatric care for bodily injury. Self-injury is associated with several mental retardation syndromes, such as Lesch-Nyhan syndrome (self-biting), Prader-Willi syndrome (skin picking), and to a lesser extent de Lange's syndrome and fragile X syndrome.

Dudley et al. (1999) sought to determine whether specific patterns of behavior distinguish persons with mental retardation and mental illness. These investigators noted that persons with mental retardation are thought to be more susceptible to mental illness than is the general population and evaluated a group of 940 patients. A factor analysis was used to determine whether distinct patterns of factors were evident. Six patterns were identified based on problem behaviors and diagnosis: 1) aggressive/disturbing behavior, 2) withdrawn/asocial behavior, 3) inappropriate behaviors, 4) sociopathic features, 5) suicidal or runaway crisis, and 6) pica disorders (more common in those with severe and profound mental retardation). The authors noted that these findings suggest that mental illness is a prominent characteristic of some of the six factors but not of others. Moreover, a mental retardation diagnosis and the particular level of mental retardation are reflected very differently among all of these factors.

Treatment

Treatment of mental retardation in children and adults must consider the complex interplay of neurobiological and psychosocial factors. Therefore, a comprehensive, interdisciplinary approach is essential. The full range of treatments used with nonretarded children and adults should be considered. In most instances, several treatment modalities are indicated. Improved environmental provisions; cognitive and educational interventions; individual, family, and group psychotherapy; family intervention; behavioral interventions; and psychopharmacology should be considered. The efficacy of each of these treatment approaches has been confirmed when the treatment was appropriately selected and implemented.

Environmental Provisions

Appropriate living conditions, vocational opportunities, and planned leisure time activities are essential environmental provisions for mentally retarded persons. It is especially important that these individuals participate in their program by expressing their preferences and making personal choices about living conditions, work, and recreational activities. When handled well, adequate provision may lead to an improved quality of life and a considerable reduction in maladaptive affective and behavioral symptoms. Environmental provisions for the child with a mentally retarded parent require particular attention (Whitman and Accardo 1990). A home program for a mentally retarded person should provide access to preferred activities, present choices with regard to household tasks, and schedule highly preferred tasks and activities immediately after nonpreferred (but essential) ones.

Educational Interventions/Skill Development

A major challenge in the care and treatment of mentally retarded persons is to assist them in developing new ways to interact appropriately with others. Emotional and behavioral disturbances are linked to the lack of self-monitoring and adaptive control over activity, emotions, impulses, and the external environment. Communication deficits, learning difficulty, and limited educational experience may have resulted in their not having the skills needed for personal competence and social responsibility. Consequently, an educationally based program should focus on the social, communication, and vocational skills needed to improve self-control and reduce maladaptive behavior. Essential elements of a social skills program include independence training (teaching self-help and leisure skills), communication training (enhancing speech and nonverbal communication [e.g., signing, gesture, picture/word boards]), and self-management skill development (teaching strategies for self-monitoring and self-reinforcement). Social skills training provides specific and concrete instructions, introduces observation and modeling of effective behavior, structures reinforcement, and focuses on teaching through simple, observable tasks. Social skills training procedures emphasize appropriate interpersonal behavior in a variety of social situations, such as being introduced to another person and properly responding, initiating and participating in social group activities, and learning to interpret and respond appropriately to verbal and nonverbal social cues. Successful social skills programs include demonstrations by instructors, modeling, role-playing, social practice, positive reinforcement, and constructive feedback. Training might include initial instruction and practice in a therapeutic environment, followed by practice in natural community settings to generalize the behavior.

Psychotherapy

Individuals with mild cognitive impairments do benefit from individual, family, and group psychotherapy. Such psychotherapeutic interventions are most effective for emotional and behavioral disturbances in individuals who have experienced traumatic psychosocial experiences that resulted in internalized conflict and maladaptive personality functioning. Continuous failure, social rejection, frequent losses, and dependency on others often lead to feelings of inferiority, ambivalence, anxiety, dysphoria, demoralization, and anger. Each of these symptoms may be targeted. Family conflicts commonly involve feelings of jealousy toward normally developing siblings and personal tension with parents regarding issues of emancipation and independence. Psychotherapeutic interventions may be underused because of misconceptions about their effectiveness for mentally retarded persons (Szymanski 1980). Persons with mental retardation can be highly motivated to establish interpersonal relationships and frequently have a strong desire for enhancing their personal competence and independence.

The goals of psychotherapeutic treatment include resolution of internalized conflict, improvement in self-esteem, and enhancement of personal competence and independence.

The usual treatment approaches may need to be modified, and such treatment is generally recommended following a multidisciplinary diagnostic evaluation that takes into account the developmental level of the patient and the nature of the disabilities and how they may limit the individual's capacity to participate in treatment; this is particularly true for communication disorders. A supportive, focused approach by the therapist and shorter, more frequent sessions may be necessary. O'Hara (1999) provided a review of recent advances in psychotherapy for mentally retarded persons.

Attachment Theory: A Basis for Psychotherapy in Developmental Disorders

Attachment theory (Holmes 1993) is pertinent to the following aspects of psychotherapy for mentally retarded persons: 1) the provision of a secure base in the therapeutic relationships, 2) the establishment of autobiographical competence, 3) the importance of affect and its processing as a central theme, 4) the role of cognition, 5) the effect of separation and loss, and 6) issues related to sexuality. Each of these areas should be considered in working with developmentally disabled persons. The implementation of psychotherapy for disabled persons requires considerable flexibility and ingenuity on the part of the therapist because of the complexity of various disabling conditions.

Orientation of the Psychotherapist

The psychotherapist working with a developmentally disabled individual must openly accept the disabled individual as a person and develop a sense of respect for his or her individuality. A developmental approach is needed that incorporates the results from cognitive, language, and other evaluations into treatment sessions. These sessions are designed to facilitate socialization and mastery of developmental challenges. The therapist appreciates the individual's relative strengths and takes satisfaction in small increments of change. He or she must be prepared to accept the dependency of the disabled person that may emerge during therapy, while concurrently providing praise and reassurance as a means of facilitating independence. In the treatment setting itself, establishing structure, offering specific suggestions, and providing direction are essential. To accomplish these goals, an accepting and receptive attitude is necessary to help the individual improve his or her communicative expression. If inappropriate expressions of aggression occur during sessions and intervention is necessary, an attitude that appreciates the need for nonpunitive intervention is required.

The therapist must be familiar with both the physical and the behavioral characteristics of particular syndromes. He or she must be comfortable in sharing information and using information provided by other professionals involved. Finally, the therapist must acknowledge and empathize with the difficulties that parents experience in raising a child or adolescent or in living with an adult with a disability and be able to offer practical advice and direction to them.

Effect of Developmental Disabilities

An important issue in the development of a psychotherapeutic relationship with a developmentally disabled person is an appreciation of the degree of his or her communication disorder. The therapist must consider the lack of communication skills in the receptive, expressive, and pragmatic language domains. Facilitating communication so that the individual may recognize, label, discriminate, and describe the various emotions becomes a starting point of therapy. In addition, the disabled person's perceptual difficulties in understanding social cues, limited ability to assume social roles, and limited understanding of the intentions of others all enter into this process.

Communication problems are linked to impaired executive functioning in self-monitoring, in abstracting, and in understanding the pragmatic subtleties of social communication with peers and caregivers. Because of these linked cognitive and affective limitations, the repertoire of social behaviors may be reduced. Limitations in communication may be most apparent when a disabled person is stressed. When the person is under stress, emotional dysregulation may lead to reduced impulse control and aggressive behavior. Moreover, cognitive and communication problems may limit the ability to abstract and generalize improved behavior and better self-awareness to new settings. Communicative devices used in treatment include, but are not restricted to, signing, communication boards, and speech synthesizers.

In addition to communication problems, limitations in life experience may influence the psychotherapeutic relationship. The therapist must take into account the lack of basic social understanding based on limited life experiences. Parental or caregiver overprotection may be an important contributing factor in limiting life experience. The overprotective parent or caregiver may limit the disabled person's social contact with peers and activities outside the home and in the community. Such caregivers may infantalize the child or adolescent by making limited demands on him or her to master age-appropriate tasks. Life experiences may be restricted in other ways—for example, being placed in self-contained classrooms or being separated from peers in other settings. The school day for mentally retarded persons tends to be very structured and involves extensive behavior management programs that may provide little free time for recreation and informal activity with peers. Such lack of support for normalized activity may extend to an absence of long-term planning for adaptation in other areas. Developmental issues such as sexuality, vocational training, and assistance in independent living may not be fully addressed.

Mentally retarded and developmentally disabled children, adolescents, and adults may be teased and stigmatized because of their disability; they may also be ignored or excluded from normative peer activities. Reiss and Benson (1984) described how stigmatization leads to labeling, segregation, peer rejection and ridicule, and restricted opportunities. Such exploitation and repeated failure in developmental tasks adversely affects self-esteem.

Overall, the effect of mental retardation can be associated with psychological problems in developmentally disabled persons. These may occur as a consequence of poor communication skills, poor self-monitoring, distorted social perception, lack of life experiences, and traumatic life experiences that lead to poor self-esteem, loneliness, compensatory denial of being disabled, and increased dependency.

Approach to Psychotherapy

The overall psychotherapeutic goals are as follows: 1) to improve adaptive functioning and help the individual to master developmental tasks and avoid stigmatization; 2) to promote resiliency in the individual and to enhance his or her ability to cope with psychosocial stressors; and 3) to prevent the emergence of symptoms during development as new capacities emerge.

In the initiation of treatment of developmentally disabled persons, the psychotherapist must address the same basic issues as with nondisabled persons. Establishing therapeutic contact may require considerable initial effort but is essential, because rapport is basic to enhancing motivation to change. As the psychotherapeutic process unfolds, the extent of communication deficits, as well as the patient's response to psychosocial stressors and the presence of co-occurring behavioral and psychiatric disorders, may become more evident. Consequently, the first phase of treatment also serves as an extended evaluation that may be used to develop a more comprehensive and realistic case formulation.

Psychotherapy with developmentally disabled children and adolescents includes an educational component that involves teaching new adaptive skills. One goal when working with parents or caregivers is to evaluate child and adolescent rearing techniques and teach these techniques, if necessary. Because the child or adolescent may not report significant life events and previous traumas, family members or other caregivers may be asked to assist in providing this information as well as information on new family problems that arise. Moreover, the parents or caregivers play a critical role in ongoing day-to-day guidance and in finding additional resources. The therapy also must be coordinated with educational, communication science, occupational therapy, behavior therapy, medical, social services, and other professionals. Group home or residential staff should be actively involved in establishing the psychotherapeutic goals.

Because multiple caregivers may be involved, interventions must be applied consistently across various settings to maintain gains across these settings. This is particularly true in the teaching of social skills. Because data gathered in one setting may require a change of program in others, communication across settings is vital. When new information comes up during psychotherapy that is pertinent to another treatment setting, there must be a means for it to be conveyed. Finally, the psychotherapist should be prepared for long-term, continuous treatment with episodic crisis management. The frequency of sessions will decrease as symptoms improve.

Adaptation of Psychotherapeutic Methods

Psychotherapeutic techniques need to be adapted when working with developmentally disabled persons. Hurley (1989) recommended six adaptations to psychotherapeutic techniques that she has culled from multiple published reports: 1) matching the technique to the child's, adolescent's, or adult's cognitive and developmental level; 2) taking a directive approach; 3) maintaining flexibility in the choice of treatment methods; 4) involving family and staff; 5) recognizing one's own interpersonal distortions and biases; and 6) providing help in acknowledging the extent of the disability. Even though these adaptations are based largely on case reports, they do offer reasonable general guidelines for clinical practice.

Matching the therapeutic intervention to the patient's cognitive and developmental level and the type of disorder requires the 1) use of syntactically simple language geared to the child's or adolescent's developmental level and 2) provision of concrete examples in an understandable context. The therapist must frequently verify that the patient has understood what has been said and repeat concepts from one session to the next until they are understood (Hurley and Hurley 1986). Hurley and Hurley (1987) suggested that clinicians who are working with older mentally retarded persons should carefully build on the relationship as they would when working with younger children. Initial sessions may be used to help the patient discriminate and label feelings before work is done to link feelings to situations.

A directive approach is needed to maintain the focus of the therapeutic interactions on pertinent issues. In the first session, the reason for the referral is clarified and a specific and concrete explanation is given about what therapy is, how often therapy sessions will occur, and what will take place in each session. The therapist must carefully explain the rules and structure for each therapy session. Firm but appropriate limits are established for aggressive, destructive, and excessively affectionate behavior. When speaking with the child, adolescent, or adult, the therapist must ask for minute particulars about events that have occurred and the mentally retarded person's responses to them. The therapist may recommend alternative means of coping with stressors and may provide alternative interpretations of life events. The person with mental retardation is encouraged to express curiosity and ask questions. This may be a new experience, because in the past he or she may not have been provided an opportunity to do so. When specific questions are posed, the therapist must consider answering them directly rather than exploring for fantasy material that may underlie them. Providing appropriate feedback for effective behavior and offering reassurance when successes are reported are crucial. Acknowledging potential doubts about handling tasks and problems and indicating that, in general, people are not always sure how to accomplish a task may be useful. Moreover, frequently reviewing alternative strategies to master a problem is one way to facilitate problem-solving ability and rational thinking.

Flexibility is needed in the choice of treatment techniques. Alternative approaches are often required when treatment is not progressing adequately. When selecting treatments and particular verbal and interpersonal play techniques, the therapist must take into account the child's cognitive, communicative, and affective developmental level. Play techniques (Chess 1962; Leland and Smith 1965) must be adapted to the person's mental age; drawings, music, and puppets are generally used. The length and frequency of therapy sessions should be based on the patient's ability to tolerate the designated length of time necessary for the therapy to be effective (Stavrakaki and Klein 1986). More frequent and briefer sessions often are necessary for developmentally disabled persons. Adaptability is particularly important to maintain continuity and establish a time perspective in crisis situations.

As noted earlier in this chapter, the family and caregiving staff must be used to provide information, to function as co-therapists when needed, and to provide support. Working with the patient in isolation can be futile (Hurley 1989) because developmentally disabled individuals may be fully dependent on others for care. This is similar to therapy with younger persons, who cannot make all their own decisions and depend on caregivers (Menolascino et al. 1986). Concurrently, family members themselves need support in accepting and adapting to the disability. However, confidentiality is also required to maintain the patient's trust. Excessive involvement by the therapist in making interpretations can make the therapy more difficult because it may reduce the patient's confidence in the therapeutic process (Szymanski 1980). Despite the involvement of others, the person must be encouraged to view himself or herself as an essential source of information.

Overprotection, interpersonal distortions, and biases on the part of the therapist may emerge in the treatment of developmentally disabled persons just as they do in therapy with persons who are not disabled. Important interpersonal issues include the therapist's own attitude toward the disability and any possible discomfort that he or she may feel in the presence of a disabled person. Minimizing or devaluing a retarded or disabled person's individuality can occur in subtle ways. It is important that the therapist acknowledge the reality, chronicity, and permanence of the patient's limitations. Recognizing and treating the disabled person at his or her own developmental level and acknowledging and encouraging mastery of his or her particular life experiences are essential to avoid infantalizing the disabled person and further increasing his or her dependency. The therapist should be aware of his or her own possible wishes to rescue the disabled person, which can lead to an overprotective attitude and a reluctance to set adequate limits (Szymanski 1980). Therefore, the therapist must not place undue emphasis on symptoms but should emphasize the person's independence and accomplishments.

From the disabled person's point of view, dependency on the therapist may result in the therapist's being idealized or considered as a parent (Szymanski 1980). This situation may arise if the therapist is the first person whom the individual can openly confide in who treats him or her in an age-appropriate way. Levitas and Gilson (1987) suggested that such idealization is not necessarily harmful and may be similar to that seen in normally developing children. However, the person in treatment may distort the interpersonal relationship (i.e., parataxic distortion) by projecting fantasies or actual previous experiences of rejection or maltreatment onto the therapist. The patient may expect that the therapist will impose severe prohibitions on him or her as others have in the past. Finally, the disabled person may develop romantic fantasies about the therapist. Mildly retarded persons may be very aware of negative interpersonal responses to them (Reiss and Benson 1984). Like other disabled persons, a mentally retarded person suffers when learning that he or she is different and is stigmatized as a member of a devalued group.

The effect of the specific disability also must be addressed. Mentally retarded persons often have not been targeted as a group who can benefit from disability counseling (Hurley 1989). Because the individual may not clearly understand the nature of his or her disability, specific problems arise in disability counseling. This is particularly true with mental retardation, in which limitations in cognitive ability themselves limit insight and reasoning about the nature of the disability. Although a mentally retarded person may have no clear-cut awareness of what "retarded" means, he or she may be sensitive to being labeled "mentally retarded" (Szymanski and Rosefsky 1980). Such anxiety may be reduced by explaining that mental retardation refers to slowed development in some areas, especially academic areas, but that there may be strengths in other areas. However the disability is described, the explanation needs to be concrete and presented at the individual's developmental level. When discussing the specific disability, the therapist may ask the disabled person 1) if he or she understands the diagnostic label, 2) why he or she is in special classes, and 3) how his or her development differs from that of a sibling.

Along with disability counseling, the therapist may provide "ability" counseling by helping the individual place his or her overall disability into perspective (Hurley 1989). For example, the individual might be taught that he or she has value as a human being that is separate and distinct from being a disabled person, that his or her abilities are important, and that he or she is unique as a person. Hurley (1989) suggested using the principles of rational-emotive therapy developed by Ellis and Bernard (1983) for children, adolescents, and adults with mental retardation. In doing so, the therapist may need to confront the child or adolescent directly regarding his or her possible unwillingness to acknowledge or accept the limitations of mental retardation or other disabilities. Care must be taken if the therapist feels that he or she is "attacking" the patient's self-esteem when asking directly about limitations (Feinstein 1993). The risk of encouraging autonomy is that the individual may be impulsive and, because of cognitive limitations, make choices that could be dangerous. Therefore, the context in which the child or adolescent might make decisions outside of therapy must be carefully understood. Moreover, in developing choices, training in appropriate social assertiveness is needed.

Self-Understanding

The capacity for self-understanding is linked to the cognitive stage of development. Higher-functioning mentally retarded persons may benefit from interpretation of their behavior and show some self-understanding (Feinstein 1993). With younger children, play, drawings, and pictures may be very useful to facilitate such understanding. Self-observation may develop in some adolescents, most commonly those in the mild to borderline range of intelligence. With ongoing therapy, the higher-functioning group may carry out self-monitoring and provide introspective responses when asked about their behavior. Moreover, some disabled persons may identify with the therapist's supportive posture and acknowledge interpretations as helpful. Others may identify with the verbal procedures of the therapy itself, may imitate the therapist's approach to them, and may internalize thinking about behavior and feelings. For example, the patient may remember the therapist's question "How are you feeling now?" and ask it of himself or herself through the use of self-talk when stressed. By the disabled person's identifying with and internalizing the therapist's approach, self-evaluation may be facilitated if the disabled person subsequently reflects on the "here and now" and identifies and discriminates feeling states before acting.

When considering the developmentally disabled person's ability to respond to and use interpretations about his or her behavior, the cognitive and linguistic capacity to talk about past events and use autobiographical memory are critical. One must ask whether the individual has reached the stage of development at which theory of mind—that is, the ability to anticipate the intentions of others and act based on these anticipations—is present. To assess this degree of awareness, the therapist might ask questions such as "What might have you been feeling when she did that?" Those individuals who tend to benefit most from therapy have the capacity to recognize the similarity of their current life situations to previous life events. Such self-understanding may lead them to make different choices based on recognition of past maladaptive patterns of behavior.

Individuals may require specific education to learn how to acknowledge and interpret feelings. They might be told that they are not alone in how they feel, that many people become angry or become jealous of their siblings, or that many people may have bad feelings toward others even though they love them. Preparation may be necessary for interpretation of feelings because those individuals who are anxious to comply and please the therapist become anxious if feelings that they consider unacceptable are attributed to them. One might use figurines in play to clarify the child's or adolescent's understanding of emotion by making statements such as "I can't see any feelings in the soldier's face when the man knocked him over, but maybe he was having some secret feelings." One might then add, "But maybe the soldier had a secret feeling of being angry or scared but thought he wasn't to tell anyone about it. What do you think?"

Group Therapy

Group therapy is a particularly useful approach for the adolescent and adult age groups, more so than for younger children. In group therapy, the patient has an opportunity to directly practice social skills and learn how to develop supportive relationships. Adolescents and adults may feel more comfortable discussing peer-related topics in a group setting with others of their own age group who have similar disabilities. In the group, the therapist actively facilitates these interactions and provides structure. The support and reassurance of group members help individuals verbalize their concerns. Specific topic areas will arise in the group that may be further pursued in individual treatment sessions.

Family Intervention

In working with developmentally disabled children, the family and other caregivers require direct support. Individual and family therapy are often combined to provide consistency in management across settings. The family serves as a therapeutic setting for change and the consolidation of new skills. As therapy progresses, parents may ask for advice on parenting. The treatment goals are positive parenting skills and improved relationships with siblings.

For the family, times of crisis include the initial diagnosis and during phases of adaptation when feelings are mixed and, if not addressed, may lead to chronic sorrow. Kanner (1953) observed that

> whenever parents are given an opportunity to express themselves, they invariably air their emotional involvements in the form of questions, utterances of guilt, open and sometimes impatient rebellion against destiny, stories of frantic search for causes, pathetic accounts of matrimonial dissensions about the child's condition, regret about the course that has been taken so far, anxious appraisals of the child's future, and tearful pleas for reassurance. (p. 375)

Families require support in identifying resources and need specific guidance in management and support techniques. Advocacy by the therapist in helping families in these ways is essential.

The family may become conflicted in coping with a developmentally disabled family member, often leading to marital discord. Commonly, maternal overinvolvement and paternal withdrawal from the therapy occur and must be addressed at the onset of treatment. If this does happen, couples therapy may be needed. Alternatively, a parent may need to be seen individually to work through his or her bereavement. When the disabled person becomes a source of displacement and scapegoating for other family issues, these issues are worked through in family therapy. Richmond (1972) identified several psychological processes in dealing with parents who are adapting to the disabled child. These include phases of denial, projection, guilt, and dependency that must be recognized and worked through.

Family interview sessions may include the developmentally disabled person, and when they do, family interactional patterns should be observed as an additional source for diagnostic information. Family therapy may provide an avenue to support new capabilities for independent functioning. When adolescents are included, it may result in better family negotiating styles if conflict exists between the adolescent and the parent(s). Family treatment may foster assertiveness in the adolescent and may lead to better relationships with siblings, who are often stressed when a child or adolescent in the family has a developmental disorder.

Behavioral Interventions

Behavior therapy has been defined by Werry and Wollersheim (1989) as "those treatments that utilize the principles and terms of learning theory and allied aspects of experimental psychology *and* that are committed to explicit specification of treatment procedures and goals and to the objective evaluation of therapeutic outcomes" (p. 2). Behavior therapy includes approaches that focus only on overt behavior (behavior modification) and others, such as cognitive-behavioral approaches, that recognize internal processes. How complex internal events, such as thinking, could fit into a behavioral model has been explored through the introduction of cognitive-behavioral approaches. With this expansion, behavioral approaches take into account not only principles derived from animal learning and conditioning but also principles derived from social and cognitive psychology.

Behavior therapies are the most commonly used and the best studied treatment approaches for behavior disorders in persons with mental retardation. The techniques of *behavior modification, contingency management,* and *applied behavioral analysis* are included in these therapies. Behavior therapy deals with the technology of behavior change (Jansen 1980). Behavioral procedures are effective for maladaptive patterns of behavior that are the result of faulty learning and also for emotional and behavioral symptoms linked to pathophysiological disorders. Behavioral treatments are used to enhance adaptive, socially desirable behavior; to reduce maladaptive behavior; and to promote habilitative skills. The behaviorist uses the term *behavior* to refer to anything that a person does, thinks, or feels (overtly or covertly) that can be counted or measured. Behavioral interventions may be specifically indicated for self-injurious behavior, self-stimulatory behavior, aggressive behavior, and habit training.

Operant behavioral approaches have continued to evolve and now incorporate functional communication training that considers behavioral responses as potentially aberrant forms of communication. Such functional communication training considers the role of communication impairments in children and adolescents with mental retardation and in their ability to make their needs known. This training is used to teach children self-direction and ways to access reinforcement through communication (Carr and Durand 1985).

Behavior Modification

The goal of behavior therapy is not only to reduce undesirable behavior but also to promote appropriate behavior and provide environments in which successful experiences can occur. Before beginning an individual behavioral treatment program, family issues and community issues must be considered. When interpersonal difficulties within the family or community have a role in the cause or in the continuation of an emotional or behavioral problem, interventions in these areas are coordinated with the behavioral program. Moreover, acknowledging the effect of the disruptive behavior on others, particularly on other family members, helps to facilitate their involvement and willingness to assist in carrying out a treatment program.

Behavior modification procedures are particularly useful in increasing desirable behaviors and reducing undesirable ones. Behavioral procedures are of paramount importance in dealing with individuals with more severe mental retardation because these interventions do not require the use of language or conscious motivation. Targets include daily activities, such as toilet training, self-help skills, and functional communication training. Behavioral methods are less successful in establishing new social skills and in generalizing behavior to other settings (Robertson et al. 1984). When a problem behavior is being addressed, a functional analysis of behavior is carried out and formulated after careful observations of behavioral antecedents, frequency and duration of behaviors, and the consequences that follow them. Target symptoms are identified, and various behavioral interventions are initiated.

One such intervention involves changing the antecedents of the behavioral difficulty, which may stop the behavior from being triggered; this technique is referred to as *stimulus control*. For example, social attention to disruptive behavior may be a prime stimulus for eliciting or maintaining such behavior. Iwata et al. (1982) developed a method to systematically manipulate environmental stimuli to clarify which are relevant in regard to self-injurious behavior. With this approach, it has been shown that some children will stop their self-injury when they receive adult attention, others may reduce the frequency of this behavior when the behavior is ignored, and still others may stop when they are provided environmental stimulation or given functional communication training.

Another approach to diminishing undesirable behavior is to facilitate its replacement with new behaviors. To do so, appropriate reinforcers must be identified. In those instances when social attention is not adequate, other primary reinforcers include tangibles such as food and drink, music, and toys. When no specific reinforcer preference is identified, the "Premack principle" (Premack 1959) can be applied through observing what the child does spontaneously when left alone and using those preferred behaviors as reinforcers. Regardless of the reinforcer that is identified, the desired behavior may need to be built up through shaping and prompting procedures, which are followed by gradual fading out of the schedule of reinforcement until new patterns of behavior are established. A common procedure in establishing new behaviors is the technique of differential reinforcement of appropriate behavior.

A third approach is to apply techniques for decreasing undesirable behavior. In this approach, extinction procedures are used that involve removing contingent rewards. If the functional analysis of behavior indicates that social attention seems to be the reward, ignoring the behavior is the first step. However, if the functional analysis shows that the reward was that the child would be allowed to stop the task when he or she cried or screamed, encouragement to continue the task would be tried. In other instances, nonaversive punishment techniques are necessary. These techniques may be indicated when 1) the consequences of the behavior are too harmful to allow even the temporary rise in frequency that might occur during extinction, as in the case of severe self-injurious behavior; 2) a rapid result is necessary; 3) control of the rewarding consequence is not possible, a situation that may occur in an institutional setting; or 4) other methods have not been successful.

The nonaversive punishment techniques include time-out procedures and response-cost procedures. The first of these refers to time out from positive reinforcement, which is carried out by removal from a socially stimulating environment (e.g., to a quiet room). In working with mentally retarded persons, the time-out period must be short—generally less than 15 minutes—and other desired behaviors must continue to be rewarded. Response cost refers to the removal of known rewards, such as tokens or stars, that have been successfully used for reinforcement. Their removal establishes a response cost for the inappropriate behavior. In using response-cost procedures, the reward system must be in place to begin with. Once established, it may be changed by taking away the rewards, which can result in considerable protest from the child.

Aversive punishment techniques, such as introducing unpleasant tastes and smells, facial screening, physical restraint, water sprays, and mild electric shock (Foxx et al. 1986), have been used in the past. These procedures are questionable ethically and may lead to abuse of the mentally retarded person. Such abuse is most likely if skilled personnel to provide alternative psychological management are lacking or when caregivers become exhausted and perhaps angry because of repeated destructive acts or aggression toward them.

In the United States, some states, such as Massachusetts and Michigan, ban the use of aversive procedures, and alternatives must be established (Nolley et al. 1982). Yet some evidence shows that in selected cases less severe aversive methods may have some benefit if properly applied (Lennox et al. 1988). Therefore, regulation of aversive techniques rather than their complete banning has been recommended (Matson and Taras 1989). The use of such procedures was the subject of a National Institutes of Health (1990) consensus conference.

A fourth approach to diminishing undesirable behavior is to combine the various behavioral procedures into more complex treatment packages. With higher-functioning children and adults, these procedures may be used with self-instruction to facilitate generalization to other settings. All of these behavior management techniques are time-consuming; therefore, there has been increasing interest in teaching caregivers and parents to be co-therapists in the use of these techniques (Baker et al. 1991). Caregiver and parent training may be carried out either individually or in group settings.

Stereotypic behaviors, psychophysiological symptoms, and noncompliance seem to be most responsive to behavioral treatment (65%–75% success rate); destructive behaviors are often responsive (45%–65% success rate), and inappropriate social interactions are the least responsive (35%–40% success rate) (Bregman and Harris 1995). Positive behavioral interventions appear to be most efficacious for the treatment of affective symptoms (e.g., depression, anxiety) and social skills deficits, whereas punishment procedures (e.g., disapproval, extinction, time-out, overcorrection) seem to be most efficacious for destructive behaviors (e.g., aggression, self-injurious behavior). Systematic research is needed to identify the specific behavioral interventions that are most effective for particular maladaptive behaviors. Most behavioral studies use single-case designs with small sample sizes and rarely report clinical variables that might affect treatment outcome (e.g., psychosocial circumstances, clinical psychiatric syndromes and disorders, family history). Data on these clinical variables are needed to properly assess future behavioral treatments.

Pharmacotherapy

Medication may be an important adjunct or a specific indicated treatment in working with mentally retarded persons (Baumeister et al. 1993). However, medication use is not the first and is not the only treatment for behavior that is difficult to manage. Drug treatment begins following careful assessment of all co-occurring conditions that may have an effect on behavior. Before beginning drug treatment, physical health and recent changes in everyday routines are considered, and appropriate environmental and psychosocial adjustments are made. Moreover, in working with mentally retarded persons, it is particularly important to do a baseline assessment—which may include the use of blood testing, baseline studies such as an electrocardiogram, and a specific review of possible side effects—before beginning drug treatment. Agreement is needed before beginning medication with regard to the assessment criteria for improvement, and continuous review is required regarding termination of drug treatment. Consultation is important in the use of medications, and physicians who are unfamiliar with working with mentally retarded persons should consider obtaining consultation because the behavioral difficulties are frequently complex. Consent for medication treatment must always be obtained. Careful follow-up for side effects is especially important because many mentally retarded persons may not be able to provide self-report of drug-related symptoms. Sprague and Werry (1971) outlined minimum design requirements for drug research for developmental disabilities. Unfortunately, few studies have followed all of these guidelines.

In 1998, an international consensus conference was held to establish recommendations for the use of psychotropic medications in mentally retarded persons with psychiatric disorders (Reiss and Aman 1998). *The International Consensus Handbook: Psychotropic Medications and Developmental Disabilities* that resulted from this meeting should be consulted for guidelines in the use of psychoactive medications. The previous year, the Health Care Financing Administration (1997) published *Psychopharmacological Medications—Safety Precautions for Persons With Developmental Disabilities*. This manual is for surveyors who access intermediate-care facilities (to determine whether a facility is in compliance with regulations for mentally retarded persons). These guidelines were written with input from the Committee on Mental Retardation and Developmental Disabilities of the American Psychiatric Association and may be helpful to consultants.

Aman and Singh (1991) suggested seven issues that should be considered that are pertinent to psychopharmacological studies with developmental disorders: 1) dual diagnoses, 2) dosage effects, 3) the limited number of studies examining learning, 4) predictors of drug response, 5) the historic emphasis on institutional settings, 6) the paucity of follow-up studies, and 7) physiological risk.

Antipsychotics

Spreat et al. (1997) conducted a population-based study to determine the use of psychoactive medications in one state—Oklahoma. The authors found that 22% of the adults with mental retardation were receiving antipsychotic medications. Although this represents a decrease in antipsychotic medication use from previous years, the continuing high prevalence of antipsychotic use indicates the importance of continued careful surveillance of medication use.

The most commonly prescribed medications in the past were haloperidol, chlorpromazine, and thioridazine. However, these medications are being replaced with the atypical antipsychotics such as risperidone (McDougle et al. 1997, 1998). Antipsychotic medications have been used in mentally retarded persons not only for psychotic symptoms but also in the management of aggression and hyperactivity, particularly in autistic mentally retarded persons. This group of medications has been used successfully to treat stereotypies. In one study, a subgroup of patients with marked stereotypy (Aman et al. 1989) showed significant improvement. Antipsychotics also may be used as part of emergency pharmacotherapy in the management of acute outbursts of violence. In using antipsychotics, it is important to consider that the drug doses of these medications that are used to treat disruptive behavior might suppress some adaptive behaviors or may reduce alertness. The effect on learning is a particular concern, so doses must be monitored carefully. Formal tests of learning and laboratory tests of attention may be used to clarify whether a drug is leading to impaired function. However, when medication is used appropriately, cognitive ability may be improved and task performance enhanced as severe behavioral difficulties are reduced.

Disorders of impulse control (e.g., self-injurious behaviors, sterotyped behaviors, and aggression) may be treated with antipsychotics (Baumeister et al. 1998). Self-injurious behavior may be suppressed by antipsychotic treatment. Risperidone was used to treat mentally retarded individuals with persistent behavioral disturbance in a double-blind, placebo-controlled crossover trial (Vanden Borre et al. 1993). Risperidone was compared with placebo and administered as an add-on treatment to existing medication in 30 mentally retarded individuals. Risperidone was found to be superior to placebo on ratings from the Aberrant Behavior Checklist and the Clinical Global Impression Checklist. No differences were found between risperidone and placebo on the Extrapyramidal Symptom Rating Scale. Sedation and drowsiness were the most frequently reported drug effects. The authors recommended continuing assessment of the effects of risperidone, both as add-on therapy and as a single treatment. McDougle et al. (1997, 1998) showed the effectiveness of risperidone in an open case study with children and adolescents (1997) and in a control study of adults (1998) with a diagnosis of pervasive developmental disorders.

All of the recognized side effects of antipsychotics may occur in persons with mental retardation. The side effect causing the most concern is tardive dyskinesia (Gualtieri et al. 1984; Kane 1991). The typical prevalence rate of tardive dyskinesia in persons with mental retardation exposed to antipsychotics has been reported to be as high as 30% (Kalachnik 1984). Although older persons may be at greater risk for these symptoms, children and adolescents also may develop tardive dyskinesia. Paulson et al. (1975) found that 20% of 11- to 16-year-olds with mental retardation were symptomatic. To date, there is no clear evidence of increased risk for tardive dyskinesia in persons with mental retardation, organic brain syndromes, or other specific diagnoses (Golden 1988). A possible exception may be phenylketonuria (M. A. Richardson et al. 1986). Female sex confers an increased risk for tardive dyskinesia, as does total lifetime dose (American Psychiatric Association 1991). Campbell et al. (1997) used haloperidol to reduce anger, lack of cooperation, hyperactivity, and maladaptive behavior in autistic persons. They reported that 40 of 118 (33.9%) of those treated with haloperidol over 15 years developed drug-related dyskinesias, most at the time of drug withdrawal.

Lithium

Because lithium has been used to treat aggression associated with labile mood in the general adult population, lithium trials in adults with mental retardation who were showing aggressive behavior have been reported (Craft et al. 1987; Spreat et al. 1989; Tyrer et al. 1984). Improvement has been reported in about two-thirds of very carefully selected patients. The authors found that blood levels need to be at the higher end of the therapeutic range (0.7–1.0 mmol/L), and treatment for 6–8 weeks was necessary before evident response was seen in these studies. However, adequate controlled trials of lithium in children with mental retardation and aggression have not been done. It should be noted that mixed results were obtained when aggressive children without mental retardation were treated with lithium. Two studies found statistical improvement (Campbell et al. 1984; Carlson et al. 1992); however, the improvement was not clinically effective enough to continue the drug. Greenhill et al. (1973) found that only two of nine children with hyperactivity and aggression improved. For bipolar disorder, lithium may be effective but not well tolerated because of associated cognitive dulling (Poindexter et al. 1998).

Stimulants

The psychostimulant drugs dextroamphetamine and methylphenidate are generally considered the drugs of choice for ADHD in children of normal intelligence. In children with ADHD, these medications improve attention span, improve impulsivity, reduce activity level, increase behavioral compliance, improve cooperativeness with peers, and improve focus on learning tasks. Stimulants may be safe and effective for hyperactive children with mild to moderate mental retardation (Aman et al. 1991a, 1991b; Gadow 1985, 1992; Handen et al. 1990; Payton et al. 1989). Side effects must be monitored carefully and may be idiosyncratic in mentally retarded persons (Handen et al. 1991, 1994, 1997).

Handen et al. (1999) carried out a double-blind, placebo-controlled study of the safety and efficacy of methylphenidate in 11 preschool children (ages 4.0–5.1 years) with ADHD and developmental disability; 8 of 11 were responders, indicating that the response rate was similar to that of school-age children with mental retardation. However, 5 of 11 had adverse side effects of social withdrawal, especially with the higher dose used (0.6 mg/kg).

Aman et al. (1991a) evaluated methylphenidate in children with mental retardation with a range of IQs from untestable to 90. Significant clinical improvement was noted in some children, but primarily those with higher cognitive function (IQ $\geq$ 46). These findings suggest that a relation exists between the effectiveness of stimulants and cognitive level. However, case selection is a major determinant of effectiveness, and profound and severely retarded persons who are carefully selected may respond to stimulants alone or in combination with other medications, such as clonidine.

Anticonvulsants

Anticonvulsant drugs may be helpful in the treatment of mood disorders and behavioral management in mentally retarded individuals. First-line medications for the treatment of bipolar disorder, particularly for rapid-cycling mood disorders, include carbamazepine and valproic acid (Poindexter et al. 1998). Moreover, these medications may have effects on behavior and cognition when prescribed specifically for control of seizures. In addition, some of the anticonvulsants may cause toxic reactions that mimic neurological disease, which may be difficult to recognize in severely and profoundly retarded individuals. The newer anticonvulsants such as gabapentin and lamotrigine might be considered, but only after the effectiveness of these medications is documented for bipolar disorder in non–mentally retarded persons. Valproic acid may be helpful in mentally retarded individuals with mood lability, aggression, and self-injurious behavior. Ruedrich and colleagues (1999) treated 28 adults ages 20–63 years with divalproex sodium and found improvement in behavior in 70%. There were co-occurring diagnoses of pervasive developmental disorder, organic mood disorder, and psychotic disorders.

Antidepressants

Selective Serotonin Reuptake Inhibitors

The selective serotonin reuptake inhibitors are increasingly used for mood disorders because of their low side-effect profile (Sovner et al. 1998). In an open trial, Masi et al. (1997) treated depression and intellectual disability in seven adolescents with paroxetine, a serotonin reuptake inhibitor, and reported a good response with mild side effects. Cook et al. (1992) reported on the use of fluoxetine in the treatment of autistic disorder and mental retardation in children and adults.

Davanzo et al. (1998) conducted an open, prospective assessment of the treatment of severe aggression and self-injurious behavior with paroxetine in 15 institutionalized persons with mental retardation. Frequency and severity of aggression and self-injurious behavior were charted by trained staff members. Only aggression severity, but not self-injury, was reduced over the entire 4-month follow-up period.

Tricyclic Antidepressants

Although tricyclic antidepressants are effective, they are used less often because of potential cardiac and cognitive effects. However, Harris (1988) evaluated the effects of amitriptyline in the treatment of depression in Down syndrome and reported positive outcome in five individuals, all of whom showed increased appetite, increased interest in activities, improved sleep, and reduction in separation anxiety. Thuppal and Fink (1999) reported that electroconvulsive therapy can be effective in mentally retarded adults but only in those whose depression did not respond to antidepressant medication. However, its use is controversial, and it is rarely used; there are difficulties with consent and there may be a perceived concern about abuse (Szymanski and King 1999).

Conclusions

Considerable progress is being made in the psychopharmacological treatment of behavioral and psychiatric disorders in persons with mental retardation. More rigorous application of appropriate experimental design in the evaluation of drug efficacy is now more common. Psychopharmacological research leads to new hypotheses, and as new drugs become available for treatment, these hypotheses are being explored. When successfully applied, new research may lead to less polypharmacy and a more rational approach to drug treatment.

References

Aman MG: Assessing psychopathology and behavior problems in persons with mental retardation: a review of available instruments (DHHS Publ No ADM-91-1712). Rockville, MD, U.S. Department of Health and Human Services, 1991a

Aman MG: Review and evaluation of instruments for assessing emotional and behavioural disorders. Australia and New Zealand Journal of Developmental Disabilities 17:127–145, 1991b

Aman MG, Singh NN: Patterns of drug use, methodological considerations, measurement techniques, and future trends, in Psychopharmacology and the Developmental Disabilities. Edited by Aman MG, Singh NN. New York, Springer-Verlag, 1988

Aman MG, Singh NN: Pharmacological intervention, in Handbook of Mental Retardation, 2nd Edition. Edited by Matson JL, Mulick JA. New York, Pergamon, 1991, pp 347–372

Aman MG, Teehan CJ, White AJ, et al: Haloperidol treatment with chronically medicated residents: dose effects on clinical behavior and reinforcement contingencies. Am J Ment Retard 93:452–460, 1989

Aman MG, Marks RE, Turbott SH, et al: Clinical effects of methylphenidate and thioridazine in intellectually subaverage children. J Am Acad Child Adolesc Psychiatry 30:246–256, 1991a

Aman MG, Marks RE, Turbott SH, et al: Methylphenidate and thioridazine in the treatment of intellectually subaverage children: effects on cognitive-motor performance. J Am Acad Child Adolesc Psychiatry 30:816–824, 1991b

American Association on Mental Retardation: Mental Retardation: Definition, Classification, and Systems of Support, Special 9th Edition. Washington, DC, American Association on Mental Retardation, 1992

American Psychiatric Association: Diagnostic and Statistical Manual of Mental Disorders, 3rd Edition. Washington, DC, American Psychiatric Association, 1980

American Psychiatric Association: Diagnostic and Statistical Manual of Mental Disorders, 3rd Edition, Revised. Washington, DC, American Psychiatric Association, 1987

American Psychiatric Association: Tardive Dyskinesia: A Task Force Report of the American Psychiatric Association. Washington, DC, American Psychiatric Press, 1991

American Psychiatric Association: Diagnostic and Statistical Manual of Mental Disorders, 4th Edition. Washington, DC, American Psychiatric Association, 1994

American Psychiatric Association: Diagnostic and Statistical Manual of Mental Disorders, 4th Edition, Text Revision. Washington, DC, American Psychiatric Association, 2000

Baker BL, Landen SJ, Kashima KJ: Effects of parent training on families of children with mental retardation: increased burden or generalized benefit? Am J Ment Retard 96:127–136, 1991

Baumeister AA, Todd ME, Sevin JA: Efficacy and specificity of pharmacological therapies for behavioral disorders in persons with mental retardation. Clin Neuropharmacol 16:271–294, 1993

Baumeister AA, Sevin JA, King BH: Neuroleptics, in Psychotropic Medication and Developmental Disabilities: The International Consensus Handbook. Edited by Reiss S, Aman MG. Columbus, OH, The Ohio State University Nisonger Center for Mental Retardation and Developmental Disabilities, 1998, pp 133–150

Benson B, Lamar D: Suicidal tendencies of mentally retarded adults in community settings. Australia and New Zealand Journal of Developmental Disabilities 14:49–54, 1988

Bouras N, Drummond C: Behavior and psychiatric disorders of people with mental handicaps living in the community. J Intellect Disabil Res 36:349–357, 1992

Bregman JD: Current developments in the understanding of mental retardation, part II: psychopathology. J Am Acad Child Adolesc Psychiatry 30:861–872, 1991

Bregman JD, Harris J: Mental retardation, in Comprehensive Textbook of Psychiatry, 6th Edition. Edited by Kaplan E, Sadock BJ. Baltimore, MD, Williams & Wilkins, 1995, pp 2207–2241

Campbell M, Small AM, Green WH, et al: Behavioral efficacy of haloperidol and lithium carbonate—a comparison in hospitalized aggressive children with conduct disorder. Arch Gen Psychiatry 41:650–656, 1984

Campbell M, Armenteros JL, Malone RP, et al: Neuroleptic-related dyskinesias in autistic children: a prospective, longitudinal study. J Am Acad Child Adolesc Psychiatry 36:835–843, 1997

Carlson GA, Rapport MD, Pataki CS, et al: Lithium in hospitalized children at 4 and 8 weeks: mood, behavior and cognitive effects. J Child Psychol Psychiatry 33:411–425, 1992

Carr EG, Durand VM: Reducing behavior problems through functional communication training. J Appl Behav Anal 18:111–126, 1985

Chess S: Psychiatric treatment of the mentally retarded child with behavior problems. Am J Orthopsychiatry 32:863–869, 1962

Clarke AM, Clarke DB, Berg JM: Mental Deficiency: The Changing Outlook, 4th Edition. New York, Free Press, 1985

Cook EH Jr, Rowlett R, Jaselskis C, et al: Fluoxetine treatment of children and adults with autistic disorder and mental retardation. J Am Acad Child Adolesc Psychiatry 31:739–745, 1992

Craft M, Ismail IA, Krishnamurti D, et al: Lithium in the treatment of aggression in mentally handicapped patients: a double-blind trial. Br J Psychiatry 150:685–689, 1987

Dana L: Personality disorder in persons with mental retardation: assessment and diagnosis, in Mental Health Aspects of Mental Retardation: Progress in Assessment and Treatment. Edited by Reiss S, Aman MG. New York, Lexington Books, 1993, pp 130–140

Davanzo PA, Belin TR, Widawski MH, et al: Paroxetine treatment of aggression and self-injury in persons with mental retardation. Am J Ment Retard 102:427–437, 1998

Dudley JR, Ahlrim-Delzell L, Calhoun ML: Diverse diagnostic and behavioral patterns amongst people with a dual diagnosis. J Intellect Disabil Res 43:70–79, 1999

Edgerton RB: The Cloak of Competence, Revised and Updated. Berkeley, University of California Press, 1993, pp 181–195

Ellis A, Bernard ME: Rational-Emotive Approaches to the Problems of Childhood. New York, Plenum, 1983

Feinstein CB: Psychotherapeutic approaches for mentally retarded children, adolescents, and their family, in Mental Retardation and Psychotherapy: The New Definitions, Assessment, and Treatment. Edited by Szymanski L, Feinstein C, Harris J. Presented at the Institute, American Academy of Child and Adolescent Psychiatry, San Antonio, TX, October 1993, pp 1–10

Feinstein CB, Reiss AL: Psychiatric disorder in mentally retarded children and adolescents: the challenges of meaningful diagnosis. Child Adolesc Psychiatr Clin N Am 5:827–852, 1996

Foxx RM, McMorrow MJ, Bittle RG, et al: The successful treatment of a dually diagnosed deaf man's aggression with a programme that included contingent electric shock. Behavior Therapy 17:170–186, 1986

Gadow KD: Prevalence and efficacy of stimulant drug use with mentally retarded children and youth. Psychopharmacol Bull 21:291–303, 1985

Gadow KD: Pediatric psychopharmacotherapy: a review of recent research. J Child Psychol Psychiatry 33:153–195, 1992

Gillberg C, Persson E, Grufman M, et al: Psychiatric disorders in mildly and severely mentally retarded urban children and adolescents: epidemiological aspects. Br J Psychiatry 149:68–74, 1986

Glue P: Rapid cycling affective disorders in the mentally retarded. Biol Psychiatry 26:250–256, 1989

Golden GS: Tardive dyskinesia and developmental disabilities, in Psychopharmacology of the Developmental Disabilities. Edited by Aman MG, Singh NN. New York, Springer-Verlag, 1988, pp 198–216

Greenhill LL, Reider RO, Wender PH, et al: Lithium carbonate in the treatment of hyperactive children. Arch Gen Psychiatry 28:636–640, 1973

Griffin JC, Ricketts RW, Williams DE, et al: A community survey of self-injurious behavior among developmentally disabled children and adolescents. Hospital and Community Psychiatry 38:959–963, 1987

Grossman HJ: Manual on Terminology and Classification in Mental Retardation, Revised Edition. Washington, DC, American Association on Mental Deficiency, 1983

Gualtieri CT, Quade D, Hicks RE, et al: Tardive dyskinesia and other clinical consequences of neuroleptic treatment in children and adolescents. Am J Psychiatry 141:20–23, 1984

Handen BL, Breaux AM, Gosling A, et al: Efficacy of methylphenidate among mentally retarded children with attention deficit hyperactivity disorder. Pediatrics 86:922–930, 1990

Handen BL, Feldman H, Gosling A, et al: Adverse side effect of methylphenidate among mentally retarded children with ADHD. J Am Acad Child Adolesc Psychiatry 30:241–245, 1991

Handen BL, Janosky J, McAuliffe S, et al: Prediction of response to methylphenidate among children with ADHD and mental retardation. J Am Acad Child Adolesc Psychiatry. 33:1185–1193, 1994

Handen BL, Janosky J, McAuliffe S: Long term follow-up of children with mental retardation/borderline intellectual functioning and ADHD. J Abnorm Child Psychol 25:287–295, 1997

Handen BL, Feldman HM, Lurier A, et al: Efficacy of methylphenidate among preschool children with developmental disabilities and ADHD. J Am Acad Child Adolesc Psychiatry 38:805–812, 1999

Harris J: Psychological adaptation and psychiatric disorders in adolescents and young adults with Down syndrome, in The Young Person With Down Syndrome: Transition From Adolescence to Adulthood. Edited by Pueschel S. Baltimore, MD, Paul H Brookes, 1988

Harris J: Neurobiological factors in self-injurious behavior, in Self-Injurious Behavior: Analysis, Assessment and Treatment. Edited by Luiselli JK, Matson JL, Singh NN. New York, Springer-Verlag, 1992, pp 59–92

Harris J: Assessment, Diagnosis, and Treatment of Developmental Disorders. New York, Oxford University Press, 1998

Harris JC, Tune LE, Allen M, et al: Management of akathisia in a severely retarded adolescent male with help of an anticholinergic drug assay (letter). Lancet 2(8243):414, 1981

Health Care Financing Administration: Psychopharmacological Medications—Safety Precautions for Persons With Developmental Disabilities. Washington, DC, Health Care Financing Administration, 1997

Holmes J: Attachment theory: a biological basis for psychotherapy? Br J Psychiatry 163:430–438, 1993

Hurley AD: Individual psychotherapy with mentally retarded individuals: a review and call for research. Res Dev Disabil 10:261–275, 1989

Hurley AD, Hurley FJ: Counseling and psychotherapy with mentally retarded clients, I: the initial interview. Psychiatric Aspects of Mental Retardation Reviews 5:22–26, 1986

Hurley AD, Hurley FJ: Counseling and psychotherapy with mentally retarded clients, II: establishing a relationship. Psychiatric Aspects of Mental Retardation Reviews 6:15, 1987

Iwata DA, Dorsey MF, Slifer KJ, et al: Toward a functional analysis of self-injury. Analysis and Intervention in Developmental Disabilities 3:1–20, 1982

Jan JE, Abroms IF, Freeman RD, et al: Rapid cycling in severely multidisabled children: a form of bipolar disorder? Pediatr Neurol 10:30–39, 1994

Jansen PE: Basic principles of behavior therapy with retarded persons, in Emotional Disorders of Mentally Retarded Persons. Edited by Szymanski LS, Tanguay PE. Baltimore, MD, University Park Press, 1980, pp 223–240

Kalachnik JE: Tardive dyskinesia and the mentally retarded: a review, in Mental Retardation and Developmental Disabilities, Vol 2. Edited by Breuning SE, Matson JL, Barrett R. Greenwich, CT, JAI Press, 1984, pp 329–356

Kane JM: Tardive Dyskinesia: A Task Force Report of the American Psychiatric Association. Washington, DC, American Psychiatric Press, 1991

Kanner L: Parents' feelings about retarded children. American Journal of Mental Deficiency 57:375–383, 1953

Kazuo N, Leland H, Lambert N: AAMR Adaptive Behavior Scale—Residential and Community, 2nd Edition. Austin, TX, Pro-Ed, 1993

Lambert N, Kazuo N, Leland H: AAMR Adaptive Behavior Scale—School, 2nd Edition. Austin, TX, Pro-Ed, 1993

Leland H, Smith DE: Play Therapy With Mentally Subnormal Children. New York, Grune & Stratton, 1965

Lennox DB, Miltenberger RG, Spengler P, et al: Decelerative treatment practices with persons who have mental retardation: a review of five years of the literature. Am J Ment Retard 92:492–501, 1988

Levitas A, Gilson S: Transference, countertransference, and resistance. National Association for the Dually Diagnosed Newsletter 1:2–7, 1987

Lund J: The prevalence of psychiatric morbidity in mentally retarded adults. Acta Psychiatr Scand 72:563–570, 1985

Masi G, Marcheschi M, Pfanner P: Paroxetine in depressed adolescents with intellectual disability. J Intellect Disabil Res 41:268–272, 1997

Masi G, Mucci M, Favilla L, et al: Dysthymic disorder in adolescents with intellectual disability. J Intellect Disabil Res 43:80–87, 1999

Matson JL: The PIMRA Manual. Orlando Park, IL, International Diagnostic Systems, 1988

Matson JL, Taras ME: A year review of punishment and alternative methods to treat problem behaviors in developmentally delayed persons. Res Dev Disabil 10:85–104, 1989

McDougle CJ, Holmes JP, Bronson MK, et al: Risperidone treatment of children and adolescents with PDD: a prospective open case study. J Am Acad Child Adolesc Psychiatry 36:685–693, 1997

McDougle CJ, Holmes JP, Carlson DC, et al: A double-blind, placebo-controlled study of risperidone in adults with autistic disorder and other pervasive developmental disorders. Arch Gen Psychiatry 55:633–641, 1998

Menolascino FJ: Mental illness in the mentally retarded: diagnostic and treatment issues, in Mental Retardation and Mental Health: Classification, Diagnosis, Treatment, Services. Edited by Stark JA, Menolascino FJ, Albarelli MH, et al. New York, Springer-Verlag, 1988, pp 109–123

Menolascino FJ, Wilson J, Golden C, et al: Medication and treatment of schizophrenia in persons with mental retardation. Ment Retard 24:277–283, 1986

Moss S, Patel P, Prosser H, et al: Psychiatric morbidity in older people with moderate and severe learning disability, I: development and reliability of the patient interview (PAS-ADD). Br J Psychiatry 163:471–480, 1993

Moss SC, Emerson E, Bouras N, et al: Mental disorders and problematic behaviors in people with intellectual disability: future directions for research. J Intellect Disabil Res 41:440–447, 1997

National Institutes of Health: Consensus Conference on Treatment of Destructive Behaviors in Persons With Developmental Disabilities. Washington, DC, U.S. Government Printing Office, 1990

Nolley D, Butterfield B, Fleming A, et al: Non-aversive treatment of severe self-injurious behavior: multiple replications with DRO and DRI, in Life-Threatening Behavior. Edited by Hollis JH, Meyers CE. Washington, DC, American Association on Mental Deficiency, 1982

O'Hara J: Advances in psychotherapy in leaning disability. Current Opinion in Psychiatry 12:555–559, 1999

Paulson GW, Rizvi CA, Crane GE: Tardive dyskinesia as a possible sequel of long-term therapy with phenothiazines. Clin Pediatr 14:953–955, 1975

Payton JB, Burkhart JE, Hersen M, et al: Treatment of ADDH in mentally retarded children: a preliminary study. J Am Acad Child Adolesc Psychiatry 28:761–767, 1989

Pearson DA, Aman MG: Ratings of hyperactivity and developmental indices: should clinicians correct for developmental level? J Autism Dev Disord 24:395–411, 1994

Poindexter AR, Cain N, Clarke DJ, et al: Mood stabilizers, in Psychotropic Medication and Developmental Disabilities: The International Consensus Handbook. Edited by Reiss S, Aman MG. Columbus, OH, The Ohio State University Nisonger Center for Mental Retardation and Developmental Disabilities, 1998, pp 215–246

Premack D: Towards empirical behaviour laws, I: positive reinforcement. Psychol Rev 66:219–233, 1959

Reid AH: The Psychiatry of Mental Handicap. Boston, MA, Blackwell Scientific, 1982

Reid AH: Schizophrenia in mental retardation: clinical features. Res Dev Disabil 10:241–249, 1989

Reid AH, Ballenger BR: Personality disorder in mental handicap. Psychol Med 17:983–987, 1987

Reiss S: Test Manual for the Reiss Screen for Maladaptive Behavior. Orland Park, IL, International Diagnostic Systems, 1988

Reiss S: Prevalence of dual diagnosis in community-based day programs in the Chicago metropolitan area. Am J Ment Retard 94:578–585, 1990

Reiss S: Handbook of Challenging Behavior: Mental Health Aspects of Mental Retardation. Worthington, OH, IDS Publishing, 1994

Reiss S, Aman MG (eds): The International Consensus Handbook: Psychotropic Medications and Developmental Disabilities. Columbus, OH, The Ohio State University Nisonger Center for Mental Retardation and Developmental Disabilities, 1998

Reiss S, Benson BA: Awareness of negative social conditions among mentally retarded, emotionally disturbed outpatients. Am J Psychiatry 141:88–90, 1984

Reiss S, Valenti-Hein D: Reiss Scales for Children's Dual Diagnosis: Test Manual. Orland Park, IL, International Diagnostic Systems, 1990

Reiss S, Valenti-Hein D: Development of a psychopathology rating scale in children with mental retardation. J Consult Clin Psychol 62:28–33, 1994

Reiss S, Levitan GW, Szysko J: Emotional disturbance and mental retardation: diagnostic overshadowing. American Journal of Mental Deficiency 86:567–574, 1982

Richardson MA, Haugland G, Pass R, et al: The prevalence of tardive dyskinesia in a mentally retarded population. Psychopharmacol Bull 22:243–249, 1986

Richardson SA, Koller H, Katz M: Continuities and change in behavior disturbance: a follow-up study of mildly retarded young people. Am J Psychiatry 55:220–229, 1985

Richmond JB: The family and the handicapped child. Clinical Proceedings of the Children's Hospital National Medical Center 8:156–164, 1972

Robertson I, Richardson AM, Youngson SC: Social skills training with mentally handicapped people: a review. Br J Clin Psychol 23:241–264, 1984

Ruedrich S, Swales TP, Fossaceca C, et al: Effect of divalproex sodium on aggression and self-injurious behavior in adults with intellectual disability: a retrospective review. J Intellect Disabil Res 43: 105–111, 1999

Rutter M: Psychiatric disorder and intellectual impairment in childhood, in Health, Education and Behaviour. London, Spastics International Medical Publications, 1970

Santosh PJ, Baird G: Psychopharmacology in children and adults with intellectual disability. Lancet 354: 233–242, 1999

Sovner R, Pary RJ: Affective disorders in developmentally disabled persons, in Psychopathology in the Mentally Retarded, 2nd Edition. Edited by Matson JL, Barrett RP. Needham Heights, MA, Allyn & Bacon, 1993, pp 87–147

Sovner R, Pary RJ, Dosen A, et al: Antidepressant drugs, in Psychotropic Medication and Developmental Disabilities: The International Consensus Handbook. Edited by Reiss S, Aman MG. Columbus, OH, The Ohio State University Nisonger Center for Mental Retardation and Developmental Disabilities, 1998, pp 179–200

Sparrow SS, Balla DA, Cicchetti DV: Vineland Adaptive Behavior Scales, Interview Edition. Expanded Form Manual. Circle Pines, MN, American Guidance Service, 1984

Sprague RL, Werry JS: Methodology of psychopharmacological studies with the retarded, in International Review of Research in Mental Retardation, Vol 5. Edited by Ellis NR. New York, Academic Press, 1971, pp 147–210

Spreat S, Behar D, Reneski B, et al: Lithium carbonate for aggression in mentally retarded persons. Compr Psychiatry 30:505–511, 1989

Spreat S, Conroy J, Jones JC: Use of psychotropic medication in Oklahoma: a statewide survey. Am J Ment Retard 102:80–85, 1997

State M, King BH, Dykens E: Mental retardation: a review of the past 10 years, part II. J Am Acad Child Adolesc Psychiatry 36:1664–1671, 1997

Stavrakaki C, Klein J: Psychotherapies with the mentally retarded. Psychiatr Clin North Am 9:733–743, 1986

Sturmey P: Suicidal threats and behavior in a person with developmental disabilities: effective psychiatric monitoring based on a functional assessment. Behavioral Interventions 9:235–245, 1994

Szymanski LS: Individual psychotherapy with retarded persons, in Emotional Disorders of Mentally Retarded Persons. Edited by Szymanski LS, Tanguay PE. Baltimore, MD, University Park Press, 1980

Szymanski LS, King BH: Practice parameters for the assessment and treatment of children, adolescents, and adults with mental retardation and comorbid mental disorders. American Academy of Child and Adolescent Psychiatry Working Group on Quality Issues. J Am Acad Child Adolesc Psychiatry 38 (12 suppl):5S–31S, 1999

Szymanski LS, Rosefsky QB: Group psychotherapy with retarded persons, in Emotional Disorders of Mentally Retarded Persons: Assessment, Treatment, and Consultation. Edited by Szymanski LS, Tanguay PE. Baltimore, MD, University Park Press, 1980, pp 173–194

Thuppal M, Fink M: Electroconvulsive therapy and mental retardation. J ECT 15:140–149, 1999

Tyrer SP, Walsh A, Edwards DE, et al: Factors associated with a good response to lithium in aggressive mentally handicapped subjects. Prog Neuropsychopharmacol Biol Psychiatry 8:751–755, 1984

Vanden Borre R, Vermote R, Buttiens M, et al: Risperidone as add-on therapy in behavioural disturbances in mental retardation: a double-blind placebo-controlled cross-over study. Acta Psychiatr Scand 87:167–171, 1993

Walters AS, Barret RP, Knapp LG, et al: Suicidal behavior in children and adolescents with mental retardation. Res Dev Disabil 16:85–96, 1995

Werry JS, Wollersheim JP: Behavior therapy with children and adolescents: a twenty-year overview. J Am Acad Child Adolesc Psychiatry 28:1–18, 1989

Whitman BY, Accardo PJ: When a Parent Is Mentally Retarded. Baltimore, MD, Paul H Brookes, 1990

Wing L, Gould J: Severe impairments of social interaction and associated abnormalities in children: epidemiology and classification. J Autism Dev Disord 9:11–29, 1979

Wolfensberger W: The Principle of Normalization in Human Services. Toronto, Ontario, National Institute on Mental Retardation, 1972

World Health Organization: The ICD-10 Classification of Mental and Behavioural Disorders: Clinical Descriptions and Diagnostic Guidelines. Geneva, Switzerland, World Health Organization, 1992

Zigler E: Familial mental retardation: a continuing dilemma. Science 155:292–298, 1967

Zigler E, Burack JA: Personality development and the dually diagnosed person. Res Dev Disabil 10:225–240, 1989

5

Learning Disorders

Arlene R. Young, Ph.D.
Joseph H. Beitchman, M.D.

What Are Learning Disorders?

Learning disorders (LDs) are often referred to as *learning disabilities,* which include a broad array of symptoms and possible causes. The definition of learning disabilities adopted into federal law in the United States in the Education for All Handicapped Children Act (1976; Public Law 94-142) was as follows:

> Specific learning disabilities means a disorder in one or more of the basic psychological processes involved in understanding or using language, spoken or written, which may manifest itself in an imperfect ability to listen, think, speak, read, write, spell, or to do mathematical calculations. The term includes such conditions as perceptual handicaps, brain injury, minimal brain dysfunction, dyslexia, and developmental aphasia. The term does not include children who have learning problems which are primarily the result of visual, hearing, or motor handicaps, of mental retardation, of emotional disturbance, or of environmental, cultural, or economic disadvantage. (Federal Register, August 1977, p. 65083)

The most widely applied criteria for LDs are likely those of DSM-IV (American Psychiatric Association 1994), which includes LDs in the section titled "Disorders Usually First Diagnosed in Infancy, Childhood, or Adolescence" in recognition of the developmental nature of these disorders and the fact that they are typically first identified during formal schooling. DSM-IV includes three subtypes of LDs: reading disorder, mathematics disorder, and disorder of written expression. The diagnostic criteria require that achievement in a specific academic area, as measured by an individually administered standardized test, is substantially below that expected given the age, grade, and intellectual ability of the individual. A fourth subtype, learning disorder not otherwise specified, is used to reflect poor academic performance that cannot be attributed to any specific learning disorder. The diagnosis also requires that other factors that may be primary contributors to the learning problems (e.g., lack of educational opportunity, poor teaching, impaired vision or hearing, and mental retardation) be ruled out.

Public Law 94-142 and its more recent revisions, referred to as the Individuals With Disabilities Education Act (IDEA; 1990, 1997), require that all states provide "free and appropriate public education" to children with exceptionalities, including those with learning disability. Given that eligibility for special education and related services is typically contingent on a formal diagnosis of LD, the specific criteria for diagnosis and assessment procedures have important implications.

Subtypes of Learning Disorders

LDs have been subtyped on the basis of symptom patterns and underlying cognitive deficits into two broad categories: verbal and nonverbal (Johnson and Myklebust 1971). In a series of well-designed studies on LD subtyping, Rourke and associates (e.g., Rourke 1985; Rourke and Finlayson 1978; Rourke and Strang 1983) determined that verbal and nonverbal LD subtypes present with distinct patterns of academic, social, and emotional functioning. Although approximately 5% of the general school-aged population are considered to have LDs (U.S. Department of Education 1991), only 10% of the LD population (between 0.1% and 1.0% of the general population) are identified as having nonverbal LDs (Pennington 1991). Children with verbally based disorders (i.e., receptive and/or expressive language dysfunction) have particular difficulties in the areas of reading, spelling, and writing skills. In contrast, nonverbal LDs are associated with problems in visuospatial skills, handwriting, and arithmetic. Children with nonverbal LDs not only have academic difficulties but also often have problems in the social/interpersonal realm, including affect perception and social skills, which can have important implications for their functioning well beyond academics. Given that these functions are typically associated with the right hemisphere, nonverbal LDs are often referred to as right hemisphere LDs, whereas the deficits attributed to verbally based LDs are thought to reflect primarily left hemisphere dysfunction.

It is important to note that although children with verbal and nonverbal LDs can both have difficulties in mathematics and handwriting, the nature of the underlying deficits associated with these difficulties may be different for these two broad LD subtypes. Thus, a child with a verbally based LD is often referred because of generally poor academic progress, with particular difficulty on language-based tasks, such as phonological processing, following verbal directions, or verbal memory. Problems in mathematics may reflect difficulties with word problems, sequencing, and/or mathematical vocabulary items. The mathematical problems of the child with nonverbal LD may reflect more fundamental conceptual problems with mathematics and deficits in spatial cognition (e.g., Pennington 1991; Rourke 1989). Similarly, whereas the social difficulties of the child with nonverbal LD are viewed as reflecting core deficits of the disorder in the social domain, those of other children with LDs may be secondary to other comorbid difficulties, such as attention-deficit/hyperactivity disorder (ADHD), or may reflect the social repercussions of language difficulties and/or academic failure.

Outcome of Learning Disorders

Given the purported "hardwired" nature of LDs, it is not surprising that these are enduring conditions that persist throughout adolescence and into adulthood. For example, in a longitudinal, community-based sample of language-impaired children (first identified at age 5 years), 27% had a reading disorder, 29% a spelling disorder, and 43% mathematics disorders at age 19 years (A. R. Young, J. H. Beitchman, C. J. Johnson, L. Atkinson, M. Escobar, L. Douglas, and B. Wilson, "Young Adult Academic Outcomes in a Longitudinal Study of Early-Identified Language-Impaired and Control Children," submitted for publication, June 2000). When they are provided with adequate support, children with LDs can make good educational progress. However, they will likely take longer to achieve the same milestones as their peers without LDs (Maughan 1995). Follow-up studies of postsecondary education among students with LDs who have graduated from high school indicate that these students are less than half as likely as students without LDs to enroll in postsecondary programs and to remain in these programs until completion (Levine and Edgar 1994; Sitlington and Frank 1990). Employment rates for young adults with LDs are also substantially lower than the national average, with rates of women with LDs significantly below those of men with LDs during young adulthood (Blackorby and Wagner 1996; Levine and Nourse 1998). Thus, LDs can have enduring effects that must be dealt with throughout the life span.

Recommended Assessment Practices

The definition and means of identifying LDs in individuals have been topics of considerable controversy, particularly with regard to whether a significant discrepancy between IQ and achievement is necessary or particularly meaningful (e.g., Fletcher et al. 1993; Siegel 1992). Nevertheless, in keeping with the federal guidelines already presented, most school systems require an ability-achievement discrepancy in their inclusion criteria for access to special programming.

In 1997, the National Joint Committee on Learning Disabilities recommended a four-step procedure for determining whether a child meets criteria for LD and, consequently, is eligible for special education services. Step one involves thoroughly describing the student's learning problems before referral for formal assessment. This may include classroom observation, discussions with parents and teachers, and review of school records. At this point, related factors that may be contributing to the learning problems other than a learning disability (e.g., social and/or emotional problems, sensory impairments) should be considered and dealt with appropriately. Interventions or accommodations should be implemented at this stage to address the student's needs. If the learning difficulties persist, step two should be initiated.

Step two involves formal and informal assessments to determine whether the student meets the criteria for a diagnosis of LD. In addition to careful review of the information collected in step one, standardized tests that are reliable, valid, and current should be used to determine the extent to which the student's current level of functioning in both academic and cognitive domains differs from that of an age-appropriate normative sample. No specific test battery is recommended, but most assessments include a valid, individually administered measure of intelligence (e.g., the Wechsler Intelligence Scale for Children, 3rd Edition [WISC-III]; Wechsler 1991) and standardized achievement tests to evaluate reading, spelling, arithmetic, and written expression. Caution is advised in using cognitive ability/achievement discrepancies because an LD can exist in the absence of such a significant numerical discrepancy between these scores (e.g., IQ scores may be depressed by the same processing difficulties that impair academic performance).

Step three involves determining the need for special education in light of the student's functioning and current demands within the classroom. Finally, in step four, an individualized educational plan (IEP) is created through the collaboration of the student, parents, teachers, and other professionals (e.g., school, clinical, or educational psychologists and/or child and adolescent psychiatrists). Once the IEP is implemented, ongoing evaluation is recommended to evaluate its effectiveness and to make modifications as needed.

Comorbidity

Children with LDs often have a host of co-occurring conditions, including emotional and/or behavioral disorders and social difficulties that interfere with their functioning in a variety of domains. Although figures vary across disorders and research samples, a recent review indicated that between 24% and 52% of children with LDs have clinically significant social, emotional, and/or behavioral disorders (Rock et al. 1997). One of the most common comorbid conditions is reading disabilities with ADHD, with rates varying from about 10% to as high as 60% depending on the specific samples examined (Beitchman and Young 1997).

Internalizing disorders, particularly anxiety and depression, also frequently co-occur with LD, although this area has received considerably less research attention than that of behavioral disorders. Adolescents with LDs have been shown to have higher levels of trait anxiety (reviewed by Huntington and Bender 1993) than adolescents without LDs, and anxiety in grade 1 has been shown to predict lower academic performance in grade 5 (Ialongo et al. 1995). Furthermore, children with an early history of speech and/or language delay, a condition often predictive of later learning disabilities, are at twice the risk of developing anxiety disorders during young adulthood than are control subjects without speech and language delays (Beitchman et al., in press).

Children in classes for the learning disabled show higher rates of depression on self-report measures, and the co-occurrence of depression and LD appears to increase during adolescence (Huntington and Bender 1993). A link between LD and adolescent suicide has been frequently suggested (e.g., Peck 1985; Pfeffer 1986), and a recent study analysis of spelling and handwriting errors in suicide notes left by adolescents (McBride and Siegel 1997) lends some support to the hypothesis that a high percentage of adolescents who commit suicide may have learning disabilities. Children with nonverbal LDs have been described as being at risk for internalizing disorders, including anxiety and depression (Bigler 1989; Rourke 1985; Rourke et al. 1989). This increased risk is in keeping with descriptions of children with nonverbal LDs as withdrawn, isolated, and shy (Voeller 1986).

A frequent source of debate is whether the overlap between emotional and behavioral disorders and LDs is a consequence of the preexisting LD or whether these comorbidities are separately determined. This issue has received particular attention in externalizing disorders (such as ADHD and conduct disorder) because the overlap with LD is sizable and has clear educational and treatment implications (Hinshaw 1992). If the symptoms of ADHD, for example, are behavioral manifestations of comprehension difficulties and frustration within the classroom setting, then treatment should focus on remediating the LD directly as well as helping children compensate for and adapt to their learning difficulties. Alternatively, direct treatment of the comorbid condition, such as with stimulant medication, is required if a true comorbidity exists. Recent trends in the research and clinical literature point to the importance of comprehensive approaches to assessing and treating concurrent LDs and emotional or behavioral disorders rather than focusing on identifying the core disability.

Rock and colleagues (1997) proposed a conceptual model that emphasizes the interaction between concomitant LD and emotional and/or behavioral disorders. They identified six critical functioning domains in which performance deficits frequently occur, including 1) cognitive processing, 2) executive functioning, 3) language functioning, 4) behavioral functioning, 5) social/emotional functioning, and 6) academic achievement. The etiology, developmental course, and prognosis of deficits in these six critical domains are affected by several mediating factors, including environmental variables (e.g., social support, economic conditions, classroom climate) and biophysical variables (e.g., prenatal exposure to toxins, genetic predispositions, temperamental characteristics). Assessing these multiple domains and mediating factors provides the basis for setting priorities, planning interventions, and coordinating services for students with comorbid LDs and emotional or behavioral disorders.

Finally, Silver (1989, 1993) noted that children and adolescents with unidentified or untreated LDs are at higher risk for developing behavioral or psychiatric disorders. Thus, early and effective intervention for both the core deficits associated with LD and the co-occurring social, emotional, or behavioral problems is essential in reducing the negative effect of LDs.

Educational Approaches to Treatment of Learning Disorders

Reading Disorders

Considerable evidence now indicates that one of the core deficits for most reading disorders is in the awareness of, and ability to manipulate the sound structure of, spoken words. Reading disabled individuals frequently have difficulty sequencing and blending individual speech sounds within spoken words and applying letter-to-sound phonological principles in decoding words in print. Problems in speech sound processing tend to persist into adulthood (e.g., Bruck 1992) and to be disappointingly stable over time (Wagner et al. 1994), especially if the reading disorder is not identified earlier than the third grade (e.g., Francis et al. 1996). Nevertheless, literacy skills can be improved throughout adolescence and into adulthood with appropriate training and practice.

Although reading instruction has been the subject of research longer than any other area of LD intervention, interpreting results from early studies was difficult because few included appropriate controls or treatment comparison designs. Recent well-controlled treatment studies (e.g., Lovett et al. 1990; Scanlon and Vellutino 1997; Vellutino et al. 1996) point to the importance of teaching phonological decoding skills. Direct letter-sound instruction (rather than indirect) also has been shown to be a superior method of instruction for early primary students (Foorman et al. 1998). Olson et al. (1997) reported on an intervention study in which phonological awareness training contributed to improvements in phonological awareness and decoding skills after the training and at 1-year follow-up. Unfortunately, this advantage did not generalize to better word reading skills at follow-up. Similarly, Torgesen et al. (1997) reported on a 2.5-year intervention study targeting kindergarten children with poor phonological skills. The children received a program rich in phonological skill training. At the end of the second grade, the intervention children were significantly better at phonological tasks than the no-treatment control group, but again, the gains did not consistently generalize to reading real words or to reading skills more generally.

A group led by Maureen Lovett focused on generalization effects in interventions with children with severe reading disabilities. Lovett et al. (1990, 1994) reported on transfer-of-learning and generalization effects from two word-identification approaches: one that used direct instructional materials focusing on phonological analysis, blending, and letter-sound association skills in the context of word recognition, and one that was based on training in metacognitive decoding strategies. Results of this line of research indicated that both interventions were effective in producing immediate gains as well as generalization of training effects. In the most recent publication, Lovett et al. (2000) reported that "severely disabled readers do not transfer new word learning unless subsyllabic segmentation is explicitly trained and practiced in interventions that effectively target core learning problems" (p. 279). They concluded that for children with a reading disorder, phonologically based approaches alone are not sufficient for achieving optimal remedial outcomes. Thus, phonological instruction is necessary but apparently not sufficient to achieve maximal generalization of gains made in training. Instead, a multidimensional approach in which children are taught to effectively use multiple decoding strategies, allowing for a flexible approach to word identification, is essential for gains to generalize to word identification skills beyond those explicitly taught.

A comprehensive reading intervention also should involve a component to improve the fluency of continuous text reading. Children with a reading disorder often read even relatively easy, familiar text in a slow, unexpressive manner (Young and Bowers 1995). Such lack of fluency has a negative effect on a child's comprehension of the text, and this has clear implications for general academic performance. An intervention approach noted to be particularly effective in remediating fluency deficits is repeated reading of text. Various methods of rereading practice have been described in the literature and applied to the classroom (see Downs and Morin 1990 for a review). Perhaps the most well known is the repeated reading method (e.g., Moyer 1982; Samuels 1979) in which children repeatedly read a short passage of text until they can do so with both speed and accuracy. Variations of rereading practice include reading silently while listening to a tape-recorded reading (McMahon 1983) and reading in unison with a skilled reader. In a study of the effectiveness of various components of rereading practice, Young et al. (1996) reported that direct reading practice with intact text, regardless of whether a model was present, produced the greatest gains. This method can be easily used by parents and others without specific training in reading remediation. Books on tape selected at an appropriate reading level may be particularly helpful in this regard.

To summarize, key components of reading intervention include direct instruction in word identification (including activities to enhance letter-sound knowledge, regular word decoding, irregular word reading, and advanced metacognitively based word analysis skills) and activities to enhance reading fluency, including repeated reading and other practice activities that stress fast and accurate text reading. Computer-assisted instruction and peer tutoring techniques (both reviewed by Mastropieri et al. 1999) are other fluency-enhancing methods that are frequently used in school-based interventions.

Mathematics Disorder

Although prevalence varies somewhat among studies and subject ages, approximately 6% of elementary school children meet criteria for mathematics disorder (e.g., Badian 1983). Disabilities of arithmetic learning ability can represent a unique subtype of LD (e.g., Rourke and Conway 1997), although coexisting disorders in reading and spelling are also often present (Kulak 1993), and children with a history of language impairment frequently encounter difficulties in mathematics (Fazio 1996). Regardless of etiology, mathematical difficulties can interfere with both academic and everyday functioning throughout elementary school and well into adulthood (Adelman and Vogel 1991).

In a comprehensive review of studies examining the neuropsychological, cognitive, and genetic correlates of mathematics disorder—in particular, disorders in acquiring basic or lower-order numerical skills—Geary (1993) identified three core deficits. It is important to note that although described separately, deficits in one area, such as math fact retrieval, can limit the development of other mathematical skills, and, conversely, strength in one area can help compensate for deficits.

The first deficit is evident in difficulties representing or retrieving arithmetic facts from long-term memory. Associated deficits include a high error rate on number facts that are retrieved and slow processing speed. Because these memory-retrieval problems often do not improve even after extensive drilling (e.g., Howell et al. 1987) and the performance deficits resemble those of individuals with acquired mathematical deficits in neuropsychological studies, Geary concluded that this deficit is fundamental and not simply a developmental delay. This type of mathematics disorder often covaries with reading disorder (Geary 1993) and has been noted to be particularly problematic for language-impaired youngsters (Fazio 1994, 1996). Thus, problems in processing and remembering phonologically stored information may be a core deficit of this type of mathematics disorder.

The second deficit associated with mathematics disorder is manifested in problems in executing arithmetic procedures, such as counting strategies for addition or borrowing for subtraction. Findings from reviewed studies were somewhat mixed as to the nature of this deficit; some research suggested a developmental delay (e.g., Geary et al. 1992), and others suggested a more fundamental, persistent difficulty indicative of a real disability (e.g., Goldman et al. 1988). Children are exposed to mathematical procedures during class instruction, so children who do not participate fully in the classroom because of comorbid attentional or conduct problems may be particularly disadvantaged in this area.

The third deficit involves problems in visuospatial representation of numerical information. This later type of difficulty is most often associated with a pattern of neuropsychological functions attributed to the right hemisphere and referred to as a right hemisphere or nonverbal learning disability (e.g., Rourke and Conway 1997; Rourke and Finlayson 1978). This type of deficit is evident in misaligned number columns and misinterpretation of numerical information dependent on spatial relations, such as problems involving place value or geometry. Social, emotional, and writing problems often co-occur with this type of mathematics disorder.

Finally, problems in metacognitive (Montague and Applegate 1993; Rivera 1997) or executive function skills (e.g., planning, self-monitoring, abstract reasoning) contribute to mathematics disorder, especially in the higher grades (A. R. Young, J. H. Beitchman, C. J. Johnson, L. Atkinson, M. Escobar, L. Douglas, and B. Wilson, "Young Adult Academic Outcomes in a Longitudinal Study of Early-Identified Language-Impaired and Control Children," submitted for publication, June 2000). This type of deficit limits the extent to which a child monitors his or her own performance and uses strategies when attempting multistage or advanced mathematical problems. Thus, these children may fail to check their own work effectively and become overly reliant on teacher feedback rather than actively seeking appropriate strategies for problem solving.

Treatment for mathematics disorder has received relatively little research attention when compared with reading intervention. Nevertheless, recent well-controlled treatment studies and reviews (e.g., Rickard et al. 1994; Van Luit and Naglieri 1999) point to characteristics of interventions that contribute to effectiveness. In particular, remedial instruction should be based on a careful analysis of the child's current level of mathematical knowledge and areas of difficulty, often best acquired through techniques such as error analysis and clinical interviewing (Ashlock 1990; Cawley et al. 1996; Fleischner and Manheimer 1997). Such techniques can identify the bases for computational errors that should be systematically targeted in remediation. Effective remedial programs include step-by-step instruction that uses techniques such as modeling, reinforcement of correct responses, corrections, feedback, and cognitive strategy training (Smith and Rivera 1991).

Self-instruction training, in which students with mathematics disorder are taught to generate and evaluate the effectiveness of their own strategies, has been shown to be more effective than a general instruction program in both strategy acquisition and the transfer of effective problem-solving strategies to new, untrained arithmetic problems (Van Luit and Naglieri 1999). Key components of such an intervention program include one-on-one or small-group settings; discussion and modeling of effective and flexible strategy, often using the "think aloud" method; and carefully chosen instructional materials emphasizing both basic procedures (e.g., number fact memorization) and their application to specific problems. Finally, given that mathematics anxiety, very common among children with mathematics disorder, is associated with poorer performance (e.g., Ashcraft and Faust 1994), this approach may be particularly helpful in increasing their sense of both competence and control in mathematics activities.

Disorder of Written Expression

Generating written text requires a number of skills beginning with the most basic level of motor control and orthographic-motor integration needed to write words and letters automatically. Language-specific processes such as phonological coding, retrieval of lexical information, and knowledge of grammatical structures are also required. Finally, higher-order, organizational, and planning skills are needed for creative and interesting translation of ideas into text, especially as the demands and difficulty level of written assignments increase. Given the multitude of skills needed for written expression, it is not surprising that children with language, reading, or mathematics disorders frequently often have pronounced difficulty with written expression. Nevertheless, disorders in writing also exist as a unique area of difficulty for some children (James and Selz 1997).

Disorders of written expression are often multiply determined and complex. Thus, a multipronged approach to treatment is recommended. It is important to determine whether fine motor and visual-orthographic skills are intact because these skills are critical in the development of all components of writing (Berninger and Swanson 1994; Jones and Christensen 1999). The slow and effortful writing of a child who struggles with the mechanics of letter production, for example, will use up cognitive resources that might otherwise be devoted to the higher-order skills needed for effective composition. Intervention to improve handwriting should, therefore, focus on developing rapid, automatic letter recognition and production. As in all areas of remediation, intervention should begin with an assessment of each child's actual performance so that specific areas of difficulty can be targeted. Direct teaching and teacher modeling of efficient letter formation are then followed by extensive independent practice so that automaticity is developed. This type of intervention is highly effective (e.g., Jones and Christensen 1999), easily integrated into the regular classroom, and particularly cost-effective when parent volunteers or teacher aides are used.

Treatment for writing disorder often also focuses on spelling instruction because this is an area of persistent difficulty throughout elementary school and into adolescence and adulthood (Adelman and Vogel 1991; Denckla 1993). Most spelling instruction focuses on teaching a basic spelling vocabulary and teaching the tools needed to spell unfamiliar words, such as basic letter-sound correspondences and spelling rules. Graham et al. (1991) reviewed typical spelling interventions and recommended that for students with LDs only a few words (6–12) be taught each week and that these words consist specifically of the 1,000 most common words supplemented by words that the students frequently misspell in their own writing. Finally, strategies should be taught to help students spell words that have not been explicitly taught, such as using analogies between the words they have already learned to spell and similar-sounding but unknown words and applying their knowledge of spelling rules or word meanings.

Writing instruction for students with LDs also often includes sentence production skills in which students are taught to recognize various parts of speech, build a variety of sentences, and combine small sentence units into larger structures. In a review by Graham et al. (1991), little support was evident for this type of intervention despite its wide use in both remedial and special education classrooms.

All of the interventions described thus far reflect a component skills approach to writing intervention. Another type of intervention focuses on writing as communication and instructs the students in specific strategies for planning, generating, and monitoring their own writing. A variety of writing strategies are taught, including initial idea planning and brainstorming about the text content, generating appropriate vocabulary words and related ideas, goal setting, monitoring the written output, and revising and editing of both the student's own and peer writing. Research (e.g., Graham and Harris 1996) has shown that this approach to writing instruction is highly effective in improving the quality and quantity of students' writing as well as the students' sense of competence when approaching writing activities.

Finally, even with appropriate intervention, writing disorders tend to persist and need to be compensated for even into adulthood (Silver 1995). Access to computers for word processing, extra time allowances for writing assignments and tests, and permission to use dictation rather than struggle with the mechanics of writing may assist students with LDs and writing difficulties.

Psychological Treatments of Learning Disorders

Children with LDs have been found to have lower self-concept and more anxiety than their peers without LDs (e.g., Grolnick and Ryan 1990). They are also frequently less well accepted by peers (e.g., Priel and Leshem 1990; Stone and LaGreca 1990) and have social skills deficits (Kavale and Forness 1996) that may hamper their ability to form and maintain satisfying friendships. For children with LDs and comorbid conditions, a multimodal treatment approach, including education and consultation, is commonly necessary. The clinician may provide direct treatment for concurrent psychiatric disorders and other emotional, behavioral, and interpersonal problems. The clinician should determine the need for and provide psychotherapy, other psychosocial interventions, and medication therapy as indicated for associated psychiatric disorders and secondary problems. Individual and/or group psychotherapy may be recommended for the peer problems and low self-esteem that may result from chronic underachievement. Children with poor peer relationships may benefit from social skills groups or individual interventions.

The feelings of isolation and low self-esteem in a child with LD can negatively affect family functioning because he or she may react negatively to parental attempts to assist with academic skill development. Often the children manage to contain their sense of frustration during the school day, but parents report frequent temper tantrums and crying spells at home with the family. Thus, children with LDs are frequently brought to the attention of mental health professionals because of concerns about their social and/or emotional functioning.

Family or parenting stress has been shown to be higher in families with a child who has LD (e.g., Christenson 1990; Dyson 1996). It is important to note, however, that family functioning is not necessarily lower in families with children who have LD despite the higher level of stress (Dyson 1996). Thus, the presence of LD alone is likely insufficient to create family dysfunction or to undermine parent effectiveness in otherwise well-functioning families. The mental health professional can assist parents and families in their efforts to cope with LD in a child by showing them how to become effective advocates for their child. Whatever approach to treatment and remediation is adopted, it is important that the child, the child's parents, and the child's teachers have a modern understanding of that child's difficulties and their presumed biological and/or genetic basis and that the child is not viewed as simply stubborn, lazy, oppositional, or "slow." The clinician can play an important corrective role in reframing the nature of the child's difficulties should any of the relevant persons in the child's life be unfamiliar with modern concepts of learning disabilities. Given the accumulating evidence on the relevance of genetic and biological factors in the development of learning disabilities (Beitchman and Young 1997), the clinician should inquire about a family history of learning disabilities. This information can be helpful in planning interventions and enlisting the child's parents in the treatment and remediation process.

Counseling parents or caregivers about their role in collaborative interventions is useful. *Informed Instruction for Reading Success: Foundations for Teacher Preparation* (Brady and Moats 1997), which summarizes modern thinking on the conceptual foundation regarding reading acquisition and the sources of reading difficulty, can serve as a useful reference for parents and professionals on the nature of reading disabilities and the requirements for reading success. This document can be especially helpful in consulting with parents about unproven but highly touted treatments for LDs.

Parent support, consultation, and management training may be needed to help the family develop a supportive home environment and a consistent home/school reinforcement program. An important corollary for successful treatment when behavioral or emotional difficulties are comorbid is to help the parents and school appreciate the intimate connections between the learning problems and the child's behavioral and emotional problems.

Finally, as the child with LD matures into adolescence, it is important to assist him or her in learning to advocate for himself or herself because these skills will increase his or her chances of success into adulthood. In treating adolescents, it is important to be aware of coexisting disruptive behavior disorders, mood and anxiety disorders, and substance use disorders, which may lead to school dropout, truancy, and delinquency. Prevocational and vocational skill development may be needed, and helping the family to evaluate the need and/or potential for post–high school education is an appropriate role for the clinician (Scott 1994).

Individual treatment of the child or adolescent should include goals of minimizing disability and maximizing potential through problem solving, social support, study habits, encouragement in extracurricular athletic or other activities, and help with further educational and career decisions. Referral to appropriate support groups for children with LDs also may be an appropriate intervention (Falik 1995). In fact, group approaches can be particularly useful in normalizing shared areas of difficulty and fostering discussion of coping strategies.

Pharmacological Considerations

When psychotropic medication is prescribed to a child with an LD, special attention must be given to the therapeutic effects and the side effects that may influence a child's cognitive function, attention, learning, and memory. No known medications are specifically indicated for the treatment of LDs. Still, removing behavioral or emotional barriers may lead to increased task time and hence improved academic progress.

Because ADHD and reading disabilities frequently co-occur, stimulant medication also has been used in the treatment of reading disabilities. In the short term, improvements in attention and concentration lead to an increase in the amount of work completed, and because much of schoolwork is cumulative, the increase in the amount of work completed leads to academic gains (Elia et al. 1993). Some evidence indicates a direct effect on verbal retrieval mechanisms, which results in improved reading vocabulary, and more general effects on reading achievement appear to be an indirect result of improved behavioral control in hyperactive children with reading disabilities (Richardson et al. 1988). The research findings in this area, however, have been mixed. Although studies of the immediate effects of methylphenidate consistently show increases in classroom productivity, evidence for the long-term academic benefits of stimulant medication is lacking (Carlson and Bunner 1993).

Youngsters with learning disabilities who are concurrently depressed and consequently may be unable to sustain their concentration over extended periods may respond to antidepressant medication with improvement in mood and sustained academic productivity. Likewise, in considering interventions with learning disabled children with comorbid anxiety disorders, social phobias, or school phobias, anxiolytic medications should be considered among the treatments available and used as appropriate.

Conclusions

A multimodal, multidisciplinary approach to treatment is recommended given that LDs can have a lasting and pervasive effect on a child's and an adolescent's development. An essential first step is to obtain a comprehensive assessment and diagnosis so that the child's unique pattern of strengths and weaknesses can be identified and capitalized on when designing educational and other treatments for LD. Evidence-based, effective educational interventions that address the core deficit of each type of LD and assist the child in developing coping strategies to help compensate for his or her areas of difficulty are of particular importance. The mental health professional can help parents and families with a child who has an LD to become effective advocates for their child within the school setting. The behavioral and interpersonal implications of certain cognitive difficulties should be outlined and discussed to help promote a positive and effective style of interaction within the family. Shifting the focus from the child's apparent disobedience to ways in which the parents can modify their requests or interactions with their child can be particularly helpful. Parents can also be assisted in setting realistic goals for their child, and contact with other parents of children with LDs can be encouraged. Areas to target in interventions for the child include self-esteem problems; feelings of helplessness to control events that are, in fact, within the child's domain of control (learned helplessness); and the child's tendency to attribute outcomes to forces outside of himself or herself (external locus of control). Individual or group therapy approaches can be helpful in this regard.

References

Adelman PB, Vogel SA: The learning-disabled adult, in Learning About Learning Disabilities. Edited by Wong BY. San Diego, CA, Academic Press, 1991, pp 563–594

American Psychiatric Association: Diagnostic and Statistical Manual of Mental Disorders, 4th Edition. Washington, DC, American Psychiatric Association, 1994

Ashcraft MH, Faust MW: Mathematics anxiety and mental arithmetic performance: an exploratory investigation. Cognition and Emotion 8:97–125, 1994

Ashlock RB: Error Patterns in Computation: A Semi-Programmed Approach, 5th Edition. Columbus, OH, Charles E Merrill, 1990

Badian NA: Dyscalculia and nonverbal disorders of learning, in Progress in Learning Disabilities, Vol 5. Edited by Mykelbust HR. New York, Grune & Stratton, 1983, pp 235–264

Beitchman JH, Young AR: Learning disorders with a special emphasis on reading disorders: a review of the past 10 years. J Am Acad Child Adolesc Psychiatry 36:1020–1032, 1997

Beitchman JH, Wilson B, Johnson CJ, et al: Fourteen-year follow-up of speech/language impaired and control children: psychiatric outcome. J Am Acad Child Adolesc Psychiatry (in press)

Berninger VW, Swanson HL: Modifying Hayes and Flower's model of skilled writing to explain beginning and developing writing, in Children's Writing: Toward a Process Theory of the Development of Skilled Writing. Edited by Butterfield EC. Hampton Hill, Middlesex, UK, JAI Press, 1994, pp 57–81

Bigler ED: On the neuropsychology of suicide. J Learn Disabil 22:180–185, 1989

Blackorby J, Wagner M: Longitudinal postschool outcomes of youth with disabilities: findings from the National Longitudinal Transition Study. Exceptional Children 62:399–413, 1996

Brady S, Moats L: Informed Instruction for Reading Success: Foundations for Teacher Preparation: A Position Paper. Baltimore, MD, International Dyslexia Association, 1997

Bruck M: Persistence of dyslexics' phonological awareness deficits. Dev Psychol 28:874–886, 1992

Carlson CL, Bunner MR: Effects of methylphenidate on the academic performance of children with attention-deficit hyperactivity disorder and learning disabilities. School Psychology Review 22:184–198, 1993

Cawley JF, Parmar RS, Yan WF, et al: Arithmetic computation abilities of students with learning disabilities: implications for instruction. Learning Disabilities Research and Practice 11:230–237, 1996

Christenson SL: Differences in students' home environments: the need to work with families. School Psychology Review 19:505–517, 1990

Denckla M: The child with developmental disabilities grown up: adult residua of childhood disorders. Behavioral Neurology 11:105–125, 1993

Downs J, Morin S: Improving reading fluency with precision teaching. Teaching Exceptional Children, Spring 1990, pp 38–40

Dyson LL: The experiences of families of children with learning disabilities: parental stress, family functioning, and sibling self-concept. J Learn Disabil 29:280–286, 1996

Education for All Handicapped Children Act (PL 94-142). Federal Register 42:42496–42497, 1976

Elia J, Welsch PA, Gullotta CS, et al: Classroom academic performance: improvement with both methylphenidate and dextroamphetamine in ADHD boys. J Child Psychol Psychiatry 34:785–804, 1993

Falik LH: Family patterns of reaction to a child with a learning disability: a mediational perspective. J Learn Disabil 28:335–341, 1995

Fazio BB: The counting abilities of children with specific language impairment: a comparison of oral and gestural tasks. Journal of Speech and Hearing Research 37:358–368, 1994

Fazio BB: Mathematical abilities of children with specific language impairment: a 2-year follow-up. Journal of Speech and Hearing Research 39:839–849, 1996

Fleischner JE, Manheimer MA: Math interventions for students with learning disabilities: myths and realities. School Psychology Review 26:397–413, 1997

Fletcher JM, Francis DJ, Rourke BP, et al: Classification of learning disabilities, in Better Understanding of Learning Disabilities. Edited by Lyon GR, Gray DB, Kavanagh JF, et al. Baltimore, MD, Paul H Brookes, 1993, pp 27–55

Foorman BR, Francis DJ, Fletcher JM, et al: The role of instruction in learning to read: preventing reading failure in at-risk children. Journal of Educational Psychology 90:37–55, 1998

Francis DJ, Shaywitz SE, Stuebing KK, et al: Developmental lag versus deficit models of reading disability: a longitudinal, individual growth curves analysis. Journal of Educational Psychology 88:3–17, 1996

Geary DC: Mathematical disabilities: cognitive, neuropsychological, and genetic components. Psychol Bull 114:345–362, 1993

Geary DC, Bow-Thomas CC, Yao Y: Counting knowledge and skill in cognitive addition: a comparison of normal and mathematically disabled children. J Exp Child Psychol 54:372–391, 1992

Goldman SR, Pellegrino JW, Mertz DL: Extended practice of basic addition facts: strategy changes in learning disabled students. Cognition and Instruction 5:223–265, 1988

Graham S, Harris KR: Addressing problems in attention, memory, and executive functioning: an example from self-regulated strategy development, in Attention, Memory and Executive Function. Edited by Lyon GR, Krasnegor NA. Baltimore, MD, Paul H Brookes, 1996, pp 349–365

Graham S, Harris KR, MacArthur C, et al: Writing instruction, in Learning About Learning Disabilities. Edited by Wong BY. San Diego, CA, Academic Press, 1991, pp 309–343

Grolnick WS, Ryan RM: Self-perceptions, motivation, and adjustment in children with learning disabilities: a multiple group comparison study. J Learn Disabil 23:177–184, 1990

Hinshaw SP: Externalizing behavior problems and academic underachievement in childhood and adolescence: causal relationships and underlying mechanisms. Psychol Bull 111:127–155, 1992

Howell R, Sidorenko E, Jurica J: The effects of computer use on the acquisition of multiplication facts by a student with learning disabilities. J Learn Disabil 20:336–341, 1987

Huntington DD, Bender WN: Adolescents with learning disabilities at risk? Emotional well-being, depression, suicide. J Learn Disabil 26:159–166, 1993

Ialongo N, Edelsohn G, Werthamer-Larsson L: The significance of self-reported anxious symptoms in first grade children: prediction to anxious symptoms and adaptive functioning in fifth grade. J Child Psychol Psychiatry 36:427–437, 1995

Individuals With Disabilities Education Act (IDEA) (PL 101-476). Federal Register 55, Oct 30, 1990

Individuals With Disabilities Education Act (IDEA) of 1997 (PL 105-17). Available at: http://www.ideapractices.org/law/ideamain.htm (accessed September 25, 2000)

James EM, Selz M: Neuropsychological bases of common learning and behavior problems in children, in Handbook of Clinical Child Neuropsychology, 2nd Edition. Edited by Reynolds CR, Fletcher-Jansen E. New York, Plenum, 1997, pp 157–179

Johnson DJ, Myklebust HR: Learning Disabilities. New York, Grune & Stratton, 1971

Jones D, Christensen CA: Relationship between automaticity in handwriting and students' ability to generate written text. Journal of Educational Psychology 91:44–49, 1999

Kavale KA, Forness SR: Social skill deficits and learning disabilities: a meta-analysis. J Learn Disabil 29:226–237, 1996

Kulak AG: Parallels between math and reading disability: common issues and approaches. J Learn Disabil 26:666–673, 1993

Levine P, Edgar E: An analysis of respondent agreement in follow-up studies of graduates of special and regular education programs. Exceptional Children 60:292–343, 1994

Levine P, Nourse SW: What follow-up studies say about postschool life for young men and women with learning disabilities: a critical look at the literature. J Learn Disabil 31:212–233, 1998

Lovett MW, Warren-Chaplin PM, Ransby MJ, et al: Training the word recognition skills of reading disabled children: treatment and transfer effects. Journal of Educational Psychology 82:769–780, 1990

Lovett MW, Borden SL, DeLuca T, et al: Treating the core deficits of developmental dyslexia: evidence of transfer-of-learning following phonologically- and strategy-based reading training programs. Dev Psychol 30:805–822, 1994

Lovett MW, Lacerenza L, Borden SL, et al: Components of effective remediation for developmental reading disabilities: combining phonological and strategy-based instruction to improve outcomes. Journal of Educational Psychology 92:263–283, 2000

Mastropieri MA, Leinhart A, Scruggs TE: Strategies to increase reading fluency. Intervention in School and Clinic 34:278–292, 1999

Maughan B: Annotation: long-term outcomes of developmental reading problems. J Child Psychol Psychiatry 36:357–371, 1995

McBride HE, Siegel LS: Learning disabilities and adolescent suicide. J Learn Disabil 30:652–659, 1997

McMahon ML: Development of reading-while-listening skills in the primary grades. Reading Research Quarterly 19:38–52, 1983

Montague M, Applegate B: Middle school students' mathematical problem solving: an analysis of think-aloud protocols. Learning Disability Quarterly 16:19–30, 1993

Moyer SB: Repeated reading. J Learn Disabil 45:619–623, 1982

National Joint Committee on Learning Disabilities: Operationalizing the NJCLD Definition of Learning Disabilities for Ongoing Assessment in Schools (1997). Available at: http://www.ldonline.org/njcld/operationalizing.html (accessed September 25, 2000)

Olson RK, Wise B, Ring J, et al: Computer-based remedial training in phoneme awareness and phonological decoding: effects on the posttraining development of word recognition. Scientific Studies of Reading 1:235–254, 1997

Peck M: Crisis intervention treatment with chronically and acutely suicidal adolescents, in Youth Suicide. Edited by Peck M, Farberow HL, Litman RE. New York, Springer, 1985, pp 112–122

Pennington BF: Diagnosing Learning Disorders: A Neuropsychological Framework. New York, Guilford, 1991

Pfeffer CR: The Suicidal Child. New York, Guilford, 1986

Priel B, Leshem T: Self-perceptions of first- and second-grade children with learning disabilities. J Learn Disabil 23:637–642, 1990

Richardson E, Kupietz SS, Winsberg BG, et al: Effects of methylphenidate dosage in hyperactive reading-disabled children, II: reading achievement. J Am Acad Child Adolesc Psychiatry 27:78–87, 1988

Rickard TC, Healy AF, Bourne LE: On the cognitive structure of basic arithmetic skills: operation, order, and symbol transfer effects. J Exp Psychol Learn Mem Cogn 20:1139–1153, 1994

Rivera DP: Mathematics education and student with learning disabilities: introduction to the special series. J Learn Disabil 30:2–19, 68, 1997

Rock EE, Fessler MA, Church R: The concomitance of learning disabilities and emotional/behavioral disorders: a conceptual model. J Learn Disabil 30:245–263, 1997

Rourke BP: Neuropsychology of Learning Disabilities: Essentials of Subtype Analysis. New York, Guilford, 1985

Rourke BP: Nonverbal Learning Disabilities: The Syndrome and the Model. New York, Guilford, 1989

Rourke BP, Conway JA: Disabilities of arithmetic and mathematical reasoning: perspectives from neurology and neuropsychology. J Learn Disabil 30:34–46, 1997

Rourke BP, Finlayson MA: Neuropsychological significance of variances in patterns of academic performance: verbal and visual-spatial abilities. J Abnorm Child Psychol 6:121–133, 1978

Rourke BP, Strang JD: Subtypes of reading and arithmetic disabilities: a neuropsychological analysis, in Developmental Neuropsychiatry. Edited by Rutter M. New York, Guilford, 1983, pp 473–488

Rourke BP, Young GC, Leenaars AA: A childhood learning disability that predisposes those afflicted to adolescent and adult depression and suicide risk. J Learn Disabil 22:169–175, 1989

Samuels SJ: The method of repeated readings. Reading Teacher 32:403–408, 1979

Scanlon DM, Vellutino FR: A comparison of the instructional backgrounds and cognitive profiles of poor, average, and good readers who were initially identified as at risk for reading failure. Scientific Studies of Reading 1:191–216, 1997

Scott SS: Determining reasonable academic adjustments for college students with learning disabilities. J Learn Disabil 27:403–412, 1994

Siegel LS: An evaluation of the discrepancy definition of dyslexia. J Learn Disabil 22:469–478, 486, 1992

Silver LB: Psychological and family problems associated with learning disabilities: assessment and intervention. J Am Acad Child Adolesc Psychiatry 28:319–325, 1989

Silver LB: Problems found with children and adolescents with learning disabilities, in Child and Adolescent Psychiatric Clinics of North America: Learning Disabilities. Edited by Silver L. Philadelphia, PA, WB Saunders, 1993, pp 295–308

Silver LB: Learning disorders, in Treatments of Psychiatric Disorders, 2nd Edition, Vol 1. Gabbard GO, Editor-in-Chief. Washington, DC, American Psychiatric Press, 1995, pp 123–140

Sitlington PL, Frank AR: Are adolescents with learning disabilities successfully crossing the bridge into adult life? Learning Disability Quarterly 13:97–111, 1990

Smith DD, Rivera DP: Mathematics, in Learning About Learning Disabilities. Edited by Wong BY. San Diego, CA, Academic Press, 1991, pp 345–374

Stone WL, LaGreca AM: The social status of children with learning disabilities: a re-examination. J Learn Disabil 23:32–37, 1990

Torgesen JK, Wagner RK, Rashotte CA: Prevention and remediation of severe reading disabilities: keeping the end in mind. Scientific Studies of Reading 1:217–234, 1997

U.S. Department of Education: Thirteenth Annual Report to Congress on the Implementation of the Education of the Handicapped Act. Washington, DC, U.S. Government Printing Office, 1991

Van Luit JE, Naglieri JA: Effectiveness of the MASTER program for teaching special children multiplication and division. J Learn Disabil 32:98–107, 1999

Vellutino FR, Scanlon DM, Sipay ER, et al: Cognitive profiles of difficult-to-remediate and readily remediated poor readers: early intervention as a vehicle for distinguishing between cognitive and experiential deficits as basic causes of specific reading disability. Journal of Educational Psychology 88:601–638, 1996

Voeller KKS: Right-hemisphere deficit syndrome in children. Am J Psychiatry 143:1004–1009, 1986

Wagner RK, Torgesen JK, Rashotte CA: Development of reading-related phonological processing abilities: new evidence of bi-directional causality from a latent variable longitudinal study. Dev Psychol 30:73–87, 1994

Wechsler D: Manual for the Wechsler Intelligence Scale for Children, 3rd Edition. San Antonio, TX, Psychological Corporation, 1991

Young AR, Bowers PG: Individual difference and text difficulty determinants of reading fluency and expressiveness. J Exp Child Psychol 60:428–454, 1995

Young AR, Bowers PG, MacKinnon GE: Effects of prosodic modeling and repeated reading on poor readers' fluency and comprehension. Applied Psycholinguistics 17:59–84, 1996

6

Autistic Disorder

Bryna Siegel, Ph.D.
Catherine Hayer, M.S.
Peter E. Tanguay, M.D.

State of the Art

In the past 10 years, much has changed in the treatment landscape for pervasive developmental disorders (PDDs). In this chapter, we review behavior- and medicine-based interventions for autism, emphasizing a model for formulating which intervention models, methods, and medicines may be most suitable for which individuals with PDDs.

One major trend is earlier intervention: earlier treatment has resulted from earlier diagnoses of developmental disorders through various child-find efforts in primary care and educational settings. Public funding of infant (birth to 3 years) services via additions to the Individuals With Disabilities Education Act (IDEA) has created impetus for both earlier diagnosis and earlier treatment. In the past, clinicians were sometimes understandably reluctant to diagnose autism or another PDD early when no substantial treatment services were available to follow the diagnosis.

A second major trend propelling treatment for PDD has been a growing understanding of early neuromaturation and neurodevelopmental factors that have special implications for early intervention through exploiting neuroplasticity and transfer of function (Minshew et al. 1997). The focus on importance of early treatment has galvanized a cadre of parents who have spearheaded advocacy activities around early treatment, resulting in wider availability of very intensive treatments focused on ages associated with most prominent neuronal growth, differentiation, and migration (Harris and Handleman 1994). There has also been a similar expansion of interest and pursuit of nonmainstream treatments, especially because of the rise of non-peer-reviewed modalities of information dissemination such as the Internet (Siegel 1996b). (Treatments not supported by generally accepted peer-reviewed empirical research are not included in this review.)

The third trend is that attention to implementation of more *autism-specific* interventions has increased. This is in contrast to earlier treatment standards for PDDs in which these disorders tended to be treated with essentially the same interventions as for other developmental, communicative, and behavior disorders. The emergence of more autism-specific treatments and an understanding of how they may be most efficiently matched to symptom profiles are discussed in the first part of this chapter. In the second part of the chapter, we review omnibus and symptom-specific treatment approaches for autism. In the third part of the chapter, we review the current state of the psychopharmacology for PDD.

Methodological Limitations in Available Treatment Research

The greatest difficulty in presenting the body of knowledge on autism treatment is that virtually no comparative empirical studies across treatment methods have been done and relatively little empirical research is available on outcome studies for either omnibus or symptom-specific treatments. Experimental designs are more readily applicable to the assessment of new psychopharmacological agents that can be administered in comparison to placebo or competing agents from the same or different class of drugs. However, behavioral interventions are not so readily isolated for experimental investigations, especially in treatment of the youngest subjects whose parents are often desperate for the "window of opportunity" not to "close" or not to leave any stone unturned. In recent years, the ethics of forgoing a treatment supported by even preliminary empirical data in favor of an alternative intervention regimen that has not been systematically studied but is believed to be effective by some consensus of clinicians and educators has posed particularly thorny legal challenges (Heflin and Simpson 1998; McIntosh 1999). Specifically, the efficacy of applied behavioral analysis approaches for children with autism has been studied in a preliminary way, although with quasi-experimental designs (Baer 1997; Gresham and MacMillian 1995) that have been subjected to significant criticisms. Other methodologies for teaching the youngest children with autism either 1) have not been subject to similar study or 2) are eclectically administered or administered on university sites and/or with special funding, rendering generalizations about efficacy of such treatments meaningless (Siegel 1996a). In addition, many different treatments and modalities of treatment are often administered at the same time, and many are simultaneously initiated around the time of diagnosis, making designs that might employ multiple baselines or partial correlations or other studies of covariance extremely difficult to interpret.

This state of affairs certainly calls for empirical research on the treatment of autism. However, in the absence of empirical treatment research to answer important questions about which treatments are most suitable for which patients with autism, other criteria must be used until better data are available. Clinical judgment about individual differences in treatment responses, as well as knowledge of a range of treatment modalities for autism, resides mainly with a few autism specialists who follow up a large clinical population.

Therefore, presented here is a theoretical framework for formulating which treatments for autism may be indicated based on the specific presentation of autistic symptoms in a given individual. This model is intended as a heuristic approach for more generalist clinicians who 1) seek to understand the relative utility of different treatment approaches and 2) need to prescribe individualized treatment for patients with PDDs without extensive previous familiarization with the PDD treatment literature and its controversies.

Autistic Learning Disability Model

"Primary Deficits" Research

Two types of descriptive literature allow the clinician-researcher to delineate the nature of autism and its related disorders and, therefore, what the target for treatment might be. The first is research that focuses on an individual variable or construct and examines the centrality or explanatory power of that construct for the syndrome as a whole. Without solid neurophysiological and neuroanatomical data, such theories remain substantially unproven and so have shifted over the years: Examples would be work in the areas of theory of mind (e.g., Baron-Cohen 1995), executive function (Rogers and Pennington 1991), and stimulus overselectivity (Lovaas et al. 1971). However, research in these areas has influenced whether we view autism as a disorder of sensory functioning (stimulus overselectivity), information processing (executive functioning), or innate social dysfunction (theory of mind), for example. Goals of various modalities of treatment also can be seen as corresponding to these hypothetically different primary deficits such as behaviorally based desensitization training for stimulus overselectivity, training of more abstract reasoning for executive function deficits, or social skills training for theory of mind deficits.

However, an overarching framework that permits a comparative assessment of the relative appropriateness of different treatment approaches and that takes into consideration the variation of expression in autism deficits across individuals is still lacking. The idea of a primary deficit implies that its remediation or amelioration will promote the remediation or amelioration of other derivative deficits, once the underlying problem is addressed. However, it is clear that, phenomenologically, 1) many kinds of deficits coexist in a given individual, and 2) it may be moot from a treatment point of view to determine which is primary if remediations for different deficits are simultaneously used and are in some way incrementally effective.

"DSM-ology": Nomenclature-Based Literature

The second type of descriptive clinical literature on autism has focused on classification and nomenclature. In the last 20 years, we have moved from the original serial case-studies-based definition of autism (Kanner 1943) to the first manualized definition of autism and related conditions as set forth in DSM-III (American Psychiatric Association 1980) and on to DSM-III-R (American Psychiatric Association 1987) and DSM-IV (American Psychiatric Association 1994). Revisions to DSM-III-R and DSM-IV were based not only on empirical field trials but also on studies that compared and contrasted various subgroups with proposed research diagnostic criteria, which subsequently refined our understanding of traits that do and do not delineate groups. This area of endeavor is propelled ever forward by a dynamism between "lumpers," who propose that autism is a spectrum-like syndrome with arbitrary boundaries between subgroups, and the "splitters," who propose that the PDDs must be subjected to rigorous empirical subgrouping if etiologically specific, treatment-response-specific, or prognosis-specific groups are to be identified (Schopler 1998). Therefore, addressing whether treatment research samples should be diagnostically homogeneous or heterogeneous is a factor in generalizability of any research conclusions.

Autistic Learning Disabilities

The autistic learning disability model (Siegel 1999, in press) was developed as a way of integrating perspectives from the primary deficits approach with the nosological debate between "lumpers" and "splitters." This was accomplished by remapping autistic symptoms onto a treatment decision-making model that permits individualized analysis of how each symptom of the autistic syndrome, when present in a given individual, can be reinterpreted in terms of specific limitations to meaningful processing of experience. The autistic learning disability model facilitates recognition of how experience and learning are altered by the presence of each symptom of autism and therefore is intended to lead directly to therapeutic training or teaching methods designed to ameliorate that symptom. The autistic learning disability model permits an analysis of omnibus treatment programs designed to be "autism-specific" and how completely each may address the symptom (e.g., learning) profile of specific patients. Reviews of model programs have noted that several factors likely influence outcome, including program factors—such as age at initiation of treatment, treatment intensity, methodology of treatment, and parent involvement—and pretreatment child characteristics—such as behavior problems, intellectual functioning, and language capacity (Dawson and Osterling 1996; Olley et al. 1993; Rogers 1998). Because these indicators are neither autism- nor symptom-specific, the autistic learning disability approach is used in this review.

Symptom-Specific Versus Diagnosis-Specific Treatment

It has long been recognized that there is no single drug to treat autism per se. Rather, psychopharmacological agents tend to be fairly specific to a range of related autistic symptoms such as repetitive behaviors or anxiety-driven avoidance and specifically recommended to those individuals with autism most impaired by such symptoms. This is discussed further in the latter part of this chapter. The autistic learning disability model similarly suggests that behaviorally based treatments should be selected and modified as needed, to include therapeutic approaches specific to corresponding autistic symptoms. Table 6–1 presents the way in which the model for autistic learning disability can be mapped onto the DSM criteria for autism as a way of generally regrouping symptoms of autism so that treatments can be selected that most specifically address the learning disabilities of a specific individual.

Omnibus Treatment Approaches for Autism

Reviewed here briefly are three different widely disseminated, behaviorally based omnibus treatments for PDDs: 1) the use of applied behavioral analysis via discrete trial training innovated by the UCLA Early Autism Project (Lovaas 1987; Lovaas and Smith 1989); 2) the structured teaching model that has been adapted for use in PDD by Project TEACCH based at the University of North Carolina (Schopler et al. 1981, 1995); and 3) integrated, inclu-

TABLE 6–1. Mapping diagnostic criteria for autism onto autistic learning disability profile

DSM-IV criteria for autistic disorder	Autistic learning disability
A. Qualitative impairments in reciprocal social interaction 1. Marked impairment in the use of multiple nonverbal behaviors such as eye-to-eye gaze, facial expression, body postures, and gestures to regulate social interaction 2. Failure to develop peer relationships appropriate to developmental level 3. Markedly impaired expression of pleasure in other people's happiness 4. Lack of socioemotional reciprocity	Social interaction–based disabilities 1. Lack of modeling/imitation (DSM-IV A1, A2) 2. Lack of drive for peer affiliation (DSM-IV A2) 3. Lack of social reference or only use of instrumental reference (DSM-IV A3) 4. Lack of response to social reward (DSM-IV A1, A4)
B. Qualitative impairments in communication 1. A delay in, or total lack of, the development of spoken language (not accompanied by an attempt to compensate through alternative modes of communication such as gesture or mime) 2. Marked impairment in the ability to initiate or sustain a conversation with others despite adequate speech 3. Stereotyped and repetitive use of language or idiosyncratic language 4. Lack of varied, spontaneous make-believe play or social imitative play appropriate to developmental level	Reception and expression of verbal and nonverbal information 1. Problems in comprehension of natural gesture and emotional expression (DSM-IV A1) 2. Problems in expression of natural gestural and facial expression (DSM-IV B1, A1) 3. Preference for visual over auditory modalities (DSM-IV B3) 4. Problems of gestalt perception and processing (DSM-IV B3)
C. Restricted, repetitive, and stereotyped patterns of behavior, interests, or activities 1. Encompassing preoccupation with one or more stereotyped and restricted patterns of interest, abnormal in either intensity or focus 2. An apparently compulsive adherence to specific nonfunctional routines or rituals 3. Stereotyped and repetitive motor mannerisms (e.g., hand or finger flapping, twisting, or complex whole-body movements) 4. Persistent preoccupation with parts of objects	Disabilities based in processing environmental stimuli 1. Stimulus overselectivity/perseveration on parts of objects (DSM-IV C1, C4) 2. Low response to novelty/preference for routines and ritual patterns of action (DSM-IV C2) 3. Sensory modulation difficulties (DSM-IV C2, C3)

sive education with an array of individualized ancillary special education support services (e.g., Odom and Strain 1984; Strain and Kohler 1988). These treatments are detailed because each is considered by some to represent an effective standard of treatment practice for PDD. Each omnibus approach is analyzed with respect to how it may address specific autistic learning disabilities by applying the autistic learning disability model—mapping autistic learning disabilities onto treatment approaches. The autistic learning disability analysis can then be used for developing or assessing an individualized treatment plan in a way that allows the clinician to move beyond the diagnosis of autism as a unitary dimension for making recommendations for treatment of PDD, using some relevant features from different treatment approaches. The autistic learning disability model also allows treatment recommendations to be autism symptom–specific rather than based on the more general indicators such as IQ, presence or absence of speech, behavior problems, or a delineation of autism versus PDD not otherwise specified. Table 6–2 provides an overview of how these three different omnibus autism treatment approaches may be characterized in terms of the autistic learning disabilities (or symptoms of autism) they purport to address. It is important to note, however, that studies showing amelioration of specific diagnostic characteristics of autism in response to specific treatments have not been carried out. Furthermore, as can be seen, no one treatment clearly targets the full range of learning difficulties that may be associated with a particular case of PDD. Possible conclusions that could be drawn from such an observation are that 1) all treatments are inadequate; 2) the treatment that addresses the most autistic learning disabilities is likely best; or 3) treatments need to be combined, based on the specific autistic learning disability of a particular patient. Given the lack of data linking symptoms to program characteristics, the third conclusion is put forward as most supportable.

Autism treatment and autism treatment research (and the lack of it) have been mired in controversy engendered by ideological purists who insist that "If it is autism, the treatment must be *X*," irrespective of how the symptoms of autism are expressed in a given individual. It is important to remember that no current body of comparative autism treatment research exists and thus little unequivocal support is found for any one treatment for every case of PDD. It is also important to keep in mind that 1) each patient's treatment consists not only of a selected program but also of other experiences throughout the day and 2) process measures of treatments (also not studied) would likely reveal both substantial similarities and differences among treatment approaches (e.g., time spent one to one; frequency of teacher to child "turns" during instruction). In addition, each omnibus treatment model promotes the importance of generalization activities, as well as parent training and participation—which should not remain unmeasured sources of variance in future treatment outcome studies.

Reviewed here first are the two most widely disseminated autism treatment models. Each is analyzed with respect to how specific autistic learning disabilities are addressed. Inclusion of children with PDD into regular education programs with or without individual instructional assistance is a third widely used treatment modality, and its relative advantages and drawbacks are examined as well. Then, in the following section, we examine other more derivative or ancillary methodologies—mainly designed around compensation for a specific symptomatic area of deficit (i.e., some area of autistic learning disability).

Applied Behavioral Analysis

The most widely researched treatment modality for young children with autism has been applied behavioral analysis. The idea that autism could be treated with the basic tenets of learning theory has been reported since the early 1960s. Most empirically based research in this realm began with the inception of the Young Autism Project in 1970 and the work

TABLE 6–2. Three omnibus treatments for autism: autistic learning disabilities/autism symptoms hypothesized to be addressed

Area of autistic learning disability	Applied behavioral analysis	Project TEACCH	Integration/full inclusion
Social interaction–based disabilities			
Lack of modeling or imitation	Yes		Yes
Lack of peer affiliation			Yes
Lack of social reference			Yes
Lack of response to social reward	Yes	Yes	Yes
Reception/expression of verbal/nonverbal communication			
Problems in comprehension of natural gesture and emotional expression	Yes		
Problems in expression of natural gesture and facial expression			
Preference for visual over auditory modalities	Yes	Yes	
Gestalt perception and processing			
Disabilities based in processing environmental stimuli			
Stimulus overselectivity/ perseveration on parts of objects	Yes	Yes	
Preference for routines/ritual over novelty		Yes	
Sensory modulation difficulties			

of O. Ivar Lovaas. In 1987, Lovaas reported results from an early intervention project comparing treatment gains between 19 children assigned to an experimental group and 19 children designated as control subjects. It was reported that the children did not differ on pretreatment variables such as chronological age, IQ, or family socioeconomic status. The study group received 40 hours/week of intensive behavioral intervention based on discrete trials methodology for 2 years. In contrast, control children received approximately 10 hours of the same intervention for the same time period. Follow-up data on these children at approximately age 7 years indicated that 47% of the children in the experimental group had achieved normal functioning as defined by performance on IQ tests and adaptive behavior measures and successful first-grade performance. This percentage is contrasted with 2% of the control children achieving this level of functioning. Follow-up data at an average age of 13 years found that 8 of 9 children in the treatment group designated as "recovered" maintained gains incurred during intervention. Although criticisms and controversy surrounding the findings of this study (to be discussed later) abound, it can be credited for being one of the few quasi-experimental and well-designed research protocols to assess the effectiveness of treatment approaches to autism in children.

Several model programs have based their treatment philosophy on the principles of applied behavioral analysis and report outcome data to varying degrees. Some of these include the May Center for Early Childhood Education (Anderson et al. 1993), the Douglass Developmental Disabilities Center (Harris et al. 1990), and the Princeton Child Development

Institute (McClanahan and Krantz 1994). These programs typically serve children between ages 2 and 5 years whose level of cognitive impairment at intake is assessed as being moderate to absent. Children receive between 20 and 30 hours/week of program time that are typically divided between home program activities and more typical preschool activities. All programs emphasize a progression from highly segregated one-to-one work in the home to gradual transitions to integrated preschool settings. Extensive intake information is obtained with a variety of standardized cognitive and adaptive behavior instruments. Outcome data are available for most children within the programs but are described differently, which makes comparisons across programs difficult. Data provided include measures of public school placements, measures of developmental gains, and measures of change in IQ and adaptive behavior functioning. Children subsequently placed in typical mainstream classrooms varied by program and ranged from 14% of the children in the Douglass Developmental Disabilities Center being "fully integrated" to 54% of the children from the May Center being "mainstreamed." (It should be noted that 50% of the mainstreamed group required some type of support, such as an instructional aide.)

The literature to date describing the efficacy of programs with a firm basis in applied behavioral analysis seems to support the utility of these programs for some children with autistic spectrum disorders during the preschool years. However, the research data thus far have several methodological difficulties, and the descriptions of which children with autistic spectrum disorders these types of programs may or may not be appropriate for are somewhat vague. The programs do not offer comparison groups of children receiving alternative therapies or in public education programs. Hence, the efficacy of these programs cannot be compared with that of the alternatives. Virtually all studies report only on preschool and early elementary age pupils. The Lovaas data do provide a control group, but their comparisons were primarily based on time intensity (40 hours vs. 10 hours), with children receiving comparable treatment regimens. Most of the literature does not describe the criteria for program inclusion. The Douglass, Princeton, and Lovaas programs included children meeting either DSM-III or DSM-III-R criteria for autistic disorder. The May program accepted children with a diagnosis of either autism or PDD. Furthermore, with the exception of the Lovaas program, the literature does not describe the exclusion criteria or child characteristics that would render a child inappropriate for the program. The Lovaas research describes the exclusion of 15% of referrals because of "profound retardation" (approximate ratio IQ of less than 36). There are numerous difficulties with the establishment of baseline IQ in these children. (We refer the reader to a comprehensive analysis by Gresham and MacMillian [1995] of the methodological concerns regarding these data.) Professionals and practitioners working with these children would agree that this type of program is not appropriate for certain children. Research should seek to identify child characteristics that indicate the likelihood that children will succeed in these types of programs as well as pretreatment characteristics or early treatment response characteristics that may make it unlikely that specific subtypes of children will benefit. In addition, future research in this area needs to provide data on process measures to ensure that treatments are administered comparably within and across studies.

Given the current state of the literature, one cannot conclude that programs based largely on applied behavioral analysis and discrete trial methodology are superior to alternative forms of treatment. Few studies used comparison groups receiving alternative forms of intervention. The highly quoted Lovaas research indicates that children receiving

40 hours/week of intervention achieved better outcomes than children receiving 10 hours of intervention. At present, few experts within the field would disagree with the assertion that 10 hours/week of treatment is inadequate. In a preliminary study of treatment intensity for home-based interventions for young children with autism, Sheinkopf and Siegel (1998) found some evidence that the number of hours greater than 27 hours/week affected neither subsequent gains in IQ nor symptom reduction.

Overall, the use of behavioral techniques in the treatment and education of children with autistic spectrum disorders has been well substantiated over the last three decades. The research, however, has not confirmed the benefit of these programs for all children who present with autistic spectrum disorders. The strongest responders to this treatment may be children with higher pretreatment cognitive and language abilities. Future research is needed to 1) better understand responder characteristics, 2) control and document the process to enable replication, and 3) better characterize outcomes in terms of standardized diagnosis and the need for continuing educational and social supports.

Project TEACCH

Treatment and Education for Autistic and Communication Handicapped Children (TEACCH) was begun in the 1960s by Eric Schopler as a psychoanalytic, relation-based approach to treating children with autism and their parents (Mesibov 1995). Schopler shifted to a more skill-based approach in the early 1970s, and TEACCH became the first statewide program for individuals with autistic spectrum disorders mandated by a state legislature. TEACCH programs are implemented throughout the special education system for persons of all ages throughout North Carolina. The program is best described as a way of thinking about children with autism (or autistic learning disabilities) rather than a unitary technique (such as applied behavioral analysis) or methodology (such as discrete trial training). The emphasis is on early identification, parent training, education, social and leisure skills development, and vocational training. TEACCH focuses on improving the adaptive and independent living skills through modifying the environment to accommodate the characteristics of persons with autistic disorders. For example, visual aids are strongly emphasized, whereby students use picture schedules and other cues to signal the beginning and ending of activities, steps in a task, and the sequence of activities in a typical day. Areas of the classroom are clearly demarcated to emphasize the particular purpose of an area and types of activities that can take place in that area. TEACCH purports to be developmentally and individually based in that it compiles an assessment of each individual's particular strengths and emerging skills to plan program curricula.

Research activities from the TEACCH founders and proponents have focused primarily on describing the efficacy of these highly structured and routine-focused teaching methods in educating autistic children as an alternative to less structured environments (Bartak 1978; Bartak and Rutter 1973; Rutter and Bartak 1973; Schopler et al. 1971). Other literature describes the effectiveness of parent training and the ability to generalize skills to the home (Marcus et al. 1978; Short 1984). Outcome has been defined as measures of parent satisfaction (Schopler et al. 1981), decrease in levels of family stress, and decreases in parental depressive symptoms (Bristol and Schopler 1983; Bristol et al. 1993). Recently, Ozonoff and Cathcart (1998) described the implementation of a home-based TEACCH program with a quasi-experimental design for young children with autism. These authors concluded that implementation of a TEACCH-based program in the home resulted in developmental gains three to four times that of a no-treatment control group. This program was implemented by the parents in the home and was provided in addition to a school-based program described as using discrete trials methodology. Ozonoff and Cathcart's study provides some evidence for the appropriateness of melding alternative forms of teaching methodology and is the first study to specifically examine TEACCH principles with a comparison group, although subjects were not randomly assigned. It is likely that positive responses in the treatment group were at least partly a result of family motivation, because these were the first families to respond to a call for subjects. Finally, this study did not directly compare teaching methods. It is difficult to ascertain how much of the gain was achieved through the implementation of the TEACCH home program specifically and how much was due to the increase in program intensity alone. The authors further noted that the children more likely to show gains were also those with higher cognitive and language abilities initially.

Although TEACCH has been used throughout the world for some 30 years and has received considerable recognition by various state, federal, and international organizations, research proving its efficacy over alternative forms of treatment is scarce. As is the case with applied behavioral analysis, TEACCH has yet to indicate the relative merits of this type of program when given a choice between TEACCH-based classrooms and alternatively designed programs and classrooms for children with autistic spectrum disorders. Similar to the Lovaas-type applied behavioral analysis program, TEACCH is relatively more efficacious in proximity to its point of origin and training supports. External validation difficulties occur when programs are implemented by poorly trained staff who "read a manual" or attended a 2- to 5-day training session. Yet, the effect of TEACCH in the design of classrooms for children with autistic spectrum disorders cannot be underestimated because most are based on a structured teaching model and use elements of TEACCH in terms of visual orientation and structuring of the environment.

Inclusion

Inclusion is a term coined to describe the political position that children with mental, physical, or emotional disabilities are entitled to an education within the mainstream of public education. Although inclusion can be implemented in varying degrees, inclusion advocates mostly support the argument that the segregation of children by diagnosis or disability is not in the children's best interest. Advocates of "full inclusion" argue that children should be integrated into regular education classrooms at all times.

The underpinnings of inclusion are based primarily on two arguments: 1) segregating children in special classes or programs denies these children access to regular classes and normal experiences, and 2) segregated services have not resulted in adequate education for disabled students (i.e., most disabled pupils remain disabled even after receiving special education). The arguments for inclusion sound similar to those for another movement—mainstreaming—but there are important differences. Mainstreaming disabled children typically has involved integrating children when the child showed that he or she could successfully participate in the regular planned activities within the regular education class. Inclusion advocates typically argue that mainstreaming efforts have forced the disabled child to "earn" time in the integrated settings. Inclusion advocates typically support the notion that each child has a right to be included and that necessary support services and accommodations to the child's disability must be made within the regular education classrooms. It is important to note that this is a political distinction rather than one that has been empirically well supported (Kaufman and Hallahan 1995).

Research regarding the efficacy of inclusion for children with disabilities is equivocal and does not support the notion that inclusion benefits all children with developmental problems (Siegel 1996a). Most of the literature consists of case reports, model program descriptions, and position papers, with few empirical studies published in scientific journals. Empirical data published to date have not shown benefit for children with severe disabilities and report more positive outcomes for children with milder impairment. Of those children with positive outcomes, gains were found not to persist beyond a short period (3–6 months) or to generalize to new settings (Hundert and Houghton 1992).

Specific (Nonpharmacological) Treatment Approaches for Autism

Other research has examined specific teaching strategies that address specific learning problems that are characteristic of children with autistic spectrum disorders, such as generalization of skills, functional communication, and social skills. Such approaches are numerous and not always specifically designed for children with autism. Reviewed here are four examples of autism-specific treatments that have received wide dissemination. This is not an exhaustive list of treatment approaches: Those lacking both confirmatory empirical data and specificity for treatment of PDDs, such as auditory integration training (Berard 1993; Tomatis 1977) or sensory integration (Ayres 1979), are not included, nor are fairly new approaches that may be promising for children with autism, such as integrated peer play groups (Wolfberg and Schuler 1993) and Fast For Word, a computer-assisted instructional method for auditory retraining (Merzenich et al. 1996). Included are examples of autism-specific treatment that have been experimentally or clinically supported. These include pivotal response training (generalization and independence), floor time (social reciprocity), the picture exchange communication system (instrumental communication), and social stories (understanding of the mental states of others).

Pivotal Response Training

Pivotal response training is designed to ameliorate some of the difficulties inherent in the assumptions about learning that are not congruent with what has been described here as social interaction–based autistic learning disabilities (see Tables 6–1 and 6–2). The large majority of the work in this area for children with autistic spectrum disorders can be attributed to the efforts of Robert Koegel and Laura Schreibman. Pivotal response training (Koegel and Schreibman 1977) involves teaching "pivotal" behaviors, or behaviors that are applicable across a wide variety of contexts with naturally occurring consequences. These procedures have proved superior to earlier implementation of principles of applied behavioral analysis in teaching students with autistic spectrum disorders appropriate skills through self-management of behaviors such as motor stereotypies and functional communication (Koegel and Frea 1993; Koegel and Koegel 1986; Koegel et al. 1994). Over time, these methods have been elaborated in related experimental studies of motivation, choice, and heuristics (Koegel and Koegel 1995).

Floor Time

The approach discussed in this section is what Stanley Greenspan termed a developmental, individual difference (DIR), relationship-based approach to intervention—also known as *floor time.* The basic premise to this approach is to build increasingly larger circles of interaction between child and adult in a developmentally based sequence (Greenspan 1992). Treatment is described as beginning with simple two-way communication and should be self-gratifying and works up to increasingly symbolic interactions as the child progresses. One underpinning for floor time is that because children with autism often have hyper- or hyposensitive sensory responses, careful building of circles should exfoliate these sensitivities to reveal a child with a capacity for more typical social reciprocity.

No empirical literature has described the utility of floor time for children with autism, however. Increasing popularity and implementation of this approach appear related to case testimonials and use by child mental health professionals who now can apply already-familiar play therapy–like techniques to the autistic population.

Greenspan and Weider (1997) provided a review of 200 charts indicating that 58% of the children achieved "very good" outcomes, although outcome was not empirically defined. Furthermore, the children studied were not necessarily classified as having PDD or autism according to any DSM criteria. Greenspan (1992) appeared to classify those with autistic spectrum disorders as falling along a spectrum with multisystem developmental disabilities and reactive attachment disorders (categories that have been neither empirically validated nor empirically delineated from autistic spectrum disorders [Siegel 1999]). Thus far, because of these difficulties, it is unclear for whom floor time may be most appropriate because it is unclear which population of children, if any, is deriving benefit.

Picture Exchange Communication System

The picture exchange communication system has proven successful in accelerating communication for young children beginning treatment and for those who are likely to remain nonverbal (Bondy and Frost 1994). The program teaches a functional communication system based on initiation of communicative interactions. Behavior-based instructional methods are used to teach students to exchange a picture of an item for the desired object or activity. This system capitalizes on the typically more developed visual skills of persons with autistic spectrum disorders. It also circumvents difficulties with abstract concept formation when persons are required to use symbolic means such as verbal language and sign to communicate. This method is designed to prime receptive and expressive communicative functions in young children who have had difficulty understanding the function of communicative exchanges and their ability to affect the behaviors of others to obtain specific and desired outcomes. For individuals who have a more difficult time learning language and are likely to remain nonverbal, it provides them with a form of functional communication and can lead to a decrease in later maladaptive behaviors that are often attributed to poor communicative effectiveness.

Social Stories

Social stories, a relatively new strategy for promoting desired social behavior, describe specific social situations along with appropriate social responses in clear, concrete terms (Gray 1995). Stories are individualized to the student and situation and typically begin with identifying a situation for the student with words or pictures, presenting the story to the student along with a model of the desired behavior. Another emphasis is on promoting the student's learning and planning for generalization. The method models social skills for those with established receptive and expressive capacities but who lack social understanding or intuition. Reports of effectiveness are limited to case presentations. This method, therefore, appears to work best with higher-functioning children with autistic spectrum disorders who want to be more successful in social interactions but are unable to do so. Thus, it is best regarded as part of an intervention program for some children and is not accessible to those with significant language understanding and use difficulties.

Behaviorally Focused Treatments

Reviewed thus far are omnibus treatments for PDDs, as well as exemplar autism-specific intervention approaches that target specific aspects of clinical presentation. Behaviorally based treatments are often combined with pharmacotherapy as part of a unified approach to addressing an individual child's full range of autism symptoms.

Pharmacotherapy

Medication should be given as part of a comprehensive program of treatment. Medications should target specific symptoms and should be chosen on the basis of what is known to be effective. The history of medication use in autism is a cautionary tale: medications that initially appear promising on the basis of a few open trials are found to be ineffective when careful work is done, or medications are touted as useful without any clinical trials at all. All too often, there seems to be an unseemly rush to try the latest psychoactive medication before adequate studies have been done to identify the proper dosage or untoward reactions and long-term effects. The goal of this section is to review those psychoactive medications that are currently available and that have undergone at least one open clinical trial, with a view to identifying which medications appear to be useful and safe in persons with autism or Asperger's disorder.

Stimulants

Stimulants are used in autism and Asperger's disorder for much the same purpose that they are used in general in child psychiatry—to decrease hyperactivity and impulsivity and to improve attention span. Most studies of stimulant use in autism date back to the previous decade (for a review, see Campbell and Cueva 1995). It appears that the indications, treatment parameters, and success rates for the use of stimulants to treat hyperactivity in autism are no different from those used to treat attention-deficit/hyperactivity disorder alone.

For many years, it has been known that many persons with autism have elevated levels of serotonin in their platelets. When it became known that fenfluramine, a medication developed as an appetite suppressant, could lower blood serotonin levels, a study was begun to learn if the medication would lower blood serotonin levels in autism and if it did so, whether social and language skills improved (Geller et al. 1982). Although fenfluramine has been shown to reduce blood serotonin in persons with autism, careful studies have found that it does not improve social or communicative skills or intellectual functioning (Campbell et al. 1988; Leventhal et al. 1993). Although modest decreases in hyperactivity resulted, fenfluramine was not considered superior to stimulants for this use.

Naltrexone

The rationale for the use of the opioid antagonist naltrexone to treat autism was based on a hypothesis by Herman and Panksepp (1978) that heightened activity in brain opioid systems could lead to an inhibition of social attachment in persons with autism. Recent studies of this hypothesis have been disappointing. Willemsen-Swinkels et al. (1999) reported that six children who received naltrexone for 6 months benefited in terms of showing a decrease in hyperactivity, but no improvements in social or adaptive functioning were noted. Double-blind studies have reported that although hyperactivity and restlessness were reduced (Campbell et al. 1990; Feldman et al. 1999; Kolmen et al. 1997; Willemsen-Swinkels et al. 1999), there was no effect on discriminative learning (Campbell et al. 1990; Willemsen-Swinkels et al. 1999), communication skills (Feldman et al. 1999), or self-injurious behaviors (Zingarelli et al. 1992). Bouvard and colleagues (1995) suggested that a small subgroup of autistic children, defined in terms of certain plasma abnormalities, might have shown some improvement in communication and sociability, but this has not been confirmed by others. No investigators have reported problems with side effects following administration of naltrexone.

Clonidine

Jaselskis et al. (1992) used a double-blind, placebo-controlled approach to administer clonidine to eight autistic subjects who also had symptoms of inattention, impulsivity, irritability, and hyperactivity. These latter symptoms improved in comparison to placebo, as did oppositional behavior. No other behavioral changes were noted. Side effects of drowsiness and hypotension in some children suggested that the use of clonidine as a treatment for attentional problems and hyperactivity might be limited.

Antidepressants

Although tricyclic antidepressants have been used in the past to treat symptoms of depression, irritability, and aggression in persons with autism, the use of imipramine and desipramine has faded in recent years, in part because of concerns of the latter's cardiac effects. Interest has shifted to clomipramine in the past several years. An early double-blind study (Gordon et al. 1993) of 30 children with autism reported that clomipramine was superior to desipramine and placebo in reducing stereotypies, anger, and compulsive ritualized behaviors. In the same study, both clomipramine and desipramine were superior to placebo in reducing hyperactivity. An open-label trial (Brodkin et al. 1997) of clomipramine in adult autistic subjects was encouraging, but some patients had clinically significant adverse effects. Eighteen of 33 subjects were classified as "very much improved" or "much improved" in terms of repetitive thoughts and behaviors and aggression. The authors also reported modest improvements in social relatedness in a few subjects. Side effects included seizures in 3 patients, 2 of whom were being treated for a known seizure disorder. Sanchez et al. (1996) reported another open study of clomipramine in 8 children that had less encouraging results. Although target symptoms were similar to those in the previous studies (stereotypies, aggression, hyperactivity), only 1 child improved (moderately) and 6 were rated as worse. They reported that 1 child developed acute urinary retention from the medication.

As might be expected, the introduction of the selective serotonin reuptake inhibitors (SSRIs) has led to studies of these medications in autism. In several open-label trials (Awad 1996; McDougle et al. 1998) the SSRIs appeared to be effective in decreasing symptoms of hyperactivity, restlessness, and agitation or in reducing obsessions and intense preoccupations. The only double-blind, placebo-controlled study of SSRIs was a study of fluvoxamine in 30 adults with autistic disorder (McDougle et al. 1996). Fifty-three percent of the subjects were categorized as responders over 12 weeks. Fluvoxamine was superior to placebo in reducing repetitive thoughts and behavior, in improving maladaptive behavior and aggression, and, to a lesser degree, in improving social relatedness. Few side effects occurred.

Antipsychotics

Although for some years, haloperidol was the antipsychotic of choice in treating autistic disorder, the modesty of the improvements attributable to haloperidol and the risk it posed for tardive dyskinesia have led clinicians to turn to the new class of "atypical" antipsychotics in their search for more effective psychopharmacological agents. Within this class, risperidone has been the most often investigated. The studies (McDougle et al. 1997; Nicolson et al. 1998; Perry et al. 1997) all have been open label and nonblinded. The results indicate that in dosages of between 1 and 2 mg/day, risperidone appears to be effective in reducing overactivity and aggression, impulsivity, and obsessive preoccupations. To a lesser degree, it may also increase socialization. The measures of socialization used in these studies do not appear to have been especially robust, or at least not as robust as those that measured hyperactivity and aggression. Except for moderate amounts of weight gain in some subjects, few side effects were noted. An open-label, 12-week study of olanzapine also has been reported (Potenza et al. 1999). Seven patients completed the study, six of whom were deemed responders. Motor restlessness and hyperactivity, self-injurious behavior, repetitive behaviors, and social relatedness and anxiety were among those symptoms reported as improved. As was found with risperidone, the main side effect of olanzapine was a moderate degree of weight gain.

Vitamin B_6 and Magnesium

Claims that high-dose vitamin B_6 and magnesium are effective in treating autism have been advocated for more than 30 years. Two reviews (Kleijnen and Knipschild 1991; Pfeiffer et al. 1995) concluded that few scientific data support such assertions, which are largely based on anecdotal accounts and open trials without placebo control. A recent double-blind, placebo-controlled study (Findling et al. 1997) concluded that the treatment was ineffective in ameliorating autistic behaviors.

Pharmacological interventions appear to have little to offer in ameliorating the social relationship disturbances that are paramount in autism. The only medications that appear to have a possibly salutary effect on social relatedness are the atypical antipsychotics, especially olanzapine. However, few studies have been done and have involved only open trials. Also, several medications can ameliorate symptoms of overactivity, impulsivity, aggressivity, stereotypies, and, in some instances, obsessional behaviors. In choosing a medication to treat these symptoms, safety and absence of serious side effects would seem to be especially important considerations. The SSRIs seem particularly well suited to fill this role. Were it not for the propensity to cause weight gain, the atypical antipsychotics also would be recommendable. However, studies to compare the relative effectiveness of the various SSRIs with that of the atypical antipsychotics are needed. Such studies may eventually be done, but they may be displaced by studies of the newer mood stabilizers, antidepressants, and antipsychotics that will soon be introduced. As more medications are developed, we will need many more studies than have been done in the past. We hope that some of the current or newly introduced medications might even help to alleviate some of the core social and interpersonal disabilities of persons with autism and Asperger's disorder. It is also worthwhile to note that pharmacological studies seldom control or report concomitant behavioral treatments. Future research will need to elucidate proportions of variance in outcomes of medical and behavior-based treatment.

Conclusions and Future Research

Review of the empirical treatment research for children with autistic disorders identifies several difficulties and several opportunities for future research. To date, no empirical studies have used the most rigorous type of experimental design—randomized assignment to experimental and control groups—either for behavior-based or for most pharmacological treatments. Realistically, this would be extremely difficult to do, although quasi-experimental procedures such as carefully yoked control subjects or multiple baseline studies might be obtained. Comparison groups are often completely missing from treatment research design in autism. Very few protocols use examiners blind to key aspects of the research. The behavior-based studies virtually never measure or control for implementation of the intervention itself (quality control). With regard to outcomes, measurements also varied widely. Behavior rating–based outcomes assessing changes in hyperactivity, sociability, irritability, aggressiveness, and so on are subject to variation according to the setting in which the child is observed, the identity of the respondent (e.g., parent or teacher), and the duration of the time sample. In behavior-based treatment research, most problematic appears to be the relative change in IQ scores, particularly when using disparate measures from pre- to posttreatment. Because of deficits and variations in "readiness to learn skills" (attending, imitation, following direction), most young autistic children will have wide discrepancies in IQ scores based on instruments that place relatively more emphasis on these skills (Bayley Scales of Infant Development, 2nd Edition; Wechsler Preschool and Primary Scale of Intelligence—Revised; Stanford-Binet Intelligence Scale, 4th Edition) than on more nonverbal instruments that require less adult directives (Merrill-Palmer Scale of Mental Tests, Leiter International Performance Scale). Our own clinical experience has indicated that children can show anywhere from 8- to 12-month discrepancies when administered Bayley and Merrill-Palmer scales on the same occasion. This can translate to an approximate 27- to 40-point IQ difference in the same child at the same point in time. Therefore, factors related to learning readiness, cooperation and motivation, receptive language, and the performance versus verbal construction of the test all can skew outcome measures. This makes comparisons across studies using different measures of IQ assessment, as well as within-subject comparisons, difficult. Other outcomes such as inclusion in mainstream education must be reported carefully along with information on use of one-to-one instructional assistance and other ancillary services.

Most important, research has not addressed which behavioral or medical interventions are effective for which children at which stage in their development. In addition, children with autism are often at different developmental stages in different domains of development simultaneously. Clinical experience in working with children with autistic spectrum disorders indicates that not all children respond to intervention in a similar manner. Future empirical research needs to provide empirical guidelines as to which behavior-based, which pharmacology-based, and which combined treatment can be best tailored to each child's specific autistic learning disabilities.

References

American Psychiatric Association: Diagnostic and Statistical Manual of Mental Disorders, 3rd Edition. Washington, DC, American Psychiatric Association, 1980

American Psychiatric Association: Diagnostic and Statistical Manual of Mental Disorders, 3rd Edition, Revised. Washington, DC, American Psychiatric Association, 1987

American Psychiatric Association: Diagnostic and Statistical Manual of Mental Disorders, 4th Edition. Washington, DC, American Psychiatric Association, 1994

Anderson SR, Campbell S, O'Malley C: The May Center for Early Childhood Education, in Preschool Education Programs for Children With Autism. Edited by Harris SL, Handleman JL. Austin, TX, Pro-Ed, 1993, pp 15–36

Awad GA: The use of selective serotonin reuptake inhibitors in young children with pervasive developmental disorders: some clinical observations. Can J Psychiatry 41:361–366, 1996

Ayres JA: Sensory Integration and the Child. Los Angeles, CA, Western Psychological Services, 1979

Baer D: Quasi-random assignment can be as convincing as random assignment. Am J Ment Retard 4:373–375, 1997

Baron-Cohen S: Mind-Blindness: An Essay on Autism and Theory. Cambridge, MA, MIT Press, 1995

Bartak L: Educational approaches, in Autism: A Reappraisal of Concept and Treatment. Edited by Rutter M, Schopler E. New York, Plenum, 1978, pp 423–438

Bartak L, Rutter M: Special educational treatment of autistic children: a comparative study. J Child Psychol Psychiatry 14:162–179, 1973

Berard G: Hearing Equals Behavior. New Canaan, CT, Keats, 1993

Bondy AS, Frost LA: The Delaware autistic program, in Preschool Education Programs for Children With Autism. Edited by Harris SL, Handleman JL. Austin, TX, Pro-Ed, 1994, pp 37–54

Bouvard MP, Leboyer M, Launay JM, et al: Low-dose naltrexone effects on plasma chemistries and clinical symptoms in autism: a double-blind, placebo-controlled study. Psychiatry Res 58:191–201, 1995

Bristol MM, Schopler E: Stress and coping in families of autistic adolescents, in Autism in Adolescents and Adults. Edited by Schopler E, Mesibov GB. New York, Plenum, 1983, pp 251–278

Bristol MM, Gallagher JJ, Holt KD: Maternal depressive symptoms in autism: response to psychoeducational intervention. Rehabilitation Psychology 38:8–10, 1993

Brodkin ES, McDougle CJ, Naylor ST, et al: Clomipramine in adults with pervasive developmental disorders: a prospective open-label investigation. J Child Adolesc Psychopharmacol 7:109–121, 1997

Campbell M, Cueva JE: Psychopharmacology in child and adolescent psychiatry: a review of the past seven years, part I. J Am Acad Child Adolesc Psychiatry 34:1124–1132, 1995

Campbell M, Adams P, Small AM, et al: Efficacy and safety of fenfluramine in autistic children. J Am Acad Child Adolesc Psychiatry 27:434–439, 1988

Campbell M, Anderson LT, Small AM, et al: Naltrexone in autistic children: a double-blind and placebo-controlled trial. Psychopharmacol Bull 26:130–135, 1990

Dawson G, Osterling J: Early intervention in autism, in The Effectiveness of Early Intervention. Edited by Guralnick MJ. Baltimore, MD, Paul H Brookes, 1996, pp 307–326

Feldman HM, Kolmen BK, Gonzaga AM: Naltrexone and communication skills in young children with autism. J Am Acad Child Adolesc Psychiatry 38:587–593, 1999

Findling RL, Maxwell K, Scotese-Wojtila L, et al: High-dose pyridoxine and magnesium administration in children with autistic disorder: an absence of salutary effects in a double-blind, placebo-controlled study. J Autism Dev Disord 27:467–478, 1997

Geller E, Ritvo ER, Freeman BJ, et al: Preliminary observations on the effects of fenfluramine on blood serotonin and symptoms in three autistic boys. N Engl J Med 307:165–169, 1982

Gordon CT, State RC, Nelson JE, et al: A double-blind comparison of clomipramine, desipramine, and placebo in the treatment of autistic disorder. Arch Gen Psychiatry 50:441–447, 1993

Gray C: Teaching children with autism to "read" social situations, in Teaching Children With Autism: Strategies to Enhance Communication and Socialization. Edited by Quill K. Albany, NY, Delmar, 1995

Greenspan SI: The traditional and developmental approaches to therapy with infants, young children, and their families: an introduction to floor time, in Infancy and Early Childhood: The Practice of Clinical Assessments and Intervention With Emotional and Developmental Challenges. Madison, CT, International Universities Press, 1992, pp 431–477

Greenspan SI, Weider S (with Simons R): The Child With Special Needs—Encouraging Intellectual and Emotional Growth. Reading, MA, Addison-Wesley, 1997

Gresham FM, MacMillian DL: Autistic recovery? An analysis and critique of the empirical evidence on the Early Intervention Project. Behavior Disorders 22:185–201, 1995

Harris SL, Handleman JS: Preschool programs for children with autism, in Preschool Education Programs for Children With Autism. Edited by Harris SL, Handleman JS. Austin, TX, Pro-Ed Press, 1994, pp 1–13

Harris SL, Handleman JS, Kristoff B, et al: Changes in language development among autistic and peer children in segregated preschool settings. J Autism Dev Disord 20:23–31, 1990

Heflin JL, Simpson RL: Interventions for children and youth with autism: prudent choices in a world of exaggerated claims and empty promises, part I: interventions and treatment option review. Focus on Autism and Other Developmental Disabilities 13(4):194–211, 1998

Herman B, Panksepp J: Effects of morphine and naloxone on social attachment in infant guinea pigs. Pharmacol Biochem Behav 9:213–220, 1978

Hundert J, Houghton A: Promoting social interaction of children with disabilities in integrated preschools: a failure to generalize. Except Child 58:311–320, 1992

Jaselskis CA, Cook EHJ, Fletcher KE, et al: Clonidine treatment of hyperactive and impulsive children with autistic disorder. J Clin Psychopharmacol 12:322–327, 1992

Kanner L: Autistic disturbances of affective contact. Nervous Child 2:217–250, 1943

Kaufman JM, Hallahan DP (eds): The Illusion of Full Inclusion: A Comprehensive Critique of a Current Special Education Bandwagon. Austin, TX, Pro-Ed, 1995

Kleijnen J, Knipschild P: Niacin and vitamin B_6 in mental functioning: a review of controlled trials in humans. Biol Psychiatry 29:931–941, 1991

Koegel RL, Frea WD: Treatment of social behaviors in autism through the modification of pivotal social skills. J Appl Behav Anal 26:369–377, 1993

Koegel RL, Koegel LK: Promoting generalized treatment gains through direct instruction of self-monitoring skills. Direct Instruction News 5:13–15, 1986

Koegel RL, Koegel LK: Teaching Children With Autism—Strategies for Initiating Positive Interactions and Improving Learning Opportunities. Baltimore, MD, Paul H Brookes, 1995

Koegel RL, Schreibman L: Teaching autistic children to respond to simultaneous multiple cues. J Exp Child Psychol 24:299–311, 1977

Koegel RL, Frea WD, Surratt AV: Self-management of problematic social behaviors, in Behavioral Issues in Autism. Edited by Schopler E, Mesibov GB. New York, Plenum, 1994, pp 81–97

Kolmen BK, Feldman HM, Handen BL, et al: Naltrexone in young autistic children: replication study and learning measures. J Am Acad Child Adolesc Psychiatry 36:1570–1578, 1997

Leventhal BL, Cook EHJ, Morford M, et al: Clinical and neurochemical effects of fenfluramine in children with autism. J Neuropsychiatry Clin Neurosci 5:307–315, 1993

Lovaas OI: Behavioral treatment and normal educational and intellectual functioning in young autistic children. J Consult Clin Psychol 55:3–9, 1987

Lovaas OI, Smith T: A comprehensive behavioral theory of autistic children: paradigm for research and practice. J Behav Ther Exp Psychiatry 20:17–29, 1989

Lovaas OI, Schreibman L, Koegel RL, et al: Selective responding by autistic children to multiple sensory input. J Abnorm Psychol 77:211–222, 1971

Marcus L, Lansing M, Andrews C, et al: Improvement of teaching effectiveness in parents of autistic children. Journal of the American Academy of Child Psychiatry 17:625–639, 1978

McClanahan L, Krantz P: The Princeton Child Development Institute, in Preschool Education Programs for Children With Autism. Edited by Harris SL, Handleman JL. Austin, TX, Pro-Ed, 1994, pp 107–126

McDougle CJ, Naylor ST, Cohen DJ, et al: A double-blind, placebo-controlled study of fluvoxamine in adults with autistic disorder (see comments). Arch Gen Psychiatry 53:1001–1008, 1996

McDougle CJ, Holmes JP, Bronson MR, et al: Risperidone treatment of children and adolescents with pervasive developmental disorders: a prospective open-label study (see comments). J Am Acad Child Adolesc Psychiatry 36:685–693, 1997

McDougle CJ, Brodkin ES, Naylor ST, et al: Sertraline in adults with pervasive developmental disorders: a prospective open-label investigation. J Clin Psychopharmacol 18:62–66, 1998

McIntosh H: Two autism studies fuel hope—and skepticism. American Psychological Association Monitor Online, September 1999. Available at: http://www.apa.org/monitor/sep99/pi3.html (accessed November 30. 2000)

Merzenich MM, Jenkins WM, Johnston O, et al: Temporal processing deficits of language-learning impaired children ameliorated by training. Science 271:77–81, 1996

Mesibov GB: A comprehensive program for serving people with autism and their families: the TEACCH model, in Autism in Children and Adults: Etiology, Assessment, and Intervention. Edited by Matson JL. Belmont, CA, Brookes/Cole, 1995, pp 85–97

Minshew N, Sweeny JA, Bauman ML: Neurological aspects of autism, in Handbook of Autism and Pervasive Developmental Disorders. Edited by Volkmar F, Cohen DJ. New York, Wiley, 1997, pp 344–369

Nicolson R, Awad G, Sloman L: An open trial of risperidone in young autistic children (see comments). J Am Acad Child Adolesc Psychiatry 37:372–376, 1998

Odom SL, Strain PS: Peer-mediated approaches to increasing children's social interaction: a review. Am J Orthopsychiatry 54:544–557, 1984

Olley JG, Robbins FR, Morelli-Robbins M: Current practices in early intervention for children with autism, in Preschool Issues in Autism. Edited by Schopler E, Van Bourgondien ME, Bristol M. New York, Plenum, 1993, pp 223–245

Ozonoff S, Cathcart K: Effectiveness of a home program intervention for young children with autism. J Autism Dev Disord 28:25–31, 1988

Perry R, Pataki C, Munoz-Silva DM, et al: Risperidone in children and adolescents with pervasive developmental disorder: pilot trial and follow-up. J Child Adolesc Psychopharmacol 7:167–179, 1997

Pfeiffer SI, Norton J, Nelson L, et al: Efficacy of vitamin B_6 and magnesium in the treatment of autism: a methodology review and summary of outcomes. J Autism Dev Disord 25:481–493, 1995

Potenza MN, Holmes JP, Kanes SJ, et al: Olanzapine treatment of children, adolescents, and adults with pervasive developmental disorders: an open-label pilot study. J Clin Psychopharmacol 19:37–44, 1999

Rogers SJ: Empirically supported comprehensive treatments for young children with autism. J Clin Child Psychol 27:168–179, 1998

Rogers SJ, Pennington BF: A theoretical approach to the deficits in infantile autism. Dev Psychopathol 3:137–162, 1991

Rutter M, Bartak L: Special educational treatment of autistic children: a comparative study, II: follow-up findings and implications for services. J Child Psychol Psychiatry 14:246–270, 1973

Sanchez LE, Campbell M, Small AM, et al: A pilot study of clomipramine in young autistic children. J Am Acad Child Adolesc Psychiatry 35:537–544, 1996

Schopler E: Premature popularization of Asperger syndrome, in Asperger Syndrome or High-Functioning Autism? Edited by Schopler E, Mesibov GB. New York, Plenum, 1998, pp 385–399

Schopler E, Brehm SS, Kinsbourne M, et al: Effects of treatment structure on development in autistic children. Arch Gen Psychiatry 24:415–421, 1971

Schopler E, Mesibov G, De Villis R, et al: Treatment outcome for autistic children and their families, in Frontiers of Knowledge in Mental Retardation, Vol 1: Social, Educational, and Behavioral Aspects. Edited by Mittler P. Baltimore, MD, University Park Press, 1981, pp 293–301

Schopler E, Mesibov GB, Hearsey KA: Structured teaching in the TEACCH system, in Learning and Cognition in Autism. Edited by Schopler E, Mesibov GB. New York, Plenum, 1995, pp 243–268

Sheinkopf S, Siegel B: Home-based behavioral treatment of young children with autism. J Autism Dev Disord 28:15–23, 1998

Short A: Short term treatment outcome using parents as cotherapists for their own autistic children. J Child Psychol Psychiatry 25:443–458, 1984

Siegel B: Is the emperor wearing clothes? Social policy and the empirical support for full inclusion of children with disabilities in the preschool and early elementary years. Society for Research in Child Development Social Policy Report 10(2–3):2–17, 1996a

Siegel B: The World of the Autistic Child: Understanding and Treating Autistic Spectrum Disorders. New York, Oxford University Press, 1996b

Siegel B: Autistic learning disabilities and individualizing treatment for autistic spectrum disorders. Infants and Young Children 12:27–36, 1999

Siegel B: Autistic Learning Disabilities: Designing, Implementing and Evaluating Programs for Children With Autistic Spectrum Disorders. New York, Oxford University Press (in press)

Strain PS, Kohler FW: Social skill intervention with young handicapped children: some new conceptualizations and directions, in Early Intervention for Infants and Children With Handicaps: An Empirical Base. Edited by Odom SL, Karnes MB. Baltimore, MD, Paul H Brookes, 1988, pp 129–143

Tomatis A: L'Oreille et la Vie. Paris, France, Laffont, 1977

Willemsen-Swinkels SH, Buitelaar JK, Berckelaer-Onnes IA, et al: Brief report: six months continuation treatment in naltrexone-responsive children with autism: an open-label case-control design. J Autism Dev Disord 29:167–169, 1999

Wolfberg PJ, Schuler AL: Integrated play groups: a model for promoting the social and cognitive dimensions of play in children with autism. J Autism Dev Disord 23:467–489, 1993

Zingarelli G, Ellman G, Hom A, et al: Clinical effects of naltrexone on autistic behavior. Am J Ment Retard 97:57–63, 1992

7

Attention-Deficit/ Hyperactivity Disorder

Joseph Biederman, M.D.
Thomas Spencer, M.D.
Timothy Wilens, M.D.
Ross Greene, Ph.D.

Attention-deficit/hyperactivity disorder (ADHD) is defined in DSM-IV (American Psychiatric Association 1994) as a behavioral disorder of childhood onset (by age 7 years) characterized by symptoms of inattentiveness and hyperactivity-impulsivity (Table 7–1). Based on the type of symptoms that predominate, DSM-IV recognizes a combined type in which both inattention and hyperactivity-impulsivity symptoms are present, a predominantly inattentive subtype, and a predominantly hyperactive-impulsive subtype. In addition, DSM-IV also recognizes the category of ADHD not otherwise specified (NOS) for individuals presenting with atypical features.

ADHD is one of the major clinical and public health problems in the United States in terms of morbidity and disability in children and adolescents. It is estimated to affect at least 5% of school-age children. Its effect on society is enormous in terms of financial cost, the stress to families, the effect on schools, and the damaging effects on self-esteem. Al-

TABLE 7–1. Pharmacotherapy for disruptive behavior disorders

Disorder	Main characteristics	Pharmacotherapy
Attention-deficit/hyperactivity disorder (ADHD)	Inattentiveness, impulsivity, hyperactivity 50% will continue to manifest the disorder into adulthood	*First line:* Stimulants (70% response; for uncomplicated ADHD; caution in patients with tic disorders) *Second line:* TCAs (70% response; first line for patients with comorbid mood or anxiety disorders and for patients with ADHD and tics). Requires serum-level and cardiovascular monitoring Bupropion *Third line:* Clonidine, guanfacine (first line for patients with ADHD and tics) *Fourth line:* MAOIs Combined pharmacotherapy for treatment-resistant patients
Conduct disorder (CD)	Persistent and pervasive patterns of aggressive and antisocial behaviors Often associated with ADHD, mood disorder, and bipolar disorder	*Core disorder:* No specific pharmacotherapy available Behavioral treatment *Comorbid Axis I disorders* (e.g., ADHD, mood disorder, mania, psychosis, anxiety): Treat the underlying disorder—anti-ADHD agents for ADHD, antimanic agents for mania, SSRIs for mood disorder, antianxiety agents for anxiety, and α-adrenergic agents and β-blockers for agitation, aggression, and self-abuse
Oppositional defiant disorder (ODD)	A pattern of persistent oppositionalism and defiance	

Note. MAOIs = monoamine oxidase inhibitors; SSRIs = selective serotonin reuptake inhibitors; TCAs = tricyclic antidepressants.

though the etiology of ADHD is unknown, data from family genetic, twin, adoption, and segregation analysis strongly suggest a genetic etiology. Indeed, the genetic contribution appears to be substantial as suggested by the very high heritability coefficients (mean = 0.8) associated with this disorder. Preliminary molecular genetic studies have implicated several candidate genes, including the dopamine D_2 and D_4 (*DRD4–7*) receptors as well as the dopamine transporter (*DAT-1*) (Faraone et al. 1999). It is of note that both dopamine and norepinephrine, neurotransmitters that are thought to mediate the response to anti-ADHD pharmacotherapy, are potent agonists of the D_4 receptor.

Data from follow-up studies indicate that children with ADHD are at risk for maintaining and developing new psychiatric disorders in adolescence and adulthood, including antisocial and substance use disorders (tobacco, alcohol, and drugs). Follow-up data also document that the disorder persists into adulthood in a substantial number of children and that ADHD may be a common adult diagnosis (Spencer et al. 1998a). In recent years, there has been an increasing recognition that ADHD is highly heterogeneous with high levels of psychiatric (disruptive [conduct and oppositional defiant disorder], mood [unipolar and bipolar], and anxiety disorders), cognitive (learning disability), and social (social disability, nonverbal learning disability) disorders. Neuroimaging studies identified subtle anomalies in the frontal cortex and in projecting subcortical structures (Faraone and Biederman 1999), and dysregulation of catecholamine neurotransmission has been posited to underlie its pathophysiology (Zametkin and Rapoport 1987).

Pharmacotherapy Treatment Literature

Stimulants

An extensive literature has clearly documented the short-term efficacy of methylphenidate treatment, mostly in latency-age Caucasian boys (Spencer et al. 1997). A much more limited literature exists for stimulants at other ages and in females and ethnic minorities. Despite small numbers, the few studies of stimulants in adolescents reported response rates highly consistent with those seen in latency-age children. In contrast, the few studies on preschoolers appeared to indicate that young children respond less well to stimulant therapy, which suggests that ADHD in preschoolers may be more refractory to treatment. The literature clearly documents that treatment with stimulants improves not only abnormal behaviors of ADHD but also self-esteem and cognitive, social, and family function, supporting the importance of treating ADHD patients beyond school or work hours to include evenings, weekends, and vacations. Three recent controlled clinical trials documented the efficacy of methylphenidate, amphetamine and dextroamphetamine, and pemoline in adults with ADHD (Spencer et al. 1995; Wilens et al. 1999a). It is remarkable not only that these trials documented a highly clinically and statistically significant separation from placebo but also that the magnitude of effects was consistent with the pediatric trials.

Treatment with stimulants improves a wide variety of cognitive abilities (Barkley 1977; Klein 1987; Rapport et al. 1988), increases school-based productivity (Famularo and Fenton 1987), and improves performance in academic testing. However, despite these beneficial cognitive effects, it is important to be aware that patients with ADHD can manifest additional learning disabilities that do not respond to pharmacotherapy (Bergman et al. 1991; Faraone et al. 1993) but may respond to educational remediation.

Although stimulants are effective in the treatment of ADHD, it is estimated that at least 30% of affected individuals do not adequately respond or cannot tolerate stimulant treatment (Barkley 1977; Gittelman 1980; Spencer et al. 1996). In addition, because stimulants are short-acting drugs, they require multiple administrations during the day, including during school or work hours, which has an attendant effect on compliance. This problem may be offset by the development of an effective long-acting stimulant. This class of drugs often adversely affects sleep, making their use in the evening hours difficult when children and adults need the ability to concentrate to help them deal with daily demands and in interactions with family members and friends. In addition to these problems, the fact that stimulants are controlled substances continues to fuel worries in children, families, and the treating community and further inhibits their use. These fears are based on lingering concerns about the abuse potential of stimulant drugs by the child, family member, or his or her associates; the possibility of diversion; and safety concerns regarding the use of a controlled substance by patients who are impulsive and frequently have antisocial tendencies (Goldman et al. 1998). Similarly, the controlled nature of stimulant drugs poses important medicolegal concerns to the treating community that further increase the barriers to treatment.

In addition to these unresolved problems, it is increasingly evident that ADHD is frequently comorbid with mood and anxiety disorders, conditions that may adversely affect responsivity to stimulant drugs. For example, of pediatric studies that examined children with ADHD and depression and anxiety, 75% (6 of 8) reported that stimulants reduced ADHD symptoms less in children with comorbid mood and anxiety disorders (DuPaul et al. 1994; Pliszka 1989; Swanson et al. 1978; Tannock et al. 1995; Taylor et al. 1987; Voelker et al. 1983). Moreover, a recent report indicated that stimulants are poorly effective in the treatment of ADHD in the context of coexisting manic symptomatology and that their use in such patients may result in worsening of mood instability (Biederman et al. 1999b).

Antidepressants

Other than the psychostimulants, noradrenergic and dopaminergic active antidepressants such as secondary amine tricyclic antidepressants (TCAs) (Biederman et al. 1989a; Donnelly et al. 1986; Wilens et al. 1993), bupropion (Barrickman et al. 1995; Casat et al. 1989; Conners et al. 1996), and monoamine oxidase inhibitors (MAOIs) (Zametkin et al. 1985) have been found to be superior to placebo in controlled clinical trials (see Table 7–3 [later in this chapter] for doses and side effects). Possible advantages of these compounds over stimulants include a longer duration of action without symptom rebound or insomnia, greater flexibility in dosage, the option of monitoring plasma drug levels (for TCAs), minimal risk of abuse or dependence, and the potential treatment of comorbid internalizing symptoms. Although one open case series reported on the beneficial effects of the selective serotonin reuptake inhibitor (SSRI) fluoxetine in the treatment of ADHD (Barrickman et al. 1991), little other clinical or scientific evidence implicates serotonergic systems in the pathophysiology of ADHD.

Tricyclic Antidepressants

Perhaps the best-established second-line treatment for ADHD is the TCAs. Out of 33 studies (21 controlled, 12 open) evaluating TCAs in children and adolescents (n = 1139), and adults (n = 78), 91% reported positive effects on ADHD symptoms (Spencer et al. 1997). Imipramine and desipramine are the most studied TCAs followed by a handful of studies on other TCAs. Although most TCA studies (73%) were relatively brief, lasting a few weeks to several months, 9 studies (27%) reported enduring effects for up to 2 years. Outcomes in both short- and long-term studies were equally positive. Although 1 study (Quinn and Rapoport 1975) reported a 50% dropout rate after 1 year, it is noteworthy that in those who continued taking imipramine, improvement was sustained. More recent studies that used aggressive doses of TCAs reported sustained improvement for up to 1 year with desipramine (>4 mg/kg) (Biederman et al. 1986; Gastfriend et al. 1985) and nortriptyline (2.0 mg/kg) (Wilens et al. 1993). Although response was equally positive in all the dose ranges, it was more sustained in those studies that used higher doses. A high interindividual variability in TCA serum levels has been consistently reported for imipramine and desipramine, with little relation between serum level and daily dose, response, or side effects. In contrast, nortriptyline appears to have a positive association between dose and serum level (Wilens et al. 1993).

In the largest controlled study of a TCA in children, our group reported favorable results with desipramine in 62 clinically referred children with ADHD, most of whom had failed to respond to psychostimulant treatment (Biederman et al. 1989a). The study was a randomized, placebo-controlled, parallel-design, 6-week clinical trial. Clinically and statistically significant differences in behavioral improvement were found for desipramine (average daily dosage = 5 mg/kg) over placebo. Although the presence of comorbidity increased the likelihood of a placebo response, neither comorbidity with conduct disorder, depression, or anxiety nor a family history of ADHD yielded differential responses to desipramine treatment. In addition, patients with ADHD who received desipramine showed a substantial reduction in depressive symptoms compared with patients who received placebo. Similar results were observed in a similarly designed controlled clinical trial of desipramine in 41 adults with ADHD (Wilens et al. 1996b). Desipramine (average daily dosage = 150 mg, average serum level = 113 ng/mL) was statistically and clinically more effective than placebo. Sixty-eight percent of the desipramine-treated patients responded compared with none of the placebo-treated patients ($P < 0.0001$). Moreover, at the end of the study, the average severity of ADHD symptoms in patients receiving desipramine was reduced to below the level required to meet diagnostic criteria. Importantly, the full desipramine dose was achieved at week 2, but clinical response improved further over the following 4 weeks, indicating a latency of response. Response was independent of dose, serum desipramine level, sex, or lifetime psychiatric comorbidity with anxiety or depressive disorders.

In a prospective placebo-controlled discontinuation trial, we recently confirmed the efficacy of nortriptyline in dosages of up to 2 mg/kg/day in 35 school-age youth with ADHD (Prince et al. 1999). In that study, 80% of the youth responded by week 6 in the open phase. During the discontinuation phase, subjects randomized to placebo lost the anti-ADHD effect, whereas those receiving nortriptyline maintained a robust anti-ADHD effect. Youth with ADHD receiving nortriptyline also had more modest but statistically significant reductions in oppositionality and anxiety. Nortriptyline was well tolerated with some weight gain. Weight gain is frequently considered a desirable side effect in this population. In contrast, a systematic study in 14 youth with treatment-refractory ADHD receiving protriptyline (mean dose = 30 mg) reported less favorable results. Only 45% of the ADHD youth responded or could tolerate protriptyline secondary to adverse effects (Wilens et al. 1996a).

Thirteen of the 33 TCA studies (39%) compared TCAs with stimulants. Four studies each reported that stimulants were superior to TCAs (Garfinkel et al. 1983; Gittelman-Klein 1974; Greenberg et al. 1975; Rapoport et al. 1974) or equal to TCAs (Gross 1973; Huessy and Wright 1970; Kupietz and Balka 1976; Rapport et al. 1993; Yepes et al. 1977), and three studies reported that TCAs were superior to stimulants (Watter and Dreyfuss 1973; Werry 1980; Winsberg et al. 1972). Analysis of response profiles indicated that TCAs consistently improve behavioral symptoms, as rated by clinicians, teachers, and parents, more than they affect cognitive function, as measured in neuropsychological testing (Gualtieri and Evans 1988; Quinn and Rapoport 1975; Rapport et al. 1993; Werry 1980). As noted earlier in this chapter, studies of TCAs have uniformly reported a robust response rate of ADHD symptoms in subjects with comorbid depression or anxiety (Biederman et al. 1993; Cox 1982; Wilens et al. 1993, 1995). In addition, studies of TCAs have consistently reported a robust response rate in subjects with ADHD and comorbid tic disorders (Dillon et al. 1985; Hoge and Biederman 1986; Riddle et al. 1988; Singer et al. 1994; Spencer et al.

1993a, 1993b). For example, in a recent controlled study, Spencer (1997) replicated data from a retrospective chart review indicating that desipramine had a robust beneficial effect on ADHD and tic symptoms. The potential benefits of TCAs in the treatment of ADHD have been clouded by concerns about their safety stemming from reports of sudden, unexplained death in four children with ADHD treated with desipramine (Riddle et al. 1991), although the causal link between desipramine and these deaths is uncertain (Biederman et al. 1995a).

Bupropion

The mixed dopaminergic/noradrenergic antidepressant bupropion has been shown to be effective for ADHD in children in a controlled multisite study ($N = 72$) (Casat et al. 1987, 1989; Conners et al. 1996) and in a comparison with methylphenidate ($N = 15$) (Barrickman et al. 1995). In an open study of adults with ADHD, sustained improvement was documented at 1 year at an average of 360 mg for 6–8 weeks (Wender and Reimherr 1990). A recent double-blind, controlled clinical trial of bupropion in adults with ADHD documented superiority over placebo (Wilens et al. 1999c), with an effect size highly consistent with the pediatric trials. Although bupropion has been associated with a slightly increased risk (0.4%) of drug-induced seizures relative to other antidepressants, this risk has been linked to high doses, a history of seizures, and eating disorders.

Monoamine Oxidase Inhibitors

Although a few studies suggested that MAOIs may be effective in juvenile and adult ADHD, their potential for hypertensive crisis associated with the irreversible MAOIs (e.g., phenelzine, tranylcypromine), with dietetic transgressions (tyramine-containing foods [e.g., most cheeses]), and with drug interactions (pressor amines, most cold medicines, amphetamines) seriously limits their use. Although MAOIs are not available in the United States, this "cheese effect" may be obviated with the reversible MAOIs (e.g., moclobemide), which have shown promise in one open trial (Trott et al. 1991). A single small open study (Barrickman et al. 1991) suggested that fluoxetine may be beneficial in the treatment of ADHD in children; however, the usefulness of SSRIs in the treatment of core ADHD symptoms is not supported by clinical experience (National Institute of Mental Health 1996). Similarly uncertain is the usefulness of the mixed serotonergic/noradrenergic atypical antidepressant venlafaxine in the treatment of ADHD. In four open studies of adults with ADHD ($N = 61$), a 77% response rate was reported in those who completed the studies, but 21% dropped out because of side effects (Adler et al. 1995; Findling et al. 1996; Hornig-Rohan and Amsterdam 1995; Reimherr et al. 1995). Additionally, a single open study of venlafaxine in 16 children with ADHD reported a 50% response rate in those who completed the study, with a 25% dropout rate because of side effects, most prominently increased hyperactivity (Luh et al. 1996).

Tomoxetine

More promising results have been associated with the experimental noradrenergic specific reuptake inhibitor tomoxetine. An initial controlled clinical trial in adults documented efficacy and good tolerability (Spencer et al. 1998b). These initial encouraging results, coupled with extensive safety data in adults, fueled efforts at developing this compound for the treatment of pediatric ADHD, and an initial open study of this compound in pediatric

ADHD documented strong clinical benefits with excellent tolerability, including a safe cardiovascular profile (T. Spencer, J. Biederman, T. Wilens, J. Heiligenstein, and J. Rea, unpublished data, October 1999).

Antihypertensives

Although clonidine is widely used in children with ADHD, only four studies (two controlled; *N* = 122 children) (Gunning 1992; Hunt 1987; Hunt et al. 1985; Steingard et al. 1993) have supported its efficacy. Treatment with clonidine appears to have mostly a behavioral effect in disinhibited and agitated youth, with limited effect on cognition. Several cases of sudden death have been reported in children treated with clonidine plus methylphenidate, raising concerns about the safety of this combination (Wilens and Spencer 1999). Even more limited is the literature on guanfacine. Only three small open studies of guanfacine in children and adolescents with ADHD have been done. In these studies, beneficial effects on hyperactive behaviors and attentional abilities were reported (Chappell et al. 1995; Horrigan and Barnhill 1995; Hunt et al. 1995).

β-noradrenergic blockers also have been studied for use in ADHD. An open study of propranolol for ADHD in adults with temper outbursts reported improvement at dosages of up to 640 mg/day (Mattes 1986). Another report indicated that β-blockers may be helpful in combination with the stimulants (Ratey et al. 1991). In a controlled study of pindolol in 52 children with ADHD, symptoms of behavioral dyscontrol and hyperactivity improved, with less apparent cognitive benefit (Buitelaar et al. 1996). However, prominent adverse effects such as nightmares and paresthesias led to discontinuation of the drug in all test subjects. An open study of nadolol in aggressive, developmentally delayed children with ADHD symptoms reported effective diminution of aggression but little apparent effect on ADHD symptoms (Connor et al. 1997).

Anxiolytics

A recent open study of 12 children with ADHD reported that the nonbenzodiazepine anxiolytic buspirone at 0.5 mg/kg/day improved both ADHD symptoms and psychosocial function (Malhotra and Santosh 1998). Buspirone has a high affinity to serotonin type 1A (5-HT_{1A}) receptors, both pre- and postsynaptic, as well as a modest effect on the dopaminergic system and α-adrenergic activity. However, a recent multisite controlled clinical trial of transdermal buspirone found that buspirone's effects were equivalent to those of placebo in a large sample of children with ADHD (Bristol-Myers Squibb, unpublished data). The old literature suggested that typical antipsychotics were effective in the treatment of ADHD in children, but their spectrum of both short-term (extrapyramidal reactions) and long-term (tardive dyskinesia) adverse effects greatly limits their usefulness. A recent meta-analysis pooling data from 10 studies provided preliminary evidence that carbamazepine may have activity in ADHD (Silva et al. 1996).

Nicotinic Drugs

In recent years, evidence has emerged that nicotinic dysregulation may contribute to the pathophysiology of ADHD. This is not surprising considering that nicotinic activation enhances dopaminergic neurotransmission (Mereu et al. 1987; Westfall et al. 1983). Independent lines of investigation have documented that ADHD is associated with an increased risk and earlier age at onset of cigarette smoking (Milberger et al. 1997; Pomerleau et al. 1995), that maternal smoking during pregnancy increases the risk for ADHD in the offspring, and that in utero exposure to nicotine in animals confers a heightened risk for an ADHD-like syndrome in the newborn (Fung 1988; Fung and Lau 1989; Johns et al. 1982; Milberger et al. 1996). In subjects without ADHD, central nicotinic activation has been shown to improve temporal memory (Meck and Church 1987), attention (Jones et al. 1992; Peeke and Peeke 1984; Wesnes and Warburton 1984), cognitive vigilance (Jones et al. 1992; Parrott and Winder 1989; Wesnes and Warburton 1984), and executive function (Wesnes and Warburton 1984).

Support for a "nicotinic hypothesis" of ADHD can be derived from a recent study that evaluated the therapeutic effects of nicotine in the treatment of ADHD in adults (Levin et al. 1996). Although this controlled clinical trial in adults with ADHD documented that a commercially available transdermal nicotine patch resulted in significant improvement of ADHD symptoms, working memory, and neuropsychological functioning (Levin et al. 1996), the trial was very short (2 days) and included only a handful of patients. More promising results supporting the usefulness of nicotinic drugs in ADHD derives from a recent controlled clinical trial of ABT-418 in adults with ADHD (Wilens et al. 1999b). ABT-418 is a central nervous system cholinergic nicotinic activating agent with structural similarities to nicotine. Phase I studies of this compound in humans indicated its low abuse liability, as well as adequate safety and tolerability in elderly adults (Abbott Laboratories, unpublished data). A double-blind, placebo-controlled, randomized crossover trial comparing a transdermal patch of ABT-418 (75 mg/day) with placebo in adults with DSM-IV ADHD showed that a significantly higher proportion of the adults were very much improved while receiving ABT-418 than while receiving placebo (40% vs. 13%; χ^2 test = 5.3, $P = 0.021$). These preliminary results suggest that nicotinic analogues may have activity in ADHD.

Other Agents

Several other compounds, including dopamine agonists (amantadine and L-dopa) (Gittelman-Klein 1987) and amino acid precursors (DL-phenylalanine and L-tyrosine) (Reimherr et al. 1987), have been evaluated and found to be ineffective in the treatment of ADHD. In addition, a controlled study failed to find therapeutic benefits in ADHD for the antiserotonergic, anorexigenic drug fenfluramine (Donnelly et al. 1989).

Other Disruptive Behavior Disorders: Conduct Disorder and Oppositional Defiant Disorder

In DSM-IV, conduct disorder is conceptualized as a childhood-onset disorder characterized by antisocial and aggressive behaviors. Children with conduct disorder are at very high risk to develop adult antisocial personality disorder and substance use disorders. As its name implies, oppositional defiant disorder is characterized by oppositional and obstinate behaviors. Although very taxing to families, oppositional defiant disorder does not share with conduct disorder its serious adult outcome. Although no specific pharmacotherapy for conduct disorder or oppositional defiant disorder is available, several controlled investigations documented the efficacy of mood stabilizers (Platt et al. 1984) and antipsychotics in reducing aggression and explosiveness (but not sociopathy) in children with conduct disorder. These findings are consistent with mounting evidence linking some forms of conduct disorder and oppositional defiant disorder with bipolar and nonbipolar mood disorders (hence dysphoric) (Biederman et al. 1999a; Frazier et al. 1999). Studies also have shown a significant decrease in aggressive behaviors as a result of treatment with behavioral management techniques, whether focused on the child's coping skills or the parents' management skills (Greene 1998; Quay 1986). When conduct disorder and oppositional defiant disorder co-occur with ADHD, mood disorders, or anxiety disorders, the treatment of the comorbid disorder can result in substantial clinical stabilization and facilitate the psychosocial treatment approach for the child with conduct disorder.

Pharmacological Treatment of Attention-Deficit/Hyperactivity Disorder

Stimulants

Stimulant drugs are the first class of compounds reported as effective in the treatment of the behavioral disturbances that are evident in children with ADHD (Table 7–2). Stimulants are sympathomimetic drugs structurally similar to endogenous catecholamines. The most commonly used compounds in this class include methylphenidate, amphetamine and dextroamphetamine, and magnesium pemoline. These drugs are thought to act both in the central nervous system and peripherally by enhancing dopaminergic and noradrenergic neurotransmission. Because the various stimulants have somewhat different mechanisms of action, some patients may respond preferentially to one or another (Greenhill et al. 1999).

Methylphenidate and amphetamine compounds are short-acting drugs with an onset of action within 30–60 minutes and a peak clinical effect usually seen between 1 and 3 hours after administration. Therefore, multiple daily administrations are required for a consistent daytime response. Slow-release preparations, with a peak clinical effect between 1 and 5 hours, are available for methylphenidate and dextroamphetamine and can often allow for a single dose to be administered in the morning that will last throughout the school day. Recent studies suggest that amphetamine and dextroamphetamine may have a somewhat longer duration of action than immediate-release methylphenidate and dextroamphetamine that could avoid in-school dosing. Similarly, magnesium pemoline is a longer-acting compound, thus allowing for effectiveness through the school day. Typically, stimulants have a rapid onset of action so that clinical response will be evident when a therapeutic dose has been obtained.

The usual daily dosage ranges from 1.0 to 2.0 mg/kg for methylphenidate and approximately half that for amphetamine compounds because they are about twice as potent as methylphenidate. The starting dosage is generally 2.5–5.0 mg/day given in the morning, and the dose is increased if necessary every few days by 2.5–5.0 mg in a divided-dose schedule. Because of the anorexigenic effects of the stimulants, it may be beneficial to administer the medicine after meals. The longer-acting magnesium pemoline is typically given once or twice daily in doses ranging from 1.0 to 2.5 mg/kg (pemoline is approximately three times less potent than methylphenidate). The typical starting dosage of pemoline is 18.75–37.5 mg/day, with increments in dose of 18.75 mg every few days thereafter until desired effects occur or side effects preclude further increments.

The early concern that optimal clinical efficacy is attained at the cost of impaired learning ability has not been confirmed (Gittelman-Klein 1987). In fact, studies indicate that

TABLE 7–2. Stimulants used in the pharmacotherapy of attention-deficit/hyperactivity disorder (ADHD)

Drug	Daily dose (mg/kg)	Daily dosage schedule	Main indications	Common adverse effects and comments
Methylphenidate	1.0–2.0	Two or three times		Available in long-acting preparation (effect less reliable)
Dextroamphetamine	0.3–1.0	Two or three times	ADHD; mental retardation + ADHD	Insomnia, decreased appetite, weight loss, depression, psychosis (rare, with very high doses), increase in heart rate and blood pressure (mild), possible reduction in growth velocity with long-term use, withdrawal effects and rebound phenomena Available in long-acting preparation (effect less reliable)
Mixed salts of levo- and dextro-amphetamine	0.5–1.5	Once or twice	Adjunct treatment in refractory depression	Long-acting
Magnesium pemoline	1.0–2.5	Once or twice		Rare serious hepatotoxicity; requires monitoring of liver function tests

Note. Doses are general guidelines. All dosages must be individualized with appropriate monitoring. Weight-corrected doses are less appropriate for obese children.

both behavior and cognitive performance improve with stimulant treatment in a dose-dependent fashion (Douglas et al. 1988; Klein 1987; Kupietz et al. 1988; Pelham et al. 1985; Rapport et al. 1987, 1989a, 1989b; Tannock et al. 1989). The literature on the association between clinical benefits in ADHD and plasma levels of stimulants has been equivocal and complicated by large inter- and intraindividual variability in plasma levels at constant oral doses (Gittelman-Klein 1987).

The most commonly reported side effects associated with the administration of stimulant medication are appetite suppression and sleep disturbances. The commonly reported sleep disturbance is delayed sleep onset, which usually accompanies late-afternoon or early-evening administration of the stimulant medications. Although less commonly reported, mood disturbances ranging from increased tearfulness to a full-blown major depression–like syndrome can be associated with stimulant treatment (Wilens and Biederman 1992). Other infrequent side effects include headaches, abdominal discomfort, increased lethargy, and fatigue.

Although the adverse cardiovascular effects of stimulants beyond heart rate and blood pressure have not been examined, mild increases in pulse and blood pressure of unclear clinical significance have been observed (Brown et al. 1984). Although less of a clinical concern in pediatric care, potential increases in blood pressure associated with stimulant drugs may be of greater clinical significance in the treatment of ADHD in adults. A stimulant-associated toxic psychosis also has been very rarely observed and usually in the context of either a rapid rise in the dosage or very high doses. The reported psychosis in children in response to stimulant medications resembles a toxic phenomenon (i.e., visual hallucinosis) and is dissimilar from the exacerbation of the psychotic symptoms present in schizophrenia. The development of psychotic symptoms in a child exposed to stimulants requires careful evaluation to rule out the presence of a preexisting psychotic disorder. Administration of magnesium pemoline has been associated with rare hypersensitivity reactions involving the liver accompanied by elevations in liver function studies (aspartate aminotransferase and alanine aminotransferase) after several months of treatment. Thus, baseline and repeat liver function studies are recommended with the administration of this compound. Because of increasing concerns about hepatotoxicity, the U.S. Food and Drug Administration (FDA) now requires biweekly liver function monitoring when pemoline is used.

Early reports indicated that children with a personal or family history of tic disorders were at greater risk for developing a tic disorder when exposed to stimulants (Lowe et al. 1982). However, more recent work has increasingly challenged this view (Comings and Comings 1988; Gadow et al. 1992, 1995). For example, in a controlled study of 34 children with ADHD and tics, Gadow et al. (1995) reported that methylphenidate effectively suppressed ADHD symptoms with only a weak effect on the frequency of tics. In a recent study of 128 boys with ADHD, Spencer et al. (1999) reported no evidence of earlier onset, greater rates, or worsening of tics in the subgroup exposed to stimulants. Although this work is reassuring, it is clear that more information is needed in larger numbers of subjects over longer periods to obtain closure on this issue. Until more is known, it seems prudent to weigh the risks and benefits on individual cases with appropriate discussion with the child and family about the benefits and pitfalls of the use of stimulants in children with ADHD and tics.

Similar uncertainties remain about the abuse potential of stimulants in children with ADHD. Despite the concern that ADHD may increase the risk of substance abuse in adolescents and young adults, to date no clear evidence indicates that children with ADHD who take stimulants abuse prescribed medication when their disorder is appropriately diagnosed and carefully monitored. Moreover, the most common abused substance in adolescents and adults with ADHD is marijuana and not stimulants (Biederman et al. 1995b). Furthermore, a recent report provided statistical evidence documenting that the use of stimulants and other pharmacological treatments for ADHD significantly decreased the risk for subsequent substance use disorders in ADHD youth (Biederman et al. 1999c).

Although concerns continue about the effect of long-term administration of stimulants on growth, recent work has begun to question this issue. Although stimulants routinely produce anorexia and weight loss, their effect on growth in height is much less certain. Initial reports suggested that a persistent stimulant-associated decrease in growth in height occurred in children (Mattes and Gittelman 1983; Safer et al. 1972), but other reports have failed to substantiate this claim (Gross 1976; Satterfield et al. 1979). Moreover, several studies showed that ultimate height appears to be unaffected if treatment is discontinued in adolescence (Gittelman and Mannuzza 1988). A recent study suggested that deficits in growth in height may be transient maturational delays associated with ADHD rather than stunting of growth in height in children with ADHD (Spencer et al. 1998c). If confirmed, this finding would not support the common practice of drug holidays in children with ADHD. However, it seems prudent to provide drug holidays or alternative treatment in children suspected of stimulant-associated growth deficits. This recommendation should be carefully weighed against the risk for exacerbation of symptoms caused by drug discontinuation. A transient behavioral deterioration can occur in some children when stimulant medications are abruptly discontinued. The prevalence of this phenomenon and the etiology are unclear. Rebound phenomena also may occur in some children between doses, creating an uneven, often disturbing clinical course. In those cases, alternative treatments should be considered.

Antidepressants

There are several main families of antidepressant medications (Table 7–3): TCAs (mixed neurotransmitter profile); MAOIs (mixed neurotransmitter profile); SSRIs (serotonergic-specific profile); atypical antidepressants such as bupropion (dopaminergic/noradrenergic profile), venlafaxine (serotonergic/noradrenergic profile), nefazodone (serotonergic/noradrenergic profile), and mirtazapine (serotonergic/noradrenergic profile); and the noradrenergic-specific reuptake inhibitors reboxetine and tomoxetine. Open and controlled studies have reported beneficial effects of noradrenergic antidepressant medications in children and adolescents with ADHD (noradrenergic agents, TCAs) (Biederman et al. 1989a) and serotonergic antidepressants in the treatment of obsessive-compulsive disorder (SSRIs) (DeVeaugh-Geiss et al. 1992; Geller et al. 1995), depression (SSRIs) (Emslie et al. 1997; Wagner et al. 1998), and enuresis (TCAs) (Gittelman 1980). Other childhood conditions that may benefit from antidepressant treatment include anxiety (serotonergic drugs) and tic disorders (TCAs, possibly other noradrenergic compounds) (Singer et al. 1994; Spencer 1997). The mechanism of action of antidepressant drugs appears to be due to various effects on pre- and postsynaptic receptors affecting the release and reuptake of brain neurotransmitters, including norepinephrine, serotonin, and dopamine. Although these agents have variable effects on various pre- and postsynaptic neurotransmitter systems, their effect and adverse-effect profiles differ greatly among the various classes of antidepressant drugs. Because a substantial interindividual variability in metabolism and elimination has been reported in children, the dose should always be individualized. Recent studies have begun to document striking similarities in pharmacokinetic profiles of children and adults for sertraline (Alderman et al. 1998), venlafaxine (Derivan 1995), and paroxetine (Findling et al. 1999).

The TCAs include the tertiary (imipramine, amitriptyline, and clomipramine) and the secondary (desipramine and nortriptyline) amine compounds. Treatment with a TCA should be initiated with a 10- or 25-mg dose and increased slowly every 4–5 days by 20%–30%. When a daily dosage of 3 mg/kg (or a lower effective dose) or 1.5 mg/kg for nortriptyline is reached, steady-state serum levels and an electrocardiogram (ECG) should be obtained. Typical dosage ranges for the TCAs are 2.0–5.0 mg/kg/day (1.0–3.0 mg/kg/day for nortriptyline). Common short-term adverse effects of the TCAs include anticholinergic effects, such as dry mouth, blurred vision, and constipation. However, no known deleterious effects are associated with chronic administration of these drugs. Gastrointestinal symptoms and vomiting may occur when these drugs are discontinued abruptly; thus, slow tapering of these medications is recommended. Because the anticholinergic effects of TCAs limit salivary flow, they may promote tooth decay.

Evaluations of short- and long-term effects of therapeutic doses of TCAs on the cardiovascular systems in children have found that TCAs are generally well tolerated, with only minor ECG changes associated with TCA treatment in daily oral dosages as high as 5 mg/kg. TCA-induced ECG abnormalities (conduction defects) have been consistently reported in children at doses higher than 3.5 mg/kg (Biederman et al. 1989b) (1.0 mg/kg for nortriptyline). Although of unclear hemodynamic significance, the development of conduction

TABLE 7–3. Antidepressants used in the pharmacotherapy of attention-deficit/hyperactivity disorder (ADHD)

Drug	Daily dose (mg/kg)	Daily dosage schedule	Main indications	Common adverse effects and comments
Tricyclic antidepressants (TCAs)				
Tertiary amines: Imipramine Amitriptyline Clomipramine *Secondary amines:* Desipramine Nortriptyline	2.0–5.0 (1.0–3.0 for nortriptyline); dose adjusted according to serum levels (therapeutic window for nortriptyline)	Once or twice	ADHD, enuresis, tic disorder, ?anxiety disorders, OCD (clomipramine)	Mixed mechanism of action (noradrenergic/serotonergic) Secondary amines are more noradrenergic Clomipramine is primarily serotonergic Narrow therapeutic index Overdoses can be fatal Anticholinergic effects (dry mouth, constipation, blurred vision) Weight loss Cardiovascular: mild increase in diastolic blood pressure and electrocardiogram (ECG) conduction parameters with daily doses > 3.5 mg/kg Treatment requires serum-level and ECG monitoring No known long-term side effects Withdrawal effects can occur (severe gastrointestinal symptoms, malaise) Risk of seizures

TABLE 7–3. Antidepressants used in the pharmacotherapy of attention-deficit/hyperactivity disorder (ADHD) *(continued)*

Drug	Daily dose (mg/kg)	Daily dosage schedule	Main indications	Common adverse effects and comments
Monoamine oxidase inhibitors (MAOIs)				
Phenelzine	0.5–1.0	Two or three times	Atypical depression, treatment-refractory depression	Difficult medicines to use in juveniles
Tranylcypromine				Reserved for refractory cases
				Severe dietary restrictions (high-tyramine foods)
Selegiline	0.2–0.4			Drug-drug interactions
				Hypertensive crisis with dietetic transgression or with certain drugs
				Weight gain
				Drowsiness
				Changes in blood pressure
				Insomnia
				Liver toxicity (remote risk)
Selective serotonin reuptake inhibitors (SSRIs)				
Fluoxetine	0.3–0.9	Once (in the A.M.)	Mood disorder, dysthymia, OCD, anxiety disorders, eating disorders, ?PTSD	Mechanism of action is serotonergic
Paroxetine				Large margin of safety
Citalopram				No cardiovascular effects
				Irritability
Sertraline	1.5–3.0			Insomnia
Fluvoxamine	1.5–4.5			Gastrointestinal symptoms
				Headaches
				Sexual dysfunction
				Withdrawal symptoms more common in short-acting
				Potential drug-drug interactions (cytochrome P450)

TABLE 7–3. Antidepressants used in the pharmacotherapy of attention-deficit/hyperactivity disorder (ADHD) *(continued)*

Drug	Daily dose (mg/kg)	Daily dosage schedule	Main indications	Common adverse effects and comments
Other new antidepressants				
Bupropion (SR)	3–6	Twice	ADHD, mood disorder, smoking cessation, ?anticraving effects, ?bipolar depression	Mixed mechanism of action (dopaminergic/ noradrenergic) Irritability Insomnia Drug-induced seizures (with doses >6 mg/kg) Contraindicated in bulimia patients
Venlafaxine (XR)	1–3	Once	Mood disorder, anxiety disorders, ?ADHD, ?OCD	Mixed mechanism of action (serotonergic/ noradrenergic) Similar to SSRIs Irritability Insomnia Gastrointestinal symptoms Headaches Potential withdrawal symptoms Blood pressure changes
Nefazodone	4–8	Once	Mood disorder, anxiety disorders, ?OCD, ?bipolar depression	Mixed mechanism of action (serotonergic/ noradrenergic) Dizziness Nausea Potential interactions with nonsedating antihistamines, cisapride (cytochrome P450) ?Less manicogenic

TABLE 7–3. Antidepressants used in the pharmacotherapy of attention-deficit/hyperactivity disorder (ADHD) *(continued)*

Drug	Daily dose (mg/kg)	Daily dosage schedule	Main indications	Common adverse effects and comments
Mirtazapine	0.2–0.9	Once (in the P.M.)	Mood disorder, anxiety disorders, ?stimulant-induced insomnia, ?bipolar depression	Mixed mechanism of action (serotonergic/noradrenergic) Sedation Weight gain Dizziness ?Less manicogenic

Note. *OCD = obsessive-compulsive disorder; PTSD = posttraumatic stress disorder.* Doses are general guidelines. All doses must be individualized with appropriate monitoring. Weight-corrected doses are less appropriate for obese children. When high doses are used, serum levels may be obtained to avoid toxicity.

defects in children receiving TCA treatment merits closer ECG and clinical monitoring, especially when relatively high doses of these medicines are used. In the context of cardiac disease, conduction defects may have potentially more serious clinical implications. When in doubt about the cardiovascular state of the patient, a more comprehensive cardiac evaluation is suggested, including 24-hour ECG and cardiac consultation, before initiating treatment with a TCA to help determine the risk-benefit ratio of such an intervention.

Several case reports in the 1980s of sudden death in children being treated with desipramine raised concern about the potential cardiotoxic risk associated with TCAs in the pediatric population (Riddle et al. 1991). Despite uncertainty and imprecise data, an epidemiological evaluation (Biederman et al. 1995a) suggested that the risk of desipramine-associated sudden death may be slightly elevated but not much greater than the baseline risk of sudden death in children not taking medication. Nevertheless, treatment with a TCA should be preceded by a baseline ECG, with serial ECGs at regular intervals throughout treatment. Because of the potential lethality of TCA overdose, parents should be advised to carefully store the medication in a place inaccessible to the children or their siblings.

The MAOIs, which include the hydrazines (phenelzine) and the nonhydrazines (tranylcypromine), have been tested in ADHD. In adults, MAOIs have been helpful in the treatment of atypical depressive disorders with reverse endogenous features and depressive disorders with prominent anxiety features (Quitkin et al. 1991). Daily dosages should be carefully titrated based on response and adverse effects and range from 0.5 to 1.0 mg/kg. Short-term adverse effects include orthostatic hypotension, weight gain, drowsiness, and dizziness. However, major limitations for the use of MAOIs in children and adolescents are the severe dietetic restrictions of tyramine-containing foods (e.g., most cheeses), pressor amines (e.g., sympathomimetic substances), and severe drug interactions (e.g., most cold medicines, amphetamines), which can induce a hypertensive crisis and a serotonergic syndrome. Although not available in the United States, a new family of reversible MAOIs has been developed and used in Europe and Canada that may be free of these difficulties.

Currently available SSRIs include fluoxetine, paroxetine, sertraline, fluvoxamine, and citalopram. At present, expert opinion does not support the usefulness of these serotonergic compounds in the treatment of core ADHD symptoms. Nevertheless, because of the high rates of comorbidity in ADHD, these compounds are frequently combined with effective anti-ADHD agents. Because many psychotropics are metabolized by the cytochrome P450 system, which in turn can be inhibited by the SSRIs, caution should be exercised when combining agents, such as the TCAs with SSRIs.

The antidepressants and many other psychotropics are metabolized in the liver by the cytochrome P450 system (DeVane 1998; Greenblatt et al. 1998; Nemeroff et al. 1996). Genetic polymorphism results in slow and rapid metabolizers. In addition, exogenous compounds can dramatically affect the efficacy of these enzymes and lead to drug-drug interactions. The coadministration of TCAs and SSRIs (paroxetine, fluoxetine, and sertraline; fluvoxamine with a weak nefazodone effect) may result in increased TCA levels. High levels of cisapride have been associated with QT prolongation and have led to potentially lethal ventricular arrhythmias (torsades de pointes). Thus, great caution should be exercised when using cisapride and the SSRIs that affect cytochrome P450 3A4 (fluvoxamine and nefazodone and, to a lesser degree, fluoxetine and sertraline). Citalopram, venlafaxine, and mirtazapine have minimal inhibition of P450 enzymes. Because levels of any drug metabolized by an isoenzyme that is inhibited by another drug can rise to dangerous levels, caution should be exercised when using combination treatments (DeVane 1998; Greenblatt et al. 1998; Nemeroff et al. 1996).

Bupropion hydrochloride, an antidepressant with a novel structure, belongs to the aminoketone class and is related to the phenylisopropylamines but is pharmacologically distinct from known antidepressants. Although its specific site or mechanism of action is unknown, bupropion seems to have an indirect mixed agonist effect on dopamine and norepinephrine neurotransmission. Bupropion is indicated for depression and smoking cessation in adults (Hunt et al. 1997). Bupropion is rapidly absorbed, with peak plasma levels usually achieved after 2 hours, with an average elimination half-life of 14 hours (8–24 hours). The usual dosage range is 4.0–6.0 mg/kg/day in divided doses. Side effects include irritability, anorexia, insomnia, and rarely edema, rashes, and nocturia. Exacerbation of tic disorders also has been reported with bupropion. It appears to have a somewhat higher (0.4%) rate of drug-induced seizures relative to other antidepressants, particularly in daily dosages higher than 6 mg/kg, and in patients with preexisting seizure disorder and those with bulimia. Bupropion also has been recently formulated into a long-acting (sustained-release [SR]) preparation that can be administered twice daily.

Other Drugs

Clonidine, a presynaptic α_2-adrenergic agonist, has been widely used in pediatric psychopharmacology despite extremely limited safety and efficacy data supporting its use (Table 7–4). Clonidine, an imidazoline derivative with α-adrenergic agonist properties, has been used primarily in the treatment of hypertension. At low doses, it appears to stimulate inhibitory, presynaptic autoreceptors in the central nervous system. The most common use of clonidine in pediatric psychiatry is the treatment of Tourette's disorder and other tic disorders (Leckman et al. 1991), ADHD, and ADHD-associated sleep disturbances (Hunt et al. 1990; Prince et al. 1996). In addition, clonidine has been reported to be useful in patients with developmental disorders to control aggression to self and others. Clonidine is a relatively short-acting compound with a plasma half-life ranging from approximately 5.5 hours (in children) to 8.5 hours (in adults). Daily doses should be titrated and individualized. The usual daily dosage ranges from 3 to 10 μg/kg generally given in divided doses two or three times a day and sometimes four times a day. Therapy is usually initiated at the lowest manufactured dose of a full or half tablet of 0.1 mg depending on the size of the child (approximately 1–2 μg/kg) and increased depending on clinical response and adverse effects. Initial dosage can be given more easily in the evening hours or before bedtime because of sedation, the most common short-term adverse effect of clonidine. It can also produce, in some cases, hypotension, dry mouth, depression, and confusion. Clonidine is not known to be associated with long-term adverse effects. In hypertensive adults, abrupt withdrawal of clonidine has been associated with rebound hypertension. Thus, it requires slow tapering when discontinued. Clonidine should not be administered concomitantly with β-blockers because adverse interactions have been reported with this combination. Recent reports of death in several children taking the combination of methylphenidate and clonidine have generated new concerns about its safety. Although more work is needed to evaluate if an increased risk exits with this combination, a cautious approach is advised, including increased surveillance and cardiovascular monitoring. Recently, anecdotal evidence has indicated that the more selective α_{2a}-agonist guanfacine may have a spectrum of benefits similar to those of clonidine with less sedation and longer duration of action (Chappell et al. 1995; Horrigan and Barnhill 1995; Hunt et al. 1995). The usual daily dosage ranges from 42 to 86 μg/kg generally given in divided doses two or three times a day.

TABLE 7–4. Noradrenergic modulators used in the pharmacotherapy of attention-deficit/hyperactivity disorder (ADHD)

Drug	Daily dosage (mg/kg)	Daily dosage schedule	Main indications	Common adverse effects and comments
α_2 Agonists				
Clonidine	0.003–0.010	Two or three times	Tourette's disorder, ADHD, aggression/self-abuse, severe agitation, withdrawal syndromes	Sedation (very frequent) Hypotension (rare) Dry mouth Confusion (with high dose) Depression Rebound hypertension Localized irritation with transdermal preparation
Guanfacine	0.015–0.05	Two or three times		Same as clonidine Less sedation, hypotension
β-Blockers				
Propranolol	1–7	Twice	Aggression/self-abuse, severe agitation, akathisia	Sedation Depression Risk for bradycardia and hypotension (dose-dependent) and rebound hypertension Bronchospasm (contraindicated in asthmatic patients) Rebound hypertension on abrupt withdrawal

Note. Doses are general guidelines. All doses must be individualized with appropriate monitoring. Weight-corrected doses are less appropriate for obese children.

Psychosocial Treatment of Attention-Deficit/Hyperactivity Disorder

Although pharmacotherapy is an important, and in many instances indispensable, form of treatment for ADHD in children, psychosocial treatment is also commonly used to treat not only the behaviors resulting from the disorder but also those associated with conditions that are often comorbid with ADHD (e.g., oppositional defiant disorder, social skills deficits). Although empirical evidence supporting the effectiveness of psychosocial treatment for ADHD is equivocal, parents and teachers often seek guidance regarding effective nonmedical management of ADHD in children. Space limitations preclude a comprehensive description of the full range of psychosocial treatment procedures and the fairly extensive research literature connected with these procedures. Thus, this section provides a general overview of such procedures and a description of findings from the Multimodal Treatment Study for ADHD (MTA), the largest-scale and most ambitious examination of their efficacy to date.

Overview of Psychosocial Models

The development and application of psychosocial treatment procedures for ADHD are grounded in theories related to 1) how human behavior is trained and maintained and 2) the core deficits underlying ADHD. Such procedures roughly fall into one of two categories. *Operant procedures* (also referred to as behavior modification procedures) flow from the notions that 1) human behavior is trained and maintained through its consequences and 2) individuals with ADHD have difficulty considering the consequences of their actions and with cause-and-effect relationships, at least at moments when such considerations are most crucial (Anastopoulos et al. 1998; Pelham and Sams 1992). Operant procedures are aimed at exerting "external control" over behaviors associated with ADHD. In contrast, *cognitive-behavioral procedures* can best be conceived as training "internal control" over behaviors associated with ADHD and flow from the notions that 1) much of human behavior is governed by cognitive processes and trained through observational learning and modeling and 2) individuals with ADHD have difficulty bringing to bear various internal controls (e.g., sustained attention, impulse control, problem solving) at moments when such controls are most crucial. Such procedures flow from the early work of Douglas (1980); Meichenbaum and Goodman (1971), and others (see Hinshaw and Erhardt 1991 for a review).

Operant Procedures (Behavior Modification)

Briefly, operant programs typically involve application of contingency management procedures at home or school, or both. Such programs vary in form and content (e.g., home-based contingency contracts, home-school daily report cards) but usually involve 1) identifying specific target behaviors (e.g., compliance with adult directives, completion of classwork and homework, on-task behavior), 2) developing a menu of specific rewards and punishments (e.g., privilege gain and loss, time-out from reinforcement), and 3) establishing a "currency" system (e.g., points, stickers, tokens) to track a child's degree of success in meeting target behaviors and thereby signal the dispensing of rewards or punishments (Abramowitz 1994; Pfiffner and O'Leary 1993).

Operant procedures have been shown to be effective in reducing some of the primary and secondary behaviors associated with ADHD but only while the procedures are actively implemented. In other words, studies have shown that, like medication, the treatment gains achieved by such procedures are not maintained once their active application ends. Treatment gains achieved by operant procedures are typically not as great as those achieved by high doses of stimulant medication. Rarely do children with ADHD treated with such procedures progress to within the "normal" range of functioning, and a meaningful percentage fail to show any improvement (Hinshaw et al. 1998; Pelham 1989). These limitations may be the result of, at least in part, the willingness (or lack thereof) of parents and teachers to implement operant programs (Pelham and Murphy 1986). Applying a goodness-of-fit model to intervention, Greene and colleagues (Greene 1995, 1996; Greene and Doyle 1999) referred to the degree to which interventions are well matched to the needs, characteristics, and capacities of those responsible for implementation as "teacher-treatment incompatibility" and "parent-treatment incompatibility" and argued that these compatibility equations are as crucial to effective treatment as the intervention ingredients themselves.

Cognitive-Behavioral Procedures

The cognitive-behavioral approach also has varied in form and content and has included the training of skills such as self-instruction, self-evaluation, self-monitoring, self-reinforcement, anger management, and social behavior. Such procedures teach children to modify, via "self-talk," the cognitions that precede and accompany overt behavior, thereby helping to orient children to the task at hand, organize a behavioral strategy, and regulate performance until completed. For example, in problem-solving training (a self-instruction strategy), children are taught to identify the problem at hand, to generate alternative solutions, to consider the likely outcomes of each solution, to monitor and evaluate such outcomes, and to self-reward or self-punish successful or unsuccessful outcomes (Hinshaw and Erhardt 1991; Hinshaw and Melnick 1992). These cognitive skills have been taught in individual and group formats, with role-playing and modeling as the primary training tools.

The limited number of studies examining the efficacy of cognitive-behavioral procedures in children with ADHD have produced disappointing findings. In general, cognitive-behavioral interventions have produced minimal, if any, change in the primary and secondary behaviors associated with ADHD (Abikoff 1985, 1987). Investigators have argued that this outcome results at least partially because cognitive-behavioral skills training has seldom been implemented in natural environments or included the training of adults in the environments where the children are most apt to experience difficulty (Greene 1996; Meichenbaum 1988; Whalen et al. 1985). However, cognitive-behavioral procedures also have fared poorly in studies in which relevant adults *were* included in treatment (Bloomquist et al. 1991; Braswell et al. 1997). Various limitations of such studies—that is, the degree to which adults were actively involved in treatment, the mechanisms by which such involvement occurred, the degree to which cognitive-behavioral treatment was individualized, and the duration of treatment—are discussed in greater detail below.

Based on recent theoretical notions of ADHD, Barkley (1997) provided a rationale for the equivocal findings regarding the effectiveness of cognitive-behavioral treatment of ADHD. Barkley noted that, because of the neurogenetic origin of ADHD, treatments are unlikely to ameliorate the disorder because they cannot correct the underlying neurological substrates or genetic mechanisms contributing to its development. Thus, Barkley argued that treatment is best understood as management of a chronic developmental condition and should therefore focus on finding the means to cope with, compensate for, and accommodate to the developmental deficiencies imposed by the disorder. Furthermore, Barkley suggested that ADHD be viewed as a disorder of performance (i.e., of doing what one knows) rather than of lacking knowledge (i.e., of knowing what to do). From this perspective, children with ADHD are conceived as unlikely to benefit from interventions aimed at the training of knowledge or skills (as occurs in cognitive-behavioral treatment) because lacking knowledge and skills are not at the core of their difficulties. Thus, training more knowledge is not as helpful as altering the motivational parameters associated with the performance of adaptive behaviors at the appropriate points of performance through operant procedures (Barkley 1997). These theoretical notions are discussed in greater detail below as well.

Multimodal Treatment Study for ADHD (MTA)

More recent studies have examined combinations of medical and nonmedical treatments for ADHD, usually in an effort to determine whether one form of treatment is superior to, or enhances the effectiveness of, another. As noted earlier in this chapter, the largest-scale study examining the relative and combined effectiveness of medical and nonmedical interventions for ADHD is the recently completed MTA. In this 5-year, six-site project, 579 elementary school–age children with ADHD were randomly assigned to one of four 14-month treatment conditions: behavioral treatment, medication management (usually methylphenidate), combined behavioral treatment and medication management, and a community comparison group (most of the children in the latter group were receiving medication for ADHD). Key outcome assessment occurred at 9 and 14 months. Children in the behavioral treatment arm received a very intensive combination of predominantly operant treatment ingredients, including school consultation, a classroom aide, an 8-week summer treatment program, and 35 sessions of parent management training. Behavioral treatment was faded before the final assessment. In contrast, pharmacotherapy—in both the medication management and the combined treatment conditions—was not tapered but rather was ongoing throughout treatment.

The rationale for the design of the behavioral treatment arm of the MTA has been described by Wells et al. (2000). Those responsible for designing this ambitious treatment protocol took into account findings from prior research, particularly that 1) the effects of behavioral treatment of ADHD tend to dissipate once such treatment is withdrawn, 2) behavioral treatment of ADHD typically does not achieve the same effect as high doses of stimulant medication, 3) combined behavioral treatment and medication generally have had equivocal effects as compared with medication alone, and 4) studies of cognitive-behavioral treatment had produced disappointing findings. It was hypothesized that a lengthier, more intensive form of (operant) treatment might provide greater benefits: "Just as the effects of medication can be enhanced by increasing the dosage, the effects of behavioral treatment can be maximized by increasing the power, intensity, and range of the treatment" (Wells et al. 2000).

In brief, initial reports of findings from the MTA indicated that, similar to prior findings, medical intervention was significantly more effective than behavioral and community treatments; behavioral treatment only modestly (and nonsignificantly) enhanced the effect of medication alone, and behavioral treatment alone was no more effective than the treatment received by children in the community comparison group (Jensen 1998). Pelham (1999) argued that these findings are at least partially attributable to the design of the MTA, namely, that behavioral treatment was faded over time, whereas medical treatment was not. Indeed, applying behavioral treatment in this manner seems inconsistent with the view of ADHD as a chronic condition that requires continuous intervention (presumably medical *and* nonmedical). Pelham (1999) also suggested that the MTA findings actually support the notion that behavioral treatment alone improves the functioning of children with ADHD because the children who received behavioral treatment alone improved at a level commensurate with those in the community comparison group, most of whom were receiving medical treatment.

Another major concern with the nonmedical treatment component of the MTA relates to what some might view as a fairly narrow range of treatment. The behavioral treatment arm (originally referred to as the "psychosocial" treatment arm) included virtually no non-operant treatments (the exception was a social skills training program delivered as part of the summer treatment program component). Thus, the MTA did not apply a full range of available psychosocial treatment options but rather an extraordinarily intensive and almost exclusively operant treatment package. There are legitimate concerns about the ecological validity of this treatment package (e.g., the lack of feasibility of 9 weeks of summer camp, a classroom aide, classroom consultation, and 35 sessions of parent management training as the standard of care for children with ADHD) and related concerns that the intensive operant program of the MTA produced effects that appear to have been no more beneficial (alone or in combination with medication) than those seen in previous studies examining far less intensive behavioral treatment programs. However, the nearly total absence of cognitive-behavioral treatment—while justifiable in light of the existing literature—is perhaps of greatest concern. The literature examining the effectiveness of cognitive-behavioral treatment of children with ADHD has a variety of important limitations that might have been well examined by the MTA. First—similar to operant procedures—most cognitive-behavioral treatment programs have been delivered as rigid treatment "packages," providing training for a fairly circumscribed set of skills over a fairly brief period, usually in treatment groups that were removed from the environments in which children were experiencing the greatest difficulties (Greene and Barkley 1996; Hinshaw 1992). In other words, cognitive-behavioral treatment has rarely been provided in an individualized fashion, matched to the specific needs and deficits of individual children. Moreover, as noted earlier, only in rare instances have important caregivers been provided with training in cognitive-behavioral procedures so as to foster the continued practicing of cognitive skills in which children were being trained. Even when such caregivers have been involved in treatment (Bloomquist et al. 1991), they also were provided with circumscribed, group training (outside the presence of their children) matched to no one. In some studies (Braswell et al. 1997), parental participation was so poor that this arm of treatment had to be eliminated from data analyses. Prior studies examining the effectiveness of cognitive-behavioral treatment have convincingly shown that it is not particularly beneficial when such treatment 1) is not matched to the specific, assessed needs of individual ADHD children; 2) does not engage relevant adults in the therapeutic process; 3) does not provide intensive, individualized training to those responsible for implementation in environments proximal to where a child has the greatest difficulties; and 4) is not provided over the long term.

Attempts to capture the "core" deficit of ADHD—for example, to characterize all children with ADHD as having a "performance" deficit rather than a "skills" deficit—inevitably belie the heterogeneity of the disorder. Although many children with ADHD do indeed appear to have a "performance" deficit, it is just as plausible that others may not have acquired requisite skills because of the developmental lag that typifies the disorder. Presumably, children with ADHD who have performance deficits might benefit maximally from a behavioral treatment approach emphasizing motivational strategies. However, those with deficits in cognitive skills might benefit more from an approach emphasizing the training of such skills. Greene and colleagues (Greene 1995, 1996; Greene and Doyle 1999) referred to the "fit" between a child's actual clinical needs and the treatments used to address those needs as "child-treatment compatibility."

For example, the social skills deficits of children with ADHD, which have extremely adverse ramifications for long-term outcomes (Greene et al. 1997, 1999), may present in diverse ways and with diverse etiologies: some ADHD children may have fairly intact social skills, but because of the poor impulse control and overactivity associated with the disorder, they have difficulty performing such skills on a consistent basis in the ongoing stream of behavior. Such children might well benefit from motivational strategies aimed at enhancing the performance of existing skills. However, other children with ADHD might have various compromised cognitive skills related to social functioning: social problem-solving skills; modulating their emotions (e.g., anger, frustration); social self-awareness (knowledge and insight about themselves in social settings); and empathy (perspective taking, awareness of others' feelings, and cognizance of the effect of their behavior on others) (Eslinger 1996). The training of some of these cognitive skills might be enhanced by medication, but this presumably occurs on a case-by-case basis as well. However, it is difficult to conceive of how operant strategies alone would be well suited to the training of such skills. It is also difficult to conceive of how these complex cognitive skills could be trained and maintained in the types of brief, nonindividualized, nonproximal cognitive-behavioral programs that have typified the literature. These issues were not addressed in the MTA and will require further study. However, it seems premature to dismiss the potential role of cognitive-behavioral treatment in children with ADHD. To do so leaves only a very narrow range of treatment options available to parents and teachers who must interact with, and improve the functioning of, such children.

Conclusions

A careful differential diagnostic assessment that assesses psychiatric, social, cognitive, educational, and medical/neurological factors that may contribute to the child's clinical presentation is essential in considering the use of pharmacotherapy and psychosocial treatments as part of a broader plan that encompasses all aspects of a child's life. Realistic expectations of interventions, careful definition of target symptoms, and careful assessment of the potential risks and benefits of each type of intervention for psychiatrically disturbed children are major ingredients for success.

References

Abikoff H: Efficacy of cognitive training intervention in hyperactive children: a critical review. Clin Psychol Rev 5:479–512, 1985

Abikoff H: An evaluation of cognitive behavior therapy for hyperactive children, in Advances in Clinical Child Psychology. Edited by Lahey B, Kazdin A. New York, Plenum, 1987, pp 171–216

Abramowitz AJ: Classroom interventions for disruptive behavior disorders. Child Adolesc Psychiatr Clin N Am 3:343–360, 1994

Adler L, Resnick S, Kunz M, et al: Open-Label Trial of Venlafaxine in Attention Deficit Disorder. Orlando, FL, New Clinical Drug Evaluation Unit Program, 1995

Alderman J, Wolkow R, Chung M, et al: Sertraline treatment of children and adolescents with obsessive-compulsive disorder or depression: pharmacokinetics, tolerability, and efficacy. J Am Acad Child Adolesc Psychiatry 37:386–394, 1998

American Psychiatric Association: Diagnostic and Statistical Manual of Mental Disorders, 4th Edition. Washington, DC, American Psychiatric Association, 1994

Anastopoulos AD, Smith JM, Wien EE: Counseling and training parents, in Attention Deficit Hyperactivity Disorder: A Handbook for Diagnosis and Treatment. Edited by Barkley RA. New York, Guilford, 1998, pp 373–393

Barkley RA: A review of stimulant drug research with hyperactive children. J Child Psychol Psychiatry 18:137–165, 1977

Barkley RA: ADHD and the Nature of Self-Control. New York, Guilford, 1997

Barrickman L, Noyes R, Kuperman S, et al: Treatment of ADHD with fluoxetine: a preliminary trial. J Am Acad Child Adolesc Psychiatry 30:762–767, 1991

Barrickman LL, Perry PJ, Allen AJ, et al: Bupropion versus methylphenidate in the treatment of attention-deficit hyperactivity disorder. J Am Acad Child Adolesc Psychiatry 34:649–657, 1995

Bergman A, Winters L, Cornblatt B: Methylphenidate: effects on sustained attention, in Ritalin: Theory and Patient Management. Edited by Greenhill L, Osman B. New York, Mary Ann Liebert, 1991, pp 223–231

Biederman J, Gastfriend DR, Jellinek MS: Desipramine in the treatment of children with attention deficit disorder. J Clin Psychopharmacol 6:359–363, 1986

Biederman J, Baldessarini RJ, Wright V, et al: A double-blind placebo controlled study of desipramine in the treatment of attention deficit disorder, I: efficacy. J Am Acad Child Adolesc Psychiatry 28: 777–784, 1989a

Biederman J, Baldessarini RJ, Wright V, et al: A double-blind placebo controlled study of desipramine in the treatment of attention deficit disorder, II: serum drug levels and cardiovascular findings. J Am Acad Child Adolesc Psychiatry 28:903–911, 1989b

Biederman J, Baldessarini RJ, Wright V, et al: A double-blind placebo controlled study of desipramine in the treatment of attention deficit disorder, III: lack of impact of comorbidity and family history factors on clinical response. J Am Acad Child Adolesc Psychiatry 32:199–204, 1993

Biederman J, Thisted RA, Greenhill LL, et al: Estimation of the association between desipramine and the risk for sudden death in 5- to 14-year-old children. J Clin Psychiatry 56:87–93, 1995a

Biederman J, Wilens T, Mick E, et al: Psychoactive substance use disorder in adults with attention deficit hyperactivity disorder: effects of ADHD and psychiatric comorbidity. Am J Psychiatry 152: 1652–1658, 1995b

Biederman J, Faraone SV, Chu MP, et al: Further evidence of a bidirectional overlap between juvenile mania and conduct disorder in children. J Am Acad Child Adolesc Psychiatry 38:468–476, 1999a

Biederman J, Mick E, Prince J, et al: Systematic chart review of the pharmacologic treatment of comorbid attention deficit hyperactivity disorder in youth with bipolar disorder. J Child Adolesc Psychopharmacol 9:247–256, 1999b

Biederman J, Wilens T, Mick E, et al: Pharmacotherapy of attention-deficit/hyperactivity disorder reduces risk for substance use disorder. Pediatrics 104:e20, 1999c

Bloomquist ML, August GJ, Ostrander R: Effects of a school-based cognitive-behavioral intervention for ADHD children. J Abnorm Child Psychol 19:591–605, 1991

Braswell L, August GJ, Bloomquist ML, et al: School-based secondary prevention for children with disruptive behavior: initial outcomes. J Abnorm Child Psychol 25:197–208, 1997

Brown RT, Wynne ME, Slimmer LW: Attention deficit disorder and the effect of methylphenidate on attention, behavioral, and cardiovascular functioning. J Clin Psychiatry 45:473–476, 1984

Buitelaar JK, van de Gaag RJ, Swaab-Barneveld H, et al: Pindolol and methylphenidate in children with attention-deficit hyperactivity disorder: clinical efficacy and side effects. Journal of Child and Adolescent Psychiatry 36:587–595, 1996

Casat CD, Pleasants DZ, Van Wyck Fleet J: A double-blind trial of bupropion in children with attention deficit disorder. Psychopharmacol Bull 23:120–122, 1987

Casat CD, Pleasants DZ, Schroeder DH, et al: Bupropion in children with attention deficit disorder. Psychopharmacol Bull 25:198–201, 1989

Chappell PB, Riddle MA, Scahill L, et al: Guanfacine treatment of comorbid attention-deficit hyperactivity disorder and Tourette's syndrome: preliminary clinical experience. J Am Acad Child Adolesc Psychiatry 34:1140–1146, 1995

Comings DE, Comings BG: Tourette's syndrome and attention deficit disorder, in Tourette's Syndrome and Tic Disorders: Clinical Understanding and Treatment. Edited by Cohen DJ, Bruun RD, Leckman JF. New York, Wiley, 1988, pp 119–136

Conners CK, Casat CD, Gualtieri CT, et al: Bupropion hydrochloride in attention deficit disorder with hyperactivity. J Am Acad Child Adolesc Psychiatry 35:1314–1321, 1996

Connor DF, Ozbayrak KR, Benjamin S, et al: A pilot study of nadolol for overt aggression in developmentally delayed individuals. J Am Acad Child Adolesc Psychiatry 36:826–834, 1997

Cox W: An indication for the use of imipramine in attention deficit disorder. Am J Psychiatry 139:1059–1060, 1982

Derivan A: Venlafaxine metabolism in children and adolescents. Scientific Proceedings of the XI Annual Meeting: American Academy of Child and Adolescent Psychiatry, New Orleans, LA, October 1995

DeVane C: Differential pharmacology of newer antidepressants. J Clin Psychiatry 59:85–93, 1998

DeVeaugh-Geiss J, Moroz G, Biederman J, et al: Clomipramine hydrochloride in childhood and adolescent obsessive-compulsive disorder—a multicenter trial. J Am Acad Child Adolesc Psychiatry 31:45–49, 1992

Dillon DC, Salzman IJ, Schulsinger DA: The use of imipramine in Tourette's syndrome and attention deficit disorder: case report. J Clin Psychiatry 46:348–349, 1985

Donnelly M, Zametkin AJ, Rapoport JL, et al: Treatment of childhood hyperactivity with desipramine: plasma drug concentration, cardiovascular effects, plasma and urinary catecholamine levels, and clinical response. Clin Pharmacol Ther 39:72–81, 1986

Donnelly M, Rapoport JL, Potter WZ, et al: Fenfluramine and dextroamphetamine treatment of childhood hyperactivity: clinical and biochemical findings. Arch Gen Psychiatry 46:205–212, 1989

Douglas VI: Treatment and training approaches to hyperactivity: establishing internal or external control, in Hyperactive Children: The Social Ecology of Identification and Treatment. Edited by Whalen C, Henker B. New York, Academic Press, 1980, pp 283–318

Douglas VI, Barr RG, Amin K, et al: Dosage effects and individual responsivity to methylphenidate in attention deficit disorder. J Child Psychol Psychiatry 29:453–475, 1988

DuPaul GJ, Barkley RA, McMurray MB: Response of children with ADHD to methylphenidate: interaction with internalizing symptoms. J Am Acad Child Adolesc Psychiatry 33:894–903, 1994

Emslie GJ, Rush AJ, Weinberg WA, et al: A double-blind, randomized, placebo-controlled trial of fluoxetine in children and adolescents with depression. Arch Gen Psychiatry 54:1031–1037, 1997

Eslinger PJ: Conceptualizing, describing, and measuring components of executive function, in Attention, Memory, and Executive Function. Edited by Lyon GR, Krasnegor NA. Baltimore, MD, Paul H Brookes, 1996, pp 367–395

Famularo R, Fenton T: The effect of methylphenidate on school grades in children with attention deficit disorder without hyperactivity: a preliminary report. J Clin Psychiatry 48:112–114, 1987

Faraone SV, Biederman J: The neurobiology of attention deficit hyperactivity disorder, in Neurobiology of Mental Illness. Edited by Charney DS, Nestler EJ, Bunney BS. New York, Oxford University Press, 1999, pp 788–801

Faraone SV, Biederman J, Lehman BK, et al: Intellectual performance and school failure in children with attention deficit hyperactivity disorder and in their siblings. J Abnorm Psychol 102:616–623, 1993

Faraone SV, Biederman J, Weiffenbach B, et al: Dopamine D_4 gene 7-repeat allele and attention deficit hyperactivity disorder. Am J Psychiatry 156:768–770, 1999

Findling RL, Schwartz MA, Flannery DJ, et al: Venlafaxine in adults with attention-deficit/hyperactivity disorder: an open clinical trial. J Clin Psychiatry 57:184–189, 1996

Findling RL, Reed MD, Myers C, et al: Paroxetine pharmacokinetics in depressed children and adolescents. J Am Acad Child Adolesc Psychiatry 38:952–959, 1999

Frazier JA, Meyer MC, Biederman J, et al: Risperidone treatment for juvenile bipolar disorder: a retrospective chart review. J Am Acad Child Adolesc Psychiatry 38:960–965, 1999

Fung YK: Postnatal behavioural effects of maternal nicotine exposure in rats. J Pharm Pharmacol 40: 870–872, 1988

Fung YK, Lau YS: Effects of prenatal nicotine exposure on rat striatal dopaminergic and nicotinic systems. Pharmacol Biochem Behav 33:1–6, 1989

Gadow KD, Nolan EE, Sverd J: Methylphenidate in hyperactive boys with comorbid tic disorder, II: short-term behavioral effects in school settings. J Am Acad Child Adolesc Psychiatry 31:462–471, 1992

Gadow KD, Sverd J, Sprafkin J, et al: Efficacy of methylphenidate for attention-deficit hyperactivity disorder in children with tic disorder [published erratum appears in Arch Gen Psychiatry 52:836, 1995]. Arch Gen Psychiatry 52:444–455, 1995

Garfinkel BD, Wender PH, Sloman L, et al: Tricyclic antidepressant and methylphenidate treatment of attention deficit disorder in children. J Am Acad Child Adolesc Psychiatry 22:343–348, 1983

Gastfriend DR, Biederman J, Jellinek MS, et al: Desipramine in the treatment of attention deficit disorder in adolescents. Psychopharmacol Bull 21:144–145, 1985

Geller DA, Biederman J, Reed ED, et al: Similarities in response to fluoxetine in the treatment of children and adolescents with obsessive-compulsive disorder. J Am Acad Child Adolesc Psychiatry 34:36–44, 1995

Gittelman R: Childhood disorders, in Drug Treatment of Adult and Child Psychiatric Disorders. Edited by Klein D, Quitkin F, Rifkin A, et al. Baltimore, MD, Williams & Wilkins, 1980, pp 576–756

Gittelman R, Mannuzza S: Hyperactive boys almost grown up, III: methylphenidate effects on ultimate height. Arch Gen Psychiatry 45:1131–1134, 1988

Gittelman-Klein R: Pilot clinical trial of imipramine in hyperkinetic children, in Clinical Use of Stimulant Drugs in Children. Edited by Conners C. The Hague, The Netherlands, Excerpta Medica, 1974, pp 192–201

Gittelman-Klein R: Pharmacotherapy of childhood hyperactivity: an update, in Psychopharmacology: The Third Generation of Progress. Edited by Meltzer HY. New York, Raven, 1987, pp 1215–1224

Goldman L, Genel M, Bezman RJ, et al: Diagnosis and treatment of attention-deficit/hyperactivity disorder in children and adolescents. Council on Scientific Affairs, American Medical Association. JAMA 279:1100–1107, 1998

Greenberg L, Yellin A, Spring C, et al: Clinical effects of imipramine and methylphenidate in hyperactive children. International Journal of Mental Health 4:144–156, 1975

Greenblatt DJ, von Moltke LL, Harmatz JS, et al: Drug interactions with newer antidepressants: role of human cytochromes P450. J Clin Psychiatry 59 (suppl 15):19–27, 1998

Greene RW: Students with ADHD in school classrooms: teacher factors related to compatibility, assessment, and intervention. School Psychology Review 24:81–93, 1995

Greene RW: Students with ADHD and their teachers: implications of a goodness-of-fit perspective, in Advances in Clinical Child Psychology. Edited by Ollendick TH, Prinz RJ. New York, Plenum, 1996, pp 205–230

Greene R: The Explosive Child: A New Approach for Understanding and Parenting Easily Frustrated, Chronically Inflexible Children. New York, Harper-Collins, 1998

Greene RW, Barkley RA: Attention deficit/hyperactivity disorder: diagnostic, developmental, and conceptual issues, in Behavioral Approach to Assessment of Youth With Emotional/Behavioral Disorders: A Handbook for School-Based Practitioners. Edited by Breen M, Fiedler C. Austin, TX, Pro-Ed, 1996, pp 413–449

Greene RW, Doyle AE: Toward a transactional conceptualization of oppositional defiant disorder: implications for treatment and assessment. Clinical Child and Family Psychology Review 2:129–148, 1999

Greene RW, Biederman J, Faraone SV, et al: Adolescent outcome of boys with attention-deficit/hyperactivity disorder and social disability: results from a 4-year longitudinal follow-up study. J Consult Clin Psychol 65:758–767, 1997

Greene RW, Biederman J, Faraone SV, et al: Further validation of social impairment as a predictor of substance use disorders: findings from a sample of siblings of boys with and without ADHD. J Clin Child Psychol 28:349–354, 1999

Greenhill LL, Halperin JM, Abikoff H: Stimulant medications. J Am Acad Child Adolesc Psychiatry 38:503–512, 1999

Gross M: Imipramine in the treatment of minimal brain dysfunction in children. Psychosomatics 14: 283–285, 1973

Gross M: Growth of hyperkinetic children taking methylphenidate, dextroamphetamine, or imipramine/desipramine. J Pediatr 58:423–431, 1976

Gualtieri CT, Evans RW: Motor performance in hyperactive children treated with imipramine. Percept Mot Skills 66:763–769, 1988

Gunning B: A controlled trial of clonidine in hyperkinetic children. Thesis, Department of Child and Adolescent Psychiatry, Academic Hospital Rotterdam–Sophia Children's Hospital, Rotterdam, The Netherlands, 1992

Hinshaw SP: Intervention for social competence and social skill. Child Adolesc Psychiatr Clin N Am 1:539–552, 1992

Hinshaw SP, Erhardt DE: Attention-deficit hyperactivity disorder, in Child and Adolescent Therapy: Cognitive-Behavioral Procedures. Edited by Kendall PC. New York, Guilford, 1991, pp 98–130

Hinshaw SP, Melnick S: Self-management therapies and attention-deficit hyperactivity disorder: reinforced self-evaluation and anger control interventions. Behav Modif 16:253–273, 1992

Hinshaw SP, Klein RG, Abikoff H, et al: Childhood attention-deficit hyperactivity disorder: nonpharmacologic and combination treatments, in Treatments That Work. Edited by Nathan PE, Gorman J. New York, Oxford University Press, 1998

Hoge SK, Biederman J: A case of Tourette's syndrome with symptoms of attention deficit disorder treated with desipramine. J Clin Psychiatry 47:478–479, 1986

Hornig-Rohan M, Amsterdam J: Venlafaxine vs. Stimulant Therapy in Patients With Dual Diagnoses of ADHD and Depression. Orlando, FL, New Clinical Drug Evaluation Unit Program, 1995

Horrigan JP, Barnhill LJ: Guanfacine for treatment of attention-deficit hyperactivity disorder in boys. J Child Adolesc Psychopharmacol 5:215–223, 1995

Huessy H, Wright A: The use of imipramine in children's behavior disorders. Acta Paedopsychiatrie 37:194–199, 1970

Hunt RD: Treatment effects of oral and transdermal clonidine in relation to methylphenidate: an open pilot study in ADD-H. Psychopharmacol Bull 23:111–114, 1987

Hunt RD, Minderaa RB, Cohen DJ: Clonidine benefits children with attention deficit disorder and hyperactivity: report of a double-blind placebo-crossover therapeutic trial. Journal of the American Academy of Child Psychiatry 24:617–629, 1985

Hunt RD, Capper L, O'Connell P: Clonidine in child and adolescent psychiatry. J Child Adolesc Psychopharmacol 1:87–102, 1990

Hunt RD, Arnsten AF, Asbell MD: An open trial of guanfacine in the treatment of attention-deficit hyperactivity disorder. J Am Acad Child Adolesc Psychiatry 34:50–54, 1995

Hunt RD, Sachs DP, Glover ED, et al: A comparison of sustained-release bupropion and placebo for smoking cessation. N Engl J Med 337:1195–1202, 1997

Jensen PS: NIMH Multimodal Treatment Study. Scientific Proceedings of the Annual Meeting: American Academy of Child and Adolescent Psychiatry, Anaheim, CA, October 1998

Johns JM, Louis TM, Becker RF, et al: Behavioral effects of prenatal exposure to nicotine in guinea pigs. Neurobehavioral Toxicology and Teratology 4:365–369, 1982

Jones GM, Sahakian BJ, Levy R, et al: Effects of acute subcutaneous nicotine on attention, information processing and short-term memory in Alzheimer's disease. Psychopharmacology (Berl) 108:485–494, 1992

Klein RG: Pharmacotherapy of childhood hyperactivity: an update, in Psychopharmacology: The Third Generation of Progress. Edited by Meltzer HY. New York, Raven, 1987, pp 1215–1225

Kupietz SS, Balka EB: Alterations in the vigilance performance of children receiving amitriptyline and methylphenidate pharmacotherapy. Psychopharmacology 50:29–33, 1976

Kupietz SS, Winsberg BG, Richardson E, et al: Effects of methylphenidate dosage in hyperactive reading-disabled children, I: behavior and cognitive performance effects. J Am Acad Child Adolesc Psychiatry 27:70–77, 1988

Leckman JF, Hardin MT, Riddle MA, et al: Clonidine treatment of Gilles de la Tourette's syndrome. Arch Gen Psychiatry 48:324–328, 1991

Levin ED, Conners CK, Sparrow E, et al: Nicotine effects on adults with attention-deficit/hyperactivity disorder. Psychopharmacology (Berl) 123:55–63, 1996

Lowe TL, Cohen DJ, Detlor J, et al: Stimulant medications precipitate Tourette's syndrome. JAMA 247: 1168–1169, 1982

Luh J, Pliszka S, Olvers R, et al: An Open Trial of Venlafaxine in the Treatment of Attention Deficit Hyperactivity Disorder: A Pilot Study. San Antonio, TX, The University of Texas Health Science Center at San Antonio, 1996

Malhotra S, Santosh PJ: An open clinical trial of buspirone in children with attention deficit/hyperactivity disorder. J Am Acad Child Adolesc Psychiatry 37:364–371, 1998

Mattes JA: Propranolol for adults with temper outbursts and residual attention deficit disorder. J Clin Psychopharmacol 6:299–302, 1986

Mattes JA, Gittelman R: Growth of hyperactive children on maintenance regimen of methylphenidate. Arch Gen Psychiatry 40:317–321, 1983

Meck W, Church R: Cholinergic modulation of the content of temporal memory. Behav Neurosci 101: 457–464, 1987

Meichenbaum D: Cognitive behavioral modification with attention deficit hyperactivity children, in Attention Deficit Disorder: Criteria, Cognition, and Intervention. Edited by Bloomingdale L, Sergeant J. New York, Pergamon, 1988, pp 127–140

Meichenbaum DH, Goodman J: Training impulsive children to talk to themselves: a means of developing self-control. J Abnorm Psychol 77:115–126, 1971

Mereu G, Yoon KW, Boi V, et al: Preferential stimulation of ventral tegmental area dopaminergic neurons by nicotine. Eur J Pharmacol 141:395–399, 1987

Milberger S, Biederman J, Faraone SV, et al: Is maternal smoking during pregnancy a risk factor for attention deficit hyperactivity disorder in children? Am J Psychiatry 153:1138–1142, 1996

Milberger S, Biederman J, Faraone SV, et al: ADHD is associated with early initiation of cigarette smoking in children and adolescents. J Am Acad Child Adolesc Psychiatry 36:37–44, 1997

National Institute of Mental Health: Alternative Pharmacology of ADHD. Rockville, MD, National Institute of Mental Health, 1996

Nemeroff CB, DeVane CL, Pollock BG: Newer antidepressants and the cytochrome P450 system. Am J Psychiatry 153:311–320, 1996

Parrott AC, Winder G: Nicotine chewing gum (2 mg, 4 mg) and cigarette smoking: comparative effects upon vigilance and heart rate. Psychopharmacology 97:257–261, 1989

Peeke S, Peeke H: Attention, memory, and cigarette smoking. Psychopharmacology 84:205–216, 1984

Pelham WE: Behavior therapy, behavioral assessment, and psychostimulant medication in the treatment of attention deficit disorders: an interactive approach, in Attention Deficit Disorders (IV): Current Concepts and Emerging Trends in Emotional and Behavioral Disorders of Childhood. Edited by Swanson J, Bloomingdale L. London, Pergamon, 1989, pp 169–195

Pelham WE: President's Message: The NIMH Multimodal Treatment Study for ADHD: just say yes to drugs? Clinical Child Psychology Newsletter, Summer 1999

Pelham WE, Murphy HA: Attention deficit and conduct disorders, in Pharmacological and Behavioral Treatments: An Integrative Approach. Edited by Hersen M. New York, Wiley, 1986, pp 108–148

Pelham WE, Sams SE: Behavior modification. Psychiatr Clin North Am 1:505–518, 1992

Pelham WE, Bender ME, Caddell J, et al: Methylphenidate and children with attention deficit disorder. Arch Gen Psychiatry 42:948–952, 1985

Pfiffner LJ, O'Leary SG: School-based psychological treatments, in Handbook of Hyperactivity in Children. Edited by Matson JL. Boston, MA, Allyn & Bacon, 1993

Platt JE, Campbell M, Green WH, et al: Cognitive effects of lithium carbonate and haloperidol in treatment-resistant aggressive children. Arch Gen Psychiatry 41:657–662, 1984

Pliszka SR: Effect of anxiety on cognition, behavior, and stimulant response in ADHD. J Am Acad Child Adolesc Psychiatry 28:882–887, 1989

Pomerleau OF, Downey KK, Stelson FW, et al: Cigarette smoking in adult patients diagnosed with attention deficit hyperactivity disorder. J Subst Abuse 7:373–378, 1995

Prince JB, Wilens TE, Biederman J, et al: Clonidine for sleep disturbances associated with attention-deficit hyperactivity disorder: a systematic chart review of 62 cases. J Am Acad Child Adolesc Psychiatry 35:599–605, 1996

Prince J, Wilens T, Biederman J, et al: A controlled study of nortriptyline in children and adolescents with attention deficit hyperactivity disorder. Scientific Proceedings of the American Academy of Child and Adolescent Psychiatrists, Chicago, IL, October 1999

Quay HC: Conduct disorder, in Psychopathologic Disorders of Childhood. Edited by Quay HC, Werry JS. New York, Wiley, 1986, pp 35–73

Quinn PO, Rapoport JL: One-year follow-up of hyperactive boys treated with imipramine or methylphenidate. Am J Psychiatry 132:241–245, 1975

Quitkin FM, Harrison W, Stewart JW, et al: Response to phenelzine and imipramine in placebo nonresponders with atypical depression: a new application of the crossover design. Arch Gen Psychiatry 48:319–323, 1991

Rapoport JL, Quinn PO, Bradbard G, et al: Imipramine and methylphenidate treatment of hyperactive boys: a double-blind comparison. Arch Gen Psychiatry 30:789–793, 1974

Rapport MD, Jones JT, DuPaul GJ, et al: Attention deficit disorder and methylphenidate: group and single-subject analyses of dose effects on attention in clinic and classroom settings. J Clin Child Psychol 16:329–338, 1987

Rapport MD, Stoner G, DuPaul GJ, et al: Attention deficit disorder and methylphenidate: a multilevel analysis of dose-response effects on children's impulsivity across settings. J Am Acad Child Adolesc Psychiatry 27:60–69, 1988

Rapport MD, DuPaul GJ, Kelly KL: Attention deficit hyperactivity disorder and methylphenidate: the relationship between gross body weight and drug response in children. Psychopharmacol Bull 25:285–290, 1989a

Rapport MD, Quinn SO, DuPaul GJ, et al: Attention deficit disorder with hyperactivity and methylphenidate: the effects of dose and mastery level on children's learning performance. J Abnorm Child Psychol 17:669–689, 1989b

Rapport MD, Carlson GA, Kelly KL, et al: Methylphenidate and desipramine in hospitalized children, I: separate and combined effects on cognitive function. J Am Acad Child Adolesc Psychiatry 32: 333–342, 1993

Ratey JJ, Greenberg MS, Lindem KJ: Combination of treatments for attention deficit disorders in adults. J Nerv Ment Dis 176:699–701, 1991

Reimherr FW, Wender PH, Wood DR, et al: An open trial of L-tyrosine in the treatment of attention deficit disorder, residual type. Am J Psychiatry 144:1071–1073, 1987

Reimherr F, Hedges D, Strong R: An Open Trial of Venlafaxine in Adult Patients With Attention Deficit Hyperactivity Disorder. Orlando, FL, New Clinical Drug Evaluation Unit Program, 1995

Riddle MA, Hardin MT, Cho SC, et al: Desipramine treatment of boys with attention-deficit hyperactivity disorder and tics: preliminary clinical experience. J Am Acad Child Adolesc Psychiatry 27: 811–814, 1988

Riddle MA, Nelson JC, Kleinman CS, et al: Sudden death in children receiving Norpramin: a review of three reported cases and commentary. J Am Acad Child Adolesc Psychiatry 30:104–108, 1991

Safer D, Allen R, Barr E: Depression of growth in hyperactive children on stimulant drugs. N Engl J Med 287:217–220, 1972

Satterfield JH, Cantwell DP, Schell A, et al: Growth of hyperactive children treated with methylphenidate. Arch Gen Psychiatry 36:212–217, 1979

Silva RR, Munoz DM, Alpert M: Carbamazepine use in children and adolescents with features of attention-deficit hyperactivity disorder: a meta-analysis. J Am Acad Child Adolesc Psychiatry 35: 352–358, 1996

Singer HS, Brown J, Quaskey S, et al: The treatment of attention-deficit hyperactivity disorder in Tourette's syndrome: a double-blind placebo-controlled study with clonidine and desipramine. Pediatrics 95:74–81, 1994

Spencer T: A double-blind, controlled study of desipramine in children with ADHD and tic disorders. Scientific Proceedings of the Annual Meeting: American Academy of Child and Adolescent Psychiatry, Toronto, ON, October 1997

Spencer T, Biederman J, Kerman K, et al: Desipramine treatment of children with attention-deficit hyperactivity disorder and tic disorder or Tourette's syndrome. J Am Acad Child Adolesc Psychiatry 32:354–360, 1993a

Spencer T, Biederman J, Wilens T, et al: Nortriptyline treatment of children with attention deficit hyperactivity disorder and tic disorder or Tourette's syndrome. J Am Acad Child Adolesc Psychiatry 32:205–210, 1993b

Spencer T, Wilens T, Biederman J, et al: A double-blind, crossover comparison of methylphenidate and placebo in adults with childhood-onset attention-deficit hyperactivity disorder. Arch Gen Psychiatry 52:434–443, 1995

Spencer T, Biederman J, Wilens T, et al: Pharmacotherapy of attention deficit hyperactivity disorder across the life cycle: a literature review. J Am Acad Child Adolesc Psychiatry 35:409–432, 1996

Spencer T, Biederman J, Wilens T, et al: Pharmacotherapy of ADHD: a life span perspective, in The American Psychiatric Press Review of Psychiatry, Vol 16. Edited by Dickstein LJ, Riba MB, Oldham JM. Washington, DC, American Psychiatric Press, 1997, pp IV-87–IV-128

Spencer T, Biederman J, Wilens TE, et al: Adults with attention-deficit/hyperactivity disorder: a controversial diagnosis. J Clin Psychiatry 59 (suppl 7):59–68, 1998a

Spencer T, Biederman J, Wilens T, et al: Effectiveness and tolerability of tomoxetine in adults with attention deficit hyperactivity disorder. Am J Psychiatry 155:693–695, 1998b

Spencer T, Biederman J, Wilens T: Growth deficits in children with attention deficit hyperactivity disorder. Pediatrics 102 (2 Pt 3):501–506, 1998c

Spencer T, Biederman J, Coffey B, et al: The 4-year course of tic disorders in boys with attention-deficit/hyperactivity disorder. Arch Gen Psychiatry 56:842–847, 1999

Steingard R, Biederman J, Spencer T, et al: Comparison of clonidine response in the treatment of attention deficit hyperactivity disorder with and without comorbid tic disorders. J Am Acad Child Adolesc Psychiatry 32:350–353, 1993

Swanson J, Kinsbourne M, Roberts W, et al: Time-response analysis of the effect of stimulant medication on the learning ability of children referred for hyperactivity. Pediatrics 61:21–29, 1978

Tannock R, Schachar RJ, Carr RP, et al: Dose-response effects of methylphenidate on academic performance and overt behavior in hyperactive children. Pediatrics 84:648–657, 1989

Tannock R, Ickowicz A, Schachar R, et al: Differential effects of methylphenidate on working memory in ADHD children with and without comorbid anxiety. J Am Acad Child Adolesc Psychiatry 34: 886–896, 1995

Taylor E, Schachar R, Thorley G, et al: Which boys respond to stimulant medication? A controlled trial of methylphenidate in boys with disruptive behaviour. Psychol Med 17:121–143, 1987

Trott GE, Menzel M, Friese HJ, et al: [Effectiveness and tolerance of the selective MAO-A inhibitor moclobemide in children with hyperkinetic syndrome]. Zeitschrift fur Kinder und Jugendpsychiatrie 19:248–253, 1991

Voelker S, Lachar D, Gdowski CL: The Personality Inventory for Children and response to methylphenidate: preliminary evidence for predictive validity. J Pediatr Psychol 8:161–169, 1983

Wagner K, Birmaher B, Carlson G, et al: Safety of Paroxetine and Imipramine in the Treatment of Adolescent Depression. Boca Raton, FL, New Clinical Drug Evaluation Unit, 1998

Watter N, Dreyfuss FE: Modifications of hyperkinetic behavior by nortriptyline. Virginia Medical Monthly 100:123–126, 1973

Wells KC, Pelham WE, Kotkin RA, et al: Psychosocial treatment strategies in the MTA study: rationale, methods, and critical issues in design and implementation. J Abnorm Child Psychol 28:483–505, 2000

Wender PH, Reimherr FW: Bupropion treatment of attention-deficit hyperactivity disorder in adults. Am J Psychiatry 147:1018–1020, 1990

Werry J: Imipramine and methylphenidate in hyperactive children. J Child Psychol Psychiatry 21:27–35, 1980

Wesnes K, Warburton D: The effects of cigarettes of varying yield on rapid information processing performance. Psychopharmacology (Berl) 82:338–342, 1984

Westfall T, Grant H, Perry H: Release of dopamine and 5-hydroxytryptamine from rat striatal slices following activation of nicotinic cholinergic receptors. Gen Pharmacol 14:321–325, 1983

Whalen CK, Henker B, Hinshaw SP, et al: Cognitive-behavioral therapies for hyperactive children: premises, problems, and prospects. J Abnorm Child Psychol 13:391–409, 1985

Wilens T, Biederman J: The stimulants. Psychiatr Clin North Am 15:191–222, 1992

Wilens TE, Spencer TJ: Combining methylphenidate and clonidine: a clinically sound medication option. J Am Acad Child Adolesc Psychiatry 38:614–622, 1999

Wilens TE, Biederman J, Geist DE, et al: Nortriptyline in the treatment of attention deficit hyperactivity disorder: a chart review of 58 cases. J Am Acad Child Adolesc Psychiatry 32:343–349, 1993

Wilens TE, Biederman JB, Mick E, et al: A systematic assessment of tricyclic antidepressants in the treatment of adult attention-deficit hyperactivity disorder. J Nerv Ment Dis 183:48–50, 1995

Wilens TE, Biederman J, Abrantes AM, et al: A naturalistic assessment of protriptyline for attention-deficit hyperactivity disorder. J Am Acad Child Adolesc Psychiatry 35:1485–1490, 1996a

Wilens TE, Biederman J, Prince J, et al: Six-week, double-blind, placebo-controlled study of desipramine for adult attention deficit hyperactivity disorder. Am J Psychiatry 153:1147–1153, 1996b

Wilens TE, Biederman J, Spencer TJ, et al: Controlled trial of high doses of pemoline for adults with attention-deficit/hyperactivity disorder. J Clin Psychopharmacol 19:257–264, 1999a

Wilens TE, Biederman J, Spencer TJ, et al: A pilot controlled clinical trial of ABT-418, a cholinergic agonist, in the treatment of adults with attention deficit hyperactivity disorder. Am J Psychiatry 156:1931–1937, 1999b

Wilens TE, Spencer TJ, Biederman J, et al: A Controlled Trial of Bupropion SR for Attention Deficit Hyperactivity Disorder in Adults. Boca Raton, FL, New Clinical Drug Evaluation Unit, 1999c

Winsberg BG, Bialer I, Kupietz S, et al: Effects of imipramine and dextroamphetamine on behavior of neuropsychiatrically impaired children. Am J Psychiatry 128:1425–1431, 1972

Yepes LE, Balka EB, Winsberg BG, et al: Amitriptyline and methylphenidate treatment of behaviorally disordered children. J Child Psychol Psychiatry 18:39–52, 1977

Zametkin AJ, Rapoport JL: Noradrenergic hypothesis of attention deficit disorder with hyperactivity: a critical review, in Psychopharmacology: The Third Generation of Progress. Edited by Meltzer HY. New York, Raven, 1987, pp 837–842

Zametkin A, Rapoport JL, Murphy DL, et al: Treatment of hyperactive children with monoamine oxidase inhibitors, I: clinical efficacy. Arch Gen Psychiatry 42:962–966, 1985

8

Conduct Disorder

Alayne Yates, M.D.

Definition and Differential Diagnosis

The term *conduct disorder* (CD) refers to a pattern of behaviors that violate the norms and rules of society or the rights of others. Vandalism, truancy, fighting, fire setting, stealing, lying, assault, and rape are examples of antisocial behaviors. Children are not considered to have a CD unless the behaviors are quite severe and/or the overall functioning is compromised. CD is a problematic diagnosis in that it is based on a collection of behaviors and does not speak to dynamic or etiological factors (Cantwell and Baker 1989). It does not make the crucial distinction between impulsive-affective aggression (sudden excessive reaction) and controlled-predatory aggression, the latter of which is of most concern in CD and delinquent youths (Vitiello and Stoff 1997). In DSM-IV (American Psychiatric Association 1994), a child must have at least 3 of 15 problematic behaviors present for at least 6 months to qualify (Table 8–1). CD is further defined as 1) mild, moderate, or severe and 2) of adolescent onset (no conduct problems before age 10) or of childhood onset (at least one conduct problem before age 10). The childhood-onset type is associated with a poorer prognosis, male gender, more aggressive behavior, development of antisocial personality disorder (Kazdin 1987; Pliszka 1998), and deficiencies in verbal skills, visual motor integration, and visuospatial skills (Moffit and Silva 1988). In childhood-onset CD, attention-deficit/hyperactivity disorder (ADHD) is almost always present (Szatmari et al. 1989) and other family members are likely to be antisocial (Lahey et al. 1988).

TABLE 8–1. DSM-IV diagnostic criteria for conduct disorder

A. A repetitive and persistent pattern of behavior in which the basic rights of others or major age-appropriate societal norms or rules are violated, as manifested by the presence of three (or more) of the following criteria in the past 12 months, with at least one criterion present in the past 6 months:

Aggression to people and animals

(1) often bullies, threatens, or intimidates others

(2) often initiates physical fights

(3) has used a weapon that can cause serious physical harm to others (e.g., a bat, brick, broken bottle, knife, gun)

(4) has been physically cruel to people

(5) has been physically cruel to animals

(6) has stolen while confronting a victim (e.g., mugging, purse snatching, extortion, armed robbery)

(7) has forced someone into sexual activity

Destruction of property

(8) has deliberately engaged in fire setting with the intention of causing serious damage

(9) has deliberately destroyed others' property (other than by fire setting)

Deceitfulness or theft

(10) has broken into someone else's house, building, or car

(11) often lies to obtain goods or favors or to avoid obligations (i.e., "cons" others)

(12) has stolen items of nontrivial value without confronting a victim (e.g., shoplifting, but without breaking and entering; forgery)

Serious violations of rules

(13) often stays out at night despite parental prohibitions, beginning before age 13 years

(14) has run away from home overnight at least twice while living in parental or parental surrogate home (or once without returning for a lengthy period)

(15) is often truant from school, beginning before age 13 years

B. The disturbance in behavior causes clinically significant impairment in social, academic, or occupational functioning.

C. If the individual is age 18 years or older, criteria are not met for antisocial personality disorder.

Code based on age at onset:

312.81 Conduct disorder, childhood-onset type: onset of at least one criterion characteristic of conduct disorder prior to age 10 years

312.82 Conduct disorder, adolescent-onset type: absence of any criteria characteristic of conduct disorder prior to age 10 years

312.89 Conduct disorder, unspecified onset: age at onset is not known

Specify severity:

Mild: few if any conduct problems in excess of those required to make the diagnosis **and** conduct problems cause only minor harm to others

Moderate: number of conduct problems and effect on others intermediate between "mild" and "severe"

Severe: many conduct problems in excess of those required to make the diagnosis ***or*** conduct problems cause considerable harm to others

CD must be differentiated from adjustment disorder, mental retardation, organic syndromes, and psychosis. CD has significant comorbidity with ADHD (Cantwell and Baker 1989), Tourette's disorder (Comings and Comings 1987), major depressive disorder (Marriage et al. 1986; Puig-Antich 1982), and substance abuse (Stowell and Estroff 1992). In younger children, CD must be differentiated from oppositional defiant disorder (ODD), which often develops into CD. A few youths with CD have bipolar disorder. However, bipolar disorder can be overdiagnosed in this population because of the irritability and sudden mood changes frequently observed.

Youths with CD feel better when they are active, and they are likely to become restless and frustrated if asked to sit still. When confined to detention, some become acutely depressed and suicidal. This immediate reaction should not be confused with major depressive disorder. When CD and major depressive disorder coexist, CD symptoms may remit when the depression is treated (Kovacs et al. 1988).

Prevalence

One-third to one-half of child and adolescent clinic referrals are initiated because of aggressive or antisocial behaviors (Robins 1981). CD is present in 4%–10% of children and adolescents, with sex-specific rates of 6%–16% for males and 2%–9% for females (American Psychiatric Association 1994). Boys are more likely to be physically aggressive, whereas girls are more likely to threaten or devalue others. Antisocial behavior is common among adolescents—60% reported having engaged in antisocial behaviors such as assault, property damage, arson, and drug abuse (Feldman et al. 1983; Kazdin 1987).

Aggressivity, negativism, and physical fighting at age 5 years are the best predictors of adolescent onset of CD. Other predictors are lower socioeconomic status, parental substance abuse, oppositional defiant disorder, and ADHD (Spender and Scott 1998). Parental criticism and harsh punishment of 5-year-old children predict the emergence of defiant, disruptive behaviors later on (Nix et al. 1999).

Outcome

The prognosis for CD is fair to poor. It is the most stable of all child psychiatric diagnoses (Offord et al. 1992; Robins 1978). As adults, most of these persons will continue to qualify for a clinical diagnosis, although it may not be CD (Rutter and Giller 1983). A few will no longer warrant any diagnosis. Early-onset antisocial behavior has the worst long-term prognosis (Kazdin 1987; Pliszka 1998). Eighteen percent become chronic offenders who commit more than half of all reported offenses (Wolfgang et al. 1972). The mortality rate for seriously disturbed delinquent youths is about 50 times that of nondelinquent youths (Yeager and Lewis 1990). Death is often by homicide, suicide, or violent accident but also may be by drug overdose.

Etiological Factors

Biological Factors

The limbic system, including the amygdala, septal area, and hypothalamus, is involved in the activation and inhibition of aggression. However, higher cortical centers interpret stimuli and mediate the aggressive response. Frontal lobe lesions decrease goal-directed activity but increase impulsive behavior, irritability, and aggression. Various researchers have postulated diminished activity in the prefrontal and premotor cortex and the left temporal and left parietal areas to explain loss of inhibition, impulsivity, and symptoms of hyperactivity (Chelune et al. 1986; Mattes 1980; Mirsky 1987). The limbic system may play a relatively greater role in the generation of affective aggression, whereas higher cortical centers are implicated in predatory aggression.

Youths with CD have a less robust autonomic sympathetic response to fear-arousing stimuli. They also show more rapid habituation in skin conductance to intense or aversive stimuli (Schmidt et al. 1985). This dampened reaction to threat suggests an impaired ability to learn from experience and a weak system of behavioral inhibition (Lytton 1990). When youngsters without CD are punished, their negative behavior diminishes, but when children with CD are punished, their negative behavior increases (Patterson 1976; Snyder 1977). A dampened reaction to threat characterizes predatory aggression, whereas excess reaction to threat characterizes affective aggression (Vitiello and Stoff 1997).

Current data are consistent with a decrease in the levels of the neurotransmitters serotonin and norepinephrine in CD (Rogeness et al. 1992; Siever and Davis 1991). Decreased serotonergic function correlates with aggressive behavior and fire setting in delinquent youngsters (Pliszka et al. 1988; Rogeness et al. 1992) and with traits such as impulsivity, sensation seeking, and proneness to alcoholism (Trimble 1996). Decreased noradrenergic function is associated with problems with attention, conditioning, internalization of values, inhibition, and conduct and with fewer symptoms of anxiety or depression (Rogeness et al. 1990). Youths with CD are more apt to have experienced early abuse with head injury, birth injury, encephalitis, and seizure disorder (Lewis et al. 1987). Early environmental adversity can permanently lower norepinephrine levels, perhaps by affecting dopamine β-hydroxylase, which is necessary for the conversion of dopamine into norepinephrine (Galvin et al. 1995). Thus, early adversity could set the stage for certain youths to develop CD.

Antisocial behaviors tend to run in families. Criminal behavior and alcoholism (especially in fathers), alcohol abuse and somatization (especially in mothers), and antisocial personality (in both) place children at risk for CD (Lahey et al. 1988; Rutter and Giller 1983). In a study of three generations, the stability of aggressive behavior was as pronounced across generations (from grandparent to parent to child) as it was across the 22 years of the children's lives (Huesmann et al. 1984). The Virginia Twin Study (Silberg et al. 1996) showed that genetic influences are strongest for youths with multiple symptoms and/or the combination of hyperactivity and conduct disturbance. Genetic influences are much less pronounced in adolescents with "pure" CD. Another study of adopted children indicated a strong genetic influence on oppositional defiant disorder but an equally strong family/environmental influence on the emergence of CD symptoms (Langbehn et al. 1998). The interaction between environmental and genetic forces is critical for the evolution of CD.

Psychosocial Factors

Severely impaired youths with CD are those most likely to present with neuropsychiatric, developmental, and psychoeducational problems. They often have cognitive limitations, such as low IQ, concrete thought processes, and impaired attention, concentration, memory, sequencing, and abstraction (Moffit and Silva 1988). They may not anticipate problems or understand the consequences of their behavior. They present additional moral limitations, such as the inability to experience guilt or remorse or to see rules as important. Additional emotional limitations include mood lability, paranoid ideation, and inability to identify affects or differentiate one affect from another (Guerra and Slaby 1989; Short and Simeonsson 1986). They are apt to confuse thought, feeling, and action, and the confusion paves the way for impulsivity and affective aggression. They have little self-reflection and often feel chronically misunderstood.

Stable parents who provide consistent structure and emotional support mediate against the development of CD. Parents who are not under stress and who do not have disorders themselves are better able to provide this (Kazdin and Wassell 1999). Parents who are inconsistent and who use harsh criticism and severe punishment promote the emergence of CD symptoms in genetically at-risk youths. The parental approach to child rearing accounts for almost 60% of the variance in adolescent antisocial behavior. The character of the parents is important also; disagreeable, anxious, or neurotic fathers and depressed, neurotic mothers foster children's antisocial behaviors (Nigg and Hinshaw 1998). However, family dynamics are far from simple: siblings who witness the harsh treatment of the CD youth seem to be somewhat protected from developing antisocial behaviors (Reiss et al. 1995).

The crucial role that the family plays underscores the importance of family intervention. However, therapists should not assume that parents willfully aggravate the problem. Youths with CD are difficult and (as any residential facility will attest) can challenge the most skillful of caregivers. Despite good intentions, the parents may not have been able to break through the self-perpetuating cycle of bad behavior leading to ever more desperate consequences.

Treatment

Although several promising treatments are described in this section, long-term follow-up studies are not available. Success is limited once the pattern of antisocial behavior is well established. Intervention is most effective when it begins before the negative, self-perpetuating behavioral patterns are well established.

General Principles

Youngsters with CD often present with bravado and/or threatening behavior. They do this to control the interview and so they will not be seen as "nuts." If the examiner does not have the time or skill to delve beneath the facade, true paranoia, organic impairment, a schizophrenic process, or episodic depression may be overlooked. For instance, when grandiose bipolar disorder adolescents steal, stay up all night, and are sexually promiscuous, this is often attributed to the CD rather than to the underlying process (Lewis 1991).

Transference issues surface rapidly with violent adolescents with CD. Those who feel the most helpless are the ones most likely to threaten, manipulate, or "stonewall" the examiner. Once the evaluation session begins, the examiner may experience anxiety, if not anger, disgust, terror, or loathing, in response to the youth's demeanor or the details of the criminal offense. It is important to deal internally with countertransference issues. If the examiner appears angry, afraid, or judgmental to the patient, this can elicit a menacing or assaultive response.

Assessment and Planning

Children and adolescents with CD rarely request treatment on their own. Schools, community agencies, and parents are more likely to contact the psychiatrist or mental health professional. Some parents come only because of pressure from the schools or juvenile court.

They may be poorly motivated to follow through with treatment plans. The clinician should find out the reasons for the referral, why the parents are seeking help now, and the history of treatment. Information should be gathered from as many sources as possible to 1) cross-check for accuracy, 2) determine whether the delinquent behavior is situation specific (e.g., occurs only when the child visits his or her grandparents), and 3) identify prosocial competencies.

The evaluation should yield a reasonably reliable estimate of the frequency and duration of the problematic behaviors. Several parent and teacher checklists are useful in this respect: the Parent Daily Report Checklist; the Eyberg Child Behavior Inventory and Sutter-Eyberg Student Behavior Inventory; the Self-Report Delinquency Measure; and the New York Teacher Rating Scale. The Connors Rating Scales also can be used. (For a description of these scales and references, see the Fall 1993 *American Academy of Child and Adolescent Psychiatry [AACAP] Research Notes,* available from the AACAP Office of Research, 3615 Wisconsin Avenue, N.W., Washington, DC 20016.)

The family's response to delinquent behavior is an important prognostic indicator. Problematic families role-model violent solutions and may under- or overreact to the child's antisocial behavior. Some families offer little structure or consistency in the home. They do not provide adequate supervision, and the child does not learn to be responsible. The child may be hit, bullied, or taken advantage of by older siblings, thus learning to do the same to younger siblings. Other families overindulge and overprotect the child and refuse to believe anything bad about the child's behavior. Some families blame the system for frustrating the child and bringing out the bad behavior.

An evaluation session with the entire family yields valuable information. Alliances, sources of frustration, and motivation to change should be assessed. Antisocial behavior in a child brings parental conflicts into focus. One or both parents may feel guilty and responsible for not having identified the problem, or one parent may blame the other for being too strict or too easy. Parents who disagree on how a child should be handled usually cannot agree on a behavioral program either.

The child must be thoroughly assessed through direct observation, interview, and a complete neurodevelopmental history. The clinician should ask the child for a narrative history of the antisocial behaviors, his or her perception of the problem, and his or her feelings about what happened and note the presence or absence of guilt and remorse. Predatory (intentional) violence must be differentiated from affective (unintentional) violence. The mental status examination may suggest a need for a full neuropsychological or psychoeducational assessment.

At the end of the evaluation, the psychiatrist will have identified the major psychiatric, neurological, educational, and social strengths and deficits so that he or she can construct a differential diagnosis that includes any possible underlying disorders. An initial treatment plan with target behaviors and contingency rewards can be constructed.

Choice of Treatment Modality

Traditional psychotherapy (Sowles and Gill 1970) and supportive case work (Romig 1976) have not proven effective in treating CD. In fact, youths with CD may become more aggressive when encouraged to express their feelings (Truax et al. 1970). Nevertheless, occasional youths have the capacity to form a meaningful relationship and may benefit from traditional psychotherapy. As DSM's ability to discriminate improves, these individuals may no longer be classified as having CD.

In the past, many youths with CD were treated in specialized inpatient programs. In general, these programs used tightly structured, long-term approaches that tried to nurture competence and a positive identity. Current psychiatric hospitalizations are for stabilization and not intended to treat the underlying process. However, brief hospitalizations can initiate treatment for major depression, organicity, psychosis, ADHD, and learning disabilities. Homicidal or suicidal youths can be stabilized and transferred to less restrictive, long-term settings.

If the family is solid, committed to following through with treatment, and able to exert some behavioral control, a youth with CD may be maintained at home, as long as his or her presence does not endanger other members of the family. Adequate support services must be available for home placements to succeed.

Multisystemic therapy is the best researched approach in use with hard-core delinquent offenders (Borduin 1999). Although the original multisystemic therapy studies need to be replicated by other groups, three randomized trials with serious juvenile offenders have shown long-term reductions in criminal activity, violent offenses, drug-related arrests, and incarceration (Henggeler 1999). The technique, which is based on social-ecological theory, is directed toward family, schools, peers, and the community. A master's-level case manager accesses and coordinates most mental health services, involving probation officers, school social workers, specialized classrooms, day treatment, and/or after school "street" programs and groups according to the particular needs of the youth. Case managers have a small caseload and are available to the family 24 hours a day. A doctoral level psychologist or psychiatrist supervises the program. Multisystemic therapy is usually funded by state or municipal agencies and is thought to be more cost-effective than institutional placement. The chief barrier to implementation is the up-front cost and the availability of suitably trained therapists.

When the youngster cannot be maintained at home, group home or residential treatment is usually the next step. These programs use a strong behavioral approach coupled with around-the-clock supervision, coordination with agencies, positive role modeling, group therapy, peer pressure, and, sometimes, vocational training. However, many programs today are severely hampered by lack of funding. Line staff bear enormous responsibility, are often in danger, and are paid little above minimum wage. This contributes to low morale and extremely high staff turnover. Under these circumstances, it may be impossible for youths to develop meaningful, therapeutic relationships with stable, caring adults.

Group therapy can help youths with CD. However, neurologically and educationally impaired youths may do poorly in groups because of their cognitive limitations and inability to comprehend social nuances. They may, however, be able to profit from a highly structured group that focuses on concrete tasks. Groups can also lead to an increase in problems, presumably because of peer influence (Dishion and Andrews 1995). Social skills training concentrates on developing problem-solving and social/conversational skills within the peer group. Improved impulse control, social competence, and a more internal locus of control can result. Studies are generally favorable (Cunliffe 1992). Anger management and 12-Step groups are also used in treating CD. These groups are highly structured, with a strong psychoeducational and social emphasis. Peer interventions are school-based programs that involve role modeling, confrontation, and social skill building. Immediate results are positive, but long-term effectiveness has not been shown (Offord and Bennett 1994).

Cognitive-Behavioral Techniques

Parent management training is based on social learning theory. It empowers parents, teaching them to establish rules, negotiate compromises, construct treatment contracts, and offer appropriate rewards for prosocial behavior (Patterson et al. 1982). Concrete rewards are used instead of social reinforcers such as approval and encouragement. Initially, parents focus on changing simple behaviors, but as they become more skilled, they address complex issues such as provocative behavior. They are taught to identify prodromata of aggression (e.g., irritability, argumentativeness, temper tantrums) and to respond rapidly and definitively with time-outs. If the youth refuses time-outs, parents withhold certain privileges.

In parent management training, parents systematically record behaviors such as lying, drug use, and stealing on the Parent Daily Report Checklist or another simple check sheet (Chamberlain and Patterson 1985). A variation of this approach uses videotaped modeling of effective approaches. Outcome studies support the use of this technique (Brestan and Eyberg 1998; Kazdin et al. 1987), especially for aggressive youths with CD (Patterson et al. 1982). However, parents must be fairly intelligent, motivated, and able to cooperate with each other and the therapist.

Functional family therapy uses behavioral, structural, and strategic techniques to improve communication and reciprocity between family members. The basic assumption is that the child's behavior has a function in the family, such as keeping family members together. Families of youths with CD learn early behavior identification, negotiation methods, problem solving, and positive reinforcement. Family members learn how to be consistent and how to resist coercion. Functional family therapy has yielded generally positive results (Tolan et al. 1986). Patient-centered and psychodynamic family therapies have not achieved the same positive effects with this population (Kazdin 1987).

The physician managing the youth with CD must be patient, supportive, and very firm. Consequences and contingencies should be outlined in advance. For example, if the program at home does not effect behavioral change, then the court must be reinvolved to consider other options such as a probation home or detention. The physician must avoid under- or overreacting to antisocial behaviors, remembering that it is the patient who must regain self-control. Individual sessions must stress the realities of life and the demands of living. Caregivers need clear direction and support.

There is limited evidence for the long-term effectiveness of treatment programs. Programs fail because 1) the situation is too volatile, 2) the behavior is already entrenched, 3) the parents covertly support the behavior, 4) the parents have already "written the youth off," 5) the parents are no match for the youth and cannot control the behavior, 6) the parents try to accomplish too much too fast, 7) the program is poorly designed or the rewards too costly, or 8) the parents have little in the way of social support.

Psychopharmacological Intervention

Ordinarily, medication can be used to control pathological anger or affective aggression, but it should not be used only to control bad behavior. Youths with CD need to take responsibility for their actions and, if possible, to develop internal controls. For these and other reasons, medication is best initiated within a restricted environment such as detention or a residential facility. If a good response is obtained and the youth appears ready to work with the therapist, medication can be maintained after discharge. Progress should be assessed with checklists, systematic behavioral observations, or other quantifiable data. Drugs with addictive potential are usually avoided, although stimulant medication is prescribed because of the proven benefits.

Pills can be sold, hoarded and taken at once, or bartered. Youths with CD like pills for these reasons, and the more intelligent youngsters are good at presenting the "right" symptoms to manipulate the examiner. Every psychiatrist working with youths who have CD has likely been "conned" more than once.

Most pharmacological agents currently in use for CD have not been adequately studied. Available evidence does support the use of stimulants, often combined with lithium, to treat symptoms of CD (Pliszka 1998). Antipsychotics, antidepressants, lithium, valproate, and clonidine are also beneficial in the treatment of aggression and coexisting disorders. Buspirone, diphenylhydantoin, carbamazepine, and naltrexone are not currently used. β-Blockers are used occasionally but without research support.

Stimulants

Stimulant medication is effective in reducing antisocial behaviors and aggression in CD in youths with and without ADHD (Klein et al. 1997; Weller et al. 1999). Stimulants are not as effective in affective aggression or high-frequency aggression as they are in aggression overall (Gadow et al. 1990). Stimulants also diminish stealing, vandalism, and fighting with peers (Hinshaw et al. 1992; Murphy et al. 1992). Stimulants are usually well tolerated, but less appreciated side effects include increased anxiety, agitation, and even depression.

Lithium

Lithium is an effective treatment for explosive behavior in CD in youths (Brizer 1988), even if it is not the panacea once thought (Weller et al. 1999). It is as effective as haloperidol and has fewer side effects (Campbell et al. 1984; Platt et al. 1984). Lithium also decreases aggressive and explosive behavior in medically or neurologically impaired patients with CD (DeLong and Aldershof 1987). Lithium does not help ADHD symptoms per se, nor does it affect antisocial behavior (Klein et al. 1997). The chief side effects of lithium are weight gain, nausea, and tremor.

Antidepressants

The efficacy of antidepressants in CD has received little attention from researchers, especially considering the substantial comorbidity with depression (Hendren 1991). Studies that do exist indicate that tricyclic medication (imipramine) is effective in diminishing antisocial behaviors (Puig-Antich 1982; Winsberg et al. 1972). Common side effects include dry mouth, dizziness, and fatigue, but the most serious problem is cardiac arrhythmia. Patients with CD may "cheek" medication and hoard and later ingest it in an attempt to commit suicide.

Selective serotonin reuptake inhibitors have not been studied in CD but have been shown to diminish hostility, irritability, and anger attacks in adults with personality disorders and depression (Fava and Rosenbaum 1998). Calming effects are likely related to modulation of serotonin. Selective serotonin reuptake inhibitors are generally safe, even in substantial overdose, but can adversely affect sexual function.

α-Adrenergic Agonists

Clonidine has successfully reduced aggressive outbursts in CD in youths with and without ADHD (Kemph et al. 1993). It is most often used in combination with stimulants but can also be used alone. Clonidine increases central γ-aminobutyric acid (GABA). As GABA levels increase, aggression tends to decrease in youths with CD.

Anticonvulsants

Although carbamazepine has antiaggressive effects that are independent of abnormalities on the electroencephalogram, a review and analysis of many studies yielded equivocal results in the treatment of aggression. Carbamazepine probably should be reserved for patients with a concomitant seizure disorder (Smith and Perry 1992). Valproate used alone or in conjunction with lithium improves aggressive symptoms. In an open trial, valproate was beneficial in 10 youths with mood lability and temper outbursts, and the gains persisted in longer-term follow-up (Donovan et al. 1997). Adolescents may respond more slowly than adults, and this may be caused by lower serum levels (West et al. 1995).

Antipsychotics

Antipsychotic agents such as haloperidol and chlorpromazine are effective in treating aggressive outbursts in CD (Campbell et al. 1984; Werry and Aman 1975). However, short-term side effects of excessive sedation and acute dystonia are frequent and troublesome. In addition, haloperidol has a significant negative effect on cognition (Platt et al. 1984), which is particularly distressing for neurologically and educationally impaired persons. These problems, together with the risk of tardive dyskinesia, limit the usefulness of antipsychotic medication for long-term treatment of CD.

Promising New Medications

Atypical antipsychotics (clozapine, risperidone, olanzapine) have fewer side effects than the older antipsychotic medications. Because the older agents were clearly effective, the newer drugs also may be effective. Novel anticonvulsants—gabapentin and lamotrigine—are effective in stabilizing mood in adults with bipolar disorder and could potentially be used to modulate affective aggression in CD. Calcium antagonists such as verapamil also might stabilize mood and diminish aggression.

Conclusions

Youths with CD present a challenge to clinicians because of their heterogeneity and resistance to intervention. Assessment and treatment by a psychiatrist are valuable additions to social and behavioral approaches commonly used. With such treatment, some extraordinarily difficult youths can be helped to live reasonably productive lives. However, treatment is often not successful because of biological predisposition, inadequate environmental controls, and family disruption.

References

American Psychiatric Association: Diagnostic and Statistical Manual of Mental Disorders, 4th Edition. Washington, DC, American Psychiatric Association, 1994

Borduin CM: Multisystemic treatment of criminality and violence in adolescents. J Am Acad Child Adolesc Psychiatry 36:242–249, 1999

Brestan EV, Eyberg SM: Effective psychosocial treatments of conduct-disordered children and adolescents: 29 years, 82 studies, and 5,272 kids. J Clin Child Psychol 27:180–189, 1998

Brizer DA: Psychopharmacology and the management of violent patients. Psychiatr Clin North Am 11:551–568, 1988

Campbell M, Small AM, Green WH, et al: Behavioral efficacy of haloperidol and lithium carbonate—a comparison in hospitalized aggressive children with conduct disorder. Arch Gen Psychiatry 41:650–656, 1984

Cantwell DP, Baker L: Stability and natural history of DSM-III childhood diagnoses. J Am Acad Child Adolesc Psychiatry 28:691–700, 1989

Chamberlain P, Patterson GR: Aggressive behavior in middle childhood, in The Clinical Guide to Child Psychiatry. Edited by Shaffer D, Ehrhardt AA, Greenhill LL. New York, Free Press, 1985, pp 229–250

Chelune GJ, Ferguson W, Koon R, et al: Frontal lobe disinhibition in attention deficit disorder. Child Psychiatry Hum Dev 16:221–232, 1986

Comings DE, Comings BG: A controlled study of Tourette syndrome, II: conduct. Am J Hum Genet 41:742–760, 1987

Cunliffe T: Arresting youth crime: a review of social skills training with young offenders. Adolescence 27:891–899, 1992

DeLong GR, Aldershof AL: Long-term experience with lithium treatment in childhood: correlation with clinical diagnosis. J Am Acad Child Adolesc Psychiatry 26:389–394, 1987

Dishion TJ, Andrews DW: Preventing escalation in problem behaviors with high risk young adolescents: immediate and one-year outcomes. J Consult Clin Psychol 63:538–548, 1995

Donovan SJ, Susser ES, Nunes EV, et al: Divalproex treatment of disruptive adolescents: a report of 10 cases. J Clin Psychiatry 58:12–15, 1997

Fava M, Rosenbaum JF: Anger attacks in depression. Depress Anxiety 8 (suppl 1):59–63, 1998

Feldman DP, Caplinger TE, Wodarski JS: The St. Louis Conundrum: The Effective Treatment of Antisocial Youths. Englewood Cliffs, NJ, Prentice-Hall, 1983, pp 54–93

Gadow KD, Nolan EE, Svered J, et al: Methylphenidate in aggressive-hyperactive boys, I: effects on peer aggression in public school settings. J Am Acad Child Adolesc Psychiatry 29:710–718, 1990

Galvin M, Ten Eych R, Shekhar A, et al: Serum dopamine beta hydroxylase and maltreatment in psychiatrically hospitalized boys. Child Abuse Negl 19:821–832, 1995

Guerra NG, Slaby RG: Evaluative factors in social problem solving by aggressive boys. J Abnorm Child Psychol 17:277–289, 1989

Hendren RL: Conduct disorder in childhood, in Textbook of Child and Adolescent Psychiatry. Edited by Wiener JM. Washington, DC, American Psychiatric Press, 1991, pp 288–297

Henggeler SW: Multisystemic therapy: an overview of clinical procedures, outcomes, and policy implications. Child Psychology and Psychiatry Review 4:2–10, 1999

Hinshaw SP, Heller T, McHale JP: Covert antisocial behavior in boys with attention-deficit hyperactivity disorder: external validation and effects of methylphenidate. J Consult Clin Psychol 60:274–280, 1992

Huesmann LR, Eron LD, Lefkowitz M, et al: Stability of aggression over time and generations. Dev Psychol 20:1120–1134, 1984

Kazdin AE: Treatment of antisocial behavior in children: current status and future directions. Psychol Bull 102:187–203, 1987

Kazdin AE, Wassell G: Barriers to treatment participation and therapeutic change among children referred for conduct disorder. J Clin Child Psychol 28:60–72, 1999

Kazdin AE, Esveldt-Dawson K, French NH, et al: Effects of parent management training and problem-solving skills training combined in the treatment of antisocial child behavior. J Am Acad Child Adolesc Psychiatry 26:416–424, 1987

Kemph JP, DeVane CL, Levin GM, et al: Treatment of aggressive children with clonidine: results of an open pilot study. J Am Acad Child Adolesc Psychiatry 32:577–581, 1993

Klein RG, Abikoff H, Klass E, et al: Clinical efficacy of methylphenidate in conduct disorder with and without attention deficit hyperactivity. Arch Gen Psychiatry 54:1073–1080, 1997

Kovacs M, Paulauskas S, Gatsonis C, et al: Depressive disorders in childhood, III: a longitudinal study of comorbidity with and risk for conduct disorders. J Affect Disord 15:205–217, 1988

Lahey BB, Piacentini JC, McBurnett K, et al: Psychopathology in the parents of children with conduct disorder and hyperactivity. J Am Acad Child Adolesc Psychiatry 27:163–170, 1988

Langbehn DR, Cadoret RJ, Yates WR, et al: Distinct contributions of conduct and oppositional defiant symptoms to adult antisocial behavior: evidence from an adoption study. Arch Gen Psychiatry 55:821–829, 1998

Lewis DO: Adolescent conduct and antisocial disorders, in Textbook of Child and Adolescent Psychiatry. Edited by Wiener JM. Washington, DC, American Psychiatric Press, 1991, pp 298–308

Lewis DO, Pincus JH, Lovely R, et al: Biopsychosocial characteristics of matched samples of delinquents and nondelinquents. J Am Acad Child Adolesc Psychiatry 26:744–752, 1987

Lytton H: Child and parent effects in boys' conduct disorder: a reinterpretation. Dev Psychol 26:683–697, 1990

Marriage K, Fine S, Moretti M, et al: Relationship between depression and conduct disorder in children and adolescents. J Am Acad Child Adolesc Psychiatry 25:687–691, 1986

Mattes JA: The role of frontal lobe dysfunction in childhood hyperkinesis. Compr Psychiatry 21:358–369, 1980

Mirsky A: Behavioral and psychophysiological markers of disordered attention. Environ Health Perspect 74:191–199, 1987

Moffit TE, Silva PA: Neuropsychological deficit and self-reported delinquency in an unselected birth cohort. J Am Acad Child Adolesc Psychiatry 27:233–240, 1988

Murphy DA, Pelham WE, Lang AR: Aggression in boys with attention deficit-hyperactivity disorder: methylphenidate effects on naturalistically observed aggression, response to provocation, and social information processing. J Abnorm Child Psychol 20:451–466, 1992

Nigg JT, Hinshaw SP: Parent personality traits and psychopathology associated with antisocial behaviors in childhood attention-deficit hyperactivity disorder. J Child Psychol Psychiatry 39:145–159, 1998

Nix RL, Pinderhughes EE, Dodge KA, et al: The relation between mother's hostile attribution tendencies and children's externalizing behavior problems: the mediating role of mother's harsh discipline practices. Child Dev 70:896–909, 1999

Offord DR, Bennett KJ: Conduct disorder: long-term outcomes and intervention effectiveness. J Am Acad Child Adolesc Psychiatry 33:1069–1078, 1994

Offord DR, Boyle MH, Racine YA, et al: Outcome, prognosis, and risk in a longitudinal follow-up study. J Am Acad Child Adolesc Psychiatry 31:916–923, 1992

Patterson GR: The aggressive child: victim and architect of a coercive system, in Behavior Modification and Families. Edited by Mash EJ, Hamerlynck L, Handy L. New York, Brunner/Mazel, 1976, pp 267–316

Patterson GR, Chamberlain P, Reid JB: A comparative evaluation of parent training procedures for families of antisocial children. Behavior Therapy 13:638–650, 1982

Platt JE, Campbell M, Green WH, et al: Cognitive effects of lithium carbonate and haloperidol on treatment-resistant aggressive children. Arch Gen Psychiatry 41:657–662, 1984

Pliszka SR: Comorbidity of attention-deficit/hyperactivity disorder with psychiatric disorder: an overview. J Clin Psychiatry 59 (suppl 7):50–58, 1998

Pliszka SR, Rogeness GA, Renner P, et al: Plasma neurochemistry in juvenile offenders. J Am Acad Child Adolesc Psychiatry 27:588–594, 1988

Puig-Antich J: Major depression and conduct disorder in prepuberty. J Am Acad Child Adolesc Psychiatry 21:118–128, 1982

Reiss D, Hetherington EM, Plomin R: Genetic questions for environmental studies: differential parenting and psychopathology in adolescence. Arch Gen Psychiatry 52:925–936, 1995

Robins LN: Sturdy childhood predictors of adult antisocial behaviour: replications from longitudinal studies. Psychol Med 8:611–622, 1978

Robins LN: Epidemiological approaches to natural history research: antisocial disorders in children. Journal of the American Academy of Child Psychiatry 20:566–580, 1981

Rogeness GA, Javors MA, Maas JW, et al: Catacholamines and diagnoses in children. J Am Acad Child Adolesc Psychiatry 29:234–241, 1990

Rogeness GA, Javors MA, Pliszka SR: Neurochemistry and child and adolescent psychiatry. J Am Acad Child Adolesc Psychiatry 31:765–781, 1992

Romig DA: Justice for Children. Lexington, MA, DC Heath, 1976

Rutter M, Giller H: Juvenile Delinquency: Trends and Perspectives. New York, Penguin, 1983

Schmidt K, Solant MV, Bridger WH: Electrodermal activity of undersocialized aggressive children: a pilot study. J Child Psychol Psychiatry 26:653–660, 1985

Short RJ, Simeonsson RJ: Social cognition and aggression in delinquent adolescent males. Adolescence 21:159–176, 1986

Siever LJ, Davis KL: A psychobiological perspective on the personality disorders. Am J Psychiatry 148:1647–1658, 1991

Silberg J, Meyer J, Pickles A, et al: Heterogeneity among juvenile antisocial behaviours: findings from the Virginia Twin Study of Adolescent Behavioural Development. Ciba Foundation Symposium 94:76–86, 1996

Smith DA, Perry PJ: Nonneuroleptic treatment of disruptive behavior in organic mental syndromes. Ann Pharmacother 26:1400–1408, 1992

Snyder JJ: Reinforcement analysis of interaction in problem and nonproblem families. J Abnorm Psychol 86:528–535, 1977

Sowles RC, Gill SH: Institutional and community adjustment of delinquents following counseling. J Consult Clin Psychol 34:378–402, 1970

Spender Q, Scott S: Conduct disorder. Current Opinion in Psychiatry 9:273–277, 1998

Stowell RJA, Estroff TW: Psychiatric disorders in substance-abusing adolescent inpatients: a pilot study. J Am Acad Child Adolesc Psychiatry 31:1036–1040, 1992

Szatmari P, Boyle M, Offord DR: ADHD and conduct disorder: degree of diagnostic overlap and differences among correlates. J Am Acad Child Adolesc Psychiatry 28:865–872, 1989

Tolan PH, Cromwell RE, Brasswell M: Family therapy with delinquents: a critical review of the literature. Fam Process 25:619–650, 1986

Trimble M: Biological Psychiatry, 2nd Edition. Chichester, England, Wiley, 1996, pp 172–173

Truax CB, Wargo DG, Volksdorf NR: Antecedents to outcome in group counseling with institutionalized juvenile delinquents: effects of therapeutic conditions, patient self-exploration, alternate sessions, and vicarious therapy pretraining. J Abnorm Psychol 76:235–242, 1970

Vitiello B, Stoff DM: Subtypes of aggression and their relevance to child psychiatry. J Am Acad Child Adolesc Psychiatry 36:307–315, 1997

Weller EB, Rowan A, Elia J, et al: Aggressive behavior in patients with attention-deficit/hyperactivity disorder, conduct disorder, and pervasive developmental disorders. J Clin Psychiatry 60 (suppl 15): 5–11, 1999

Werry JS, Aman MG: Methylphenidate and haloperidol in children: effects on attention, memory, and activity. Arch Gen Psychiatry 32:790–795, 1975

West SA, Keck PEJ, McElroy SL: Oral loading doses in the valproate treatment of adolescents with mixed bipolar disorder. J Child Adolesc Psychopharmacol 5:225–231, 1995

Winsberg BG, Bialer I, Kupietz S, et al: Effects of imipramine and dextroamphetamine on behavior of neuropsychiatrically impaired children. Am J Psychiatry 128:1425–1431, 1972

Wolfgang ME, Figlio RM, Sellin T: Delinquency in a Birth Cohort. Chicago, IL, University of Chicago Press, 1972

Yeager CA, Lewis DO: Mortality in a group of formerly incarcerated juvenile delinquents. Am J Psychiatry 147:612–614, 1990

9

Tic Disorders

Kenneth E. Towbin, M.D.
Donald J. Cohen, M.D.
James F. Leckman, M.D.

Definitions

DSM-IV criteria for Tourette's disorder (American Psychiatric Association 1994; Table 9–1) mirror the description offered by Gilles de la Tourette (1885) more than 100 years ago. DSM-IV departs from DSM-III-R (American Psychiatric Association 1987) by integrating a definition of tics into the criteria, reducing the latest age at onset from 21 to 18 years, and specifying the duration of active and symptom-free periods. Symptoms should be present continuously for at least 1 year and never absent for longer than 3 months. When one or more episodes of transient tics are followed months or years later by typical tics lasting a year or more, Tourette's disorder is still the appropriate diagnosis.

For uniformity, DSM-IV introduced an impairment criterion requiring that tic symptoms produce significant distress or impairment; obvious but unimpairing symptoms would not justify a diagnosis. It did not indicate how much distress was required or whose distress was relevant. This criterion created problems for genetic research, epidemiology, and determination of family history. It has been eliminated in DSM-IV-TR (American Psychiatric Association 2000); however, whether for clinical or research work, it may still be prudent to regard "subclinical" chronic symptoms as part of Tourette's disorder.

DSM-IV criteria for the tic disorders are shown in Table 9–1 and compared in Table 9–2. The maximum age at onset is 18 years also for chronic tic disorders (motor or vocal) and transient tic disorder. The minimum duration of symptoms necessary to warrant a diagnosis of transient tic disorder was increased to 4 weeks.

TABLE 9–1. Differences in DSM-IV tic disorders

				Tics during active phase permitted by definition		
Tic disorder	Minimum duration	Maximum duration	Longest interval without tics	Motor only	Vocal only	Concurrent motor and vocal
Transient	4 weeks	<12 months	None	Yes	Yes	Yes
Chronic motor	12 months	None	3 months	Yes	No	No
Chronic vocal	12 months	None	3 months	No	Yes	No
Tourette's disorder	12 months	None	3 months	Yes	Yes	*Required* at some time

Clinical Features

Tics may be differentiated from other repetitive movements by characteristic features of suppressibility, premonitory urges, and variability (Fahn 1993; Towbin et al. 1999). *Suppressibility* is the capacity to delay making movements. *Premonitory urges* are sensations or mental experiences that immediately precede a tic and localize to the same body part as the movement (Leckman et al. 1993). *Variability* refers to the continual changes in location, duration, intensity, complexity, and frequency that are characteristic of tics. Tics arise in one body part or muscle group and then move to another; the speed, intensity, and frequency fluctuate over hours, days, and weeks. Generally, tics arise abruptly and are short-lived, in contrast to dystonic and tonic tics, which begin more gradually and last longer.

Diagnosing tic disorders can be uncomplicated, but some patients' movements defy classification. Other diagnoses to be considered are myoclonus, chorea, seizures, dystonia, athetosis, mannerisms, stereotypies, and restless legs (Jankovic 1992; Towbin et al. 1999). Observing the movements, obtaining a detailed history of the movements and their evolution, and acquiring a detailed family history usually are enough to determine whether the patient has another syndrome or a tic disorder. Occasionally, more time and observations are needed before a diagnosis can be made. When movements are ambiguous, supplementary characteristics should be considered (Towbin et al. 1999): How are the symptoms influenced by distraction? Is there a subjective experience of relief after the movement? How are movements affected by relaxation or intentional effort? Tics also can be observed while the patient sleeps.

Tics may be grouped into different types based on their complexity and origin, as shown in Table 9–3. The groupings can be helpful in tracking the course and frequency of symptoms. Complex tics may be difficult to recognize and mistaken for misbehaviors; sometimes they are thought to be compulsions. Tic disorders rarely begin with only complex tics. When only complex tics are present, the disorder most likely has been present for some time.

Natural History

The three tic disorders probably have different natural histories. However, no systematic studies of the course of chronic or transient tics have been done to prove this. Movements

TABLE 9–2. Examples of tics

Tics	Examples
Simple motor	Blinking eyes; grimacing; thrusting tongue; widening eyes; jerking jaw, head, shoulder, stomach; nodding; turning head; moving arms, fingers, legs; kicking; tensing body parts
Complex motor	Holding funny expressions, squinting, grooming hair, cracking joints, stretching neck or arms, touching body parts, tapping, hopping, stomping, picking at things (self, clothes), pushing on eyes, hitting self, slamming things, making obscene gestures such as giving the finger (copropraxia)
Simple vocal	Coughing, emitting "hawwwwk" noises, squeaking, saying "aaaaaa" or "tttttuh," clearing throat, saying "uh, uh, uh," blowing across upper lip, making popping sounds, snorting, gnashing teeth, swishing
Complex vocal	Repeatedly saying "uh huh," "you bet," "all right," "yeah"; repeating one's own words, phrases, sentences (palilalia); repeating others' words, phrases, sentences (echolalia); swearing; using obscene language or making obscene noises; making racial or colloquial insults

TABLE 9–3. DSM-IV diagnostic criteria for tic disorders

307.22 Chronic motor or vocal tic disorder

A. Single or multiple motor or vocal tics (i.e., sudden, rapid, recurrent, nonrhythmic, stereotyped motor movements or vocalizations), but not both, have been present at some time during the illness.

B. The tics occur many times a day nearly every day or intermittently throughout a period of more than 1 year, and during this period there was never a tic-free period of more than 3 consecutive months.

C. The onset is before age 18 years.

D. The disturbance is not due to the direct physiological effects of a substance (e.g., stimulants) or a general medical condition (e.g., Huntington's disease or postviral encephalitis).

E. Criteria have never been met for Tourette's disorder.

307.21 Transient tic disorder

A. Single or multiple motor and/or vocal tics (i.e., sudden, rapid, recurrent, nonrhythmic, stereotyped motor movements or vocalizations)

B. The tics occur many times a day, nearly every day for at least 4 weeks, but for no longer than 12 consecutive months.

C. The onset is before age 18 years.

D. The disturbance is not due to the direct physiological effects of a substance (e.g., stimulants) or a general medical condition (e.g., Huntington's disease or postviral encephalitis).

E. Criteria have never been met for Tourette's disorder or chronic motor or vocal tic disorder.

Specify if:

Single episode or **recurrent**

of Tourette's disorder typically appear in early to middle childhood. The peak age at incidence is between 5 and 8 years (Leckman et al. 1998). Usually, Tourette's disorder commences with eye or facial tics (see Table 9–3). Commonly, it advances to grimacing and other facial movements. Sometimes shoulders, arms, trunk, legs, and feet are affected. Patients usually do not have involvement of every extremity or body part, but a sequence of rostral to caudal progression is common. Virtually all Tourette's disorder patients have waxing and waning of tics throughout the day and over months. The morphology, intensity, and frequency of movements generally change.

Bursts of tics are not random events; they cluster together in "bouts" (Peterson and Leckman 1998). These bouts also erupt in a pattern that produces "bouts of bouts," and the "bouts of bouts" bunch together. The clinical observations of more and less severe periods during the illness are supported by methodical research (Peterson and Leckman 1998).

At least 50% of the patients who are referred for treatment of Tourette's disorder have a prodrome of inattention, decreased concentration, and excessive motor restlessness (Bornstein et al. 1990; Caine et al. 1988). In nonclinical community samples, this fraction shrinks to 8% (Apter et al. 1993). Symptoms such as these may result in a diagnosis of attention-deficit/hyperactivity disorder (ADHD). Similarly, children with a diagnosis of ADHD are much more likely to develop tic disorders when compared with the general population (Spencer et al. 1999). At present, the association between Tourette's disorder and ADHD can be interpreted in two ways. The co-occurrence of hyperactivity and tics may be the simultaneous expression of two different disorders or two different features of one disorder (Pauls et al. 1993; Spencer et al. 1999). It now appears that treating ADHD with stimulants is not the cause of Tourette's disorder. However, stimulants produce tics in some individuals, and medication-induced movements typically disappear when stimulants are stopped (Barkley 1990; Bocherding et al. 1990). Tics persisting after cessation of stimulants are now understood to be the hastened or coincidental expression of an underlying tic disorder in a vulnerable individual.

Obsessions and compulsions usually emerge long after the onset of tics in Tourette's disorder. Symptoms of obsessive-compulsive disorder (OCD) are reported by 40% of the patients who have had Tourette's disorder for 10 years or longer (Frankel et al. 1986; Robertson et al. 1988). Family genetic studies suggest that OCD in persons with Tourette's disorder *and* a significant percentage of OCD without concurrent tics have the same genetic etiology (Pauls and Leckman 1986). Furthermore, obsessive-compulsive symptoms in Tourette's disorder may be as pernicious as severe primary OCD (George et al. 1993).

Transient tics usually emerge during early or middle childhood and then disappear. Chronic motor tics or vocal tics also emerge during this time and typically fluctuate over long periods, changing in morphology, location, frequency, and intensity. Chronic motor tic disorder probably is a variant of Tourette's disorder and confers roughly equivalent recurrence risk in successive generations for either Tourette's disorder or chronic motor tics. Evidence indicates that associated symptoms are as common in chronic motor tic disorder as in Tourette's disorder, but this has not been studied methodically.

Epidemiology

The lifetime prevalence of tic disorders may be as high as 20%. Among tic disorders, the largest lifetime prevalence is for transient tics (15%). Three-month prevalence rates for chronic multiple tics are estimated to be 3%–4% (Costello et al. 1996a, 1996b). Estimates of the general population point prevalence of tic disorders are 2.9–9.3 per 10,000. Boys carry a greater risk for tics; measured sex ratios range from 1.6:1 (Tanner 1993) to nearly 3:1 (Shapiro et al. 1988). The prevalence rate for children may be as much as 12 times the adult rate (Burd et al. 1986). For Tourette's disorder specifically, the estimated point prevalence is 4 per 10,000, with a point prevalence of 5 per 10,000 for males and 3 per 10,000 for females (Apter et al. 1993).

Initiating Treatment

Treatment of Tourette's disorder relies on an awareness of development, neurobiology, life events, and intrapsychic processes. Ordinarily, successful treatment hinges on the clinician's ability to manage and participate in different simultaneous interventions that target these elements. For this reason, the assessment of patients for Tourette's disorder should go beyond determining the mere presence or severity of tics and draw upon multiple strategies.

The Interview

Interviewing the child and his or her parents is critical to a complete evaluation. The goals are to gather a thorough history and learn about the child and his or her family. It is important to consider domains of school, peers, self-image, future aspirations, and relationships with family members. It is useful to ascertain the location, frequency, and intensity of tics; the impairment they produce; and whether premonitory urges occur with movements. During the interview, the clinician can observe movements directly.

However, the objectives of the interview go beyond basic data. As a part of a complete assessment, the interview gives the examiner an opportunity to learn about associated conditions and the child's affective state, coping styles, capacities, and current level of adaptation. The interview permits the examiner to evaluate the relationship between the child and his or her parents: how successfully they cooperate, the intensity and valence of their interactions, and the methods they use to resolve their conflicts and worries. The examiner can perceive how the child's parents regard the movements and any associated conditions. Discussion with family members can uncover other sources of family tension or impairment that precipitate or aggravate distress. The genetics of Tourette's disorder suggest that one or both parents also may have a tic spectrum disorder. The emergence of a child's symptoms can produce immense anguish for these parents. How they manage this anxiety can strongly influence further conflict.

Multiple Data Sources: Raters, Sites, and Times

The diversity of symptoms and their fluctuation place unusual demands on the evaluator. No single gauge of impairment exists. Impairment may correlate best with the magnitude, duration, and circumstances at the peak (worst) or modal (most common) levels of severity rather than the average level. Consequently, direct observation in the consulting room has limited value in determining symptom severity; any single hour of observation is an unreliable measure of impairment. Conversely, general levels of symptom severity may be equally erroneous; very severe short outbursts may demand treatment nevertheless. An evaluator should discover the settings, times of day, and situations that aggravate or ameliorate symptoms because symptoms may change so much within a short time.

The goal of assessment is to learn as much as possible about factors that influence the patient's symptoms. It relies on multiple objective measures of symptom severity and determining which symptoms or features are the most onerous. For some patients, tics are the greatest burden; for others, coexisting psychological or familial difficulties are the most disabling (Dooley et al. 1999). Knowing this is essential when selecting and monitoring treatment interventions.

Assessment Instruments

A comprehensive evaluation of tic disorders in children and adolescents is as intricate as for any serious neurological or psychiatric symptom. Standardized instruments are based on either clinician or patient ratings for tics and associated phenomena such as ADHD and OCD. General screening tools offer a "review of systems" for comorbid conditions. Also, instruments are available for use with videotapes (Chappell et al. 1994; Goetz et al. 1999); some of these can be completed by parents or teachers.

Standard Scales for Tics and Associated Disorders

Most instruments for assessing tic severity are completed by clinicians. The Yale Global Tic Severity Scale (YGTSS; Leckman et al. 1988, 1989; Scahill et al. 1999) probes number, frequency, intensity, complexity, and interference of motor and vocal tics. There are separate global severity estimates of motor tics, vocal tics, and overall impairment. The YGTSS is valid and reliable (Leckman et al. 1989) and includes an index checklist of movements. By organizing observations, the YGTSS can complement a complete examination record. The scale may be used as a semistructured interview to obtain observations from anxious parents. Its disadvantages are its length, detail, and time requirements and the need for training and practice to achieve interrater reliability.

The Hopkins Motor and Vocal Tic Scale (HMVTS; Walkup et al. 1992) is another valid and reliable clinician-rated instrument. It uses visual analog scales grouped by the anatomical area affected by each tic symptom. It, too, contains global ratings of motor and vocal tic severity on an interval scale of 1 (absent) to 5 (severe) and an overall global impairment rating (best ever to worst ever) on a visual analog scale. Its advantages are its high specificity and simplicity. The HMVTS also may be used to assess treatment progress. However, it does not provide measures of tic complexity or simplicity.

Clinicians, teachers, and/or parents may find the Tourette Syndrome Symptom List (TSSL; Scahill et al. 1999) helpful. This checklist informs the clinician about the variety of movements and associated symptoms that patients show outside the consulting room. It can be valuable for obtaining information from teachers about symptoms that are visible in the classroom.

A consensus scale has recently been adopted for measuring severity and lifetime likelihood of tic disorders (Robertson et al. 1999).

The evaluator should determine whether symptoms or disorders coexist with tics. General behavior scales that review a variety of symptoms can help. A common scale is the Child Behavior Checklist (CBCL; Achenbach and Edelbrock 1981). Symptoms of depression may be elucidated by self-assessments, such as the Children's Depression Inventory (CDI; Kovacs and Beck 1977). In addition, symptoms of excessive motor activity and inattention warrant specific measures of severity. For screening, the more specific and shorter Child Attention Problems Scale (CAPS; Barkley 1990) is supplanting the Conners Rating Scales (Goyette et al. 1978). Once ADHD is diagnosed, treatment efficacy can be monitored by the ADHD Rating Scale (Barkley 1990). The Conners Parent Rating Scale can help in monitoring symptoms at home (Goyette et al. 1978).

Laboratory Studies

The proper laboratory evaluation depends on the history, neurological examination, and treatment plan. A routine extensive laboratory evaluation is not necessary. Before medication is started, complete blood counts and liver function studies (alanine aminotransferase [ALT], aspartate aminotransferase [AST]) should be obtained. Electrocardiograms (ECGs) can be postponed until the clinician plans to start medicines that pose a cardiac conduction risk. If anxiety or depression is present, thyroid function studies should be included. Computed tomography (CT) or magnetic resonance imaging (MRI) scans are indicated clinically only if focal neurological signs or obvious central nervous system abnormalities are present. MRI investigations suggested that differences in the structure of the basal ganglia occur in Tourette's disorder (Peterson et al. 1993; Singer et al. 1993). In the absence of a sudden onset of symptoms or a family history of rheumatic heart disease or Sydenham's chorea, routine throat cultures, anti-DNAase, and anti-streptolysin O (ASO) titers are unnecessary for the general evaluation of new-onset tics.

Academic Achievement and Standardized Psychological Testing

Learning problems influence emotional adjustment and life trajectory. Coexisting learning problems are common in persons with Tourette's disorder who present for treatment, especially the subgroup with ADHD and tics (Schultz et al. 1998). Deficits in arithmetic skills (Como 1993; Dykens et al. 1990) and visual motor integration also are seen (Dykens et al. 1990; Schultz et al. 1998). Standardized psychological evaluations help identify these problems (Carter et al. 1999b). Cognitive tests add information about the patient's intellectual and verbal capacities, and projective assessments can make emotional struggles clearer. Children with tic disorders may have social immaturity or problems in social adjustment. They may be ostracized by their peers. Social adjustment measures such as the Vineland Scales of Adaptive Functioning may help ascertain these difficulties (Dykens et al. 1990; Stokes et al. 1991).

Treatment Interventions

The primary goal of treatment is to facilitate general developmental progress and adaptation; symptom reduction is only relevant in the context of this primary objective. The primary goal is accomplished by both active support and reducing as many impediments to healthy developmental progress as possible. Treatment should avert interjecting additional impairment from other sources such as medication side effects, spiraling family anxiety, and social isolation. The clinician must be alert to the demands that these chronic disorders place on patients and families. The fluctuating symptoms and the influence of development create varying conditions. For example, during the course of the illness, serious new symptoms may arise or the introduction of new demands can overwhelm previously successful adaptations.

Psychological and Environmental Interventions

Patient and Family Education

The mainstay of treatment of tic disorders is patient and family education. Education about the etiology and natural history of the disorder, the assessment of severity, treatment alternatives, and the variety of other interventions is imperative. Education can reduce anxiety, put symptom severity in perspective, and lay the groundwork for later treatment. It also cements the relationship between the clinician and the patient. Such a relationship is critical during difficult periods when symptoms have worsened or treatment results are disappointing.

Behavioral and Other Interventions at School

Adaptation to school is among the most important developmental tasks that children and adolescents face. Those with Tourette's disorder confront difficulties in academic, behavioral, social, and intrapsychic domains. Many individuals with Tourette's disorder also have significant learning problems. Interventions must be tailored to the symptoms and requirements of each patient. This demands that clinicians work closely with school staff. Educating teachers and school nurses about Tourette's disorder can be a vital first step in the care of an individual patient. For those children with high levels of impulsivity, inattention, and restlessness, programming that is predictable, articulates clear expectations, has low pupil-to-teacher ratios, and contracts for rewards within time frames that are consonant with the patient's limitations may be extremely useful (Denkla and Reader 1993). For children and adolescents with severe motor tics, introducing flexibility into the program often can permit the pupil's strengths to emerge. Use of word processors, permission to take extra time for examinations, time each day away from the class, and other interventions can be important (Carter et al. 1999a). In addition to academic needs, attention to relationships with classmates and subtle or overt exclusion is important. Social isolation and ostracism should be a focus of intervention for teachers and guidance counselors as well. Sometimes social exclusion can be reduced by talking with students in small groups or an entire class.

Behavioral and Other Interventions at Home

Severe symptoms often create a vicious cycle of increasing stress, increasingly severe symptoms, and increasing impairment. Home can contribute to this cycle as much as school. Many of the strategies that are useful in school may be applied at home, especially those for impulsivity, inattention, and hyperactivity. Taking the time to develop behavioral programs with clear expectations, predictability, and appropriate and timely rewards for achievement can be extremely helpful.

The genetic transmission of Tourette's disorder has immediate clinical relevance. The chances are that one of the child's parents has or has had symptoms in the spectrum of tics or OCD. When ADHD is present, it is also likely that a parent experienced similar difficulties during childhood. How the parent managed or is managing symptoms and the adaptation to his or her disorder may be a factor in his or her relationship with the child. As a result, work with parents, siblings, and even extended family members may be critical to dampening anxiety and frustration (Cohen et al. 1988). Sometimes a parent's experience may offer a model of adaptation and provide endless reassurance to the child. The converse may also occur: a parent's precarious adjustment to his or her condition may be played out with the child in ways that impede the child's adaptation.

Psychotherapy

Tic disorders can exert harmful psychological effects at any point along the continuum of development. Tourette's disorder can amplify a minor imbalance between drives and defenses into a significant conflict. Self-esteem, identifications, and self-perception may be powerfully influenced by a tic disorder. Destructive ego defenses and impaired interpersonal relationships may result. These types of problems are especially suited to psychotherapeutic intervention (Cohen 1980; Cohen et al. 1982).

The choice of which psychotherapeutic modality should be used—psychodynamic, cognitive, behavioral, or interpersonal—will depend on patient characteristics and symptoms (Cohen 1995). A variety of defenses can emerge to cope with a chronic condition that forces one to act involuntarily. Dynamic or cognitive psychotherapy offers patients an understanding of the vicissitudes of these destructive defenses or reactions and of their effect on the illness. These modalities provide opportunities to employ alternative coping strategies or more adaptive defenses (Cohen 1995).

Serious comorbid conditions, such as anxiety or depression, may aggravate a tic disorder. Interpersonal or cognitive psychotherapy may be quite useful in reducing sources of depression or anxiety and in helping the patient understand how the two disorders aggravate each other.

The adaptation some patients make to their symptoms may have dramatic effects on interpersonal relationships. Battles over dependency and autonomy, oppositional behaviors, risk taking, and investment in being seen as "sick" or helpless are examples of detrimental patterns that can entangle others. Individual psychodynamic psychotherapy may be uniquely suited to assisting patients who develop such highly maladaptive concessions to their illness.

Support groups sponsored by the Tourette Syndrome Association or clinical centers specializing in tic disorders also can be quite helpful. The Tourette Syndrome Association has a readily accessible Web site: http://tsa.mgh.harvard.edu.

Family Therapy

In addition to a patient's personal struggles, Tourette's disorder can place an extraordinary burden on his or her family and closest relationships. Tourette's disorder symptoms influence and are influenced by the family system; recognizing this reciprocal relationship between symptoms and family functioning is important. Impaired family relationships can fuel stress at home. Destructive parent-child dynamics can crystallize around the nidus of tic symptoms. These kinds of relationships can limit or thwart improvement.

Reciprocally, parents and siblings may be affected by their family member's symptoms (Cohen et al. 1988). The family may become overwhelmed by the additional demands of a troubled member. Severe symptoms may transform preexisting, previously manageable family conflicts into relentless antagonism. The patient's impairment or treatment requirements may widen long-standing discord in a marriage, magnify dysfunctional patterns of family adaptation, or overwhelm the stability of a fragile parent. Family therapy may be very useful in absorbing and treating these additional demands at two critical points: initially, when the diagnosis is made, and later, when clinical or family crises occur. Sometimes individual treatment for family members is crucial.

Pharmacological Therapies

The use of pharmacological agents in the treatment of tics and associated symptoms has received extensive attention over the last decade. It must be underscored that medications should be prescribed in the context of a therapeutic relationship in which the patient understands targets for which the drug is being used and is able to talk openly about any side effects or concerns he or she may have. Medication is a sound choice only when the level of impairment, risks, and benefits have been carefully weighed (Carpenter et al. 1999). Important principles that should be heeded when using any of the agents outlined in the following subsections are presented in Table 9–4 (Towbin 1995).

TABLE 9–4. Basic principles of pharmacotherapy of Tourette's disorder

Start patients on the lowest doses of medication possible.
Slowly increase dose in the smallest increments.
Ensure adequate duration of a drug trial before changing to a new medication.
Use sufficient doses before changing to a different medication.
Maintain the lowest effective dose.
Minimize polypharmacy.
If you must change medications, add or discontinue one medication at a time.

Pharmacotherapy for Tics

Pharmacological agents that have been shown to be useful in the treatment of tics are presented in Table 9–5. Because clonidine exerts powerful effects on blood pressure, it must be initiated at very low doses and increased gradually. The minimum time necessary to determine whether clonidine has been ineffective may be as long as 12 weeks. This is a disadvantage when a patient has severe tics and is in crisis. Clonidine may not fulfill the requirement for rapid improvement. For some clinicians, α_2-noradrenergic agents are the first choice in pharmacological treatment because they are safer for chronic use and have fewer side effects than the more potent dopamine-blocking agents (e.g., haloperidol). The primary disadvantage of these agents is that fewer patients will respond to clonidine, and perhaps guanfacine. The long minimum duration of treatment requires patience and no more than moderate impairment.

For the treatment of Tourette's disorder, haloperidol and pimozide have been studied more than any other agents. Some clinicians also use fluphenazine. Perhaps 80% of Tourette's disorder patients will benefit from haloperidol or pimozide, with a reduction of symptoms by at least 25%. However, haloperidol, fluphenazine, and pimozide produce significant adverse effects. As many as 50% of patients develop side effects (Shapiro and Shapiro 1993). For some patients, the side effects are as intolerable as their tic symptoms. In addition, the risks of long-term administration, especially tardive dyskinesia but also weight gain, problems with memory, and dulling of emotions, require that children receive regular, thoughtful monitoring while taking medication for chronic tics.

Risperidone is a benzisoxazole with antagonistic action against both serotonergic and dopaminergic receptors. Risperidone has not been marketed for tic disorders, but several reports now suggest that it may help patients with Tourette's disorder or comorbid Tourette's disorder and OCD (Bruun and Budman 1996; Lombroso et al. 1995). Some controlled investigations suggested that risperidone may have a more desirable profile than haloperidol with regard to learning and memory in schizophrenic patients (Kern et al. 1999). Risperidone can produce tardive dyskinesia, although the risk may be lower than with conventional agents. In about 30% of risperidone-treated patients, weight gain has been a problem (Wirshing et al. 1999). Risperidone also can produce significant prolonga-

TABLE 9–5. Drugs used in the treatment of tics

Type of agent	Drug	Dosage range (mg/day)	Noteworthy side effects
Dopaminergic blocking agents	Haloperidol	0.5–6.0	Sedation, drug-induced parkinsonism, akathisia, emotional blunting, weight gain, tardive dyskinesia, dysphoria, acute dystonia, endocrine changes
	Fluphenazine and others	0.5–6.0	
	Pimozide	1.0–8.0	All the above; also possible QTc prolongation
	Risperidone	0.25–4.0	All the above, including QTc prolongation
α_2-Noradrenergic agonists	Clonidine	0.1–0.3	Sedation, dry mouth, headache, postural hypotension, ordinary hypotension, dizziness, rebound hypertension with abrupt withdrawal
Benzodiazepines	Clonazepam	1.0–4.0	Sedation

tion of the QTc interval; cardiac monitoring is advised. Studies comparing risperidone and haloperidol in the treatment of schizophrenic patients have reported mixed results on the relative frequency and severity of side effects (Rosebush and Mazurek 1999). Nevertheless, when carefully monitored, risperidone may be an appropriate alternative to haloperidol for the treatment of tics.

Clonazepam is a benzodiazepine conventionally used as an anticonvulsant. It has not been extensively investigated, but it has been useful for a small minority of Tourette's disorder patients (Gounce and Barbeau 1977). Positive characteristics of clonazepam are that it is safe in long-term use and has few serious side effects. Many patients taking clonazepam will find that sedation is a problem, and it is less likely than other agents to be helpful to those persons with Tourette's disorder. Steingard et al. (1994) suggested an adjunctive role for clonazepam in otherwise refractory patients.

Reports on the use of injected botulinum toxin suggest some benefit (Awaad 1999; Jankovic 1994; Scott et al. 1996). This treatment may be appropriate for the very few isolated, extremely severe single tics that are highly refractory, although other experience suggests that the benefits are marginal at best.

Pharmacotherapy for Obsessive-Compulsive Symptoms

The treatment of OCD is reviewed elsewhere in this volume (see Chapters 14 [in children and adolescents] and 50 [in adults]). Several studies suggest that a variety of agents that share properties of inhibiting the presynaptic reuptake of serotonin can be helpful (Table 9–6). Selective serotonin reuptake inhibitors (SSRIs) may successfully reduce obsessive-compulsive symptoms in patients with Tourette's disorder and aggression (Bruun and Budman 1998), but these agents seem to have little effect on typical complex tics (King et al.

1992). An unsatisfactory response to SSRIs in persons with tics or with a family history of tics plus disabling obsessive-compulsive symptoms warrants consideration of augmentation techniques. Adding agents that block dopamine, such as haloperidol, pimozide, or risperidone, may be helpful (McDougle et al. 1990, 1994) but carries an increased risk of parkinsonian side effects (Kurlan 1998).

TABLE 9–6. Drugs used in the treatment of obsessive-compulsive symptoms with Tourette's disorder

Type of agent	Drug	Dosage range (mg/day)	Common or noteworthy side effects
Tricyclic antidepressants	Clomipramine	50–250	Sedation, dry mouth, postural hypotension, tachycardia, hypotension, constipation, QTc prolongation
Selective serotonin reuptake inhibitors	Fluoxetine Fluvoxamine Paroxetine Sertraline	5–80 25–300 20–60 25–200	Restlessness, insomnia, agitation, sedation, nausea, microsomal enzyme induction, anorexia, akathisia, sexual dysfunction, gastric upset, weight gain
Augmentation agents (used in conjunction with above)	Haloperidol	0.5–3.0	Sedation, drug-induced parkinsonism, akathisia, emotional blunting, weight gain, tardive dyskinesia, dysphoria, acute dystonia, endocrine effects
	Pimozide	1–6	As above, plus possible QTc prolongation
	Risperidone	0.5–5.0	As above, plus possible QTc prolongation
	Buspirone	15–45	Nausea, vomiting, dizziness

Pharmacotherapy for Impulsivity, Inattention, and Hyperactivity

The medications that have been studied for the pharmacological treatment of inattention, hyperactivity, *and* tics in children are listed in Table 9–7. The treatment of ADHD-like symptoms in children with tics has been modified significantly by clinical research over the last 5 years. Among individuals with ADHD-like symptoms and tics, evidence indicates that tics will worsen during stimulant treatment in 15%–36% (Castellanos et al. 1997) as a result of the stimulant (Riddle et al. 1995). Other data suggest that stimulants may not increase tics (Erenberg et al. 1985; Gadow et al. 1999). These studies have different interpretations; thus, preferences differ for the first-line pharmacotherapy of ADHD symptoms. An emerging body of literature suggests that the increase in tic symptoms may be time-limited and that patients' tic symptoms return to baseline after several months (Castellanos et al. 1997; Gadow et al. 1999). Consequently, some clinicians reason that stimulant-induced worsening of tics may not occur or may be temporary. They choose stimulants as the first-line intervention. There is uncertainty about whether dextroamphetamine and methylphenidate are equally benign; some investigators believe methylphenidate produces shorter-lived, less severe increases in tic symptoms (Castellanos et al. 1997).

TABLE 9–7. Drugs used in the treatment of hyperactivity with tics

Type of agent	Drug	Dosage range (mg/day)	Common side effects
α_2-Noradrenergic agonists	Clonidine Guanfacine	0.1–0.3 0.5–2.5	Sedation, dry mouth, headache, postural hypotension, ordinary hypotension, dizziness, rebound hypertension with abrupt withdrawal
Tricyclic antidepressants	Desipramine Nortriptyline	25–250 25–125	Sedation, hypotension, tachycardia, fatigue, dry mouth, QTc prolongation (especially desipramine)
Stimulants	Methylphenidate D-amphetamine Adderall®	5–60 2.5–50 5–50	Increased tics, insomnia, weight loss, anorexia, headache, tachycardia, irritability, dysphoria
	Magnesium pemoline	37.5–112.5	Significantly elevated risk of hepatotoxicity with pemoline

Some patients will develop unendurable worsening of symptoms or emotional side effects while taking stimulants. Parents and the patient worry that the medication may be causing harm. Stimulants are impractical under these circumstances; uncertainty over whether the worsening symptoms are emanating from acute stressors, natural waxing and waning, or the medication cannot be resolved.

Other clinicians view any increase in tics as undesirable and prefer to begin with medications that will not produce this. They reason that if more "tic-benign" agents fail to control ADHD symptoms or produce other intolerable side effects, then stimulants can be considered because the alternatives have been eliminated. This approach is based on observations that some patients will have a marked reduction in ADHD-like symptoms with α_2-noradrenergic agonists (Chappell et al. 1995; Leckman et al. 1991; Steingard et al. 1993). These agents pose a negligible risk of drug-induced worsening of tics and are often well tolerated in low doses. Sedation can be a problem as the dose increases. Clonidine and guanfacine have similar mechanisms of action, although guanfacine may have greater affinity than clonidine for critical frontal region receptors (Aoki et al. 1994; Arnsten et al. 1996). Both agents may require observations for up to 12 weeks to determine their efficacy. Some clinicians also prefer to first use nonstimulant medications such as these in children with ADHD symptoms without tics if they have a family history of tics.

If α_2-noradrenergic agents are not successful, then the patient and physician face a series of dilemmas. Evidence indicates that desipramine is beneficial in the control of hyperactivity and impulsivity, but it also may pose a serious risk of cardiac arrhythmia (Biederman 1991; Riddle et al. 1991). Some investigators propose that desipramine can be prescribed safely with close follow-up of ECGs and attention to drug-drug interactions (Biederman 1991). Nortriptyline appears to convey less cardiac risk and may be beneficial, but it has been studied only minimally for this condition (Spencer et al. 1993). Some clinicians advocate combinations of tricyclic medications and α_2-noradrenergic agents. Frequent blood pressure monitoring becomes critical when these agents are used together.

Pharmacological intervention becomes pivotal when tics and ADHD-like symptoms are both severe. In some patients, α_2-noradrenergic agonists alone may reduce both tics and ADHD-like symptoms; it may be prudent to try this medication first. Other patients can have a similar response with dopaminergic blocking agents alone. For others, stimulants are the only agents that will effectively reduce the ADHD-like symptoms. Hyperactivity and inattention may diminish without worsening tics, but close monitoring is recommended. Some patients are forced to confront worsening tics when stimulants are the only agents that reduce their ADHD-like symptoms; the addition of dopamine blocking agents temporarily may be necessary under these circumstances (Golden 1993). This approach can help some patients, but it should be regarded as the last resort for those in whom adequate trials of other measures have been unsuccessful.

Pharmacotherapy for Self-Injurious Behaviors

Repetitive self-injurious behaviors are the most distressing and dangerous symptoms. Often these behaviors respond to medications that are used for tics. Dopaminergic blocking agents are prescribed first because they are more likely to work and because of the speed of their action. Yet some clinicians will turn to α_2-noradrenergic agonists if dopaminergic blocking agents are ineffective or if side effects develop. SSRIs in doses similar to those used in the treatment of compulsions have been suggested. Sometimes it is impossible to determine whether a self-injurious behavior is a compulsion or a complex tic. Because one cannot predict which repetitive self-injurious behaviors will respond to SSRIs, when other agents are ineffective, SSRIs should be tried.

Pharmacological treatments for self-injurious behaviors in conditions such as autism, habit disorders, or organic brain disorders warrant consideration for Tourette's disorder as well. No controlled studies have been done, but case reports do exist in which these agents, including lithium (Luchins and Dojka 1989) and β-adrenergic blocking agents such as propranolol and atenolol (Luchins and Dojka 1989), were used for self-injurious behaviors.

Conclusions

Each decade finds investigators closer to learning essential truths about the etiology, natural history, associated features, and useful treatments of tic disorders. With recent research that links cortico-striato-thalamo-cortical pathways with the basal ganglia (Leckman et al. 1992), MRI scanning data that suggests changes in the basal ganglia (Peterson et al. 1993), and the progressive elaboration of the human genome, we are on the threshold of discovering basic relationships between genes, neurotransmitters, and clinical symptoms. Work exploring risk factors that influence genetic expression has highlighted important environmental mechanisms that affect adaptation and impairment (Carter et al. 1994; Leckman et al. 1990). For persons with Tourette's disorder, these are early steps toward the discovery of more specific medications, treatment techniques, and accurate genetic counseling (Cohen et al. 1992).

Clinicians, families, and patients must wrestle with the day-to-day influence of symptoms. But now they can turn to an ever larger repertoire of interventions and medications prescribed by a clinical community that is more knowledgeable than ever. Forming and maintaining a close physician-patient relationship, educating the patient and his or her family about Tourette's disorder, and implementing school-based interventions continue to be critical. Physicians have an expanding variety of medications that are helpful to patients and produce fewer burdensome side effects. There has been great progress in the development of new medications and methods of intervening. Nevertheless, the cornerstone of treatment firmly remains with the clinician acquiring an understanding of the person with the disorder and being mindful of his or her specific talents, aspirations, and needs.

References

Achenbach TM, Edelbrock CS: Behavioral problems and competencies reported by parents of normal and disturbed children aged 4 through 16. Monogr Soc Res Child Dev 46:1–82, 1981

American Psychiatric Association: Diagnostic and Statistical Manual of Mental Disorders, 3rd Edition, Revised. Washington, DC, American Psychiatric Association, 1987

American Psychiatric Association: Diagnostic and Statistical Manual of Mental Disorders, 4th Edition. Washington, DC, American Psychiatric Association, 1994

American Psychiatric Association: Diagnostic and Statistical Manual of Mental Disorders, 4th Edition, Text Revision. Washington, DC, American Psychiatric Association, 2000

Aoki C, Go CG, Venkatesan C, et al: Perikaryal and synaptic-localization of $alpha_{2A}$-adrenergic receptor-like immunoreactivity. Brain Res 306:9–18, 1994

Apter A, Pauls DL, Bleich A, et al: An epidemiologic study of Gilles de la Tourette's syndrome in Israel. Arch Gen Psychiatry 50:734–738, 1993

Arnsten A, Steere J, Hunt R: The contribution of alpha 2-noradrenergic mechanisms of prefrontal cortical cognitive function: potential significance for attention-deficit hyperactivity disorder. Arch Gen Psychiatry 53:448–455, 1996

Awaad Y: Tics in Tourette syndrome: new treatment options. J Child Neurol 14:316–319, 1999

Barkley RA: Attention Deficit Hyperactivity Disorder: A Handbook for Diagnosis and Treatment. New York, Guilford, 1990, pp 304, 311

Biederman J: Sudden death in children treated with a tricyclic antidepressant. J Am Acad Child Adolesc Psychiatry 30:495–497, 1991

Bocherding BG, Keysor CS, Rapoport JL, et al: Motor/vocal tics and compulsive behaviors on stimulant drugs: is there a common vulnerability? Psychiatry Res 33:83–94, 1990

Bornstein RA, Stefl ME, Hammond L: A survey of Tourette syndrome patients and their families: the 1987 Ohio Tourette survey. J Neuropsychiatry Clin Neurosci 2:275–281, 1990

Bruun RD, Budman CL: Risperidone as a treatment for Tourette's syndrome. J Clin Psychiatry 57:29–31, 1996

Bruun RD, Budman CL: Paroxetine treatment of episodic rages associated with Tourette's disorder. J Clin Psychiatry 59:581–584, 1998

Burd L, Kerbeshian J, Wikenheiser M, et al: Prevalence of Gilles de la Tourette syndrome in North Dakota adults. Am J Psychiatry 143:787–788, 1986

Caine ED, McBride MC, Chiverton P, et al: Tourette's syndrome in Monroe County school children. Neurology 38:472–475, 1988

Carpenter LL, Leckman JF, Scahill L, et al: Pharmacological and other somatic approaches to treatment, in Tourette's Syndrome—Tics, Obsessions, Compulsions: Developmental Psychopathology and Clinical Care. Edited by Leckman JF, Cohen DJ. New York, Wiley, 1999, pp 370–398

Carter A, Pauls DL, Leckman JF, et al: A prospective longitudinal study of Gilles de la Tourette's syndrome. J Am Acad Child Adolesc Psychiatry 33:377–385, 1994

Carter AS, Fredine NJ, Findley D, et al: Recommendations for teachers, in Tourette's Syndrome—Tics, Obsessions, Compulsions: Developmental Psychopathology and Clinical Care. Edited by Leckman JF, Cohen DJ. New York, Wiley, 1999a, pp 360–369

Carter AS, Fredine NJ, Schultz RA, et al: Comprehensive psychological and educational assessment, in Tourette's Syndrome—Tics, Obsessions, Compulsions: Developmental Psychopathology and Clinical Care. Edited by Leckman JF, Cohen DJ. New York, Wiley, 1999b, pp 325–337

Castellanos FX, Giedd JN, Elia J, et al: Controlled stimulant treatment of ADHD and comorbid Tourette's syndrome: effects of stimulant and dose. J Am Acad Child Adolesc Psychiatry 36:589–596, 1997

Chappell PB, McSwiggan-Hardin MT, Scahill L, et al: Videotape counts in the assessment of Tourette's syndrome: stability, reliability, and validity. J Am Acad Child Adolesc Psychiatry 33:386–393, 1994

Chappell P, Riddle MA, Scahill L, et al: Guanfacine treatment of comorbid attention-deficit hyperactivity disorder in Tourette's syndrome: preliminary clinical experience. J Am Acad Child Adolesc Psychiatry 34:1140–1146, 1995

Cohen DJ: The pathology of the self in primary childhood autism and Gilles de la Tourette syndrome. Psychiatr Clin North Am 3:383–402, 1980

Cohen DJ: Psychosocial therapies for children and adolescents: overview and future directions. J Abnorm Child Psychol 23:141–156, 1995

Cohen DJ, Detlor J, Shaywitz B, et al: Interaction of biological and psychological factors in the natural history of Tourette's syndrome: a paradigm for childhood neuropsychiatric disorders, in Gilles de la Tourette Syndrome. Edited by Friedhoff A, Chase T. New York, Raven, 1982, pp 31–40

Cohen DJ, Ort SI, Leckman JF, et al: Family functioning in Tourette syndrome, in Tourette's Syndrome & Tic Disorders: Clinical Understanding and Treatment. Edited by Cohen DJ, Bruun RD, Leckman JF. New York, Wiley, 1988, pp 179–197

Cohen DJ, Friedhoff A, Leckman JF, et al: Tourette syndrome: extending basic research to clinical care, in Tourette Syndrome: Genetics, Neurobiology and Treatment. Edited by Chase T, Friedhoff A, Cohen D. New York, Raven, 1992, pp 341–362

Como P: Neuropsychological testing, in The Handbook of Tourette's Syndrome and Related Tic and Behavioral Disorders. Edited by Kurlan R. New York, Marcel Dekker, 1993, pp 221–239

Costello EJ, Angold A, Burns BJ, et al: The Great Smoky Mountains Study of Youth: goals, design, methods, and the prevalence of DSM-III-R disorders. Arch Gen Psychiatry 53:1129–1136, 1996a

Costello EJ, Angold A, Burns BJ, et al: The Great Smoky Mountains Study of Youth: functional impairment and serious emotional disturbance. Arch Gen Psychiatry 53:1137–1143, 1996b

Denkla MB, Reader MJ: Education and psychosocial interventions: executive dysfunction and its consequences, in The Handbook of Tourette's Syndrome and Related Tic and Behavioral Disorders. Edited by Kurlan R. New York, Marcel Dekker, 1993, pp 431–453

Dooley JM, Brna PM, Gordon KE: Parent perceptions of symptom severity in Tourette's syndrome. Arch Dis Child 81:440–441, 1999

Dykens E, Leckman J, Riddle M, et al: Intellectual, academic, and adaptive functioning of Tourette syndrome children with and without attention deficit disorder. J Abnorm Child Psychol 18:607–615, 1990

Erenberg G, Cruse RP, Rothner AD: Gilles de la Tourette's syndrome: effects of stimulant drugs. Neurology 35:1346–1348, 1985

Fahn S: Motor and vocal tics, in The Handbook of Tourette's Syndrome and Related Tic and Behavioral Disorders. Edited by Kurlan R. New York, Marcel Dekker, 1993, pp 3–17

Frankel M, Cummings JL, Robertson MM, et al: Obsessions and compulsions in Gilles de la Tourette's syndrome. Neurology 36:378–382, 1986

Gadow KD, Sverd J, Sprafkin J, et al: Long-term methylphenidate therapy in children with attention-deficit hyperactivity disorder and chronic multiple tic disorder. Arch Gen Psychiatry 56:330–336, 1999

George MS, Trimble MR, Ring HA, et al: Obsessions in obsessive-compulsive disorder with and without Gilles de la Tourette syndrome. Am J Psychiatry 150:93–97, 1993

Gilles de la Tourette G: Etude sur une affection nerveuse caracterisee par de l'incoordination motrice accompagnee d'echolalie et de coprolalie. Archives de Neurologie 9:19–42, 158–200, 1885

Goetz CG, Pappert EJ, Louis ED, et al: Advantages of a modified scoring method for the Rush Video-Based Tic Rating Scale. Mov Disord 14:502–506, 1999

Golden GS: Treatment of attention deficit hyperactivity disorder, in The Handbook of Tourette's Syndrome and Related Tic and Behavioral Disorders. Edited by Kurlan R. New York, Marcel Dekker, 1993, pp 423–431

Gounce M, Barbeau A: Seven cases of Gilles de la Tourette's syndrome: partial relief with clonazepam—a pilot study. Can J Neurol Sci 4:279–283, 1977

Goyette CH, Conners CK, Ulrich RF: Normative data on Revised Conners Parent and Teacher Rating Scales. J Abnorm Child Psychol 6:221–236, 1978

Jankovic J: Diagnosis and classification of tics and Tourette's syndrome, in Tourette Syndrome: Genetics, Neurobiology and Treatment (Advances in Neurology Series, Vol 58). Edited by Chase TN, Friedhoff AJ, Cohen DJ. New York, Raven, 1992, pp 7–14

Jankovic J: Botulinum toxin in the treatment of dystonic tics. Mov Disord 9:347–349, 1994

Kern RS, Green MF, Marshall BD Jr, et al: Risperidone versus haloperidol on secondary memory: can newer medications aid learning? Schizophr Bull 25:223–232, 1999

King R, Riddle MA, Goodman WK: Psychopharmacology of obsessive compulsive disorder in Tourette's syndrome, in Tourette Syndrome: Genetics, Neurobiology and Treatment (Advances in Neurology Series, Vol 58). Edited by Chase TN, Friedhoff AJ, Cohen DJ. New York, Raven, 1992, pp 283–291

Kovacs M, Beck A: An empirical-clinical approach toward a definition of childhood depression, in Depression in Childhood: Diagnosis, Treatment, and Conceptual Models. Edited by Schulterbrandt J, Raskin A. New York, Raven, 1977, pp 1–25

Kurlan R: Acute parkinsonism induced by the combination of a serotonin reuptake inhibitor and a neuroleptic in adults with Tourette's syndrome. Mov Disord 13:178–179, 1998

Leckman JF, Towbin KE, Ort SI, et al: Clinical assessment of tic disorder severity, in Tourette's Syndrome and Tic Disorders: Clinical Understanding and Treatment. Edited by Cohen DJ, Bruun RD, Leckman JF. New York, Wiley, 1988, pp 55–79

Leckman JF, Riddle A, Hardin MT, et al: The Yale Global Tic Severity Scale (YGTSS): initial testing of a clinician rated scale of tic severity. J Am Acad Child Adolesc Psychiatry 28:566–574, 1989

Leckman JF, Dolnansky ES, Hardin MT, et al: Perinatal factors in the expression of Tourette's syndrome: an exploratory study. J Am Acad Child Adolesc Psychiatry 29:220–226, 1990

Leckman JF, Hardin MT, Riddle MA, et al: Clonidine treatment of Gilles de la Tourette's syndrome. Arch Gen Psychiatry 48:324–328, 1991

Leckman JF, Pauls DL, Peterson BS, et al: Pathogenesis of Tourette syndrome: clues from the clinical phenotype and natural history, in Tourette Syndrome: Genetics, Neurobiology and Treatment (Advances in Neurology Series, Vol 58). Edited by Chase TN, Friedhoff AJ, Cohen DJ. New York, Raven, 1992, pp 15–24

Leckman JF, Walker DE, Cohen DJ: Premonitory urges in Tourette's syndrome. Am J Psychiatry 150:98–102, 1993

Leckman JF, Zhang H, Vitale A, et al: Course of tic severity in Tourette syndrome: the first two decades. Pediatrics 102 (1 pt 1):14–19, 1998

Lombroso PJ, Scahill L, King RA, et al: Risperidone treatment of children and adolescents with chronic tic disorders: a preliminary report. J Am Acad Child Adolesc Psychiatry 34:1147–1152, 1995

Luchins DJ, Dojka D: Lithium and propranolol in aggression and self-injurious behavior in the mentally retarded. Psychopharmacol Bull 25:556–563, 1989

McDougle C, Goodman WK, Price L, et al: Neuroleptic addition in fluvoxamine-refractory obsessive compulsive disorder. Am J Psychiatry 147:652–654, 1990

McDougle CJ, Goodman WK, Leckman JF, et al: Haloperidol addition in fluvoxamine-refractory obsessive compulsive disorder: a double-blind, placebo-controlled study of fluvoxamine in patients with and without tics. Arch Gen Psychiatry 51:302–308, 1994

McDougle CJ, Epperson CN, Pelton GH, et al: A double-blind, placebo-controlled study of risperidone addition in serotonin reuptake inhibitor-refractory obsessive-compulsive disorder. Arch Gen Psychiatry 57:794–801, 2000

Pauls DL, Leckman JF: The inheritance of Gilles de la Tourette syndrome and associated behaviors: evidence for an autosomal dominant transmission. N Engl J Med 315:993–997, 1986

Pauls DL, Leckman JF, Cohen DJ: Familial relationship between Gilles de la Tourette syndrome, attention deficit disorder, learning disabilities, speech disorders, and stuttering. J Am Acad Child Adolesc Psychiatry 32:1044–1050, 1993

Peterson BS, Leckman JF: The temporal dynamics of tics in Gilles de la Tourette syndrome. Biol Psychiatry 44:1337–1348, 1998

Peterson BS, Riddle MA, Cohen DJ, et al: Reduced basal ganglia volumes in Tourette's syndrome using three-dimensional reconstruction techniques from magnetic resonance images. Neurology 43: 941–949, 1993

Riddle M, Nelson JC, Kleinman CS, et al: Sudden death in children receiving norpramine: a review of three reported cases and commentary. J Am Acad Child Adolesc Psychiatry 30:104–108, 1991

Riddle MA, Lynch L, Scahill L, et al: Methylphenidate discontinuation and re-initiation during long term treatment of children with Tourette's disorder and attention-deficit hyperactivity disorder. J Child Adolesc Psychopharmacol 5:205–214, 1995

Robertson MM, Trimble MR, Lees AJ: The psychopathology of the Gilles de la Tourette syndrome: a phenomenological analysis. Br J Psychiatry 152:383–390, 1988

Robertson MM, Banerjee S, Kurlan R, et al: The Tourette Syndrome Diagnostic Confidence Index: development and clinical associations. Neurology 53:2108–2112, 1999

Rosebush PI, Mazurek MF: Neurologic side effects in neuroleptic-naive patients treated with haloperidol or risperidone. Neurology 52:782–785, 1999

Scahill L, King RA, Schultz RT, et al: Selection and use of diagnostic and clinical rating instruments, in Tourette's Syndrome—Tics, Obsessions, Compulsions: Developmental Psychopathology and Clinical Care. Edited by Leckman JF, Cohen DJ. New York, Wiley, 1999, pp 310–324

Schultz RT, Carter AS, Bladstone M, et al: Visual motor, visuoperceptual and fine motor functioning in children with Tourette syndrome. Neuropsychology 12:134–145, 1998

Scott BL, Jankovic J, Donovan DT: Botulinum toxin injection into vocal cord in the treatment of malignant coprolalia associated with Tourette's syndrome. Mov Disord 11:431–433, 1996

Shapiro AK, Shapiro E: Neuroleptic drugs, in The Handbook of Tourette's Syndrome and Related Tic and Behavioral Disorders. Edited by Kurlan R. New York, Marcel Dekker, 1993, pp 347–377

Shapiro AK, Shapiro ES, Young JG, et al: Gilles de la Tourette Syndrome. New York, Raven, 1988

Singer HS, Reiss AL, Brown JE, et al: Volumetric MRI changes in basal ganglia of children with Tourette's syndrome. Neurology 43:950–956, 1993

Spencer T, Biederman J, Wilens T, et al: Nortriptyline treatment of children with attention deficit disorder and tic disorder or Tourette's syndrome. J Am Acad Child Adolesc Psychiatry 32:205–210, 1993

Spencer T, Biederman J, Coffey B, et al: The 4-year course of tic disorders in boys with attention-deficit/hyperactivity disorder. Arch Gen Psychiatry 56:842–847, 1999

Steingard R, Biederman J, Spencer T, et al: Comparison of clonidine response in the treatment of attention-deficit hyperactivity disorder with and without comorbid tic disorder. J Am Acad Child Adolesc Psychiatry 32:350–353, 1993

Steingard RJ, Goldberg M, Lee D, et al: Adjunctive clonazepam treatment of tic symptoms in children with co-morbid tic disorders and ADHD. J Am Acad Child Adolesc Psychiatry 33:394–399, 1994

Stokes A, Bawden HN, Camafield PR, et al: Peer problems in Tourette's disorder. Pediatrics 87:936–942, 1991

Tanner CM: Epidemiology, in The Handbook of Tourette's Syndrome and Related Tic and Behavioral Disorders. Edited by Kurlan R. New York, Marcel Dekker, 1993, pp 337–346

Towbin KE: Evaluation, establishing the therapeutic alliance, and informed consent in child and adolescent psychopharmacology. Child Adolesc Psychiatr Clin N Am 4:1–15, 1995

Towbin KE, Peterson BS, Cohen DJ, et al: Differential diagnosis, in Tourette's Syndrome—Tics, Obsessions, Compulsions: Developmental Psychopathology and Clinical Care. Edited by Leckman JF, Cohen DJ. New York, Wiley, 1999, pp 118–139

Walkup JT, Rosenberg LA, Brown J, et al: The validity of instruments measuring tic severity in Tourette's syndrome. J Am Acad Child Adolesc Psychiatry 30:472–477, 1992

Wirshing DA, Wirshing WC, Kysar L, et al: Novel antipsychotics: comparison of weight gain liabilities. J Clin Psychiatry 60:358–363, 1999

10

Elimination Disorders

David Shaffer, M.B., B.S.,
F.R.C.P., F.R.C.Psych.

Enuresis

Definitions

Functional enuresis is defined by DSM-IV (American Psychiatric Association 1994, p. 109) as the "repeated voiding of urine into bed or clothes (whether involuntary or intentional)" in children who have achieved a chronological age of at least 5 years (or an equivalent developmental level) (Table 10–1). The wetting must be considered clinically significant, as evidenced by a frequency of two episodes per week for at least 3 consecutive months or by the presence of distress or impairment in social, academic (occupational), or other important areas of functioning. Further, the wetting must not occur exclusively as the result of the physiological effect of a substance such as a diuretic or a general medical condition. This criterion would not exclude the frequent occurrence of nocturnal incontinence that occurs during treatment with antipsychotics. A distinction is made in DSM-IV between *nocturnal enuresis,* in which the wetting occurs only at night, and daytime, or *diurnal,* enuresis. A combination of these conditions, termed *nocturnal and diurnal enuresis,* also may be present.

Preparation of this chapter was made possible by National Institute of Mental Health (NIMH) Research Training Grant T32 MH16434 and NIMH Intervention Research Center Grant 1 P30 MH60570.

TABLE 10–1. DSM-IV diagnostic criteria for enuresis

A. Repeated voiding of urine into bed or clothes (whether involuntary or intentional).

B. The behavior is clinically significant as manifested by either a frequency of twice a week for at least 3 consecutive months or the presence of clinically significant distress or impairment in social, academic (occupational), or other important areas of functioning.

C. Chronological age is at least 5 years (or equivalent developmental level).

D. The behavior is not due exclusively to the direct physiological effect of a substance (e.g., a diuretic) or a general medical condition (e.g., diabetes, spina bifida, a seizure disorder).

Specify type:

Nocturnal only

Diurnal only

Nocturnal and diurnal

Natural History and Epidemiology

Enuresis has historically been classified as a primary subtype if the person has never been continent for a significant period and as a secondary subtype if a child has been dry for a period of time before the onset of incontinence. However, these distinctions have not proved helpful clinically or etiologically and are not recognized in DSM-IV.

Bladder control is acquired in most children by age 4 years. Children who are not dry at night by age 4 years acquire continence relatively slowly (Kaffman and Elizur 1977; F. J. W. Miller et al. 1960; Oppel et al. 1968; Verhulst et al. 1985). At age 5 years, between 5% and 10% of children are enuretic, decreasing to about 1% by age 18. About 1% of children have an onset of enuresis after age 7 (Essen and Peckham 1976; McGee et al. 1984; F. J. W. Miller et al. 1960; Oppel et al. 1968); onset after age 11 is exceedingly rare. Spontaneous remission of the disorder at any age is generally preceded by intermittent or sporadic wetting, often followed by a period during which the child wets only when ill or during cold weather (F. J. W. Miller et al. 1960).

Enuresis is equally common in males and in females until age 5 years, but by age 11, males with enuresis outnumber females with this disorder two to one (Essen and Peckham 1976; Oppel et al. 1968; Rutter et al. 1973). In early childhood, males appear to be both less likely to remit spontaneously and more likely to develop secondary enuresis (Essen and Peckham 1976). Diurnal enuresis occurs at least weekly in about 3% of children ages 5–7 years and at least once a month in 8% (Dejonge 1973). Diurnal enuresis occurs more commonly in girls (Blomfield and Douglas 1956; Hallgren 1956; Jarvelin et al. 1988) and is associated with higher rates of psychiatric disturbance (Rutter et al. 1973) and urinary tract abnormalities and urinary tract infections (Hansson 1992) than is nocturnal enuresis.

Etiology

The etiology of enuresis is not completely understood. The disorder commonly runs in families (Bakwin 1961; Fergusson et al. 1986; Jarvelin et al. 1988). Family aggregation studies of nocturnal enuresis suggest an autosomal dominant mode of inheritance with variable degrees of penetrance (Arnell et al. 1997). Molecular genetic studies have implicated DNA polymorphisms on chromosomes 8, 12, and 13 (Arnell et al. 1997; Dahl et al. 1995; Eiberg et al. 1995; Hollmann et al. 1998), but as yet no evidence indicates that clinically distinct subtypes are associated with one or another location (von Gontard et al. 1998, 1999a). Cases of monozygotic twins with only one enuretic child suggest that not all enuresis has a genetic cause.

An unknown but substantial proportion of enuretic persons have functional urinary tract abnormalities, variously referred to as detrusor instability or unstable bladder syndrome (Hellstrom et al. 1990; Jarvelin et al. 1990, 1991; Starfield 1967; Van Gool and de Jonge 1989). Abnormal diurnal rhythms of urine production have been noted in enuretic patients with nocturnal polyuria. This has been attributed to abnormalities of central vasopressin receptor activity (Norgaard et al. 1985; Rittig et al. 1989). No evidence indicates that enuresis is related to disorders of sleep or sleep architecture (Mikkelsen and Rapoport 1980). Other biological correlates of the disorder include early developmental delays (Essen and Peckham 1976; Fergusson et al. 1986; Steinhausen and Göbel 1989), minor neurological abnormalities (Mikkelsen et al. 1980; Shaffer et al. 1984), and low IQ (Jarvelin et al. 1988).

Associations between enuresis and several psychosocial factors have been noted. These include a delay in starting toilet training until after age 18 months (Fergusson et al. 1986; Kaffman and Elizur 1977), stressful events in early childhood such as hospitalizations (Douglas 1973; Fergusson et al. 1986), the birth of a younger sibling (Werry and Cohrssen 1965), and serious trauma (Chadwick 1985).

Associated Conditions

As noted earlier in this chapter, urinary tract infections are found more frequently in children with diurnal enuresis (Hansson 1992; Kunin et al. 1962). Treatment of the infection rarely cures the enuresis (Jones et al. 1972). Enuresis may facilitate ascending urinary tract infection (Dodge et al. 1970), or the association may reflect a third factor such as structural abnormalities of the urinary tract and/or incomplete bladder voiding (Jarvelin et al. 1990; Sujka et al. 1991). Infection should always be ruled out by urine microscopy and culture. Chronic constipation has been reported to be associated with enuresis (Jarvelin et al. 1990; O'Regan et al. 1986), and a loaded rectum could be expected to reduce bladder capacity, leading to detrusor muscle irritability and wetting behavior.

Enuresis has traditionally been regarded as a symptom of an underlying psychological disturbance. Psychiatric disorder is more frequent in enuretic than in nonenuretic persons, with the highest rates in children with mixed or diurnal enuresis (von Gontard et al. 1999b). However, no specific associated disorders have been identified in epidemiologically based studies (Rutter et al. 1973). Treatment of enuresis is associated with an improvement in well-being (Baker 1969; Behrle et al. 1956; Hagglof et al. 1998; Longstaffe et al. 2000; Lovibond 1964; Moffatt et al. 1987), but it generally does not result in a "cure" of the associated psychiatric disorder (Moffatt 1994; Moffatt et al. 1987; Shaffer et al. 1984).

Assessment

Assessment should include determination of associated pathological conditions, including day wetting, learning and behavior problems, encopresis, urinary tract infection, and constipation. The assessment should include a urine culture and microscopy to rule out urinary tract infection.

Treatment

Night Wetting

Only a minority of enuretic persons are ever evaluated (Foxman et al. 1986), and many who see a physician do not receive any treatment. Many families appear to accept bed-wetting as an unavoidable part of growing up.

Initial steps. The child's wetting behavior should be charted over the course of 2 weeks to establish a baseline against which the effects of future treatment can be judged. Keeping this baseline assessment may reduce symptoms in up to 20% of enuretic persons (Devlin and O'Cathain 1990; Schmitt 1986). Fluid restriction before bed and night lifting (i.e., waking the child at night and bringing him or her to the toilet to empty the bladder) are commonsense measures that may lead to a small initial reduction in wetting frequency, but their effectiveness is usually short-lived (Fournier et al. 1987; Hagglund 1965; Roberts and Schoellkopf 1951). More specific interventions are almost always required.

Night alarm. Treatment with the night alarm is more likely to result in permanent remission than are pharmacological interventions (Houts et al. 1994), but weeks or months and whole-hearted participation by the parents are required. Most alarms link an auditory signal to a sensor that is triggered by the presence of urine. The sensor may be placed in the bed or attached to the child's pants. The alarm may be carried on a wristband or in a pocket or placed on the side of the bed. The effect of alarm treatment has variously been attributed to classical conditioning (Collins 1973; Finley et al. 1973; Young and Morgan 1972), operant conditioning (De Leon and Mandell 1966; Hansen 1979; Lovibond 1964), avoidant learning (Houts 1995; Lovibond 1972), and social learning theory (Turner 1973).

"Cure," defined as 14 consecutive dry nights (Butler 1991), is effected in between 50% and 100% of cases. Most studies report a cure rate of approximately 80% (Forsythe and Butler 1989; von Gontard 1998). Factors relating to less successful outcomes include day wetting (Fielding 1985), presence of an associated psychiatric disorder, family stress, and lack of concern in the child about the symptom. Mentally retarded children, institutionalized children, and children with diabetes mellitus are often thought to be difficult to treat; however, enuresis in all may respond to the night alarm (Boggs et al. 1992; Hanson et al. 1988; Sloop and Kennedy 1973; Smith 1981), but more slowly than in other children. Cure, when achieved, usually occurs in the second month of treatment (Kolvin et al. 1972), but it may occur sooner with the body-worn alarm (Butler et al. 1990). Treatment should continue for at least 12 weeks before being abandoned.

Premature termination rates run as high as 48% (Turner 1973; Turner et al. 1970). Significant relapse occurs in about one-third of the children who initially achieve cure, within 6 months of completion of initial treatment (Doleys 1977). No clear predictors of relapse have been identified (Butler et al. 1990; Doleys 1977; Fielding 1985; Turner 1973; Young and Morgan 1973). Strategies that have been developed to reduce the relapse rate include intermittent reinforcement (Finley et al. 1973) and overlearning (Houts 1995; Houts et al. 1984; Young and Morgan 1972).

Drug treatment. Medication is less likely to result in permanent cure than is night alarm treatment. However, because of its convenience, medication is almost certainly the most commonly offered treatment for enuresis by practitioners (Foxman et al. 1986). The most frequently prescribed medicines are the synthetic antidiuretics and the antidepressants.

Synthetic antidiuretics. Randomized, double-blind, placebo-controlled clinical trials have shown that desamino-D-arginine vasopressin (DDAVP) may be effective in the short-term treatment of enuresis (Dimson 1986; K. Miller and Klauber 1990; Terho and Kekomaki 1984) and, when combined with a night alarm, may be more effective than either treatment alone (Bradbury 1997; Sukhai et al. 1989). The mechanism of action is thought to involve a reduction of nocturnal urine flow. Administered either intranasally with a dose-metered pump or orally, in doses of 20–40 μg, before bedtime, DDAVP exerts an effect for 6–12 hours (Ramsden et al. 1982; Richardson and Robinson 1985). Fifty percent of enuretic persons stop wetting completely with this treatment, whereas another 40% show a marked reduction in wetting frequency. Most children relapse when the treatment is stopped (K. Miller et al. 1989), so that in the long run the effect of treatment with DDAVP is inferior to that with the night alarm (Wille 1986). The most common side effects are nasal pain, nasal congestion, rhinitis, and conjunctivitis. Hyponatremia is a rare complication, especially if water intake is controlled. Long-term suppression of endogenous antidiuretic hormone secretion is not thought to occur (Rew and Rundle 1989).

Tricyclic antidepressants. Since the first report by MacLean (1960) of the use of tricyclic antidepressants (TCAs) in the treatment of enuresis, many randomized, double-blind, placebo-controlled studies have confirmed the efficacy of these agents. Imipramine reduces wetting frequency in 85% of enuretic children and suppresses wetting completely in 30%, but most children relapse within 3 months of discontinuing treatment (Rapoport et al. 1980; Shaffer et al. 1968). Response is dose related, and a single nighttime dose of between 1.0 and 2.5 mg/kg is usually effective (Jorgensen et al. 1980). There appears to be no benefit in exceeding a combined desipramine-imipramine serum level of 60 ng/mL (De Gatta et al. 1984, 1990; Rapoport et al. 1980). Common side effects include dry mouth, dizziness, headache, and constipation. There is the potential for severe, even lethal, toxicity from accidental or intentional overdoses. The mechanism of action of the TCAs in enuresis is not clear but may be related to noradrenergic reuptake inhibition (Rapoport et al. 1980).

Other drug treatments. Anticholinergic medications that increase functional bladder capacity, reduce neurogenic bladder contractions, and delay the desire to void (e.g., belladonna, propantheline, oxybutynin chloride, and terodiline) do not appear to reduce night wetting (Baigrie et al. 1988; Elmer et al. 1988; Lovering et al. 1988; Rapoport et al. 1980; Wallace and Forsythe 1969).

Antipsychotic-induced enuresis. Most antipsychotics may induce enuresis, the management of which should be determined by the intended course of treatment. Patients who are taking antipsychotics (particularly adolescents) should be asked about the onset of enuresis, because embarrassment over the condition may lead to underreporting or noncompliance with antipsychotic treatment. If the need for antipsychotics is marginal, discontinuation should be considered. If antipsychotics are needed but the duration of treatment is likely to be no more than 6–12 months, then treatment with desmopressin or a TCA should, if not contraindicated by the underlying psychiatric condition, be tried. If longer-term antipsychotic treatment is envisaged, a course of treatment with the alarm system should be used.

Day Wetting

Diurnal enuresis occurs, usually but not invariably, with night wetting. Diurnal enuresis is more likely to be associated with bladder instability and the presence of an associated urinary tract infection, and these should be ruled out. Persons with diurnal enuresis feel the urge to micturate but defer a response (using the toilet) either because their irritable bladder does not give them time or because they are anxious about asking the teacher or other caregiver if they can use the toilet.

Behavioral treatment requires ascertaining the timing and circumstances of the enuretic incidents and then helping the child to plan and to reinforce use of the toilet (Berg et al. 1982). The most common time of the day for enuretic incidents is in the early afternoon, so treatment will often require enlisting the cooperation of a teacher. Foxx and Azrin (1973) developed an intensive treatment involving copious fluid intake to increase the number of toileting responses available for reinforcement or punishment. A portable alarm is worn and is set to sound at predetermined intervals to remind the child to toilet (Halliday et al. 1987). Imipramine has been found to be ineffective in the treatment of day wetting (Meadow and Berg 1982), but anticholinergics such as oxybutynin and terodiline may reduce daytime wetting frequency (Baigrie et al. 1988; Elmer et al. 1988).

Encopresis

Definitions

Functional encopresis is the repeated passage of stool in inappropriate places whether intentional or involuntary. A DSM-IV diagnosis is made only in persons who have a chronological and mental age of at least 4 years, who inappropriately stool at least once per month for at least 3 months, and who are taking no substance that would lead to unwanted stooling (i.e., laxatives) and have no underlying causative medical disorder. A further distinction is drawn in DSM-IV (Table 10–2) between *encopresis with constipation and overflow incontinence* and *encopresis without constipation and overflow incontinence*. Constipation can be assumed to be present if a large stool mass can be palpated or if the child passes fewer than three stools per week.

TABLE 10–2. **DSM-IV diagnostic criteria for encopresis**

A. Repeated passage of feces into inappropriate places (e.g., clothing or floor) whether involuntary or intentional.

B. At least one such event a month for at least 3 months.

C. Chronological age is at least 4 years (or equivalent developmental level).

D. The behavior is not due exclusively to the direct physiological effects of a substance (e.g., laxatives) or a general medical condition except through a mechanism involving constipation.

Code as follows:

787.6 **With constipation and overflow incontinence**

307.7 **Without constipation and overflow incontinence**

Natural History and Epidemiology

Fewer than one-third of the children in the United States are completely toilet trained by age 2 years (Stephens and Silber 1974); the average age of attaining continence is 27.7 months (Brazelton 1962). Fecal retention or abnormally decreased defecation frequency occurring between ages 1 and 2 years is predictive of later encopresis (Levine 1975). Encopresis also may occur as the result of an acute episode of constipation following a medical illness or a change in diet (Pettei and Davidson 1988). Anal fissures or irritation may lead the child to withhold stool to avoid painful defecation, leading to impaired bowel evacuation and constipation. By age 8, only 1.5% of children have not established adequate bowel control (Bellman 1966). This percentage decreases with advancing age until it is rare to find a child at age 16 who is still soiling.

Bellman (1966) found that the prevalence of encopresis in children ages 7 and 8 was 1.5%, with a male-to-female ratio of 3.4 to 1. Rutter et al. (1970/1981) studied an older sample and reported that approximately 1.0% of 10- to 12-year-olds were encopretic, with a male-to-female ratio of about 5 to 1.

Etiology

Several factors have been implicated in the etiology of encopresis. Twin studies suggest a role for genetic factors (Bakwin and Davidson 1971). Levine (1982) suggested that "colonic inertia" may have been present in some encopretic persons since infancy and that this may be genetically determined. Many abnormalities of anorectal physiology have been described in encopretic children with underlying constipation (Loening-Baucke 1984; Loening-Baucke and Younoszai 1982; Loening-Baucke et al. 1987; Wald et al. 1986).

Stressful events are often associated with the onset of an episode of encopresis (Levine 1975), but it is not clear whether the stress led to constipation and subsequent encopresis or whether the fecal soiling was a direct consequence.

Historically, early single case studies concluded that "coercive" and "neglectful" toilet-training techniques and specific patterns of family psychopathology were causal (Anthony 1957; Bemporad et al. 1971). No evidence shows that any particular pattern of family structure or function or economic circumstance is systematically associated with the disorder (Hersov 1985; Levine 1975).

Associated Conditions

Constipation is found in most, but not all, children presenting with encopresis (Levine 1975; Loening-Baucke 1984). Enuresis occurs in approximately one-third of encopretic children (Loening-Baucke 1992, 1997). The relation between encopresis and other psychiatric disturbance is controversial. Although encopretic children are often believed to have many other behavior problems, studies have not convincingly demonstrated that these children have specific psychiatric disorders (Gabel et al. 1986; Loening-Baucke et al. 1987).

Assessment

Medical assessment, including rectal examination, is important because most children presenting with encopresis have concurrent fecal impaction. The psychiatrist may choose to do this himself or herself or refer the child to a pediatrician. Under no circumstances should a course of extensive psychological treatment be begun before such an evaluation.

Treatment

Behavioral-Educational Therapy

In most instances, treatment of underlying constipation will lead to a remission. A behavioral-educational approach to treatment of encopresis should be started if constipation is not present. A randomized controlled comparison of behavioral treatment and multimodality treatment (behavioral techniques combined with laxative therapy) showed the superiority of multimodality management (Nolan et al. 1991). Successful multimodality therapy, indicated by a marked improvement in symptoms after 1–2 years of follow-up, can be expected in approximately 70%–80% of patients (Levine and Bakow 1976; Loening-Baucke 1992). Behavioral-educational treatment of encopresis comprises 1) educating both child and parents about the disorder and its relation to regular bowel action, 2) designing a feasible program of consistent toilet use, and 3) providing the child with a system of positive reinforcements for, at first, any use and, subsequently, for successful use of the toilet (Boon and Singh 1991). Most practitioners advocate repeated scheduled toileting for the child (Howe and Walker 1992), usually shortly after meals to take advantage of the "gastrocolic reflex." Charting the child's toileting and successful defecation attempts serves as a means of following the symptoms over time and assessing the child's progress. Rewards for toileting behavior and successful defecation act as positive reinforcements for the child. Some investigators advocate mild punishment techniques, such as requiring the child to clean his or her clothes after a soiling episode (Doleys et al. 1977).

Medical Management

Various forms and regimens of laxative therapy are the mainstay of the treatment of retentive encopresis. Most regimens divide medical treatment into different phases (Levine 1982). The initial phase includes the aggressive use of suppositories and enemas to remove the underlying impaction and to decompress the bowel. The precise method for accomplishing this goal varies among clinics (Howe and Walker 1992; Levine 1982; Loening-Baucke 1992). After clean-out has been achieved, maintenance therapy is started, using mineral oil, milk of magnesia, senna derivatives, and/or a high-fiber diet. All these may encourage regular defecation and prevent the reoccurrence of fecal accumulation and impaction (Loening-Baucke 1992). The child is gradually weaned off this maintenance treatment only after a significant improvement in symptoms has been maintained for a substantial period of time. The child should be followed up regularly so that any recurrence of symptoms may be detected.

Approximately 20% of children respond inadequately to the treatment (Levine 1982), and a larger percentage relapse after initially achieving remission of symptoms. Some children require maintenance laxative therapy for years because of the tendency to relapse whenever laxatives are discontinued. In one series, a successful response to psychotherapy in patients for whom medical treatment had failed was seen in only 1 of 11 patients (Levine and Bakow 1976).

Biofeedback Therapy

In a proportion of treatment-refractory cases of retentive encopresis, it appears that the child involuntarily contracts the muscles of the pelvic floor and the external anal sphincter during defecation attempts, thus interfering with fecal expulsion (Loening-Baucke and

Cruikshank 1986). Loening-Baucke (1993) investigated a biofeedback technique in children who showed this pattern of response and who failed to respond to standard multimodality treatment. A series of six sessions of biofeedback training was effective in 86% of the patients and was associated with both short- and long-term symptom reduction.

References

American Psychiatric Association: Diagnostic and Statistical Manual of Mental Disorders, 4th Edition. Washington, DC, American Psychiatric Association, 1994

Anthony EJ: An experimental approach to the psychopathology of childhood: encopresis. Br J Med Psychol 30:146–175, 1957

Arnell H, Hjalmass K, Jagervall M, et al: The genetics of primary nocturnal enuresis: inheritance and suggestion of a second major gene on chromosome 12q. J Med Genet 34:360–365, 1997

Baigrie RJ, Kelleher JP, Fawcett DP, et al: Oxybutynin: is it safe? Br J Urol 62:319–322, 1988

Baker BL: Symptom treatment and symptom substitution in enuresis. J Abnorm Psychol 74:42–49, 1969

Bakwin H: Enuresis in children. J Pediatr 58:806–819, 1961

Bakwin H, Davidson M: Constipation in twins. Am J Dis Child 121:1179–1181, 1971

Behrle FC, Elkin MT, Laybourne PC: Evaluation of a conditioning device in the treatment of nocturnal enuresis. Pediatrics 17:849–855, 1956

Bellman M: Studies on encopresis. Acta Paediatr Scand Suppl 170:1–150, 1966

Bemporad JR, Pfeifer CM, Gibbs L, et al: Characteristics of encopretic patients and their families. Journal of the American Academy of Child Psychiatry 10:272–292, 1971

Berg L, Forsythe I, McGuire R: Response of bedwetting to the enuresis alarm: influence of psychiatric disturbance and maximal functional bladder capacity. Arch Dis Child 57:394–396, 1982

Blomfield JM, Douglas JWB: Bedwetting—prevalence among children aged 4–7 years. Lancet 1:850–852, 1956

Boggs SR, Geffken GR, Johnson SB, et al: Behavioral treatment of nocturnal enuresis in children with insulin-dependent diabetes mellitus. J Pediatr Psychol 17:111–118, 1992

Boon FFL, Singh NN: A model for the treatment of encopresis. Behav Modif 15:355–371, 1991

Bradbury M: Combination therapy for nocturnal enuresis with desmopressin and an alarm device. Scand J Urol Nephrol 31 (suppl 183):61–63, 1997

Brazelton TB: A child oriented approach to toilet training. Pediatrics 29:121–128, 1962

Butler RJ: Establishment of working definitions in nocturnal enuresis. Arch Dis Child 66:267–271, 1991

Butler RJ, Forsythe WI, Robertson J: The body-worn alarm in treatment of childhood enuresis. British Journal of Child Psychiatry 44:237–241, 1990

Chadwick O: Psychological sequelae of head injury in children. Dev Med Child Neurol 27:69–79, 1985

Collins RW: Importance of the bladder-cue buzzer contingency in the conditioning treatment for enuresis. J Abnorm Psychol 82:299–308, 1973

Dahl N, Arnell H, Hjalmaas K, et al: Primary nocturnal enuresis: linkage to chromosome 12q and evidence for genetic heterogeneity (abstract). Am J Hum Genet 57:A190, 1995

De Gatta MM, Garcia MJ, Acosta A, et al: Monitoring of serum levels of imipramine and desipramine and individualization of dose in enuretic children. Ther Drug Monit 6:438–443, 1984

De Gatta MM, Galindo P, Rey F, et al: The influence of clinical and pharmacological factors on enuresis treatment with imipramine. Br J Clin Pharmacol 30:693–698, 1990

Dejonge GA: A survey of the literature, in Bladder Control and Enuresis (Clinics in Developmental Medicine, Vol 48/49). Edited by Kolvin I, MacKeith R, Meadow SR. London, Heinemann/Spastics International Medical Publications, 1973, pp 39–46

De Leon G, Mandell W: A comparison of conditioning and psychotherapy in the treatment of functional enuresis. J Clin Psychol 22:326–330, 1966

Devlin JB, O'Cathain C: Predicting treatment outcome in nocturnal enuresis. Arch Dis Child 65:1158–1161, 1990

Dimson SB: DDAVP and urine osmolality in refractory enuresis. Arch Dis Child 49:375–382, 1986

Dodge WF, West EF, Bridgforth MS, et al: Nocturnal enuresis in 6- to 10-year-old children. Am J Dis Child 120:32–35, 1970

Doleys DM: Behavioral treatments for nocturnal enuresis in children: a review of the recent literature. Psychol Bull 84:30–54, 1977

Doleys DM, McWhorter MS, Williams SC, et al: Encopresis: its treatment and relation to nocturnal enuresis. Behavior Therapy 8:77–82, 1977

Douglas J: Early disturbing events and later enuresis, in Bladder Control and Enuresis (Clinics in Developmental Medicine, Vol 48/49). Edited by Kolvin I, MacKeith R, Meadow SR. London, Heinemann/Spastics International Medical Publications, 1973, pp 109–117

Eiberg H, Berendt I, Mohr J: Assignment of dominant inherited nocturnal enuresis (ENUR1) to chromosome 13q. Nat Genet 10:354–356, 1995

Elmer M, Norgaard JP, Djurhuus JC, et al: Terodiline in the treatment of diurnal enuresis in children. Scand J Prim Health Care 6:119–124, 1988

Essen J, Peckham C: Nocturnal enuresis in childhood. Dev Med Child Neurol 18:577–589, 1976

Fergusson DM, Horwood LJ, Shannon FT: Factors related to the age of attainment of nocturnal bladder control: an 8-year longitudinal study. Pediatrics 78:884–890, 1986

Fielding D: Factors associated with drop out, relapse and failure in the conditioning treatment of nocturnal enuresis. Behavioural Psychotherapy 13:174–185, 1985

Finley WW, Besserman RL, Clapp RK, et al: The effect of continuous, intermittent and placebo reinforcement on the effectiveness of the conditioning treatment for enuresis nocturna. Behav Res Ther 11:289–297, 1973

Forsythe WI, Butler RJ: Fifty years of enuretic alarms. Arch Dis Child 64:879–885, 1989

Fournier J-P, Garfinkel BD, Bond A, et al: Pharmacological and behavioral management of enuresis. J Am Acad Child Adolesc Psychiatry 26:849–853, 1987

Foxman B, Valdez RB, Brook RH: Childhood enuresis: prevalence, perceived impact, and prescribed treatments. Pediatrics 77:482–487, 1986

Foxx RM, Azrin NH: Dry pants: a rapid method of toilet training children. Behav Res Ther 11:435–442, 1973

Gabel S, Hegedus AM, Wald A, et al: Prevalence of behavior problems and mental health utilization among encopretic children: implications for behavioral pediatrics. J Dev Behav Pediatr 7:293–297, 1986

Hagglof B, Andren O, Bergstrom E, et al: Self-esteem in children with nocturnal enuresis and urinary incontinence: improvement of self-esteem after treatment. Eur Urol 33 (suppl 3):16–19, 1998

Hagglund TB: Enuretic children treated on fluid restriction or forced drinks: a clinical and cystometric study. Ann Paediatr Fenn 11:84–90, 1965

Hallgren B: Enuresis: a study with reference to certain physical, mental and social factors possibly associated with enuresis. Acta Psychiatrica et Neurologica Scandinavica 31:405–436, 1956

Halliday S, Meadow SR, Berg I: Successful management of daytime enuresis using alarm procedures: a randomly controlled trial. Arch Dis Child 62:132–137, 1987

Hansen GD: Enuresis control through fading, escape and avoidance training. J Appl Behav Anal 12: 303–307, 1979

Hanson RH, Thompson T, Wieseler NA: Methodological considerations in enuresis—treatment research: a three-treatment comparison. Behav Modif 12:335–352, 1988

Hansson S: Urinary incontinence in children and associated problems. Scand J Urol Nephrol Suppl 141: 47–55, 1992

Hellstrom AL, Hanson E, Hansson S, et al: Micturition habits and incontinence in 7-year-old Swedish school entrants. Eur J Pediatr 149:434–437, 1990

Hersov L: Faecal soiling, in Child and Adolescent Psychiatry: Modern Approaches, 2nd Edition. Edited by Rutter M, Hersov L. Oxford, UK, Blackwell Scientific, 1985, pp 482–489

Hollmann E, Von Gontard A, Eiberg H, et al: Molecular genetic, clinical and psychiatric associations in nocturnal enuresis. Br J Urol 81 (suppl 3):37–39, 1998

Houts AC: Behavioural treatment for enuresis. Scand J Urol Nephrol Suppl 173:83–86, 1995

Houts AC, Peterson JK, Liebert RM: The effect of prior imipramine treatment on the results of conditioning therapy in children with enuresis. J Pediatr Psychol 9:505–509, 1984

Houts AC, Berman JS, Abramson H: Effectiveness of psychological and pharmacological treatments for nocturnal enuresis. J Consult Clin Psychol 62:737–745, 1994

Howe AC, Walker CE: Behavioral management of toilet training, enuresis, and encopresis. Pediatr Clin North Am 39:413–432, 1992

Jarvelin MR, Vikevainen-Tervonen L, Moilanen I, et al: Enuresis in seven-year-old children. Acta Paediatr Scand 77:148–153, 1988

Jarvelin MR, Huttunen NP, Seppanen J, et al: Screening of urinary tract abnormalities among day and nightwetting children. Scand J Urol Nephrol 24:181–189, 1990

Jarvelin MR, Moilanen I, Kangas P, et al: Aetiological and precipitating factors for childhood enuresis. Acta Paediatr Scand 80:361–369, 1991

Jones B, Gerrard JW, Shokeir MK, et al: Recurrent urinary infection in girls: relation to enuresis. Can Med Assoc J 106:127–130, 1972

Jorgensen OS, Lober M, Christiansen J, et al: Plasma concentration and clinical effect in imipramine treatment of childhood enuresis. Clin Pharmacokinet 5:386–393, 1980

Kaffman M, Elizur E: Infants who become enuretics: a longitudinal study of 161 kibbutz children. Monogr Soc Res Child Dev 42:1–53, 1977

Kolvin I, Taunch J, Currah J, et al: Enuresis: a descriptive analysis and a controlled trial. Dev Med Child Neurol 14:715–726, 1972

Kunin CM, Zacha E, Paquin AJ Jr: Urinary tract infections in school children: an epidemiologic, clinical and laboratory study. N Engl J Med 266:1287–1296, 1962

Levine MD: Children with encopresis: a descriptive analysis. Pediatrics 56:412–416, 1975

Levine MD: Encopresis: its potentiation, evaluation and alleviation. Pediatr Clin North Am 29:315–330, 1982

Levine MD, Bakow H: Children with encopresis: a study of treatment outcome. Pediatrics 58:845–852, 1976

Loening-Baucke VA: Sensitivity of the sigmoid colon and rectum in children treated for chronic constipation. J Pediatr Gastroenterol Nutr 3:454–459, 1984

Loening-Baucke VA: Elimination disorders, in Behavioral Pediatrics. Edited by Greydanus DE, Wolraich M. New York, Springer-Verlag, 1992, pp 280–297

Loening-Baucke VA: Modulation of abnormal defecation dynamics by biofeedback treatment in chronically constipated children with encopresis. J Pediatr 116:214–222, 1993

Loening-Baucke V: Urinary incontinence and urinary tract infection and their resolution with treatment of chronic constipation of child. Pediatrics 100:228–232, 1997

Loening-Baucke VA, Cruikshank B: Abnormal defecation dynamics in chronically constipated children with encopresis. J Pediatr 108:562–566, 1986

Loening-Baucke VA, Younoszai MK: Abnormal anal sphincter response in chronically constipated children. Pediatrics 100:213–218, 1982

Loening-Baucke VA, Cruikshank B, Savage C: Defecation dynamics and behavior profiles in encopretic children. Pediatrics 80:672–679, 1987

Longstaffe S, Moffatt ME, Whalen JC: Behavioral and self-concept changes after six months of enuresis treatment: a randomized, controlled trial. Pediatrics 105:935–940, 2000

Lovering JS, Tallett SE, McKendry JBJ: Oxybutynin efficacy in the treatment of primary enuresis. Pediatrics 82:104–106, 1988

Lovibond SH: Conditioning and Enuresis. Oxford, UK, Pergamon, 1964

Lovibond SH: Critique of Turner, Young and Rachman's conditioning treatment for enuresis. Behav Res Ther 10:287–289, 1972

MacLean REG: Imipramine hydrochloride (Tofranil) and enuresis. Am J Psychiatry 117:551, 1960

McGee R, Makinson T, Williams S, et al: A longitudinal study of enuresis from five to nine years. Australian Paediatric Journal 20:39–42, 1984

Meadow R, Berg I: Controlled trial of imipramine in diurnal enuresis. Arch Dis Child 57:714–716, 1982

Mikkelsen EJ, Rapoport JL: Enuresis: psychopathology sleep stage and drug response. Urol Clin North Am 7:361–377, 1980

Mikkelsen EJ, Rapoport JL, Nee L, et al: Childhood enuresis, I: sleep patterns and psychopathology. Arch Gen Psychiatry 37:1139–1144, 1980

Miller FJW, Court SDM, Walton WS, et al: Growing Up in Newcastle-Upon-Tyne. London, Oxford University Press, 1960

Miller K, Klauber GT: Desmopressin acetate in children with severe primary nocturnal enuresis. Clin Ther 12:357–366, 1990

Miller K, Goldberg S, Atkin B: Nocturnal enuresis: experience with long-term use of intranasally administered desmopressin. J Pediatr 14:723–726, 1989

Moffatt MEK: Nocturnal enuresis: is there a rationale for treatment? Scand J Urol Nephrol Suppl 163: 55–66, 1994

Moffatt MEK, Kato C, Pless IB: Improvements in self-concept after treatment of nocturnal enuresis: randomized control trial. J Pediatr 110:647–652, 1987

Nolan T, Debelle G, Oberflaid F, et al: Randomised trial of laxatives in treatment of childhood encopresis. Lancet 338:523–527, 1991

Norgaard JP, Pedersen EB, Djurhuus JC: Diurnal anti-diuretic hormone levels in enuretics. J Urol 134: 1029–1031, 1985

Oppel WC, Harper PA, Rider RV: Social, psychological and neurological factors associated with enuresis. Pediatrics 42:627–641, 1968

O'Regan S, Yazbeck S, Hamberger B, et al: Constipation: a commonly unrecognized cause of enuresis. Am J Dis Child 140:260–261, 1986

Pettei M, Davidson M: Constipation, in Textbook of Pediatric Gastroenterology. Edited by Siverberg M, Daum F. Chicago, IL, Year Book Medical, 1988, pp 180–188

Ramsden P, Hindmarsh JR, Price D, et al: DDAVP for adult enuresis: a preliminary report. Br J Urol 54:256–258, 1982

Rapoport JL, Mikkelsen EJ, Zavadil A, et al: Childhood enuresis, II: psychopathology, tricyclic concentration in plasma, and antienuretic effect. Arch Gen Psychiatry 37:1146–1152, 1980

Rew DA, Rundle JSH: Assessment of the safety of regular DDAVP therapy in primary nocturnal enuresis. Br J Urol 63:352–353, 1989

Richardson DW, Robinson AG: Desmopressin. Ann Intern Med 103:228–239, 1985

Rittig S, Knudsen U, Norgaard J, et al: Abnormal diurnal rhythm of plasma vasopressin and urinary output in patients with enuresis. Am J Physiol 256:664–671, 1989

Roberts KE, Schoellkopf JA: Eating, sleeping and elimination practices in a group of 2½-year-olds. Am J Dis Child 82:144–152, 1951

Rutter M, Tizard J, Whitmore K (eds): Education, Health and Behaviour. London, Longmans, 1970 [Reprinted Melbourne, FL, Krieger, 1981]

Rutter ML, Yule W, Graham PJ: Enuresis and behavioural deviance: some epidemiological considerations, in Bladder Control and Enuresis (Clinics in Developmental Medicine, Vol 48/49). Edited by Kolvin I, MacKeith R, Meadow SR. London, Heinemann/Spastics International Medical Publications, 1973, pp 137–147

Schmitt BD: New enuresis alarms: safe, successful and child operable. Contemporary Pediatrics 3:1–6, 1986

Shaffer D, Costello AJ, Hill JD: Control of enuresis with imipramine. Arch Dis Child 43:666–671, 1968

Shaffer D, Gardner A, Hedge B: Behavior and bladder disturbance in enuretics: the rational classification of a common disorder. Dev Med Child Neurol 26:781–792, 1984

Sloop EW, Kennedy WA: Institutionalized retarded nocturnal enuretics treated by a conditioning technique. American Journal of Mental Deficiency 77:717–721, 1973

Smith LJ: Training severely and profoundly mentally handicapped nocturnal enuretics. Behav Res Ther 19:67–74, 1981

Starfield SB: Functional bladder capacity in enuretic and non-enuretic children. J Pediatr 70:777–781, 1967

Steinhausen H-C, Göbel D: Enuresis in child psychiatric clinic patients. J Am Acad Child Adolesc Psychiatry 28:279–281, 1989

Stephens JA, Silber DL: Parental expectations vs outcome in toilet training. Pediatrics 54:493–495, 1974

Sujka SK, Piedmonte MR, Greenfield SP: Enuresis and the voiding cystourethrogram: a re-evaluation. Urology 38:139–142, 1991

Sukhai RN, Mol J, Harris AS: Combined therapy of enuresis alarm and desmopressin in the treatment of nocturnal enuresis. Eur J Pediatr 148:465–467, 1989

Terho P, Kekomaki M: Management of nocturnal enuresis with a vasopressin analogue. J Urol 131:952–957, 1984

Turner RK: Conditioning, treatment of nocturnal enuresis: present studies, in Bladder Control and Enuresis (Clinics in Developmental Medicine, Vol 48/49). Edited by Kolvin I, MacKeith R, Meadow SR. London, Heinemann/Spastics International Medical Publications, 1973, pp 195–210

Turner R, Young G, Rachman S: Treatment of nocturnal enuresis by conditioning techniques. Behav Res Ther 8:367–381, 1970

Van Gool JD, de Jonge GA: Urge syndrome and urge incontinence. Arch Dis Child 64:1629–1634, 1989

Verhulst FC, van der Lee JH, Akkerhuis GW, et al: The prevalence of nocturnal enuresis: do DSM III criteria need to be changed? A brief research report. J Child Psychol Psychiatry 26:989–993, 1985

von Gontard A: Annotation: day and night wetting in children—a paediatric and child psychiatric perspective. J Child Psychol Psychiatry 39:439–451, 1998

von Gontard A, Eiberg H, Hollmann E, et al: Molecular genetics of nocturnal enuresis: clinical and genetic heterogeneity. Acta Paediatr 87:571–578, 1998

von Gontard A, Eiberg H, Hollmann E, et al: Molecular genetics of nocturnal enuresis: linkage to a locus on chromosome 22. Scand J Urol Nephrol Suppl 202:76–80, 1999a

von Gontard A, Mauer-Mucke K, Pluck J, et al: Clinical behavioral problems in day- and night-wetting children. Pediatr Nephrol 13:662–667, 1999b

Wald A, Chandra R, Chiponis D, et al: Anorectal function and continence mechanisms in childhood encopresis. J Pediatr Gastroenterol Nutr 5:346–351, 1986

Wallace IR, Forsythe WI: The treatment of enuresis: a controlled clinical trial of propantheline, propantheline and phenobarbitone, and placebo. Br J Clin Pract 23:207–210, 1969

Werry JS, Cohrssen J: Enuresis: an etiologic and therapeutic study. J Pediatr 67:423–431, 1965

Wille S: Comparison of desmopressin and enuresis alarm for nocturnal enuresis. Arch Dis Child 61:30–33, 1986

Young GC, Morgan RTT: Overlearning in the conditioning treatment of enuresis. Behav Res Ther 10:147–151, 1972

Young GC, Morgan RTT: Rapidity of response to the treatment of enuresis. Dev Med Child Neurol 15:488–496, 1973

11

Anxiety Disorders in Children and Adolescents

Tami Benton, M.D.
Laura E. Sanchez, M.D.

Anxiety disorders are one of the most prevalent categories of psychopathology in children and adolescents, affecting as many as 10% of youths (Bell-Dolan et al. 1990; Bernstein and Borchardt 1991; Kashani and Orvaschel 1990). These disorders are frequently associated with psychosocial difficulties; school difficulties; and an increased risk for other, more serious conditions, including depression, suicide, and substance abuse. Despite several well-designed studies documenting the high prevalence of anxiety disorders in children and adolescents (Anderson et al. 1987; Bird et al. 1988; Costello 1989; McGee et al. 1990), these disorders are frequently unrecognized and underdiagnosed. Some of the diagnostic difficulties may be related to the anxiety disorders' high degree of comorbidity with other disorders, particularly depression and attention-deficit/hyperactivity disorder (ADHD), and to the problems in defining what constitutes an anxiety disorder in comparison with normal anxiety. Children appear to undergo what are considered developmentally "sanctioned" progressions in anxiety symptoms (Last et al. 1987a; Silverman et al. 1995). Some childhood fears may be viewed as adaptive protective mechanisms. Differentiation of normal anxiety from pathological anxiety requires consideration of sex, race, and age norms, because developmental physiological and developmentally specific environmental factors affect the clinical presentation of anxiety disorders. Only when anxiety is considered excessive or the context is developmentally inappropriate does it become clinically significant.

Definition

In DSM-IV (American Psychiatric Association 1994), children and adolescents may be diagnosed with the following anxiety disorders: separation anxiety disorder, generalized anxiety disorder, social phobia, specific phobia, panic disorder, obsessive-compulsive disorder, and posttraumatic stress disorder. The specific features of each disorder are defined in DSM-IV.

The essential feature of *separation anxiety disorder* is excessive anxiety about separation from attachment figures. The reaction to separation from an attachment figure must cause some clinically significant distress and must interfere with important areas of functioning such as school (American Psychiatric Association 1994). Early onset is defined as onset before age 6 years.

Generalized anxiety disorder is characterized by chronic excessive worries and anxiety that are difficult to control and are associated with physiological symptoms of hyperarousal. Children need to endorse only one of six symptoms of hyperarousal, whereas adults must endorse at least three to meet diagnostic criteria.

Social phobia is characterized by marked, persistent fear of social or performance situations in which embarrassment may occur. Although adults and adolescents may recognize the fear as excessive, this may not be the case with children. There is an emerging viewpoint that selective mutism, characterized by the failure to speak in specific social situations but the ability to talk in other situations, is a form of social phobia. *Specific phobia* is defined as marked and persistent fear of clearly discernable, circumscribed objects or situations.

Panic disorder is characterized by recurrent spontaneous episodes of panic that are associated with physiological and psychological symptoms of anxiety. *Posttraumatic stress disorder* and *obsessive-compulsive disorder,* both of which are classified as anxiety disorders, are discussed separately in this section (see Chapters 13 and 14).

Assessment

The diagnosis of anxiety disorders can be difficult at times for the reasons stated earlier in this chapter. Thus, specific questions to screen for symptoms of anxiety disorders must be included in the clinical interview. Important areas to assess include the history of onset and development of the anxiety symptoms, the degree of impairment, associated stressors, medical history, school history, psychiatric history, family psychiatric history, and mental status examination. A comprehensive evaluation may include structured or semistructured diagnostic interviews and symptom rating scales to aid in the assessment of anxiety in children and adolescents. Because of the subjective nature of anxiety symptoms, it is important to question the child or adolescent directly about his or her anxiety symptoms because children report internal states best, whereas parents describe behaviors best. Detailed guidelines for the assessment of children and adolescents with anxiety disorders are available elsewhere (American Academy of Child and Adolescent Psychiatry 1997) and are not repeated here.

Anxious children should receive a comprehensive medical evaluation if they present with somatic complaints or if they have not had a comprehensive physical examination in the last 12 months. If pharmacotherapy is to be initiated, an electrocardiogram, renal and hepatic screens, and pregnancy test are indicated.

Differential Diagnosis and Comorbidity

The anxiety disorders manifest physiologically, psychologically, and socially. Patients frequently present with somatic symptoms such as abdominal pain, diarrhea, headache, or panic episodes, which can disrupt academic and social development.

Many physical conditions can mimic anxiety disorders and should be considered as part of the differential diagnosis. These include hypoglycemic episodes, hyperthyroidism, cardiac arrhythmias, caffeinism, pheochromocytoma, seizure disorders, migraine, and other central nervous system disorders. If the initial history and physical examination suggest that an endocrine, cardiac, or neurological condition may be responsible for the onset or exacerbation of anxiety symptoms in a child, the appropriate workup to rule out these conditions should be included as part of the assessment. Excessive or invasive procedures should be used only if clearly indicated for objective signs of illness.

Untoward effects from prescription or over-the-counter medications can precipitate or exacerbate anxiety symptoms in children and adolescents. Thus, the clinician should obtain a detailed medication history. In particular, patients and their families should be questioned about the child's use of antihistamines, antiasthmatics, sympathomimetics, steroids, antipsychotics, serotonin reuptake inhibitors, diet pills, and cold medications. For children who present with somatic complaints that originate with anxiety, the history, physical examinations, and laboratory assessments obtained at follow-up will help detect any emerging medical disorder and provide reassurance for both the child and the family.

Comorbidity with other psychiatric disorders is extremely common in anxious children and adolescents (Kashani and Orvaschel 1990; Strauss and Last 1993). At least one-third of the children with anxiety disorders meet criteria for two or more anxiety disorders. Children with anxiety disorders commonly have comorbid major depression (Bernstein and Borchardt 1991; Kashani and Orvaschel 1988; Strauss et al. 1988). Also, an association is found between ADHD and anxiety disorders (Anderson et al. 1987; Biederman et al. 1991; Bird et al. 1988; Last et al. 1987b, 1987c; Strauss et al. 1988).

Other disorders that are comorbid with or misdiagnosed as anxiety disorders include adjustment disorders, substance use disorders, some personality disorders, eating disorders, somatoform disorders, tic disorders, trichotillomania, reactive attachment disorder, pervasive developmental disorders, schizophrenia, and sleep terror disorder (American Academy of Child and Adolescent Psychiatry 1997).

In the initial assessment, these disorders should be considered, with a focus on the chronology of symptom development. If one symptom complex precedes another, it should be noted. All symptoms meeting the criterion level for an Axis I or Axis II diagnosis should be identified. Diagnosing the specific type of anxiety disorder (recognizing that there may be more than one present) is important to determine the best treatment approach.

Rating Scales

Use of a structured or semistructured psychiatric interview in combination with anxiety symptom rating scales is often helpful in the evaluation and treatment of disorders in children and adolescents. Structured and semistructured diagnostic interviews that may be used to establish or confirm an anxiety disorder diagnosis and to identify comorbid psychiatric disorders are listed in Table 11–1. Several clinician rating scales, self-report instruments, and parent report measures are available to assess the severity of symptoms at baseline and to monitor target symptoms over time (Table 11–2). Information must be obtained from both parent and child because parent and child reports of anxiety are often discordant (American Academy of Child and Adolescent Psychiatry 1997; D. F. Klein et al. 1992). Limitations of these rating scales include overlap of symptoms on the self-report measures of anxiety and depression (Brady and Kendall 1992) and the limited availability of scales that examine both state and trait anxiety (Stallings and March 1995).

TABLE 11–1. Instruments for diagnostic assessment of anxiety in children and adolescents

Measure	Type of measure	Informant
Schedule for Affective Disorders and Schizophrenia for School-Age Children (Chambers et al. 1985)	Semistructured psychiatric interview; information from all available sources used to derive a summary score	Parent and child versions; epidemiological version available (K-SADS-E) (Orvaschel et al. 1982)
Anxiety Disorders Interview Schedule for Children (Silverman and Nelles 1988)	Semistructured psychiatric interview that includes other disorders but focuses on anxiety disorders	Parent and child versions
Diagnostic Interview for Children and Adolescents—Revised (Welner et al. 1987)	Structured psychiatric interview	Parent, child, and adolescent versions
NIMH Diagnostic Interview Schedule for Children (Shaffer et al. 1996)	Highly structured psychiatric interview; designed for lay interviewers	Parent and child versions
Children's Interview for Psychiatric Syndromes (Weller et al. 2000)	Highly structured psychiatric interview; designed for lay interviewers	Parent and child versions

Note. NIMH = National Institute of Mental Health.

Goals of Treatment

Children with anxiety disorders show a wide range of symptoms ranging from mild worries to overwhelming distress. The goals of treatment are to alleviate overwhelming, incapacitating anxiety that interferes with functioning in social or academic spheres and to prevent a chronic course of remissions and exacerbations that continues into adulthood (Bernstein et al. 1990; Keller et al. 1992). Common complications that warrant the treatment of anxiety symptoms include

- Disrupted academic and vocational progress caused by school refusal, poor attendance, and/or poor concentration

TABLE 11–2. Common rating scales for children and adolescents with anxiety disorders

Measure	Type of measure	Informant
State-Trait Anxiety Inventory for Children (Spielberger 1973)	Severity measure; assesses state and trait anxiety	Self-report
Revised Children's Manifest Anxiety Scale (Reynolds and Richmond 1978)	Severity measure with three anxiety subscales and a Lie subscale	Self-report
Revised Fear Survey Schedule for Children (Ollendick 1983)	Severity measure; examines fears	Self-report
Visual Analogue Scale for Anxiety—Revised (Bernstein and Garfinkel 1992)	Visual analogues to quantify anxiety related to anxiety-producing situations	Self-report
Social Anxiety Scale for Children—Revised (LaGreca and Stone 1993)	Severity measure of social anxiety	Self-report
Multidimensional Anxiety Scale for Children (March 1996)	Severity measure with four main anxiety factors	Self-report
Hamilton Anxiety Rating Scale (Hamilton 1959)	Clinician rating scale for adults that has been validated for adolescents (Clark and Donovan 1994)	Clinician rating using the adolescent's report
Anxiety Rating for Children—Revised (Bernstein et al. 1996)	Clinician rating scale; assesses severity; has Anxiety subscale and Physiological subscale	Clinician rating using the child's or adolescent's report
Personality Inventory for Children (Wirt et al. 1977)	Multiple scales, including Anxiety scale	Parent report
Child Behavior Checklist (Achenbach 1991)	Multiple scales, including Anxious/Depressed scale	Parent report
Screen for Child Anxiety-Related Emotional Disorders (SCARED) (Birmaher et al. 1997)	Self-report measure for children and parents screening for identification of anxiety disorders	Parent and child versions

Source. Adapted from Bernstein et al. 1996.

- Social isolation due to phobic avoidance
- Impaired self-esteem and self-concept that affect social development
- Somatization that results in unnecessary medical procedures, hospitalizations, or treatments
- Sleep disturbance causing daytime fatigue and somnolence
- Onset or exacerbation of comorbid disorders (i.e., onset of depression or exacerbation of ADHD)
- Family problems that are created or exacerbated by the child's anxiety

It is important to explain to both the parents and the child the goals of treatment because many times their initial expectations are neither realistic nor ultimately helpful to the child. The goal of treatment should never be the complete elimination of the subjective symptoms of anxiety in the child. The ability to experience anxiety under appropriate circumstances is adaptive and protective. Anxiety heightens a child's alertness and can enhance a child's ability to respond to environmental threats. Furthermore, children who develop anxiety disorders tend even after treatment to be more anxious rather than less anxious in novel situations. Thus, appropriate goals for treatment are 1) to diminish the child's anxiety and its associated symptoms to the point that they no longer interfere with either the child's functioning in social and academic spheres, the family's functioning, or normal development; 2) to improve the child's and the family's ability to identify and manage unproductive harmful worrying; and 3) to maximize the child's ability to experience anxiety without having to express the anxiety in dysfunctional ways.

Formulation of the Treatment Plan

Symptom severity and its associated disability, the presence of any comorbid medical or psychiatric conditions, and the distress of the child and family should guide a clinician's decision to treat. The recommendations for treatment should be based on the level of distress, severity of symptoms, and disability caused by these symptoms. When treatment is recommended, the diagnosis, reasons for treatments, goals of treatment, target symptoms, potential interventions, expected response to treatment, and prognosis should be clearly explained to the parents and child or adolescent. The discussion about treatment, including all of the above elements and the parents' and patients' acceptance of treatment, should be clearly documented in the chart.

A biopsychosocial-developmental understanding of the patient and the family should form the basis for the development of a treatment plan because these factors influence a child's response to treatment and the child's and family's compliance with treatment. Comorbid diagnoses and psychosocial, genetic, and socioeconomic factors that may contribute to the development and maintenance of anxiety symptoms in the child should be considered in relation to the primary diagnosis. Strengths in the child, the family, and the environment also should be considered and discussed with the family.

The treatment plan for primary anxiety disorder should be comprehensive and include all comorbid diagnoses, target symptoms, interventions that will be used to ameliorate specific target symptoms, methods that will be used for continued symptom assessment, criteria for improvement (i.e., which rating scale will be used for follow-up), and clearly specified frequency of evaluations. Documenting the potential effects of comorbidity on the prognosis for the principal diagnosis, if known, is important. For example, if an anxiety disorder precedes the onset of a depressive disorder and the depressive symptoms are related to the disability caused by the anxiety disorder, then successful treatment of the anxiety disorder may improve the depressive symptoms (Livingston et al. 1995).

Collaboration with school personnel and the primary care physician should be considered and initiated as appropriate. A multimodal treatment program with a biopsychosocial-developmental approach, in partnership with the child and the family, the school, and other providers, is recommended by the American Academy of Child and Adolescent Psychiatry (1997).

Therapeutic Alliance With Patients and Families

The key to successful treatment of anxiety disorders is the ability to form a working relationship with the patient and family. This therapeutic alliance begins with the first contact.

When a child's psychiatric disorder is serious enough for a family to seek treatment, parents may appear anxious and skeptical. In some circumstances, the referral was not initiated by the family but was made at the insistence of the primary care provider who has completed exhaustive medical tests to evaluate somatic complaints or was in response to concerns of the schools or the courts. Under such circumstances, families often feel less than hopeful about psychiatric treatment. Thus, the provider must make an extra effort to ensure the development of a therapeutic alliance. Establishing a therapeutic alliance will require empathic support for the patient and family, recognition and support of their legitimate concerns, and reinforcement and support of their appropriate coping skills.

Educating parents and other significant persons about symptoms, clinical course, treatment options, and prognosis aids tremendously in establishing a therapeutic alliance. Children also must be informed about their illness in a developmentally appropriate fashion. Many children experience an exacerbation of symptoms as treatment is initiated. This should be explained to the family. They should also be provided with specific techniques to aid with the management of their child's symptoms. The family and child must understand the disorder and the factors that predispose to, precipitate, and perpetuate symptoms. They must view the physician as one who has the child's and the family's best interests in mind and who wants to relieve their discomfort. Finally, because anxious children often have anxious parents, the family must be educated as to the familial nature of these disorders. Parents should be supported in seeking treatment as necessary for themselves. A recent study suggested that children with at least one anxious parent respond less favorably to treatment than children whose parents are not anxious (Cohen et al. 1998).

Parental anxiety is an important consideration when beginning treatment of anxiety in a child. Parents who are themselves anxious or depressed may be unable to provide the structure and support necessary to facilitate the treatment. This may interfere with the establishment of a therapeutic alliance. If a parent has a psychiatric disorder, that disorder must be treated before the child's treatment can be successful. Thus, the parent should be referred for treatment. If the parent is only mildly anxious, then support, education, and reassurance by the child's therapist may be sufficient. If family dysfunction appears to be a factor in the maintenance of the anxiety symptoms, then family therapy is indicated. The family should be reassured that appropriate interventions can lead to a favorable outcome for the child and family.

Treatment Modalities

The treatment of anxiety disorders in children and adolescents requires a multimodal approach. The "Practice Parameters for the Assessment and Treatment of Anxiety Disorders" (American Academy of Child and Adolescent Psychiatry 1997) recommends that a clinician who is developing a treatment plan should consider the following components: providing feedback to and educating the parents and child about the specific disorder; consulting with primary care physicians and school personnel; and using pharmacotherapy, cognitive-behavioral interventions, psychodynamic psychotherapy, and family therapy.

This section begins with a review of pharmacotherapeutic interventions for anxiety disorders in childhood followed by an overview of cognitive-behavioral approaches with anxiety disorders. A review of traditional psychodynamic psychotherapies and family therapy follows.

Use of Pharmacotherapy

Noradrenergic, serotonergic, and γ-aminobutyric acid (GABA) dysfunction has been associated with anxiety disorders in adults and underlies the rationale for the use of pharmacological agents in their treatment. Presumed continuity between adult- and childhood-onset anxiety disorders and the proven efficacy of psychopharmacological agents for the treatment of anxiety disorders in adults suggest that psychopharmacological agents also may be useful in the treatment of anxiety in children and adolescents.

In contrast to the adult literature, research on the pharmacological treatment of anxiety disorders in children and adolescents is limited. Many of the existing studies are methodologically flawed. This makes it difficult to draw conclusions about efficacy and safety. Furthermore, no studies have systematically compared pharmacotherapy or combined pharmacotherapy and psychotherapy with nonpharmacological interventions.

Systematic evaluation of the role of pharmacotherapy in the treatment of anxiety in children and adolescents awaits further research.

Initiation of Pharmacotherapy

Pharmacotherapy should not be the only intervention initiated to manage anxiety in children but should be part of a comprehensive and individualized treatment program (American Academy of Child and Adolescent Psychiatry 1997). A general strategy is to use medication to help ameliorate the child's subjective anxiety while working with the child and the family to modify the child's avoidance behaviors. Psychoactive agents should be administered only after a careful workup of the patient and an adequate baseline assessment period during which the frequency and intensity of target symptoms and baseline somatic complaints are documented. Before starting medication, the clinician must assess patients for somatic symptoms that might resemble untoward effects of the medication being prescribed. In addition, the parents and child must be educated about the benefits and the risks associated with medication treatment. It is important to explain to the family that symptoms may actually get worse before they get better. Children and adolescents with anxiety disorders are frequently somatically preoccupied. Therefore, it is important to instruct families to monitor but not focus on non-life-threatening untoward effects. The clinician should also provide education about available and alternative treatments, expected onset of therapeutic effects, and common side effects of the medication.

Benzodiazepines

Benzodiazepines are agonists of the GABA-benzodiazepine-chloride receptor complex and have been reported to have anxiolytic, sedative, anticonvulsant, and muscle relaxant properties. Most studies on the use of benzodiazepines in children and adolescents report on their use in seizure disorders. Reports on their use in the treatment of anxiety disorders in children and adolescents are scant. Results are mixed as to efficacy and are limited by small sample sizes.

Benzodiazepines have been widely studied in adults, but only a few controlled studies in children and adolescents have been reported. Benzodiazepines have been studied for panic symptoms, general anxiety, social phobia, separation anxiety disorder, and school refusal in youth. However, conclusions are limited by small sample sizes, short duration of medical trials, low dosages, and high placebo response rates.

An open trial of alprazolam involving 18 children and adolescents with separation anxiety disorder found significant improvement on clinician, parent, teacher, and self-report measures (Kutcher et al. 1992). An open study of clonazepam in adolescents with panic disorder found improvement in somatic and psychological symptoms of anxiety. Improvement in somatic symptoms occurred more quickly than improvement in psychological symptoms of anxiety (Kutcher and MacKenzie 1988).

An open-label study of alprazolam administered to pediatric oncology patients found an effective decrease in anticipatory and acute situational anxiety associated with bone marrow aspiration and spinal taps (Pfefferbaum et al. 1987b).

A double-blind, placebo-controlled study comparing alprazolam, imipramine, and placebo in children and adolescents with school refusal showed a favorable response in both medication groups (Bernstein et al. 1990). A 4-week trial of alprazolam versus placebo did not show statistically significant improvement in children with overanxious disorder or avoidant disorders (Simeon et al. 1992).

A double-blind crossover study of clonazepam versus placebo in 15 children, most of whom had diagnoses of separation anxiety disorder, found no significant difference between treatment groups (Graae et al. 1994). A double-blind, placebo-controlled study of clonazepam for adolescents with panic disorders showed improvement in measures of generalized anxiety, frequency of panic attacks, and social disability (Kutcher and Reiter, cited in Riddle et al. 1999).

Clinical trials indicate that benzodiazepines are generally well tolerated by children (Bernstein et al. 1990; Biederman 1987, 1990; Simeon and Ferguson 1987; Simeon et al. 1992). As in adults, sedation, drowsiness, and decreased mental acuity are the most common side effects (Biederman 1991). Other potential side effects include poor coordination, diplopia, and tremor (Biederman 1991). Behavioral disinhibition in children manifested as irritability, tantrums, and aggression (Graae et al. 1994) and in adolescents as irritability and behavioral outbursts (Reiter and Kutcher 1991) can be a particularly troubling untoward effect of these medications. Psychotic reactions or exacerbation of psychotic symptoms also have been reported (Pfefferbaum et al. 1987a). Tolerance to and dependence on benzodiazepines occur in adults (Salzman 1989). No data have been published regarding the risk of physiological and psychological dependence in children and adolescents. However, cognitive untoward effects and the risk of dependence limit the use of benzodiazepines in the treatment of anxiety in children and adolescents.

When selecting a benzodiazepine for the treatment of an anxiety disorder, factors such as the patient's age, patient's health, patient's ability to comply, family lifestyle, and side-effect profiles will contribute to a physician's choice of agent. Benzodiazepines are most frequently used as a temporary measure when rapid reduction of anxiety symptoms is necessary to aid the child in quickly resuming developmentally appropriate behavior (i.e., return child to school and reduce child's initial resistance to other treatment modalities). Often another medication such as a selective serotonin reuptake inhibitor (SSRI) is initiated concurrently, with the expectation that the benzodiazepine will be tapered as the other medication begins to exert its effects. Long-acting agents such as clonazepam can be given less frequently and are less likely to cause withdrawal symptoms. Short-acting benzodiazepines are less likely to accumulate, and side effects may be more transient when they occur. Benzodiazepines with a rapid onset of action, such as diazepam and triazolam, may be more likely to create a transient euphoric effect, which may be associated with increased abuse potential (American Psychiatric Association 1990). Substance abuse is a relative contraindication for use of benzodiazepines in children and adolescents.

Benzodiazepines are, in general, absorbed and metabolized more rapidly in children than in adults (Simeon 1993). Thus, children may need higher milligram-per-kilogram doses as well as more frequent doses than adults do. Pharmacokinetic data exist only for children and adolescents treated with diazepam (D. F. Klein and Riddle 1995). Recommendations for starting dosages and maximum daily doses for several benzodiazepines are summarized in Table 11–3.

TABLE 11–3. Dosing guidelines for the use of anxiolytic agents in children and adolescents

	Starting dose (mg)		
Agent	Preadolescent	Adolescent	Maximum daily dose (mg/kg)
Alprazolam	0.125 two or three times a day	0.25 two or three times a day	0.005–0.05
Clonazepam	0.25 once a day	0.5 four times a day	0.02–0.1
Lorazepam	0.25 two or three times a day	0.5 mg two or three times a day	0.02–0.1

Discontinuation of benzodiazepines can be associated with recurrence of anxiety, rebound anxiety, and withdrawal symptoms such as anxiety, malaise, irritability, headache, sweating, gastrointestinal symptoms, insomnia, and muscle tension (Coffey 1993; Salzman 1990). Abrupt discontinuation of benzodiazepines can result in seizures, especially in children with a history of seizures. Gradual tapering of benzodiazepines is recommended. For clonazepam, a discontinuation rate of less than 0.04 mg/kg/week was found to be safe in one prospective study (Sugai 1993).

Buspirone and Other Serotonin Type 1A Receptor Agonists

Agonists of the serotonin type 1A (5-HT_{1A}) receptor enhance the tonic activity of postsynaptic serotonin receptors by acting to desensitize the 5-HT_{1A} receptor located on the somatodendritic portion of the presynaptic neuron (Blier et al. 1990). The 5-HT_{1A} receptor is part of a negative feedback loop and limits release of serotonin from the presynaptic neuron as synaptic serotonin concentrations rise. Buspirone is the only 5-HT_{1A} agonist currently marketed in the United States (for generalized anxiety disorder in adults). Despite the lack of controlled studies, buspirone is used in children and adolescents for conditions as diverse as oppositional behavior, anxiety, and depression. This is probably due in part to the belief that it is remarkably free of side effects (Kutcher et al. 1995). Other compounds active at presynaptic and postsynaptic serotonin receptors are also under development (Dubovsky 1993; Mosconi et al. 1993). For example, flesinoxan (Rodgers et al. 1994), gepirone (McGrath et al. 1994), ipsapirone (Cutler et al. 1994), and tandospirone (Evans et al. 1994) have shown promise in adults.

No pharmacokinetic, dose-finding, or controlled safety and efficacy studies of buspirone or any other 5-HT_{1A} agonist in mentally ill children or adolescents have been reported (Hughes and Preskorn 1994; Kutcher et al. 1995). Based on open trials, case reports, clinical experience, and age-downward extension of studies in adults, buspirone has been used in children with generalized anxiety (Coffey 1990; Kutcher et al. 1992, 1995; Popper 1993).

An open trial by Simeon (1993) found significant improvement in anxiety, behavior, and hyperactivity in 15 children with various anxiety disorders treated with buspirone. Adverse events were infrequent and mild. Case reports involving children and adolescents suggest benefit in overanxious disorder (Kranzler 1988) and social phobia (Zwier and Rao 1994).

Buspirone is commonly associated with few and mild side effects, including lightheadedness, stomach upset, dizziness, sedation, asthenia, and headaches. Also, buspirone has no withdrawal symptoms even after prolonged administration (Rakel 1990) and has no addictive potential (Murphy et al. 1989). In a recent open-label study of 25 prepubertal children with anxiety and aggression, test dosages up to 50 mg/day for up to 9 weeks revealed the following: 6 children showed increased aggression or mania; of the 19 who completed the study, only 3 had sufficient benefit to continue buspirone after the study (Pfeffer et al. 1997).

Buspirone is usually started at 2.5 mg twice daily for children and 5 mg twice daily for adolescents. The dosage may be gradually increased every 2 weeks in two to three divided doses up to a maximum daily dosage of 20 mg in children and 60 mg in adolescents. The need for three-times-a-day dosing limits feasibility and compliance.

Tricyclic Antidepressants

The therapeutic effects of tricyclic antidepressants (TCAs) are believed to be due to their ability to block the reuptake of the neurotransmitters serotonin and norepinephrine in nerve terminals, resulting in alterations in the sensitivity of various neuroreceptors. The use of TCAs in the treatment of anxiety disorders in children and adolescents is not clearly supported by the literature (Geller et al. 1999). Imipramine was reported to be significantly superior to placebo in 35 children ages 6–12 years with school refusal and associated anxiety disorders (Gittelman-Klein and Klein 1973). The efficacy of imipramine was not replicated in a smaller study involving 21 children with separation anxiety disorder (R. Klein et al. 1992). Furthermore, clomipramine was reported to be no better than placebo in 51 children with a variety of anxiety disorders (Berney et al. 1981).

Clinical experience, however, suggests that TCAs may be helpful for some children with separation anxiety as well as other anxiety disorders. Case reports suggest that TCAs may be helpful in the treatment of panic disorder in children and adolescents (Ballenger et al. 1989; Black and Robbins 1990; Garland and Smith 1990). Studies involving children with diagnoses of ADHD and comorbid anxiety disorders suggest a role for TCAs in the treatment of this condition; reports suggest that children with ADHD and comorbid anxiety respond better to treatment with TCAs than to treatment with stimulants (Biederman et al. 1989a, 1989b; Garfinkel et al. 1983).

The most common side effects associated with the TCAs include dry mouth, transient blurred vision, sedation, constipation, urinary hesitancy, dizziness, and tremor. Behavioral untoward effects have been observed and are most commonly associated with desipramine (Leonard et al. 1989). TCAs lower the seizure threshold and should be used with caution in children with seizure disorders. Cardiac side effects are not uncommon and include prolongation of the PR interval, widening of the QRS complex, inversion or flattening of the T waves, tachycardia, and postural hypotension. In several case reports, sudden, unexplained death occurred in children stable on TCA medication (Abramowicz 1990; Biederman 1991; Riddle et al. 1993; Varley and McClellan 1997). This phenomenon has been the focus of an epidemiological study (Biederman et al. 1995).

The potential arrhythmogenicity of TCAs and the risk for sudden death require further investigation. Heart rate variability has been reported to be higher in children than in adults. Desipramine was noted to reduce the beat-to-beat variability in children; reduction of beat-to-beat variability has been suggested as a possible arrhythmogenic mechanism in children (Walsh et al. 1994).

Because of unresolved issues of possible sudden, unexplained cardiac fatalities, the use of TCAs for the treatment of anxiety disorders remains controversial. Before TCAs are initiated in a child, the parent and child must be carefully informed about risks, including the risk of death versus the benefit of treatment. Furthermore, the family should be carefully questioned about familial cardiac history and familial history of sudden death. Although the amount of risk is unclear, the current recommendation is that a baseline electrocardiogram, pulse rate, and blood pressure measures be obtained before treatment. Patients should be followed up with serial electrocardiograms. Any significant change from baseline electrocardiogram warrants a cardiology consultation and potential discontinuation of the medication.

TCAs should be initiated at low dosages to minimize both side effects and risk of exacerbation of anxiety. Recommended starting doses for imipramine range from 10 to 25 mg. In adolescents, TCAs are usually prescribed in once-a-day bedtime doses; because children metabolize medications faster than adults do, prepubertal children usually require twice-a-day dosing. Dosages may be increased every week by 25 mg/day until either symptoms resolve or untoward effects limit further dosage increase. The recommended maximum daily dosage for imipramine, desipramine, amitriptyline, and clomipramine is 5 mg/kg. The maximum daily dosage for nortriptyline is 2.5 mg/kg. Withdrawal effects occur with discontinuation of TCAs, and withdrawal should occur slowly over weeks. Detailed guidelines for the use of TCAs are reviewed elsewhere in this book (see Chapter 39).

Selective Serotonin Reuptake Inhibitors

SSRIs inhibit serotonin reuptake into the presynaptic terminal, which results in increased serotonin concentration at the synaptic cleft of neurons. Serotonin reuptake inhibition, however, is not thought to explain their therapeutic effects. Therapeutic effects, which are seen only after several weeks of administration, are postulated to involve neuroadaptive change of specific receptors. Reports suggest that SSRIs are safer in overdose than TCAs (Riddle et al. 1989), are not addictive, and are associated with fewer cognitive untoward effects than benzodiazepines. This provides the rationale behind the popularity of these agents in the treatment of anxiety disorders in adults and children and adolescents (Emslie et al. 1999). The safety and efficacy of SSRIs in adults who have obsessive-compulsive disorder, panic disorder, generalized anxiety disorder, and phobias have been well established. With the exception of obsessive-compulsive disorder, however, few controlled studies involving SSRIs in the treatment of anxiety in children and adolescents have been published.

Open studies of SSRIs in children with anxiety disorders are encouraging. In open trials, five children received fluoxetine for anxiety disorders or anxiety-related problems (Manassis and Bradley 1994). Anxiety symptoms remitted in all of the children after 6 weeks of treatment, as documented by parent and self-report. Fluoxetine seemed to be effective in the treatment of anxiety disorders in 21 children and adolescents in an open-label study by Birmaher et al. (1994). Moderate to marked improvements were manifested in 81% of the subjects, as measured on a global impression scale.

An open trial (Dummit et al. 1996) and a controlled study (Black and Uhde 1994) suggested that fluoxetine may be beneficial in the treatment of selective mutism. Selective mutism is conceptualized as a variant of social phobia (Black and Uhde 1995). Twenty-four children with selective mutism received 9 weeks of fluoxetine treatment in an open trial. At the end of the treatment, 76% showed benefits, with decreased anxiety and increased speech in social settings (Dummit et al. 1996). In a 12-week double-blind, placebo-controlled study of fluoxetine in children with selective mutism, children taking fluoxetine showed significantly greater improvement than those taking placebo. Both groups remained symptomatic at the end of the study.

In an open trial of fluoxetine in 21 children and adolescents with overanxious disorder plus a variety of other anxiety disorders (but not obsessive-compulsive disorder or panic disorder), 17 patients had moderate to marked improvement (Birmaher et al. 1994).

Transient anxiety and agitation may occur when initiating or increasing the dosage of SSRIs, but tolerance generally develops. Behavioral activation, including motor restlessness and behavioral disinhibition, has been described (Riddle et al. 1990–1991). As with other antidepressants, SSRIs have been reported to induce mania (Geller et al. 1993, 1994; Riddle et al. 1990–1991). It is unclear whether treatment-induced mania in this age group occurs only in children who would have ultimately developed bipolar disorder.

Other side effects include gastrointestinal symptoms, insomnia or hypersomnia, tremor, diaphoresis, and headache, including migraines in patients with a positive family history. However, these side effects rarely cause discontinuation of medication. Sexual side effects, such as anorgasmia, delayed orgasm, and ejaculatory delay, may occur. These side effects are particularly likely to interfere with compliance in adolescents. SSRIs should be initiated at a low dosage and gradually increased. For example, recommended dosing guidelines for fluoxetine are that it should be started at a dosage of 5 mg/day and increased every 7 days until a level of 20 mg is reached. The recommended maximum daily dosage of fluoxetine is 80 mg. Paroxetine should be started at a dosage of 10 mg/day and increased every 7 days up to a maximum dosage of 60 mg/day. Sertraline should be started at 25 mg/day and increased every 7 days up to a maximum dosage of 200 mg/day, which should be given in divided doses. Fluvoxamine should be started at 25 mg/day and increased every 4–7 days by 25-mg increments. The recommended maximum daily dosage of fluvoxamine is 200 mg.

When SSRIs are discontinued, a gradual withdrawal over at least 1 week is preferred.

Antihistamines

Diphenhydramine and hydroxyzine have been used to treat anxiety symptoms in children with various psychiatric disorders (Effron and Freedman 1953; Fish 1968). One controlled study reported that diphenhydramine at 1 mg/kg was effective in decreasing sleep latency and midsleep awakenings in 50 children ages 2–12 years during a 1-week period (Russo et al. 1976). These medications can have a paradoxical stimulation or disinhibition effect and are generally not recommended for the treatment of anxiety disorders in children and adolescents (Coffey 1990). The only use for which antihistamines might be indicated in anxiety disorders would be as a temporary aid for inducing sleep. The dose for treatment of initial insomnia would be 12.5–50.0 mg at bedtime.

β-Blockers

β-Blockers block the physiological symptoms of anxiety. They have been used in children and adolescents with anxiety disorders and episodic rage episodes. However, systematic studies have not been done (Riddle et al. 1999). There are essentially no pharmacokinetic data in children. β-Blockers differ in type (specificity) of β-receptor blockade, lipophilicity, and elimination half-life. Propranolol and nadolol are nonselective β-blockers (at β_1 and β_2 receptors), whereas atenolol and metoprolol are selective for β_1 receptors. These drugs differ with respect to central and peripheral effects. However, it is not clear which may play a role in moderating anxiety symptoms. Propranolol and metoprolol undergo hepatic metabolism, whereas atenolol and nadolol are cleared by renal elimination.

Studies in adults have not shown significant effects of β-blockers over placebo in the treatment of social phobia, panic disorder, performance anxiety, or posttraumatic stress disorder (Liebowitz et al. 1992; Turner et al. 1994), yet these agents are commonly prescribed for such disorders. Data in children are even more limited.

An open-label study by Famularo et al. (1988) reported some improvement in 11 children with posttraumatic stress disorder treated with propranolol up to 2.5 mg/kg/day. Joorabchi (1977) reported that propranolol (up to 30 mg/day) helped 13 of 14 adolescents with hyperventilation syndrome and suggested that this drug might be effective in treating panic disorder.

Side effects in children are similar to those in adults. These effects include sedation, mild hypotension, decreased heart rate, bronchoconstriction, hypoglycemia (in diabetic patients), dizziness, Raynaud's phenomenon, and sleep disruption (Coffey 1990). Potential for bradycardia, hypotension, and bronchoconstriction limit their use in asthmatic patients. Rebound hypertension can occur with abrupt withdrawal.

Asthma, heart failure, and diabetes mellitus are general contraindications for use of propranolol. Pulse and blood pressure should be monitored closely in all children taking these agents.

β-Blockers have been reported to affect growth hormone. β-Blockers do not appear to stimulate growth hormone when given alone, but a controlled study found that long-term administration of atenolol potentiated the growth-promoting effects of growth hormone–releasing hormone therapy in growth-deficient children (Cassorla et al. 1995). β-Blockers can also suppress melatonin (Riddle et al. 1988). The long-term effects of these neuroendocrine manipulations in children are unknown, and additional studies are needed.

Antipsychotics

Because of the risks of impaired cognitive functioning and tardive dyskinesia, antipsychotics are not recommended for treating anxiety symptoms in children and adolescents in the absence of specific indications such as Tourette's disorder or psychosis. Pimozide and haloperidol have been reported to induce separation anxiety in some patients (Linet 1985; Mikkelson et al. 1981).

Monoamine Oxidase Inhibitors

Monoamine oxidase inhibitors (MAOIs) have been shown to be efficacious for adults with panic disorder and social phobia, but there are no systematic studies involving children. Liebowitz et al. (1992) compared phenelzine, alprazolam, and placebo as treatments for social phobia in a double-blind trial. The response rate was clinically significant for phenelzine. Gelernter et al. (1991) compared the efficacy of phenelzine, alprazolam, and placebo in a parallel-design study and reported greater improvements in those patients who received phenelzine. Van Winter and Stickler (1984) reported a case series suggesting that phenelzine reduces panic symptoms in children. At this time, the child psychiatrist is left to extrapolate from these adult data.

The new reversible MAOIs show promise in adults. Brofaromine has been found to be superior to placebo (Van Vliet et al. 1996) and as effective as clomipramine (Bakish et al. 1993) for panic disorder and social phobia. Furthermore, the maladaptive personality traits associated with social phobia, such as avoidant behavior and depressive anxious profile, have been reported to normalize during treatment with brofaromine (Fahlen 1995).

If one extrapolates from the adult literature, phenelzine may, at times, be an appropriate choice in children and adolescents, especially when alternative treatments have failed or are contraindicated (Livingston 1995). Concurrent treatment with sympathomimetic drugs, SSRIs, or TCAs is a relative contraindication (Allen et al. 1993).

Barriers to clinical use in children are worries of hypertensive crisis and the difficulty of enforcing a tyramine-free diet. Careful instructions, a list of foods to avoid, and instructions on what to do if tyramine-containing foods are ingested should be provided to families. Health status, blood pressure, and dietary compliance must be monitored often. Phenelzine can be started at 15 mg once daily and increased slowly to the point at which the diastolic blood pressure is maintained at 5–10 mm Hg lower than normal. The adult maximum daily dosage is 90 mg. Tapering is required to discontinue medication.

Psychotherapeutic Treatments

In this section, we review the use of cognitive-behavioral interventions, psychotherapies, and family therapy in the treatment of anxiety disorders in children and adolescents. This section is not a detailed analysis of the literature but rather a summary of selected reports by type of therapeutic intervention.

Cognitive-Behavioral Therapy

Behavioral therapies target the patient's overt behaviors and emphasize treatment in the context of family and school instead of focusing on intrapsychic conflicts (Bernstein et al. 1996). The focus is not on etiology (Kazdin 1991). Cognitive-behavioral therapies integrate a behavioral management approach with an emphasis on changing the cognitions associated with the patient's anxiety (Kendall et al. 1991). This technique instructs patients to restructure their thoughts into a more positive framework, resulting in more assertive and adaptive behaviors (Bernstein et al. 1996).

Despite considerable interest in behavioral strategies for the treatment of anxiety disorders, the literature is sparse and consists primarily of case reports and single case studies (March et al. 1997). Cognitive-behavioral treatment strategies are based on models of learning. Principles of classical conditioning, operant conditioning, cognitive learning theory, and social learning theory are the underpinnings of cognitive-behavioral strategies used to treat childhood anxiety.

Classical conditioning or respondent conditioning occurs when two stimuli become paired to elicit the same response. In classical conditioning, stimuli evoke reflex responses. If an organism receives an electrical shock each time it hears the sound of a bell, after a time, the bell alone will elicit the same response as does the shock. Thus, the organism will become phobic of the bell (Livingston 1995). Operant conditioning is based on the understanding that the frequencies of specific behaviors can be influenced by consequences. This approach can be used to increase or decrease desired or undesired behaviors in a planned manner.

Some cognitive-behavioral strategies, including exposure-based interventions such as systematic desensitization, gradual exposure, and flooding, as well as contingency management, modeling, and cognitive strategies, have been used to treat childhood anxiety. Cognitive-behavioral strategies are the cornerstone of treatment for anxious children and adolescents.

Exposure-based strategies. Exposure-based treatments require that the child approach anxiety-provoking situations. This can be done via either imagery or direct exposure to the anxiety-provoking situation. For example, using gradual exposure, the child and therapist generate a list of feared situations in a hierarchy from least to most anxiety-provoking situations. The child then approaches each situation sequentially, moving up the hierarchy as his or her anxiety level permits. The patient starts with situations that provoke only minimal anxiety to facilitate success.

Systematic desensitization. Systematic desensitization consists of three steps: 1) relaxation training, 2) construction of the anxiety hierarchy, and 3) pairing of relaxation with gradual presentation of anxiety-provoking situations (Wolpe 1958).

Relaxation training decreases nervousness and promotes sleep at night. Progressive muscle relaxation scripts have been developed for use with children. Koeppen (1974) produced a script that teaches progressive muscle relaxation by using imagery. For example, a child is taught to tense and relax muscles in the hands by imagining that he or she is squeezing the juice from a lemon and to tense and relax muscles in the feet and legs by imagining that he or she is stepping into a big gooey mud puddle. Audiotapes of progressive muscle relaxation scripts can be purchased or devised by clinicians. The narrative should be age appropriate and presented in a soothing, monotonous voice with ample repetition. Practice should lead to more rapid relaxation (Livingston 1995).

Relaxation training is followed by in vitro exposure to the anxiety-provoking stimulus, beginning with the least distressing stimulus and working hierarchically toward the most distressing. Exposure can occur through imagery, photographs, or other substitutes for the anxiety-provoking stimulus. The child's tolerance of the anxiety-provoking situations can be measured by observing the child's affect and autonomic state. Increased tolerance is accompanied by the maintenance of baseline affect and autonomic symptoms in the face of the anxiety-provoking stimulus or a rapid return to baseline. Relaxation followed by exposure should continue until tolerance develops. Once in vitro exposure is well tolerated, in vivo exposure can be attempted as necessary. These exercises should be repeated frequently (daily) until tolerance develops. The frequency should then decrease as the child masters the techniques.

Flooding. Flooding involves repeated and prolonged exposure to the feared stimulus with the goal of extinguishing the anxiety response. Such exposure can be conducted either imaginally or in vivo. This method uses the same techniques as gradual exposure but with increased intensity and more rapid response. Throughout the flooding process, the child provides anxiety ratings and remains in the presence of the anxiety-provoking stimulus until his or her self-reported anxiety level diminishes. Flooding is generally used in conjunction with response prevention, which requires that the child not engage in avoidance responses. More so than some of the other interventions, flooding and response prevention are usually associated with more initial distress. Because of the degree of distress that can be generated initially, it is very important that the child and the parents have a clear understanding of the rationale for this procedure. Additionally, the degree of impairment must be severe enough to justify use of this technique in children. This technique has been used successfully primarily to treat obsessive-compulsive disorder and some phobic conditions and posttraumatic fear (Blagg and Yule 1984; Foa and Wilson 1991; Harris and Wiebe 1992).

Contingency management. Contingency management procedures are used to modify antecedent and consequent events that may influence the acquisition and/or maintenance of fearful or anxious behavior. Operant strategies such as positive reinforcement, shaping, extinction, and punishment are examples of contingency management.

Positive reinforcement. Positive reinforcement provides a desirable consequence to a given behavior. For an anxious child, an adaptive behavior can be positively reinforced by providing a reward (positive reinforcer). These reinforcers can be provided according to several schedules, at fixed or variable intervals of time, and with fixed or variable behaviors. The most powerful schedule for increasing the frequency of a given behavior is the variable ratio schedule, in which the individual cannot predict positive reinforcement. Contingency management is most effective when the child participates in the development of the plan and helps choose the reinforcer. Contingency management programs are often used in conjunction with systematic desensitization techniques.

In general, the reinforcement schedule is regular and predictable at the start of treatment to help initiate the desired behaviors. Then it is adjusted to the child's progress. Primary reinforcers have inherent value, such as praise, play time, and food. Secondary reinforcers can be exchanged for something with value (i.e., token economies). Both types of reinforcers are useful in particular situations, but secondary reinforcers may be less effective with younger children. Younger children respond better to immediate reinforcement than to delayed reinforcement.

Negative reinforcement. Negative reinforcement is the withholding or removal of positive reinforcement to modify behavior. Time-out from positive reinforcement is an example of negative reinforcement. Livingston (1995) identified two circumstances in which these methods are particularly useful in anxious children: 1) to reduce unwanted behaviors that are reinforced by "secondary gains" and 2) to reduce anxiety-driven oppositional behaviors. In secondary gain, it is assumed that some reinforcer is the main reason for the unwanted behaviors and that removal of that reinforcer would result in resolution of that behavior.

Punishment. Punishment—noxious consequences for undesirable behaviors—is generally less powerful than the other operant methods. Anxious children, who are already sensitive, may become more anxious and fearful as a result of this intervention. Although useful in certain situations, it should be used with caution.

Modeling. Social learning theory indicates that children can learn an enormous amount by watching others (Bandura 1977). Modeling has been most successful in children undergoing medical and dental procedures. Modeling also has been used to treat common childhood fears (Graziano and Mooney 1982). Anxious children can benefit from watching a model approach and cope with a feared situation. Ideally, the model should be similar in age, sex, and cultural background to the patient. This technique has been especially successful in older children. Variants of modeling include

- *Filmed*—the child watches a videotape of the model.
- *Live*—the model is in the presence of the child.
- *Participant modeling*—the live model interacts with the child and guides the child through the anxiety-provoking stimulus.

Cognitive strategies. Cognitive therapies attempt to reduce symptoms by identifying and correcting the unexamined or inaccurate cognitions that produced the symptoms. Cognitive procedures include a variety of techniques, such as self-instruction training, problem solving, and altering maladaptive self-talk. These strategies are taught by using modeling, exposure, and behavioral rehearsal. Self-instruction training for anxious children was described by Ollendick and Cerney (1981) and incorporates the following steps:

1. The therapist approaches the feared stimulus while talking aloud about coping.
2. The child approaches the feared stimulus and verbalizes the coping statements at the direction of the therapist.
3. The child approaches the feared stimulus while saying the coping statements aloud.
4. The child approaches the feared stimulus while whispering the coping statements.
5. The child approaches the feared stimulus while thinking about the coping statements.

Problem-solving training involves teaching the patient to define a problem, to determine an approach to solving the problem, to focus his or her attention on mastering the problem, and to repeat coping statements to himself or herself while attempting to master the problem (Kendall and Braswell 1986).

To modify maladaptive self-talk, the child first must learn to identify and monitor self-statements associated with anxiety and avoidance behaviors. Once maladaptive self-talk is identified, the child works with the therapist to generate alternative self-statements that serve to decrease anxiety, facilitate appropriate behaviors, and improve coping (Kendall et al. 1992). The use of cognitive strategies to treat childhood anxiety is relatively new and generally used in combination with other forms of behavior therapy.

Cognitive-behavioral therapies can be done in a fairly standardized way and usually can be completed in 10–20 sessions if used in a prescribed way for problems that are mutually identified, listed, and prioritized. This standardized approach makes this technique amenable to good studies of treatment outcomes. Several well-controlled studies have confirmed the efficacy of cognitive-behavioral therapy for anxiety in children and adolescents.

The first controlled study of cognitive-behavioral therapy in children and adolescents was published by Kendall (1994) and involved children ages 9–13 years with a variety of anxiety disorders, including overanxious, avoidant, and separation anxiety disorders. In this study, 16 sessions of cognitive-behavioral therapy were reported to be significantly superior to an 8-week, waiting-list control in decreasing the severity of anxiety and depressive symptoms. Cognitive interventions were aimed at helping the child identify anxious feelings and somatic reactions to anxiety and devising strategies to cope with them; behavioral techniques included role-playing, relaxation, exposure, and modeling. Importantly, treatment gains were maintained on long term follow-up 2–5 years later, as measured by self-report and parent report, indexes of anxiety and depression, and absence of anxiety diagnosis in the children (Kendall and Southam-Gerow 1996). A recent replication of this study, involving 94 children ages 9–13 years with mixed anxiety disorders, confirmed that cognitive-behavioral therapy was significantly better than wait-list control in decreasing symptoms of anxiety and depression and in resolving anxiety diagnoses. Treatment gains were maintained at 1-year follow-up (Kendall et al. 1997).

King et al. (1988) evaluated the efficacy of a 4-week trial of a cognitive-behavioral intervention program involving cognitive-behavioral therapy plus parent/teacher training in child behavioral management compared with wait-list control in 34 children ages 5–15 years with school refusal. The active treatment group reported significant improvement in school attendance and on self-reports and parent and/or clinician measures of symptoms, relative to wait-list control subjects. These gains were maintained at 3-month follow-up.

A recent study suggested that traditional educational and supportive treatment may be as effective as highly structured cognitive-behavioral treatment in returning school phobic children to school (Last et al. 1988). In this study, 56 children ages 6–17 years with school phobia were randomized to 12 weeks of either cognitive-behavioral therapy or an educational-supportive therapy control condition. Both treatments were equally effective in increasing school attendance and in reducing anxiety and depressive symptoms in these children. Treatment gains for both groups were maintained at 4-week follow-up.

Psychoanalysis

Limited systematically collected data have evaluated the utility of long-term psychoanalytic treatment in children with anxiety disorders. Most of the reports on the effects of long-term psychoanalytic treatment of children with anxiety disorders consist of case reports on the treatment of phobias, school refusal, or anxiety symptoms comorbid with other problems (Bornstein 1949; Fraiberg 1987; Pearson 1968; Tyson 1978). Although these reports have been favorable, they must be considered in light of the absence of comparison groups, lack of standardized pretreatment and posttreatment measures, and incomplete description and standardization of interventions (Marans 1989).

One of the larger systematic studies of child psychoanalysis compared the effects of 1) one session per week, 2) one session per week followed by four sessions per week, and 3) four sessions per week in 12 boys ages 7–10 years with DSM-III (American Psychiatric Association 1980) diagnoses of overanxious disorder and learning disabilities. Boys receiving sessions more than once a week showed significantly greater improvement in their capacity for relationships, greater frustration tolerance, more balanced use of defenses, and improved reading in comparison with boys receiving less frequent treatment. Gains were maintained at 2-year follow-up. Psychodynamic psychotherapy consisting of one session per week produced significant improvement in anxiety. Fewer characterological changes were reported for this treatment group than for the other treatment groups (Heinicke and Ramsey-Klee 1986).

Target and Fonagy (1994) reviewed the Anna Freud Centre's records of 352 children who were retrospectively assigned DSM-III-R (American Psychiatric Association 1987) diagnoses of anxiety and depressive disorders. All children received either 4–5 sessions per week of psychoanalysis or 1–3 sessions per week of psychodynamic therapy. Children receiving 6 months or more of either treatment had a 72% improvement in adaptation. Predictors of improvement were greater frequency of sessions, longer period of treatment, phobic symptomatology, and younger age.

Psychodynamic Psychotherapies

Psychodynamic psychotherapy is a derivative of child psychoanalysis (Bemporad 1991). Differences between psychodynamic psychotherapy and child psychoanalysis include (for the former) less-frequent appointments, greater participation of the parents in the treatment, and more explicit use of active support, practical guidance, and environmental interventions (American Academy of Child and Adolescent Psychiatry 1997).

Psychodynamic therapies assume that the origins of the presenting symptom lie within internal conflicts that are outside of the individual's consciousness and must be brought to consciousness—verbally or through play—by the therapist. The neutral therapist serves as a model for important relationships that may be the context in which the symptom developed. Additionally, psychodynamic psychotherapies involve identification of the patient's defenses or characteristic ways of coping, which may be ineffective. Defenses commonly identified in anxious patients are displacement, somatization, and repression. Psychodynamic psychotherapies attempt to help the child develop new and better ways of coping by replacing those immature defenses with more mature ones. Anxiety disorders frequently involve issues of separation, independence, and self-esteem (Leonard and Rapoport 1991). Parents are frequently involved in the treatment so they learn to understand the patient's need for reassurance and encouragement and what to expect as therapy progresses.

Many of the difficulties inherent in the study of psychoanalysis also pertain to the study of psychodynamic psychotherapy. Few systematic studies have shown the efficacy of psychodynamic psychotherapy in the treatment of anxiety disorders in children and adolescents. Many case reports have documented its usefulness in individual cases (Gardner 1977; McDermott et al. 1989; Sarnoff 1987). Several meta-analytic studies of clinically heterogeneous groups provide some support for the effectiveness of psychodynamic psychotherapies in children (Casey and Berman 1985; Weiss and Weisz 1990; Weisz et al. 1987).

Family Therapy

Children with anxiety disorders often have family members who have anxiety disorders and depression (Last et al. 1987c, 1991; Livingston 1985; Weisman et al. 1984). These family studies do not provide information about mode of transmission, whether environmental or genetic, although it is presumed to be both. Anxiety can be contagious within families (Eisenberg 1958), as the anxious child's distress is exacerbated by anxious parents. In a recent study, Manassis and Hood (1998) evaluated predictors of impairment in childhood anxiety disorders in 74 families; they identified parental anxiety and behavior management difficulties as possible predictors of impaired functioning in addition to children's depression and developmental and psychosocial adversity.

The possible benefits of family therapies have only begun to be systematically evaluated. Despite the dearth of studies in the literature, family therapy is recommended when serious systematic abnormalities of family functioning are noted. Family characteristics that have been associated with anxiety include high levels of expressed emotion, inconsistency, poor family boundaries and enmeshment, role reversals, unrealistic expectations, and excessive power on the part of the children in the family system.

Several recent studies have begun to examine the role of family-based treatments in the management of anxiety disorders in children. Mendlowitz et al. (1999) examined the effect of a cognitive-behavioral group intervention on anxiety, depression, and coping strategies in school-age children (7–12 years) with Axis I anxiety disorders and the effect of parental involvement in outcomes. Children (N = 62) were randomly assigned to 1) parent-child intervention groups, 2) child-only intervention groups, or 3) parent-only intervention groups. All treatment groups reported fewer symptoms of anxiety and depression posttreatment and changes in their use of coping strategies. The children in the parent-child group reported the most improvement in symptoms, active coping strategies, and emotional well-being. A limitation of this study was the lack of follow-up to determine whether gains were maintained.

Barrett et al. (1996) used cognitive-behavioral strategies in a controlled trial of family treatment in children with anxiety disorders. Subjects were 79 children ages 7–14 years who had diagnoses of various anxiety disorders. They were randomly allocated to three treatment conditions: 1) cognitive-behavioral therapy for the child alone, 2) cognitive-behavioral therapy and family management training, and 3) a waiting-list control group. Effectiveness of these interventions were evaluated immediately posttreatment and at 6- and 12-month follow-up. The results showed that 69.8% of the children no longer met criteria for an anxiety disorder compared with 26% of the waiting-list control subjects at follow-up. At 12-month follow-up, 95.6% of the children who were randomized to the cognitive-behavioral therapy and family management training group continued not to meet criteria for an anxiety disorder, whereas only 70.3% of children who were randomized to cognitive-behavioral therapy without family management continued not to meet criteria for an anxiety disorder.

Cobham et al. (1998) similarly evaluated 67 children ages 7–14 years with anxiety disorders. Anxious children whose parents were not anxious were as likely to benefit from individual cognitive-behavioral therapy as they were from the combined treatment (cognitive-behavioral therapy with parental anxiety management). Anxious children whose parents were also anxious, however, were significantly more likely to benefit from the combined treatment approach; 77% responded to the combined treatment approach, whereas only 39% responded to cognitive-behavioral therapy alone. Treatment response was maintained over time. This emerging body of literature shows support for the utility of parent management training and family treatment in the treatment of anxiety in children and adolescents.

Conclusions

The number of well-designed studies evaluating the efficacy of treatment strategies for anxiety disorders in children and adolescents has been steadily increasing. The available data have provided strong support for the effectiveness of cognitive-behavioral strategies for children and their families and promising data for the effectiveness of some pharmacotherapeutic strategies. A rational, well-developed treatment plan using a multimodal, biopsychosocial approach will produce a favorable outcome for these children and their families.

References

Abramowicz M: Sudden death in children treated with a tricyclic antidepressant (letter). Med Lett Drugs Ther 32:53, 1990

Achenbach TM: Manual for the Child Behavior Checklist/4–18 and 1991 Profile. Burlington, VT, University of Vermont Department of Psychiatry, 1991

Allen AJ, Rapoport JL, Swedo SE: Psychopharmacologic treatment of childhood anxiety disorders. Child Adolesc Psychiatr Clin N Am 2:795–817, 1993

American Academy of Child and Adolescent Psychiatry: AACAP Official Action Practice Parameters for the Assessment and Treatment of Anxiety Disorders. J Am Acad Child Adolesc Psychiatry 32:1089–1098, 1997

American Psychiatric Association: Diagnostic and Statistical Manual of Mental Disorders, 3rd Edition. Washington, DC, American Psychiatric Association, 1980

American Psychiatric Association: Diagnostic and Statistical Manual of Mental Disorders, 3rd Edition, Revised. Washington, DC, American Psychiatric Association, 1987

American Psychiatric Association: Benzodiazepine Toxicity and Abuse: A Task Force Report of the American Psychiatric Association. Washington, DC, American Psychiatric Association, 1990

American Psychiatric Association: Diagnostic and Statistical Manual of Mental Disorders, 4th Edition. Washington, DC, American Psychiatric Association, 1994

Anderson JC, Williams S, McGee R, et al: DSM-III disorders in preadolescent children: prevalence in a large sample from the general population. Arch Gen Psychiatry 44:69–76, 1987

Bakish D, Saxena BM, Bowen R, et al: Reversible monoamine oxidase–A inhibitors in panic disorders. Clin Neuropharmacol 16 (suppl 12):577–582, 1993

Ballenger JC, Carek DJ, Steele JJ, et al: Three cases of panic disorder with agoraphobia in children. Am J Psychiatry 146:922–924, 1989

Bandura A: Social Learning Theory. Englewood Cliffs, NJ, Prentice-Hall, 1977

Barrett PM, Dodds MR, Rapee RM: Family treatment of childhood anxiety: a controlled trial. J Consult Clin Psychol 64:333–342, 1996

Bell-Dolan DJ, Last CG, Strauss CC: Symptoms of anxiety disorders in normal children. J Am Acad Child Adolesc Psychiatry 29:759–765, 1990

Bemporad J: Psychoanalysis and psychodynamic therapy, in Textbook of Child and Adolescent Psychiatry. Edited by Weiner JM. Washington, DC, American Psychiatric Press, 1991, pp 571–575

Berney T, Kolvin I, Bhate SR, et al: School phobia: a therapeutic trial with clomipramine and short-term outcome. Am J Psychiatry 138:110–118, 1981

Bernstein GA, Borchardt CM: Anxiety disorders of childhood and adolescence: a critical review. J Am Acad Child Adolesc Psychiatry 30:519–532, 1991

Bernstein GA, Garfinkel BD: The Visual Analogue Scale for Anxiety—Revised: psychometric properties. J Anxiety Disord 6:223–239, 1992

Bernstein GA, Shaw K: Practice parameters for the assessment and treatment of children and adolescents with anxiety disorders. American Academy of Child and Adolescent Psychiatry. J Am Acad Child Adolesc Psychiatry 36 (10 suppl):69S–84S, 1997

Bernstein GA, Garfinkel B, Borchardt C: Comparative studies of pharmacotherapy for school refusal. J Am Acad Child Adolesc Psychiatry 29:773–781, 1990

Bernstein GA, Borchardt CM, Perwien AR: Anxiety disorders in children and adolescents: a review of the past 10 years. J Am Acad Child Adolesc Psychiatry 35:1110–1119, 1996

Biederman J: Clonazepam in the treatment of prepubertal children with panic like symptoms. J Clin Psychiatry 48 (suppl):38–41, 1987

Biederman J: The diagnosis and treatment of adolescent anxiety disorders [discussion, pp 50–53; erratum, p 440]. J Clin Psychiatry 51 (suppl):20–26, 1990

Biederman J: Sudden death in children treated with tricyclic antidepressant. J Am Acad Child Adolesc Psychiatry 30:495–497, 1991

Biederman J, Baldessarini RJ, Wright V, et al: A double-blind placebo controlled study of desipramine in the treatment of ADD, I: efficacy. J Am Acad Child Adolesc Psychiatry 28:777–784, 1989a

Biederman J, Baldessarini RJ, Wright V, et al: A double-blind placebo controlled study of desipramine in the treatment of ADD, II: serum drug levels and cardiovascular findings. J Am Acad Child Adolesc Psychiatry 28:903–911, 1989b

Biederman J, Faraone SV, Keenan K, et al: Familial association between attention deficit disorder and anxiety disorders. Am J Psychiatry 148:251–256, 1991

Biederman J, Thisted RA, Greenhill LL, et al: Estimation of the association between desipramine and the risk for sudden death in 5- to 14-year-old children. J Clin Psychiatry 56:87–93, 1995

Bird, HR, Canino G, Rubio-Stipic M, et al: Estimates of the prevalence of childhood in a community survey in Puerto Rico. Arch Gen Psychiatry 45:1120–1126, 1988

Birmaher B, Waterman GS, Ryan N, et al: Fluoxetine for childhood anxiety disorders. J Am Acad Child Adolesc Psychiatry 33:993–999, 1994

Birmaher B, Brent DA, Chiapetta L, et al: Psychometric properties of the Screen for Child Anxiety-Related Emotional Disorders (SCARED): scale construction and psychometric characteristics. J Am Acad Child Adolesc Psychiatry 36:545–553, 1997

Birmaher B, Khetarpal S, Bunt D, et al: The Screen for Child Anxiety-Related Emotional Disorders (SCARED): a replication study. J Am Acad Child Adolesc Psychiatry 38:1230–1236, 1999

Black B, Robbins DR: Panic disorder in children and adolescents. J Am Acad Child Adolesc Psychiatry 29:36–44, 1990

Black B, Uhde TW: Treatment of elective mutism with fluoxetine: a double-blind placebo-controlled study. J Am Acad Child Adolesc Psychiatry 33:1000–1006, 1994

Black B, Uhde TW: Psychiatric characteristics of children with selective mutism: a pilot study. J Am Acad Child Adolesc Psychiatry 34:847–856, 1995

Blagg NR, Yule W: The behavioral treatment of school refusal—a comparative study. Behav Res Ther 22:119–127, 1984

Blier P, de Montigny C, Chaput Y: A role for the serotonin system in the mechanism of action of antidepressant treatments: preclinical evidence. J Clin Psychiatry 51 (suppl):14–20, 1990

Bornstein B: The analysis of a phobic child: some problems of theory and technique in child analysis. Psychoanal Study Child 3:181–226, 1949

Brady EU, Kendall PC: Comorbidity of anxiety and depression in children and adolescents. Psychol Bull 3:244–255, 1992

Casey RJ, Berman JS: The outcome of psychotherapy with children. Psychol Bull 98:388–400, 1985

Cassorla F, Mericq V, Garcia H, et al: The effects of beta 1-adrenergic blockade on the growth response to growth hormone (GH)-releasing hormone therapy in GH-deficient children. J Clin Endocrinol Metab 80:2997–3001, 1995

Chambers WJ, Puig-Antich J, Hirsch M, et al: The assessment of affective disorders in children and adolescents by semistructured interview. Arch Gen Psychiatry 42:696–702, 1985

Clark DB, Donovan JE: Reliability and validity of the Hamilton Anxiety Scale in an adolescent sample. J Am Acad Child Adolesc Psychiatry 33:354–360, 1994

Cobham VE, Dodds MR, Spence SH: The role of parental anxiety in the treatment of childhood anxiety. J Clin Child Psychol 27:459–468, 1998

Coffey BJ: Anxiolytics for children and adolescents: traditional and new drugs. J Child Adolesc Psychopharmacol 1:57–83, 1990

Coffey BJ: Review and update: benzodiazepines in childhood and adolescence. Psychiatric Annals 23:332–339, 1993

Cohen P, Kasen S, Brook JS, et al: Behavior patterns of young children and their offspring: a two-generation study. Dev Psychol 34:1202–1208, 1998

Costello EJ: Child psychiatric disorders and their correlates: a primary care pediatric sample. J Am Acad Child Adolesc Psychiatry 28:851–855, 1989

Cutler NR, Hesselink JM, Sramek JJ: A phase II multicenter dose-finding, efficacy and safety trial of ipsapirone in outpatients with generalized anxiety disorder. Prog Neuropsychopharmacol Biol Psychiatry 18:447–463, 1994

Dubovsky SL: Approaches to developing new anxiolytics and antidepressants. J Clin Psychiatry 54 (suppl):75–83, 1993

Dummit SE, Klein RG, Tancer NK, et al: Fluoxetine treatment of children with selective mutism: an open trial. J Am Acad Child Adolesc Psychiatry 35:615–621, 1996

Effron AJ, Freedman AM: The treatment of behavior disorders in children with Benadryl. J Pediatr 42:261–266, 1953

Eisenberg L: School phobia: a study in the communication of anxiety. Am J Psychiatry 114:712–718, 1958

Emslie GJ, Walkup JT, Pliszka SR, et al: Nontricyclic antidepressants: current trends in children and adolescents. J Am Acad Child Adolesc Psychiatry 38 (suppl):517–528, 1999

Evans SM, Troisi JR, Griffiths RR: Tandospirone and alprazolam: comparison of behavioral effects and abuse liability in humans. J Pharmacol Exp Ther 271:683–694, 1994

Fahlen T: Personality traits in social phobia, II: changes during drug treatment. J Clin Psychiatry 56:569–573, 1995

Famularo R, Kinsherff R, Fenton T: Propranolol treatment for childhood post traumatic stress disorder, acute type: a pilot study. Am J Dis Child 142:1244–1247, 1988

Fish B: Drug use in psychiatric disorders of children. Am J Psychiatry 124:31–36, 1968

Foa EB, Wilson R: Stop Obsessing! How to Overcome Your Obsessions and Compulsions. New York, Bantam Books, 1991

Fraiberg S: Selected Writings. Columbus, OH, Ohio State University Press, 1987

Gardner RA: Therapeutic Communication With Children. New York, Jason Aronson, 1977

Garfinkel BD, Wender PH, Sloman L, et al: Tricyclic antidepressant and methylphenidate treatment of attention deficit disorder in children. J Am Acad Child Adolesc Psychiatry 22:343–348, 1983

Garland EJ, Smith DH: Case study: panic disorder on a child psychiatric consultation service. J Am Acad Child Adolesc Psychiatry 29:785–788, 1990

Gelernter CS, Uhde TW, Cimbolic P, et al: Cognitive-behavioral and pharmacological treatments of social phobia: a controlled study. Arch Gen Psychiatry 48:938–945, 1991

Geller B, Fox LW, Fletcher M: Effect of tricyclic antidepressants on switching to mania and on the onset of bipolarity in depressed 6- to 12-year-olds. J Am Acad Child Adolesc Psychiatry 32:43–50, 1993

Geller B, Fox LW, Clark KA: Rate and predictors of prepubertal bipolarity during follow-up of 6- to 12-year-old depressed children. J Am Acad Child Adolesc Psychiatry 33:461–468, 1994

Geller B, Reising D, Leonard HL, et al: Critical review of tricyclic antidepressant use in children and adolescents. J Am Acad Child Adolesc Psychiatry 38:513–516, 1999

Gittelman-Klein R, Klein DF: School phobia: diagnostic considerations in the light of imipramine effects. J Nerv Ment Dis 156:199–215, 1973

Graae F, Milner J, Rizzotto L, et al: Clonazepam in childhood anxiety disorders. J Am Acad Child Adolesc Psychiatry 33:372–376, 1994

Graziano AM, Mooney KC: Behavioral treatment of "nightfears" in children: maintenance of improvement at 2½- to 3-year follow-up. J Consult Clin Psychol 50:598–599, 1982

Hamilton M: The assessment of anxiety states by rating. Br J Med Psychol 32:50–55, 1959

Harris CV, Wiebe DJ: An analysis of response prevention and flooding procedures in the treatment of adolescent obsessive compulsive disorder. J Behav Ther Exp Psychiatry 23:107–115, 1992

Heinicke CM, Ramsey-Klee DM: Outcome of child psychotherapy as a function of frequency of session. J Am Acad Child Psychiatry 25:247–253, 1986

Hughes CW, Preskorn SH: Pharmacokinetics in child/adolescent psychiatric disorders. Psychiatric Annals 24:76–82, 1994

Joorabchi B: Expression of the hyperventilation syndrome in childhood: studies in the management, including an evaluation of the effectiveness of propranolol. Clin Pediatr (Phila) 16:1110–1115, 1977

Kashani JH, Orvaschel H: Anxiety disorders in mid-adolescence—a community sample. Am J Psychiatry 145:960–964, 1988

Kashani JH, Orvaschel H: A community study of anxiety in children and adolescents. Am J Psychiatry 147:313–318, 1990

Kazdin AE: Behavior modification, in Textbook of Child and Adolescent Psychiatry. Edited by Weiner JM. Washington, DC, American Psychiatric Press, 1991, pp 576–593

Keller MB, Lavori P, Wunder J, et al: Chronic course of anxiety disorders in children and adolescents. J Am Acad Child Adolesc Psychiatry 31:595–599, 1992

Kendall PC: Treating anxiety disorders in children: results of a randomized clinical trial. J Consult Clin Psychol 62:100–110, 1994

Kendall PC, Braswell L: Medical application of cognitive behavioral interventions with children. J Dev Behav Pediatr 7:257–264, 1986

Kendall PC, Southam-Gerow MA: Long-term follow-up of a cognitive behavioral therapy for anxiety disordered youth. J Consult Clin Psychol 64:724–730, 1996

Kendall PC, Chansky TE, Friedman M, et al: Treating anxiety disorders in children and adolescents, in Child and Adolescent Therapy—Behavioral Procedures. Edited by Kendall PC. New York, Guilford, 1991, pp 131–164

Kendall PC, Kortlander E, Chansky TE, et al: Comorbidity of anxiety and depression in youth: treatment implications. J Consult Clin Psychol 60:869–880, 1992

Kendall PC, Flannery-Schroeder E, Panichelli-Mindel SM, et al: Therapy for youth with anxiety disorders: a second randomized trial. J Consult Clin Psychol 65:366–380, 1997

King NJ, Tonge BJ, Heyne DM, et al: Cognitive-behavioral treatment of school refusing children: a controlled evaluation. J Am Acad Child Adolesc Psychiatry 37:395–403, 1988

Klein DF, Riddle MA: Pharmacokinetics in children and adolescents. Child Adolesc Psychiatr Clin N Am 4:59–75, 1995

Klein DF, Mannuzza S, Chapman T, et al: Child panic revisited. J Am Acad Child Adolesc Psychiatry 31:112–116, 1992

Klein R, Kopelwicz H, Kanner A: Imipramine treatment of children with separation anxiety disorder. J Am Acad Child Adolesc Psychiatry 31:21–28, 1992

Koeppen AS: Relaxation training for children. Elementary School Guidance and Counseling 9:14–21, 1974

Kranzler HR: Use of buspirone in an adolescent with overanxious disorder. J Am Acad Child Adolesc Psychiatry 27:789–790, 1988

Kutcher SP, MacKenzie S: Successful clonazepam treatment of adolescents with panic disorder. J Clin Psychopharmacol 8:299–301, 1988

Kutcher SP, Reiter S, Gardner DM, et al: The pharmacotherapy of anxiety disorders in children and adolescents. Psychiatr Clin North Am 15:41–67, 1992

Kutcher S, Reiter S, Gardner D: Pharmacotherapy: approaches and applications, in Anxiety Disorders in Children and Adolescents. Edited by March JS. New York, Guilford, 1995, pp 341–385

LaGreca AM, Stone WL: Social Anxiety Scale for Children—Revised: factor structure and concurrent validity. J Clin Child Psychol 22:17–27, 1993

Last CG, Francis G, Hersen M, et al: Separation anxiety and school phobia: a comparison using DSM-III criteria. Am J Psychiatry 144:653–657, 1987a

Last CG, Hersen M, Kazdin AE, et al: Comparison of DSM-III separation anxiety and overanxious disorders: demographic characteristics and patterns of comorbidity. J Am Acad Child Adolesc Psychiatry 26:527–531, 1987b

Last CG, Strauss CC, Francis G: Comorbidity among childhood anxiety disorders. J Nerv Ment Dis 175:726–730, 1987c

Last CG, Hansen C, Franco N: Cognitive-behavioral treatment of school phobia. J Am Acad Child Adolesc Psychiatry 37:404–411, 1988

Last CG, Hersen M, Kazdin AE, et al: Anxiety disorders in children and their families. Arch Gen Psychiatry 48:928–934, 1991

Leonard HL, Rapoport JL: Separation anxiety, overanxious, and avoidant disorders, in Textbook of Child and Adolescent Psychiatry. Edited by Weiner JM. Washington, DC, American Psychiatric Press, 1991, pp 311–322

Leonard HL, Swedo SE, Rapoport JL, et al: Treatment of obsessive-compulsive disorder with clomipramine and desipramine in children and adolescents: a double-blind crossover comparison. Arch Gen Psychiatry 46:1088–1092, 1989

Liebowitz MR, Schnier F, Campeas R, et al: Phenelzine vs atenolol in social phobia. Arch Gen Psychiatry 49:290–300, 1992

Linet LS: Tourette syndrome, pimozide, and school phobia: the neuroleptic separation anxiety syndrome. J Am Acad Child Adolesc Psychiatry 142:613–615, 1985

Livingston R: Anxiety and anxiety disorders, in Treatments of Psychiatric Disorders, 2nd Edition, Vol 1. Gabbard GO, Editor-in-Chief. Washington, DC, American Psychiatric Press, 1995, pp 230–252

Livingston R, Nugent H, Rader L: Family histories of depressed and severely anxious children. Am J Psychiatry 142:1497–1499, 1995

Manassis K, Bradley S: Fluoxetine in anxiety disorders (letter). J Am Acad Child Adolesc Psychiatry 33:761–762, 1994

Manassis K, Hood J: Individual and familial predictors of impairment in childhood anxiety disorders. J Am Acad Child Adolesc Psychiatry 37:428–434, 1998

Marans S: Psychoanalytic psychotherapy with children: current research trends and challenges. J Am Acad Child Adolesc Psychiatry 28:669–674, 1989

March JS: Manual for the Multidimensional Anxiety Scale for Children (MASC). Toronto, ON, Multi-Health Systems, 1996

March JS, Sullivan K: Test-retest reliability of the Multidimensional Anxiety Scale for Children. J Anxiety Disord 13:349–358, 1999

March JS, Parker JD, Sullivan K, et al: The Multidimensional Anxiety Scale for Children (MASC): factor structure, reliability and validity. J Am Acad Child Adolesc Psychiatry 36:554–565, 1997

McDermott JF, Werry J, Petti T: Anxiety disorders of childhood and adolescence, in Treatments of Psychiatric Disorders: A Task Force Report of the American Psychiatric Association, Vol 1. Washington, DC, American Psychiatric Association, 1989, pp 401–446

McGee R, Feehan M, Williams S, et al: DSM-III disorders in a large sample of adolescents. J Am Acad Child Adolesc Psychiatry 29:611–619, 1990

McGrath PJ, Stewart JW, Quitkin FM, et al: Gepirone treatment of atypical depression: preliminary evidence of serotonergic involvement. J Clin Psychopharmacol 14:347–352, 1994

Mendlowitz SL, Manassis K, Bradley S, et al: Cognitive-behavioral group treatments in childhood anxiety disorders: the role of parental involvement. J Am Acad Child Adolesc Psychiatry 38:1223–1229, 1999

Mikkelson EJ, Detlor J, Cohen DJ: School avoidance and school phobia triggered by haloperidol in patients with Tourette's disorder. J Am Acad Child Adolesc Psychiatry 138:1572–1576, 1981

Mosconi M, Chiamuleva C, Recchia G: New anxiolytics in development. Int J Clin Pharmacol Res 13:331–344, 1993

Murphy SM, Owen R, Tyrer P: Comparative assessment of efficacy and withdrawal symptoms after 6 and 12 weeks' treatment with diazepam or buspirone. Br J Psychiatry 154:529–534, 1989

Ollendick TH: Reliability and validity of the Revised Fear Surgery Schedule for Children (FSSC-R). Behav Res Ther 21:685–692, 1983

Ollendick TH, Cerney JA: Clinical Behavior Therapy With Children. New York, Plenum, 1981

Orvaschel H, Puig-Antich J, Chambers W, et al: Retrospective assessment of prepubertal major depression with the Kiddie-SADS-e. Journal of the American Academy of Child Psychiatry 21:392–397, 1982

Pearson A: Handbook of Psychoanalysis. New York, Basic Books, 1968

Pfeffer CR, Jiang H, Domeschek LJ: Buspirone treatment of psychiatrically hospitalized prepubertal children with symptoms of anxiety and moderately severe aggression. J Child Adolesc Psychopharmacol 7:145–155, 1997

Pfefferbaum B, Butler PM, Mullins D, et al: Two cases of benzodiazepine toxicity in children. J Clin Psychiatry 38:450–452, 1987a

Pfefferbaum B, Overall JE, Boren HA, et al: Alprazolam in the treatment of anticipatory and acute situational anxiety in children with cancer. J Am Acad Child Adolesc Psychiatry 26:532–535, 1987b

Popper CW: Psychopharmacologic treatment of anxiety disorders in adolescents and children. J Clin Psychiatry 54 (5, suppl):52–63, 1993

Rakel RE: Long term buspirone therapy for chronic anxiety: a multicenter international study to determine safety. South Med J 83:194–198, 1990

Reiter S, Kutcher S: Disinhibition and anger outbursts in adolescents treated with clonazepam (letter). J Clin Psychopharmacol 11:268, 1991

Reynolds CR, Richmond BO: What I think and feel: a revised measure of children's manifest anxiety. J Abnorm Child Psychol 6:271–280, 1978

Riddle MA, Leckman JF, Anderson GM, et al: Tourette's syndrome: clinical and neurochemical correlates. J Am Acad Child Adolesc Psychiatry 27:409–412, 1988

Riddle MA, Brown N, Dzubinski D, et al: Case study: fluoxetine overdose in an adolescent. J Am Acad Child Adolesc Psychiatry 28:587–588, 1989

Riddle MA, King RA, Hardin MT, et al: Behavioral side effects of fluoxetine in children and adolescents. J Am Acad Child Adolesc Psychiatry 1:193–198, 1990–1991

Riddle MA, Geller B, Ryan N: Case study: another sudden death in a child treated with desipramine. J Am Acad Child Adolesc Psychiatry 32:792–797, 1993

Riddle MA, Bernstein GA, Cook EH, et al: Anxiolytics, adrenergics, and naltrexone. J Am Acad Child Adolesc Psychiatry 38 (suppl):546–556, 1999

Rodgers RJ, Cole JC, Davies A: Antianxiety and behavioral suppressant actions of the novel 5HT1A receptor agonist, flesinoxan. Pharmacol Biochem Behav 48:959–963, 1994

Russo RM, Gururaj VJ, Allen J: The effectiveness of diphenhydramine HCl in pediatric sleep disorder. J Child Adolesc Psychopharmacol 16:284–288, 1976

Salzman C: Treatment with antianxiety agents, in Treatments of Psychiatric Disorders: A Task Force Report of the American Psychiatric Association, Vol 3. Washington, DC, American Psychiatric Association, 1989, pp 2036–2092

Salzman C: Benzodiazepine dependency: summary of the APA Task Force on Benzodiazepines. Psychopharmacol Bull 26:61–62, 1990

Sarnoff CA: Psychotherapeutic Strategies in the Latency Years. Northvale, NJ, Jason Aronson, 1987

Shaffer D, Fisher P, Dulcan MK, et al: The NIMH Diagnostic Interview Schedule for Children Version 2.3 (DISC-2.3): description, acceptability, prevalence rates, and performance in the MECA Study. Methods for the Epidemiology of Child and Adolescent Mental Disorders Study. J Am Acad Child Adolesc Psychiatry 35:865–877, 1996

Silverman WK, Nelles WB: The Anxiety Disorders Interview Schedule for Children. J Am Acad Child Adolesc Psychiatry 27:772–778, 1988

Silverman WK, La Greca AM, Wasserstein S: What do children worry about? Worries and their relation to anxiety. Child Dev 66:671–686, 1995

Simeon JG: Use of anxiolytics in children. Encephale 19:71–74, 1993

Simeon JG, Ferguson HB: Alprazolam effects in children with anxiety disorders. Can J Psychiatry 32:570–574, 1987

Simeon JG, Ferguson HB, Knott V, et al: Clinical, cognitive and neuropsychological effects of alprazolam in children and adolescents with overanxious and avoidant disorders. J Am Acad Child Adolesc Psychiatry 31:29–33, 1992

Spielberger C: Manual for State-Trait Anxiety Inventory for Children. Palo Alto, CA, Consulting Psychologists Press, 1973

Stallings P, March JS: Assessment, in Anxiety Disorders in Children. Edited by March JS. New York, Guilford, 1995, pp 125–147

Strauss CC, Last CG: Social and simple phobias in children. Anxiety Disorders 7:141–152, 1993

Strauss CC, Lease CA, Last CG, et al: Overanxious disorder: an examination of developmental differences. J Abnorm Child Psychol 16:433–443, 1988

Sugai K: Seizures with clonazepam: discontinuation and suggestions for safe discontinuation rates in children. Epilepsia 34:1089–1097, 1993

Target M, Fonagy P: Efficacy of psychoanalysis for children with emotional disorders. J Am Acad Child Adolesc Psychiatry 33:361–371, 1994

Turner SM, Beidel DC, Jacob RG: Social phobia: a comparison of behavior therapy and atenolol. J Consult Clin Psychol 62:350–358, 1994

Tyson RL: Notes on the analysis of a prelatency boy with a dog phobia. Psychoanal Study Child 33:427–460, 1978

Van Vliet IM, den Boer JA, Westenberg HG, et al: A double blind comparative study of brofaromine and fluvoxamine in outpatients with panic disorder. J Clin Psychopharmacol 16:299–306, 1996

Van Winter JT, Stickler GB: Panic attack syndrome. J Pediatr 105:661–665; 1984

Varley CK, McClellan J: Case study: two additional sudden deaths with tricyclic antidepressants. J Am Acad Child Adolesc Psychiatry 36:390–394, 1997

Walsh BT, Giardina EGV, Sloan RP, et al: Effects of desipramine on autonomic control of the heart. J Am Acad Child Adolesc Psychiatry 38:179–186, 1994

Weisman NM, Leckman JF, Merikangos KR, et al: Depression and anxiety disorders in parents and children: results from the Yale Family Study. Arch Gen Psychiatry 41:845–847, 1984

Weiss B, Weisz JR: The impact of methodological factors on child psychotherapy outcome research: a meta-analysis for researchers. J Abnorm Child Psychol 18:639-670, 1990

Weisz JR, Weiss B, Alicke MD, et al: Effectiveness of psychotherapy with children and adolescents: a meta-analysis for clinicians. J Consult Clin Psychol 55:542–549, 1987

Weller EB, Weller RA, Fristad MA, et al: Children's Interview for Psychiatric Syndromes (ChIPS). J Am Acad Child Adolesc Psychiatry 39:76–84, 2000

Welner Z, Reich W, Herjanic B, et al: Reliability, validity, and parent-child agreement studies of the Diagnostic Interview for Children and Adolescents (DICA). J Am Acad Child Adolesc Psychiatry 26:649–653, 1987

Wirt RD, Lachar D, Klinedinst JK, et al: Multidimensional Description of Child Personality: A Manual for the Personality Inventory for Children. Los Angeles, CA, Western Psychological Services, 1977

Wolpe J: Psychotherapy by Reciprocal Inhibition. Stanford, CA, Stanford University Press, 1958

Zwier KJ, Rao U: Buspirone use in adolescents with social phobia and mixed personality disorder (Cluster A type). J Am Acad Child Adolesc Psychiatry 33:1007–1011, 1994

12

Mood Disorders and Suicidal Behavior

Gabrielle A. Carlson, M.D.
Joan Rosenbaum Asarnow, Ph.D.

Treatment of any disorder is obviously predicated on thorough assessment and accurate diagnosis. We feel that this consists of three components: 1) a clinical developmental interview that allows the clinician to understand the historical, psychosocial, and contextual/temporal events that are relevant and to understand the onset of the mood disorder in relation to other disorders and problems; 2) a semistructured interview that allows the clinician to assess systematically the presence and absence of target symptoms and other relevant psychiatric disorders; and 3) rating scales that provide cross-sectional severity information and place the information in the context of norms and cutoff scores.

Although the focus of this chapter is not on diagnosis and assessment, several issues must be kept in mind in order to provide responsible and responsive treatment.

1. Although our knowledge base about mood disorders in youth has grown enormously over the past 25 years, it is still evolving. Until we have definitive validators, we are still dealing with descriptive data and best-estimate diagnostic procedures. Child and adolescent depression is essentially how we define it.
2. The DSM criteria that are used for adults "work" for children and adolescents in that they describe a population of youth whose clinical pictures look like those of adults

with the same disorder. However, as shown in Table 12–1, the clinician must be aware of several age-related differences and associated features in order to identify, as accurately as possible, children with mood disorders. There may be an age-related response to different kinds of treatment as well, but that has not been proven as yet.

3. Mood disorders in children and adolescents often co-occur with other psychiatric disorders, most notably other internalizing (anxiety) and externalizing disorders (Angold and Costello 1993). (This may be the case in many adults as well, but because structured interviews for adults do not ascertain the presence of childhood disorders, it is impossible to address the issue [Carlson 1993a].) Evidence to date suggests that the comorbid disorders usually remain despite successful treatment of the mood disorder. This is important because one is supposed to be treating people as well as disorders. Successful treatment of the child, therefore, may depend on addressing several different psychiatric disorders, not just the mood disorder.
4. In addition to the variation typically seen in the diagnostic presentation of depressed children, children vary in their competencies and level of impairment. Current evidence indicates that depressive episodes are associated with impairments in social and interpersonal functioning (e.g., Puig-Antich et al. 1985a, 1985b). Thus, the level of competence that a child has achieved prior to a depressive episode, in conjunction with the duration and severity of the episode itself, is likely to affect both therapeutic goals and treatment response. For example, social skills training in a child with premorbid social skills deficits might aim to build his or her social skill repertoire. On the other hand, social skills training in a youth with a high level of premorbid social skills competence would activate dormant skills through increased social reinforcement and activity level.

In summary, we underscore the need to consider the full child or adolescent and his or her environment, as well as diagnosis in generating optimal treatment plans.

TABLE 12–1. Frequency (%) of DSM-III/DSM-III-R "age-specific symptoms" of mood disorder in youth and adults

	Adult (n = 54)	Adolescent (n = 92)	Child (n = 95)	Preschool (n = 9)
Felt sad	93	99	95	100
Sad appearance	74	47	64	89
Crying	50	NA	NA	89
Irritability	67	83	83	78
Social withdrawal	78	73	64	89
Anxiety	30	59[a]	78[a]	67[a]
Somatic complaints	74	66	83	100
Sulkiness	NA	NA	NA	67
Conduct disorder/fighting	NA	5	38	11
Mood-congruent hallucinations	2	10	22	NA

Note. NA = not available. [a]Separation anxiety.
Source. Compiled from Carlson and Kashani 1988; D. W. Goodwin and Guze 1979; Ryan et al. 1987.

Since this chapter appeared in the previous edition of this book, a number of open trials and chart reviews of antidepressant medications have been conducted. Although several studies with tricyclic antidepressants (TCAs) have been published since the review by Ambrosini et al. (1993) (e.g., see review by Geller et al. 1999), data are consistent on the TCAs' lack of efficacy versus placebo for treatment of depression in youth. However, these studies continue to have very small sample sizes and certainly do not show complete lack of response to TCAs. Nonetheless, given their unimpressive results compared with placebo and the significant morbidity and mortality that can occur with overdose, TCAs have become second or third lines of treatment in children.

On the other hand, studies of selective serotonin reuptake inhibitors (SSRIs), whether open studies or chart reviews (e.g., Ambrosini et al. 1999; review by Emslie et al. 1999) or double-blind, placebo-controlled trials (Emslie et al. 1997a; M.B. Keller, N. Ryan, M. Strober, R. Klein, S. Kutcher, B. Birmaher, H. Kopelwicz, J. Armenteros, G. Carlson, G. Clarke, G. Emslie, D. Feinberg, B. Geller, V. Kusumaker, G. Papatheodorou, W. Sack, K. Wagner, E. Weller, R. Oakes, and J.P. McCafferty, "Efficacy of Paroxetine But Not Imipramine in the Treatment of Adolescent Major Depression: A Randomized, Controlled Trial" [submitted for publication]; Simeon et al. 1990), are more positive. The pharmaceutical industry has been mandated to include children and adolescents in trials of developing drugs and has the incentive of extending the patent life of its drugs by conducting postmarketing studies and by developing child and adolescent indications for already-approved drugs. However, although there are a plethora of controlled studies of different medications in depressed adults indicating an overall efficacy rate of about 70% (compared with a placebo response rate of about half that), double-blind, controlled treatment studies in youth remain uncommon.

Given this state of affairs, we believe that treatment of mood disorders in youth should be as systematic as possible with as much dialogue as possible between parent/child and clinician (see Table 12–2). One should be knowledgeable about the child and family, about the disorders being treated, about the environmental situation that may be exacerbating or mitigating symptoms, and, in the case of psychopharmacological intervention, about the drug—what is known in adults and the limitations of such knowledge for children. Finally, accumulating evidence documenting the high recurrence risk among depressed youth (e.g., Kovacs et al. 1984; McCauley et al. 1993) emphasizes the need to employ monitoring and intervention strategies beyond the acute phase. As we have learned from adults, treatment plans for depressed youth must include maintenance strategies and strategies aimed at preventing relapse and recurrence. Thus, treatment of depression is usually broken down into three phases: 1) the acute phase, which brings the patient into treatment and lasts until symptom remission; 2) the continuation phase, which lasts an additional 6–12 months to prevent relapse; and 3) the maintenance phase, during which the clinician needs to decide whether ongoing treatment is still necessary.

TABLE 12–2. Basic goals of psychiatrist-mediated psychoeducation

1. Educate family members and patient about the nature of the disorder(s) being treated.
2. Focus on aspects of the disorder on which family, child, or school may have an effect and for which they therefore have responsibility.
3. Discuss advantages, limitations, and risks of medication use as well as consequences of no use.
4. Help the family begin the process of accepting a youngster with a chronic disorder or problems that may have better and worse times but for which short-term "cure" is unlikely.

Decisions About Type of Treatment

Although considerably more research is available on the treatment of depression in children and adolescents than existed a few years ago, no definitive guidelines are available to help determine whether to begin with medication or psychotherapy. There are several commonsense ways to help the clinician decide which type of treatment to begin first. For instance, patients who do not appear interested in thinking psychologically about problems, are cognitively limited, are severely depressed with vegetative symptoms, have not responded to 8 weeks of psychotherapy, have had more than two prior episodes of depression, or cannot regularly get to therapy sessions should probably begin treatment with an antidepressant medication. Conversely, patients who are afraid of medication, do not like swallowing pills or liquid medicines, are pregnant or lactating, prefer talking about problems, or have complex life stressors that need sorting out may be candidates for psychotherapy first.

Psychopharmacological Interventions: How to Proceed

Information Gathering

Basic information, such as age, weight, intelligence, drug history (including problems with compliance, hypersensitivity, hyposensitivity, and allergic responses), presence of other diseases, other prescription medications, and likelihood of a placebo response or psychological dependency, should initially be gathered. The clinician also should document whether the child has received treatment for psychiatric disorder in the past, how the disorder was treated, and whether treatment has affected the course of the symptoms in question. In the case of medications, the clinician needs to know which have been used, what dose was given, and how long they were used. Ideally, one should know how specific symptom complexes have responded (e.g., insomnia, irritability, anxiety), not just whether the child "improved" or not. Finally, the clinician should obtain 1) baseline rating scales from the parents and school for all the major child psychiatric disorders and self-rating scales from the child for depression and anxiety and a side-effect rating scale; 2) baseline vital signs and weight; and 3) baseline laboratory work (complete blood count, blood studies that include liver, kidney, electrolyte, and thyroid function), so that one can minimize the number of venipunctures the child needs, and an electrocardiogram (ECG) to identify at the outset any abnormalities that would preclude specific interventions (e.g., an arrhythmia that rules out the use of a TCA).

In a medically healthy child, most guidelines do not recommend obtaining baseline laboratory tests. However, children who have abnormal chemistries (usually liver or kidney function tests) after starting medication run the risk of having the abnormalities attributed to the medication, and frequently there is great pressure to discontinue medication to the exclusion of pursuing other reasons for the abnormal findings. In addition, during the evaluation phase of treatment, child and family are more disposed to having procedures done. Therefore, it makes sense, when possible, to procure baseline blood work and an ECG so that all bases are covered for medication changes that may be needed in the future.

Psychoeducation

The medication administration procedure described in Table 12–3 provides a format to follow in undertaking a medication trial. Establishing a relationship with the patient and family is critical to the success of treatment and the decisions that go into treatment. It is especially relevant in discussing the risk-benefit ratio to be able to discuss the natural history of mood disorders in children. As noted earlier in this chapter, short-term studies indicate a substantial level of chronicity (it takes almost a year for 80%–90% of youth to recover), relapse rate is high (one-third to two-thirds will relapse over the following 3 years), dysthymia is even more tenacious, and in the case of an acute, severe depression characterized by psychosis and psychomotor retardation in adolescents, a manic/hypomanic episode may occur within 4 years in at least 20% (Kovacs et al. 1984; Strober and Carlson 1982; Strober et al. 1993).

TABLE 12–3. Medication administration procedure

1. Decide whether problems are amenable to drug treatment.
2. Establish risk-benefit ratio—consider patient and environmental variables.
3. Inform parents and patients about the importance of following the exact prescription and of keeping medications secure.
4. Obtain baselines.
5. Have separate baselines for the major symptom areas being addressed to track time and response.
6. Keep as many other variables as constant as possible.
7. Set up a priority of drugs for trial and prepare staff, patient, and family. In outpatient settings, go from least complicated to most complicated. In inpatient settings, especially if duration of hospitalization is limited, consider the more complicated drug that needs closer observation or the highest-risk treatments first.
8. Give each dose adequate time to work. Sometimes it is necessary to overshoot and then back off.

Choice of Medication

Given the relative success of SSRIs in both double-blind, placebo-controlled studies and open studies noted earlier in this chapter, guidelines for treatment of acute depression in adolescents are advocating the use of SSRIs as first-line agents (American Academy of Child and Adolescent Psychiatry 1998). In fact, a trial of two different SSRIs for at least 6 weeks is suggested before proceeding to another type of antidepressant. Although none of the published placebo-controlled studies have as yet included children younger than 12, in the absence of data, the field generalizes studies from adolescents. No data suggest better response to one or another of the medications. All appear to have a relatively flat dose-response curve. For children, young adolescents, and/or apprehensive families, treatment should begin with half the adult dose. It should continue for about 4 weeks, and if no improvement has been observed, the dose should be increased.

The most commonly used antidepressant medications are described in Table 12–4 (see articles cited in Findling et al. 1999). Data that have been available on pharmacology in youth are included in the table. SSRIs have obvious advantages. Cardiotoxic effects are minimal, and the drugs appear to be relatively safe in overdose situations. Sedation, weight

TABLE 12–4. Psychopharmacology of newer antidepressants

	Fluoxetine	Sertraline	Paroxetine	Venlafaxine	Bupropion	Nefazodone
Parent drug half-life	2–4 days	15–26 hours	3 hours–2.7 days	4 hours	14 hours	2–4 hours
Metabolite half-life	4–15 days	2.6–4.5 days	No clinically active metabolite	10 hours		
Steady state	5 weeks	7 days	10 days	3 days	8 days for sustained-release form	4–5 days
Starting dose:						
Child	5 mg	25 mg	10 mg	12.5 mg	1.5–3 mg/kg/day	50 mg bid
Teen	5 mg	50 mg	10 mg	37.5 mg		
Usual dose	20 mg	100 mg	20 mg	75–150 mg	3–5 mg/kg/day; not over 150 mg/dose	100 mg bid 300 mg bid
Dose range:						
Child	5–40 mg	50–150 mg	10–30 mg	75–150 mg	6 mg/kg/day; maximum not over 450 mg/day	?50 mg bid
Teen	10–60 mg	50–200 mg	20–40 mg	150–300 mg		
Time of administration	Morning	With food	Morning	bid or tid	bid	bid, especially at bedtime; food decreases absorption
Side effects	Activation Nausea Nervousness Insomnia Headache Serotonin syndrome Lowest rate of sexual dysfunction	Activation Nausea Headache Loose stools Insomnia Somnolence Usually transient and mild	Dizziness Headache Sedation Insomnia Dry mouth Highest rate of sexual dysfunction in adults; no data in children	Nausea Headache Somnolence Dry mouth Insomnia Sexual dysfunction	Restlessness Anxiety Agitation Insomnia Seizures at high doses Tics in Tourette's disorder	Somnolence Dry mouth Nausea Dizziness Constipation Asthenia Blurred vision

TABLE 12–4. Psychopharmacology of newer antidepressants *(continued)*

	Fluoxetine	Sertraline	Paroxetine	Venlafaxine	Bupropion	Nefazodone
Time to switch to monoamine oxidase inhibitor (weeks)	5	2	2	1	2	2
Enzyme inhibition	P450 2D6+++, 3A4+	2D6+, 3A4+	2D6+++	Weak 2D6 effects		3A4, 2D6
Available formulations	10-, 20-mg caplets; oral suspension 20 mg/5 mL	25-, 50-, 100-mg tablets	10-, 20-, 30-, 40-mg tablets; oral suspension	25-, 37.5-, 50-, 75-, 100-mg tablets 37.5-, 75-, 150-mg extended-release caplets	75-, 100-mg tablets 100-, 150-mg sustained-release caplets	50-, 100-, 150-, 200-, 250-mg tablets
Cost/day ($)	2.00	3.00	2.00	Variable	Variable	Variable
Advantage(s)	Long half-life useful for forgetful patients	Fewer drug interactions				
Disadvantage(s)	Drug remains in body a long time		Higher rate of sexual dysfunction High rate of withdrawal symptoms			

gain, and anticholinergic effects are rare. Because of their long half-life, only one daily dose is needed. Patients taking medications with shorter half-lives (e.g., paroxetine) may experience withdrawal symptoms. The advantages conferred by fluoxetine's very long half-life are also a disadvantage (e.g., one would need to wait at least 5 weeks before starting a monoamine oxidase inhibitor [MAOI] after fluoxetine). Drug interactions may occur in people at any age, so parents should be warned to tell their pharmacist that their child is taking an antidepressant whenever prescription or nonprescription drugs are purchased.

Although there has been considerable publicity about the induction of suicidal behavior with fluoxetine (R. A. King et al. 1991), careful study has not substantiated that fluoxetine incites any more suicidal behavior than might be expected given its use in a disorder in which suicidal ideation is a symptom and compared with other antidepressants (Mann and Kapur 1991).

The major disadvantage of SSRIs in youths in our opinion is the frequent occurrence of behavioral activation (e.g., Riddle et al. 1991) and, in some cases, the precipitation of a manic or hypomanic episode (Venkataraman et al. 1992 and numerous letters to editors). Virtually every antidepressant has been reported to precipitate mania in vulnerable populations. The onset of restlessness, agitation, irritability, or euphoria may occur within days to weeks of starting the drug or increasing the dose. Similarly, symptoms may abate when the dose is lowered or the drug is stopped. The difference between an activation state and a true manic episode induction may be the dose-response–time relationship (Bond 1998). If symptoms begin early in the course of dose initiation or increase and disappear quickly on lowering the dose, it is fair to say that activation or drug-induced behavioral disinhibition has taken place. However, the ultimate diagnostic significance (i.e., does the youth actually have a bipolar disorder) is unclear. The clinical implications are twofold. First, does a disinhibitory response preclude further use of that particular class of medication (i.e., if one gets an activated state with fluoxetine, does it mean that no other SSRI should be used), and second, are there implications for a future bipolar course in that individual? It is certainly true that many people become euphoric, irritable, and unmanageable with excessive alcohol ingestion, and that is not considered a "bipolar" manifestation. On the other hand, bipolar disorder often has its onset in adolescence, and the propensity to develop a manic syndrome with mood-elevating agents may have a different meaning in youth than it does in adults.

It would appear that disinhibitory states (which some choose to call secondary mania) can occur in subjects regardless of what diagnosis is being treated (e.g., Levy et al. 1998). However, evidence is not consistent about whether this implies a bipolar diathesis. In addition, even in a vulnerable population (e.g., patients with bipolar II disorder), SSRIs do not invariably produce switches to mania (Amsterdam et al. 1998). Nonsystematic 8-year follow-up by the author of several children who appeared to become manic while taking 20-mg doses of fluoxetine has found that none of the patients has yet developed autonomous bipolar disorder. This does not rule out the disorder or state that the chances are greater in such a population, but it does suggest that not every child who develops manic symptoms subsequent to ingestion of an SSRI develops bipolar disorder.

The dose-response relation in youth for depression has not been studied. However, it appears that trials must be continued for at least 8–12 weeks before concluding that medication has not worked.

The efficacy of other medications with different receptor blockades and affinities has been shown in adults, and double-blind studies are being planned in children and adolescents. Because less information is available, these medications usually are considered when first-line medications fail or when a comorbid condition is present that might respond. For instance, bupropion has been used with some success in the treatment of attention-deficit/hyperactivity disorder (ADHD) (Greenhill 1992), so some clinicians have chosen to use this medication in youth with comorbid ADHD and depression. For ADHD, a maximum dose of 6 mg/kg was recommended, achieved over a 6-week period. In adults whose depression was treated with bupropion, the response rate was comparable to that for other antidepressants. The advantages of bupropion, as with the other second-generation antidepressants, are the low side-effect profile (agitation, insomnia, headache, nausea, and vomiting are reported but at rates lower than with the TCAs), absence of weight gain, and minimum cardiotoxicity (Tollefson 1993). The disadvantages, besides the low but notable rate of seizure induction, are that until recently, the pills were available in only 75- and 100-mg tablets and, thus, it was difficult to titrate the medication in children. Extended-release forms are now available that decrease the frequency of dosing but do not solve the problem of needing a smaller dose size for some children.

Mirtazapine and nefazodone are very sedating and have been used in youths for whom insomnia is very troubling. Controlled trials of these medications are as yet lacking in young people.

The major advantage of the TCAs is their long track record in adults and, although anecdotal, in youth. Regardless of the unimpressive results of controlled studies, many clinicians have found TCAs to be helpful with their patients. The major disadvantages are the very rare but still unaccountable reports of sudden death (e.g., Riddle et al. 1993), the costly and inconvenient cardiac monitoring that is now required (see Table 12–5), the lethality of this class of drugs in an overdose situation, the withdrawal symptoms that may occur if doses are missed or if the drug is precipitously stopped, and the lack of demonstrated efficacy compared with placebo even when plasma levels have been controlled (Ambrosini et al. 1993; Geller et al. 1999).

TCAs have sometimes been used to treat comorbid ADHD and major depression in children because of their demonstrated efficacy in treating ADHD (Biederman et al. 1989) and the hope that depressive symptoms also will be helped. In a small double-blind, crossover study of hospitalized children with comorbid ADHD and depression, Carlson et al. (1995) administered a combination of desipramine and methylphenidate. Combined desipramine and methylphenidate (20 mg) was most effective compared with placebo at improving self-control and reducing inattention, hyperactivity, and aggressive behavior. Nonetheless, overall clinical improvement was modest. No drug regimen was successful in reducing mood problems. There was no differential efficacy of desipramine for children with major depressive disorder. There was no evidence that stimulant medication potentiated desipramine response.

The amount of cardiovascular supervision necessary to prevent accidental death is simply unknown. Ryan (1992) published parameters even more conservative than those noted in Table 12–5—that is, baseline ECG plus rhythm strip after *every* dosage increase (not just when dose exceeds 3 mg/kg). Also recommended is reduction or discontinuation of the TCA 1) if PR interval is greater than 0.18 seconds in children younger than 10 or greater than 0.20 seconds in children age 10 years or older, 2) if QRS interval is greater than 0.12 seconds or widens more than 50% over baseline, 3) if resting heart rate is greater than 110 beats/minute in children younger than 10 or greater than 100 beats/minute in children age 10 years or older).

TABLE 12–5. Cardiac monitoring in children taking tricyclic antidepressants

Cardiovascular parameters in children	
PR interval	≤210 ms
QRS interval	Change ≤30% baseline
QTc interval	≤450 ms
Heart rate	≤130 beats/min
Systolic blood pressure	≤130 mm Hg
Diastolic blood pressure	≤85 mm Hg
Electrocardiogram parameters in children	
PR interval	From onset of atrial activation to ventricular activation (i.e., atrioventricular conduction time) Normal range is 100–200 ms; greater values indicate atrioventricular conduction problem
QRS interval	Duration of ventricular activity Normally does not exceed 100 ms; greater values indicate intraventricular conduction problem
QT interval	Entire cycle of electrical polarization and depolarization Varies with age, sex, and heart rate When adjusted for heart rate, it is reported as QTc Normal rate is 340–425 ms

The most commonly reported TCA side effects are either sedative (drowsiness, lethargy, feeling drugged) or anticholinergic (dry mouth, nausea, constipation, blurred vision, dizziness). Withdrawal effects may be mitigated by gradually reducing the dose of medication over several weeks, the decrements used depending on the dose from which withdrawal is started (i.e., 25-mg decrements can be used if the dose is greater than 100 mg/day). The time taken depends on whether one notes problems with a dose reduction occurring every 2 days.

If, after pondering these considerations, one still has the nerve to use medications that are widely prescribed despite the above concerns, we suggest the following scheme:

1. Obtain a baseline ECG.
2. Obtain baseline pulse and blood pressure measurements (blood pressure should be measured at several different times if possible). Teach parent(s) how to take the child's pulse and have the parent obtain pulse rate *on several occasions* at rest and after exercise. This is necessary because children's heart rate and blood pressure fluctuate, and one may have an occasional resting blood pressure of 140/85 mm Hg off medication. If parameters fall within accepted guidelines,
3. Begin dosing at 1–2 mg/kg at bedtime.
4. After 2 weeks, if no untoward effects occur, depending on the age and size of the child, increase the dosage by either 10 or 25 mg every 4–5 days to 5 mg/kg. Obtain a repeat rhythm strip at doses greater than 3 mg/kg. Doses should be divided be-

tween dinner time and bedtime initially, then at breakfast time, dinner time, and bedtime, with a minimum of 2 hours between doses. Have parent check pulse at rest and after exercise several times after each dosage increment; parents should call the physician if the pulse begins to rise to greater than 110 beats/minute at rest. If this problem persists,

5. Obtain a rhythm strip and blood level. If the rhythm strip is normal and the blood level is low, one can proceed to increase medication cautiously, continuing to monitor pulse and blood pressure closely. If plasma level is within or at the upper limits of acceptable range, there is not much to be gained with increasing the dose. One should maintain that dose for several weeks until response occurs, cardiovascular parameters worsen, or the decision is made to discontinue the drug because of lack of response.

It makes sense to obtain plasma levels 1) if a child is experiencing side effects but has not had a response (if levels are at the upper limits of normal, it suggests that not much more will be gained by pushing the dose), 2) if the child is taking more than 3 mg/kg and is experiencing neither side effects nor response (to ensure he or she is taking the drug and to gauge whether a considerably higher dose will be needed), and 3) when the child has had a response to provide guidance if a relapse occurs (i.e., how much higher can the dose be pushed) or another occasion in which medication may need to be resumed because relapse has occurred on discontinuation.

Trazodone is less well studied in youth but is relative safe in an overdose situation. It has no serious anticholinergic effects, and its significant sedating property can be an advantage if used at bedtime and a disadvantage if sedation is unwanted. It must be taken with meals because of problems with nausea and headaches if the drug is taken on an empty stomach. To mitigate noncompliance due to oversedation, dosage increments may need to be undertaken more slowly than is done with TCAs. Priapism has been rarely reported in adult men. Male patients should be warned of this possibility and told to seek emergency treatment immediately if this should occur (Tollefson 1993).

MAOIs have been used in adolescent depression (see review by Emslie et al. 1999). They also might offer potential advantages in adolescents with atypical depression (depression characterized by hypersomnia, overeating, rejection sensitivity, reactive mood, and leaden paralysis), which seems to respond better to MAOIs than to TCAs in adults (Stewart et al. 1993). The disadvantages are better known and include the dietary restrictions, interaction with other drugs, hypotension, and weight gain. The dietary proscription may be somewhat moot in adolescents, because many of the foods most rich in tyramine are not high on the list of favorite teenage foods (e.g., aged cheeses, brewer's yeast, liver, smoked fish, fava beans). More relevant are the possible effects of mozzarella cheese and pepperoni (found in pizza), beer, and red wine (which all too often are consumed by adolescents) and stimulant drugs (e.g., decongestants taken for upper respiratory infections, street drugs). Patients should be advised to report to a local emergency room to rule out a hypertensive crisis if they develop a violent headache while taking an MAOI.

Because of their long bioavailability (up to 14 days) and the length of time needed to regenerate the enzyme monoamine oxidase, a 10- to 14-day hiatus is needed between cessation of one MAOI and initiation of another, initiation of another antidepressant, or discontinuation of the tyramine-free diet. The length of time needed to switch from another antidepressant to an MAOI varies and is noted in Table 12–4.

Treatment of Bipolar Depression

A major problem in treating a bipolar depression in youth is distinguishing it from a non-bipolar depression because early in the course of a chronic disorder, it is not always clear whether one is, in fact, treating a unipolar or a bipolar disorder. Some evidence indicates that some depressions occurring in childhood may be an early manifestation of bipolar disorder (Geller et al. 1993). The veracity of this supposition depends, in part, on how narrowly or broadly one defines bipolar disorder and whether one is dealing with a primary or an uncomplicated bipolar disorder or one that has been preceded by another disorder (usually a disruptive behavior disorder) (Carlson 1990). In a previously well-functioning adolescent with an acute, psychotic, psychomotor retarded depression, the likelihood of a subsequent manic episode is as high as 20%–30% (Strober and Carlson 1982). Needless to say, however, a careful history that reveals the existence of a prior hypomanic or manic episode is much more helpful.

If it is determined that a hypomanic or manic episode has occurred before the depression for which treatment is sought, or if a strong family history of bipolar disorder is present, the clinician has several options:

1. Warn the patient and family about the risk of precipitating another manic episode, but use conventional antidepressant medication. SSRIs, (Amsterdam et al. 1998), bupropion (Goodnick et al. 1998), and venlafaxine (Amsterdam 1998) all have been used with success in bipolar II depression.
2. "Cover" the patient with a mood stabilizer before starting another antidepressant and, hopefully, control or avoid the onset of a manic episode.
3. Use a mood-stabilizing drug as an antidepressant and add another antidepressant only if the symptoms do not improve with the mood stabilizer alone.

There are accumulating data in adults that the anticonvulsant lamotrigine is somewhat effective in bipolar I depression (Calabrese et al. 1999) (response rates of 41% and 51% with 50 mg/day and 200 mg/day, respectively), but the higher incidence of serious rashes in young people has excluded this age group from studies in the United States.

Treatment of Bipolar Disorder

General Considerations

Guidelines published elsewhere for the use of mood-stabilizing drugs (American Academy of Child and Adolescent Psychiatry 1997) include both clear and experimental indications. Clear indications comprehend definitive history of both major depression and mania or hypomania. Less clear indications include acute, psychotic depression with a family history of bipolar disorder or an acute psychotic disorder with affective features. Finally, in hopes of disclosing previously undetected cases of bipolar disorder, clinicians are increasingly using mood stabilizers in children to treat disruptive behavior disorders, positive family histories of mood disorder (among other psychiatric disorders), and emotional lability defined as cyclothymia or bipolar II disorder. Our experience in this latter population with lithium under double-blind, controlled conditions (Carlson et al. 1992) has not been encouraging. However, studies in adults with similar clinical pictures (Black et al. 1988) have not found a great response to mood-stabilizing drugs either. The current DSM-IV (American Psychiatric Association 1994) definition of a manic episode, especially a mixed manic syndrome, likely subsumes heterogeneous agitated states that are not responsive to mood stabilizers alone (see Table 12–6). It is also clear that patients with a particularly severe form of bipolar disorder are not successfully treated by current therapies alone and often need multiple medications to achieve some stability (Post et al. 1998).

TABLE 12–6. Adolescents with bipolar disorder

	Kafantaris et al. 1998 (*n* = 48)	Strober et al. 1998 (*n* = 60)	Kutcher et al. 1998 (*n* = 28)	Carlson et al. 1999 (*n* = 23)
Source of sample	Teens specifically recruited for drug study of lithium	Clinical "historical" sample, case controlled; drug study of lithium	Clinical sample specifically defined to be bipolar	Community sample hospitalized with first psychosis; naturalistic follow-up
Mean age at diagnosis	16	Mid-teens	16.7 (mania)	18.3 (mania), 17.7 (depression)
% Male	43.7	66.7	50.0	69.6
% Externalizing	29.2	30.0	22.0	60.9
% Substance use disorders	Excluded from study	0	Not stated	65.2 at onset
% Mixed episodes	77% with HAM-D ≥18	0	74	26 (SCID criteria)
% Psychosis	48 (73 in teen onset; 36 in ADHD onset)	32	57	100 (by definition)
% No child comorbidity	31	70	61	13
Treatment history	53.5%, ADHD made no difference; 26.1% psychotic; antipsychotics also needed in these	80.6%, non-ADHD, lithium responsive; 57.7%, comorbid ADHD, lithium responsive; 33% adjunctive antipsychotics	46%, lithium; stable; 33% taking antipsychotics, 57% divalproex, 14% carbamazepine	At 4-year follow-up, 45.5% were not taking medications, 70% recurrence; 54.5% taking medications, 67% recurrence

Note. HAM-D = Hamilton Rating Scale for Depression; SCID = Structured Clinical Interview for DSM-IV; ADHD = attention-deficit/hyperactivity disorder.

Although lithium has been used in children (for a review, see Alessi et al. 1994), no double-blind, placebo-controlled studies of bipolar I disorder have been completed (although several are in progress), and data gathered to date are somewhat conflicting (for reviews, see Carlson 1998 and Ryan et al. 1999). For instance, Strober et al. (1998) reported a high rate of response of hospitalized manic adolescents to lithium, although the response of bipolar adolescents with comorbid externalizing disorders was less robust (see Table 12–6). On the other hand, Kafantaris et al. (1998) reported about a 50% response rate to lithium, and most of those adolescents needed adjunctive haloperidol. The presence of comorbid ADHD did not affect drug response. Open trials of valproate in hospitalized adolescents (Deltito et al. 1998; Papatheodorou et al. 1995) and anecdotal reports of other medications have been successful. Finally, a recently published randomized open trial of divalproex, lithium, and carbamazepine in 41 child and adolescent (ages 6–17 years) patients with bipolar I and II disorder demonstrated a 40%–50% response rate, as assessed by a drop in the Young Mania Rating Scale (Young et al. 1978) score (Kowatch et al. 2000).

The prevailing assumption of child and adolescent psychiatrists has been to keep track of drug studies in adult bipolar subjects and extrapolate those results to their younger patients (for a review, see Ryan et al. 1999). Depending on how loosely one defines bipolar disorder in adults, that extrapolation is fair. That is, early age at onset of mania is associated with increased comorbidity. In fact, youths designated as having prepubertal-onset bipolar disorder apparently never have classical histories of premorbid good function followed by episodes of mania, depression, and a return to euthymia (for a review, see Carlson 1998). It may be appropriate, then, to equate very early onset bipolar disorder in which comorbid ADHD and conduct disorder are the rule to bipolar spectrum disorders (including mixed mania, bipolar II disorder, and bipolar disorder not otherwise specified) in adults, who also have considerable comorbidity, usually with substance abuse and treatment resistance (Strakowski et al. 1992). Under those circumstances, low response to lithium is not surprising because predictors of poor lithium response include variables such as dysphoric or mixed mania, comorbidity with anxiety or obsessive-compulsive traits, rapid cycling, slow onset, family history of disorders other than uncomplicated manic depression, and many psychosocial stressors (Abou-Saleh 1993; Solomon et al. 1995). Data from adult studies appear to indicate that valproate may be more effective in these cases (Bowden et al. 1994; Greil et al. 1998).

Maintenance treatment with lithium shows a decided advantage over placebo in adults (F. K. Goodwin and Jamison 1990). Similarly, adolescents who discontinue maintenance treatment have a high (92%) rate of relapse compared with those who maintain lithium treatment (37%) (Strober et al. 1990). Patients with mixed episodes, rapid cycling, inter-episode personality disorder, and/or substance abuse have poor prophylactic response to lithium, and some respond better to anticonvulsants (Keck et al. 1998).

A particularly vexing question in young people is how long to continue maintenance medication. With adults who have experienced several episodes, one can use the life experience to help decide the relative merits of long-term continuation. For young people taking mood stabilizers after only one or at most two episodes, and for whom the specter of taking a drug for "the rest of one's life" is particularly awesome, the issue is even more complex. Data from adult studies regarding recurrence of major depression in both non bipolar and bipolar patients suggest that continuation for up to 2 years is preferable to shorter maintenance periods. Our strategy has been to encourage the young person to continue medication until completion of high school in a younger adolescent, or college or trade school in an older adolescent, or past a major life stressor that is anticipated (e.g., starting a new job, getting married). Discontinuation, if it is insisted on, should come at a time when the least effect on life is likely and when as much observation and social support as possible is available to abort an episode, with prompt referral if one starts to occur. Discontinuation should be undertaken very gradually because evidence indicates an increased likelihood of mania on rapid discontinuation of lithium (Suppes et al. 1991).

Young people seem to present with particularly psychotic-appearing episodes of depression and mania such that the diagnosis is initially unclear (Carlson 1993b). Traditionally, such patients were given antipsychotics. Increasingly, they are given mood stabilizers and atypical antipsychotics or benzodiazepines in an attempt to avoid older antipsychotics. After several weeks of stabilization, if the clinical picture indicates that the episode (both the mood component and the psychosis) has remitted, it is worth trying to gradually withdraw the antipsychotic under controlled conditions. This may not be successful, however (Kafantaris et al. 1998). Patients otherwise are likely to withdraw themselves under less optimal conditions. Persistence of compelling psychotic symptoms long after mood symptoms have abated suggests a more schizoaffective course and the need for chronic antipsychotics.

Breakthrough of either manic or depressive symptoms in a person stabilized on lithium is a reason to add another mood-stabilizing medication such as valproate.

Specific Treatment Strategies

Lithium

The pharmacokinetics of lithium in children and adolescents are similar to those in adults, with the exception of a higher glomerular filtration rate that sometimes necessitates a higher dose of lithium to achieve the same serum level of drug. Otherwise, the dose-response and time-action data can be extrapolated from those in adults. Specific issues for children include side effects, drug interactions, and long-term effects. Major side effects are outlined in Table 12–7. In our experience, polydipsia and polyurea (with resumption of bed-wetting) may be more troubling in children. The most noteworthy drug interaction for otherwise healthy adolescents occurs with nonsteroidal anti-inflammatory agents (except for aspirin). These drugs may increase serum lithium levels by reducing renal clearance (Jefferson 1993). Little information is available on long-term renal or bone effects in children, although nothing suggests long-term harm. There have been a few studies of cognitive effects of lithium in children (Carlson et al. 1992), and these suggest that lithium is neither helpful nor harmful.

Lithium has the advantage of being the best studied of the mood-stabilizing drugs (Ryan et al. 1999). Although only approved for patients older than 12, it has been used in young children, even though they may be prone to more side effects (Hagino et al. 1995). Lithium levels are a problem in youths with needle phobias. In those cases, saliva lithium levels may be worth investigating. Because of the potential difficulties with electrolyte imbalance, parents and youths must be informed about the need for adequate hydration and prompt medical and psychiatric attention in the case of vomiting and diarrhea (which will change hydration and lithium levels). Dose may be determined by trial and error (starting with 300–600 mg), by weight (Weller et al. 1986), or most promptly and accurately by use of a loading dose (Fetner and Geller 1992). Lithium levels should be drawn 10–12 hours after the last dose, which can be either early in the morning (before school) or late in the afternoon (after school) and repeated weekly until stable. After that, levels may be repeated every few months and when there is any suggestion of symptom recurrence. Laboratory data should be repeated at least yearly. Lithium has been combined with methylphenidate in children with comorbid ADHD and manic symptoms with some suggestion of synergistic effect (Carlson et al. 1992).

TABLE 12–7. Mood stabilizers and aggression

	Dose range	Side effects	Comments
Lithium	30 mg/kg/day; not >1.2 mEq/day	In teens/older children: enuresis, fatigue, nausea, vomiting, tremor, acne; increased "confused/ bewildered" and "tension/ anxiety" symptoms In children ages 4–6: 50% had tremor, drowsiness, ataxia, or confusion; 25% had gastrointestinal problems; 10% had enuresis, polydipsia; 10% had blurred vision; 20% had serious side effects	Measure level often until stable Be especially cautious during medical illness In two double-blind, controlled trials of inpatient children ages 6–12, 68% showed marked to moderate improvement; positive effect on bullying, temper outbursts over 6 weeks
Carbamazepine	400–800 mg Serum levels 5–9 μg/mL Enzyme induction requires reestablishing blood levels after several weeks	Transient but marked leukopenia, rash, dizziness, diplopia, headache	Open study (10 patients): 80% improved; controlled study (11 carbamazepine patients) showed 85% moderate or marked improvement but no difference from placebo (65% with improvement)
Divalproex/ valproic acid	"Therapeutic levels" (>50 μg/mL) 5 days to reach steady state Levels 8–12 hours after administration	Stomach upset, nausea/ vomiting, weight gain, drowsiness, skin rash, muscle weakness, hair loss	Open trial only 10 adolescents with "explosive aggression" much improved Anecdotal: worth a try with emotional storms
Lamotrigine	25 mg bid × 1 week 25 mg A.M., 50 mg at bedtime × 1 week 50 mg bid (up to 6 mg/kg/day)—60% respond in 10–21 days (0.1–0.2 mg/kg/ day start if taking valproic acid) ?5–15 mg/L blood levels	Rashes, Stevens-Johnson syndrome with rapid early increase in dosing, tremors, poor coordination, blurred vision	Experimental in mood disorders Some experience as anticonvulsant in children Currently not approved for youth younger than 16; rash in 1/50 to 1/100 children vs. 1/1000 adults Multicenter trial ongoing; greater efficacy in bipolar depression?
Gabapentin	900–2,400 mg/day Blood levels 3.5–15 mL/L, although >10 not usually therapeutic	Sedation, irritability	7-hour half-life tid administration ? Use in rapid cycling Multicenter trial ongoing

Valproate/Divalproex Sodium

Valproate has been used extensively in adults, both alone and with lithium (for a review, see Bowden 1998 and Keck et al. 1998). It appears to be useful in mixed mania and is an easier drug to use than carbamazepine because enzyme induction does not occur. No controlled studies have been completed in adolescents, but open studies suggest that adolescents' response is similar to that in adults. Valproate has relatively few side effects (gastrointestinal effects are less troublesome with divalproex sodium than with valproic acid), and those that occur include nausea, thinning hair, and sedation. Hepatotoxicity seems to occur in children younger than 2 years who are taking other anticonvulsants or other medication. Therefore, liver function must be monitored. Given its short half-life, at least two daily doses are needed. The contribution of blood levels is unclear (see Table 12–7), although levels between 50 and 120 μg/mL are generally recommended. Finally, the U.S. Food and Drug Administration has recently mandated that a "black box warning" of an increased risk for pancreatitis be added to the labeling of divalproex sodium and valproate to alert clinicians that symptoms of abdominal pain, nausea, and vomiting that could be associated with pancreatitis should receive prompt medical attention.

Recent concern has surfaced with regard to the development of polycystic ovary disease (characterized by truncal obesity, hyperandrogenism, hyperinsulinemia, and lipid abnormalities). Although this has been observed only in patients taking divalproex as an anticonvulsant (Isojarvi et al. 1993, 1998), the fact that subjects were young women who had taken the medication for several years has raised concern about the long-term implications of this drug for pubertal bipolar women. As of this writing, given the severity of early-onset bipolar disorder, in young women being prescribed medications for which weight gain is a problem, it is prudent to obtain a baseline weight, baseline waist and hip measurements, and a good menstrual history and to inquire about symptoms of hirsutism. If changes in those findings occur after several months of treatment, gynecological consultation and possible discontinuation of medication is warranted.

Carbamazepine

Carbamazepine is used primarily as a treatment for generalized, simple, and complex partial seizures in both children and adults but also has mood-stabilizing properties. This aspect, however, has not been examined in youth other than in case reports. Data from research on adults suggest that its primary advantage is in rapid cycling or mixed bipolar disorders or in situations such as chronic renal disease in which lithium may present problems. Carbamazepine may enhance lithium as well as have its own independent value. It is more complicated to use than lithium or valproate because it induces its own metabolic enzymes. This means that the initial half-life (between 20 and 30 hours) and dose are likely to change after several weeks (see Table 12–7). Carbamazepine also interacts with many other drugs, potentiating them and altering their efficacy (because of changed metabolism) and being altered by them such that neurotoxicity can be potentiated. The *Physicians' Desk Reference* should be consulted any time a drug is used for any reason in a person taking carbamazepine. Finally, the significance of blood levels in treatment of mood disorders is not as clear for carbamazepine as it is for lithium. At minimum, blood levels are monitored to prevent toxicity and check compliance. Dosing is approached by gradually increasing the dose until response, side effects, or unacceptable blood levels are achieved.

For both carbamazepine and valproate, when white blood cell counts and platelets may decrease, close follow-up of those variables is warranted for any decline to below 25% of baseline.

Medication should be discontinued if the absolute neutrophil count decreases to less than 1,000 or the platelet count decreases to less than 100,000.

Other Medications

Anecdotal experience is accumulating on the use of other medications—most notably, the benzodiazepines, atypical antipsychotics, calcium channel blockers, and, of course, other anticonvulsants. Combinations of medications, especially different anticonvulsants or anticonvulsants and benzodiazepines or atypical antipsychotics, appear most frequently in the literature.

Algorithms for adult bipolar disorder advocate beginning with lithium in uncomplicated bipolar disorder and with divalproex in mixed or rapid-cycling bipolar disorder. In the event of a partial response, these medications may be combined. Beyond that advice, alternatives appear to include adding other anticonvulsants, adding an atypical antipsychotic, or, in the case of a severely manic patient, adding a benzodiazepine (see Suppes et al. 1998 for a review)

Electroconvulsive Therapy

As noted in the American Psychiatric Association's "Practice Guidelines for Major Depressive Disorder in Adults" (American Psychiatric Association 1993, p. 16),

> Electroconvulsive therapy (ECT) has a high rate of therapeutic success, relative speed in inducing improvement in depressive symptoms, and an excellent safety profile. Nevertheless, except in special circumstances, ECT is not generally regarded as a first-line treatment for uncomplicated major depression. This is in part a result of an undeserved reputation among the lay public that the treatment is "dangerous" and induces "brain damage."

It is not surprising that this attitude has limited the use of ECT in youth. However, the recent literature has been replete with increased numbers of positive anecdotal reports and literature reviews (e.g., Rey and Walter 1997; Schneekloth et al. 1993; Walter et al. 1999) on the effectiveness of ECT in depressed and bipolar youth. Rey and Walter (1997) found 154 case reports in the literature in which enough information had been presented to allow diagnosis and outcome to be ascertained. They reported that 19 of 26 (73%) teens with major depression, 6 of 14 (43%) with psychotic depression, 16 of 20 (80%) with a manic episode, and 37 of 51 (73%) with bipolar disorder experienced remission or marked improvement. In a separate study of patient attitudes, 88% of those assessed believed ECT was a legitimate treatment, 62% said that it was humane, 23% said that it was cruel, and 19% said that it was outdated. Compared with psychopharmacology, rates of side effects were similar (rates of confusion from ECT vs. medication: 46% vs. 42%), except that memory impairment was much greater in patients with ECT (62% vs. 35%). It would appear that both indications and response to treatment *are* similar in adolescents and adults. Other than the observation that seizure threshold in adolescents is often quite low (M. Fink, personal communication, August 1999), number of treatments and aftercare are *also* similar in youth and adults. Fink (1999) recommended that use of ECT in adolescents parallel the use of clozapine in schizophrenia (i.e., the use of a somewhat complicated alternative after failure of two adequate medication trials with different classes of medication).

Psychosocial Interventions

Since this chapter appeared in the previous edition of this book, major advances have been made in our knowledge of psychosocial treatments for depression in youth. Several major clinical trials have documented the efficacy of psychosocial treatment strategies, and solid data exist to guide the evaluation and development of treatment plans for depressed youth. Psychosocial interventions may be used before medication, in addition to medication, or instead of medication. Clinicians today have a diverse range of psychosocial interventions with some demonstrated efficacy that they can use in relieving depressive symptoms and promoting adaptive growth.

Issues that remain to be resolved include 1) the advantages and disadvantages of beginning treatment with a trial of psychosocial therapy as opposed to medication, 2) how to identify those youth who are most likely to be responsive to psychosocial as opposed to pharmacological treatment, and 3) the advantages of combined pharmacological and psychosocial treatment. In addition, most extant data focus on acute treatment, and limited data are available on treatment strategies following the acute phase. The need for greater attention to strategies for continuation treatment is underscored by observations that relapse rates following acute treatment have been reported to be in the range of 30%–40% (Birmaher et al. 2000; Emslie et al. 1997b).

Although these issues require additional research, indications for a trial of psychosocial therapy appear to be as follows: 1) youth and/or family who prefer psychosocial treatment, 2) youth who cannot swallow pills, 3) contraindications to medication (such as pregnancy or breast-feeding), 4) complex life stressors, and 5) a failure to respond to medication (Asarnow et al. 1999). Results of randomized clinical trials suggest generally comparable effects for medications and psychotherapies with demonstrated efficacy. Consequently, when no clear preferences or contraindications guide therapy choice, clinicians should explain the treatment options and assist youth and families in making a decision about treatment. The advantages of adding or switching to pharmacological treatment should be considered when individuals have no response or only a partial response to psychosocial treatment. Results from the National Institute of Mental Health (NIMH) Multisite Treatment of Adolescent Depression Study (J. March, personal communication, April 1999)—which will directly compare medication, cognitive-behavioral therapy (CBT), combined medication plus CBT, and placebo—will provide critical information to guide such treatment decisions in the future.

Psychosocial interventions provide a means of addressing several characteristics and sequelae of depressive episodes. First, acute and chronic depression can affect how a person thinks, relates, and views the world. Psychosocial interventions, such as CBT, that target these "depressotypic" cognitive and behavioral patterns are likely to yield improved outcome. Second, considerable evidence indicates that some level of disability may remain even when the depression remits (e.g., Klein et al. 1997; Rohde et al. 1994). These data have been interpreted as supporting the hypothesis that depressive episodes are associated with "psychosocial scars," or difficulties that are present after but not before the episode. Such difficulties or "scars" identified in adolescents following episodes of major depression include internalizing behavior problems, stressful life events, excessive emotional reliance on others, cigarette smoking, and subsyndromal depressive symptoms (Rohde et al. 1994). Psychosocial interventions may be necessary to help youths to recover from this "psychosocial scarring." Third, as noted previously, depression in youths is associated with a high level of comorbidity. Psychosocial treatment strategies can be developed for each youth that specifically address comorbid disorders and psychosocial stressors.

Information Gathering

As in the guidelines offered with respect to psychopharmacological interventions, the clinician needs to clarify the child's treatment history, the kinds of psychosocial interventions that have been attempted in the past and their efficacy, the barriers that arose with respect to the delivery of treatment (e.g., missed appointments, noncompliance), and treatment efficacy. For example, a child may have been responding to treatment, showing a remission of target symptoms and improved psychosocial adjustment, until his or her parents announced that they were going to divorce. This example underscores the crucial importance of evaluating and anticipating stressors in the child's environment that may moderate the effects of any intervention. Thus, in addition to the baseline information on major childhood disorders and symptoms suggested earlier in this chapter, it is important to collect more detailed information about 1) the family environment (who lives in the home, what types of stresses and supports exist within the family); 2) the child's school history, adjustment, and academic achievement; 3) the child's peer relationships, adjustment, and influences; 4) the kinds of social and community supports available to the child; 5) the child's strengths and competencies, and 6) the child's health and physical functioning.

Before selecting an intervention strategy, it is also useful to examine how the child and key family members view his or her difficulties and what their expectations and beliefs are regarding various treatment alternatives. A common clinical dilemma, for example, involves the depressed teenager who contends that the problem is with his or her parents and believes that their behavior is causing the depression. This information would argue for some family-based intervention rather than one that simply focuses primarily on the teenager. As with psychopharmacological treatment, taking a family history of response to psychosocial treatment strategies is also helpful because family members are likely to have more confidence and hope for treatments that they have found to be successful. For instance, if a depressed mother has had a positive response to cognitive therapy, she is more likely to have confidence in a cognitive treatment approach with her child and provide a more optimal treatment environment.

Systems-level interventions need to be considered in some cases when psychotherapy and/or medication are insufficient to promote recovery. Wraparound services, residential treatment, and partial or full hospitalization are needed for some youth and should be considered when safety or severity of dysfunction dictates the need for more intensive services. Clinicians also should consider the need for ancillary educational services (e.g., tutoring, special education) as well as recreational (e.g., sports activities, clubs, scouts) and/or social service (e.g., housing, food, job training) interventions that are likely to be helpful to the youth and family.

Choice of Psychosocial Intervention

Various psychosocial treatment strategies (Table 12–8) are available for treating depression in youth. Because of the breadth of this literature, it is beyond the scope of this chapter to review all of the approaches described in the literature. Consequently, we emphasize those approaches that are supported by clinical trials among youth with depressive disorders and highlight those areas where additional research is needed to inform treatment decisions.

Interested readers are referred to other sources for more extensive discussion of treatment approaches that are supported primarily by clinical reports (e.g., Bemporad 1988; Kestenbaum and Kron 1987) and for more detailed reviews of the research on psychosocial treatments and interventions with youth with depressive symptoms but not necessarily depressive disorders (Asarnow et al., in press).

TABLE 12–8. Overview of systematic psychosocial interventions

Individual interventions
Interpersonal psychotherapy
Cognitive/cognitive-behavioral therapy
Group interventions
Coping with depression course
Social skills and problem solving
Self-control interventions
Family interventions
Cognitive-psychoeducational approaches
Cognitive-behavioral family therapy
Parent training

At the start, it is important to consider several caveats:

- The field is advancing rapidly, and other treatment strategies will be shown to be effective with time.
- The most marked improvements generally have been found on measures of depression. Improvements in functioning outcomes have been more difficult to show and may require more extended treatment or alternative approaches.
- Most extant data emphasize adolescents. This is not surprising given the increased rate of depressive disorders in adolescence. However, additional work is needed to clarify optimal treatment strategies for younger children with depressive disorders.
- The psychosocial treatments tested to date with clinically depressed youths have shown efficacy relative to control conditions and/or comparison interventions. However, within clinically depressed samples, about 40% of the sample failed to show significant recovery or remission as defined in each study. This rate is consistent with the recovery rate observed in pharmacological trials (Ambrosini et al. 1993; Emslie et al. 1997a). Thus, although the tested treatments have shown promise, a substantial proportion of youths fail to respond, underscoring the need for tests of combination treatments and/or algorithms for guiding treatment decisions over time.
- Despite the rapid advances in knowledge regarding the treatment of depression during the acute phase and the relatively high risk of relapse found in child and adolescent depression, the data on continuation treatment are very limited.

The conceptual frameworks on which theorists base ultimate interventions may superficially seem quite different depending on whether one has a psychodynamic, behavioral, social learning, or family interactional approach. However, some common threads run through these theories explaining the origins of depression. Each seems to target (to a greater or lesser extent) 1) psychosocial stresses (e.g., family problems, losses, or other psychiatric or medical disorders); 2) a chasm between the way a person thinks things should be and the way he or she thinks they are; 3) attention to negative events that only confirm how bad the situation is; 4) the overly high ideals or the person's pitting himself or herself against impossible goals that can reinforce his or her sense of helplessness; 5) the pessimistic, angry, sullen, and/or anergic interpersonal style (symptoms of depression) that diminishes the likelihood of positive relationships and positive reinforcement and increases the likelihood of object loss, 6) inadequate social supports (sometimes due to the presence of psychiatrically disturbed family members) that limit the sources of positive attachment, attention, and comfort; and 7) behaviors that contribute to cycles of increasing stress, social isolation, and dysphoric reactions. The sections below review general approaches to treatment during the acute phase, continuation treatment strategies, and preventive interventions.

Acute-Phase Treatment

Cognitive-Behavioral Therapy

Accumulating data support the efficacy of both individual and group CBT for the treatment of depression in adolescents and, to a lesser extent, in children. Six groups have completed treatment studies with youth meeting diagnostic criteria for depressive disorders. First, Lewinsohn et al. (1990) and Clarke et al. (1999) reported a significant advantage for group CBT for the treatment of major depression or dysthymic disorder in adolescents, as compared with a wait-list control condition, in two independent studies. Results across the two studies showed a recovery rate of about 60.8% at the end of CBT.

Second, Brent and colleagues (1997) examined the relative efficacy of 12–16 sessions of individual CBT, systemic behavioral family therapy, and individual nondirective supportive therapy. Results indicated a higher rate of remission (60%) among adolescents who received CBT compared with those who received either family therapy (29%) or supportive therapy (36.4%).

Third, Wood et al. (1996) compared six to eight sessions of individual CBT for depression with relaxation training among youth meeting DSM-III-R (American Psychiatric Association 1987) criteria for major depression or Research Diagnostic Criteria for minor depression. Results after treatment indicated significantly higher remission rates for youth in the CBT condition (54%) as compared with those in the relaxation condition (21%).

Fourth, Vostanis et al. (1996) found substantial recovery (87%) following brief two- to nine-session CBT (mean = six sessions, similar to the Wood et al. CBT) among 8- to 17-year-olds with major depression, dysthymic disorder, or minor depression. Gains were generally maintained at the 9-month follow-up. High recovery rates also were observed among youths in a comparison nonfocused intervention condition (75% recovery rate), suggesting that the nonfocused intervention had either only a somewhat weaker psychotherapy effect or a high placebo response rate. It is important to note, however, that this study included many youths with mild depression severity (54.4% with minor depression) who may have responded to nonspecific therapy factors.

Fifth, Rosello and Bernal (1999) found that both CBT and interpersonal psychotherapy (IPT) led to significant reductions in depressive symptoms as compared with a wait-list control condition in a sample of Puerto Rican adolescents meeting criteria for major depression and/or dysthymic disorder.

CBT for depression aims to relieve depressive symptoms and prevent future depressive episodes by changing cognitive, attributional, and behavioral patterns that contribute to depressive tendencies. The groups described in this section developed and tested manuals for cognitive-behavioral treatments for depression in youth, and these approaches vary somewhat. However, common themes are found across the various approaches. Major themes or components of cognitive-behavioral treatments for depression in youth are reviewed below and examples provided to illustrate the approach.

Therapeutic Relationship

The therapeutic relationship is based on "collaborative empiricism," in which therapist and youth work as a team to understand the youth's thoughts, the basis for his or her thinking, and the practical positive and negative consequences of this thinking style. The youth's contribution to the relationship is to bring in raw data on his or her thoughts and feelings, whereas the therapist's role is to guide the youth about what data to collect and how to assess the data. Relatively structured techniques are used, such as mood monitoring. In this activity, the youth rates his or her mood on a daily basis. These ratings are then used as data to help the youth and therapist identify factors that influence the youth's mood and those strategies that are most helpful for interrupting depressive tendencies.

Psychoeducation

CBT for depression generally begins with the presentation of a conceptual model for understanding the nature of depression as well as how treatment will help the youth to recover. In general, cognitive-behavioral psychoeducational models emphasize interactions between 1) feelings or emotions, 2) thoughts, and 3) behaviors or actions. Because how one feels is influenced by how one thinks about things as well as what one does, treatment is conceptualized as a learning process through which the youth examines different strategies for developing behavioral and cognitive responses that interrupt depressive spirals and enhance coping. These skills or strategies are hypothesized to be useful for coping with depression as well as preventing future depressive episodes (see Clarke et al. 1990 for more detail).

Thoughts/Cognitions

The cognitive component of cognitive-behavioral treatment emphasizes helping youth to identify and interrupt negative and pessimistic thoughts, beliefs, biases, and causal attributions and to substitute more positive and optimistic thought patterns. Cognitive theory postulates that stressful events themselves do not cause depressed mood, but rather the negative or dysfunctional interpretations that are made about such events create and maintain depressed mood. Thus, the cognitive model views depressive symptoms as consequences of the activation of negative cognitive patterns involving 1) negative thoughts about the self, world, and future (the cognitive triad, Beck et al. 1979); 2) negative schemas, or patterns of processing information; and 3) cognitive errors that serve to maintain negative beliefs despite the presence of contradictory evidence. The emphasis in the cognitive component of CBT is on teaching youths to monitor and evaluate thinking patterns, evaluate the validity of automatic thoughts, and develop alternative thinking patterns.

Various techniques are used to help youths learn to identify and dispute dysfunctional automatic thoughts. One technique, for example, is to have youths use a "dysfunctional thoughts record" that has four columns describing 1) the situation, 2) the emotion experienced, 3) the automatic thought, and 4) the evidence for and against the thought. This technique is used to help the therapist and adolescent work as a team in examining the evidence for and against automatic thoughts, identifying logical errors such as dichotomous thinking and overgeneralization, and developing more adaptive cognitive patterns. Questions are asked, such as 1) What is the evidence? 2) What are the errors in my thinking? 3) What is the worst thing that could happen? 4) What are the alternative ways of viewing this situation? (D.A. Brent and K. Poling, "Cognitive Therapy Manual for Depressed and Suicidal Youth," unpublished manual, 1997). Homework and guided experiments aimed at testing the validity of automatic thoughts and assumptions are also used. For example, a youth who felt humiliated and stigmatized by receiving a poor grade on an examination might be asked to make a list of successful people who have received similar grades on examinations.

Behavior

The behavioral component of cognitive-behavioral treatment emphasizes increasing positive behavioral patterns such as social skills and pleasant activity scheduling, which are likely to lead to an increased rate of positive reinforcement and a decreased rate of negative reinforcement in the youth's environment. Social problem-solving and communication skills are also emphasized as a means of decreasing interpersonal stresses, strengthening social support systems, and promoting more reinforcing social environments. More behavioral techniques often take priority over cognitive interventions in patients with severe depressions, in which the initial goal is to increase motivation and activity level. Behavioral techniques, such as social skills training, role-playing, and social problem-solving interventions, also may be more effective than more conceptual approaches such as cognitive restructuring with younger children because of their more limited abstract thinking skills.

Interpersonal Psychotherapy

IPT is based on the assumptions that depression evolves in a social context, and, consequently, the onset, response to treatment, and outcome of depressive episodes are influenced by interpersonal relationships with significant others. Major goals are to decrease depressive symptoms and to improve interpersonal functioning by enhancing communication skills in major interpersonal relationships.

Consistent with the extensive literature documenting the efficacy of IPT with depressed adults (e.g., Elkin et al. 1989; Frank et al. 1990), data from two recent trials support the efficacy of IPT for depression in adolescents. First, in a sample of clinic-referred adolescents with major depression, Mufson et al. (1999) found that IPT was associated with greater improvements in depressive symptoms, social functioning, and problem-solving skills as compared with a control clinical monitoring condition. Second, as noted earlier in this chapter, Rosello and Bernal (1999) found a significant advantage for IPT as well as CBT, when compared with a wait-list condition, among Puerto Rican adolescents meeting criteria for major depression and/or dysthymic disorder. Youths who received IPT showed greater gains in social functioning and self-esteem when compared with the wait-list group, and the effect size for IPT (0.73) exceeded that for CBT (0.43). These two studies underscore the promise of IPT for adolescent depression. Note, however, that both of the completed studies evaluating IPT with adolescents included largely Latino samples, underscoring the importance of testing the efficacy of all interventions in different cultural groups.

A treatment manual is available for a 12-week trial of IPT for adolescents (IPT-A; see Mufson et al. 1993). IPT-A is conceptualized as appropriate for adolescents (ages 12–18) with DSM-III-R–defined major depression, normal intellectual functioning, and no active suicidal risk. Psychotic symptoms and primary diagnoses of bipolar disorder, substance abuse, anxiety disorders, or conduct disorders generally have been viewed as contraindications for a trial of IPT-A.

IPT involves three phases: The first phase (sessions 1–4) emphasizes diagnosis of depression, review of significant interpersonal relationships and how they relate to depression, identification of one or more current problem areas, and negotiation of the therapeutic contract. In sessions 1 and 2, the therapist specifically focuses on diagnosis, educating the youth and parent(s) about depression and treatment strategies, and providing reassurance and guidance about symptom management. A major message conveyed to the youth and parents is that depressive symptoms are time-limited and reflect a treatable disorder and that the depressed youth will function better with treatment. In session 3, the therapist focuses on a comprehensive review of significant interpersonal relationships that is used to identify one or more current problem areas for emphasis from one of the following areas: grief; interpersonal role disputes; role transitions; interpersonal deficits; and single-parent families. During session 4, the therapist presents the interpersonal assessment to the adolescent, and an agreement is reached about the primary problem area(s) that will serve as the focus of treatment.

Another component of the initial phase of IPT is educating the adolescent about being a "patient." The adolescent is allowed to assume a limited "sick role" in order to provide some relief from the strains of usual social roles and allow him or her to receive some time-limited special care. Although adolescents are encouraged to maintain their usual social roles, it is recognized that they may have difficulties performing at their best. Discussing the "sick role" with parents and reframing problematic behaviors as symptoms of depression assist parents in being supportive and nonpunitive as they gently encourage their children to participate in social activities. At the end of this phase of IPT, the therapist should have developed collaborative relationships with the adolescent and parents and established a shared therapeutic contract.

In the middle phase of treatment (sessions 5–8), the therapist focuses on the primary identified problem area(s) and strategies for resolving the adolescent's problems. A major shift in the roles of the adolescent and therapist occurs during this phase of IPT, with adolescents assuming more responsibility for actively contributing information relevant to the identified problems and searching for problem solutions. The therapist remains active but assumes the role of a "team facilitator" who assists the adolescent in formulating and addressing problem areas and clarifying feelings. Parents or other significant persons in the adolescent's life may be asked to participate in some sessions during this phase of IPT in order to assist in negotiations and/or clarify expectations. The expectation of brief, time-limited treatment is emphasized as the adolescent is reminded of the number of remaining sessions.

In the termination phase of IPT (sessions 9–12), the therapist emphasizes conclusion of work on the specified problems and a review of the course of treatment, including strategies learned, changes that have been achieved, and future applications of the skills learned in treatment. Therapists help adolescents recognize their competence by highlighting accomplishments achieved during treatment and foster the expectancy that this competence will be maintained following termination. Therapists assist adolescents in addressing their feelings about termination and, when possible, try to link feelings about termination with the problem area (e.g., feelings about termination may resemble feelings experienced before a role transition or during a grief reaction).

Typically, final termination sessions are conducted with the adolescent alone and with the adolescent and his or her family. During the family termination session, the therapist reviews the presenting symptoms, treatment goals, changes resulting from therapy, and the possibility that some symptoms may recur shortly after termination. When indicated, management of further treatment and future recurrent depressive episodes is discussed.

Family Interventions

The need to consider the family in treatment strategies for depressed youths is underscored by accumulating studies documenting the importance of family attitudinal and interaction patterns for depressed youth (for a review, see McCauley and Myers 1992). Indeed, Kazdin and Weisz (1998) suggested that "child and adolescent therapy is often de facto 'family context' therapy" (p. 20).

Several research findings point to the importance of a "family context" approach for the treatment of depression in youths. First, data indicate that family stress is associated with poor outcomes (e.g., Asarnow et al. 1993; McCauley et al. 1993). Second, during depressive episodes, children have high rates of negative and guilt-inducing behavior in laboratory-based family interactional tasks when compared with nondepressed psychiatric and control subjects (Hamilton et al. 1999), underscoring the high level of stress experienced by families of depressed children. Finally, findings of high rates of mood disorders among first-degree relatives of depressed youth (Kovacs et al. 1997; Kutcher and Marton 1991), in conjunction with data indicating that maternal and child depressive episodes may be temporally linked such that symptoms in one member of the dyad potentiate symptoms in the other (Hammen et al. 1991), underscore the treatment needs of both children and parents. Collectively, these data support an interactional model whereby family stress increases the risk of depression in children and other family members, which in turn fuels family stress and dysfunction.

Current data on family-based treatments for depression in youth are limited. Approaches that have been tested to date can be grouped into two general categories: 1) brief family education interventions and 2) more extended family interventions.

Brief Family Education Interventions

There is emerging support for the value of brief psychoeducational family programs. Brent et al. (1993c) examined the effect of family education on depression in youth. They reported that following a 2-hour psychoeducation session, participants showed greater knowledge about depression and fewer dysfunctional beliefs about depression and the treatment of depression. Participants almost uniformly rated the program as worthwhile (97%) and felt that they had learned a lot (98%). Additionally, in perhaps the largest adolescent depression treatment study completed to date, Brent et al. (1997) added a brief family psychoeducation component across all treatment conditions as a means of minimizing dropout and promoting a family atmosphere that would support treatment gains.

Additionally, our group (J. R. Asarnow, C. V. Scott, and J. Mintz, "A Combined Cognitive-

Behavioral Family Education Intervention for Depression in Children: A Treatment Development Study," unpublished manuscript, April 2000) tested a combined cognitive-behavioral and family education intervention in fourth through sixth graders with depressive symptoms. The family education session followed nine sessions of group CBT, during which children produced a videotape to help them practice and consolidate the skills introduced in each CBT session. The family education session was designed to promote generalization of skills to key environmental contexts (home, school, community). A major part of the session was a brief parent-only segment, in which the emphasis was on 1) the importance of helping the children to generalize the skills to real-world contexts and problems, 2) the fact that children would be more likely to use the skills if they felt good about what they had accomplished in the group, and 3) the value of the family session as a means of helping parents to help their children to feel positively about the CBT skills and to use the CBT skills in real-world settings. After this introduction, parents and children were brought together for a multiple family meeting, during which the children's videotape illustrating the treatment model was presented and children were given awards for their accomplishments during the CBT. Parents and their children then engaged in a series of structured games designed to teach the parents the skills emphasized in the group CBT and promote generalization to critical life settings. The session ended with each child presenting his or her parent(s) with an award for their participation in the family session. Results indicated that the intervention was associated with greater reductions in depressive symptoms than in a wait-list control group. Additionally, children and parents almost uniformly rated the intervention as helpful. When asked about the family component, all of the parents rated this intervention as useful. However, only 40% of the parents felt that more extended family sessions would be helpful, underscoring the potential utility of including some family education as well as the potential difficulties with lengthy family interventions.

Extended Family Interventions

Results of extant studies on the efficacy of extended family interventions are not encouraging. As noted earlier in this chapter, Brent et al. (1997) found that systemic-behavioral family therapy was significantly less effective than individual CBT and comparable in efficacy to nondirective supportive therapy for the treatment of major depression in adolescents. The family treatment used a combination of reframing and communication and problem-solving skills training to alter family interaction patterns. It is important to note, however, that all groups in this study received the brief family psychoeducation intervention described in the previous subsection.

Lewinsohn and colleagues (Clarke et al. 1999; Lewinsohn et al. 1990) compared adolescent-only group CBT, adolescent group CBT plus parallel parental group CBT, and a wait-list control condition. The addition of the parental component offered no clear advantage over adolescent group CBT alone. However, note that the Lewinsohn et al. (1990) group CBT focused on family interactions by teaching communication, negotiation, and conflict resolution skills for use with parents and peers and including homework assignments to practice these skills with parents.

The depression-specific treatment used in the Wood et al. (1996) study, which encouraged parents to help in the CBT, was significantly superior to relaxation training in reducing depression. However, the design of the study does not permit evaluation of the specific effect of family involvement per se.

Fristad et al. (1998) provided preliminary data on a six-session multifamily psychoeducational group for child and adolescent mood disorders. Although these group sessions begin and end with both the parents and the adolescent or child, "breakout sessions" are used in which parallel parent and child groups are conducted. Topics addressed in the groups include education about mood disorders, medication and medication side effects, interpersonal factors, communication skills, and stress reduction. Initial data indicate that families are satisfied with the intervention, and parents report positive changes in their interactions with their child following the intervention. However, the effect of the intervention on clinical symptoms remains to be evaluated.

Two additional groups have developed family treatment models that are currently being evaluated. First, Diamond and Siqueland (1995, 1998) developed a family treatment model for adolescent depression based on attachment theory. The emphasis in this model is on reestablishing the family as a secure base for the adolescent by building the bond between the adolescent and his or her parents. Once this secure base is established, the focus shifts to the adolescent's autonomy and competence outside of the home. Treatment strategies include shifting the focus of therapy to improving family relationships as opposed to "fixing" the patient; establishing therapeutic alliances with both the adolescent and the parent(s); encouraging the adolescent to disclose vulnerable feelings and describe core interpersonal conflicts, leading to mutual acceptance and a shared commitment to communicate and respect each other in the future; and assisting the adolescent in rebuilding his or her life at school and relationships with peers. Early results from an ongoing treatment trial highlight the promise of this approach, with initial results indicating greater recovery rates for youth in the family-treated group than for those in a wait-list control group (G. Diamond, personal communication, December 1999).

Second, Schwartz et al. (1998) described an interpersonal family therapy model that integrates theory and techniques from family systems perspectives, cognitive-behavioral approaches, attachment theory, interpersonal therapy, and developmental psychopathology. This approach focuses on decreasing depressive symptoms through changing maladaptive cognitive patterns, improving family affective communication, increasing adaptive behavior, and improving both interpersonal and family functioning. Work with each family is individually tailored to focus on identifying and intervening in areas of particular need within each family.

Collectively, the data reviewed in this section highlight the potential advantages and disadvantages of adding a family component to the intervention. From a positive perspective, current data indicate that families tend to view brief family educational interventions as helpful, no data indicate that these interventions are detrimental, and some data from the adult literature indicate that family interventions are associated with improved outcome/course in unipolar and bipolar mood disorders (e.g., Jacobson et al. 1991; Rea et al. 1998). Alternatively, to our knowledge, no data demonstrate that family treatments are more effective than other forms of treatment for depression in youth. Insisting on family treatment models also appears to result in a sizable proportion of families refusing treatment. Nine of the 15 families (60%) refusing randomization in the Brent et al. (1997) study did so because they did not want family treatment, an observation that is consistent with results from our pilot study indicating that families preferred a brief as opposed to more extended family intervention. It is important to note, however, that studies examining family interventions have emphasized adolescents rather than younger children, who may be particularly likely to benefit from family-based treatment (Barrett et al. 1996).

Other Treatment Approaches

Psychodynamic Approaches

Psychodynamic psychotherapy has as its overall goal returning disturbed children to normal developmental paths by improving the young person's ability to deal with unconscious thoughts and feelings that have been linked to maladaptive behaviors. Play, drawings, dream interpretation, and free association are the techniques commonly used in young children. The child is encouraged to play out the problems within the confines of a safe, trusting therapeutic relationship. More direct discussion of issues is possible in more cognitively mature children and adolescents. In either case, a major goal is interpretation of the child's fantasies and behaviors and, ultimately, helping him or her verbalize and understand these attempts at mastering the conflicts. Note that psychodynamic theory has contributed to the development of some of the family approaches discussed earlier in this chapter and IPT.

Self-Control Interventions

The self-control model of depression emphasizes links between depression and deficits in self-monitoring, self-evaluation, and self-reinforcement. Depression is characterized as associated with tendencies to selectively attend to both negative events and immediate as opposed to delayed consequences, overly stringent criteria for self-evaluation, negative attributional patterns, insufficient self-reinforcement, and excessive self-punishment. Studies of self-control therapy for adult depression and more recent studies with children have reported superior efficacy to wait-list control conditions (Kaslow and Rehm 1983; Reynolds and Coats 1986; Stark et al. 1987). Interventions emphasized in self-control therapies for depressed youths include skills for self-monitoring (attend to good things that happen, enjoyable things, positive thoughts, and delayed as well as immediate consequences), "self-consequation" (reward yourself more and punish yourself less), self-evaluation (set less perfectionistic standards), and goal-setting (set realistic and attainable subgoals and goals as part of a self-change plan).

Continuation Treatment

The high relapse rate seen in naturalistic follow-up studies of depressed youth underscores the need for continuation treatment strategies. To date, the data to guide clinicians in this area are very limited, but these limited data suggest the value of continuation treatment. Notably, Clarke et al. (1999) showed that the addition of a continuation treatment at the end of acute CBT involving booster sessions every 4 months was associated with accelerated recovery among youth who were still depressed at the end of acute treatment but not with a decrease in rates of recurrence. Similarly, in a small pilot study, Kroll et al. (1996) found that youths receiving continuation CBT about monthly over a 6-month period were less likely to have depression as compared with youths who did not receive continuation treatment.

Prevention

Increasing recognition of the negative effect of depression on development has led to interest in the development of preventive interventions. Three groups testing preventive interventions for youth "at risk for depression" based on the presence of high levels of depressive symptoms have reported promising results for cognitive-behavioral preventive interventions. These interventions are based on the notion that youth can be inoculated against depression by teaching and/or reinforcing the same skills and strategies that are emphasized in treatments for depressive disorders. First, Clarke et al. (1995) used a variation of their group CBT for the treatment of adolescent depression and reported a significantly lower rate of onset of major depression or dysthymia over a 12-month period and improved psychosocial functioning for youth receiving the preventive intervention as compared with a no-intervention comparison group. Second, Jaycox et al. (1994) selected children at risk for depression by virtue of subthreshold depressive symptoms or a high degree of family conflict at home and randomized schools to CBT or wait-list control conditions. CBT was associated with lower levels of depressive symptoms and better classroom behavior as compared with a no-treatment condition. These gains were generally sustained at a 2-year follow-up assessment (Gillham et al. 1995). Third, C.A. King and Kirschenbaum (1990) found that a preventive intervention emphasizing social skills training and consultation with parents resulted in better outcomes than a consultation-only comparison group.

Another approach to preventive interventions has been tested by Beardslee et al. (1996). Two preventive interventions have been developed and evaluated: 1) a clinician-based psychoeducational intervention and 2) a lecture-based approach. Both interventions target children and adolescents who are at risk for depression by virtue of having a parent with a mood disorder, and target their parents as well. The general approach, however, is applicable to families with depressed children and is particularly relevant given the high rate of parental mood disorder reported for parents of depressed youths and evidence documenting more protracted depressive episodes among depressed youths whose parents also have depression (e.g., Warner et al. 1992).

The clinician-based intervention includes 6–10 sessions composed of individual sessions with parents, an individual session with each child, and one or two family meetings. Clinicians are available to the family both during the intervention and afterward by telephone. Major components of the intervention are 1) assessing all family members, 2) teaching family members about mood disorder and risks and resilience in children, 3) linking this information to the family's experience with mood disorder, and 4) enhancing the child's understanding of mood disorder and developing concrete plans for helping the child cope.

The intervention involves the presentation of didactic information about mood disorders, with an emphasis on discussion of risks to children, ways of enhancing resilience, and linking the didactic information with the family's experience with illness. A plan is made for each child that anticipates potential problems related to parental illness and identifies coping strategies for the children. Strategies that encourage children to view themselves as separate from their parents and to seek out relationships outside of the home are emphasized. Couples sessions are used to help parents develop a shared understanding of the illness, which they present to the children in a subsequent family session. Individual sessions with children focus on assessing the children and helping them to identify questions and concerns that can be addressed in the family meeting.

The less intensive, lecture-based intervention includes two 1-hour lectures designed to provide families with information about depression and address major concerns and misunderstandings. However, unlike the clinician-based psychoeducational intervention, the lecture-based intervention does not provide a direct link to the individual experience of each family. Comparison of the two interventions found that children receiving the more intensive clinician-based psychoeducational intervention reported greater understanding of parental mood disorder and had better adaptive functioning as compared with children in a lecture-only comparison group. Parents receiving the more intensive intervention also reported significantly more change. The differences between the two groups were sustained over the course of a 2-year follow-up period. It is important to note that both interventions were perceived as helpful with concerns and resulted in changes in behavior and attitudes that were sustained over time. Thus, although the lecture-based approach was less effective than the more intensive clinician-based psychoeducational intervention, lecture-based psychoeducational interventions are a relatively efficient and cost-effective approach that can be included as one component of a treatment plan.

Treatment of Suicidal Behavior

Suicidal behavior (ideation, threats, gestures, attempts) and completed suicide are multidetermined phenomena. They may be associated with a variety of diagnoses, with depression (major depressive disorder, bipolar disorder and dysthymia singly or comorbid with externalizing and internalizing disorders), substance/alcohol abuse, schizophrenia, and impulse disorders being the most notable (Brent et al. 1993b). For some youth, suicidal behavior erupts as part of low frustration tolerance and rage. The combination of impulsivity and an accessible, lethal means can be fatal. For others, as with adults, suicidal behavior may occur at the nadir of a hopeless, despairing depressive illness. Finally, for some adolescents, suicidal behavior is a lifestyle. It is kept, like a sword of Damocles, over the "head" of the adolescent's environment. It is clear that there is no single, overall treatment for suicidal behavior.

Interventions

Figure 12–1 outlines our model for ultimate suicide. It delineates a number of points at which intervention can take place. Given that suicide is a relatively rare event but the "predictors" that numerous studies have evolved are not uncommon, many people feel that an underlying abnormality exists that distinguishes those with a suicidal propensity from those without. Whether this abnormality is genetic, biochemical, or caused by another unknown mechanism remains to be elucidated and is the impetus for research.

Mental Illness

The most commonly addressed area is that of the mental illnesses associated with suicidal behavior (Brent et al. 1993b). Certainly, the most expedient approach to suicidal behavior is to treat the disorders that have suicidal behavior as a symptom. In this chapter, we have discussed depressive disorders. However, substance/alcohol abuse, which co-occurs with depression and which may either arise from untreated depression or be part of the natural history of disruptive behavior disorders, also needs to be addressed.

The current consensus of suicide prevention efforts is that it is better to concentrate one's resources on identifying those at risk for suicide by identifying those with diagnosable depression or alcohol abuse problems and those who have made previous suicide attempts (Shaffer 1993). The assumption is that treating these otherwise undetected psychiatrically ill youth will reduce suicidal behavior.

- "Perturbation"/neurotransmitter abnormality???
  - Mental illness (usually depression and/or substance/alcohol misuse)
    - Immediate stressor or precipitant
      - No environmental deterrent (friend, therapist, circumstance)
        - No lethal means
        - Inadequate knowledge
        - Good luck

SUICIDE ATTEMPT

- Adequate knowledge
- Lethal means
- Bad luck

SUICIDE

FIGURE 12–1. Pathway to suicide.

Postvention efforts that take place after a youth suicide are valuable treatment measures insofar as they help schools organize an intelligent response to announcing the suicide, help students grieve, dampen destructive rumors, and maintain school security dealing with media intrusion. Postvention mental health efforts appear to be best directed at youth who have the aforementioned suicide risk factors (Brent et al. 1993a). In addition, close friends of the suicide victim appear to be particularly vulnerable to grief reactions that appear, for all intents and purposes, to be major depressive episodes (Brent et al. 1993a). Providing short-term group treatment that has both a psychoeducational and a cathartic goal may diminish long-term pathological grief. Maintaining and following up those youth most at risk by virtue of their relationship to the victim and previous psychopathology at least ensures that referral and treatment will be made available sooner than might otherwise be the case.

Stressors

The next possible intervention point, immediate stressors or precipitants, is helpful only in a patient who is known to be easily upset by stress. Otherwise, the stressors identified in suicidal youth are so ubiquitous that it is naive to assume much can be done to eliminate them. However, treatments such as those mentioned earlier in this chapter, which include intervention components designed to enhance stress management and coping strategies, are clearly useful in youth with suicidal tendencies. Additionally, family interventions that aim to enhance family coping and support provide another strategy for increasing the youth's stress resilience. For example, Rotheram-Borus and colleagues (1994) developed a six-session family treatment for adolescent suicide attempters (most of whom were depressed) and their parents. Successful Negotiation Acting Positively (SNAP) uses the following intervention strategies: 1) exercises designed to establish a positive family climate, such as complimenting one another and noticing positive family events; 2) exercises designed to help family members recognize and label their feelings, describe and assess the intensity of feelings, and manage and control highly charged emotional reactions; 3) practice applying a basic problem-solving approach to solving family problems through role-playing, scripts, and observed interactions with feedback; 4) negotiation skills training and practice; and 5) practice enjoying pleasant activities and showing positive feelings.

Each therapy session includes exercises aimed at creating a positive family atmosphere, followed by a focus on specific skills training. A "tell, show, and do" model is employed. Each skill is introduced with a description of what will be learned and why it is important. Next, the therapist shows family members the skill by modeling, vicarious learning, and scripts. Finally, role-playing and other active methods are used to practice the targeted skill.

Initial results provide some support for the value of this intervention with Latina adolescent suicide attempters (Rotheram-Borus et al. 1994). However, treatment adherence was poor, leading to the development of an emergency room intervention aimed at addressing problematic attitudes, expectations, and behaviors of emergency room staff and families about adolescents who attempt suicide and their treatment. This emergency room intervention led to enhanced treatment adherence (Rotheram-Borus et al. 1996). This finding underscores the need to consider systems interventions to increase the likelihood that youth will actually receive treatment.

Environmental Deterrents

Environmental deterrents are another point at which intervention is possible. The most obvious deterrent is psychiatric hospitalization. This presumably offers supervision and protection as well as treatment. As hospitalization becomes something to be avoided at almost all costs, one of the costs likely will be a life or two. That is simply unacceptable. Although many more youths attempt suicide than complete it, and suicide among children younger than 15 is particularly a very rare event, we have no perfect way to predict who is actually going to succeed. "No-suicide contracts" are suggested as one means of trying to ascertain whether the person is willing to try to control his or her impulses. (However, if a person is determined to kill himself or herself, nothing will prevent him or her from lying about keeping the contract). If the youth will not engage in that contract, hospitalization is unavoidable. For some children, responsible adults may provide around-the-clock, one-on-one supervision until hospitalization is arranged. That cannot be maintained for extended periods, however. It also may be necessary to medicate suicidal youth in protected settings. Although some of the newer antidepressants are less toxic when ingested in large quantities, the TCAs, MAOIs, lithium, and carbamazepine can be fatal if used to overdose.

Beyond its protective aspects, hospitalization is still an important assessment tool. The level of chaos and/or impaired communication in some families and the difficulties many people have in understanding, let alone explaining, their own feelings and behaviors may make an accurate assessment of suicidal behavior on an outpatient basis impossible. Hospitalization has proven vital in two situations: 1) paranoid youth whose "blaming" behavior had been assumed to be part of an externalizing behavior disorder and 2) situations in which families seemed to be covertly giving their children messages to end their lives by making lethal weapons and pills available despite repeated requests to get rid of these items.

Other environmental deterrents are therapists, caring relatives and friends, and adequate supervision. Public education (e.g., health classes in high schools) has not provided a measurable benefit in educating youths about what to do if a friend is suicidal (Shaffer et al. 1988). This is probably because the information seems irrelevant to most youths when disseminated, and when they really need the information, either they have forgotten it or they do not recognize that they need it. Nonetheless, it is useful information in specific contexts such as postvention educational efforts or day treatment settings where suicidal behavior is more frequent.

Lethal Means

Although some suicides are well planned and executed, many are impulsive and had there not been a convenient method available, the suicidal urge would have passed before the person managed the wherewithal to kill himself or herself. Guns are the quickest, most thorough, most readily available means of suicide in our culture. They simply do not belong in households with depressed family members. Although owners repeatedly respond that the guns are not loaded or that ammunition is locked up elsewhere in the house, somehow they manage to kill the very people they were supposed to protect (Brent et al. 1991). If the family is unwilling to get rid of the weapon permanently, they should be told to have another family hold onto weapon until suicide is no longer a risk.

Other obvious lethal means are pills with known toxicity. Interestingly, household poisons usually are not used for suicide and are most evident as means of accidental deaths in small children.

One cannot purge the household (where most suicides occur) of rafters, upper-story windows, garages (for carbon monoxide poisoning), and so forth. However, the more complicated and time-consuming the actual task of suicide is, the more likely the potential victim is to change his or her mind or perhaps be discovered before it is too late.

Adequate Knowledge

It is difficult to advocate promotion of ignorance. However, insofar as publicity about suicide and specifics about circumstances contribute to a contagion effect, conventional wisdom supports downplaying the sensational aspects of teen suicide. Trying to keep media away from such stories, however, is almost impossible. Those professionals dealing with the aftermath of such tragedies would be well advised to figure out ways of working with media and collaborating with more responsible reporters to effect some level of damage control. Families and friends also should be given ways of dealing with the press to mitigate the consequences of publicity.

The other major area in which knowledge control can play a part in suicide is promulgating the fact that most mental illness, if not always curable, is certainly treatable and that, in most cases, the person does not have to contemplate a lifetime of whatever misery is prompting the suicidal alternative. Such information can help instill hope and shift the focus to reasons for living rather than the hopelessness and helplessness that so often characterize depressed youth.

Conclusions

Children with depressive disorders present a complicated array of problems that have to be addressed, with both the disorder and the child and family in mind. It is unlikely that one strategy will work. Clinical care will require the knowledgeable and artful combination of guidance, therapy, and psychopharmacology.

References

Abou-Saleh MT: Who responds to prophylactic lithium therapy? Br J Psychiatry 163 (suppl 21):20–26, 1993

Alessi N, Naylor MW, Ghaziuddin M, et al: Update on lithium carbonate therapy in children and adolescents. J Am Acad Child Adolesc Psychiatry 33:291–304, 1994

Ambrosini J, Bianchi MD, Rabinovitch H, et al: Antidepressant treatments in children and adolescents, I: affective disorders. J Am Acad Child Adolesc Psychiatry 32:1–6, 1993

Ambrosini J, Wagner KD, Biederman J, et al: Multicenter open-label sertraline study in adolescent outpatients with major depression. J Am Acad Child Adolesc Psychiatry 38:566–573, 1999

American Academy of Child and Adolescent Psychiatry: Practice parameters for the assessment and treatment of children and adolescents with bipolar disorder. J Am Acad Child Adolesc Psychiatry 36 (10 suppl):157S–176S, 1997

American Academy of Child and Adolescent Psychiatry: Practice parameters for the assessment and treatment of children and adolescents with depressive disorders. J Am Acad Child Adolesc Psychiatry 37 (10 suppl):63S–83S, 1998

American Psychiatric Association: Diagnostic and Statistical Manual of Mental Disorders, 3rd Edition, Revised. Washington, DC, American Psychiatric Association, 1987

American Psychiatric Association: Practice guidelines for major depressive disorder in adults. Am J Psychiatry 150 (10 suppl), April 1993

American Psychiatric Association: Diagnostic and Statistical Manual of Mental Disorders, 4th Edition. Washington, DC, American Psychiatric Association, 1994

Amsterdam J: Efficacy and safety of venlafaxine in the treatment of bipolar II major depressive episode. J Clin Psychopharmacol 18:414–417, 1998

Amsterdam JD, Garcia-Espana F, Fawcett J, et al: Efficacy and safety of fluoxetine in treating bipolar II major depressive episode. J Clin Psychopharmacol 18:435–440, 1998

Angold A, Costello EJ: Depressive comorbidity in children and adolescents: empirical, theoretical, and methodological issues. Am J Psychiatry 150:1779–1791, 1993

Asarnow JR, Goldstein MJ, Tompson M, et al: One-year outcomes of depressive disorders in child psychiatric inpatients: evaluation of the prognostic power of a brief measure of expressed emotion. J Child Psychol Psychiatry 34:129–137, 1993

Asarnow JR, Carlson G, Schuster M, et al: Youth Partners in Care: Clinician Guide to Depression Assessment and Management Among Youth in Primary Care Settings: A Guide for Primary Care Providers and Care Managers (adapted for youth from Rubenstein L, Unutzer J, Miranda J, et al: Partners in Care: Clinician Guide to Depression Assessment and Management in Primary Care Settings. Santa Monica, CA, RAND, 1996). Los Angeles, CA, UCLA, 1999

Asarnow JR, Jaycox LH, Tompson MC: Depression in youth: psychosocial interventions. J Clin Child Psychol (in press)

Barrett PM, Dadds MR, Rapee RM: Family treatment of childhood anxiety: a controlled trial. J Consult Clin Psychol 64:333–342, 1996

Beardslee WR, Wright E, Rothberg PC, et al: Response of families to two preventive intervention strategies: long-term differences in behavior and attitude change. J Am Acad Child Adolesc Psychiatry 35:774–782, 1996

Beck AT, Rush AJ, Shaw BF, et al: Cognitive Therapy of Depression. New York, Guilford, 1979

Bemporad JR: Psychodynamic treatment of depressed adolescents. J Clin Psychiatry 49 (suppl):26–31, 1988

Biederman J, Baldessarini R, Wright V, et al: A double-blind, placebo controlled study of desipramine in the treatment of attention deficit disorder, I: efficacy. J Am Acad Child Adolesc Psychiatry 28: 777–784, 1989

Birmaher B, Brent DA, Kolko D, et al: Clinical outcome after short-term psychotherapy for adolescents with major depressive disorder. Arch Gen Psychiatry 57:29–36, 2000

Black DW, Winokur G, Bell S, et al: Complicated mania—comorbidity and immediate outcome in the treatment of mania. Arch Gen Psychiatry 45:232–236, 1988

Bond AJ: Drug induced behavioral disinhibition: incidence, mechanisms and therapeutic implications. CNS Drugs 9:41–57, 1998

Bowden CL: Key treatment studies of lithium in manic-depressive illness: efficacy and side effects. J Clin Psychiatry 59 (suppl 6):13–19, 1998

Bowden CL, Brugger AM, Swann AC, et al: Efficacy of divalproex vs lithium and placebo in the treatment of mania. The Depakote Mania Study Group. JAMA 271:918–924, 1994

Brent DA, Perper JA, Allman CJ, et al: The presence and accessibility of firearms in the homes of adolescent suicides: a case-control study. JAMA 266:2989–2995, 1991

Brent DA, Perper J, Moritz G, et al: Bereavement or depression? The impact of the loss of a friend to suicide. J Am Acad Child Adolesc Psychiatry 32:1189–1198, 1993a

Brent DA, Perper JA, Moritz G, et al: Psychiatric risk factors for adolescent suicide: a case-control study. J Am Acad Child Adolesc Psychiatry 32:521–529, 1993b

Brent DA, Poling K, McKain B, et al: A psychoeducational program for families of affectively ill children and adolescents. J Am Acad Child Adolesc Psychiatry 32:770–774, 1993c

Brent DA, Holder, D, Kolko, D, et al: A clinical psychotherapy trial for adolescent depression comparing cognitive, family and supportive therapy. Arch Gen Psychiatry 54:877–885, 1997

Calabrese JR, Bowden CL, Sachs GS, et al: A double-blind, placebo-controlled study of lamotrigine monotherapy in outpatients with bipolar I depression. J Clin Psychiatry 60:79–88, 1999

Carlson GA: Child and adolescent mania—diagnostic considerations. J Child Psychol Psychiatry 31: 331–341, 1990

Carlson GA: Can we validate childhood psychiatric disorders in adults? Am J Psychiatry 150:1763–1766, 1993a

Carlson GA: Psychosis and mania in adolescents, in Current Psychiatric Therapy. Edited by Dunner DL. Philadelphia, PA, WB Saunders, 1993b, pp 427–431

Carlson GA: Bipolar disorder and attention deficit disorder—comorbidity or confusion? J Affect Disord 51:177–189, 1998

Carlson GA, Kashani JH: Phenomenology of major depression from childhood through adulthood: analysis of three studies. Am J Psychiatry 145:1222–1225, 1988

Carlson GA, Rapport MD, Pataki CS, et al: Lithium in hospitalized children at 4 and 8 weeks: mood, behavior and cognitive effects. J Child Psychol Psychiatry 33:411–425, 1992

Carlson GA, Rapport MD, Kelly K, et al: Methylphenidate and desipramine effects on children's behavior and mood. J Child Adolesc Psychopharmacol 5:191–204, 1995

Carlson GA, Lavelle J, Bromet EJ: Medication treatment in adolescents vs adults with psychotic mania. J Child Adolesc Psychopharmacol 9:221–231, 1999

Clarke GN, Lewinsohn PM, Hops H, et al: Leader's Manual, Adolescent Coping With Depression Course. Eugene, OR, Castalia, 1990

Clarke GN, Hawkins W, Murphy M, et al: Targeted prevention of unipolar depressive disorder in an at-risk sample of high school adolescents: a randomized trial of a group of cognitive intervention. J Am Acad Child Adolesc Psychiatry 34:312–321, 1995

Clarke GN, Rohde P, Lewinsohn PM, et al: Cognitive-behavioral treatment of adolescent depression: efficacy of acute group treatment and booster sessions. J Am Acad Child Adolesc Psychiatry 38: 272–279, 1999

Deltito AJ, Levitan J, Damore J, et al: Naturalistic experience with the use of divalproex sodium on an in-patient unit for adolescent psychiatric patients. Acta Psychiatr Scand 97:236–240, 1998

Diamond G, Siqueland L: Family therapy for the treatment of depressed adolescents. Psychotherapy 32:77–90, 1995

Diamond G, Siqueland L: Emotions, attachment and the relational reframe: the first session. Journal of Systemic Therapies 17(2):36–50, 1998

Elkin I, Shea T, Watkins J, et al: National Institute of Mental Health Treatment of Depression Collaborative Research Program. Arch Gen Psychiatry 46:971–982, 1989

Emslie GJ, Rush AJ, Weinberg WA, et al: A double-blind, randomized placebo-controlled trial of fluoxetine in depressed children and adolescents. Arch Gen Psychiatry 54:1031–1037, 1997a

Emslie GJ, Rush AJ, Weinberg WA, et al: Recurrence of major depressive disorder in hospitalized children and adolescents. J Am Acad Child Adolesc Psychiatry 36:785–792, 1997b

Emslie GJ, Rush AJ, Weinberg WA, et al: Fluoxetine in child and adolescent depression: acute and maintenance treatment. Depress Anxiety 7:32–39, 1998

Emslie GJ, Walkup JT, Pliszka SR, et al: Nontricyclic antidepressants: current trends in children and adolescents. J Am Acad Child Adolesc Psychiatry 38:517–529, 1999

Fetner HH, Geller B: Lithium and tricyclic antidepressants. Psychiatr Clin North Am 15:223–242, 1992

Findling RL, Reed MD, Blumer JL: Pharmacological treatment of depression in children and adolescents. Paediatr Drugs 1:161–182, 1999

Fink M: Electroconvulsive Therapy: Restoring the Mind. New York, Oxford University Press, 1999

Frank E, Kupfer DJ, Perel JM, et al: Three year outcomes for maintenance therapies in recurrent depression. Arch Gen Psychiatry 48:1053–1059, 1990

Fristad MA, Gavazzi SM, Soldano KW: Multi-family psychoeducation groups for childhood mood disorders: a program description and preliminary efficacy data. Contemporary Family Therapy 20:385–402, 1998

Geller B, Fox LW, Fletcher M: Effect of tricyclic antidepressants on switching to mania and on the onset of bipolarity in depressed 6- to 12-year-olds. J Am Acad Child Adolesc Psychiatry 32:43–50, 1993

Geller B, Reising D, Leonard HL, et al: Critical review of tricyclic antidepressant use in children and adolescents. J Am Acad Child Adolesc Psychiatry 38:513–517, 1999

Gillham J, Reivich KJ, Jaycox LH, et al: Prevention of depressive symptoms in schoolchildren: two year follow-up. Psychological Science 6:343–351, 1995

Goodnick PJ, Dominguez RA, DeVane CL, et al: Bupropion slow-release response in depression: diagnosis and biochemistry. Biol Psychiatry 44:629–632, 1998

Goodwin DW, Guze SB: Psychiatric Diagnosis, 2nd Edition. New York, Oxford University Press, 1979

Goodwin FK, Jamison KR: Manic-Depressive Illness. New York, Oxford University Press, 1990

Greenhill L: Pharmacologic treatment of attention deficit disorder. Psychiatr Clin North Am 15:1–27, 1992

Greil W, Kleindienst N, Erazo N, et al: Differential response to lithium and carbamazepine in the prophylaxis of bipolar disorder. J Clin Psychopharmacol 18:455–460, 1998

Hagino OR, Weller EB, Weller RA, et al: Untoward effects of lithium treatment in children aged four through six years. J Am Acad Child Adolesc Psychiatry 34:1584–1590, 1995

Hamilton EB, Asarnow JR, Tompson MC: Family interaction styles of children with depressive disorder, schizophrenia-spectrum disorder and normal controls. Fam Process 38:463–476, 1999

Hammen C, Burge K, Adrian C: Timing of mother and child depression in a longitudinal study of children at risk. J Consult Clin Psychol 59:341–345, 1991

Isojarvi JI, Laatikainen TJ, Pakarinen AJ, et al: Polycystic ovaries and hyperandrogenism in women taking valproate for epilepsy. N Engl J Med 329:1383–1388, 1993

Isojarvi JIT, Ratrya J, Myllyla W, et al: Valproate, lamotrigine and insulin-mediated risks in women with epilepsy. Ann Neurol 43:446–451, 1998

Jacobson NS, Dobson K, Fruzzetti AE, et al: Marital therapy as a treatment for depression. J Consult Clin Psychol 59:547–557, 1991

Jaycox LH, Reivich KJ, Gillham JE, et al: Prevention of depressive symptoms in school children. Behav Res Ther 32:801–816, 1994

Jefferson JW: Mood stabilizers: a review, in Current Psychiatry Therapy. Edited by Dunner DL. Philadelphia, PA, WB Saunders, 1993, pp 246–254

Kafantaris V, Coletti DJ, Dicker R, et al: Childhood psychiatric histories of bipolar adolescent: association with family history, psychosis and response to lithium treatment. J Affect Disord 51:153–164, 1998

Kaslow NJ, Rehm LP: Childhood depression, in The Practice of Child Therapy. Edited by Morris RJ, Kratochwill TR. New York, Guilford, 1983, pp 27–52

Kazdin AE, Weisz JR: Identifying and developing empirically supported child and adolescent treatments. J Consult Clin Psychol 66:19–36, 1998

Keck PJ Jr, McElroy SL, Strakowski SM: Anticonvulsants and antipsychotics in the treatment of bipolar disorder. J Clin Psychiatry 59 (suppl 6):74–81, 1998

Kestenbaum CJ, Kron L: Psychoanalytic intervention with children and adolescents with affective disorders: a combined treatment approach. J Am Acad Psychoanal 5:153–174, 1987

King CA, Kirschenbaum DS: An experimental evaluation of a school-based program for children at-risk: Wisconsin early intervention. Journal of Community Psychology 18:167–177, 1990

King RA, Riddle MA, Chappell PB, et al: Emergence of self-destructive phenomenology in children and adolescents during fluoxetine treatment. J Am Acad Child Adolesc Psychiatry 30:179–186, 1991

Klein DL, Lewinsohn PM, Seeley JR: Psychosocial characteristics of adolescents with a past history of dysthymic disorder: comparison with adolescents with past histories of major depressive and non-affective disorders, and never mentally ill controls. J Affect Disord 42:127–135, 1997

Kovacs M, Feinbert TL, Crouse MA, et al: Recovery in childhood depressive disorders: a longitudinal prospective study. Arch Gen Psychiatry 41:229–237, 1984

Kovacs M, Delvin B, Pollock M, et al: A controlled family history study of childhood-onset depressive disorder. Arch Gen Psychiatry 54:613–623, 1997

Kowatch RA, Suppes T, Carmody TJ, et al: Effect size of lithium, divalproex sodium, and carbamazepine in children and adolescents with bipolar disorder. J Am Acad Child Adolesc Psychiatry 39:713–720, 2000

Kroll L, Harrington R, Jayson D, et al: Pilot study of continuation cognitive-behavioral therapy for major depression in adolescent psychiatric patients. J Am Acad Child Adolesc Psychiatry 35: 1156–1161, 1996

Kutcher S, Marton P: Affective disorders in first-degree relatives of adolescent onset bipolars, unipolars, and normal controls. J Am Acad Child Adolesc Psychiatry 30:75–78, 1991

Kutcher S, Robertson HA, Bird D: Premorbid functioning in adolescent onset bipolar I disorder: a preliminary report from an ongoing study. J Affect Disord 51:137–144, 1998

Levy D, Kimhi R, Barak Y, et al: Antidepressant-associated mania: a study of anxiety disorders patients. Psychopharmacology 136:243–246, 1998

Lewinsohn PM, Clarke GN, Hops H, et al: Cognitive-behavioral treatment for depressed adolescents. Behavior Therapy 21:385–401, 1990

Mann JJ, Kapur S: The emergence of suicidal ideation and behavior during antidepressant pharmacotherapy. Arch Gen Psychiatry 48:1027–1033, 1991

McCauley E, Myers K: The longitudinal clinical course of depression in children and adolescents. Child Adolesc Psychiatr Clin N Am 1:183–196, 1992

McCauley E, Myers K, Mitchell J, et al: Depression in young people: initial presentation and clinical course. J Am Acad Child Adolesc Psychiatry 32:714–722, 1993

Mufson L, Moreau D, Weissman MM, et al: Interpersonal Psychotherapy for Depressed Adolescents. New York, Guilford, 1993

Mufson L, Weissman MM, Moreau D, et al: Efficacy of interpersonal psychotherapy for depressed adolescents. Arch Gen Psychiatry 56:573–579, 1999

Papatheodorou G, Kutcher SP, Katic M, et al: The efficacy and safety of divalproex sodium in the treatment of acute mania in adolescents and young adults: an open clinical trial. J Clin Psychopharmacol 15:110–116, 1995

Post RM, Frye MA, Leverich GS, et al: The role of complex combination therapy in the treatment of refractory bipolar illness. CNS Spectrums 3:66–86, 1998

Puig-Antich J, Lukens E, Danes M, et al: Psychosocial functioning in prepubertal depressive disorders, I: interpersonal relationships during the depressive episode. Arch Gen Psychiatry 42:500–507, 1985a

Puig-Antich J, Lukens E, Danes M, et al: Psychosocial functioning in prepubertal depressive disorders, II: interpersonal relationships after sustained recovery from affective episode. Arch Gen Psychiatry 42:511–517, 1985b

Rea MM, Goldstein MJ, Tompson MC, et al: Family and individual treatment in bipolar disorder: outline and first results of the UCLA Study. Paper presented at the World Association for Psychosocial Rehabilitation, Hamburg, Germany, May 1998

Rey JM, Walter G: Half a century of ECT use in young people. Am J Psychiatry 154:595–602, 1997

Reynolds WM, Coats KI: A comparison of cognitive-behavioral therapy and relaxation training for the treatment of depression in adolescents. J Consult Clin Psychol 54:653–660, 1986

Riddle MA, King RA, Hardin MT, et al: Behavioral side effects of fluoxetine in children and adolescents. J Child Adolesc Psychopharmacol 1:193–198, 1991

Riddle MA, Geller B, Ryan N: Another sudden death in a child treated with desipramine. J Am Acad Child Adolesc Psychiatry 32:792–797, 1993

Rohde P, Lewinsohn PM, Seeley JR: Are adolescents changed by an episode of major depression? J Am Acad Child Adolesc Psychiatry 33:1289–1298, 1994

Rosello J, Bernal G: Treatment of depression in Puerto Rican adolescents: the efficacy of cognitive-behavioral and interpersonal treatments. J Consult Clin Psychol 67:734–745, 1999

Rotheram-Borus MJ, Piacentini J, Miller S, et al: Brief cognitive-behavioral treatment for adolescent suicide attempters and their families. J Am Acad Child Adolesc Psychiatry 33:508–517, 1994

Rotheram-Borus MJ, Piacentini J, Van Rossem R, et al: Enhancing treatment adherence with a specialized emergency room program for adolescent suicide attempters. J Am Acad Child Adolesc Psychiatry 35:654–663, 1996

Ryan ND: The psychopharmacologic treatment of child and adolescent depression. Psychiatr Clin North Am 15:29–40, 1992

Ryan ND, Puig-Antich J, Ambrosini P, et al: The clinical picture of major depression in children and adolescents. Arch Gen Psychiatry 44:854–861, 1987

Ryan ND, Rhatara VS, Perel JM: Mood stabilizers in children and adolescents. J Am Acad Child Adolesc Psychiatry 38:529–538, 1999

Schneekloth TD, Rummans TA, Logan KM: Electroconvulsive therapy in adolescents. Convuls Ther 9:158–166, 1993

Schwartz JAJ, Kaslow NJ, Racusin GR, et al: Interpersonal family therapy for childhood depression, in Handbook of Psychological Treatment Protocols for Children and Adolescents. Edited by Van Hasselt VB, Hersen M. Mahwah, NJ, Lawrence Erlbaum, 1998, pp 109–151

Shaffer D: Advances in youth suicide—research update. Lifesavers: Newsletter of the American Suicide Foundation 5:4, 1993

Shaffer D, Garland A, Gould M, et al: Preventing teenage suicide: a critical review. J Am Acad Child Adolesc Psychiatry 27:675–688, 1988

Simeon JG, Dinicola VF, Ferguson BH, et al: Adolescent depression: a placebo controlled fluoxetine treatment study and follow-up. Prog Neuropharmacol Biol Psychiatry 14:791–795, 1990

Solomon DA, Keitner GI, Miller IW, et al: Course of illness and maintenance treatments for patients with bipolar disorder. J Clin Psychiatry 56:5–13, 1995

Stark KD, Livingston RB, Kaslow NJ: A comparison of the relative efficacy of self-control therapy and a behavioral problem-solving therapy for depression in children. J Abnorm Child Psychol 15:91–113, 1987

Stewart JW, Rabkin JG, Quitkin FM, et al: Atypical depression, in Current Psychiatric Therapy. Edited by Dunner DL. Philadelphia, PA, WB Saunders, 1993, pp 215–220

Strakowski SM, Tohen M, Stoll AL, et al: Comorbidity in mania at first hospitalization. Am J Psychiatry 149:554–556, 1992

Strober M, Carlson GA: Bipolar illness in adolescents with major depression: clinical, genetic and psychopharmacologic predictors. Arch Gen Psychiatry 39:549–555, 1982

Strober M, Morrell N, Lampert C, et al: Lithium carbonate in prophylactic treatment of bipolar I illness in adolescents: a naturalistic study. Am J Psychiatry 147:457–461, 1990

Strober M, Lampert C, Schmidt S, et al: The course of major depressive disorder in adolescents: recovery and risk of manic switching in a 24-month prospective, naturalistic follow-up of psychotic and nonpsychotic subtypes. J Am Acad Child Adolesc Psychiatry 32:34–42, 1993

Strober M, DeAntonio M, Schmidt-Lackner S, et al: Early childhood attention deficit hyperactivity disorder predicts poorer response to acute lithium therapy in adolescent mania. J Affect Disord 51:145–151, 1998

Suppes T, Baldessarini RJ, Faedda GL, et al: Risk of recurrence following discontinuation of lithium treatment in bipolar disorder. Arch Gen Psychiatry 48:1082–1088, 1991

Suppes T, Rush AJ, Kraemer HC, et al: Treatment algorithm use to optimize management of symptomatic patients with a history of mania. J Clin Psychiatry 59:89–96, 1998

Tollefson GD: Major depression, in Current Psychiatric Therapy. Edited by Dunner DL. Philadelphia, PA, WB Saunders, 1993, pp 196–203

Venkataraman S, Naylor MW, King CA: Mania associated with fluoxetine treatment in adolescents. J Am Acad Child Adolesc Psychiatry 31:276–281, 1992

Vostanis P, Feehan C, Grattan E, et al: A randomized controlled out-patient trial of cognitive-behavioural treatment for children and adolescents with depression: 9-month follow-up. J Affect Disord 40:105–116, 1996

Walter G, Koster K, Rey JM: Electroconvulsive therapy in adolescents: experience, knowledge and attitudes of recipients. J Am Acad Child Adolesc Psychiatry 38:594–599, 1999

Warner V, Weissman MM, Fendrich M, et al: The course of major depression in the offspring of depressed parents: incidence, recurrence, recovery. Arch Gen Psychiatry 49:795–801, 1992

Weller EB, Weller RA, Fristad MA: Lithium dosage guide for prepubertal children: a preliminary report. J Am Acad Child Adolesc Psychiatry 25:92–96, 1986

Wood A, Harrington R, Moore A: Controlled trial of a brief cognitive-behavioural intervention in adolescent patients with depressive disorders. J Child Psychol Psychiatry 37:737–746, 1996

Young RC, Biggs JT, Ziegler VE, et al: A rating scale for mania: reliability, validity and sensitivity. Br J Psychiatry 133:429-435, 1978

13

Childhood Posttraumatic Stress Disorder

Lenore Terr, M.D.

Because posttraumatic stress disorder (PTSD) of childhood is relatively new to the psychiatric diagnoses of children and adolescents, the treatment approaches to this condition have not yet been completely standardized. Moreover, rigorously designed studies have not yet proved any of these therapies to be effective in children. The information in this chapter, therefore, must be seen as preliminary. With those medications that are mentioned, appropriate precautions must be taken with a pediatric population. In this chapter, I review the possibilities for individual psychotherapy, medications, family therapy, group therapy, and large-scale preventive strategies. In almost every instance, treatment for childhood PTSD should consist of a combination of the various treatment modalities.

Individual Psychotherapy

The most important and most commonly used treatment for PTSD in children is psychotherapy. Psychotherapy is capable of modifying the internal changes a child has made to cope with the externally generated trauma. Because of the traumatic experience, a youngster may have abandoned all trust in key individuals and institutions, or the child may have stopped believing in his or her own personal autonomy and in the future. In the unconscious attempt to master what was once perceived as an overwhelming force coming from the outside, the child may have been forced to repeat again and again in behavior, play, creative efforts, and physiological states the horrors that were originally attached to the event. The traumatic experience, if repeated or if connected with serious loss or disfiguring or limiting injury, may also have led to massive defensive patterns that robbed the child of verbal memory and/or the subjective feelings connected with the trauma (Terr 1991). These defenses may have set the groundwork for a personality disorder. Repeatedly traumatized children may also have become chronically depressed or, even worse, almost entirely numb to their own feelings, as well as to the feelings of others. It is the therapist's task to help such children modify these changes and go on to more normal development.

Phases of Individual Psychotherapy

Beginning Phase

In most instances, individual psychotherapy for a traumatized child requires an early, full recital by the child of everything that he or she can remember about the event(s) that precipitated the condition (Pynoos and Eth 1985, 1986). A psychiatrist cannot spare the child or the psychiatrist this recitation of old, traumatic history. Although the child may not want to tell the story the first or the second time he or she is evaluated, the child's verbal tale—even if consisting of only a few words—must come out at some point close to the beginning of therapy. The child needs to abreact about his or her experiences (Levy 1939). And the psychiatrist will not fully understand the nature of the child's symptoms and will not be able to explain or interpret them to the young patient without a full recital of the events. In the absence of a request for a story, the child also may conclude that the therapist feels afraid to really know about the event(s) or the connected feelings. In the case of the traumatized toddler or preschooler who cannot form a full verbal memory of what took place, it may be helpful for the child to hear from the psychiatrist that the story has already been conveyed by the child's parents or guardian. It is highly recommended that parents, guardians, babysitters, social workers, and others who were in contact with the child around the time of the event(s) be interviewed early in the course of the evaluation so that the psychiatrist can understand as much as possible about the child's exposure to the event and about the event itself (Black and Kaplan 1988; Bloch et al. 1956; Terr 1989a, 1989b). A young child should not be told, however, at this beginning phase of his or her treatment what social workers, visiting nurses, parents, or therapists have guessed or reconstructed about the child's nonverbal ordeals (Ceci and Bruch 1995).

The child's telling of a traumatic experience points to the particular, individual terrors inspired by the event—usually terrors of death or nonbeing, terrors of the loss of loved ones, and terrors of more terror to come (Terr 1979). The child should be asked what his or her most intense fear was at the time of the event and what the most intense fear is now. Because traumas involve such an admixture of feelings, the child also should be asked if he or she can remember feeling sadness, rage, confusion, and/or excitement connected with the experience. Careful observations and notation of these affects—as told by the child in the consulting room—are very helpful. Many times the child must be helped to develop a rudimentary vocabulary of emotions (e.g., "sad," "angry," "excited," "scared") before he or she can proceed with treatment.

An important part of the early individual therapy for the traumatized child is the establishment of trust (Herman 1992). Because adults or "Mother Nature" herself has usually conspired in some way against the child, the traumatized child has little initial reason to form a therapeutic alliance. The therapist must offer a friendly, truthful, steady, humor-filled, and extraordinarily reliable behavior pattern. He or she must be willing, if necessary, to see the child with the child's parents present (Terr 1990). The therapist may gain the child's trust by getting on the floor and playing directly with the child or by sharing a joke or two with him or her. If possible, the therapist is careful to keep secret the details of what the child tells (but only if there is no pending lawsuit or criminal action relating to the trauma). The therapist must stringently keep whatever word has been originally given to the child. True empathy must be shown for the child's predicament. Even if the therapist himself or herself has experienced a personal trauma in childhood, however, it is better to withhold this information from the child. Sharing traumas may add to the child's fears.

It is often helpful to traumatized children, however, to eventually hear more distant, inspirational stories or to watch television tapes of others who overcame similar ordeals (Terr 1990). One example would be a girl preschooler who had both feet amputated and was given (through the therapist's intervention) the tape of a television commercial about a male basketball player with artificial limbs. Watching this tape enabled the very young, inexperienced toddler to see the future possibility of living a normal life with artificial feet. It broadened the context of her trauma, educated her, and increased her confidence in her own future.

Early in therapy, the psychiatrist encourages the child to play or to render whatever artwork, poetry, music, or dramatic scenarios he or she prefers (Terr 1983, 1990; Webb 1999; Winnicott 1971). The child almost inevitably produces trauma-inspired art. Notes are kept of what the child says about these artistic renderings. Several repetitions of play are allowed so that the therapist is fully aware of repetitive themes before intervening. Children of any age (and for that matter, adults) can be encouraged to play or to produce artwork related to their traumas. As opposed to ordinary pretend play, which dwindles off as preadolescence approaches, posttraumatic play appeals to many adolescents and adults (Terr 1981). Older children should be encouraged to discuss their play and to bring play products (e.g., poetry, sketches) to their therapy sessions (Terr 1999). Play that is encouraged early in the course of a patient's psychotherapy gives the therapist an extremely powerful tool with which to later modify the course of the PTSD.

However, one does not want the child to experience therapy as tremendously anxiety-provoking, and posttraumatic play without therapeutic intervention is extremely provocative of anxiety. Except in cases of stress that can be worked out in a child's mind from play unmodified by words (Levy 1939), the psychiatrist must begin to enter into the child's play to help the child to reinterpret it and to modify it, once the psychiatrist has observed enough repetitions to detect the theme (Terr 1990). Eventually the therapist will instill "corrective dénouements" into this play (Terr 1983).

Behavior modification and cognitive approaches are very useful to young patients early in the course of their individual therapy. One early option of this type is "corrective dreaming." If a child has been recently traumatized and has developed repetitive nightmares of the traumatic event with relatively little symbolic elaboration or disguise, the child may be able to decide at night before falling asleep to redream the recurring dream but with a planned corrective ending. (This process is sometimes called "lucid dreaming" [Gackenback and Schillig 1983; LaBerge et al. 1986].) For example, a teenage girl who ate poisoned pizza and later dreamed of a man's head blowing up into pieces willed herself to dream this same nightmare, this time with the man picking up all of his pieces and reconstructing an intact head. By using planned corrective dreaming, this teenager was able to stop dreaming her nightmare and also to stop visualizing it by day. A younger girl, who, by luck and extraordinary willpower, was able to wiggle away from a man who had snatched her from a city sidewalk and was trying to force her into his car, dreamed the first night after the attempted abduction that the man had successfully put her into his car trunk, had opened it, and was now coming at her with a knife. After a crisis intervention the next day, this child willed herself that evening to dream the same dream. She decided to finish with her actual escape from the man and her possible future courtroom testimony against him. Because the young girl was able to quickly master a new psychotherapeutic technique, the intensity and frequency of her nightmares diminished. This technique also occasionally works for adults suffering from very old childhood traumas. It is a positive suggestion that the psychiatrist can offer a patient early in the course of therapy, and it gives the patient hope of later overcoming many other related problems.

A second early and often successful brief psychotherapeutic approach to childhood trauma is behavior modification (Kipper 1976; Silverman and Geer 1968). The child attacked by a large dog, for instance, might go early in the course of treatment to a pet store to play with puppies of the same breed as the dog that attacked him or her. The child would then be exposed, according to his or her own pacing, to small adult dogs of the same breed, muzzled and leashed. Eventually the child would encounter a trained, well-behaved, unleashed animal of the same breed. Learned relaxation techniques aid children in facing feared objects. It is helpful and often necessary for the child's parent or guardian to accompany the child through these trials, holding hands or otherwise providing physical reassurance to the youngster.

Middle Phase

After a child patient has spent four to six sessions telling and playing out a fearful experience, the therapist begins more actively to intervene. These interventions are geared to help the child discover new modes of control over what previously had been uncontrollable. They are also planned to give the child a new, larger context in which to place his or her trauma. Children need to realize that bad luck is not a lifelong pattern. They need to know that traumatic events occur at random. They also need to realize that they are not responsible for the actions of the adults who perpetrated horrible events on them. They need to know that they will eventually be able to go on in life and control things the way anyone else would. These realizations must come from within the child, not from the therapist. So a child must play these things out—chant about them, draw them, write poems, or somehow set up new scenarios that prove these empowerments. The therapist can talk about a possibility that a certain doll might take into account—screaming when the kidnapper comes, for instance, or yelling "Stay!" to the ferocious dog. Children who were abused at home can be informed about dialing "911" in the middle of the night to get help while everyone sleeps or telling a teacher what has been happening.

Most children automatically go to the toys or the drawing materials in a psychiatrist's office. In thousands of ways, they set up the little cats on the doctor's desk to attack one another, the family of dolls in the dollhouse to experience a death, the baby china dog to endure the sexual attack from the fully grown dog, the dinosaurs to pursue the babies. If a child experienced a specific horror—for instance, enduring an alligator attack—the psychiatrist may purchase an alligator puppet, along with two or three other similarly made animal puppets, such as a rabbit and a raccoon. This kind of specific toy often speeds the treatment along (Maclean 1977; Shapiro 1973). Specific toys depict specific ordeals. To start, the child may ask the psychiatrist to hold the "offending" toy, refusing to touch it himself or herself. "*You* take the alligator," she says, for instance. After taking the alligator, the psychiatrist might suggest, "*You* tell my alligator what to do." Eventually the alligator must be subdued. But this conquest may take several attempts on the child's part. If the child becomes inordinately excited or frightened, the psychiatrist makes suggestions—for instance, "Let's put him in a pen" or "Let's hit him with a tranquilizer gun."

When posttraumatic play occurs in the doctor's office with miniaturized toy symbols (e.g., a little girl doll or a tiny doll-family set), much of the therapeutic work is accomplished by talking about "that" symbol (e.g., the girl doll), not about the child herself. "How does that girl feel?" "What can that little girl do to escape?" the therapist asks, eventually suggesting things such as screaming very loudly, calling the police, or learning karate. Even if the child never actually screamed or called the police at the time of the trauma(s), she becomes aware of her new options. She is gradually becoming reempowered, and her world begins to broaden. Sometimes the therapist introduces his or her own game in this new phase of therapy. "Tea party," for instance, is a very useful piece of pretend because the child decides whom to invite and what conditions to impose on any offending guests (the "abuser"). For example, what would the alligator need to do in order to attend the bitten girl's party? Occasionally, the therapist turns to the child to ask what he or she might do if an uninvited snake insists on coming to the party. "Do you know how to call '911'? Let's try." But this is not always necessary. Play itself can be curative. The lessons are carried inside of the play metaphor itself. "What does the doll do after her attacker is subdued?" The child's future must be reconceptualized as the youngster plays.

Middle-phase cognitive-behavioral therapeutic approaches can be very helpful to traumatized children. Mapping out imaginary scenarios of what a boy could say when, for example, confronting the abuser in jail or running into the kidnapper again makes the lad feel more potent. Seeing a series of actions as potentially useful helps a girl to rebuild confidence. Facing feared items whenever possible in real life minimizes the fear of other such items. Realizing that growing older creates new alternatives for control brings the child a number of philosophical benefits. Again, these realizations must be integrated into the young person's mentality; they do not ordinarily enter the child's mind through anyone's reassurances. Scenario making and actual practice at facing feared objects—first with help and later alone—are particularly useful to children.

In the middle phase of psychotherapy, the therapist works with not only the miniaturized pretend world of play, a world dedicated to the child's past and future, but also the child's "here and now." Can he or she take over in some productive way at school? Can he or she learn self-defense or animal training? Mastery techniques are invaluable to previously overpowered youngsters. Can the child's social ties be expanded? Can he or she do something exemplary? Is there a hobby that could become something with which the child achieves excellence? And how does the child modify personality patterns that have been maladaptively set up to meet repeated or long-standing traumas? One boy whose father died in an airplane crash improved his outlook in life by taking over his school snack-bar business and making more money for his school than had ever been made by a child before. The boy's enthusiasm and pride improved each day that he excelled at this job. A girl who had become angry, irritable, and hypersexual after long-standing exposure to sexual abuse at nursery school regained her originally sweet demeanor once she practiced corrective dénouements in play and worked actively with her therapist in learning to refrain from her urges to sexually overcome other children. She talked at length in therapy about her disappointment in her parents' failure to protect her. The girl's own future as a mother and wife was extraordinarily important to her and remained a key ingredient in her play and talk during this middle phase of her psychotherapy.

The object of therapeutic interpretations of play, of artwork, and of the child's behaviors and symptoms is to demonstrate that the child was not personally responsible for the trauma, to modify any pathological defenses (e.g., identification with the aggressor or dissociation), to introduce a wider context within which to view the trauma (that the trauma is just a moment in a long, productive life), and to give the child new options for future behaviors. By the end of the middle phase of treatment, the child's trauma-specific fears should be resolved, nightmares should be on the wane, and repetitive behaviors should be virtually absent. The personality should be organized into stable, nonpathological patterns. Development should be progressing again at a normal rate and along normal lines.

End Phase

Toward the end of a child's psychotherapy, if the therapist has outside documentation and/or proof of the traumatic event, he or she often chooses to review these facts with the child, even if the child was too young to have formed a full verbal memory at the time that the event originally took place. Because children are known to retain implicit memories of their ordeals, making the story explicit toward the end of therapy helps a child to realize what future problems may relate to his or her experience. The child can become a conscious observer of the "self." The child's play can be linked by the psychiatrist to the child's reality. Discussion of the future can now deal directly with what happened to the child, not just as expressed through the activities of the dolls or in the drawings. Questions about sexuality can be linked by the therapist to the child's own experience. The therapist helps the child to form conscious, verbal memories of the trauma so that the context of the trauma can be understood within other contexts—the child's past life, present situation, and future life as an adult (Terr 1990).

I have often found that traumatized children, too young to have formed explicit memories of their traumas, become "stuck" in therapy toward the end phase of treatment if they are not given a narrative event by which to understand what happened, why they misbehaved afterward, and why they have been receiving treatment. Obviously, the real story cannot be offered to a child who is serving as a criminal witness or a child whose parents are considering a lawsuit on the child's behalf (Brown et al. 1999; Ceci and Bruch 1995; Terr 1994). But many of these young patients come to therapy entirely clear of any legal action, or the legal action is over. In these cases, presenting an unadulterated story to the child toward the end of treatment often stimulates progress in the child. Children must see their traumas in the context of their own lives before they can be released from the pressing requirements of those traumas: to behave in a fixed pattern (repetition) and to fear (avoidance and hyperalertness). They must gain perspective, considering their past in the course of a long, rich lifetime. Life books or scrapbooks that show snapshots and information about the child from as early as possible to the present are often useful in achieving perspective.

At the termination of therapy, most posttraumatic play should receive healthy endings that are nontraumatic and corrective. The young protagonist should survive in his or her play and master the events that he or she imagines. Gardner (1971) sees these dénouements as most easily arranged by "mutual storytelling." Play and art, however, flow as naturally as tale-telling in psychotherapy with traumatized children. Any creative technique allows children to find fuller contexts and meaningful corrections. The new endings encouraged in psychotherapy should not deny the awfulness of a traumatic event. Instead, they should include the event but go on to tell a tale of the child's ultimate survival and growth.

In all therapies for trauma, the therapist should use the principles of abreaction, context, and correction. These most often are respectively placed in beginning, middle, and end stages of treatment but can be handled out of order (e.g., the toddler who was given a tape of the basketball player with artificial legs *before* she was told of her amputated feet by the psychiatrist). In the end phase of trauma therapy, all sorts of corrections are in order—altruistic thoughts, stories of heroism, statements of faith or spirituality, ceremonies, uplifting poetry, and humor. Children who spontaneously offer such materials are well on their way to a resolution of their disorder.

Medication as an Adjunct to Individual Psychotherapy

Medication is useful in any of the phases of individual psychotherapy for childhood trauma. But medication is not a sole treatment for childhood trauma. Reempowerment and the achievement of context and perspective are too important in curing childhood traumas to be bypassed by treatments that consist of medications alone. Medications, however, can be used successfully for symptomatic or for more general relief.

Early in the course of childhood PTSD, a youngster may have difficulty going to school or playing outside because of fears of the traumatically offending object (e.g., a yellow taxi or a pit bull). In these situations, the β-blocking agent propranolol may be used at a dosage level calculated according to the child's size. It is administered approximately 40 minutes before an expected meeting with such an object. The physician also might consider propranolol divided in three doses throughout the day. In a small, uncontrolled study, propranolol (starting at 0.8 mg/kg/day and increased to 2.5 mg/kg/day over a 2-week period) was found to be useful (Famularo et al. 1988).

Clonidine, a central-acting agent (α_2-adrenergic presynaptic agonist), has long been used in the treatment of childhood Tourette's disorder and has recently been suggested for the treatment of PTSD. Although the only controlled study thus far has been on adult war veterans (Kolb et al. 1984), clonidine is said to generally increase the traumatized child's sense of well-being, helping especially with fears and hyperarousal. In a similar way, the tricyclic antidepressants imipramine and desipramine or a selective serotonin reuptake inhibitor (e.g., sertraline or fluoxetine) is sometimes given to children with PTSD to achieve a better sense of well-being and to mediate against the depression and/or panic that often accompanies trauma. The tricyclic antidepressant medications have been relatively well studied in children, although their use for PTSD has not been worked out. Fluoxetine and paroxetine have been administered separately to adults with PTSD, with some amelioration of symptoms (e.g., Nagy et al. 1993). They continue to be relatively untested in children, particularly for PTSD.

A benzodiazepine tranquilizer, especially diazepam or lorazepam, is very occasionally given at night to children with PTSD who are having so many nightmares or sleep interruptions that they cannot function at school the following day. These medications can also be given in the early stages of trauma to modify the extreme anxiety that occurs on coming home from the hospital or trying to go back to school. They work best when given on a daily basis and for no longer than 2–3 weeks running. A second 2- to 3-week course of this kind of tranquilizer can be administered during a different period of the child's recovery to treat another run of nightmares or to facilitate a new and difficult, but necessary, life adjustment.

Some children who have been sexually abused or otherwise repeatedly traumatized have the compulsive need to masturbate, to involve other children in sex, or to otherwise repeat their traumas in socially unacceptable ways. There may be some benefit in these instances to considering clomipramine (Flament et al. 1985) or fluvoxamine at the same dose schedule recommended for compulsive behaviors in children. Another possibility would be to consider using the selective serotonin reuptake inhibitors that have the potential side effect of loss of sexual interest (e.g., fluoxetine or paroxetine). This side effect might be the primary purpose for administrating such a drug, but again, its effectiveness in quieting the sexual behaviors of PTSD has not been studied in a controlled fashion.

Carbamazepine may be effective in children who have been repeatedly traumatized and show acting-out behaviors or unstable moods. In an open trial, Lipper et al. (1986) reported that carbamazepine was effective in adult PTSD. Carbamazepine has long been used for childhood seizures and thus is recognized as a standard medication in the pediatric population. When traumatized children engage in frequent self-mutilation, trichotillomania, or compulsive eating disturbances, carbamazepine may be of some use.

Eye Movement Desensitization and Restructuring as an Adjunct to Individual Psychotherapy

Eye movement desensitization and restructuring (EMDR), as developed by psychologist Francine Shapiro, has gained numbers of enthusiastic advocates in recent times (Greenwald 1999; Lovett and Shapiro 1999; Tinker et al. 1999). The therapist who uses this technique asks the child to follow the therapist's finger in a back-and-forth, straight pattern at about the pace of the tick of a clock. Patients who are very young may, instead, be given an alternating snap of the fingers at the side of the head (making a click sound and not touching the subject's ear). The youngster is encouraged to relax, to talk about the trauma, and to remember parts of it as the eyes (or the ears) experience this back-and-forth alternating stimulation. Many trauma therapists are enthusiastic about the results that are possible in connection with this technique (Scheck et al. 1998). Most, however, suggest EMDR as an adjunct to, not as a substitute for, the individual treatment of trauma. The biology of EMDR has not been clearly worked out. If, as some claim, trauma can be internally integrated and resolved simply by moving the eyes back and forth, this theory is clinically and biologically unproven at this time.

Further Courses of Psychotherapy

During development, a posttraumatic problem is likely to reemerge in certain phases (James 1989). A 6-year-old traumatized in an automobile accident, for example, may have a resurgence of symptoms at age 16 when the family car becomes available for driving. A sexually abused 3-year-old boy may experience a new outbreak of symptomatology when he begins to attend slumber parties or to date, or when he gets married. An adult who was traumatized early in childhood may encounter new outbreaks of symptomatology when his or her children reach the same age that he or she was when the traumatic event(s) occurred. Ordinarily, if a child was treated successfully at the time of the trauma, this later course of treatment is not as long or as intensive as the first.

New meanings are applied to old traumas by children as they develop cognitively (Terr

1990). In adolescence, negative attitudes about an event may fester and grow over months or years (Terr et al. 1997). When these changing ideas and philosophies are evident, it is often helpful for child patients to have a few psychotherapy sessions during adolescence in order to verbalize their newly forming ideas, to consider them in the context of the trauma and their future, and to work out new corrections for them.

Therapeutic Work With Parents and Families

If a parent is the perpetrator of a trauma against a child, that parent (and the nonperpetrating parent) must be worked with therapeutically to stop the abuses. Safeguards, such as temporary court custody and visits from social workers and nurses, are absolutely essential if the child is to remain at home (Terr and Watson 1968). Further safeguards of the child, such as frequent pediatric checkups, are also important. The nonabusing parent must become an active observer of and advocate for the child if the child is to continue living with the parents.

Most parents who abuse their child never fully admit to what they do to their child. This lack of admission is an issue for the courts, not for the psychotherapy session. Acceptance of responsibility for a crime is not absolutely necessary to the treatment process. One looks instead for parental attitudes toward the child that must change, small interactions that can be used as models for change, new interventions by the "observing" parent, and positive changes in the child's relationship with both parents. If there is little to no movement in a positive direction following a good course of parental therapy, the treating mental health professional may have to consider recommending permanent termination of parental rights (Terr and Watson 1968). If further abuses occur while a child and parents are receiving treatment, the above option must be seriously deliberated.

In cases in which the parents did not perpetrate any crimes against the traumatized child, these parents should be involved in any treatment efforts with the child. Parents are needed to report on the child's recent behaviors, to modify their own behaviors and words in order to handle the child therapeutically, to administer medications, and to provide ongoing help to the suffering child. Many times the parents are experiencing extreme anxiety of their own (Terr 1989b).

One option would be to see one or both parents for 10–15 minutes at the beginning of the child's session. Often, parents must undergo their own psychotherapeutic sessions every week or every few weeks. They also may be asked to attend all or some of the child's interviews. The bulk of the time when parents attend their child's psychotherapy is spent with the child, but the parents may offer their own observations (in the child's presence) of the child's behavior at home and school so that the child can hear how he or she is doing. The therapist also may show in such sessions how the child is being handled in treatment (to inform the parents about what they might observe and/or how they might respond).

Erna Furman (1957, 1979) developed a treatment technique called "filial therapy," in which the therapist offers interpretations to nonabusing parents, who then impart these interpretations at home to their child. This technique applies to either single-incident or long-standing childhood trauma, although it is unlikely that an entire treatment of PTSD could be accomplished this way. Another technique, child-centered family treatment, developed by Anna Ornstein (1981), has potential applications to long-standing childhood trauma, even in cases in which the parent(s) brought on the trauma. In the course of learning how to relate better to the youngster, parents may be able to alter their potential for sexual or physical abuse. Or they may be able to stop forcing a child into silence about his or her trauma and to facilitate a child's verbal expressions.

Group Psychotherapy

To complete psychotherapy—individual or group—with children, the youngsters must experience abreaction, context, and correction. Group psychotherapies for traumatized children can be close-ended or open-ended, but they must include these processes. Many outpatient groups for children with PTSD begin on a set day and end on another prearranged day (i.e., close-ended). Hence, a group for children who endured the suicide of a parent would begin once enough such children have been signed up and may last for 20 weeks or so. Many groups for sexually abused boys, for instance, would have to wait to begin until six to eight such boys were available to start the group. Some groups with definite cognitive-behavioral agendas (e.g., 12 sessions for physically abused children of the ghetto) operate almost like "classes," with a certain number of topics to be covered and a preordained order in which these topics will be introduced. Groups of this type may offer children an opportunity to work together on a large art project, a piece of rap music, poems, or psychodrama, as part of the process of expressing trauma and then giving it context.

Open-ended groups are more often seen in inpatient settings where children are being discharged and admitted; in generalized trauma groups in which all sorts of traumas are discussed in a mixed, open forum; and in those instances in which traumatized children are put into groups with children who have other diagnoses.

Group therapies are potentially very helpful and are far less costly than the long-term individual treatments. They carry, however, two serious risks: contagion and worsening of the child's traumatic condition. Trauma is one of the most contagious of psychiatric disorders. It is, therefore, important for the leader of the group of sexually traumatized children, for instance, to organize the group according to only one type of sexual trauma or to minimize the details that the children tell one another about their own particular experiences. It should be made clear to the children in such a group that they will be able to express their individual stories in individual sessions. The group will be reserved for sharing of creative expressions of the trauma, for helping one another recognize maladaptive personality patterns, for using the group process itself to aid participants in gaining control over the previously uncontrollable, and for exploring displacements and transferences of personal problems into the group at large.

Those persons running therapeutic groups for children must be mental health or educational professionals who have taken courses or have received individual supervision about the group process. Group psychotherapy is a potentially helpful and very strong "medicine" for children. There are beginning, middle, and end phases of group therapy that correspond to the beginning, middle, and end phases of individual treatment of PTSD, as discussed earlier in this chapter. Children who have been seriously traumatized often need both individual therapy and group work. Groups, however, can be important outlets for songs, poetry, drama, and art inspired by trauma as well as an environment that facilitates acquisition of more socially acceptable behaviors and better management of fears (through group-engendered behavior modification techniques). This approach is an excellent adjunct to outpatient therapy or to the more intensive residential treatments of traumatized children.

Preventive Strategies

One cannot stop natural disasters from happening, but earlier warnings may eventually lead to more effective evacuations of people who face volcanic eruptions, earthquakes, floods, and so forth. Thorough treatment of childhood traumas also may stop certain reenactment-based human disasters from occurring to others. Dorothy Otnow Lewis's group, for instance, found that delinquent children who went on to commit murder had, among other factors, backgrounds of childhood trauma (Lewis et al. 1985). Reenactment is a powerful unconscious incentive to violence. Early treatment during childhood very likely would have helped the juvenile offenders in Lewis's group. By quickly and effectively treating all children who are victims of violence, we may be able to reduce the numbers of abuses, attacks, and mayhem in the generation to come. Child victims tend to be the next generation's victimizers as well as its victims. Spousal abuse, drug misuse, hospitalizations for psychiatric illnesses of all types, and a variety of very-difficult-to-treat mental disorders, including dissociation, multiple personality disorder, borderline personality disorder, and antisocial personality disorder, often spring from childhood trauma. It certainly appears that effective treatment of PTSD *in childhood* is the best possible prevention for these problems in adult life.

Children are potentially traumatically affected by the unexpected deaths of their peers or of their peers' parents, attacks on classmates, kidnappings in the neighborhood, and any death or disfigurement involving someone from their school. They also may be affected by the shocking real-life events they see on television or even the fictional programming that they encounter. An activity book for children includes suggested drawings and essays that may help a child work out feelings around violence (Garbarino 1993). Students also need an opportunity to discuss shocking matters at school with teachers, social workers, psychiatrists, and others who have learned group techniques for childhood trauma. Often, play, artwork, drama, poetry, or music, when combined with an opportunity to talk over this kind of frightening event, leads to some closure and sense of relief.

Grouping is very important in large-scale interventions. If an elementary school, for instance, were to organize prevention groups following the hit-and-run death of one of its students, that student's closest friends would be placed in a small group of six to eight who would be treated for several weeks by a mental health professional. The student's classmates (other than the closest friends) would have, perhaps, two 90-minute sessions with a teacher to make drawings about and to speak about their dead peer. The rest of the school might have an assembly to speak of their schoolmate's life, how it feels to grieve for a person you once knew, and how accident prevention might be a suitable memorial for the child. Students could participate and offer comments into microphones spaced about the auditorium. Prepared poetry could be read by a few students who knew the child who was killed. Very strong leadership is necessary in such large interventions, but mental health problems may be prevented in this way.

The objectives of large-scale interventions for children are similar to the objectives of "mini-marathon groups" for all ages (Terr 1992b). First, the story is shared by various members of the group, each of whom expresses how he or she experienced the event. From this telling of stories, the group members learn that each person experiences a traumatic event differently. The leader emphasizes the individuality of experience. No two people go through the same happening in the same way. Next, symptoms are shared—for example, having to sleep in a bed with someone else, having frightening repeated dreams, fearing similar stimuli. Here, shows of hands along with the individual testimonies confirm to the group that most everyone is "in the same boat." The presence of a symptom or two is very common in persons shortly after traumatic events. Various self-help techniques may abate these symptoms. The leader tells the group how to try possibilities such as corrective re-dreaming and behavior modification. Participants are urged to tell a few stories about how these things may already have worked for them. The type of symptoms and the number of symptoms that would necessitate a "checkup" at the pediatrician's or the psychiatrist's office are noted. Possible future problems, such as listlessness, withdrawal, or futurelessness, are brought up as reasons to seek help. Finally, the group shares stories of heroism and of overcoming. If a child died, good things that the child did and the love that the child showed to others are emphasized. Ways to prevent further such tragedies are also discussed.

Many more large-scale group techniques will be worked out within the next few years. Any way to provide simultaneous prevention for large numbers of children will be welcomed. The general aims are abreaction, context, and correction. Television has already experimented with large-group presentations for children during the Gulf War (Terr 1992a). We expect improvement and increased sophistication of these techniques, as well as of Internet use for children, over time.

References

Black D, Kaplan T: Father kills mother: issues and problems encountered by a child psychiatric team. Br J Psychiatry 153:624–630, 1988

Bloch DA, Silber E, Perry SE: Some factors in the emotional reaction of children to disaster. Am J Psychiatry 113:416–422, 1956

Brown D, Scheflin A, Hammond DC: Memory, Trauma, Treatment, and the Law. New York, WW Norton, 1999

Ceci S, Bruch M: Jeopardy in the Courtroom: A Scientific Analysis of Children's Testimony. Washington, DC, American Psychological Association, 1995

Famularo R, Kinscherff R, Fenton T: Propranolol treatment for childhood posttraumatic stress disorder, acute type—a pilot study. American Journal of Diseases of Children 142:1244–1247, 1988

Flament MF, Rapoport JL, Berg CJ, et al: Clomipramine treatment of childhood obsessive-compulsive disorder: a double-blind controlled study. Arch Gen Psychiatry 42:977–983, 1985

Furman E: Treatment of under-fives by way of their parents. Psychoanal Study Child 12:250–262, 1957

Furman E: Filial therapy, in Basic Handbook of Child Psychiatry (Noshpitz JD, Editor-in-Chief), Vol 3: Therapeutic Interventions. Edited by Harrison SI. New York, Basic Books, 1979, pp 149–158

Gackenback J, Schillig B: Lucid dreams: the content of conscious awareness of dreaming during the dream. Journal of Mental Imagery 7:1–13, 1983

Garbarino J: Let's Talk About Living in a World With Violence. Chicago, IL, Erikson Institute, 1993

Gardner RA: Therapeutic Communication With Children: The Mutual Storytelling Technique. New York, Science House, 1971

Greenwald R: Eye Movement Desensitization and Reprocessing (EMDR) in Child and Adolescent Psychiatry. New York, Jason Aronson, 1999

Herman JL: Trauma and Recovery. New York, Basic Books, 1992

James B: Treating Traumatized Children: New Insights and Creative Interventions. Lexington, MA, Lexington Books, 1989

Kipper DA: The desensitization of war-induced fears. Current Psychiatric Therapies 16:41–47, 1976

Kolb LC, Burris BC, Griffiths S: Propranolol and clonidine in the treatment of post-traumatic stress disorders of war, in Post-Traumatic Stress Disorder: Psychological and Biological Sequelae. Edited by van der Kolk BA. Washington, DC, American Psychiatric Press, 1984, pp 97–107

LaBerge S, Levitan L, Dement WC: Lucid dreaming: physiological correlates of consciousness during REM sleep. Journal of Mind and Behavior 7:251–258, 1986

Levy DM: Trends in therapy, III: release therapy. Am J Orthopsychiatry 9:713–736, 1939

Lewis DO, Moy E, Jackson LD, et al: Biopsychosocial characteristics of children who later murder: a prospective study. Am J Psychiatry 142:1161–1167, 1985

Lipper S, Davidson JRT, Grady TA, et al: Preliminary study of carbamazepine in post-traumatic stress disorder. Psychosomatics 27:849–854, 1986

Lovett J, Shapiro F: Small Wonders: Healing Childhood Trauma With EMDR. New York, Free Press, 1999

Maclean G: Psychic trauma and traumatic neurosis: play therapy with a four-year-old boy. Canadian Psychiatric Association Journal 22:71–76, 1977

Nagy LM, Morgan CA, Southwick SM, et al: Open prospective trial of fluoxetine for posttraumatic stress disorder. J Clin Psychopharmacol 13:107–113, 1993

Ornstein A: Self-pathology in childhood: developmental and clinical considerations. Psychiatr Clin North Am 4:435–453, 1981

Pynoos RS, Eth S: Children traumatized by witnessing acts of personal violence: homicide, rape, and suicide behavior, in Post-Traumatic Stress Disorder in Children. Edited by Eth S, Pynoos RS. Washington, DC, American Psychiatric Press, 1985, pp 17–43

Pynoos RS, Eth S: Witness to violence: the child interview. Journal of American Academy of Child Psychiatry 25:306–319, 1986

Scheck MM, Schaeffer JA, Gillette C: Brief psychological intervention with traumatized young women: the efficacy of eye movement desensitization and reprocessing. J Trauma Stress 11:25–44, 1998

Shapiro SH: Preventive analysis following a trauma: a 4½-year-old girl witnesses a stillbirth. Psychoanal Study Child 28:249–285, 1973

Silverman I, Geer J: The elimination of a recurrent nightmare by desensitization of a related phobia. Behav Res Ther 6:109–111, 1968

Terr LC: Children of Chowchilla: a study of psychic trauma. Psychoanal Study Child 34:547–623, 1979

Terr LC: "Forbidden games": post-traumatic child's play. Journal of the American Academy of Child Psychiatry 20:741–760, 1981

Terr LC: Play therapy and psychic trauma: a preliminary report, in Handbook of Play Therapy. Edited by Schaefer CE, O'Connor KJ. New York, Wiley, 1983, pp 308–319

Terr LC: Family anxiety after traumatic events. J Clin Psychiatry 50 (11, suppl):15–19, 1989a

Terr LC: Treating psychic trauma in children: a preliminary discussion. J Trauma Stress 2:3–10, 1989b

Terr LC: Too Scared to Cry: Psychic Trauma in Childhood. New York, Harper & Row, 1990

Terr L: Childhood trauma: an outline and overview. Am J Psychiatry 148:10–20, 1991

Terr LC: Large-group preventive treatment techniques for use after disaster, in Responding to Disaster: A Guide for Mental Health Professionals. Edited by Austin LS. Washington, DC, American Psychiatric Press, 1992a, pp 81–99

Terr LC: Mini-marathon groups: psychological "first aid" following disasters. Bull Menninger Clin 56:76–86, 1992b

Terr LC: Unchained Memories: True Stories of Traumatic Memories, Lost & Found. New York, Basic Books, 1994

Terr L: Beyond Love and Work: Why Adults Need to Play. New York, Scribner, 1999

Terr LC, Watson AS: The battered child rebrutalized: ten cases of medical-legal confusion. Am J Psychiatry 124:1432–1439, 1968

Terr LC, Bloch DA, Michel BA, et al: Children's symptoms in the wake of Challenger. Am J Psychiatry 154:744–751, 1997

Tinker RH, Wilson SA, Dutton R, et al: Through the Eyes of a Child: EMDR With Children. New York, WW Norton, 1999

Webb NB (ed): Play Therapy With Children in Crisis: Individual, Family, and Group Treatments. New York, Guilford, 1999

Winnicott DW: Playing and Reality. New York, Basic Books, 1971

14

Obsessive-Compulsive Disorder in Children

Jennifer B. Freeman, Ph.D.

Henrietta L. Leonard, M.D.

Douglas Beer, M.D.

John March, M.D., M.P.H.

Susan E. Swedo, M.D.

Although it has been almost a century since obsessive-compulsive disorder (OCD) was first described in children and adolescents (Janet 1903), only recently has the illness been systematically studied to elucidate its phenomenology, neurobiology, and treatment in younger populations. The issue of potential subtypes of OCD within the pediatric age group also is receiving increasing attention. In this chapter, we address the assessment and treatment of OCD in children and adolescents, including investigational interventions. In addition, the American Academy of Child and Adolescent Psychiatry's (AACAP; 1998) "Practice Parameters for the Assessment and Treatment of Children and Adolescents With Obsessive-Compulsive Disorder" and the "Expert Consensus Guidelines: Treatment of Obsessive-Compulsive Disorder" (March et al. 1997) are presented in the context of this discussion.

Epidemiological findings suggest that childhood OCD affects approximately 1 in 200 children (Douglas et al. 1995; Flament et al. 1990; Valleni-Basile et al. 1994). For many children, the disorder significantly impairs academic, social, and family functioning yet is often underdiagnosed and undertreated (Leonard et al. 1993). On a global level, the same categories of obsessions and compulsions appear to extend across both the life span and cultures (Hanna 1995; Thomsen 1995). Despite an apparent core set of symptoms, however, systematic studies have found considerable heterogeneity in the onset, course, and specific symptom picture among children and adolescents with OCD (Flament et al. 1990; Hanna 1995; Swedo et al. 1989; Thomsen 1995).

Subtypes

Most early attempts to develop subtypes of OCD were based on the specific content of the obsessions and compulsions experienced by a patient. However, as is the case with adults, 90% of the children in the National Institute of Mental Health (NIMH) study reported that their obsessions and compulsions changed in both content and severity over time (Rettew et al. 1992; Swedo et al. 1989). Thus, it appears unlikely that consideration of the content of obsessions or compulsions alone will lead us to identify specific disorder subtypes.

The clinical description of children and adolescents with OCD characterized by an episodic course with dramatic and acute symptom exacerbations interspersed with periods of relative symptom quiescence has led to further exploration of potential subtypes (Leonard et al. 1993; Swedo et al. 1989, 1998). The proposal is that a distinctive subgroup of patients with neuropsychiatric disorders exists who could be identified by the following criteria: 1) presence of OCD or a tic disorder; 2) prepubertal onset of symptoms; 3) episodic course of symptom severity; 4) association with group A β-hemolytic streptococcal (GABHS) infection; and 5) association with neurological abnormalities (Swedo et al. 1997, 1998). Additionally, in these cases, the comorbid symptoms of emotional lability, acute separation anxiety, motoric hyperactivity, impulsivity, and distractibility are often episodic and related to GABHS infections (Swedo et al. 1998). These criteria reflect an underlying hypothesis that autoimmunity mediates the neuropsychiatric symptoms; hence, the group was designated as pediatric autoimmune neuropsychiatric disorders associated with streptococcal infections (PANDAS) (Swedo et al. 1997, 1998).

Comorbidity

The assessment of comorbidity is crucial for effective treatment planning because other diagnoses are common in children and adolescents with OCD (Geller et al. 1996; Swedo et al. 1989; Thomsen 1995). Diagnoses that commonly co-occur with OCD include major depression and other mood disorders, multiple anxiety disorders, tic disorders, and disruptive behavior disorders, particularly attention-deficit/hyperactivity disorder and oppositional defiant disorder. Of these, only tic disorders are thought to have a shared genetic etiology with OCD (Leonard et al. 1992; Pauls et al. 1995), and the relation with attention-deficit/hyperactivity disorder merits further study (Pauls et al. 1993). Several studies have reported that, compared with OCD without tics, tic-associated OCD may be different with regard to specific obsessions and compulsions, more familial, and more common in boys and early-onset cases (Holzer et al. 1994; Leckman et al. 1995, 1997). Tic-associated OCD also may constitute a potential subtype of the disorder. Thus, comorbidity in OCD is common and frequently requires its own diagnostic and treatment interventions.

Clinical Assessment

Because of the secretiveness of many patients with OCD, the interviewer must consider the diagnosis and ask specifically about obsessions or compulsions, particularly when depression or anxiety is evident. Suspicions should be raised by children or adolescents who start to spend excessive amounts of time in grooming, washing, or dressing rituals or in doing homework. Additionally, because young children sometimes do not identify their obsessions and compulsions as excessive or unreasonable (Swedo et al. 1989), this part of the criteria set does not have to be applied to children.

Differential Diagnosis

When evaluating a child with recurrent thoughts or repetitive behaviors, it is important to consider whether the symptoms are developmentally appropriate. Developmental rituals of childhood are normal at certain ages, although they may be performed in a stereotypic or rule-bound fashion. Additionally, OCD rituals are associated with a later age at onset and are usually more dramatic, persistent, and distressing than developmental rituals (Evans et al. 1997; Leonard et al. 1990).

The differential diagnosis of OCD includes several disorders with obsessional features and compulsive behaviors. These include depressive and anxiety disorders, eating disorders, somatoform disorders, impulse-control disorders, and tic disorders (Francis and Gragg 1996). If the obsessions or compulsions are particularly bizarre, and seen by the patient as reasonable, a diagnosis of psychosis should be considered.

Stereotypies in developmentally delayed children may resemble OCD rituals in that the former are repetitive formalized behaviors. However, stereotypies are usually simple and do not appear to be preceded by an obsession; they are not ego-dystonic, although it is difficult to assess this because of verbal skills disabilities in these patients. Reports suggest that autistic stereotypies may respond to the serotonin reuptake inhibitor (SRI) clomipramine (Gordon et al. 1992; McDougle et al. 1996), which raises some theoretical questions about the underlying etiology of repetitive behaviors.

The frequent association of OCD and tic disorders (Holzer et al. 1994; Leckman et al. 1994; Leonard et al. 1992; Pauls et al. 1986) requires that rituals and tics be distinguished because each requires different treatments. Although motor tics can be preceded by a sensation or an "urge," they are not typically initiated by a thought or accompanied by anxiety (Leckman et al. 1993). Behaviors such as touching, tapping, spitting, or skipping may represent either a tic or a ritual, so careful assessment is required. For an excellent review of Tourette's disorder, the reader is directed to Cohen and Leckman (1994).

Assessment Techniques

In addition to completing developmental, personal, and family medical and psychiatric histories, and a current assessment of social, academic, and family functioning, a comprehensive evaluation (American Academy of Child and Adolescent Psychiatry 1997) should identify the full range of current and past symptoms of OCD and comorbid diagnoses. Detailed information about onset and course of symptoms also may assist in identifying subtypes. Two valuable resources provide guidelines for the assessment of children and adolescents with OCD. The "Expert Consensus Guidelines: Treatment of Obsessive-Compulsive Disorder" (March et al. 1997) and the AACAP "Practice Parameters for the Assessment and Treatment of Children and Adolescents With Obsessive-Compulsive Disorder" (American Academy of Child and Adolescent Psychiatry 1998) both present detailed reviews of the literature and expert advice on a broad range of practical clinical issues.

In combination with a clinical interview, several diagnostic interviews and rating scales often used in research studies are available to assess OCD in children and adolescents. Rating scales, such as the widely used Children's Yale-Brown Obsessive Compulsive Scale (CY-BOCS; Scahill et al. 1997b), are also important for a complete assessment. Part of that scale, the CY-BOCS Symptom Checklist, is particularly useful in a clinical interview to elicit specific symptoms. It is relatively easy for the clinician to administer and also can be used to document baseline severity of symptoms and change in severity over time.

A child presenting with an acute onset or significant, dramatic, unexplained clinical exacerbation of OCD, with or without tics, requires a thorough assessment of recent or concomitant medical illnesses, including seemingly benign upper respiratory tract infections (American Academy of Child and Adolescent Psychiatry 1998; March et al. 1997). The clinician should inquire about any bacterial or viral illnesses in the last several months and whether the patient has a family history of rheumatic fever or Sydenham's chorea. Laboratory studies such as throat culture, antistreptolysin O (ASO) titer, and antistreptococcal deoxyribonuclease B (anti-DNase B) titer may aid in the diagnosis (American Academy of Child and Adolescent Psychiatry 1998).

Treatment

Selection of Treatment(s)

Treatment planning for children and adolescents with OCD requires consideration of not just the diagnosis but also comorbidity and psychosocial factors. Family and sociocultural factors, specific OCD symptoms, developmental level, and adaptive functioning all can influence compliance and/or treatment response, and no simple prescription from this chapter can take the place of individualized assessment. Treatment of OCD may incorporate several different techniques depending on the specifics of the child.

The "Expert Consensus Guideline" series (March et al. 1997) and the AACAP (1998) "Practice Parameters for the Assessment and Treatment of Children and Adolescents With Obsessive-Compulsive Disorder" also provide important information about treatment. Based on these guidelines, only two treatment modalities have been shown empirically to be effective in treating OCD symptomatology: 1) cognitive-behavioral therapy (CBT; specifically the technique of exposure with response prevention) and 2) pharmacological treatment with SRIs. No clear empirical data currently exist to determine whether one should begin with CBT, medication, or both. However, the AACAP practice parameters favor CBT as the initial treatment of choice for younger children as well as for children and adolescents with milder symptoms and without significant comorbidity. Cognitive-behavioral treatment has the advantages of apparent durability of treatment effects and avoidance of potential side effects of medication. In specific cases, however, an antiobsessional medication may be the initial treatment method because of concerns with urgency, expense, anxiety associated with behavioral treatment, lack of trained clinicians, insufficient cognitive ability to participate in CBT, lack of family support, or individual factors.

In the following section, we review a variety of treatments for pediatric OCD, with special emphasis on CBT and SRIs. It should be recognized, however, that other types of individual and family psychotherapy may play an important organizing role in the overall treatment plan for children and adolescents with OCD. These treatments are briefly discussed as well.

Cognitive-Behavioral Treatment

As is common in other areas of child and adolescent psychopathology, research into the effectiveness of various treatment methodologies for OCD in children and adolescents has lagged behind similar research with adults. It has been recognized for some time that CBT may be the most effective long-term treatment for adults with OCD (Foa and Kozak 1996). A number of controlled studies with adults have found that treatment with exposure with response prevention leads to higher rates of positive response, more durable treatment gains, and greater symptom reduction (Foa et al. 1984; Greist 1994; Steketee 1993). There are, however, methodological concerns with some of these studies. Only more recently has the effectiveness of CBT in children and adolescents been more carefully reviewed and studied (March 1995; Piacentini 1999). Despite this gradual advancement in the literature and expert consensus about using CBT as a first-line treatment of choice in children and adolescents, empirical studies with younger populations continue to lag behind. The following review of CBT includes 1) a more specific description of exposure with response prevention; 2) a brief overview of existing standardized/manualized protocols, open trials, and controlled trials of CBT for pediatric OCD; and 3) a description of other relevant cognitive-behavioral techniques.

Overview of Exposure With Response Prevention

In exposure with response prevention, the patient is exposed to the feared situation, and the response (i.e., the ritual or avoidance behavior) is prevented until anxiety decreases on its own. For example, the child with contamination fears and washing rituals may be asked to touch items in the garbage and then not be allowed to wash his or her hands. The effectiveness of exposure with response prevention is most often attributed to the theoretical concepts of habituation and extinction. Patients gradually learn that their anxious response decreases over time and that with prolonged exposure to the stimulus the anxiety can be reduced without performing compulsions (Francis and Gragg 1996). By combining exposure with response prevention, the patient learns both that the feared consequences do not take place and that the resultant anxiety diminishes on its own (leading to the cessation of the obsessive-compulsive symptom) (Foa and Kozak 1986). With regard to the mechanism of action in exposure with response prevention, adult OCD research suggests that both exposure and response prevention are "active" ingredients in treatment (Foa and Kozak 1996).

Treatment with exposure with response prevention generally involves a three-phase approach composed of information gathering, therapist-assisted exposure with response prevention, and homework assignments (March and Mulle 1998). Exposure most commonly progresses in a graded manner according to a symptom hierarchy of increasingly anxiety-producing stimuli. The patient and therapist work together in early sessions to generate items for the hierarchy (e.g., by listing all symptoms) and rate the severity of anxiety on a scale that the child can comprehend. This collaboration serves to decrease the child's fear of the unknown and allows him or her to gain mastery. Although new items are frequently added to the hierarchy and anxiety ratings altered, the list ideally represents the total picture of the patient's OCD symptomatology and provides a model of how treatment will progress over time.

Exposure itself can be either imaginal or in vivo. Imaginal exposure may be used first because it is less anxiety-producing for the patient (e.g., imagining yourself touching items in the garbage before actually trying it). However, imaginal exposure is also necessary for obsessions that occur in the absence of corresponding rituals or cannot be enacted in vivo (e.g., harming another person). The relative ease of implementing in vivo exposure depends on the nature of the patient's symptoms. For example, touching a contaminant such as dirt or garbage is easily completed in the office, whereas fears and rituals specific to the home or school setting will be more difficult to practice in a typical treatment session. As a result, exposure may need to take place in the community or via homework assignments. Overall, it is extremely important that exposures continue until anxiety is significantly reduced and that children and adolescents feel control over progression through their hierarchies. It is crucial to gain the child's cooperation and willingness to participate because the child has to tolerate the significant stress of implementing the program.

Overview of Cognitive-Behavioral Therapy Trials for Pediatric Obsessive-Compulsive Disorder

Only a few years ago, a review of the behavioral treatment literature for childhood OCD yielded primarily single case studies. March (1995) found 32 investigations—25 were single case reports and the rest were single case studies—and all but 1 reported benefit. Most of this early literature, however, was limited by significant methodological concerns (Piacentini 1999). Taking into consideration these concerns, March (1995) summarized, "Although empirical support remains weak, CBT may be the psychotherapeutic treatment of choice for children and adolescents with OCD" (p. 7). Overall, this early literature provided necessary support for the more recent development of standardized protocols and controlled trials.

Recently, several researchers have begun to develop and test manualized treatment programs, based on exposure with response prevention, for the treatment of pediatric OCD (for an excellent review, see Piacentini 1999). These protocols allow for systematic application of treatment but also have included some important adaptations to address developmental issues, comorbid emotional and behavioral disturbances, and family involvement (Piacentini 1999). Preliminary open-trial research suggests that these treatment programs are indeed quite promising (Franklin et al. 1998; March et al. 1994; Scahill et al. 1996).

Perhaps the best-known CBT protocol for children and adolescents with OCD is that of March et al. (1994) titled "How I Ran OCD Off My Land." This program is based on a framework of exposure with response prevention but also includes cognitive interventions. The treatment, which consists of 16 weekly sessions, places OCD in a neurobehavioral medical context and attempts to externalize the OCD symptoms for both children and their parents. In addition to graded exposure with response prevention, the program incorporates family psychoeducation (e.g., discussing OCD as a medical illness, disengaging family members from the child's symptoms), cognitive training (e.g., constructive self-talk, coping thoughts, self-administered positive reinforcement), and "mapping OCD" (e.g., developing an exposure hierarchy within a narrative context). Systematic trials are ongoing, and the manual is currently used throughout the United States. For more specific information about treatment implementation, the reader is referred to the published manual (March and Mulle 1998).

No other treatment manuals have been published, but some research groups are currently testing variations on the protocol by March and Mulle. For example, Franklin et al. (1998) tested a simplified version of the March et al. (1994) treatment by omitting anxiety management training and focusing on only the exposure with response prevention component of therapy. Additionally, the authors compared the efficacy of weekly and intensive treatment (or treatment "dose"). Overall, the treatment was highly effective, and there were no effects of either treatment "dose" or baseline medication status.

In the only controlled study to date of CBT for OCD in children and adolescents, De Haan et al. (1998) compared exposure with response prevention plus cognitive restructuring with clomipramine in 22 youngsters for a 12-week period. Both treatments produced positive effects, but the exposure with response prevention was significantly more effective than clomipramine in terms of both response rate and reduction of symptom severity. Several large-scale controlled trials of CBT for childhood OCD are currently being completed across the United States (Piacentini 1999). These results are expected to provide important new information for clinicians treating OCD in children and adolescents.

The role of the family in the individual behavior therapy of patients with OCD is particularly important and only recently has received empirical attention (Piacentini et al. 1994; Scahill et al. 1996). Frequently, parents participate in rituals in response to their child's requests or distress (e.g., providing reassurances, tying "dirty" shoelaces) and sometimes overreact to the child's behavior. The extent to which they need to interrupt or prevent rituals may vary among individual families. Although ultimate treatment success is dependent on the child's cooperation, recent studies suggest that concurrent family intervention focused on removing parents from their children's rituals is important. Interestingly, preliminary evidence also suggests that parents can play a role as co-therapists in the behavioral treatment and still not be "overinvolved" or "enabling" (Knox et al. 1996). Developmental differences (particularly with regard to understanding cognitive techniques) and family involvement are particularly relevant to the treatment of OCD in children during the early childhood years. Despite the great increase in treatment research, no psychotherapy trials have focused on children who are younger than 8 years. This remains a significant gap in the literature.

Overall, research done to date supports the efficacy of exposure with response prevention–based methods for pediatric OCD. However, much remains unknown. Improvement tends to be largely maintained at follow-up, but more data and longer-term follow-up are clearly needed. The role of combined psychopharmacological treatment also needs more intensive study. Because relapse commonly follows medication discontinuation (Leonard et al. 1989), March et al. (1994) suggested that booster behavior therapy may prevent relapse when medications are discontinued.

The above-reviewed research evidence also underscores the need for developmentally sensitive interventions when implementing CBT. Often the child may view his or her own symptoms, and may experience his or her distress or interference, very differently than the parents do (Berg et al. 1989). For example, a younger child may not identify his or her obsessions as distressing, even if they appear that way to others. The younger child also may have difficulty rating his or her own symptoms and accurately reporting (particularly historical information), which creates unique obstacles for the therapist.

Other Cognitive-Behavioral Interventions

As described earlier in this chapter, other cognitive-behavioral techniques play a significant role in many exposure with response prevention–based treatment programs for children and adolescents. The program designed by March et al. (1994) combines exposure with response prevention with anxiety management techniques or a "tool kit" that the youngster can use to manage thoughts and feelings related to exposure tasks. Techniques such as relaxation training, breathing-control training, and cognitive restructuring have all proven effective with other child anxiety disorders (Kendall 1994). Interestingly, however, these added components do not appear to affect directly obsessions or compulsions (Piacentini 1999). Instead, relaxation and other techniques are thought to help children cope with the high anxiety produced by exposure with response prevention tasks (Kearney and Silverman 1990).

Although one recent study suggested that cognitive therapy alone may be as effective as exposure with response prevention in adults, this has not been shown with a younger population or replicated in adults (Abramowitz 1997; Kearney and Silverman 1990). Other cognitive therapy techniques (e.g., satiation, hypnosis) have been tried in children with varying success (March 1995). Notably, thought stopping has been included in the treatments of obsessions only or obsessional slowness (March 1995). Additional behavioral techniques (e.g., flooding, extinction, habit reversal) also may play some role in an overall treatment package. Flooding (i.e., prolonged exposure to the most anxiety-provoking stimuli) has been used successfully in adolescents with OCD (Harris and Wiebe 1992); however, expert consensus is that children should receive graded exposure with response prevention with goals under the control of the patient (March and Mulle 1998). Extinction (i.e., the removal of positive reinforcement) may play a role in specific situations (Francis 1988). Habit reversal may have a role for patients with comorbid tic or trichotillomania symptoms or complex ticlike rituals (March 1995). Children and adolescents with obsessional slowness or primarily obsessions without rituals also may respond to techniques such as modeling or shaping (Ratnasuriya et al. 1991).

Conclusions Regarding Cognitive-Behavioral Therapy

Clearly, and as recommended by expert consensus guidelines (American Academy of Child and Adolescent Psychiatry 1998; March et al. 1997), CBT should be considered, either with or without pharmacotherapy, in the child or adolescent with OCD. As with any other disorder, the unique issues of the individual child and family play a role in weighing which specific combination of modalities is important. In general, patients with rituals who are motivated and able to monitor and report symptoms and who do not have significant comorbidity are the most likely to show a good response to CBT (American Academy of Child and Adolescent Psychiatry 1998). Unfortunately, despite its applicability in a majority of cases, behavior therapy is frequently not implemented for OCD when appropriate.

Individual and Family Psychotherapy

Freud's famous psychoanalysis of the "Rat Man," a description of which was published in 1909, illustrated how obsessive-compulsive neurosis was the manifestation of an unconscious dynamic conflict and that the specific obsessive-compulsive symptom had meaning that was theoretically understandable (Esman 1989; Freud 1909/1955). Although Freud did not treat any children with this disorder, he emphasized the importance of recalling the obsessions and compulsive behaviors of childhood in the analyses of adults. Whether the specific obsessive-compulsive symptoms have unique meaning to the person has come into debate with the understanding that a finite number of symptom constellations exist and that they are quite similar from patient to patient. Although insight-oriented dynamic psychotherapy has historically been the primary intervention for the obsessional patient, the disorder has, for the most part, been refractory to this approach regardless of patient age, and this therapy would no longer be considered the primary or sole treatment of choice (March et al. 1995a; Salzman and Thaler 1981).

Individual psychotherapy may play an important role in treating the accompanying anxiety and depressive symptoms of OCD, in teaching coping skills, in addressing comorbid diagnoses and family issues, and in helping to improve peer and family relationships. Typically, OCD has affected the child's life in many ways, such that a comprehensive psychotherapeutic approach becomes necessary. Additionally, the issue of obsessional defenses, obsessive-compulsive personality disorder, and perfectionism may be more amenable to insight-oriented psychotherapy. Although their relation to OCD is not well understood, they are believed to constitute different phenomena.

As noted in the earlier discussion of standardized CBT programs, systematic family intervention has become a recognized component of OCD treatment for children and adolescents (Knox et al. 1996; Piacentini et al. 1994). Although there are no efficacy data for children and adolescents, a multifamily group behavioral treatment (in which patients and family members jointly participate in group sessions) was shown to be effective with adults (Van Noppen et al. 1997). Less is known, however, about the efficacy of non-CBT-based family treatment models. These models, however, deserve further study, particularly in the area of early-onset/early-childhood OCD.

For example, family therapy may be required to delineate boundaries of the various members and to understand how the illness affects others. The effect of the child's symptoms on the family is usually significant. Parents and siblings may have wondered why the child just cannot stop the behavior. Siblings may be affected by the disturbance in the family and may be unfairly expected to understand why their sibling is getting so much attention. Extended family members may impose their own interpretation of the behaviors and be critical of the child and the family.

Additionally, parents who have had OCD themselves at some point (Lenane et al. 1990) may experience guilt about "transmitting" the illness and may want to acquiesce to their child's demands so that he or she will not experience any pain. Often parents need help in balancing being empathic against becoming overinvolved in their child's rituals.

Patient Advocacy and Support Groups

The patient self-help/support movement has been extremely effective in helping to destigmatize OCD and provide educational information. Support groups serve numerous functions, including updating families and patients about availability of treatments and providing a "consumer network" in their community. Patients should contact the Obsessive Compulsive Foundation, P.O. Box 70, Milford, CT 06460 (telephone: 203-878-5669, Web site: www.ocfoundation.org), to locate appropriate therapists in their area and obtain educational materials. Also, the Obsessive Compulsive Information Center, Madison Institute of Medicine, 7617 Mineral Point Road, Suite 300, Madison, WI 53717-1914 (telephone: 608-836-8070, Web site: www.healthtechsys.com/mimocic.html), will provide educational and informational services.

Pharmacotherapy

Systematic studies have reported that the SRIs are effective in treating OCD symptoms in adults and that this class of medications is superior to placebo and to drugs that are not specific for the serotonergic system (Greist et al. 1995; March et al. 1995b). The SRI clomipramine and the selective serotonin reuptake inhibitors (SSRIs) fluoxetine, paroxetine, sertraline, citalopram, and fluvoxamine are available commercially in the United States. Currently, the medications with a U.S. Food and Drug Administration (FDA)–approved indication for OCD include clomipramine (in children 10 years or older), fluoxetine (in adults), sertraline (in children 6 years or older), paroxetine (in adults), and fluvoxamine (in children 8 years or older).

Clomipramine

Clomipramine, a tricyclic and a potent SRI, was the first and probably the most thoroughly studied of the antiobsessional agents. Clomipramine was the first medication to have been systematically studied in pediatric OCD, and Flament et al. (1985) reported that clomipramine was superior to placebo in a double-blind crossover study of 19 subjects. Seventy-five percent of the patients had a moderate to marked improvement at 5 weeks, and only 16% were unchanged. These results were confirmed by a large 8-week multicenter, double-blind parallel comparison of clomipramine and placebo. DeVeaugh-Geiss et al. (1992) concluded that clomipramine was effective; the patients receiving clomipramine had a mean reduction in their OCD severity score of 37% compared with 8% in those receiving placebo. To assess the effectiveness of clomipramine over other antidepressants, it was compared with desipramine because desipramine, although more noradrenergic, has antidepressant and anxiolytic effects similar to those of clomipramine (Leonard et al. 1989). Forty-eight children and adolescents completed a 12-week controlled trial, with 2 weeks of placebo and 5 weeks of double-blind trials of clomipramine and desipramine. Clomipramine was superior to desipramine in ameliorating the OCD symptoms at 5 weeks of treatment (Leonard et al. 1989).

Clomipramine is generally well tolerated in children (controlled trials in age 6 and older) and adolescents, and an anticholinergic side-effect profile was reported (DeVeaugh-Geiss et al. 1992; Leonard et al. 1989). The most common side effects were dry mouth, constipation, tiredness, sweating, stomachache, and tremor. In general, a therapeutic trial of clomipramine would be a dosage of 3 mg/kg/day for up to 3 months. Dosages should not exceed 5 mg/kg/day or 250 mg/day because of risks of toxicity, including seizures and electrocardiogram (ECG) changes. Because of the potentially cardiotoxic effects of all the tricyclic antidepressants (Elliott and Popper 1991), baseline and periodic ECGs are suggested. Tachycardia, change in axis, or prolongation of intervals should be noted. Particular attention to the QT corrected interval is recommended (Riddle et al. 1993).

Clinical discussion has focused on whether clomipramine is more effective than the SSRIs and whether it should be used with patients who have more severe symptoms. Initial meta-analysis (Greist et al. 1995) had indicated that clomipramine was somewhat more effective for the treatment of adult OCD than any of the SSRIs. Additionally, although clomipramine had more anticholinergic side effects than the SSRIs, the dropout rate was similar in those treated with clomipramine and in those treated with SSRIs. Recent reanalysis of the data suggests that such results may have been confounded by treatment order effects: the SSRI trials may have included previous nonresponders to clomipramine, whereas nonresponse to an SSRI was not an issue for participants in the earlier clomipramine trials. Additionally, the few head-to-head comparisons of SSRIs with clomipramine, although methodologically limited by small sample size, have found them to be equally efficacious. The "Expert Consensus Guidelines" (March et al. 1997) suggest that it be used when a patient has failed two or three adequate trials of an SSRI in combination with CBT.

Selective Serotonin Reuptake Inhibitors

Fluoxetine, a bicyclic SSRI, was superior to placebo in a controlled trial of children and adolescents with OCD (Riddle et al. 1992). (Fluoxetine is currently approved by the FDA for the treatment of depression and OCD in adults.) Two small controlled trials of fluoxetine in children with OCD and Tourette's disorder reported a modest effect on OCD symptoms (improvement from baseline but not superior to placebo), and it did not exacerbate the tics (Kurlan et al. 1993; Scahill et al. 1997a). A large trial in children is under way. Although large systematic studies of children with OCD have not been published, fluoxetine is widely used (American Academy of Child and Adolescent Psychiatry 1998), and it was the first SSRI commercially available in the United States.

Fluoxetine is reasonably well tolerated in children and adolescents (Riddle et al. 1992), and the most common side effects include nervousness, insomnia, and restlessness. To minimize side effects, lower initial dosages are used, sometimes 2.5–5.0 mg/day, depending on the child's age and weight. Geller et al.'s (1995) open trial of fluoxetine in children used an average of 1 mg/kg/day, and the therapeutic effect was sustained over time (mean follow-up of 19 months). One must bear in mind that with the long half-life of the parent drug and its metabolite, steady state is not reached for 2–3 weeks, and the drug is not completely eliminated from the system for up to 6 weeks after discontinuation.

Fluvoxamine, a unicyclic SRI, has been approved for the treatment of OCD in adults and children 8 years and older. The most common side effects of fluvoxamine include sedation, nausea, anorexia, tremor, and sexual dysfunction, and its side-effect profile is clearly less anticholinergic than that of the tricyclics. The trials of its safety and efficacy in children and adolescents with OCD leading to FDA approval were completed, and preliminary data have been published (Riddle et al. 1996).

Sertraline is currently approved by the FDA for the treatment of depression in adults and for OCD in children 6 years and older. The recent multisite placebo-controlled trial of 187 children and adolescents reported the superiority of sertraline over placebo. The most common side effects of sertraline include nausea, dyspepsia, and agitation (March et al. 1998).

A large multisite study of paroxetine in the treatment of OCD in children and adolescents is under way, and an open study has been published (Rosenberg et al. 1999). Citalopram, the most recently introduced SSRI in the United States, has been studied in 23 subjects in an open fashion. Thomsen (1997) reported a generally favorable response: 11 of the 23 subjects improved, and only 5 had little or no response. Larger trials are needed to study its safety and efficacy in the pediatric population.

Choice of Medication

In general, the SSRIs have become the first-line medication for the treatment of OCD in children. The specific choice of agents requires consideration of the risk-benefit ratio, side-effect profile, comorbid diagnoses, and use of concomitant medications. Although information about the pharmacokinetics of the SSRIs in children is limited, a consideration of whether a relatively longer half-life (fluoxetine) or a shorter half-life (paroxetine, fluvoxamine, and sertraline) is needed is relevant for some. Behavioral activation has been reported with fluoxetine (Riddle et al. 1991). It can be seen with the other SSRIs, although perhaps at a slightly lower rate.

The SSRIs can inhibit one or more of the cytochrome P450 enzyme systems; therefore, drug-drug interactions are possible. The clinician should inquire about all prescriptions, over-the-counter medications, and health supplements that the patient may take. Although each SSRI may primarily inhibit one subsystem over another, it becomes very cumbersome for the clinician to identify the systems that may be affected. The reader is referred to reviews in the literature for potential interactions (Jefferson 1998; Mitchell 1997). In general, combinations of the SRIs are rarely used in children because the metabolism of one medication is often inhibited, leading to increased serum levels (Szegedi et al. 1996). In general, ethnicity and diet may affect drug metabolism, although it is not well studied in children (Jefferson 1998). The reader is directed to a review of the pharmacology of the SSRIs in children (DeVane and Sallee 1996; Leonard et al. 1997).

Augmentation Strategies

For patients who have had a partial response to an SRI, augmentation trials with an additional agent are receiving attention. Goodman et al. (1993) reviewed these strategies in adults, and similar plans are considered in children. Although many medications have been reported to augment SRIs successfully, only clonazepam and haloperidol have proved effective in systematic studies in adults (McDougle et al. 1994; Pigott et al. 1992). McDougle et al. (1990) noted that the augmentation was particularly successful if patients had a comorbid tic disorder or schizotypal personality disorder. Based on these systematic trials in adults, we have used clonazepam augmentation for partial responders to SRIs and have noted significant improvement in several patients (Leonard et al. 1994). Because of the long-term risks of antipsychotic treatment, an antipsychotic would be the second choice for augmentation strategies, unless the patient has the profile described by McDougle et al. (1990). Obviously, the risk-benefit ratio of prescribing either a benzodiazepine or an antipsychotic must be weighed.

Maintenance Therapy

Long-term maintenance may be required for the medication-responsive patient. The medication should be periodically tapered to assess whether it is still required. In a double-blind desipramine substitution study of long-term clomipramine-maintained patients, however, 8 of the 9 substitution patients but only 2 of the 11 nonsubstitution patients relapsed (Leonard et al. 1991). Even those receiving long-term clomipramine maintenance, however, manifested some continued OCD symptoms, which waxed and waned over time. Based on clinical observations, if clomipramine is tapered and discontinued, patients do not typically experience an immediate increase in their symptoms but rather may manifest a gradual return of symptoms over time (e.g., 1–3 months later).

Investigational Treatments

With the discussion of a potential subgroup of children with streptococcal-precipitated OCD, an entire new direction in treatment has been opened. The most critical issue is obtaining a detailed clinical history of onset and course of symptoms. A child presenting with an acute onset or a significant, dramatic, unexplained clinical exacerbation of OCD, with or without tics, requires a thoughtful assessment of possible streptococcal infection. A documented positive throat culture usually would be treated with antibiotics or as per general community standards. Serologic titers must be interpreted in the clinical context and are particularly useful if results from multiple time points are available. Serologic titers are expensive and may not be warranted, however, because a positive titer is not sufficient to justify antibiotic use.

Without a positive throat culture result, antibiotics are not indicated. Of specific note, the presence of frank chorea would suggest a diagnosis of Sydenham's chorea rather than PANDAS. This distinction is clinically important because Sydenham's chorea is a known variant of rheumatic fever and requires cardiological evaluation and prophylaxis against GABHS, whereas the PANDAS diagnosis does not. A placebo-controlled, double-blind crossover trial of oral penicillin prophylaxis in children with PANDAS was conducted at NIMH. No significant difference was found between phase differences in OCD or tic symptom severity ratings, although 15 of 20 parents who could detect an improvement between the phases identified improvement in the penicillin phase. During data analysis, it was noted that 14 GABHS infections occurred during the penicillin phase and 21 during the placebo phase. Several children received antibiotic treatment multiple times during the placebo phase (Garvey et al. 1999). Thus, the study yielded information important for the design of future antibiotic prophylactic trials but did not provide justification for penicillin prophylaxis in the ongoing care of children with PANDAS. For the most severe cases, investigational intravenous immunoglobulin or plasmapheresis trials should be considered (Perlmutter et al. 1999). The reader is directed to a recent review for a more detailed discussion (Leonard et al. 1999).

Prognosis

Follow-up studies of children and adolescents with OCD have noted a range of outcomes: a significant percentage of patients have continued difficulties, and some are severely disabled (Leonard et al. 1993). With the new treatment interventions of the SRIs and exposure with response prevention, it was hoped that the long-term outcome might be improved for children and adolescents with OCD. A prospective follow-up study (Leonard et al. 1993), completed after these new treatment interventions became available, reported that 81% of the subjects were improved at follow-up, although only 6% were in true remission. Seventy percent were taking medication specifically for OCD symptomatology at the time of follow-up. These results would suggest that most children with OCD could expect significant improvement, but probably not remission, over time. The study is consistent with early reports that significant difficulties remained in a small group of patients despite treatment interventions (Pleeter et al. 1996). Further research is needed to determine whether certain treatment interventions offer long-term benefits that are greater than those offered by other interventions. Investigators hope that as neurobiological research leads to new understandings and treatment interventions for OCD, long-term outcome can be improved.

Conclusions

OCD can be a chronic, debilitating disorder even with the treatments outlined in this chapter. Nevertheless, what follow-up has been done indicates that there have been true advances in available treatments (Flament et al. 1990; Leonard et al. 1993). Most patients will require some combination of behavioral and pharmacological therapies, and the art of treatment will be in balancing the timing of and focus on any one treatment over time.

References

Abramowitz JS: Effectiveness of psychological and pharmacological treatments for obsessive-compulsive disorder: a quantitative review. J Consult Clin Psychol 65:44–52, 1997

American Academy of Child and Adolescent Psychiatry: Practice parameters for the psychiatric assessment of children and adolescents. J Am Acad Child Adolesc Psychiatry 36:4S–20S, 1997

American Academy of Child and Adolescent Psychiatry: Practice parameters for the assessment and treatment of children and adolescents with obsessive-compulsive disorder. J Am Acad Child Adolesc Psychiatry 37:27S–45S, 1998

Berg CZ, Rapoport JL, Wolff RP: Behavioral treatment for obsessive-compulsive disorder in childhood, in Obsessive-Compulsive Disorder in Children and Adolescents. Edited by Rapoport JL. Washington, DC, American Psychiatric Press, 1989, pp 169–188

Cohen DJ, Leckman JF: Developmental psychopathology and neurobiology of Tourette's syndrome. J Am Acad Child Adolesc Psychiatry 33:2–15, 1994

De Haan E, Hoogduin KA, Buitelaar J, et al: Behavior therapy versus clomipramine for the treatment of obsessive-compulsive disorder. J Am Acad Child Adolesc Psychiatry 37:1022–1029, 1998

DeVane CL, Sallee FR: Serotonin selective reuptake inhibitors in child and adolescent psychopharmacology. J Clin Psychiatry 57:55–66, 1996

DeVeaugh-Geiss GJ, Moroz G, Biederman J, et al: Clomipramine hydrochloride in childhood and adolescent obsessive-compulsive disorder: a multicenter trial. J Am Acad Child Adolesc Psychiatry 31:45–49, 1992

Douglas HM, Moffitt TE, Dar R, et al: Obsessive-compulsive disorder in a birth cohort of 18-year-olds: prevalence and predictors. J Am Acad Child Adolesc Psychiatry 34:1424–1431, 1995

Elliott GR, Popper CW: Tricyclic antidepressants: the QT interval and other cardiovascular parameters (editorial). J Child Adolesc Psychopharmacol 1:187–191, 1991

Esman AH: Psychoanalysis and general psychiatry: obsessive-compulsive disorder as paradigm. J Am Psychoanal Assoc 37:319–336, 1989

Evans D, Leckman J, Carter A, et al: Ritual, habit and perfectionism: the prevalence and development of compulsive-like behavior in normal young children. Child Dev 68:58–68, 1997

Flament MF, Rapoport JL, Berg C, et al: Clomipramine treatment of childhood obsessive-compulsive disorder. Arch Gen Psychiatry 42:977–983, 1985

Flament MF, Koby E, Rapoport JL, et al: Childhood obsessive compulsive disorder: a prospective follow-up study. J Child Psychol Psychiatry 31:363–380, 1990

Foa E, Kozak M: Emotional processing of fear: exposure to corrective information. Psychol Bull 99:20–35, 1986

Foa E, Kozak M: Psychological treatment for obsessive-compulsive disorder, in Long-Term Treatments of Anxiety Disorders: Psychological and Pharmacological Approaches. Edited by Mavissakalian M, Prien R. Washington, DC, American Psychiatric Press, 1996, pp 285–309

Foa E, Steketee G, Grayson J, et al: Deliberate exposure and blocking of obsessive compulsive rituals: immediate and long-term effects. Behavior Therapy 15:450–472, 1984

Francis G: Childhood obsessive-compulsive disorder: extinction of compulsive reassurance seeking. J Anxiety Disord 2:361–366, 1988

Francis G, Gragg RA: Developmental Clinical Psychology and Psychiatry, Vol 35: Childhood Obsessive Compulsive Disorder. Thousand Oaks, CA, Sage, 1996

Franklin M, Kozak M, Cashman L, et al: Cognitive behavioral treatment of pediatric obsessive compulsive disorder: an open clinical trial. J Am Acad Child Adolesc Psychiatry 37:412–419, 1998

Freud S: Notes upon a case of obsessional neurosis (1909), in Standard Edition of the Complete Psychological Works of Sigmund Freud, Vol 10. Translated and edited by Strachey J. London, Hogarth, 1955, pp 151–318

Garvey MA, Perlmutter SJ, Allen AJ, et al: A pilot study of penicillin prophylaxis for neuropsychiatric exacerbations triggered by streptococcal infections. Biol Psychiatry 45:1564–1571, 1999

Geller D, Biederman J, Reed ED, et al: Similarities in response to fluoxetine in the treatment of children and adolescents with obsessive-compulsive disorder. J Am Acad Child Adolesc Psychiatry 34:36–44, 1995

Geller D, Biederman J, Griffin S, et al: Comorbidity of juvenile obsessive-compulsive disorder with disruptive behavior disorders: a review and report. J Am Acad Child Adolesc Psychiatry 35:1637–1646, 1996

Goodman WK, McDougle CJ, Barr LC, et al: Biological approaches to treatment-resistant obsessive compulsive disorder. J Clin Psychiatry 54 (6, suppl):16–26, 1993

Gordon CT, Rapoport JL, Hamburger SD, et al: Differential response of seven subjects with autistic disorder to clomipramine and desipramine. Am J Psychiatry 149:363–366, 1992

Greist JH: Behavior therapy for obsessive compulsive disorder. J Clin Psychiatry 55 (10, suppl):60–68, 1994

Greist JH, Jefferson JW, Kobak KA, et al: Efficacy and tolerability of serotonin transport inhibitors in obsessive-compulsive disorder: a meta-analysis. Arch Gen Psychiatry 52:53–60, 1995

Hanna GL: Demographic and clinical features of obsessive-compulsive disorder in children and adolescents. J Am Acad Child Adolesc Psychiatry 34:19–27, 1995

Harris CV, Wiebe DJ: An analysis of response prevention and flooding procedures in the treatment of adolescent obsessive compulsive disorder. J Behav Ther Exp Psychiatry 23:107–115, 1992

Holzer JC, Goodman WK, McDougle CJ, et al: Obsessive-compulsive disorder with and without a chronic tic disorder: a comparison of symptoms in 70 patients. Br J Psychiatry 164:469–473, 1994

Janet P: Les Obsessions et la Psychasthenie, Vol 1. Paris, France, Felix Alcan, 1903

Jefferson JW: Drug interactions—friend or foe? J Clin Psychiatry 59 (suppl 4):37–47, 1998

Kearney CA, Silverman WK: Treatment of an adolescent with obsessive-compulsive disorder with alternating response prevention and cognitive therapy: an empirical analysis. J Behav Ther Exp Psychiatry 21:39–47, 1990

Kendall PC: Treating anxiety disorders in children: results of a randomized clinical trial. J Consult Clin Psychol 61:235–247, 1994

Knox L, Albano A, Barlow D: Parental involvement in the treatment of childhood OCD: a multiple-baseline examination involving parents. Behavior Therapy 27:93–114, 1996

Kurlan R, Como PG, Deeley C, et al: A pilot controlled study of fluoxetine for obsessive-compulsive symptoms in children with Tourette's syndrome. Clin Neuropharmacol 16:167–172, 1993

Leckman JF, Walker DE, Cohen DJ: Premonitory urges in Tourette's syndrome. Am J Psychiatry 150:98–102, 1993

Leckman JF, Walker DE, Goodman WK, et al: "Just right" perceptions associated with compulsive behavior in Tourette's syndrome. Am J Psychiatry 151:675–680, 1994

Leckman JF, Grice DE, Barr LC, et al: Tic-related vs non-tic-related obsessive-compulsive disorder. Anxiety 1:208–215, 1995

Leckman J, Grice D, Boardman J, et al: Symptoms of obsessive compulsive disorder. Am J Psychiatry 154:911–917, 1997

Lenane MC, Swedo SE, Leonard H, et al: Psychiatric disorders in first-degree relatives of children and adolescents with obsessive compulsive disorder. J Am Acad Child Adolesc Psychiatry 29:407–412, 1990

Leonard HL, Swedo SE, Rapoport JL, et al: Treatment of obsessive-compulsive disorder with clomipramine and desipramine in children and adolescents: a double-blind crossover comparison. Arch Gen Psychiatry 46:1088–1092, 1989

Leonard HL, Goldberger EL, Rapoport JL, et al: Childhood rituals: normal development of obsessive-compulsive symptoms? J Am Acad Child Adolesc Psychiatry 29:17–23, 1990

Leonard HL, Swedo SE, Lenane MC, et al: A double-blind desipramine substitution during long-term clomipramine treatment in children and adolescents with obsessive-compulsive disorder. Arch Gen Psychiatry 48:922–927, 1991

Leonard HL, Lenane MC, Swedo SE, et al: Tics and Tourette's disorder: a 2- to 7-year follow-up of 54 obsessive-compulsive children. Am J Psychiatry 149:1244–1251, 1992

Leonard HL, Swedo SE, Lenane M, et al: A 2- to 7-year follow-up study of 54 obsessive-compulsive disorder children and adolescents. Arch Gen Psychiatry 50:429–439, 1993

Leonard HL, Topol D, Swedo SE, et al: Clonazepam as an augmenting agent in the treatment of childhood onset obsessive-compulsive disorder. J Am Acad Child Adolesc Psychiatry 33:792–794, 1994

Leonard HL, March J, Rickler KC, et al: Pharmacology of the selective serotonin reuptake inhibitors in children and adolescents. J Am Acad Child Adolesc Psychiatry 36:725–736, 1997

Leonard HL, Swedo SE, Garvey M: Postinfectious and other forms of obsessive compulsive disorder. Child Adolesc Psychiatr Clin N Am 8:497–511, 1999

March JS: Cognitive-behavioral psychotherapy for children and adolescents with OCD: a review and recommendations for treatment. J Am Acad Child Adolesc Psychiatry 34:7–18, 1995

March JS, Mulle K: OCD in Children and Adolescents: A Cognitive Behavioral Treatment Manual. New York, Guilford, 1998

March J, Mulle K, Herbel B: Behavioral psychotherapy for children and adolescents with obsessive compulsive disorder: an open trial of a new protocol-driven package. J Am Acad Child Adolesc Psychiatry 33:333–341, 1994

March JS, Leonard HL, Swedo SE: Obsessive compulsive disorder, in Anxiety Disorders in Children and Adolescents. Edited by March JS. New York, Guilford, 1995a, pp 251–275

March JS, Leonard HL, Swedo SE: Pharmacotherapy of obsessive-compulsive disorder, in Child and Adolescent Psychiatric Clinics of North America: Pediatric Pharmacology I. Edited by Riddle M. Philadelphia, PA, WB Saunders, 1995b, pp 217–236

March J, Frances A, Carpenter D, et al: Expert consensus guidelines: treatment of obsessive-compulsive disorder. J Clin Psychiatry 58 (suppl 4):1–72, 1997

March JS, Biederman J, Wolkow R, et al: Sertraline in children and adolescents with obsessive-compulsive disorder: a multicenter randomized controlled trial. JAMA 280:1752–1756, 1998

McDougle CJ, Goodman WK, Price LH, et al: Neuroleptic addition in fluvoxamine-refractory obsessive-compulsive disorder. Am J Psychiatry 147:652–654, 1990

McDougle CJ, Goodman WK, Leckman JF, et al: Haloperidol addition in fluvoxamine-refractory OCD: a double-blind placebo controlled study in patients with and without tics. Arch Gen Psychiatry 51:302–308, 1994

McDougle CJ, Naylor ST, Cohen DJ, et al: A double-blind, placebo-controlled study of fluvoxamine in adults with autistic disorder. Arch Gen Psychiatry 53:1001–1008, 1996

Mitchell PB: Drug interactions of clinical significance with selective serotonin reuptake inhibitors. Drug Saf 17:390–406, 1997

Pauls DL, Towbin KE, Leckman JF, et al: Gilles de la Tourette's syndrome and obsessive-compulsive disorder: evidence supporting a genetic relationship. Arch Gen Psychiatry 43:1180–1182, 1986

Pauls DL, Leckman JF, Cohen DJ: Familial relationship between Gilles de la Tourette's syndrome, attention deficit disorder, learning disabilities, speech disorders, and stuttering. J Am Acad Child Adolesc Psychiatry 32:1044–1050, 1993

Pauls DL, Alsobrook JP II, Goodman W, et al: A family study of obsessive compulsive disorder. Am J Psychiatry 152:76–84, 1995

Perlmutter SJ, Leitman SF, Garvey MA, et al: Therapeutic plasma exchange and intravenous immunoglobulin for obsessive-compulsive disorder and tic disorders in childhood. Lancet 354:1153–1158, 1999

Piacentini J: Cognitive behavioral therapy of childhood OCD. Child Adolesc Psychiatr Clin N Am 8: 599–616, 1999

Piacentini J, Gitow A, Jaffer M, et al: Outpatient behavioral treatment of child and adolescent obsessive-compulsive disorder. J Anxiety Disord 8:277–289, 1994

Pigott TA, L'Heureux F, Rubenstein CS, et al: A controlled trial of clonazepam augmentation in OCD patients treated with clomipramine or fluoxetine (NR144), in 1992 New Research Program and Abstracts, American Psychiatric Association 145th Annual Meeting, Washington, DC, May 2–7, 1992. Washington, DC, American Psychiatric Association, 1992, p 82

Pleeter J, Lenane MC, Leonard HL: Long-term outcome of children and adolescents with obsessive-compulsive disorder, in Do They Grow Out of It? Long-Term Outcomes of Childhood Disorders. Edited by Hechtman L. Washington, DC, American Psychiatric Press, 1996, pp 481–490

Ratnasuriya RH, Marks IM, Forshaw DM, et al: Obsessive slowness revisited. Br J Psychiatry 159:273–274, 1991

Rettew DC, Swedo SE, Leonard HL, et al: Obsessions and compulsions across time in 79 children and adolescents with obsessive compulsive disorder. J Am Acad Child Adolesc Psychiatry 31:1050–1056, 1992

Riddle MA, King RA, Hardin MT, et al: Behavioral side effects of fluoxetine in children and adolescents. J Child Adolesc Psychopharmacol 1:193–198, 1991

Riddle MA, Scahill L, King R, et al: Double-blind, crossover trial of fluoxetine and placebo in children and adolescents with obsessive-compulsive disorder. J Am Acad Child Adolesc Psychiatry 31: 1062–1069, 1992

Riddle MA, Geller B, Ryan N: Case study: another sudden death in a child treated with desipramine. J Am Acad Child Adolesc Psychiatry 32:792–797, 1993

Riddle MA, Walkup J, Claghorn J, et al: Fluvoxamine for OCD in children and adolescents: a controlled trial. Poster presented at the annual meeting of the American Academy of Child and Adolescent Psychiatry, Philadelphia, PA, October 1996

Rosenberg DR, Stewart CM, Fitzgerald KD, et al: Paroxetine open-label treatment of pediatric outpatients with obsessive-compulsive disorder. J Am Acad Child Adolesc Psychiatry 38:1180–1185, 1999

Salzman L, Thaler F: Obsessive-compulsive disorders: a review of the literature. Am J Psychiatry 138:286–296, 1981

Scahill L, Vitulano LA, Brenner EM, et al: Behavioral therapy in children and adolescents with obsessive-compulsive disorder: a pilot study. J Child Adolesc Psychopharmacol 6:191–206, 1996

Scahill L, Riddle MA, King RA, et al: Fluoxetine has no marked effect on tic symptoms in patients with Tourette's syndrome: a double-blind placebo-controlled study. J Child Adolesc Psychopharmacol 7:75–85, 1997a

Scahill L, Riddle MA, McSwiggan-Hardin MT, et al: The Children's Yale-Brown Obsessive Compulsive Scale: preliminary report of reliability and validity. J Am Acad Child Adolesc Psychiatry 36:844–853, 1997b

Steketee G: Treatment of Obsessive Compulsive Disorder. New York, Guilford, 1993

Swedo SE, Rapoport JL, Leonard HL, et al: Obsessive-compulsive disorder in children and adolescents: clinical phenomenology of 70 consecutive cases. Arch Gen Psychiatry 46:335–341, 1989

Swedo SE, Leonard HL, Mittleman BB, et al: Identification of children with pediatric autoimmune neuropsychiatric disorders associated with streptococcal infections by a marker associated with rheumatic fever. Am J Psychiatry 154:110–112, 1997

Swedo SE, Leonard HL, Garvey M, et al: Pediatric autoimmune neuropsychiatric disorders associated with streptococcal infections: clinical description of the first 50 cases. Am J Psychiatry 155:264–271, 1998

Szegedi A, Wetzel H, Leal M, et al: Combination treatment with clomipramine and fluvoxamine. J Clin Psychiatry 57:257–264, 1996

Thomsen PH: Obsessive-compulsive disorder in children and adolescents: predictors in childhood for long-term phenomenological course. Acta Psychiatr Scand 92:255–259, 1995

Thomsen PH: Child and adolescent obsessive-compulsive disorder treated with citalopram: findings from an open trial of 23 cases. J Child Adolesc Psychopharmacol 7:157–166, 1997

Valleni-Basile LA, Garrison CZ, Jackson KL, et al: Frequency of obsessive-compulsive disorder in a community sample of young adolescents. J Am Acad Child Adolesc Psychiatry 33:782–791, 1994

Van Noppen B, Steketee G, McCorkle BH, et al: Group and multifamily behavioral treatment for obsessive compulsive disorder: a pilot study. J Anxiety Disord 4:431–446, 1997

15

Substance Abuse and Substance Use Disorders

Heather J. Walter, M.D., M.P.H.

The use of psychoactive substances remains a common behavior among American youths. The most recent (Centers for Disease Control and Prevention 1998) of a series of national surveys of high school students found the 30-day prevalence of substance use to be 51% for alcohol, 36% for smoked tobacco, 26% for marijuana, and 3% for cocaine. Lifetime prevalence rates were much higher, suggesting that by age 18, the great majority of students in the United States experiment at least once with legal or illegal substances. Analyses of trends over the past two decades show that, after a decade of decline, adolescent substance use began to rise in the early 1990s, and for several drugs, use is now higher than at any time since the mid-1980s.

For many young people, experimentation with psychoactive substances may be short-lived and have no serious sequelae. Even experimental drug use, however, can result in serious morbidity or mortality from unintentional overdose, infection from the route of administration or from unsafe sexual behaviors (DiClemente and Ponton 1993), substance-induced psychiatric disorders (Bukstein et al. 1989), homicide (Bukstein 1995), suicide (Bukstein et al. 1993), and accidents (Milstein and Irwin 1988). In other cases, experimental drug use may escalate into an entrenched, destructive drug-taking pattern of abuse or dependence, in which role-fulfillment, legal, medical, and interpersonal problems mount, control over drug use is lost, and the adolescent becomes alienated from the nonusing world.

The author wishes to acknowledge the contribution of Gregory Cote to the preparation of this chapter.

Stages of Substance Use

The progression from drug experimentation to abuse or dependence may follow a characteristic pattern (Muramoto and Leshan 1993).

Experimental Stage

In the experimental stage, the adolescent has made the decision to try drugs and has experienced the altered perceptions and feeling states associated with drug use, generally in the context of social situations in which peers supply the drugs. Few behavioral signs of drug use are present. The substances most commonly used at this stage are tobacco, alcohol, and marijuana, the so-called gateway drugs (Kandel 1975).

Early Regular Use

In the stage of early regular use, the adolescent actively seeks the drug-induced perceptions and feeling states. Use is more frequent, situational, and solitary, and the user has his or her own supply of drugs. Mood, cognitive, and behavioral signs may appear and may include impaired concentration; a decline in academic or athletic performance; loss of interest in hobbies or extracurricular activities; mood swings; rebellious attitude, dress, or behavior; antisocial behavior; social withdrawal or a change in the circle of friends; and changes in daily routine or sleep and eating patterns (Jaffe 1990).

Late Regular Use

In the stage of late regular use, the adolescent plans his or her daily activities around opportunities to use drugs. The user experiences marked dysphoria or withdrawal when not using and begins to question his or her control over use. As the frequency of drug use increases, unpleasant feeling states may worsen, leading to more drug use, often with more powerful substances. Self-destructive and risk-taking behaviors increase, psychosocial and academic function is further impaired, and the adolescent retreats further into the drug-using world.

End Stage

In the end stage of drug use, the adolescent needs drugs to avoid nearly constant dysphoria. He or she turns to more potent substances and takes larger amounts. Drug use is nearly constant as the adolescent user becomes less selective, using any and all drugs available and obtaining them by whatever means necessary. Increasing physical and mental deterioration becomes obvious.

Most adolescents in the general population do not progress beyond the experimental stage of psychoactive substance use. Among the minority who progress to higher stages of use, many cease abusing substances in early adulthood. Jessor (1985) described a process of "maturing out" of drug use, in which the assumption of new life roles in work and family and the occupancy of new social contexts other than school constitute conventionalizing influences (Newcomb and Bentler 1988). Adolescents who struggle to assume adult roles because of difficult psychosocial circumstances may have much higher rates of persistent drug use. Early initiation of substance use and rapid progression through the stages of drug use convey heightened risk for the development of substance use disorders (Robins and McEvoy 1991; Robins and Przybeck 1985).

Epidemiology

Prevalence

Few data on the prevalence of substance abuse and dependence in the general population of adolescents are currently available. In community surveys, the lifetime prevalence of alcohol abuse or dependence has ranged from 5.3% in 15-year-olds to 32.4% in 17- to 19-year olds, and the lifetime prevalence of drug abuse or dependence has ranged from 3.3% in 15-year-olds to 9.8% in 17- to 19-year-olds (Kashani et al. 1987; Reinherz et al. 1993). The prevalence of substance use disorders is substantially higher in specific populations, such as males (Reinherz et al. 1993), runaways (Greene et al. 1997), abuse victims (Harrison et al. 1997), and juvenile delinquents (Milan et al. 1991).

Etiology

The etiology of substance abuse and dependence is complex and multifactorial, involving biological, psychological, social, and cultural factors (Glantz and Pickens 1992; Newcomb 1995). In the early stages of use, the easy availability of substances coupled with sociocultural norms and values that promote substance experimentation are thought to be the predominant etiological factors. In the later stages of use, biological and psychological factors may play the more powerful etiological role.

Comorbidity

Both population-based (Cohen et al. 1993; Kessler et al. 1996; Lewinsohn et al. 1993) and clinic-based studies (Bukstein et al. 1992; Clark et al. 1995; Greenbaum et al. 1991; Riggs et al. 1995; Stowell and Estroff 1992) suggest high rates of psychiatric comorbidity with substance abuse and dependence, particularly for conduct disorder (Huizinga and Elliot 1981; Loeber 1988; Milan et al. 1991). Associations with mood (Bukstein et al. 1992; Deykin et al. 1987, 1992; Hovens et al. 1994), anxiety (Clark and Sayette 1993; Clark et al. 1995; Kushner et al. 1990; Van Hasselt et al. 1992), attention-deficit/hyperactivity (Barkley et al. 1990), eating (Bulik et al. 1992), and psychotic (Kutcher et al. 1992; Regier et al. 1990) disorders also have been found. The association of other psychiatric disorders with substance abuse and dependence is complicated: psychopathology may precede substance use, may develop as a consequence of substance use, may moderate the severity of substance use, or may originate from a common vulnerability (Hovens et al. 1994).

Assessment

Interviews

The assessment of substance use should begin with an analysis of the extent to which substance use has resulted in problems and, if so, whether these problems satisfy diagnostic criteria (American Psychiatric Association 1994) for abuse or dependence. It must be remembered, however, that the diagnostic criteria for abuse and dependence were developed for adults and have not been proven applicable to adolescents. Thus, tolerance may have low diagnostic specificity, withdrawal symptoms may be much less common, and blackouts, craving, and impulsive sexual behavior may be prominent characteristics of maladaptive use (Martin et al. 1995).

Parents often are unaware of their children's substance use; accordingly, interviews should be conducted separately with the adolescent and parent(s). An explicit statement about confidentiality should be made to the adolescent; but he or she must be advised that if the evaluation reveals imminent danger to self or others, parents will be so informed.

An assessment of the teenager's personal involvement with drugs can be approached in a nonthreatening way by placing questions in the context of the adolescent's environment (e.g., drug use among peers). As rapport develops, the interviewer can inquire about the details of the adolescent's personal use of substances. Questions should focus on the identification of the drug or drugs used, the route of administration, the duration (age at initiation) and frequency of use, and the usual setting. It is critical to assess the adolescent's beliefs about the physical, psychological, and social benefits of drug use, the adolescent's experiences with the negative consequences of use, and whether the adolescent's drug use has ever resulted in his or her entering into risky situations. It also is important to ascertain how much time the adolescent spends getting, using, and thinking about drugs and whether the adolescent believes that his or her drug use is out of control.

To ascertain the degree to which drug use is maladaptive, the interviewer should inquire in detail about family and peer relationships, school or work performance, extracurricular activities, financial or legal difficulties, and other adverse life circumstances. To assess possible comorbidity with other psychiatric disorders, the clinician should take a detailed psychiatric history. Eliciting an accurate chronology of the onset of drug use and other psychiatric symptoms is particularly important in distinguishing primary from secondary substance abuse. A careful assessment of maltreatment (e.g., physical or sexual abuse or neglect) also should be conducted. Finally, it is important to assess familial attitudes toward and patterns of substance use and whether drug use is modeled by parents, older siblings, or other key adults as a way of coping with problems. Whenever possible, all historical information should be corroborated by adults who know the adolescent well, including family members, teachers, counselors, and friends.

Screening

Clinicians may elect to use screening instruments or laboratory tests to aid in the assessment process. Several psychometrically sound self-report instruments are available to assess adolescent substance use (G. Miller 1990; Rahdert 1991; Weed et al. 1994; Winters 1991; Winters and Henly 1989). The primary limitation of these instruments is that, like adults, adolescents tend to underreport their substance use (Winters et al. 1992). Urine and blood toxicology screens may be used to validate self-reports of use. Except for blood alcohol, urine drug screens are more sensitive than serum tests (Cone 1997). Sensitivity and specificity of urine screens vary with the drug being tested for and the laboratory method used. In addition, the approximate length of time a drug test will have a positive result after a patient's last use varies with the pharmacological properties of the drug: 1–3 days for heroin, amphetamine, and cocaine and up to 30 days after chronic use of marijuana. Hair, saliva, and sweat analyses represent promising alternatives (Cone 1997). Clinical indicators for using toxicology screens may include the following: 1) all adolescents with new psychiatric symptoms; 2) high-risk adolescents (e.g., children of substance-abusing parents; runaways; delinquents); 3) adolescents with changes in mental status or physical performance; 4) adolescents with unexplained behavior changes; 5) adolescents with recurrent respiratory ailments; 6) adolescents with recurrent accidents or unexplained somatic symptoms; and 7) adolescents for whom abstinence is to be monitored (Gold and Dackis 1986).

Medical Issues

Clinicians must be alert to medical complications that may arise in the context of drug use. Accidents and trauma (e.g., drownings; motor vehicle, bicycle, and skateboard accidents; use of deadly weapons) often occur when individuals are under the influence of substances (Milstein and Irwin 1988). High-risk sexual behavior also is common (DiClemente and Ponton 1993), resulting in unintended pregnancies and sexually transmitted diseases. Any substance use by an adolescent, and especially use of intravenous drugs or crack cocaine, should prompt an inquiry into specific human immunodeficiency virus (HIV) risk factors and consideration of appropriate testing. Clinicians should be aware of the immediate psychoactive and physiological effects of common substances of abuse and know how and in what setting to treat intoxication and withdrawal states (Cambor and Millman 1996). Long-term sequelae of substance use may not become apparent until adulthood; the severe medical sequelae of inhalant use are a notable exception (Sharp and Rosenberg 1992).

Treatment

Goals

The first task of treatment planning is to select an appropriate treatment goal. In most cases, the goal will be achieving and maintaining abstinence from substance use. However, given the self-limiting nature of substance use in most populations and the chronicity of substance use in others, harm reduction (i.e., reducing the potential for unintended adverse consequences of drug use) may be an appropriate interim goal. Achieving motivation for abstinence may be a difficult first step that, among adult substance abusers, is increasingly informed by motivational theory.

Prochaska and DiClemente (1992) have proposed what has become known as the "stages of change" model. This model views the process of change in drug-related behavior as a series of stages of readiness. In the first stage, the "precontemplation" stage, drug users are unwilling to change their drug use because of factors such as lack of insight, rebelliousness, enjoyment of drug use, or lack of self-efficacy. However, as the negative consequences of drug use accrue, precontemplators may move into the "contemplation" stage, in which the positive and negative consequences of drug use are finely balanced. As the costs of drug use rise, contemplators may become ready for change ("determination"). From determination, "action" emerges, in which a plan for change is formulated and implemented. Following the action stage is the fifth and final stage, which is "maintenance." Individuals in this stage have taken effective action and have achieved sustained change.

The importance of this model, according to its originators, is that different therapeutic strategies need to be deployed at different stages in the change process. For example, with the precontemplator, the aim is to increase perceptions of the risks associated with substance use by providing information. With the contemplator, the aim is to explore the positive and negative consequences of drug use and attempt to tip the balance toward change. In the determination stage, the aim is to strengthen the commitment to change by determining a sound course of action that has a high perceived likelihood of success. It is important to recognize that ambivalence to change will persist through the action stage and that it will be important for the clinician to instill a sense of accomplishment for any degree of success. In the maintenance stage, the aim is to minimize problems associated with a lapse or relapse by helping to renew the commitment to change and thus reinitiate the cycle. Key principles underlying motivational strategies are to express understanding and acceptance of the patient's position in the stages of change hierarchy, to make manifest the discrepancies between the current drug use behavior and personal goals or beliefs about oneself, to avoid arguments, to view resistance as a mismatch between the patient's stage of change and the focus of therapy, and to build the patient's confidence that his or her own course of action will achieve the desired outcome (W.R. Miller and Rollnick 1991).

Setting

A second key task of treatment planning is to select the appropriate treatment setting. Levels of care that have been used for the treatment of adolescent substance abuse or dependence include community treatment (e.g., self-help groups), outpatient treatment, partial hospitalization or day treatment, residential treatment (e.g., group homes, therapeutic communities), and inpatient treatment (e.g., hospital-based or free-standing rehabilitation centers) (American Academy of Child and Adolescent Psychiatry 1997). These levels represent successively increasing intensity and restrictiveness of care. In adolescents, as with adults, treatment should be provided in the least restrictive setting that is safe and effective. Outpatient treatment is appropriate for motivated adolescents who have strong, stable environmental support; no significant comorbid psychiatric disorders; and little functional impairment. Partial or day hospitalization can serve as a step-up or step-down service for adolescents who need intensive services but not the level of restrictiveness associated with residential or inpatient treatment. Appropriate candidates for residential treatment are adolescents who have failed in a less restrictive treatment setting, who are transitioning from inpatient treatment, who have poor environmental supports, or who have severe personality disorders or functional impairment. Inpatient treatment should be considered for adolescents who have moderate to severe psychiatric disturbance with functional impairment, who are at risk for withdrawal, who present a danger to themselves or others, or who have failed in less restrictive treatment settings.

Modality

A third key task of treatment planning is to select the appropriate treatment modality. Until the mid-1970s, treatment for all substance abuse or dependence largely was uniform. Patients abusing substances other than opiates typically were referred to inpatient settings, where they would undergo a 28-day program of detoxification and psychoeducation, followed by discharge to a 12-Step-based self-help group. Patients abusing opiates typically were referred for a longer period of treatment in inpatient settings that functioned as therapeutic communities. Today, at least six theoretically and operationally distinct treatment strategies—12-Step, cognitive-behavioral, psychodynamic, family, group, and community-based—are dominant in the United States. Although they are described separately here, in practice, most treatments integrate multiple strategies. Each of these strategies, originally developed for adults, must be modified to meet the developmental needs of adolescents.

12-Step Therapy

The 12-Step strategy was one of the first to conceptualize substance abuse and dependence as a biopsychosocial or spiritual phenomenon (Wallace 1989). This model asserts that excessive drug use leads to profound biological (e.g., altered brain chemistry), psychological (e.g., negative psychological states), social (e.g., deterioration of personal relationships), and spiritual (e.g., lack of purpose) negative consequences. The distress associated with these negative consequences leads to further excessive drug use, which leads to more negative consequences and more distress. Thus, a vicious cycle is established that maintains abuse and dependence.

The 12-Step strategy can be thought of as a fellowship of peers who can provide the means (e.g., knowledge, beliefs, skills, and supports) necessary to break this cycle. The role of the clinician in the 12-Step strategy typically is to help the patient begin the process of recovery by facilitating his or her entry into and increasing his or her involvement with this fellowship of peers (Nowinski and Baker 1992).

In early recovery, the clinician focuses on two primary therapeutic goals: the patient's acceptance of the belief that he or she can no longer exert consistent control over drug use and his or her surrender to the strength of the fellowship. The clinician works toward acceptance by examining with the patient the progressive pattern of unmanageable and destructive drug-taking behavior and the proven limitations of personal willpower. The patient must come to believe that complete abstinence is the only way to achieve and maintain recovery and that he or she is incapable of achieving abstinence on his or her own. Once the patient is ready to accept the need for a power greater than his or her own, the clinician works toward surrender by facilitating active involvement (e.g., attending "90 meetings in 90 days," assuming responsibility for some aspect of the meetings, building a support network, obtaining a sponsor, reading self-help literature, giving up friends and situations that might represent a threat to recovery) in a carefully selected 12-Step fellowship that includes a critical mass of similar-age peers. In the context of the fellowship, the patient gradually comes to eschew the pattern of solving problems with substances and to apply new knowledge, beliefs, skills, and support to the achievement of personal emotional, cognitive, social, and spiritual development. During this process, the clinician consistently advises the patient to focus on "1 day at a time" and encourages the patient to solicit and follow practical advice from fellowship members. If early recovery has been successful, termination consists of turning the patient over to the care of the 12-Step fellowship for maintenance of recovery.

Cognitive-Behavioral Therapy

The cognitive-behavioral strategy views substance abuse and dependence as arising from a combination of social learning (adopting substance use behaviors as a way to gain admission to a desired peer group), operant conditioning (experiencing powerful reinforcing contingencies for substance use), cognitions (adopting expectancies that substance use will result in highly positive outcomes), and classical conditioning (creating multiple environmental cues for substance use). In the beginning stages of use, social learning, operant conditioning, and cognitions are thought to play the prominent etiological role. In later stages of use, classical conditioning begins to assume greater importance, with both conditioned craving and withdrawal effects leading to severe dependence in some individuals.

Cognitive-behavioral treatment begins with a thorough functional analysis of the cognitive, behavioral, social, psychological, and environmental factors that trigger and maintain substance use. Then, work focuses on developing with the patient an individualized repertoire of skills aimed at the triggering and maintaining factors identified in the functional analysis. Finally, the patient develops a plan for relapse prevention in which he or she identifies potential high-risk situations and develops strategies for effectively coping with those situations.

Skills training strategies may include those derived from classical conditioning theory (e.g., cue exposure [Childress et al. 1993] and stimulus control [Bickel and Kelly 1988] skills, relaxation training [Monti et al. 1989], stress and anger management skills [Marlatt and Gordon 1985], and covert sensitization [Rimmele et al. 1989]); operant conditioning theory (e.g., contingency management [W.R. Miller and Munoz 1982; Monti et al. 1989]); social learning theory (e.g., identification with abstinent peers [Bandura 1977], refusal skills [Monti et al. 1989], and social skills [Chaney 1989]); and cognitive theory (e.g., challenging "automatic" thoughts about expectancies [Beck et al. 1993]). Common to each of these approaches are using the skills of self-awareness and behavioral monitoring, rehearsing cognitive and behavioral skills, developing an abstinent social support group, and planning for high-risk situations. During the maintenance phase of treatment, external controls are gradually faded and the patient is exposed to progressively more risky and varied substance use situations and helped to develop and use alternative coping strategies.

Psychodynamic Therapy

Advances in the psychodynamic treatment of substance abuse have paralleled shifts in emphasis with psychoanalytic theory. Thus, whereas early psychodynamic treatment of substance abuse focused on the analysis of libidinal and aggressive drives, later treatment strategies emphasized the role of ego defenses and deficits. For example, Krystal (1982) emphasized the use of substances to defend against the onslaught of overwhelming painful affects. Meissner (1986) pointed to the role of narcissistic wounds in the etiology of substance abuse. Kohut and Wolf (1978) suggested that drugs serve as substitute idealized selfobjects that were not available in early development. Khantzian (1980) emphasized the lack of an internal, comforting sense of self-validation. Luborsky (1984) and Klerman et al. (1984) suggested the importance of clarifying the role of substances in the context of interpersonal relationships.

Despite the theoretical usefulness of such conceptualizations, however, clinicians who advocate psychodynamic treatment of substance use disorders seldom recommend it as the sole treatment modality. Psychodynamic techniques aimed at conflict resolution and increased self-awareness can be combined with cognitive-behavioral approaches, psychoeducation, and provision of active support and reassurance as indicated. For example, Kaufman (1994) begins with an initial (1–2 years) phase of treatment, which focuses on achieving and maintaining abstinence through 12-Step, cognitive-behavioral, family, group, or multisystemic treatments. Early therapeutic objectives (Frances et al. 1999) include obtaining a complete developmental history of the patient; evaluating temperament in the patient and significant others; examining the patient's capacity to identify with and separate from important figures of identification; and exploring the patient's capacity to recognize and tolerate painful affects. Confrontation focuses on the denial surrounding addictive behaviors, and interpretations are aimed at increasing the patient's awareness of feeling states and their relation to substance use. In more advanced phases of treatment, more expressive psychodynamic treatment may emerge, in which relevant conflicts and defenses are analyzed within a traditional transference-countertransference framework. From early in treatment, issues of trust, dependency, separation, loss, disappointment, and truthfulness are frequent themes (Frances et al. 1999).

Family Therapy

Family therapy is indicated when dysfunctional relationships within the family are contributing directly to substance abuse or when family members are directly or indirectly enabling the substance abuser. Family therapy also can be used to help other family members who have been adversely affected by the behaviors of the substance abuser. Three models currently serve as the basis for family approaches to substance abuse treatment: the disease model, structural-strategic models, and the behavioral model.

In the disease model (Cermak 1986), family members are helped to recognize the codependent characteristics in each member that enable the substance abuser to perpetuate use. The primary goals of treatment are to help family members recognize that they all have a disease that contributes to substance abuse, appropriately detach from the abuser, and become involved with 12-Step or other treatment programs. In structural-strategic models (Lewis et al. 1990; Stanton et al. 1982), the various functions that substance abuse serves for the family are examined and explained. Once the focus is shifted from the substance abuser to the central issue or crisis within the family, a process is begun in which dysfunctional roles, rules, and boundaries can be reshaped to enable the abuser to relinquish his or her symptom. Behavioral models (Bry 1988; O'Farrell and Cowles 1989) examine family behaviors as cues and reinforcers for substance use and focus on eliminating cues and replacing rewards with consequences. Common to all family approaches are certain techniques and therapeutic goals: 1) fostering a belief that the clinician and family must work together on the problem, 2) eliciting each family member's personal experience of the substance abuser's behavior, 3) identifying central areas of interpersonal dysfunction, 4) improving communication of thoughts and feelings, and 5) addressing enabling (McKay 1996).

Group Therapy

In group therapy, therapeutic use is made of the natural inclination of youths to form peer relationships. Groups can serve to provide a nurturing situation in which adolescents experience a sense of belonging and common interest and gain support and understanding through sharing thoughts and feelings. Groups also can serve as a restraining force, as group members monitor one another's activities within and outside the group. Groups also afford adolescents the opportunity to gain insight through the reflective, confronting, and clarifying aspects of the group process. The focus of the group generally reflects the problems of its members and, as such, can address parent-child problems, social skills training, academic tutoring, and vocational planning. Preparing adolescents to cope with situations involving social pressure to use drugs may play a particularly important role in preventing relapse (Myers and Brown 1990) and should be a major focus of group therapy sessions.

Community-Based Therapy

Similar in theoretical orientation to family treatments but broader in scope are ecologically integrative treatment strategies such as Liddle's (Liddle and Diamond 1991) multidimensional family therapy and Henggeler's (Pickrel and Henggeler 1996) multisystemic family therapy. Each of these strategies broadens the scope of treatment from individuals and families to include multiple sources of potential influence on drug-taking behaviors, such as teachers, neighbors, clergy, police, and peers. School-based counseling, drug-free peer groups and recreational activities, and community campaigns are some of the treatment modalities used in multidimensional strategies. Case managers typically are used to coordinate treatments across community service groups.

Pharmacotherapy

Pharmacotherapy may be indicated for the treatment of adolescent substance abuse in the following situations (American Academy of Child and Adolescent Psychiatry 1997): detoxification, treatment of withdrawal effects, substitution of a similar drug for prolonged withdrawal or maintenance, countering of the physiological and subjective effects of abused substances, and treatment of comorbid psychiatric disorders. Detoxification and treatment of withdrawal effects should proceed as with adults. Substitution pharmacotherapies such as methadone are used infrequently and may be prohibited by law. Countering the physiological and subjective effects of substances, such as with methadone or naltrexone, has received far less research and clinical attention among adolescents than among adults. Until the safety and efficacy of such pharmacotherapies have been confirmed, the use of such agents should be reserved for those adolescents who have severe dependence and are resistant to other forms of treatment. Before pharmacotherapy for psychiatric comorbidities is initiated, a period of abstinence or limited use should be observed by the adolescent to clarify the comorbid diagnoses. Pharmacotherapy should then proceed according to standard guidelines.

Effectiveness

The effectiveness of specific treatments for adolescent substance use has not been extensively examined. In one review, Catalano et al. (1990–1991) concluded that, in general, some treatment is better than no treatment, no single treatment approach is clearly superior to another, and alcohol and marijuana use are much less effectively treated than other drug use. Relapse rates posttreatment are high, ranging from 35% to 85% (Catalano et al. 1990–1991). These rates are consistent with those reported for adult treatment programs; approximately two-thirds of adults completing treatment for alcohol or drug dependence relapse within 90 days of discharge from treatment (U.S. Surgeon General 1988). Factors associated with relapse include younger age at onset of drug use; more extensive involvement with drugs; antisocial behavior; comorbid psychiatric disorders; more frequent and intense thoughts and feelings about drugs; less involvement in school, work, or drug-free recreational activities; and less support from drug-free family and peers.

Conclusions

Psychoactive substance abuse and dependence continue to pose immediate and long-term threats to the health and well-being of American youth. Despite massive sums spent on prevention and treatment, the number of substance-abusing adolescents in the United States has not appreciably declined. Clinicians who provide services to children and adolescents should be familiar with the etiology, natural history, diagnosis, and treatment of maladaptive drug use. The development of more effective prevention and treatment methods should be a public health research priority.

References

American Academy of Child and Adolescent Psychiatry: Practice parameters for the assessment and treatment of children and adolescents with substance use disorders. J Am Acad Child Adolesc Psychiatry 36 (10 suppl):140S–156S, 1997

American Psychiatric Association: Diagnostic and Statistical Manual of Mental Disorders, 4th Edition. Washington, DC, American Psychiatric Association, 1994

Bandura A: Social Learning Theory. Englewood Cliffs, NJ, Prentice-Hall, 1977

Barkley RA, Fischer M, Edelbrock CS, et al: The adolescent outcome of hyperactive children diagnosed by research criteria, I: an 8-year prospective follow-up study. J Am Acad Child Adolesc Psychiatry 29:546–557, 1990

Beck AT, Wright FD, Newman CF, et al: Cognitive Therapy of Substance Abuse. New York, Guilford, 1993

Bickel WK, Kelly TH: The relationship of stimulus control to the treatment of substance abuse, in Learning Factors in Substance Abuse (NIDA Research Monograph 84). Edited by Ray BA. Washington, DC, U.S. Government Printing Office, 1988

Bry BH: Family-based approaches to reducing adolescent substance use: theories, techniques and findings, in Adolescent Drug Abuse: Analyses of Treatment Research (NIDA Research Monograph 77, Publ No ADM-88-1523). Edited by Rahdert ER, Grabowski J. Rockville, MD, U.S. Department of Health and Human Services, 1988, pp 39–68

Bukstein OG: Adolescent Substance Abuse. New York, Wiley, 1995

Bukstein OG, Brent DA, Kaminer Y: Comorbidity of substance abuse and other psychiatric disorders in adolescents. Am J Psychiatry 146:1131–1141, 1989

Bukstein OG, Glancy LJ, Kaminer Y: Patterns of affective comorbidity in a clinical population of dually diagnosed adolescent substance abusers. J Am Acad Child Adolesc Psychiatry 31:1041–1045, 1992

Bukstein OG, Brent DB, Perper JA, et al: Risk factors for completed suicide among adolescents with a lifetime history of substance abuse: a case control study. Acta Psychiatr Scand 88:403–408, 1993

Bulik CM, Sullivan PF, Epstein LH, et al: Drug use in women with anorexia and bulimia. Int J Eat Disord 11:213–225, 1992

Cambor RL, Millman RB: Alcohol and drug abuse in adolescents, in Child and Adolescent Psychiatry: A Comprehensive Textbook. Edited by Lewis M. Baltimore, MD, Williams & Wilkins, 1996, pp 736–752

Catalano RF, Hawkins JD, Wells EA, et al: Evaluation of the effectiveness of adolescent drug abuse treatment, assessment of risks for relapse, and promising approaches for relapse prevention. Int J Addict 25 (9A–10A):1085–1140, 1990–1991

Centers for Disease Control and Prevention: Youth risk behavior surveillance, United States, 1997. MMWR Morb Mortal Wkly Rep 47 (No SS-3):1–89, 1998

Cermak T: Diagnosing and Treating Co-Dependence. Minneapolis, MN, Johnson Institute, 1986

Chaney EF: Social skills training, in Handbook of Alcoholism Treatment Approaches: Effective Alternatives. Edited by Hester RK, Miller WR. Elmsford, NY, Pergamon, 1989, pp 206–221

Childress AR, Hole AV, Ehrman RN, et al: Cue reactivity and cue reactivity interventions in drug dependence, in Behavioral Treatments for Drug Abuse and Dependence (NIDA Research Monograph 137). Edited by Onken LS, Blaine JD, Boren JJ. Washington, DC, U.S. Government Printing Office, 1993

Clark DB, Sayette MA: Anxiety and the development of alcoholism. Am J Addict 2:56–76, 1993

Clark DB, Bukstein OG, Smith MG, et al: Identifying anxiety disorders in adolescents hospitalized for alcohol abuse or dependence. Psychiatr Serv 46:618–620, 1995

Cohen P, Cohen J, Kasen S, et al: An epidemiological study of disorders in late childhood and adolescence, I: age- and gender-specific prevalence. J Child Psychol Psychiatry 34:851–867, 1993

Cone EJ: New developments in biological measures of drug prevalence, in The Validity of Self-Reported Drug Use: Improving the Accuracy of Survey Estimates (NIDA Research Monograph 167). Edited by Harrison G, Hughes A. Rockville, MD, U.S. Department of Health and Human Services, 1997, pp 108–129

Deykin EY, Levy JC, Wells V: Adolescent depression, alcohol, and drug abuse. Am J Public Health 77:178–182, 1987

Deykin EY, Buka SL, Zeena TH: Depressive illness among chemically dependent adolescents. Am J Psychiatry 149:1341–1347, 1992

DiClemente RJ, Ponton LE: HIV-related risk behaviors among psychiatrically hospitalized adolescents and school-based adolescents. Am J Psychiatry 150:324–325, 1993

Frances R, Frances J, Franklin J, et al: Psychodynamics, in The American Psychiatric Press Textbook of Substance Abuse Treatment, 2nd Edition. Edited by Galanter M, Kleber HD. Washington, DC, American Psychiatric Press, 1999, pp 309–322

Glantz MD, Pickens RW: Vulnerability to drug abuse: introduction and overview, in Vulnerability to Drug Abuse. Edited by Glantz MD, Pickens RW. Washington, DC, American Psychological Association, 1992, pp 1–14

Gold MS, Dackis CA: Role of the laboratory in the evaluation of suspected drug abuse. J Clin Psychiatry 42 (1, suppl):17–23, 1986

Greenbaum PE, Prange ME, Friedman RM, et al: Substance abuse prevalence and comorbidity with other psychiatric disorders among adolescents with severe emotional disturbances. J Am Acad Child Adolesc Psychiatry 30:575–583, 1991

Greene JM, Ennett ST, Ringwalt CL: Substance use among runaway and homeless youth in three national samples. Am J Public Health 87:229–235, 1997

Harrison PA, Fulkerson JA, Beebe TJ: Multiple substance use among adolescent physical and sexual abuse victims. Child Abuse Neglect 21:529–539, 1997

Hovens JG, Cantwell DP, Kiriakos R: Psychiatric comorbidity in hospitalized adolescent substance abusers. J Am Acad Child Adolesc Psychiatry 33:476–483, 1994

Huizinga D, Elliot DS: A Longitudinal Study of Drug Use and Delinquency in a National Sample of Youth: An Assessment of Causal Order, Project Report No 16, A National Youth Study. Boulder, CO, Behavioral Research Institute, 1981

Jaffe J: Drug addiction and drug abuse, in The Pharmacological Basis of Therapeutics. Edited by Goodman GA. New York, Macmillan, 1990, pp 522–573

Jessor R: Adolescent problem drinking: psychosocial aspects and developmental outcomes, in Proceedings of the NIAAA–WHO Collaborating Center Designation Meeting and Alcohol Research Seminar. Washington, DC, U.S. Government Printing Office, 1985, pp 104–143

Kandel D: Stages in adolescent involvement in drug use. Science 190:912–914, 1975

Kashani JH, Beck NC, Hoeper EW, et al: Psychiatric disorders in a community sample of adolescents. Am J Psychiatry 144:584–589, 1987

Kaufman E: Psychotherapy of Addicted Persons. New York, Guilford, 1994

Kessler RC, Nelson CB, McGonagle KA, et al: The epidemiology of co-occurring addictive and mental disorders: implications for prevention and service utilization. Am J Orthopsychiatry 66:17–31, 1996

Khantzian EJ: An ego-self theory of substance dependence, in Theories of Addiction (NIDA Research Monograph 30, DHHS Publ No ADM-80-967). Washington, DC, U.S. Government Printing Office, 1980

Klerman GL, Weissman MM, Rounsaville BH, et al: The Theory and Practice of Interpersonal Psychotherapy for Depression. New York, Basic Books, 1984

Kohut H, Wolf ES: The disorders of the self and their treatment: an outline. Int J Psychoanal 59:413–425, 1978

Krystal H: Alexithymia and the effectiveness of psychoanalytic treatment. International Journal of Psychoanalytic Psychotherapy 9:353–388, 1982

Kushner MG, Sher KJ, Beitman BD: The relation between alcohol problems and anxiety disorders. Am J Psychiatry 147:685–695, 1990

Kutcher S, Kachur E, Marton P: Substance use among adolescents with chronic mental illness: a pilot study of descriptive and differentiating features. Can J Psychiatry 37:428–431, 1992

Lewinsohn PM, Hops H, Roberts RE, et al: Adolescent psychopathology, I: prevalence and incidence of depression and other DSM-III-R disorders in high school students. J Abnorm Psychol 102:133–144, 1993

Lewis RA, Piercy FP, Sprenkle DH, et al: The Purdue brief family therapy model for adolescent substance abusers, in Family Therapy With Adolescent Substance Abusers. Edited by Todd T, Selekman M. New York, Allyn & Bacon, 1990

Liddle HA, Diamond G: Adolescent substance abusers in family therapy: the critical initial phase of treatment. Family Dynamics of Addiction Quarterly 1:55–68, 1991

Loeber R: Natural histories of conduct problems, delinquency and associated substance use, in Advances in Clinical Child Psychology, Vol 11. Edited by Lahey BB, Kazdin AE. New York, Plenum, 1988, pp 73–124

Luborsky L: Principles of Psychoanalytic Psychotherapy: A Manual for Supportive-Expressive Treatment. New York, Basic Books, 1984

Marlatt GA, Gordon JR (eds): Relapse Prevention: Maintenance Strategies in the Treatment of Addictive Behaviors. New York, Guilford, 1985

Martin CS, Kaczynski NA, Maisto SA, et al: Patterns of alcohol abuse and dependence symptoms in adolescent drinkers. J Stud Alcohol 56:672–680, 1995

McKay JR: Family therapy techniques, in Treating Substance Abuse. Edited by Rotgers F, Keller DS, Morgenstern J. New York, Guilford, 1996

Meissner WW: Psychotherapy and the Paranoid Process. New York, Jason Aronson, 1986

Milan R, Halikas JA, Meller JE, et al: Psychopathology among substance abusing juvenile offenders. J Am Acad Child Adolesc Psychiatry 30:569–574, 1991

Miller G: The Substance Abuse Subtle Screening Inventory—Adolescent Version. Bloomington, IN, SASSI Institute, 1990

Miller WR, Munoz RF: How To Control Your Drinking: A Practical Guide to Responsible Drinking, Revised Edition. Albuquerque, NM, University of New Mexico Press, 1982

Miller WR, Rollnick S: Motivational Interviewing: Preparing People to Change Addictive Behavior. New York, Guilford, 1991

Milstein SG, Irwin CE: Accident-related behaviors in adolescents: a biopsychosocial view. Alcohol, Drugs and Driving 4(1):21–29, 1988

Monti PM, Abrams DB, Kadden RM, et al: Treating Alcohol Dependence: A Coping Skills Training Guide. New York, Guilford, 1989

Muramoto ML, Leshan L: Adolescent substance abuse: recognition and early intervention. Prim Care 20:141–154, 1993

Myers MG, Brown SA: Coping responses and relapse among adolescent substance abusers. J Subst Abuse 2:177–189, 1990

Newcomb MD: Identifying high-risk youth: prevalence and patterns of adolescent drug abuse, in Adolescent Drug Abuse: Clinical Assessment and Therapeutic Interventions (NIDA Research Monograph 156). Edited by Rahdert E, Czechowicz D. Rockville, MD, U.S. Department of Health and Human Services, 1995, pp 7–38

Newcomb MD, Bentler PM: Consequences of Adolescent Drug Use. Beverly Hills, CA, Sage, 1988

Nowinski J, Baker S: The Twelve-Step Facilitation Handbook: A Systematic Approach to Early Recovery from Alcohol and Addiction. New York, Lexington Books, 1992

O'Farrell TJ, Cowles KS: Marital and family therapy, in Alcoholism Treatment Approaches. Edited by Hester RK, Miller WR. New York, Pergamon, 1989

Pickrel SG, Henggeler SW: Multisystemic therapy for adolescent substance abuse and dependence. Child Adolesc Psychiatr Clin N Am 5:201–211, 1996

Prochaska JO, DiClemente CC: Stages of change in the modification of problem behaviors, in Progress in Behavior Modification. Edited by Hersen M, Eisler RM, Miller PM. Newbury Park, CA, Sage, 1992

Rahdert E: The Adolescent Assessment and Referral Manual (DHHS Publ ADM-91-1735). Rockville, MD, National Institute on Drug Abuse, 1991

Regier DA, Farmer ME, Rae DS, et al: Comorbidity of mental disorders with alcohol and other drug abuse. JAMA 264:2511–2518, 1990

Reinherz HZ, Giaconia RM, Lefkowitz ES, et al: Prevalence of psychiatric disorders in a community population of older adolescents. J Am Acad Child Adolesc Psychiatry 32:369–377, 1993

Riggs PD, Baker S, Milulich SK, et al: Depression in substance-dependent delinquents. J Am Acad Child Adolesc Psychiatry 34:764–771, 1995

Rimmele CT, Miller WR, Dougher MJ: Aversion therapies, in Handbook of Alcoholism Treatment Approaches: Effective Alternatives. Edited by Hester RK, Miller WR. New York, Pergamon, 1989

Robins LN, McEvoy L: Conduct problems as predictors of substance abuse, in Straight and Deviant Pathways From Childhood to Adulthood. Edited by Robins LN, Rutter M. Cambridge, MA, Cambridge University Press, 1991, pp 182–204

Robins LN, Przybeck TR: Age of onset of drug use as a risk factor in drug and other disorders, in Etiology of Drug Abuse: Implications for Prevention. Edited by Jones CL, Battjes RJ. Rockville, MD, U.S. Department of Health and Human Services, 1985, pp 178–192

Sharp CW, Rosenberg NL: Volatile substances, in Substance Abuse: A Comprehensive Textbook. Edited by Lowinson JH, Ruiz P, Millman RB. Baltimore, MD, Williams & Wilkins, 1992, pp 303–327

Stanton MD, Todd TC & Associates: The Family Therapy of Drug Abuse and Addiction. New York, Guilford, 1982

Stowell RJA, Estroff TW: Psychiatric disorders in substance-abusing adolescent inpatients: a pilot study. J Am Acad Child Adolesc Psychiatry 31:1036–1040, 1992

U.S. Surgeon General: The Health Consequences of Smoking: Nicotine Addiction. A Report of the Surgeon General. Atlanta, GA, Centers for Disease Control, Center for Health Promotion and Education, 1988

Van Hasselt VB, Ammerman RT, Glancy LJ, et al: Maltreatment in psychiatrically hospitalized dually diagnosed adolescent substance abusers. J Am Acad Child Adolesc Psychiatry 31:868–874, 1992

Wallace J: Ideology, belief, and behavior: Alcoholics Anonymous as a social movement, in Writings: The Alcoholism Papers of John Wallace. Newport, RI, Edgehill, 1989, pp 335–352

Weed NC, Butcher JN, Williams CL: Development of MMPI-A Alcohol/Drug Problem Scales. J Stud Alcohol 55:296–302, 1994

Winters KC: The Personal Experience Screening Questionnaire and Manual. Los Angeles, CA, Western Psychological Services, 1991

Winters KC, Henly GA: The Personal Experiences Inventory Test and User's Manual. Los Angeles, CA, Western Psychological Services, 1989

Winters KC, Stinchfeld RD, Henly GA, et al: Validity of adolescent self-report of alcohol and other drug involvement. Int J Addict 25:1379–1395, 1992

16

Childhood-Onset Schizophrenia

Andrew T. Russell, M.D.

Schizophrenia with onset in childhood and adolescence has been noted since the earliest descriptions of the syndrome (De Sanctis 1906/1971). Kraepelin found, in his series of 1,054 cases of schizophrenia, that 3.5% of the patients had an onset before age 10 and 6.2% before age 15 (Green et al. 1984; Kraepelin 1919). Although onset before age 12 is rare, the incidence of schizophrenia increases significantly in adolescence (Remschmidt et al. 1994). In fact, schizophrenia can be characterized as a disorder with modal onset in late adolescence or young adulthood (Hafner and Nowotny 1995; Loranger 1984).

Given the importance of schizophrenia as a clinical disorder and the frequency of onset in adolescence, it would follow that treatment research leading to appropriate clinical guidelines for management could be found throughout the child psychiatry literature. This is not the case. Although the literature concerning the phenomenology, course, neurobiology, and genetics of schizophrenia with onset in childhood and adolescence is growing, there is a dearth of controlled treatment research (Asarnow 1994; Campbell et al. 1999; Jacobsen and Rapoport 1998; McClellan and Werry 1994). For example, although well over 100 controlled studies of the use of antipsychotic agents in schizophrenia can be found in the general psychiatry literature, a 1999 review found one controlled study involving adolescents and one report in children younger than 12 (Campbell et al. 1999), both of which used traditional antipsychotics. At that time, only one controlled study used the newer "atypical" antipsychotics, involving treatment-resistant adolescents with an onset of psychosis before age 12 (Kumra et al. 1996). Apparently, only one study of controlled psychosocial interventions with adolescents has been reported (Rund et al. 1994).

This paucity of treatment research with children and adolescents forces the clinician to extrapolate from the results of adult treatment studies. On the face of it, this would seem a logical alternative, because the preponderance of evidence suggests that schizophrenia, at any age of onset, is one and the same disorder (Asarnow 1994; Beitchman 1985; Jacobson and Rapoport 1998; Kolvin and Berney 1990; Russell 1994; Werry 1992). Yet, assuming that treatment will be similar for adults and children may be unwise. For example, the phenomenology of major depression is similar in adolescents and adults, but several studies have shown that antidepressant medication may be significantly less effective in treating symptoms of depression in adolescents (Geller et al. 1999; Strober et al. 1990). Similarly, effective antipsychotic dosages and sensitivity to side effects may be rather different in juvenile populations with schizophrenia as compared with adults (Lewis 1998; Mandoki 1995). On the other hand, no convincing empirical evidence suggests that medications and other intervention modalities used in adults are *not* effective in children with a schizophrenic disorder. We simply do not have enough information.

Therefore, much of what is discussed about the treatment of schizophrenia with onset in childhood is, out of necessity, an extrapolation of our knowledge of intervention strategies with adults, combined with clinical experience. It is hoped that the continued excitement surrounding the introduction and use of atypical antipsychotics and the use of systematic psychosocial interventions in schizophrenia will be extended to new research efforts focusing on children and adolescents. Until this occurs, much of what follows should be considered with appropriate clinical skepticism but not an attitude of therapeutic nihilism.

Differential Diagnosis

Effective treatment depends on accurate diagnosis. Although my focus in this chapter is on treatment, special issues regarding the diagnosis of schizophrenia in children and adolescents must be briefly addressed. There are ongoing debates about the boundaries of schizophrenia, and the diagnostic dilemmas in children and adolescents are even greater than those found with adults (Armenteros et al. 1995; Kumra et al. 1998a; Maziade et al. 1996; McKenna et al. 1994; Towbin et al. 1993; Volkmar 1996). Where does a vivid fantasy life end and delusional thinking begin? How does one distinguish between, on the one hand, illogical thinking that may be developmentally appropriate for a young child and, on the other, formal thought disorder? Is the young child who carries on a spirited dialogue with an imaginary companion hallucinating? How can one distinguish between schizophrenia and bipolar illness in the floridly psychotic adolescent who is hospitalized for the first time?

Correctly answering these questions is more than an academic exercise. In one of the few longitudinal studies conducted with psychotic children and adolescents, Werry and colleagues (1991) found that out of 48 children (mean age = 13.9 years) who had initially been given a diagnosis of schizophrenia or schizophreniform disorder, 12 were diagnosed with bipolar disorder and 6 with schizoaffective disorder on follow-up. Interestingly, the converse was not true. Children initially given a diagnosis of bipolar illness did not go on to develop a clinical picture resembling schizophrenia. This difficulty in diagnosis has important treatment implications. If a first episode of psychosis is misdiagnosed as schizophrenia, the patient may be subjected to long trials of antipsychotic medication with the associated risks of tardive dyskinesia; even more important, the patient may be denied antimanic medication that may be critical for the prevention of relapse (Werry et al. 1991).

The differential diagnosis of schizophrenia in children and adolescents is particularly challenging for several reasons (McClellan and Werry 1994; Russell 1992). First, developmental issues and cognitive factors are particularly important in the differential diagnosis of childhood-onset schizophrenia. For example, Caplan (1994a, 1994b) systematically explored the nature of formal thought disorder in young schizophrenic and nonschizophrenic children, noting that distinguishing clinically significant thought disorder from normal language development is more problematic in the younger age group. The clinician also must distinguish clinically significant symptoms from phenomena normal to childhood. For example, Egdell and Kolvin (1972) discussed the differential diagnosis of hallucinations in children, which must be distinguished from hypnagogic experiences, imaginary companions, and so forth.

Second, the core symptoms of schizophrenia (i.e., hallucinations, delusions, thought disorder, and disturbance of affect) all are seen in other psychopathological disorders in childhood, adolescence, and adulthood. No symptoms are pathognomonic for schizophrenia. Carlson (1990) reviewed the differential diagnosis of mania in children and adolescents, noting that prominent psychotic features may be present in this age group, often leading to a misdiagnosis of schizophrenia. Hallucinations are also relatively common in major depressive disorder in children (Ryan et al. 1987; Tumuluru et al. 1996) and are reported by some children with "nonpsychotic" emotional and behavioral disorders (Altman et al. 1997; Del Beccaro et al. 1988; Garralda 1985). Posttraumatic stress disorder and dissociative disorders also must be considered in the differential diagnosis of children reporting hallucinations and related psychotic symptoms (Famularo et al. 1992). Kluft (1985) noted that dissociative identity disorder often has an onset in childhood, may be familial, and particularly is associated with severe abuse and neglect, especially of a sexual nature. In dissociative disorders or early forms of dissociative identity disorder, auditory hallucinations may be reported, resulting in an incorrect diagnosis of schizophrenia (Hornstein and Putnam 1992; Malenbaum and Russell 1987).

A number of other disorders also must be considered in the differential diagnosis of psychosis in children and adolescents. A wide variety of organic mental conditions may present with symptoms suggestive of schizophrenia (McClellan and Werry 1994). Although the predominance of evidence clearly has established schizophrenia and autism as separate disorders (Beitchman 1985; Green et al. 1984; Kolvin 1971; Kolvin and Berney 1990; Volkmar and Cohen 1991), a minority of children with onset of schizophrenia in childhood have symptoms and developmental abnormalities in their early years that are also seen in children with autism and pervasive developmental disorders (Alaghband-Rad et al. 1995; Hollis 1995; Petty et al. 1984; Russell et al. 1989; Watkins et al. 1988).

These differential diagnostic concerns all have clinical implications. Obviously, the diagnosis of schizophrenia must be made with great care. As noted earlier, rates of misdiagnosis, particularly in regard to initial onset of bipolar illness, might be significant. A premature diagnosis can lead to great anguish in patients and their families and result in misguided treatment. A definitive diagnosis of schizophrenia in a young person may require several years of close observation before the clinical picture is incontrovertible (Werry 1992). On the other hand, errors in the other direction can occur. Clinicians are often reluctant to include schizophrenia in a differential diagnosis even when the symptoms are clearly present and well described by the patient. Such reluctance may lead to a delay in effective treatment.

Assessment

How are symptoms of schizophrenia best assessed in children? Given the aforementioned differential diagnosis problems, it is critical to clearly elicit specific symptoms and to be able to view those symptoms from a developmental perspective. Asarnow (1994) described available structured clinical interviews and rating scales to assist in establishing an accurate and complete differential diagnosis. Detailed inquiries made to the parents must be followed by systematic interviews of the children, because parents are often unaware of internalized phenomena. In this regard, children who have had psychotic symptoms for many months or even years may not experience them as particularly distressing or ego dystonic (Russell 1994). Indirect assessment of children and adolescents (e.g., play, drawings, projective psychological testing) cannot replace the need for direct, careful, and extensive questioning about the nature of specific symptoms (e.g., auditory hallucinations) and their frequency. It is especially important to elicit specific examples. Several interviews, over time, may be required to establish a differential diagnosis (Volkmar 1996). Information from other sources (e.g., teachers) should also be obtained. The assessment of particular symptoms may be assisted by more specialized tools. Caplan et al. (1989) developed special techniques for assessing formal thought disorder in young children. Fields et al. (1994) adapted an instrument to assess positive and negative symptoms in children.

Other components of a complete clinical assessment of children and adolescents with a possible diagnosis of schizophrenia have been summarized elsewhere (McClellan and Werry 1994) and are only briefly considered here. Needless to say, a comprehensive history and family history are required. Of particular importance is the assessment of sometimes subtle developmental and social dysfunction. A complete physical and medical evaluation is important for any child presenting with psychotic symptoms (Clark and Lewis 1998). As noted previously, many organic disorders may mimic the presentation of schizophrenia (McClellan and Werry 1994). Appropriate toxicology screening is probably indicated in every adolescent who presents with a very acute onset of psychosis, even if he or she denies associated drug use. Persons with already developed psychosis are also at risk for comorbid alcohol and substance abuse (Selzer and Lieberman 1993). An electroencephalogram (EEG) and neuroimaging studies should also be carefully considered for every young patient presenting with an initial episode of psychosis. Although these tests are probably not "cost-effective"—the yield of finding a treatable disorder is low unless clear signs of organic disorder exist—I usually recommend such studies in children and adolescents presenting with a first episode of psychosis. It would be tragic to overlook a central nervous system lesion or seizure focus, especially when the clinical picture may be confusing or standard treatments are ineffective. Further justification comes from data that show a high rate of EEG abnormalities in persons with schizophrenia (Blanz and Schmidt 1993; Green et al. 1992) and from the fact that some antipsychotics (especially clozapine) lower the seizure threshold.

Treatment

General Principles

Some aspects of a basic clinical assessment, which should precede any therapeutic intervention, have been outlined in the previous section. In any child with a serious psychiatric disorder, it is essential to proceed with treatment interventions in a logical and systematic manner. After a comprehensive history is taken and a physical examination is conducted, a differential diagnosis should be established, documented in the medical record, and discussed with the family and, in the case of older patients, with the patient. Target symptoms should be identified and documented, regardless of the treatment modalities selected. Informed consent should be obtained and the cooperation of the family solicited. Informed consent, at a minimum, includes discussion of diagnosis, the nature of the proposed treatment and the likelihood of success, the risks associated with the treatment, and alternative treatments and prognosis (with and without treatment) (Schouten and Duckworth 1999). Carefully documented informed consent is particularly critical when psychotropic medications are to be used outside the approved guidelines established by the U.S. Food and Drug Administration (FDA).

There is general agreement that a comprehensive approach to treatment of schizophrenia incorporates several modalities. These modalities include psychopharmacological management in all phases of the illness, psychoeducation with the patient and family, cognitive-behavioral approaches including social skills training, supportive psychotherapy rehabilitative approaches, and special education (American Psychiatric Association 1997; Asarnow 1994; Clark and Lewis 1998; McClellan and Werry 1994; Penn and Mueser 1996; Remschmidt et al. 1994). Unfortunately, little information about the relative effectiveness of these various approaches is available, especially in children and adolescents.

Psychopharmacological Management

Antipsychotic medication is the mainstay of treatment in adult-onset schizophrenia (American Psychiatric Association 1997; Kane and Marder 1993; Marder et al. 1993). Numerous controlled studies have demonstrated its efficacy in reducing and controlling the symptoms of the disorder, especially positive symptoms such as hallucinations, delusions, and formal thought disorder. The antipsychotics have been shown to be helpful in the acute phase of the disorder and in preventing or reducing the frequency of relapse. However, approximately one-third of persons with schizophrenia do not have a beneficial response to the standard antipsychotic medications, and these medications are far less effective in modifying the negative symptoms of the disorder compared with the positive symptoms (Marder et al. 1993). In addition, all of the standard antipsychotics have a side-effect profile that is troublesome to most patients, leading to high rates of noncompliance. The introduction of the so-called atypical antipsychotics (clozapine, risperidone, olanzapine, quetiapine) has been based on the hope that these drugs may be equally or even more effective and have an improved profile of side effects, especially a lower risk for tardive dyskinesia (American Psychiatric Association 1997; Meltzer et al. 1994; Toren et al. 1998).

Much less is known about the use and effectiveness of antipsychotics in the treatment of schizophrenia with onset in childhood or adolescence. On the basis of clinical experience, some investigators have concluded that schizophrenia with onset in childhood is less responsive to antipsychotic medication, although limited empirical evidence, which is discussed below, does not necessarily support this observation. What *may* be true is that individuals with very-early-onset schizophrenia are more likely to have more severe forms of the disorder (and thus the early onset). If this is the case, it stands to reason that these persons may more closely resemble the non-drug-responsive adults who also have more severe and chronic forms of schizophrenia.

The use of the new atypical antipsychotic drugs for treatment of psychosis has increased dramatically. Some data and experience suggest that many practitioners now consider these drugs as the first choice for treatment of schizophrenia with onset in childhood or adolescence (Jensen et al. 1999). Yet their extensive use is based on very limited research data concerning efficacy and side effects (Jensen et al. 1999; Lewis 1998). Because of this discrepancy between research and practice, the following review begins with the standard antipsychotics but then focuses on these newer medications.

As noted in Campbell and colleagues' (1999) review, up to that time only three controlled studies of antipsychotic medication for the treatment of schizophrenia—two with adolescents and one with children—had been reported in the entire child psychiatry literature. In a 4-week double-blind study, Pool et al. (1976) compared loxapine, haloperidol, and placebo in 75 inpatients (43 males, 32 females) between ages 13 and 18 years inclusive (mean age = approximately 15.5 years). The adolescents were randomly assigned to the loxapine, haloperidol, or placebo groups. The average daily dosage for loxapine was 87.5 mg, and for haloperidol, 9.8 mg. Interestingly, at week 4 all three groups had improved, with no significant differences between groups on a rating of global improvement. However, for those patients identified as "severely ill" or "very severely ill" at baseline, there was a strong trend ($P = .06$) in favor of the drug treatment group, with 87.5% improved on loxapine, 70% improved on haloperidol, and only 36.4% improved on placebo (Pool et al. 1976). There were few differences between the loxapine and the haloperidol groups. Almost 75% of the subjects in both drug groups showed extrapyramidal side effects, and 81% of the loxapine group experienced sedation as compared with 52% of the haloperidol group. This study showed that loxapine and haloperidol were at least moderately effective in treating schizophrenia in adolescents but also emphasized the high frequency of side effects associated with antipsychotics in this population. The modest global gains at 4 weeks suggested the need for a more extended drug trial before full benefits might be achieved.

Useful information about dosage and side effects in adolescents with schizophrenia can also be gleaned from a non-placebo-controlled, modified single-blind study comparing a low-potency antipsychotic, thioridazine, with a high-potency drug, thiothixene (Realmuto et al. 1984). Nine boys and four girls (mean age = 15.1 years) were treated with thiothixene, and four boys and four girls (mean age = 16.1 years) were treated with thioridazine. These adolescents had been ill for an average of 3 years before the medication trial. Improvement (as measured by the Brief Psychiatric Rating Scale) was significant for both groups, with no difference in efficacy between the two drugs. The thiothixene mean optimum dosage (determined retrospectively) was 16.2 mg (0.30 mg/kg), with a range of 4.8–42.6 mg. The thioridazine mean optimum dosage was 178 mg (3.3 mg/kg), with a range of 91–228 mg. The authors emphasized that sedation was the limiting side effect in a number of cases, precluding a higher dose of medication: 75% of the thioridazine group reported drowsiness, as did 54% of the thiothixene group, and 54% of the thiothixene group also had extrapyramidal symptoms.

The single controlled study of antipsychotic medication in young children with schizophrenia is a report from an ongoing study at New York University's Bellevue Hospital (Spencer and Campbell 1994; Spencer et al. 1992). Twelve children (none boys, three girls), ranging in age from 5.5 to 11.75 years (mean age = 8.78 years), participated in a double-blind, crossover design study of haloperidol. The protocol consisted of a 2-week placebo baseline followed by either haloperidol or placebo for 4 weeks, which was then followed by the alternative regimen for 4 additional weeks. Optimum dosages ranged from 0.5 to 3.5 mg/day (0.02–0.12 mg/kg/day). All 12 children taking haloperidol showed improvement, rated as "marked" in 9, "moderate" in 2, and "mild" in 1. With placebo, 1 child was rated as markedly improved, 10 were rated as mildly improved, and 1 was rated as having mild worsening compared with baseline. These differences were highly significant in favor of the haloperidol treatment condition. Positive symptoms were more responsive to antipsychotic treatment than were negative symptoms. Of note are the relatively low dosages of medication required for optimum response, supporting findings from several studies in adult patients (Kane and Marder 1993). Two children had an acute dystonic reaction, and eight reported drowsiness. Response to haloperidol was inversely related to duration of illness (Spencer and Campbell 1994).

What can be learned from these extremely limited findings? First, it appears that standard antipsychotic medication is at least modestly effective in controlling the symptoms of schizophrenia in children and adolescents. As with adults, treatment response in children and adolescents varies markedly among individuals. When effective, standard antipsychotic medication seems to have its primary effect on positive symptoms and less effect on disturbance of affect and related negative symptoms. It appears that children and adolescents are at least as sensitive as adults to extrapyramidal side effects and sedation and, indeed, may be more sensitive (Lewis 1998). Given the high levels of sedation reported, Campbell et al. (1993) have recommended higher-potency agents as the first choice in children and adolescents. However, Green et al. (1992) found that lower-potency antipsychotics were often effective and led to better compliance. With children and adolescents, as with adults, the clinician, when prescribing and monitoring antipsychotic medications, may need to maintain a fine balance between excessive sedation and the risk for extrapyramidal side effects. Perhaps the most encouraging news is that most of the children with schizophrenia appear to be responsive to antipsychotic medication and that the most effective dosages may be in the moderate to low range. Converting to chlorpromazine equivalents, the optimum dosage in Pool et al.'s (1976) study for loxapine was 580 mg equivalents, and for haloperidol, 490 mg equivalents. In Realmuto et al.'s (1984) study, the titrated dosage for thiothixene was 324 mg chlorpromazine equivalents, and for thioridazine, 178 mg (not chlorpromazine equivalents). In Spencer et al.'s (1992) study with young children, the haloperidol dosage was only 101 mg chlorpromazine equivalents. Green et al. (1992) reported somewhat higher optimum dosages for haloperidol (50–300 mg chlorpromazine equivalents) in a similar age group, although mean dosages were not reported. Taken as a whole, the above findings suggest that clinicians treating schizophrenia in children should begin with low dosages and carefully titrate upward until an optimum balance between response and side effects is obtained. The findings argue against the need for high-dosage strategies in most children and adolescents.

The sometimes limited efficacy of typical antipsychotic drugs and their disturbing side-effect profiles, particularly their role in causing tardive dyskinesia, have stimulated the development of so-called atypical antipsychotic drugs. Typical antipsychotic agents have as their primary pharmacological action dopamine type 2 (D_2) receptor antagonism. The atypical antipsychotics effect a broader range of receptor sites, in differing combinations (Lieberman 1993). These drugs, which are under continued development, represent the first really new pharmacological tools for the treatment of schizophrenia in more than 30 years. As mentioned earlier in this chapter, the use of atypical antipsychotics in children and adolescents has been growing rapidly; what little we know about their use in children is reviewed below. The reader is also referred to two recent comprehensive reviews for additional information (Lewis 1998; Toren et al. 1998).

Clozapine was the first atypical antipsychotic introduced in the United States, and a handful of reports suggest that it has efficacy in treatment-resistant schizophrenia in adolescents and children. Clozapine in adults has been shown to be effective in about one-third of formerly nonresponsive patients, and apparently little risk of tardive dyskinesia is associated with its use (American Psychiatric Association 1997). However, clozapine has been used cautiously in patients refractory to standard treatments because of a 1%–2% incidence of potentially irreversible agranulocytosis and a dosage-related risk of the induction of seizures ranging from 1% to 5% (Kane and Marder 1993; Wahlbeck et al. 1999).

Clozapine has been used in one double-blind, controlled trial comparing clozapine and haloperidol (Kumra et al. 1996). The sample consisted of 21 young adolescent subjects, all referred to the National Institute of Mental Health and meeting strict DSM-III-R (American Psychiatric Association 1987) criteria for schizophrenia. All subjects were refractory to prior treatment and had an onset of schizophrenia prior to 12 years. Mean age was 14 years (±2.3 years). Duration of the treatment was 6 weeks, and a parallel design was used. Clozapine doses were gradually increased to a mean of 176 mg (±149 mg), and haloperidol doses were 16 mg (±8 mg). Benztropine was used prophylactically in the haloperidol group. The results "strikingly" favored clozapine on all measures of psychosis. However, the clinical effectiveness of clozapine was tempered by significant side effects. Of the 21 patients who were involved in either the double-blind or the open phases of the trial, 8 had to discontinue clozapine treatment. Three patients were discontinued for seizures, two for hematological abnormalities, and three for treatment nonresponse. Five of the 21 patients (24%) experienced mild to moderate neutropenia, and 6 patients (29%) required concomitant treatment with an anticonvulsant. The frequency of these side effects was higher than has been reported in adult populations. Despite these side effects, clozapine was clearly effective in this treatment-resistant population; 13 of the 21 patients were rated as very much improved, 7 were minimally improved, and 1 was worse.

Clozapine has also been used in a small number of open clinical trials with adolescents and in two trials with younger children. The largest open trial with adolescents was conducted in Germany. Blanz and Schmidt (1993) reported on the effects of clozapine in a population of 57 patients between ages 10 and 21 years (mean = 16.8 years); 53 of the 57 patients received a diagnosis of schizophrenia, with 41 having been hospitalized previously. Reasons for inclusion in the trial were "danger of chronification," "uncontrolled excitation," or "intolerable side effects of other neuroleptic drugs" (p. 223). The average daily dosage ranged from 75 to 800 mg (mean = 265 mg/day). The authors found that 67% of the patients improved significantly, and 21% showed partial improvement. Severe side effects requiring withdrawal from clozapine occurred in three patients and included cholinergic delirium, seizure, and significant decline in erythrocyte count. Of note, 55% of the patients showed "pathological EEG findings (sharp biphasic waves)" during clozapine treatment compared with 30% before treatment.

In an example of an open trial with younger patients, Turetz et al. (1997) reported on 11 children (mean age = 11.3, range = 9–13 years) with diagnoses of treatment-resistant schizophrenia. The mean clozapine dosage was 227 mg/day. Four of the 11 patients improved, most within the first 4–6 weeks. EEG changes were seen in 82%, but none developed seizures. No agranulocytosis occurred. Preexisting extrapyramidal symptoms improved. Sedation and drooling were reported in virtually all the children.

The reader is referred to Toren et al. (1998) and Lewis (1998) for a description of other open trials and case reports. The current consensus in general psychiatry is that clozapine has the best demonstrated effectiveness for treatment-resistant cases of schizophrenia and presents virtually no risk for tardive dyskinesia (Wahlbeck et al. 1999). However, its use remains limited in all populations because of its important side effects and need for extensive monitoring (American Psychiatric Association 1997; Clark and Lewis 1998; McClellan and Werry 1994).

Risperidone, the second atypical antipsychotic released in the United States, differs from traditional antipsychotics in that it strongly blocks serotonin type 2 (5-HT_2) receptors and dopamine type 2 (D_2) receptors. The lower incidence of extrapyramidal side effects reported with risperidone (at lower dosages only) is thought to be a result of its modulating effect on the 5-HT_2 receptor (Lewis 1998). Toren et al. (1998) summarized the open trial and case studies in children and adolescents with schizophrenia. No controlled trials have been done. For example, Armenteros et al. (1995) enrolled 10 adolescents (ages 11–18 years) with a DSM-IV (American Psychiatric Association 1994) diagnosis of schizophrenia in an open 6-week trial. Dosages were titrated to a mean of 6.6 mg/day (range = 4–10 mg/day). On a global rating, three subjects were rated very much improved, three were much improved, three were minimally improved, and one was rated as showing no change. The most significant side effects were extrapyramidal side effects (two subjects experienced an acute dystonic reaction, and four required treatment with benztropine). Eight subjects gained weight. The investigators concluded that risperidone was effective and well tolerated. Other side effects noted in other case reports are summarized in Ernst et al. 1999, Lewis 1998, and Toren et al. 1998. Probable tardive dyskinesia associated with risperidone has been reported in two cases, one in an adolescent (Feeney and Klykylo 1996). One report documented hepatotoxicity, and the authors recommended liver function monitoring (Kumra et al. 1996).

Important recent studies from the adult literature include a report that compared risperidone and haloperidol in treatment-resistant adults; risperidone was better tolerated (fewer extrapyramidal side effects) and more effective than haloperidol (Wirshing et al. 1999). In another double-blind adult study, risperidone efficacy was equivalent to that of clozapine in patients with treatment-resistant schizophrenia (Bondolfi et al. 1998). Somewhat in contrast, Rosebush and Mazurek (1999) found that extrapyramidal symptoms were comparable in neuroleptic-naïve patients treated with risperidone or haloperidol, even though low doses were used (mean = 3.2 mg and 3.7 mg, respectively). This suggests that extrapyramidal symptoms may be a more important and more frequent accompaniment of risperidone treatment than previously thought, especially if a rapid titration is used (Luchins et al. 1998).

There is very little information about the use of the newer atypical antipsychotics—olanzapine and quetiapine—in juvenile populations. Kumra and colleagues (1998b) reported an open trial with olanzapine in one child and seven adolescents (mean age 15.25 ± 2.31 years), four of whom had previously been treated with clozapine as part of the National Institute of Mental Health study discussed earlier in this chapter. Of the eight patients, three were rated much improved, two were minimally improved, one had no change, one was minimally worse, and one was much worse at 8 weeks. The magnitude of improvement was somewhat less than had been observed with clozapine, but the drug was fairly well tolerated. However, most patients reported various side effects, including increased appetite, weight gain, gastrointestinal problems, sedation, insomnia, agitation, sustained tachycardia, and sustained elevation of liver transaminase. No seizures or EEG abnormalities were noted, and extrapyramidal side effects were minimal.

Mandoki (1997) also reported a retrospective study of eight children and adolescents who were successfully switched from clozapine to olanzapine, but only after being stable on clozapine. Somewhat in contrast, Krishnamoorthy and King (1998) found olanzapine to be poorly tolerated in five preadolescent children.

One positive open trial with quetiapine fumarate has been presented in a poster session (McConville et al. 1998), and a case report has been published (Szigethy et al. 1998). Clearly, much more clinical information about these agents is needed, especially in children and adolescents.

For further discussion of side effects of the atypical antipsychotics, readers are again referred to recent reviews (Ernst et al. 1999; Lewis 1998; Toren et al. 1998). It must be noted that neuroleptic malignant syndrome has been reported in juveniles, and all clinicians should be aware of its presentation (Silva et al. 1999).

In summary, antipsychotic medication is the mainstay of treatment in schizophrenia with onset in childhood and adolescence as in adult schizophrenia. Although anecdotal reports based on clinical experience indicate that childhood-onset schizophrenia is less responsive to standard antipsychotic treatment, little controlled evidence shows that this is indeed the case. Unwarranted pessimism is therefore not in order. Dosages equivalent to those used in adults, or somewhat lower, seem to be effective. High-dosage strategies have no empirical support. Atypical antipsychotics may have particular promise in children and adolescents, because younger patients seem particularly sensitive to extrapyramidal side effects (Lewis 1998). Recent clinical guidelines for the treatment of schizophrenia still suggest that atypical antipsychotics be used after a trial of a standard antipsychotic, but this view may be changing (Clark and Lewis 1998). However, with increased use, more awareness of their side effects has emerged. For example, weight gain is common with all the atypical antipsychotics and may be a significant barrier to their acceptance, especially with adolescents. Clozapine is an important alternative in treatment-resistant cases, but its safety profile requires careful monitoring. Overall, there is a dearth of methodologically sound research on the pharmacological treatment of schizophrenia in children and adolescents. Answers to many key questions about, for example, dosage strategies, maintenance medication, adjunctive pharmacology, and the effects of chronic antipsychotic use on cognitive and physical development await further research.

Psychosocial Interventions

There is a long tradition of psychosocial intervention in schizophrenia that is based on a stress-vulnerability model. The model recognizes that persons with schizophrenia have a variety of psychophysiological, cognitive, and interpersonal deficits that make them highly vulnerable to stress (Liberman and Corrigan 1993). Sources of stress may be their environment, family, or interpersonal relationships. High levels of stress and/or an inability to cope with typical levels of stress may lead to exacerbation of psychosis and relapse. In their review of psychosocial interventions for schizophrenia, Bellack and Mueser (1993) noted that "compelling data demonstrate that the course of the illness is substantially affected by environmental events and that modification of the environment can have profound effects on the patient" (p. 317). This factor has led to a variety of psychosocial intervention strategies designed either to reduce environmental stress (e.g., family interventions) or to strengthen the patient's coping skills (e.g., social skills training). There is also ample evidence that no psychosocial strategy is sufficient in itself and that multimodality interventions combining biological interventions (medications) and psychosocial treatment constitute the most effective treatment strategy (American Psychiatric Association 1997; Falloon et al. 1998). It is beyond the scope of this chapter to review in detail the various intervention strategies designed for adults with schizophrenia and the effect of these interventions on the course of the disorder. The reader is referred to other reviews for this purpose (American Psychiatric Association 1997; Bellack 1989, 1992; Bellack and Mueser 1993; Brenner et al. 1992; Dixon and Lehman 1995; Falloon et al. 1998; Goldstein et al. 1986; Liberman and Green 1992; Penn and Mueser 1996).

Unfortunately, there is a serious lack of research concerning the use of psychosocial strategies in children or adolescents with schizophrenia. This lack of research is of concern in that developmental factors suggest that interventions such as reducing stress and increasing coping within families may be especially powerful in treating children and adolescents as opposed to young adults, who may already be outside direct family influence. Therefore, appropriate intervention strategies for children and adolescents often must be inferred from the adult literature and clinical experience.

A well-controlled study by Hogarty et al. (1986, 1991) is illustrative of this work. These authors examined the degree to which relapse in an adult population was prevented by medication alone, medication plus individual social skills training, medication plus family psychoeducation, and medication plus both social skills training and family psychoeducation. Relapse rates at 1 year were 35.7%, 21.1%, 19%, and 0%, respectively. At 2 years, medication plus family psychoeducation and medication plus both social skills training and family psychoeducation remained superior to medication alone or medication plus social skills training alone. These and other findings underscore the relative consensus in the adult literature that the ideal treatment program for persons with schizophrenia consists of continuous medication management coupled with other psychosocial interventions designed to reduce stress and improve coping skills. There is every reason to suppose that children and adolescents also need a similarly comprehensive multimodality treatment program.

What are the necessary components of a comprehensive treatment program? Bellack (1989) described an intervention model as consisting of treatment (medication, family therapy, social skills training, medical care, crisis intervention), rehabilitation, social services, and continuity of care. Medication interventions were discussed earlier in this chapter. The following review, focusing on treatment suggestions for children and adolescents, emphasizes family therapy, individual psychotherapy, social skills training, and educational intervention (the corollary of rehabilitation in Bellack's model).

Family Therapy

Direct intervention with families is an essential component of the effective treatment of a schizophrenic child or adolescent. Such intervention is critical if the child is to remain at home, but it is also of great importance even if the decision has been made to have the child treated in a long-term residential program or other facility outside the home. Much of the impetus for the development of family interventions derives directly from the stress-vulnerability model of schizophrenia and a large, if controversial, body of research concerning high "expressed emotion" (EE) in families as a predictor of relapse (Asarnow 1994; Vaughn and Leff 1976). Even though it is unclear why family intervention "works," there is little doubt that it is effective in reducing relapse in schizophrenic patients (Bellack and Mueser 1993; Penn and Mueser 1996).

Although various family interventions have been described, most include an educational component coupled with more focused behavioral techniques emphasizing the modeling and acquisition of new communication and problem-solving skills (Bellack 1989). The formal educational component usually consists of one or two sessions with the family in which a variety of topics are discussed (Cozolino and Goldstein 1986). Topics include diagnosis and basic epidemiological data with an emphasis on discussion of common "myths" about schizophrenia. The variable course of the disorder and the difficulty in predicting long-term outcome should also be reviewed. With families of children and adolescents, I also explain that some time may be required to clarify the diagnosis (see discussion of differential diagnosis earlier in this chapter). Medications and their side effects are thoroughly reviewed. Important issues include differential effects on positive and negative symptoms and the role of the family in helping with drug compliance. Critical family issues such as limit setting while allowing developmentally appropriate independence (especially for adolescents) are discussed, setting the stage for many more such discussions in the future. It is usually inappropriate for child patients to attend, but these meetings may be beneficial for mature adolescents who are not overtly psychotic. The overall goals are to provide a knowledge base to the family, reduce guilt and anger, establish a positive working relationship, and lay the foundation for further family interventions concentrating on improving communication and problem-solving skills (Bellack and Mueser 1993; Lam 1991).

A second component of family intervention programs emphasizes the development of specific communication and problem-solving skills. A program focusing on this component has been developed and implemented by Falloon (1986). In Falloon's protocol, families meet weekly for 3 months and then with gradually decreasing frequency for 1 or 2 years. The families work on specific aspects of communication, including empathic listening, expression of feelings (both positive and negative), and requests to change behavior (Falloon 1986). A second feature of this protocol is training in problem resolution (i.e., identifying a problem and solving it in a systematic matter). The family sessions are based on behavioral interventions similar to those used in social skills training—that is, identification of specific topics, modeling, rehearsal, and homework (Bellack and Mueser 1993). This model has been tested with in-home sessions with striking results. Over a 2-year period, the control group (medication management) had a relapse rate of 83%, whereas the group receiving the family interventions had a cumulative relapse rate of 17% (Bellack and Mueser 1993; Falloon 1986). Improvements were also found in social functioning and in the amount of family distress in the family treatment group.

I am aware of only one study focusing on adolescents with schizophrenia and their families. Rund et al. (1994) reported on 12 adolescents in Norway who were treated on an inpatient service and followed up for 2 years. The comparison group was a retrospectively selected sample of adolescents who had been treated in the same facility earlier but had not been part of the research treatment protocol, which used medication management in combination with several psychoeducational approaches. Outcome was measured by the number of relapses and changes in Global Assessment Scale scores over the 2-year period. Changes in EE and treatment cost also were assessed.

The experimental treatment model consisted of three phases:

1. In the *hospitalization phase*, optimal medication management was emphasized. Family treatment took place every other week, and parent seminars to teach families about the nature of schizophrenia and general approaches to its management were initiated.

2. In the *intensive rehabilitative phase,* additional seminars were held, and highly structured "problem-solving" sessions took place in the patient's home once a month.
3. In the *third phase,* these approaches were continued for 2 years but at a reduced frequency.

Another feature of the program included the establishment of community "networks," especially with the schools where training and advice were provided, and special school arrangements were created as needed. The results were encouraging. Only one patient in the experimental group had two or more rehospitalizations. Global Assessment Scale scores improved more in the experimental group but fell just short of statistical significance. Seven families in the experimental group moved from high to low EE ratings, whereas all the families in the comparison group continued to have high EE scores. A cost analysis also favored the experimental treatment program.

What can be concluded from this and other promising studies in regard to treatment of schizophrenia in children and adolescents? Although an individual child psychiatrist outside of a specialized clinic is unlikely to implement a formal family training protocol, it is clear that sustained work with families should be part of any treatment plan. The family treatment should include an educational component about the nature of schizophrenia and the role of families in prevention of relapse and maintaining compliance. Time should be devoted to finding ways to increase the quality of family communication and to providing practical techniques for problem solving and decision making within the family structure. The treatment should focus on reducing stress and improving coping in the present as opposed to making interpretations of past dysfunction. The goal of these interventions should be not only to reduce psychopathology in the patient but also to alleviate the "family burden" of caring for a chronically ill child.

Individual Psychotherapy

What is the role of individual psychotherapy in the treatment of a psychotic child or adolescent? Although many children receive such intervention, often on a weekly basis, virtually no evidence supports the effectiveness of traditional psychodynamic "investigative" approaches in schizophrenia in either adults or children (Kane 1987; Kolvin and Berney 1990). However, supportive psychotherapy enhancing coping skills and using psychoeducational approaches is often helpful. In my experience, especially if treatment is being provided outside of a specialized clinic with other support services, regular contact with an individual therapist is required to provide appropriate case management; assist the patient in coping with day to day, "here and now" issues; monitor medication compliance; and provide a constant relationship for the patient who may become increasingly isolated from others. An additional goal for such intervention is the monitoring of possible suicide intent, because suicide rates are disturbingly high in adolescents and young adults with schizophrenia (Werry et al. 1991). Such supportive therapy often combines family interventions and social skills training techniques.

Social Skills Training

Social skills training has gradually established itself as an important component of a comprehensive treatment program for schizophrenic adults (Bellack 1989; Penn and Mueser 1996). Although no studies of the use of similar techniques in the treatment of schizophrenic children and adolescents have been done, such methods have been applied to children with other disorders. Social skills training for persons with schizophrenia is important because social dysfunction is one of the hallmarks of the disease and may persist even if positive and negative symptoms are controlled (Bellack 1989; Bellack and Mueser 1993). Social skills training can be used to teach children how to approach and play appropriately with other children and how to develop friendships. Tasks for adolescents may include talking with their psychiatrist about medication, using the telephone for social purposes, or finding a summer job (Falloon 1992; Liberman and Corrigan 1993). After specific deficits are defined and assessed, interventions commonly include rehearsing (with coaching) interpersonal strategies and practicing them in real life, suggesting homework, problem-solving around obtaining access to community resources, and training family members to provide continued reinforcement (Falloon 1992). An important development in the field has been the design and implementation of training modules that can be used independently of one another and repeated as necessary (Liberman and Corrigan 1993). It is hoped that this development may eventually be extended for use with children and adolescents with chronic psychiatric disorder. In any case, child and adolescent psychiatrists working with schizophrenic patients should strive to incorporate social skills training techniques into the ongoing treatment of their patients and their patients' families.

Special Education

Another critical component of a comprehensive treatment program is special education. Most children and adolescents with schizophrenia require specialized education services, including small structured classrooms with individual educational plans (Kolvin and Berney 1990; McClellan and Werry 1994). The educational handicaps of these children are complex and may involve behavioral disturbance, impaired attention, thought disorder, cognitive handicaps, social impairments, and increased vulnerability to stress. Individual variations in handicaps require tailored educational programs. Small classrooms are often essential to decrease the level of environmental and social stimuli. Day hospital programs with a strong educational focus may be particularly helpful.

Continuity of Care

In my experience, many children with schizophrenia receive a series of uncoordinated and even chaotic interventions. Medications are changed for unclear reasons, often after inadequate trials. Hospitalizations often occur at locations away from the local treatment program and may disrupt as much as enhance the continuity of care. Patients may move from psychiatrist to psychiatrist, often with dramatic changes in the course of treatment. Specialized services, when needed, are often unavailable. Treatment compliance problems, especially among adolescents, are legion. In short, the patient suffers because of a lack of coordination of care. What can be done? A case manager system with a single individual or team monitoring and coordinating treatment often facilitates quality care. Lacking such a system, the treating psychiatrist must strive to coordinate treatment and establish effective communication with other agencies and professionals involved in the care of his or her patient. Finally, all parents of a schizophrenic child, adolescent, or young adult should be referred to self-help organizations such as the National Alliance for the Mentally Ill (NAMI). Parents have founded such organizations precisely because of the lack of treatment resources (and of coordination of available resources) for their children, and these organizations can be of invaluable assistance to other families facing similar situations.

Conclusions

Schizophrenia in children and adolescents is a devastating disorder for most young patients and their families. Limited outcome data suggest that the prognosis at best may be similar to that for schizophrenia of adult onset (Asarnow and Ben-Meir 1988; Asarnow et al. 1994; Eggers and Bunk 1997). Every child and adolescent patient with schizophrenia requires a comprehensive treatment plan that includes medication management and a variety of other interventions, emphasizing family intervention, psychoeducational, and social skills training approaches. Special education is generally required. Current approaches, including the use of antipsychotic medications, all have significant limitations, and a significant number of children do not seem to respond to interventions. Improved treatment approaches and technologies are therefore desperately needed.

Although the research on treatment of schizophrenia in children and adolescents is limited, there is a growing optimism that new medications and more sophisticated psychosocial intervention strategies being pioneered with adult populations will prove equally useful in children and adolescents. The testing of more detailed treatment protocols with appropriate controls, as has recently occurred in adult populations, should be extended to child and adolescent patients.

References

Alaghband-Rad J, McKenna K, Gordon CT, et al: Childhood-onset schizophrenia: the severity of premorbid course. J Am Acad Child Adolesc Psychiatry 34:1273–1283, 1995

Altman H, Collins M, Mundy P, et al: Subclinical hallucinations and delusions in nonpsychotic adolescents. J Child Psychol Psychiatry 38:413–420, 1997

American Psychiatric Association: Diagnostic and Statistical Manual of Mental Disorders, 3rd Edition, Revised. Washington, DC, American Psychiatric Association, 1987

American Psychiatric Association: Diagnostic and Statistical Manual of Mental Disorders, 4th Edition. Washington, DC, American Psychiatric Association, 1994

American Psychiatric Association: Practice guidelines for the treatment of patients with schizophrenia. Am J Psychiatry 154 (suppl 4):1–63, 1997

Armenteros JL, Fennelly BW, Hallin A, et al: Schizophrenia in hospitalized adolescents: clinical diagnosis, DSM-III-R, DSM-IV, and ICD-10 criteria. Psychopharmacol Bull 31:383–387, 1995

Asarnow JR: Annotation: childhood-onset schizophrenia. J Child Psychol Psychiatry 35:1345–1371, 1994

Asarnow JR, Ben-Meir S: Children with schizophrenia spectrum and depressive disorders: a comparative study of premorbid adjustment, onset pattern, and severity of impairment. J Child Psychol Psychiatry 29:477–488, 1988

Asarnow JR, Tompson MC, Hamilton EB, et al: Childhood-onset schizophrenia: a follow-up study. Schizophr Bull 20:599–618, 1994

Beitchman JH: Childhood schizophrenia: a review and comparison with adult onset cases. Psychiatr Clin North Am 8:793–814, 1985

Bellack AS: A comprehensive model for the treatment of schizophrenia, in a Clinical Guide for the Treatment of Schizophrenia. Edited by Bellack AS. New York, Plenum, 1989, pp 1–22

Bellack AS: Cognitive rehabilitation for schizophrenia: is it possible? Is it necessary? Schizophr Bull 18:43–50, 1992

Bellack AS, Mueser KT: Psychosocial treatment for schizophrenia. Schizophr Bull 19:317–336, 1993

Blanz B, Schmidt MH: Clozapine for schizophrenia (letter). J Am Acad Child Adolesc Psychiatry 31: 223–224, 1993

Bondolfi G, Dufour H, Patris M: Risperidone versus clozapine in treatment-resistant chronic schizophrenia: a randomized double-blind study. Am J Psychiatry 155:449–504, 1998

Brenner HD, Hodel B, Roder V, et al: Treatment of cognitive dysfunctions and behavioral deficits in schizophrenia. Schizophr Bull 18:21–26, 1992

Campbell M, Gonzales NM, Ernst M, et al: Antipsychotics, in Practitioner's Guide to Psychoactive Drugs for Children and Adolescents. Edited by Werry JS, Aman MG. New York, Plenum, 1993, pp 269–296

Campbell M, Rapoport J, Simpson G: Antipsychotics in children and adolescents. J Am Acad Child Adolesc Psychiatry 38:537–545, 1999

Caplan R: Communication deficits in childhood schizophrenia spectrum disorders. Schizophr Bull 20:671–683, 1994a

Caplan R: Thought disorder in childhood. J Am Acad Child Adolesc Psychiatry 33:605–614, 1994b

Caplan R, Guthrie D, Fish B, et al: The Kiddie Formal Thought Disorder Scale (K-FTDS): clinical assessment, reliability, and validity. Journal of the American Academy of Child Psychiatry 28:408–416, 1989

Carlson GA: Annotation: child and adolescent mania—diagnostic considerations. J Child Psychol Psychiatry 31:331–341, 1990

Clark AF, Lewis SW: Treatment of schizophrenia in childhood and adolescence. J Child Psychol Psychiatry 39:1071–1081, 1998

Cozolino LJ, Goldstein MJ: Family education as a component of extended family-oriented treatment programs for schizophrenia, in Treatment of Schizophrenia: Family Assessment and Intervention. Edited by Goldstein MJ, Hahlweg K. Berlin, Springer-Verlag, 1986, pp 117–128

Del Beccaro MA, Burke P, McCauley E: Hallucinations in children: a follow-up study. J Am Acad Child Adolesc Psychiatry 27:462–465, 1988

De Sanctis S: On some varieties of dementia praecox (1906), in Modern Perspective in International Child Psychiatry. Translated by Osborn ML. Edited by Howells JG. New York, Brunner/Mazel, 1971, pp 590–609

Dixon L, Lehman AF: Family interventions for schizophrenia. Schizophr Bull 21:631–643, 1995

Egdell HG, Kolvin I: Childhood hallucinations. J Child Psychol Psychiatry 13:279–287, 1972

Eggers C, Bunk D: The long-term course of childhood-onset schizophrenia: a 42-year follow-up. Schizophr Bull 23:105–117, 1997

Ernst M, Malone RP, Rowan AB, et al: Antipsychotics (Neuroleptics), in Practitioner's Guide to Psychoactive Drugs for Children and Adolescents, 2nd Edition. Edited by Werry JS, Aman MG. New York, Plenum, 1999, pp 297–328

Falloon IRH: Behavioral family therapy for schizophrenia: clinical, social, family and economic benefits, in Treatment of Schizophrenia: Family Assessment and Intervention. Edited by Goldstein MJ, Hand I, Hahlweg K. Berlin, Springer-Verlag, 1986, pp 171–184

Falloon IRH: Psychotherapy for schizophrenic disorders: a review. Br J Hosp Med 48:164–170, 1992

Falloon IRH, Held T, Roncone R, et al: Optimal treatment strategies to enhance recovery from schizophrenia. Aust N Z J Psychiatry 32(1):43–49, 1998

Famularo R, Kinscherff R, Fenton T: Psychiatric diagnosis of maltreated children: preliminary findings. J Am Acad Child Adolesc Psychiatry 31:863–867, 1992

Feeney DJ, Klykylo W: Risperidone and tardive dyskinesia (letter). J Am Acad Child Adolesc Psychiatry 35:1421–1422, 1996

Fields JH, Grochowski S, Lindenmayer JP, et al: Assessing positive and negative symptoms in children and adolescents. Am J Psychiatry 151:249–253, 1994

Garralda ME: Characteristics of the psychoses of late onset in children and adolescents: a comparative study of hallucinating children. J Adolesc 58:195–207, 1985

Geller MD, Reising MD, Henrietta L, et al: Critical review of tricyclic antidepressant use in children and adolescents. J Am Acad Child Adolesc Psychiatry 38:513–516, 1999

Goldstein MJ, Hand I, Hahlweg K: Treatment of Schizophrenia: Family Assessment and Intervention. Berlin, Springer-Verlag, 1986

Green WH, Campbell M, Hardesty AS, et al: A comparison of schizophrenic and autistic children. Journal of the American Academy of Child Psychiatry 23:399–409, 1984

Green WH, Padron-Gayol M, Hardesty AS, et al: Schizophrenia with childhood onset: a phenomenological study of 38 cases. Journal of the American Academy of Child Psychiatry 31:968–976, 1992

Hafner H, Nowotny B: Epidemiology of early onset schizophrenia. Eur Arch Psychiatry Clin Neurosci 245:80–92, 1995

Hogarty GE, Anderson CM, Reiss DJ, et al: Family psychoeducation, social skills training, and maintenance chemotherapy in the aftercare treatment of schizophrenia, I: one-year effects of a controlled study on relapse and expressed emotion. Arch Gen Psychiatry 43:633–642, 1986

Hogarty GE, Anderson CM, Reiss DJ, et al: Family psychoeducation, social skills training, and maintenance chemotherapy in the aftercare treatment of schizophrenia, II: two-year effects of a controlled study on relapse and expressed adjustment. Arch Gen Psychiatry 48:340–347, 1991

Hollis C: Child and adolescent (juvenile onset) schizophrenia: a case control study of premorbid developmental impairments. Br J Psychiatry 166:489–495, 1995

Hornstein JL, Putnam FW: Clinical phenomenology of child and adolescent dissociative disorders. J Am Acad Child Adolesc Psychiatry 31:1077–1085, 1992

Jacobsen LK, Rapoport JL: Research update; childhood-onset schizophrenia: implications of clinical and neurobiological research. J Child Psychol Psychiatry 39:101–113, 1998

Jensen P, Bhatara VS, Vitiello B, et al: Psychoactive medication prescribing practices for U.S. children: gaps between research and clinical practice. J Am Acad Child Adolesc Psychiatry 38:557–565, 1999

Kane JM: Treatment of schizophrenia. Schizophr Bull 13:133–156, 1987

Kane JM, Marder SR: Psychopharmacologic treatment of schizophrenia. Schizophr Bull 19:287–302, 1993

Kluft R (ed): Childhood Antecedents of Multiple Personality. Washington, DC, American Psychiatric Press, 1985

Kolvin I: Studies in the childhood psychoses, I: diagnostic criteria and classification. Br J Psychiatry 118:381–384, 1971

Kolvin I, Berney TP: Childhood schizophrenia, in Handbook of Studies of Child Psychiatry. Edited by Tonge BJ, Burrows GD, Werry JS. Amsterdam, Elsevier, 1990, pp 123–135

Kraepelin E: Dementia Praecox and Paraphrenia. Translated by Barclay RM. Edited by Robertson GM. Edinburgh, Scotland, E&S Livingston, 1919

Krishnamoorthy J, King BH: Open-label olanzapine treatment in five preadolescent children. J Child Adolesc Psychopharmacol 8:107–113, 1998

Kumra S, Frazier JA, Jacobsen LK, et al: Childhood-onset schizophrenia: a double-blind clozapine-haloperidol comparison. Arch Gen Psychiatry 53:1090–1097, 1996

Kumra S, Jacobsen LK, Lenane M, et al: "Multidimensionally impaired disorder": is it a variant of very early-onset schizophrenia? J Am Acad Child Adolesc Psychiatry 37:91–99, 1998a

Kumra S, Jacobsen LK, Lenane M, et al: Case series: spectrum of neuroleptic-induced movement disorders and extrapyramidal side effects in childhood-onset schizophrenia. J Am Acad Child Adolesc Psychiatry 37:221–227, 1998b

Lam DH: Psychosocial family intervention in schizophrenia: a review of empirical studies. Psychol Med 21:423–441, 1991

Lewis R: Typical and atypical antipsychotics in adolescent schizophrenia: efficacy, tolerability, and differential sensitivity to extrapyramidal symptoms. Can J Psychiatry 43:596–604, 1998

Liberman RP, Corrigan PW: Designing new psychosocial treatments for schizophrenia. Psychiatry 56: 238–249, 1993

Liberman RP, Green MF: Whither cognitive-behavioral therapy for schizophrenia? Schizophr Bull 18: 27–35, 1992

Lieberman JA: Understanding the mechanism of action of atypical antipsychotic drugs: a review of compounds in use and development. Br J Psychiatry 163 (suppl 22):7–18, 1993

Loranger AW: Sex differences in age at onset of schizophrenia. Arch Gen Psychiatry 41:157–161, 1984

Luchins DJ, Klass D, Hanrahan P: Alteration in the recommended dosing schedule for risperidone. Am J Psychiatry 155:365–366, 1998

Malenbaum R, Russell A: Multiple personality disorder in a 10 year old boy and his mother. J Am Acad Child Adolesc Psychiatry 26:436–439, 1987

Mandoki MW: Risperidone treatment of children and adolescents: increased risk of extrapyramidal side effects. J Child Adolesc Psychopharmacol 5:49–67, 1995

Mandoki M: Olanzapine in the treatment of early-onset schizophrenia in children and adolescents (abstract). Biol Psychiatry 41 (suppl 7s):22s, 1997

Marder SR, Ames D, Wirshing WC, et al: Schizophrenia. Psychiatr Clin North Am 16:567–587, 1993

Maziade M, Gingras N, Rodriguez C, et al: Long-term stability of diagnosis and symptom dimensions in a systematic sample of patients with onset of schizophrenia in childhood and early adolescence, I: nosology, sex and age of onset. Br J Psychiatry 169:361–370, 1996

McClellan JM, Werry JS: Practice parameters for the assessment and treatment of children and adolescents with schizophrenia. J Am Acad Child Adolesc Psychiatry 33:616–635, 1994

McConville B, Arvantis L, Wong J, et al: Quetiapine fumarate: clinical effectiveness, tolerability and pharmacokinetics in psychotic adolescents (abstract), in Scientific Proceedings of the Annual Meeting of the American Academy of Child and Adolescent Psychiatry, Anaheim, CA, October 1998, p 124

McKenna K, Gordon CT, Lenane M, et al: Looking for childhood-onset schizophrenia: the first 71 cases screened. J Am Acad Child Adolesc Psychiatry 33:636–644, 1994

Meltzer HY, Lee MA, Ranjan R: Recent advances in the pharmacotherapy of schizophrenia. Acta Psychiatr Scand 90 (suppl 384):95–101, 1994

Penn DL, Mueser KT: Research update on the psychosocial treatment of schizophrenia. Am J Psychiatry 153:607–617, 1996

Petty LLK, Ornitz EM, Michelman JD, et al: Autistic children who become schizophrenic. Arch Gen Psychiatry 41:129–135, 1984

Pool D, Bloom W, Mielke DH, et al: A controlled evaluation of loxitane in seventy-five adolescent schizophrenia patients. Current Therapeutic Research 19:99–104, 1976

Realmuto GM, Ericson WD, Yellin AM, et al: Clinical comparison of thiothixene and thioridazine in schizophrenic adolescents. Am J Psychiatry 141:440–442, 1984

Remschmidt HE, Schulz E, Martin M, et al: Childhood-onset schizophrenia: history of the concept and recent studies. Schizophr Bull 20:727–745, 1994

Rosebush P, Mazurek F: Neurologic side effects in neuroleptic-naïve patients treated with haloperidol or risperidone. Neurology 52:782–785, 1999

Rund BR, Sollien T, Fjell A, et al: The Psychosis Project: outcome and cost-effectiveness of a psychoeducational treatment programme for schizophrenic adolescents. Acta Psychiatr Scand 89:211–218, 1994

Russell AT: Schizophrenia, in Child Psychopathology: Diagnostic Criteria and Clinical Assessment. Edited by Hooper SR, Hynd GW, Mattison RE. Hillsdale, NJ, Lawrence Erlbaum, 1992, pp 23–63

Russell AT: The clinical presentation of childhood-onset schizophrenia. Schizophr Bull 20:631–646, 1994

Russell AT, Bott L, Sammons C: The phenomenology of schizophrenia occurring in childhood. J Am Acad Child Adolesc Psychiatry 28:399–407, 1989

Ryan ND, Puig-Antich J, Ambrosini P, et al: The clinical picture of major depression in children and adolescents. Arch Gen Psychiatry 44:854–861, 1987

Schouten R, Duckworth K: Medicolegal and ethical issues in the pharmacologic treatment of children, in Practitioner's Guide to Psychoactive Drugs for Children and Adolescents, 2nd Edition. Edited by Werry JS, Aman MG. New York, Plenum, 1999, pp 165–181

Selzer JA, Lieberman JA: Schizophrenia and substance abuse. Psychiatr Clin North Am 16:401–412, 1993

Silva RR, Munoz DM, Alpert M, et al: Neuroleptic malignant syndrome in children and adolescents. J Am Acad Child Adolesc Psychiatry 38:187–194, 1999

Spencer EK, Campbell M: Children with schizophrenia: diagnosis, phenomenology, and pharmacotherapy. Schizophr Bull 20:713–725, 1994

Spencer EK, Kafantaris V, Padron-Gayol MV, et al: Haloperidol in schizophrenic children: early findings from a study in progress. Psychopharmacol Bull 28:183–186, 1992

Strober M, Freeman R, Rigali J: The pharmacotherapy of depressive illness in adolescents, I: an open label trial of imipramine. Psychopharmacol Bull 26:80–84, 1990

Szigethy E, Brent S, Findling R: Quetiapine for refractory schizophrenia (letter). J Am Acad Child Adolesc Psychiatry 37:1127–1128, 1998

Toren P, Laor N, Weizman A: Use of atypical neuroleptics in child and adolescent psychiatry. J Clin Psychiatry 59:644–656, 1998

Towbin KE, Dykes EM, Pearson GS, et al: Conceptualizing "borderline syndrome of childhood" and "childhood schizophrenia" as a developmental disorder. J Am Acad Child Adolesc Psychiatry 32:775–782, 1993

Tumuluru S, Yaylayan RV, Weller EB, et al: Affective psychoses, I: major depression with psychosis, in Psychoses and Pervasive Developmental Disorders in Childhood and Adolescence. Edited by Volkmar F. Washington, DC, American Psychiatric Press, 1996, pp 49–69

Turetz M, Mozes T, Toren P, et al: An open trial of clozapine in neuroleptic-resistant childhood-onset schizophrenia. Br J Psychiatry 170:501–510, 1997

Vaughn C, Leff J: The influence of family and social factors in the course of psychiatric illness. Br J Psychiatry 129:125–137, 1976

Volkmar FR: Childhood and adolescent psychosis: a review of the past 10 years. J Am Acad Child Adolesc Psychiatry 35:843–851, 1996

Volkmar FR, Cohen DJ: Comorbid association of autism and schizophrenia. Am J Psychiatry 148:1705–1707, 1991

Wahlbeck K, Cheine M, Essali A: Evidence of clozapine's effectiveness in schizophrenia: a systematic review and meta-analysis of randomized trials. Am J Psychiatry 156:990–999, 1999

Watkins JM, Asarnow RF, Tanguay P: Symptom development in childhood onset schizophrenia. J Child Psychol Psychiatry 29:865–878, 1988

Werry JS: Child and adolescent (early onset) schizophrenia: a review in light of DSM-II-R. J Autism Dev Disord 22:601–625, 1992

Werry JS, McClellan JM, Chard L: Childhood and adolescent schizophrenic, bipolar, and schizoaffective disorders: a clinical and outcome study. J Am Acad Child Adolesc Psychiatry 30:457–465, 1991

Wirshing D, Marshall BD, Green MF: Risperidone in treatment-refractory schizophrenia. Am J Psychiatry 156:1374–1379, 1999

17

Childhood Sleep Disorders

Thomas F. Anders, M.D.

In this chapter, I review some of the common sleep disorders of childhood and how they affect families. Developmental failures in achieving consolidated nighttime sleep and daytime wakefulness, in going to bed and falling asleep easily, in maintaining continuity of sleep, and in circadian regulation of sleep-wake cycles are significant risk factors for potential sleep disorders in infants, children, and adolescents. An understanding of childhood sleep disorders is facilitated by knowledge about the development of both sleep-state architecture and sleep-wake–state temporal organization. The maturation of sleep-wake states has been reviewed elsewhere (Anders and Eiben 1997; Coons and Guilleminault 1982), and only a summary is provided here.

Developmental Aspects of Sleep-Wake Organization

Newborns spend 50% of their sleep time in rapid eye movement (REM) sleep (also known as active sleep or dreaming sleep) and 50% of their sleep time in non-REM (NREM) sleep (also known as quiet sleep or slow-wave sleep). By adolescence, the relative proportion of REM sleep during sleep time has diminished to 20%, whereas NREM sleep has increased proportionally to 80% of sleep time. Four stages of NREM sleep (Stages 1–4) can begin to be differentiated from patterns on the electroencephalogram (EEG) by age 3–4 months. REM and NREM periods alternate with each other in 50- to 60-minute (i.e., ultradian) sleep cycles. A period of 30 minutes of REM sleep is followed by 30 minutes of NREM sleep in a sleep cycle, and three to four sleep cycles constitute a 4-hour episode of sleep for the newborn. At age 3 months, diurnal influences begin to affect sleep-cycle organization (Ferber 1999). Early sleep cycles have 40–50 minutes of NREM sleep and 10–20 minutes of REM sleep; in sleep cycles later in the night, the reverse is true. Thus, NREM sleep, especially Stage 4 NREM sleep, shifts to the beginning of a sleep period, and REM sleep predominates later in the sleep period. As the continuous periods of sleep consolidate and lengthen, the number of REM-NREM sleep cycles increases. However, the 50- to 60-minute sleep cycle itself does not lengthen until adolescence, when the 90-minute sleep cycle of mature adults is achieved. Another noteworthy developmental landmark occurs at sleep onset. When young infants make the transition from wakefulness to sleep at the beginning of their night, their initial sleep-onset state is typically REM sleep. By age 3 months, sleep-onset REM periods begin to be replaced by sleep-onset NREM periods. By the time the child is 1 year old, transitions from waking directly to REM sleep are rare. Appreciating these maturational changes is useful for clinicians in differentiating many of the common sleep disorders that affect infants, children, and adolescents.

Classification of Sleep Disorders

In the revised *International Classification of Sleep Disorders Diagnostic and Coding Manual* (ICSD-DCM), the American Sleep Disorders Association (ASDA; 1990) broadly classifies three categories of disordered sleep: 1) dyssomnias, 2) parasomnias, and 3) sleep disorders associated with medical and psychiatric conditions. In general, the categories of sleep disorders in the DSM-IV (American Psychiatric Association 1994) classification system are consistent with the ICSD-DCM categories. In ICSD-DCM, *dyssomnias* are defined as disorders of insufficient (in duration and quality), excessive, or inefficient sleep characterized by either difficulty in initiating and/or maintaining sleep or, in contrast, excessive sleepiness. The disorders of initiating and maintaining sleep, generically referred to as the *insomnias,* are associated with sleep that is insufficient to support good daytime functioning. The disorders of excessive somnolence, also known as the *hypersomnias,* are characterized by a persistent need for sleep that is excessive and leads to impaired daytime functioning. The ASDA coding manual further subclassifies dyssomnias into *intrinsic* (i.e., those that originate from causes within the body), *extrinsic* (i.e., those that require external factors to produce and maintain the disorder), and *circadian* (i.e., those characterized by inappropriate timing of sleep within the 24-hour day). A partial list of ICSD-DCM and DSM-IV dyssomnias that are commonly observed in children and adolescents is presented in Tables 17–1 and 17–2, respectively.

The *parasomnias* are defined by behaviors that intrude into the sleep process as a result of central or autonomic nervous system activation. Parasomnias are not primary disorders of sleep-wake organization. Rather, they represent disruptions of sleep continuity. In earlier nosologies, parasomnias were limited to disruptions that were most likely to occur during the early part of the night when Stage 4 NREM sleep was prominent. In both ICSD-DCM and DSM-IV, parasomnias have been expanded to include disruptions that occur in all states of sleep. The ICSD-DCM classification includes NREM sleep parasomnias, sleep-wake transition parasomnias, and REM sleep parasomnias, whereas the DSM-IV classification does not emphasize the sleep state in which the parasomnias occur. The ICSD-DCM and DSM-IV parasomnias that most commonly affect children and adolescents are listed in Tables 17–3 and 17–4, respectively. Again, concordance between the two systems is good.

TABLE 17–1. ICSD-DCM dyssomnias (selected)

Dyssomnia	ICSD-DCM code
Extrinsic sleep disorders	
Inadequate sleep hygiene	307.41-1
Environmental sleep disorder	780.52-4
Insufficient sleep syndrome	307.49-4
Limit setting sleep disorder	307.42-4
Sleep-onset association disorder	307.24-5
Food allergy insomnia	780.52-2
Circadian rhythm sleep disorders	
Time zone change (jet lag syndrome)	307.45
Delayed sleep phase syndrome	780.55-1
Advanced sleep phase syndrome	780.55-2
Intrinsic sleep disorders	
Psychophysiological insomnia	307.42-0
Narcolepsy	347.
Post-traumatic hypersomnia	780.54-8
Obstructive sleep apnea	780.53-0
Central sleep apnea syndrome	780.51-0
Central alveolar hypoventilation	780.51-1
Restless legs syndrome	780.52-5

Note. ICSD-DCM = *International Classification of Sleep Disorders Diagnostic and Coding Manual, Revised* (American Sleep Disorders Association 1990).

The ICSD-DCM sleep disorders that co-occur most commonly with medical and psychiatric disorders of children and their DSM-IV equivalents are listed in Tables 17–5 and 17–6, respectively. (The DSM-IV criteria for substance-induced sleep disorder are presented in Table 17–7.) There are some differences in this category of disorder in the two nosologies in that DSM-IV maintains the multiaxial classification system originated in DSM-III (American Psychiatric Association 1980).

General Evaluation of Childhood Sleep-Wake Disorders

Parental concerns about sleep are common, even though youngsters may not complain themselves. Young children never seem tired and typically resist going to bed. Adolescents, in contrast, can sleep anywhere, anytime. Many become difficult to arouse on school mornings and sleep excessively on weekends. Rarely do either children or adolescents seek treatment for these behaviors. Thus, distinguishing among genuine sleep disorders, transient sleep problems, behavior problems associated with poor sleep hygiene, and parental concerns about sleep may be difficult, especially in children whose daytime functioning is minimally or not at all impaired by sleepiness.

TABLE 17–2. DSM-IV diagnostic criteria for primary sleep disorders: dyssomnias

307.42 Primary insomnia

A. The predominant complaint is difficulty initiating or maintaining sleep, or nonrestorative sleep, for at least 1 month.

B. The sleep disturbance (or associated daytime fatigue) causes clinically significant distress or impairment in social, occupational, or other important areas of functioning.

C. The sleep disturbance does not occur exclusively during the course of narcolepsy, breathing-related sleep disorder, circadian rhythm sleep disorder, or a parasomnia.

D. The disturbance does not occur exclusively during the course of another mental disorder (e.g., major depressive disorder, generalized anxiety disorder, a delirium).

E. The disturbance is not due to the direct physiological effects of a substance (e.g., a drug of abuse, a medication) or a general medical condition.

307.44 Primary hypersomnia

A. The predominant complaint is excessive sleepiness for at least 1 month (or less if recurrent) as evidenced by either prolonged sleep episodes or daytime sleep episodes that occur almost daily.

B. The excessive sleepiness causes clinically significant distress or impairment in social, occupational, or other important areas of functioning.

C. The excessive sleepiness is not better accounted for by insomnia and does not occur exclusively during the course of another sleep disorder (e.g., narcolepsy, breathing-related sleep disorder, circadian rhythm sleep disorder, or a parasomnia) and cannot be accounted for by an inadequate amount of sleep.

D. The disturbance does not occur exclusively during the course of another mental disorder.

E. The disturbance is not due to the direct physiological effects of a substance (e.g., a drug of abuse, a medication) or a general medical condition.

Specify if:

Recurrent: if there are periods of excessive sleepiness that last at least 3 days occurring several times a year for at least 2 years

347 Narcolepsy

A. Irresistible attacks of refreshing sleep that occur daily over at least 3 months.

B. The presence of one or both of the following:

(1) cataplexy (i.e., brief episodes of sudden bilateral loss of muscle tone, most often in association with intense emotion)

(2) recurrent intrusions of elements of rapid eye movement (REM) sleep into the transition between sleep and wakefulness, as manifested by either hypnopompic or hypnagogic hallucinations or sleep paralysis at the beginning or end of sleep episodes

C. The disturbance is not due to the direct physiological effects of a substance (e.g., a drug of abuse, a medication) or another general medical condition.

780.59 Breathing-related sleep disorder

A. Sleep disruption, leading to excessive sleepiness or insomnia, that is judged to be due to a sleep-related breathing condition (e.g., obstructive or central sleep apnea syndrome or central alveolar hypoventilation syndrome).

B. The disturbance is not better accounted for by another mental disorder and is not due to the direct physiological effects of a substance (e.g., a drug of abuse, a medication) or another general medical condition (other than a breathing-related disorder).

Coding note: Also code sleep-related breathing disorder on Axis III.

TABLE 17–2. DSM-IV diagnostic criteria for primary sleep disorders: dyssomnias *(continued)*

307.45 Circadian rhythm sleep disorder

A. A persistent or recurrent pattern of sleep disruption leading to excessive sleepiness or insomnia that is due to a mismatch between the sleep-wake schedule required by a person's environment and his or her circadian sleep-wake pattern.

B. The sleep disturbance causes clinically significant distress or impairment in social, occupational, or other important areas of functioning.

C. The disturbance does not occur exclusively during the course of another sleep disorder or other mental disorder.

D. The disturbance is not due to the direct physiological effects of a substance (e.g., a drug of abuse, a medication) or a general medical condition.

Specify if:

Delayed sleep phase type: a persistent pattern of late sleep onset and late awakening times, with an inability to fall asleep and awaken at a desired earlier time

Jet lag type: sleepiness and alertness that occur at an inappropriate time of day relative to local time, occurring after repeated travel across more than one time zone

Shift work type: insomnia during the major sleep period or excessive sleepiness during the major awake period associated with night shift work or frequently changing shift work

Unspecified type

It is important to obtain a careful sleep history when evaluating children whose parents describe sleep problems. In addition to assessing sleep, the clinician in his or her evaluation needs to determine the degree of impairment of the child's daytime functioning and the degree of general family distress caused by the sleep disturbance. However, because sleep symptoms may not be prominent, it is equally important to inquire about sleep hygiene in children who present with behavior problems. Important areas about which to inquire in an evaluation of sleep are presented in Table 17–8.

The sleep-wake history can be divided into several domains:

General

- Does the child's schedule conform to the family's schedule in a socially appropriate way?
- How regular are the child's sleep habits?
- What are the sleeping arrangements? With whom does the child share a room or bed?
- Are bedtime routines present?
- Whom do the child's symptoms disturb most?

Sleep Organization

- How many hours does the child sleep in each 24-hour day?
- Does the amount of sleep meet the child's developmental needs?
- Is the sleep-wake cycle structured in an age-appropriate way? That is, do bedtimes and rise times occur at customary clock times?

Sleep Disorder

Questions should focus on specific categories of dyssomnia or parasomnia such as difficulties in falling asleep or maintaining sleep, or disruptions and intrusions into sleep.

TABLE 17–3. ICSD-DCM parasomnias (selected)

Parasomnia	ICSD-DCM code
Arousal disorders	
Sleep walking	307.46-0
Sleep terrors	307.46-1
Sleep-wake transition disorders	
Rhythmic movement disorders	307.3
Sleep starts	307.42-2
Sleep talking	307.47-3
Nocturnal leg cramps	729.82
Parasomnias usually associated with REM sleep	
Nightmares	307.47-0
Sleep paralysis	780.56-2
REM-sleep behavior disorder	780.59-0
Miscellaneous parasomnias	
Sleep bruxism	306.8
Sleep enuresis	780.56-0
Nocturnal paroxysmal dystonia	780.59-1
Primary snoring	780.53-1
Infant sleep apnea	770.80
Congenital central hypoventilation	770.81
Sudden infant death syndrome	798.0

Note. ICSD-DCM = *International Classification of Sleep Disorders Diagnostic and Coding Manual, Revised* (American Sleep Disorders Association 1990).

- Are there breathing difficulties manifested by snoring, noisy breathing, or mouth breathing during sleep?
- What was the child's age at onset of the symptom or problem?
- What is the frequency of the symptom in terms of events per week or per night, and what has been its course (stable, worsening, improving)?

Timing

- What time of night or day does the symptom occur? For events occurring after sleep onset, ascertain both the actual clock time and the amount of time after falling asleep that the event occurred.

Daytime Sleepiness

- Does the child complain of being too sleepy or weary during the day?
- Is there any evidence of daytime sleepiness, such as excessive or inappropriate napping? Or, paradoxically, are there symptoms of inattention, poor concentration, and hyperactivity?
- Are school functioning, cognitive performance, or peer relationships compromised?

TABLE 17–4. DSM-IV diagnostic criteria for primary sleep disorders: parasomnias

307.47 Nightmare disorder

A. Repeated awakenings from the major sleep period or naps with detailed recall of extended and extremely frightening dreams, usually involving threats to survival, security, or self-esteem. The awakenings generally occur during the second half of the sleep period.

B. On awakening from the frightening dreams, the person rapidly becomes oriented and alert (in contrast to the confusion and disorientation seen in sleep terror disorder and some forms of epilepsy).

C. The dream experience, or the sleep disturbance resulting from the awakening, causes clinically significant distress or impairment in social, occupational, or other important areas of functioning.

D. The nightmares do not occur exclusively during the course of another mental disorder (e.g., a delirium, posttraumatic stress disorder) and are not due to the direct physiological effects of a substance (e.g., a drug of abuse, a medication) or a general medical condition.

307.46 Sleep terror disorder

A. Recurrent episodes of abrupt awakening from sleep, usually occurring during the first third of the major sleep episode and beginning with a panicky scream.

B. Intense fear and signs of autonomic arousal, such as tachycardia, rapid breathing, and sweating, during each episode.

C. Relative unresponsiveness to efforts of others to comfort the person during the episode.

D. No detailed dream is recalled and there is amnesia for the episode.

E. The episodes cause clinically significant distress or impairment in social, occupational, or other important areas of functioning.

F. The disturbance is not due to the direct physiological effects of a substance (e.g., a drug of abuse, a medication) or a general medical condition.

307.46 Sleepwalking disorder

A. Repeated episodes of rising from bed during sleep and walking about, usually occurring during the first third of the major sleep episode.

B. While sleepwalking, the person has a blank, staring face, is relatively unresponsive to the efforts of others to communicate with him or her, and can be awakened only with great difficulty.

C. On awakening (either from the sleepwalking episode or the next morning), the person has amnesia for the episode.

D. Within several minutes after awakening from the sleepwalking episode, there is no impairment of mental activity or behavior (although there may initially be a short period of confusion or disorientation).

E. The sleepwalking causes clinically significant distress or impairment in social, occupational, or other important areas of functioning.

F. The disturbance is not due to the direct physiological effects of a substance (e.g., a drug of abuse, a medication) or a general medical condition.

Concomitant with a thorough sleep-wake history, a structured 24-hour log of sleep-wake patterns filled in by parents or, in the case of adolescents, by the adolescents themselves over a 1- to 2-week baseline period helps to substantiate information obtained from the history. In addition to nightly bedtimes, sleep-onset times, middle-of-the-night awakening times, and morning rising times, the diary should provide information about bedtime routines, sleeping arrangements, parent and sibling sleep patterns, and associated daytime stresses. To save time and to focus the clinician's initial evaluation, the log may be completed in advance of the first visit. Sleep-wake logs maintained during and after treatment are useful in follow-up visits to evaluate the efficacy of treatment.

TABLE 17–5. ICSD-DCM medical and psychiatric sleep disorders (selected)

Associated with mental disorders	
	Alcoholism
	Anxiety disorders
	Mood disorders
	Psychosis
Associated with neurological disorders	
	Sleep-related epilepsy
	Sleep-related headaches
Associated with other medical disorders	
	Sleep-related asthma
	Sleep-related gastroesophageal reflux
	Fibrositis syndrome

Source. *International Classification of Sleep Disorders Diagnostic and Coding Manual, Revised* (American Sleep Disorders Association 1990).

To further substantiate history and sleep logs, more objective, technical methods of assessment are available. Referrals to accredited sleep disorders centers, directed by certified specialists in sleep disorders medicine and staffed by certified clinical polysomnographic technicians, can provide detailed information about REM and NREM sleep-state and waking-state organization. Polysomnographic recording is recommended when clinicians have reason to suspect an intrinsic cause for a sleep disorder or when severe daytime sleepiness occurs with no reasonable explanation. Polysomnography usually requires the child to sleep all night in a sleep laboratory, although ambulatory polysomnography in the home is becoming more popular for young infants and children.

For dyssomnias that are related more to extrinsic causes, and for which polysomnography is not indicated, alternative methods of objectively recording sleep in the home are available. These methods include time-lapse video recording (Anders and Sostek 1976), pressure-sensitive mattress recording of motility and respiration (Thoman and Glazier 1987), and limb actigraph recording (Sadeh et al. 1991). Each of these methods has advantages and limitations, but each generally provides clinicians with valid and reliable information, derived from algorithms that approximate polysomnographic sleep-wake state scoring regarding sleep quality, sleep efficiency, and age-appropriate level of sleep-wake state maturation. With the increasing popularity of camcorders and home video systems, many parents are able to document their child's sleep disruptions on their own. Such methods are particularly well suited for parasomnias, which usually do not occur nightly and, therefore, are likely to be missed on a scheduled laboratory or home recording session. The parent's videotape, in direct response to the sleep disruption, is useful in capturing episodic events such as night terror attacks, sleepwalking, nightmares, and seizures during sleep.

Dyssomnias

Extrinsic Dyssomnias

Night waking and/or reluctance to go to bed are the most common sleep complaints of parents about their infants and young children. These disruptions in sleep might better be

TABLE 17–6. DSM-IV diagnostic criteria for sleep disorders related to another mental disorder or a general medical condition

307.42 Insomnia related to . . . ***[indicate the Axis I or Axis II disorder]***

A. The predominant complaint is difficulty initiating or maintaining sleep, or nonrestorative sleep, for at least 1 month that is associated with daytime fatigue or impaired daytime functioning.

B. The sleep disturbance (or daytime sequelae) causes clinically significant distress or impairment in social, occupational, or other important areas of functioning.

C. The insomnia is judged to be related to another Axis I or Axis II disorder (e.g., major depressive disorder, generalized anxiety disorder, adjustment disorder with anxiety) but is sufficiently severe to warrant independent clinical attention.

D. The disturbance is not better accounted for by another sleep disorder (e.g., narcolepsy, breathing-related sleep disorder, a parasomnia).

E. The disturbance is not due to the direct physiological effects of a substance (e.g., a drug of abuse, a medication) or a general medical condition.

307.44 Hypersomnia related to . . . ***[indicate the Axis I or Axis II disorder]***

A. The predominant complaint is excessive sleepiness for at least 1 month as evidenced by either prolonged sleep episodes or daytime sleep episodes that occur almost daily.

B. The excessive sleepiness causes clinically significant distress or impairment in social, occupational, or other important areas of functioning.

C. The hypersomnia is judged to be related to another Axis I or Axis II disorder (e.g., major depressive disorder, dysthymic disorder) but is sufficiently severe to warrant independent clinical attention.

D. The disturbance is not better accounted for by another sleep disorder (e.g., narcolepsy, breathing-related sleep disorder, a parasomnia) or by an inadequate amount of sleep.

E. The disturbance is not due to the direct physiological effects of a substance (e.g., a drug of abuse, a medication) or a general medical condition.

780.xx Sleep disorder due to . . . ***[indicate the general medical condition]***

A. A prominent disturbance in sleep that is sufficiently severe to warrant independent clinical attention.

B. There is evidence from the history, physical examination, or laboratory findings that the sleep disturbance is the direct physiological consequence of a general medical condition.

C. The disturbance is not better accounted for by another mental disorder (e.g., an Adjustment Disorder in which the stressor is a serious medical illness).

D. The disturbance does not occur exclusively during the course of a delirium.

E. The disturbance does not meet the criteria for breathing-related sleep disorder or narcolepsy.

F. The sleep disturbance causes clinically significant distress or impairment in social, occupational, or other important areas of functioning.

Specify type:

.52 Insomnia type: if the predominant sleep disturbance is insomnia

.54 Hypersomnia type: if the predominant sleep disturbance is hypersomnia

.59 Parasomnia type: if the predominant sleep disturbance is a parasomnia

.59 Mixed type: if more than one sleep disturbance is present and none predominates

Coding note: Include the name of the general medical condition on Axis I, e.g., 780.52 sleep disorder due to chronic obstructive pulmonary disease, insomnia type; also code the general medical condition on Axis III (see Appendix G for codes).

TABLE 17–7. DSM-IV diagnostic criteria for substance-induced sleep disorder

A. A prominent disturbance in sleep that is sufficiently severe to warrant independent clinical attention.

B. There is evidence from the history, physical examination, or laboratory findings of either (1) or (2):
   (1) the symptoms in criterion A developed during, or within a month of, substance intoxication or withdrawal
   (2) medication use is etiologically related to the sleep disturbance

C. The disturbance is not better accounted for by a sleep disorder that is not substance induced. Evidence that the symptoms are better accounted for by a sleep disorder that is not substance induced might include the following: the symptoms precede the onset of the substance use (or medication use); the symptoms persist for a substantial period of time (e.g., about a month) after the cessation of acute withdrawal or severe intoxication or are substantially in excess of what would be expected given the type or amount of the substance used or the duration of use; or there is other evidence that suggests the existence of an independent non-substance-induced sleep disorder (e.g., a history of recurrent non-substance-related episodes).

D. The disturbance does not occur exclusively during the course of a delirium.

E. The sleep disturbance causes clinically significant distress or impairment in social, occupational, or other important areas of functioning.

Note: This diagnosis should be made instead of a diagnosis of substance intoxication or substance withdrawal only when the sleep symptoms are in excess of those usually associated with the intoxication or withdrawal syndrome and when the symptoms are sufficiently severe to warrant independent clinical attention.

Code [Specific substance]–induced sleep disorder:

(291.89 alcohol; 292.89 amphetamine; 292.89 caffeine; 292.89 cocaine; 292.89 opioid; 292.89 sedative, hypnotic, or anxiolytic; 292.89 other [or unknown] substance)

Specify type:

Insomnia type: if the predominant sleep disturbance is insomnia

Hypersomnia type: if the predominant sleep disturbance is hypersomnia

Parasomnia type: if the predominant sleep disturbance is a parasomnia

Mixed type: if more than one sleep disturbance is present and none predominates

Specify if (see table on p. 193 [DSM-IV-TR] for applicability by substance):

With onset during intoxication: if the criteria are met for intoxication with the substance and the symptoms develop during the intoxication syndrome

With onset during withdrawal: if criteria are met for withdrawal from the substance and the symptoms develop during, or shortly after, a withdrawal syndrome

TABLE 17–8. Screening for sleep-wake problems

Regularity and consistency of sleep habits (e.g., usual bedtimes, rise times)

Use of sleep aids, routines, rituals, eating-drinking

Sleep location (e.g., own room, own bed)

Circumstances of sleep onset (both daytime and nighttime)

Sleep interruptions (e.g., waking, crying, walking, confusional states)

Snoring

Daytime sleepiness, naps

classified as extrinsic "proto" or "potential" dyssomnias. Night-waking problems begin to cause concern in the last 3 months of the child's first year of life and become more prominent in the second year (Anders et al. 2000). Before the child is 9 months old, night waking is tolerated as "normal" (Ferber 1999; Goodlin-Jones et al. 2000). Moore and Ucko (1957) defined night waking as a "disorder" when a child awakens and cries one or more times between midnight and 5 A.M. on at least 4 of 7 nights, for at least 4 consecutive weeks. By age 1 year, 50% of infants who had previously slept through the night were reported as experiencing night waking. Moore and Ucko reported a further transient increase in problem night awakenings during the second year of life. In other studies, nearly 20% of toddlers were described as experiencing night waking (Bernal 1973; Jenkins et al. 1980). The prevalence decreases to 1%–5% in school-age children (Gass and Straugh 1984; Richman et al. 1982).

In this regard, it is important to acknowledge that there are significant family, community, and cultural determinants in the definitions of infant sleep problems. Some families and some cultures tolerate sleep disruptions better for longer periods (Lee 1992). Similarly, some families and cultures are more flexible in devising workable solutions. For example, having an infant sleep alone seems to be highly valued in our culture. Yet, infants' sleeping alone is a custom that is relatively new in the span of human evolution and is characteristic of only a small segment of our global society (Caudill and Plath 1966; Lozoff et al. 1984; McKenna et al. 1990; Thevenin 1987). The use of a sleep aid has cultural, community, and family implications as well. For some parents, use of sleep aids is viewed as unhealthy and is discouraged. Community and family values must be considered in evaluating problems and prescribing treatments.

Little is known about the outcomes of "proto" dyssomnias in regard to their progression to genuine dyssomnias with daytime impairment. Zuckerman and colleagues (1987) followed up 8-month-old infants with sleep problems and found that 41% of them still had problems when they were 3 years old. Only 26% of the children with sleep problems at age 3 years had not manifested them when they were 8 months old. Kataria and colleagues (1987) found that in their sample, 84% of 3-year-olds still had their sleep problems 3 years later. Richman and colleagues (1982) found that almost half of 3-year-old children who experienced night waking had had their problem from birth, and 40% of the children who had sleep problems at 8 years had had problems at least from the time they were 3 years old. Although some studies attribute the origins of these problems to intrinsic factors related to temperament (Carey 1974; Schaefer 1990; Weissbluth et al. 1984), others have emphasized the importance of extrinsic factors such as nutritional and allergenic factors, stress, and states of physical discomfort (Beal 1969; Kahn et al. 1989; Wright et al. 1983). Parental conflict, maternal personality, and maternal depression have also been identified as contributing factors (Field 1994; Guedeney and Kreisler 1987; Zuckerman et al. 1987). When the disturbance is severe, ICSD-CDM diagnostic labels such as "inadequate sleep hygiene," "environmental sleep disorder," "insufficient sleep syndrome," "limit setting sleep disorder," "sleep-onset association disorder," and "food allergy insomnia" may be appropriate (see Table 17–1).

Treatment

Pharmacological and behavioral regimens, alone or in combination, are the most commonly used approaches to treating extrinsic dyssomnias. Hypnotics are prescribed most often by pediatricians and family physicians for both night waking and problems in falling asleep, and behavioral interventions are attempted more by mental health professionals. Ounsted and Hendrick (1977) summarized survey data that indicated that 25% of children had received a sleep medication by age 18 months. The widespread use of medication persists even though research conducted to test efficacy has been limited and support for the therapeutic benefit of such medication is marginal. Positive benefits have been short-lived. Moreover, evidence from studies with adults shows significant negative effects from long-term use of sedating medication.

Behavioral interventions derive from the hypothesis that sleep problems result from habitual, learned, interactional patterns involving child and caregiver. Extinction attempts to eliminate the positive reinforcement of the parent's presence by instructing the parent to ignore attention-seeking behaviors. These instructions are applicable to both night-waking problems and protests around going to bed. Such an intervention may be too difficult for some parents, and some children do not return to sleep even after exhausting bouts of crying. A less abrupt variant prescribes gradual withdrawal of parental involvement by incremental periods of longer waiting following response to the child's crying (Ferber 1999).

Another approach to treating night waking is to schedule awakenings before the time of the expected spontaneous awakening (Rickert and Johnson 1988). This approach, too, is aimed at preventing the rewarding association between night waking, crying, and parental intervention. The method has been difficult for many parents to follow. Conjoint sleeping, as an approach to treatment, derives from the cross-cultural observations that co-sleeping is common in most non-Western societies. Conjoint sleeping provides the continuous presence of a parent sleeping on a cot in the child's bedroom without direct parental contact (Sadeh 1990).

The behavioral technique of reframing attempts to shift the focus of the intervention (Sadeh and Anders 1993). For example, night awakenings that occur several times each night are frequently associated with difficulties in separating from the parent at sleep onset. Even though the parent's concern may be directed at the nightly awakenings, the intervention focuses on presleep interaction at bedtime and naptime, and not on the symptom of night waking. The parent is instructed to develop a consistent ritual around bedtime or naptime that avoids feeding or rocking to sleep. A bedtime ritual such as reading, singing, or playing a quiet game is often suggested. Then, the parent is encouraged to put the child in his or her own bed while the child is still awake and to remain in close proximity until the child falls asleep. It may be necessary, at first, for the parent to sit by the bedside, in physical contact with the child, or even lying next to the child on an adjacent bed (conjoint sleeping). Subsequently, after the child is able to fall asleep on his or her own, the parent gradually moves ever farther away during sleep onset. Finally, the parent is instructed to leave the child's bedroom following the bedtime ritual but before the child is asleep. If the child protests or cries, the parent responds, after a brief wait, by reentering and restoring the child to a sleeping position. Such reentries are repeated at brief intervals as long as the child protests.

During the time that the intervention focuses on going to bed, parents should respond to night awakenings in their customary manner. They comfort their crying infant and sometimes return to conjoint sleeping. Ferber (1985), in a modification of this procedure, recommends a gradual, progressive lengthening of the period between times of reentering. If the separation problem at naptime and bedtime can be resolved, the awakenings in the middle of the night most often end.

In general, behavioral strategies have been reported to be effective in treating most extrinsic, some intrinsic, and most sleep-wake schedule dyssomnias of infants, children, and adolescents, even in severe cases of retardation and autism (Howlin 1984). Jones and Verduyn (1983) reported an 84% success rate in 19 children with sleep problems treated with behavioral methods. These results were maintained during a follow-up period 6 months after termination of treatment. Graziano and Mooney (1982) were successful in using behavioral methods with children who had nighttime fears. Richman et al. (1985) reported a 77% improvement in 35 children ages 1–5 years. Treatment was based on training the parents in the use of behavioral strategies tailored specifically to the individual needs or problems of their child. Sadeh (1990) used an activity monitor to objectively measure changes in sleep patterns of sleep-disturbed infants. He reported that the "checking" procedure (Richman et al. 1985) and conjoint sleeping for a defined period were equally effective in producing a marked improvement in sleep.

Intrinsic Dyssomnias

The two *intrinsic* dyssomnias that most commonly affect children and adolescents are both disorders of excessive somnolence: obstructive sleep apnea syndrome and narcolepsy. In the former, children may be sleepy during the daytime because of the multiple brief obstructive apneas that arouse them repeatedly from sleep. Over time, they become significantly sleep deprived and show compensatory daytime sleepiness. In narcolepsy, irresistible attacks of REM sleep interrupt wakefulness.

Sleep Apnea Syndromes

A sleep apnea event is an interruption of breathing during sleep that exceeds 10 seconds; a hypopnea is a period of reduced ventilation below 50% of waking ventilation (Krieger 1990). Sleep apnea syndromes are characterized by an apnea index greater than 5 apneas or 10 apnea/hypopnea combinations per hour of sleep. Apneas can last from 10 seconds to 3 minutes, usually having a duration of 30–40 seconds. Three types of sleep apneas have been described (Guilleminault and Ariagno 1989):

1. *Obstructive sleep apnea* is characterized by persistent diaphragmatic respiratory movements without passage of air through a hypopharyngeal-glottal obstruction.
2. *Central sleep apnea* is characterized by absent respiratory movements and no airflow.
3. *Mixed sleep apnea* begins with no observable respiration or airflow followed by vigorous thoracic and abdominal efforts to move air against an obstructed glottis.

Apneas may be triggered by immaturities or dysfunction of the respiratory center (central apneas) or by collapse of the airway so that glottal airflow is regularly obstructed during sleep (obstructive apneas). In children, obstructive sleep apnea syndrome may result from mechanical obstruction of the upper airway related to enlarged tonsils and adenoids or to excessive obesity; central apneas may be related to medical and neurological conditions of the lungs or of the respiratory control systems in the central nervous system.

When apneas occur during sleep, blood and brain oxygen saturation may fall to dangerous levels. A brief arousal to waking restores breathing and oxygenation, and the subject then returns to sleep. The arousal is most often a microarousal, lasting 1–2 seconds, too short to be remembered by the sleeper in the morning. Microarousals after sleep apneas may recur 200–300 times nightly in serious disorders. Because of the cumulative loss of sleep, these children may present with symptoms of daytime sleepiness, chronic fatigue, and cognitive and attention deficits. The presenting complaint may be deteriorating school performance. Sometimes children do not recognize or acknowledge their sleepiness; rather, they react by fidgeting and squirming to "fight" sleepiness to remain awake. Such children may be mistakenly identified by teachers and professionals as having attention-deficit/hyperactivity disorder (ADHD). When the multiple awakenings from sleep at night also interrupt the normal secretion of growth hormone during Stage 4 NREM sleep, a child may present initially with mild growth retardation or, in extreme cases, a full-blown failure-to-thrive syndrome. In other words, all children who present with ADHD or a failure-to-thrive syndrome should be evaluated for possible obstructive sleep apnea syndrome.

Sleep apnea must be investigated by polysomnography in a sleep laboratory. Only this technique provides an accurate description of the type of apnea episode and its association with REM or NREM sleep. The degree of oxygen desaturation, the presence of secondary cardiac arrhythmias, and the amount of sleep fragmentation (arousal) are further indicators of the severity of the condition. Another diagnostic procedure, the Multiple Sleep Latency Test (MSLT), may be indicated. This test is a standardized daytime polysomnographic procedure that attempts to elicit daytime naps at regular intervals so that the amount of daytime sleepiness or sleep debt that has accumulated can be assessed.

Until recently, medical practice in the United States advocated the routine removal of children's tonsils and adenoids. With a change in practice patterns over the past two decades, obstructive sleep apnea syndrome has become common, although epidemiological data are not available. Characteristically, children with this syndrome are referred for fragmented sleep, mouth breathing and snoring during sleep, daytime fatigue, or daytime ADHD. A careful history confirms the symptom of noisy breathing. When questioned, parents may also recognize a verbal description of "stopped" breathing during sleep. The physical examination may reveal hypertrophied tonsils, but retropharyngeal adenoidal enlargement is not always obvious without a more formal ear, nose, and throat evaluation. Surgical removal of obstructing tonsils and adenoids usually is curative. Occasionally, regeneration of obstructive tissue postoperatively necessitates a second surgical intervention. Children with craniofacial abnormalities are likely to have obstructive sleep apnea syndrome that does not respond to tonsil and adenoid surgery. Other surgical treatments for severe, refractory cases include uvulopalatopharyngoplasty, mandibular and maxillary advancement, and tracheostomy.

Narcolepsy

Narcolepsy is a REM sleep hypersomnia of unknown etiology that is attributed to dysfunction of brain-stem mechanisms associated with sleep-wake regulation (Broughton 1990). Epidemiological studies have reported the prevalence of narcolepsy at 0.04%–0.07%, making narcolepsy twice as common as multiple sclerosis and half as common as Parkinson's disease. The peak age at onset is in adolescence and young adulthood, although cases of childhood onset have been reported (Guilleminault and Pelayo 1998; Wise 1998). Genetic factors are important. First-degree probands of narcoleptic patients are at eight times greater risk of having some disorder of excessive sleepiness than are individuals in the general population. Speculation regarding pathophysiology has recently focused on genetically mediated dysfunction in cholinergic-dopaminergic interactions (Guilleminault et al. 1998). Human leukocyte antigen (HLA) testing is essentially 85% positive for the HLA-DQB1*0602 and HLA-DR2 alleles for patients with narcolepsy compared with 12%–38% of the general population. Genetic factors other than HLA are also likely to be involved. In narcoleptic dogs, a specific narcolepsy gene has been identified, and the human gene(s) will likely be discovered soon (Takahashi 1999). Nevertheless, the importance of environmental factors is evidenced by the reported 25%–30% of monozygotic twins who are concordant for narcolepsy (Honda and Matsuki 1990; Mignot 1998).

The narcoleptic tetrad of symptoms includes 1) excessive daytime sleepiness with sleep attacks, 2) cataplexy, 3) sleep paralysis, and 4) vivid hypnagogic and hypnopompic hallucinations. The excessive sleepiness of narcolepsy leads to irresistible sleep attacks in situations in which sleep normally never occurs. The narcoleptic patient naps repeatedly for 20- to 40-minute periods, awakening refreshed. He or she then becomes sleepy again within 2–3 hours. Cataplexy is characterized by sudden loss of bilateral peripheral muscle tone, often provoked by strong affect. This condition reflects the peripheral muscle inhibition of REM sleep. Consciousness and memory remain intact. Cataplectic attacks are brief, rarely more than several minutes, with immediate and complete recovery. Attacks may occur only several times a year or as frequently as many times in one day. Both sleep paralysis and hypnagogic hallucinations similarly represent REM sleep concomitants, occurring during sleep onset, when REM sleep normally is not prominent. Although cataplexy, sleep paralysis, and hypnagogic hallucinations diminish in frequency over time, narcolepsy, once present, is a lifelong, chronic condition.

The treatment of narcolepsy is symptomatic and must be individualized depending on the severity of specific symptoms (Thorpy and Goswami 1990). Stimulant medications are used most commonly for the treatment of excessive daytime sleepiness, and tricyclic antidepressant medications are used for the treatment of cataplexy. Because psychostimulants are often used in the treatment of ADHD, children who combat sleep attacks with fidgetiness and motor restlessness often receive the proper treatment for the wrong reason. In a retrospective study of adult patients with narcolepsy, a significant number had been misdiagnosed as having ADHD in adolescence but had been treated appropriately with amphetamines or methylphenidate, with good symptom improvement (Navelet et al. 1976). Clomipramine, 10–20 mg/day in divided doses, has been used successfully to manage cataplexy. Monoamine oxidase inhibitors may be used to manage both cataplexy and the REM sleep–onset symptoms of sleep paralysis and hypnagogic hallucinations. A new wake-promoting drug, modafinil, which activates orexin-containing neurons, is reported to be more effective and to have fewer side effects than the traditional stimulants (Chemelli et al. 1999; Fry 1998).

Patients with narcolepsy usually adjust poorly to their disorder. They have problems in school, at work, and in social relationships. Associated psychiatric disorders include major depression, generalized anxiety, and substance abuse. Behavioral management with psychosocial support and counseling is an essential component of treatment. Patients must be encouraged to follow regular bedtimes and rise times. Regularly scheduled naps for 20–30 minutes, two to three times daily, should be encouraged. School and work schedules need to be designed to accommodate the sleep needs of the patient. Patients are advised to attend self-help support groups. The American Narcolepsy Association publishes a newsletter that keeps members informed of recent advances.

Circadian Rhythm Dyssomnias in Adolescence

Normally, our sleep-wake cycle approximates a 24-hour diurnal rhythm. We sleep during the dark part of the day and are awake during the light part. When studied in an artificial time-isolation environment, however, most humans demonstrate a free-running, endogenous rhythm of 25 hours. The 1-hour discrepancy each day requires that our biological clocks be reset by "zeitgebers," or stimuli that entrain our natural rhythm to a shorter period. The process is called *phase delay* and is accomplished by exposure to exogenous light, dark, and social interactions occurring at particular points in the 24-hour day (Wagner 1990). That is, both our sleeping and waking lives are regulated by a variety of time cues designed to enhance good sleep hygiene and the regular resetting of our biological clock. Within limits, schedule irregularities, such as staying up later or arising earlier by 1–2 hours, can be tolerated for short periods without upsetting the phase of the clock. However, prolonged periods of sleep deprivation or persistent irregularity in sleep hygiene inevitably leads to circadian rhythm disorders. Jet lag syndromes resulting from rapid time zone changes and the dyssomnias of shift workers resulting from continuously changing schedules are typical examples.

Adolescence is also a time of disrupted schedules. Pressures at school and new social obligations cause adolescents to stay up late. Many adolescents have additional work demands, either athletic or occupational, that entail an extra commitment of hours (Carskadon 1990). Therefore, adolescence is a period when persons begin to stay up later and later. During the week, however, school schedules continue to require that adolescents rise early. Soon they become significantly sleep deprived. The problem is compounded when they "sleep in" on weekends, further disrupting their biological clock. Approximately 30% of adolescents report falling asleep in school. Many more complain of tiredness. Because adolescence is also the period for learning to drive motor vehicles and for experimenting with drugs and alcohol, the public health and personal safety issues involved in excessive sleepiness in adolescence are significant (Carskadon 1990).

The typical delayed sleep phase syndrome of adolescence is characterized by an inability to fall asleep at a usual bedtime and an inability to get up at a reasonable hour in the morning. The sleep log reveals bedtimes that do not result in rapid sleep onsets, sleep-onset times that are intractably later than the social norm (usually after 2:00 A.M.), little difficulty in maintaining sleep once asleep, and difficulty awakening at an appropriate hour in the morning. The total number of hours of sleep per night is reduced sharply, although on weekends, total sleep time is lengthened, with awakenings in the late morning or early afternoon. Once the biological clock is disrupted, the delayed sleep phase syndrome frequently persists during vacations, even when normal amounts of sleep are obtained and sleep debt is no longer significant. Similarly, when bedtime is regularly enforced, such as in a summer camp, the adolescent with delayed sleep phase syndrome typically cannot fall asleep until after midnight.

Treatment of this disorder is difficult, requiring a highly motivated adolescent and a supportive family. A careful profile of all of the adolescent's social and academic demands needs to be obtained. Assistance with stress reduction and daytime scheduling needs to be provided. Treatment may be easier to institute during vacation. A regular, more normal bedtime must be set and a daily sleep log kept. An MSLT may be necessary to assess the amount of sleep debt. Treatment should focus both on eliminating the sleep debt and on restoring a more normal sleep-onset time and waking time.

If supportive approaches directed toward stress reduction, better daytime scheduling, and improved nightly sleep hygiene are not successful, chronotherapy, or resetting of the biological clock, may be indicated. Most often, further phase delay is prescribed. A regimen of delaying both sleep times and rise times by 1–2 hours each day attempts to shift sleep onset to a more appropriate time. The treatment is stopped when bedtime and sleep-onset times approximate 10:00 to 11:00 P.M. Subsequently, this schedule needs to be maintained rigidly or the delayed sleep phase syndrome will progressively return.

Phase-advancing the clock also has been reported to be successful in some adolescents. This procedure requires that the adolescent go to bed 15–30 minutes earlier each night. The advance needs to be gradual, with small shifts instituted every few nights. Phase advance is a slower process than phase delay. Weekly improvements of 15–30 minutes may be all that is possible. Antipsychotic and hypnotic medications are not helpful in promoting sleep onset. The duration of delayed sleep phase syndrome symptoms varies from months to decades. Adolescents appear to be particularly vulnerable to the development of this syndrome.

Parasomnias

The parasomnias are characterized by undesirable physical events that disrupt sleep. Parasomnias are subdivided in the ICSD-DCM into disorders of arousal, sleep-wake transition disorders, REM parasomnias, and miscellaneous parasomnias (Table 17–3) (Thorpy 1990). Most of the symptoms are manifestations of central nervous system activation, specifically motor and autonomic discharge. All parasomnias are more common in males than in females, and persons with one type of parasomnia are more likely to manifest symptoms of another. Children with sleep terrors usually sleepwalk when they reach an older age. Positive family histories of parasomnias are common.

Disorders of Arousal

Disorders of arousal, first described by Broughton (1990), have certain features in common during an episode: mental confusion and disorientation, automatic behaviors, relative nonreactivity to external stimuli, difficulty in being fully awakened, and fragmentary or absent dream recall. The next morning, the person has amnesia for the episode. Most characteristic of the disorders of arousal is their occurrence at a typical point in the sleep cycle, usually in the first third of the sleep period, at the point of transition from Stage 4 NREM sleep to REM sleep. Instead of the usual smooth transition to the lighter state of REM sleep, the person with a parasomnia arouses suddenly and manifests symptoms of autonomic discharge.

The onset of arousal disorders follows a developmental sequence. Sleep terrors appear in 2-year-olds. Attacks are usually frightening to parents, who may seek professional help. Typically, the attack begins 60–120 minutes after sleep onset, at the point in the sleep cycle when Stage 4 NREM sleep transitions to REM sleep. The child appears awake, with eyes open, and is screaming and seemingly frightened and agitated. Pounding heart, tachypnea, diaphoresis, and general disorientation reflect autonomic nervous system activation. In fact, the child is not awake, but is deeply asleep in Stage 4 NREM sleep. The child is difficult to soothe and is unaware of his or her surroundings. He or she may fight with the person who is trying to console him or her. Although attacks are difficult to predict and patterns of occurrence are usually irregular, excessive fatigue or unusual stresses during the daytime have been noted to precipitate nighttime occurrences. Because sleep terror is not likely to occur when studied in a sleep laboratory, it may be more relevant to ask parents to use a camcorder to record episodes at home.

Sleepwalking begins in slightly older children of preschool and school age. Like sleep terrors, sleepwalking is associated with autonomic activation at the point of transition in the sleep cycle from Stage 4 NREM sleep to REM sleep, typically 60–120 minutes after sleep onset. Instead of screaming, the child sits upright in bed or walks. Behaviors are automatic and purposeless, and body movements are poorly coordinated. The sleepwalking child is difficult to arouse and, when awakened, is confused and disoriented. Sleepwalking is dangerous, because the child may injure him- or herself by falling or crashing into objects. In contrast, children and adolescents who present with "sleep" behaviors characterized by complex, purposeful actions, such as leaving the home at night to rendezvous with friends or preparing nighttime snacks, are generally not exhibiting disorders of arousal. More psychological explanations, including malingering, conduct disorder, and dissociative states, need to be considered.

Unless the parasomnia is intractable in terms of frequency and persistence, special intervention is not needed. Reassurance and explanation often provide sufficient support for the child and family. Parents should try to guide the sleepwalking child back to bed or provide comfort to the child in the midst of a sleep terror attack. Awakening the child from either is difficult and does not shorten the attack. It is important to safe-proof the environment for children who walk in their sleep. Setting alarms that trigger when the child rises from bed, sealing windows, and locking doors may be necessary to avoid the child's injuring himself or herself.

Another treatment strategy involves late-afternoon or early-evening naps. A brief 30- to 60-minute nap at that time is likely to reduce the amount of Stage 4 NREM sleep later at bedtime. The nap should not be prolonged, however, because then falling asleep at bedtime may be difficult.

Pharmacological treatment may be indicated when episodes are frequent and disruptive. One measure of severity is the degree to which the nighttime problem interferes with daytime functioning. A comprehensive neurological examination to rule out a sleep-related seizure disorder is warranted in severe cases. Similarly, arousal disorders after puberty are rare, and, when they do persist, a complete neurological evaluation for the presence of seizures is indicated. Benzodiazepines have been used successfully to reduce both the frequency and the intensity of attacks in severe intractable cases. However, tolerance develops, and when the drug is withdrawn, the disorder frequently reappears. Children normally "outgrow" their attacks as they mature.

Sleep-Wake Transition Disorders

Sleep-wake transition disorders occur in the transition from wakefulness to sleep or vice versa. Because these disorders most often occur in otherwise healthy persons, they are considered variants of normal physiology rather than indicators of pathophysiology. The term *rhythmic movement disorders* is preferred to the term *head banging*. Sleep starts, body rocking, sleep talking, and nocturnal leg cramps also are included in this category. Klackenberg (1982) reported that at age 9 months, 58% of infants exhibited at least one of these repetitive behaviors (head turning, head banging, or rocking). The prevalence of these activities decreased to 33% by age 18 months and to 22% by age 2 years. When intense rocking or head banging persists and is disruptive, parents may view the behavior as a problem. Most often, providing guidance and support for the parent suffices. The only concern should be in securing the child's safety from self-injury.

REM Parasomnias

The most common REM parasomnia is the nightmare. Nightmares are frightening awakenings from REM sleep associated with dream reports that are typically anxiety-laden. Stress of various kinds, and especially traumatic experiences, increases the frequency and severity of nightmares. Certain medications, including β-adrenergic blockers, and the withdrawal of REM suppressants can induce or increase the incidence of nightmares. Nightmares usually start between ages 3 and 6 years and affect 10%–50% of children in that age group severely enough to disturb their parents. Nightmares are easily differentiated from sleep terrors. Nightmares occur later in the night, usually in the last third of the sleep period, when REM sleep predominates. Nightmares characteristically are more organized, in terms of frightening dream reports, than sleep terrors. The child is fully awake and oriented when recounting a nightmare. The child usually has good recall of the nightmare in the morning. Nightmares also need to be differentiated from REM sleep behavior disorder described below. Treatment of nightmares consists of providing comfort at the time of occurrence and reducing precipitating daytime stressors when possible. For children with serious behavioral disruption associated with regularly recurring nightmares, often seen in association with acute or posttraumatic stress disorder, individual and/or family psychotherapy may be indicated.

REM sleep behavior disorder (Schenck et al. 1986) is characterized by the intermittent absence of the normal muscle inhibition of REM sleep and by the appearance of elaborate motor behaviors associated with dream mentation. Punching, kicking, leaping, and running from bed during an attempted dream enactment are typical manifestations. The behaviors usually correlate with reported dream imagery. REM sleep behavior disorder rarely occurs in childhood. More typically, it begins in late adulthood and may be associated with Parkinson's disease or dementia. In the few cases reported in childhood, a neurological lesion has been identified. A complete neurological evaluation, including brain imaging, is warranted. An evaluation in a sleep disorders center is also important. Excessive augmentation of submental electromyographic activation and exaggerated limb movements during REM sleep are observed polygraphically and on videotape. The beneficial response to clonazepam is impressive. Only case reports have been reported in childhood, but in one series of 55 adult patients treated with clonazepam, 76% of the patients responded favorably, with 88% of this group having a partial response and 12% having a substantial response (Mahowald and Schenck 1990).

Conclusions

In this chapter I have attempted to describe the assessment, phenomenology, and treatment of the more common childhood sleep disorders. The disorders have been viewed in a developmental framework from infancy to adolescence and placed in the structure of sleep-wake state organization. The large majority of dyssomnias that affect infants, children, and adolescents can be diagnosed from a careful history and physical examination. Sleep logs are useful to place a disorder in a temporal and chronological context as well as to gauge severity and the efficacy of treatment. Sleep laboratory investigations should be considered for all dyssomnias that are characterized by excessive somnolence. The dyssomnias associated with some neurological diseases and with developmental delay often respond better to behavioral management strategies than to hypnotic medications. Those sleep disorders that are associated with primary psychiatric or medical conditions have not been reviewed specifically. Treatment of the primary condition often leads to improvement of the sleep problem. The principles reviewed for the management of primary dyssomnias also can be useful for such secondary dyssomnias.

References

American Psychiatric Association: Diagnostic and Statistical Manual of Mental Disorders, 3rd Edition. Washington, DC, American Psychiatric Association, 1980

American Psychiatric Association: Diagnostic and Statistical Manual of Mental Disorders, 4th Edition. Washington, DC, American Psychiatric Association, 1994

American Sleep Disorders Association: The International Classification of Sleep Disorders: Diagnostic and Coding Manual. Lawrence, KS, Allen Press, 1990

Anders T, Eiben L: Pediatric sleep disorders: a review of the past 10 years. J Am Acad Child Adolesc Psychiatry 36:1–12, 1997

Anders T, Sostek A: The use of time lapse video recording of sleep-wake behavior in human infants. Psychophysiology 13:155–158, 1976

Anders T, Goodlin-Jones B, Sadeh A: Sleep disorders, in Handbook of Infant Mental Health, 2nd Edition. Edited by Zeanah C. New York, Guilford, 2000, pp 326–338

Beal V: Termination of night feeding in infancy. J Pediatr 75:690–692, 1969

Bernal J: Night waking in infants during the first fourteen months. Dev Med Child Neurol 15:760–769, 1973

Broughton R: Narcolepsy, in Handbook of Sleep Disorders. Edited by Thorpy MJ. New York, Marcel Dekker, 1990, pp 197–216

Carey W: Night waking and temperament in infancy. J Pediatr 84:756–758, 1974

Carskadon M: Adolescent sleepiness: increased risk in a high-risk population. Alcohol, Drugs, and Driving 6:317–328, 1990

Caudill W, Plath DW: Who sleeps by whom? Parent-child involvement in urban Japanese families. Psychiatry 29:344–366, 1966

Chemelli R, Willie J, Sinton C, et al: Narcolepsy in orexin knockout mice: molecular genetics of sleep regulation. Cell 98:47–51, 1999

Coons S, Guilleminault C: Development of sleep-wake patterns and non–rapid eye movement sleep stages during the first six months of life in normal infants. Pediatrics 69:793–798, 1982

Ferber R: Solve Your Child's Sleep Problem. New York, Simon & Schuster, 1985

Ferber R: Sleep disorders in childhood, in Sleep Disorders Medicine: Basic Science, Technical Considerations and Clinical Aspects, 2nd Edition. Edited by Chokroverty S. Boston, MA, Butterworth Heineman, 1999, pp 683–696

Field T: Infants of depressed mothers. Infant Behavior and Development 18:1–13, 1994

Fry J: Treatment modalities in narcolepsy. Neurology 50 (suppl 1):S43–S48, 1998

Gass E, Straugh I: The development of sleep behavior between 3 and 11 years, in Proceedings of the 7th European Sleep Congress. Munich, 1984

Goodlin-Jones B, Burnham M, Anders T: Sleep and sleep disturbances: regulatory processes in infants, in Handbook of Developmental Psychopathology, 2nd Edition. Edited by Lewis M, Sameroff A. New York, Plenum, 2000, pp 309–325

Graziano AM, Mooney KC: Behavioral treatment of "nightfears" in children: maintenance of improvement at 2½- to 3-year follow-up. J Consult Clin Psychol 50:598–599, 1982

Guedeney A, Kreisler L: Sleep disorders in the first 18 months of life: hypothesis on the role of mother-child emotional exchanges. Infant Mental Health Journal 8:307–318, 1987

Guilleminault C, Ariagno R: Apnea during sleep in infants and children, in Principles and Practice of Sleep Medicine. Edited by Kryger M, Roth T, Dement W. Philadelphia, PA, WB Saunders, 1989, pp 655–664

Guilleminault C, Pelayo R: Narcolepsy in prepubertal children. Ann Neurol 43:135–142, 1998

Guilleminault C, Heinzer R, Mignot E, et al: Investigations into the neurologic basis of narcolepsy. Neurology 50 (suppl 1):S8–S15, 1998

Honda Y, Matsuki K: Genetic aspects of narcolepsy, in Handbook of Sleep Disorders. Edited by Thorpy MJ. New York, Marcel Dekker, 1990, pp 217–234

Howlin P: A brief report on the elimination of long-term sleeping problems in a 6-year-old autistic boy. Behavioural Psychotherapy 12:257–260, 1984

Jenkins S, Bax M, Hart H: Behavior problems in preschool children. J Child Psychol Psychiatry 21:5–17, 1980

Jones D, Verduyn C: Behavioral management of sleep problems. Arch Dis Child 58:442–444, 1983

Kahn A, Mozin MJ, Rebuffat E, et al: Milk intolerance in children with persistent sleeplessness: a prospective double-blind crossover evaluation. Pediatrics 84:595–603, 1989

Kataria S, Swanson M, Trevarthin G: Persistence of sleep disturbances in preschool children. J Pediatr 110:642–646, 1987

Klackenberg G: Sleep behavior studied longitudinally: data from 4–16 years in duration, night awakening and bedtime. Acta Paediatr 71:501–506, 1982

Krieger J: Obstructive sleep apnea: clinical manifestations and pathophysiology, in Handbook of Sleep Disorders. Edited by Thorpy MJ. New York, Marcel Dekker, 1990, pp 259–284

Lee K: Pattern of night waking and crying of Korean infants from 3 months to 2 years old and its relation with various factors. J Dev Behav Pediatr 13:326–330, 1992

Lozoff B, Wolff A, Davis N: Cosleeping in urban families with young children in the United States. Pediatrics 74:171–182, 1984

Mahowald M, Schenck C: REM-sleep behavior disorder, in Handbook of Sleep Disorders. Edited by Thorpy MJ. New York, Marcel Dekker, 1990, pp 567–593

McKenna J, Mosko S, Dungy C, et al: Sleep and arousal patterns of co-sleeping human mother/infant pairs: a preliminary physiological study with implications for the study of Sudden Infant Death Syndrome (SIDS). Am J Phys Anthropol 83:331–347, 1990

Mignot E: Genetic and familial aspects of narcolepsy. Neurology 50 (suppl 1):S16–S22, 1998

Moore T, Ucko L: Night waking in early infancy, part 1. Arch Dis Child 32:333–342, 1957

Navelet Y, Anders TF, Guilleminault C: Narcolepsy in children, in Narcolepsy: Proceedings of the First International Symposium on Narcolepsy (Advances in Sleep Research, Vol 3). Edited by Guilleminault C, Dement WC, Passouant P. New York, Spectrum, 1976, pp 171–177

Ounsted M, Hendrick A: The first-born child: patterns of development. Dev Med Child Neurol 19:446–453, 1977

Richman N, Stevenson J, Graham P: Preschool to School: A Behavioral Study. London, Academic, 1982

Richman N, Douglas J, Hunt H, et al: Behavioural methods in the treatment of sleep disorders—a pilot study. J Child Psychol Psychiatry 26:581–590, 1985

Rickert V, Johnson C: Reducing nocturnal awakening and crying episodes in infants and young children: a comparison between scheduled awakenings and systematic ignoring. Pediatrics 81:203–212, 1988

Sadeh A: Actigraphic home-monitoring of sleep-disturbed infants: comparisons to controls and assessment of intervention, in Sleep '90. Edited by Horne J. Bochum, Germany, Pontenagal Press, 1990, pp 469–470

Sadeh A, Anders TF: Infant sleep problems: origins, assessment, intervention. Infant Mental Health Journal 14:17–34, 1993

Sadeh A, Lavie P, Scher A, et al: Actigraphic home monitoring of sleep-disturbed and control infants and young children: a new method for pediatric assessment of sleep-wake patterns. Pediatrics 87:494–499, 1991

Schaefer C: Night waking and temperament in early childhood. Psychol Rep 67:192–194, 1990

Schenck C, Bundlie S, Ettinger M, et al: Chronic behavioral disorders of human REM sleep: a new category of parasomnia. Sleep 9:293–308, 1986

Takahashi J: Narcolepsy genes wake up the sleep field. Science 285:2076–2077, 1999

Thevenin T: The Family Bed, An Age Old Concept in Child Rearing. Minneapolis, MN, Tine, Thevenin, 1987

Thoman E, Glazier R: Computer scoring of motility patterns for states of sleep and wakefulness: human infants. Sleep 10:122–129, 1987

Thorpy MJ: Disorders of arousal, in Handbook of Sleep Disorders. Edited by Thorpy MJ. New York, Marcel Dekker, 1990, pp 531–549

Thorpy MJ, Goswami M: Treatment of narcolepsy, in Handbook of Sleep Disorders. Edited by Thorpy MJ. New York, Marcel Dekker, 1990, pp 235–259

Wagner D: Circadian rhythm sleep disorders, in Handbook of Sleep Disorders. Edited by Thorpy MJ. New York, Marcel Dekker, 1990, pp 493–525

Weissbluth M, Davis A, Poucher J: Night waking in 4- to 8-month-old infants. J Pediatr 104:477–480, 1984

Wise M: Childhood narcolepsy. Neurology 50 (suppl 1):S37–S42, 1998

Wright P, Macleod H, Cooper M: Waking at night: the effect of early feeding. Child Care Health Dev 9:309–319, 1983

Zuckerman B, Stevenson J, Baily V: Sleep problems in early childhood: predictive factors and behavioral correlates. Pediatrics 80:664–671, 1987

SECTION 3

Delirium, Dementia, and Amnestic and Other Cognitive Disorders

Section Editors

Stuart C. Yudofsky, M.D.

Robert E. Hales, M.D.

Introduction

As indicated in the introduction to DSM-IV, the term *mental disorder* tacitly and misleadingly "implies a distinction between 'mental' disorders and 'physical' that is a reductionistic anachronism of mind/body dualism" (American Psychiatric Association 1994, p. xxi). This perpetuation of the historical mind-body dualism in psychiatry commonly leads to diagnostic and therapeutic mistakes as well as to the stigmatization of those who have so-called mental disorders. Members of the American Psychiatric Association's Task Force on DSM-IV acknowledge that the term *mental disorder* is an imperfect one and state that "a compelling literature documents that there is much 'physical' in 'mental' disorders and much 'mental' in 'physical' disorders" (American Psychiatric Association 1994, p. xxi). The term *mental disorder* persists in DSM-IV, the task force members point out, "because it is as useful as any other available definition and has helped to guide decisions regarding which conditions on the boundary between normality and pathology should be included in DSM-IV" (American Psychiatric Association 1994, p. xxi).

The topics subsumed in Section 3—delirium, dementia, amnestic disorders, cognitive disorders not otherwise specified, mental disorders due to a general medical condition, and substance-related disorders—constitute an important effort of DSM-IV to address this nosological challenge. In DSM-III-R (American Psychiatric Association 1987), most of these topics were categorized under the section titled "Organic Mental Syndromes and Disorders," which, appropriately, has been abandoned because of the inaccurate implication that so-called nonorganic mental disorders do not have biological bases. We view this conceptual change as a useful transitional step that reflects the current level of the medical profession's understanding of the indelible inseparability of brain and thought, of mind and body, and of the mental and physical.

Approximately 15 years have passed since it was our privilege to participate in the preparation of the DSM-III-R edition of *Treatments of Psychiatric Disorders*. During this time, the field of psychiatry's recognition of the relevance and psychosocial effect of conditions that previously were termed *organic mental disorders* has increased dramatically. Associated with this greater recognition has been the reemergence of neuropsychiatry as an integrating conceptual focus for both psychiatrists and neurologists. As revealed in the chapters of this section, the neuropsychiatric paradigm has energized both fields by enlarging clinicians' conceptual understanding, knowledge base, diagnostic acumen, and therapeutic armamentaria of the multifarious brain-related dysfunctions of mood, thought, perception, and behavior.

The neuropsychiatric paradigm has important implications for the understanding and treatment of the conditions reviewed in the chapters of this section for the following reasons:

Neuropsychiatry provides the means to assess and treat patients with symptoms and disorders at the interface between psychiatry and neurology.

In hospitals, academic centers, and outpatient facilities throughout the United States, "turf battles" are being waged among neurologists, psychiatrists, and medical practitioners of other disciplines over the authority for caring for patients with all of the conditions discussed in the chapters in this section. This interaction between specialties is partially the result of brain-related functions—such as attention, alertness, perception, memory, language and speech, intelligence, cognition, and motivation—that reside at the interface between neurology and psychiatry. Controversies emerge as to which specialty holds primary responsibility for caring for patients with Alzheimer's disease and other dementias, for treating traumatic brain injury, and even for assessing and treating sleep disorders or substance use disorders. Not surprisingly, the result of such territorial struggles is the fragmentation of care along conventional specialty lines.

Neuropsychiatry provides the means to reduce stigma.

Prior to the twentieth century, seizure disorders and paralysis agitans (Parkinson's disease) were considered to be predominantly mental disorders with disparaging religious and legal overtones. Following neuropathological and neurophysiological advances of the early part of the twentieth century, the stigma associated with these conditions was reduced. As more is understood about the role of the brain in the etiology and expression of disorders such as schizophrenia, bipolar disorder, obsessive-compulsive disorder, panic disorder, and attention-deficit/hyperactivity disorder, the shaming, blaming, and defaming that have historically characterized our field are being reduced. We foresee a future wherein neuropsychiatry will also encompass conditions such as violence and substance abuse. Through the neuropsychiatric paradigm, solutions for violent behavior and chemical dependency that are often punitive will be replaced with preventive and therapeutic opportunities paved by biopsychosocial research and clinical neuropsychiatry.

Neuropsychiatry provides the means to improve the clinical effectiveness of the practitioner.

Currently, residency training of psychiatrists does not sufficiently emphasize basic neuroscience, neurobiology, neuropathology, or neurology. The education of neurologists does not sufficiently focus on psychodynamics, psychotherapeutics, family treatment, and psychopharmacology. Inequalities in reimbursements for the treatment of all mental disorders from almost all payers—whether government, managed care organizations, or indemnity insurance companies—are, in part, the result of a historical demedicalization of psychiatry and our failure to consider and apply neurobiology to the therapeutic approaches to the so-called mental disorders.

Neuropsychiatry provides conceptual integrity.

Neuropsychiatry not only obviates the mind-body dualism as reflected by the limitations of the term *mental illness* but also accommodates the increasing porosity of the boundaries between psychiatry and neurology. As neuroscience expands and uncovers more associations between the brain and psychopathology, traditional boundaries between psychiatry and neurology will increasingly become constraining and artificial. The conceptual overlap between psychiatry and neurology as represented by symptomatologies that are clinical foci shared by both fields can be schematically represented as shown in Figure 1.

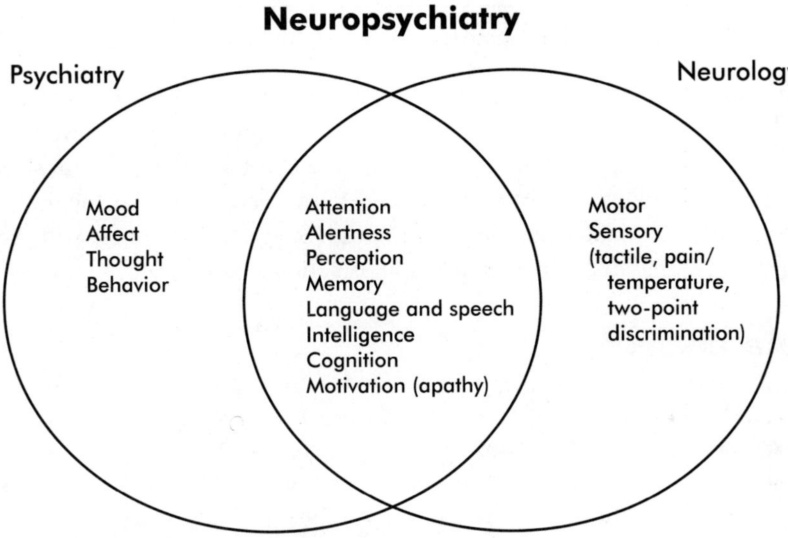

FIGURE 1. Current interface of psychiatry and neurology.

The forces driving the fields of psychiatry and neurology closer together in a fashion best integrated through the neuropsychiatric paradigm can be conceptualized as shown in Figure 2.

In addition, over the 15 years since the publication of the first edition of *Treatments of Psychiatric Disorders*, there has been extraordinary growth in both the basic science and the translational clinical research related to neuropsychiatry. The annual meetings of the American Neuropsychiatric Association, whose membership has increased by 17% over the past 2 years, provide a yearly review of progress in these basic science discoveries as well as the translational advances of basic research into the understanding and treatment of brain-based disorders of cognition, behavior, and emotion. Finally, one important measure of the

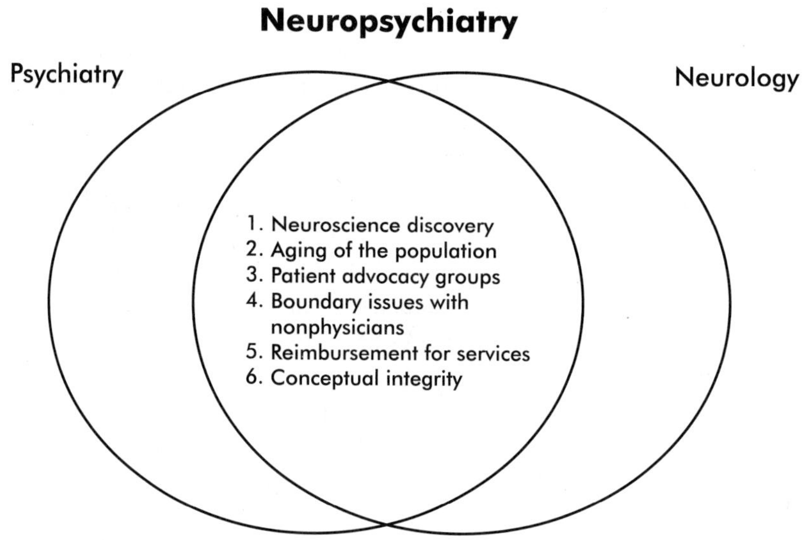

FIGURE 2. Six factors increasing future interface of psychiatry and neurology.

growth in the database and interest in neuropsychiatry since the publication of the second edition of *Treatments of Psychiatric Disorders* in 1995 is the publication of many outstanding comprehensive textbooks—in both the basic and the clinical realms of neuroscience and neuropsychiatry. For those readers whose interests are "merely whetted" by the outstanding chapters that follow, the textbooks listed in the "Suggested Readings" will provide an even deeper and more satisfying reservoir of information.

References

American Psychiatric Association: Diagnostic and Statistical Manual of Mental Disorders, 3rd Edition, Revised. Washington, DC, American Psychiatric Association, 1987

American Psychiatric Association: Diagnostic and Statistical Manual of Mental Disorders, 4th Edition. Washington, DC, American Psychiatric Association, 1994

Suggested Readings

Charney DS, Nestler EJ, Bunney BS (eds): Neurobiology of Mental Illness. New York, Oxford University Press, 1999

Coffey CE, Brumback RA (eds): Textbook of Pediatric Neuropsychiatry. Washington, DC, American Psychiatric Press, 1998

Coffey CE, Cummings JL (eds): The American Psychiatric Press Textbook of Geriatric Neuropsychiatry. Washington, DC, American Psychiatric Press, 2000

Gazzaniga MS (editor-in-chief): The New Cognitive Neurosciences, 2nd Edition. Cambridge, MA, Massachusetts Institute of Technology, 2000

Kandel ER, Schwartz JH, Jessell TM (eds): Principles of Neural Science, 4th Edition. New York, McGraw-Hill, 2000

Yudofsky SC, Hales RE (eds): The American Psychiatric Press Textbook of Neuropsychiatry, 3rd Edition. Washington, DC, American Psychiatric Press, 1997

18

Delirium Due to a General Medical Condition, Delirium Due to Multiple Etiologies, and Delirium Not Otherwise Specified

Michael G. Wise, M.D.
Donald M. Hilty, M.D.
Gabrielle M. Cerda, M.D.

Delirium occurs in 10%–15% of patients on medical and surgical wards. The frequency of delirium increases with advanced age—persons older than 80 are the fastest-growing age group in the population—and in persons with existing brain disease (e.g., dementia of the Alzheimer's type) (Kolbeinsson and Jónsson 1993; Lipowski 1990). Therefore, as life expectancy increases, the prevalence of delirium also will increase. The mortality associated with this psychiatric disorder is sobering: delirium "is a sign of impending death in 25% of cases" (Folstein et al. 1991, p. 169). Only dementia, when followed up for several years, has a higher mortality rate (Francis and Kapoor 1992; Roth 1955). Besides an increased mortality rate, patients with delirium have longer lengths of hospital stay (Francis et al. 1990; Inouye et al. 1998; Marcantonio et al. 1994), greater future cognitive decline (Francis and Kapoor 1992), higher use of hospital resources (Kane et al. 1993), an increased frequency of major postsurgical complications (Marcantonio et al. 1994), poorer functional recovery (Cole and Primeau 1993; Marcantonio et al. 1994; Murray et al. 1993), and an increased risk for nursing home placement (Inouye et al. 1998; O'Keefe and Lavan 1997) in comparison with patients without delirium. The treatment of delirium, a syndrome commonly diagnosed by consultation psychiatrists and underdiagnosed by primary care physicians, remains an underresearched phenomenon and a clinical art. This is especially true for delirium in children.

A wide variety of physiological insults produce the delirium syndrome. This multiple causality helps to explain the high prevalence of the syndrome, the extensive differential diagnosis, and the reluctance of some physicians to investigate multiple possible etiologies for an acute alteration in mental status. Delirium can manifest clinically as a hypoactive state (decreased arousal), as a hyperactive state (increased arousal), or as a mixed state with fluctuations between hypoactive and hyperactive forms (mixed variant). Accurate diagnosis must precede treatment. Without proper diagnosis and treatment, the prognosis for the delirious patient is poor.

Definition and Diagnostic Criteria

The DSM-IV (American Psychiatric Association 1994) diagnostic criteria for delirium are presented in Table 18–1. The core symptoms are impairment of consciousness with reduced ability to focus, sustain, or shift attention; acute changes in cognition (onset usually over hours to days) that are not better accounted for by dementia; and fluctuations in the mental status throughout the day. When delirium is present, a more specific diagnosis is made based on etiology. If an etiology is determined, the delirium is classified as either delirium due to a general medical condition (e.g., delirium due to hepatic encephalopathy or delirium due to hypoglycemia), substance-induced delirium (including medication side effects), or delirium due to multiple etiologies. If the clinician is unable to determine a specific etiology, a diagnosis of delirium not otherwise specified (NOS) is made.

In DSM-IV, various disturbances of psychomotor activity are noted to be associated with delirium, including hypoactive, hyperactive, and mixed behavioral states. Three lines of evidence support this subtyping: 1) the finding of equivalent degrees of cognitive impairment in hypoactive and hyperactive delirium (Ross et al. 1991); 2) the finding of diffuse electroencephalogram (EEG) slowing for both hypoactive and hyperactive variants (Trzepacz 1994), with the exception of delirium tremens (DTs); and 3) the finding of comparable responsiveness of subtypes to antipsychotic medication (Platt et al. 1994). Some neurologists divide the concept of delirium into two types: an acute confusional state and an acute agitated delirium (Adams and Victor 1989; Mesulam 1985; Mori and Yamadori 1987). DTs is the conceptual model these investigators use for delirium. Patients who are acutely confused, incoherent, and disoriented, but without autonomic instability and hallucinations, are given the diagnosis of an "acute confusional state," not delirium. The historical roots of this disparity in the concept of delirium are discussed by Lipowski (1980, 1990) and Berrios (1981). This disparity in terminology is especially notable in the limited literature on delirium in children.

TABLE 18–1. DSM-IV diagnostic criteria for delirium

Delirium due to...*[Indicate the general medical condition]*

A. Disturbance of consciousness (i.e., reduced clarity of awareness of the environment) with reduced ability to focus, sustain, or shift attention.

B. A change in cognition (such as memory deficit, disorientation, language disturbance) or the development of a perceptual disturbance that is not better accounted for by a preexisting, established, or evolving dementia.

C. The disturbance develops over a short period of time (usually hours to days) and tends to fluctuate during the course of the day.

D. There is evidence from the history, physical examination, or laboratory findings that the disturbance is caused by the direct physiological consequences of a general medical condition.

Coding note: If delirium is superimposed on a preexisting vascular dementia, indicate the delirium by coding 290.41 vascular dementia, with delirium.

Coding note: Include the name of the general medical condition on Axis I, e.g., 293.0 delirium due to hepatic encephalopathy; also code the general medical condition on Axis III (see Appendix G for codes).

Substance-induced delirium

See Chapter 19 in this volume for diagnostic criteria.

Delirium due to multiple etiologies

A. Disturbance of consciousness (i.e., reduced clarity of awareness of the environment) with reduced ability to focus, sustain, or shift attention.

B. A change in cognition (such as memory deficit, disorientation, language disturbance) or the development of a perceptual disturbance that is not better accounted for by a preexisting, established, or evolving dementia.

C. The disturbance develops over a short period of time (usually hours to days) and tends to fluctuate during the course of the day.

D. There is evidence from the history, physical examination, or laboratory findings that the delirium has more than one etiology (e.g., more than one etiological general medical condition, a general medical condition plus substance intoxication or medication side effect).

Coding note: Use multiple codes reflecting specific delirium and specific etiologies, e.g., 293.0 delirium due to viral encephalitis; 291.0 alcohol withdrawal delirium.

Delirium not otherwise specified

This category should be used to diagnose a delirium that does not meet criteria for any of the specific types of delirium described above. Examples include

1. A clinical presentation of delirium that is suspected to be due to a general medical condition or substance use but for which there is insufficient evidence to establish a specific etiology.
2. Delirium due to causes not listed above (e.g., sensory deprivation).

Epidemiology

Within the last few years, systematic research into the prevalence, incidence, and risk factors for delirium has provided valuable insight into this disorder. The frequency of delirium varies depending on the type of insult and the predisposition of the person involved. Engel (1967) estimated that 10%–15% of patients on acute medical and surgical wards have delirium. Lipowski (1990), although agreeing with this estimate, noted that the increasing age of the population may make this estimate low. Recent research on the prevalence (i.e., cases identified at a particular point in time, usually on admission to a hospital) and incidence (i.e., new cases that develop over a specified period, usually during hospitalization) of delirium indicates that the prevalence across many studies ranges from 10% to 51% (Table 18–2) and the incidence ranges from 4% to 31%. Recent cross-sectional studies of patients in emergency departments indicated a prevalence of delirium between 10% and 14% (Lewis et al. 1995; Naughton et al. 1995). Of these patients, only 17% are recognized (defined by chart notation) by the emergency physician as having delirium (Lewis et al. 1995).

TABLE 18–2. Prevalence of delirium

Population	Prevalence
Hospitalized medically ill	10%–30%
Hospitalized elderly	10%–40%
Cancer patients	25%
Acquired immunodeficiency syndrome (AIDS) patients	30%–40%
Postoperative patients	10%–51%
Terminally ill patients	Up to 80%
Coexistent structural brain disease	Up to 81%

Predisposing Factors

Five groups of patients are at increased risk to develop delirium: 1) elderly patients; 2) patients with a decreased "cerebral reserve," such as would result from dementia, strokes, and human immunodeficiency virus (HIV) infection; 3) postcardiotomy patients; 4) burn patients; and 5) patients with drug dependency who are experiencing withdrawal (Table 18–3). Advancing age increases the risk, with those persons age 60 or older usually cited as constituting the group at highest risk (Lipowski 1980, 1990). If children are excluded, the incidence of delirium increases with the age of the patient population studied. Sir Martin Roth (1955), while studying the natural history of mental disorders in older people, reported acute confusional states among psychiatric patients in 7.5% of patients ages 60–69, 9% in patients ages 70–79, and 12% in patients older than 80 years. Inouye et al. (1989) and Francis et al. (1988) reported that 23% and 25.3%, respectively, of patients older than age 70 were delirious during hospitalization. Increasing age is also a risk factor for dementia.

TABLE 18–3. Patients at high risk for delirium

Elderly patients
Patients with decreased "cerebral reserve" (e.g., as a result of dementia, human immunodeficiency virus [HIV] infection, stroke)
Postcardiotomy patients
Burn patients
Patients in drug withdrawal

Many patients, particularly as they grow older, have less cerebral reserve and are more likely to develop delirium with medical illness or surgical procedures. These persons, when faced with a relatively minor physiological stress such as a urinary tract infection, are more likely to develop a delirium. This decreased threshold for delirium results from declining cognitive function or from central nervous system (CNS) injury. For example, preexisting brain damage, whether preoperative CNS neurological abnormalities (Koponen and Riekkinen 1993; Marcantonio et al. 1994) or dementia (Kolbeinsson and Jónsson 1993), lowers the patient's threshold for developing a delirium. Koponen and Riekkinen (1993), in their study, found that 81% of delirious patients had "coexistent structural brain disease." Symptomatic HIV-1-seropositive persons also typically have significant cognitive deficits (Maj et al. 1994). Perry (1990) reported a 90% frequency of organic mental disorders in patients with far-advanced acquired immunodeficiency syndrome (AIDS). In another study, the most frequent neuropsychiatric complication of AIDS was delirium (Fernandez et al. 1989).

Postcardiotomy delirium has been the focus of considerable research. Dubin et al. (1979), in their thorough review of postcardiotomy delirium, reported that its frequency across studies varied from 13% to 67%. In a more recent study, Nussmeier et al. (1986) reported a lower frequency of delirium. They noted that 8.6% of the patients who received narcotic anesthesia and 5.6% who underwent barbiturate coma developed delirium. A number of factors in addition to increased age and preexisting brain damage may increase the risk for postcardiotomy delirium. These include time on bypass (Heller et al. 1970; Kornfeld et al. 1974), severity of postoperative illness (Kornfeld et al. 1974), serum levels of anticholinergic drugs (Tune et al. 1981), increased levels of CNS adenylate kinase and subclinical brain injury (Aberg et al. 1982, 1984), decreased cardiac output (Blachly and Kloster 1966), complexity of the surgical procedure (Dubin et al. 1979), degree of complement activation (Chenoweth et al. 1981), presence of an embolism (Nussmeier et al. 1986), and nutritional status as measured by albumin levels.

According to Andreasen et al. (1972), about 30% of adult burn patients have symptoms of delirium, and the "frequency increases with both the age of the patient and the severity of the burn" (p. 68). Blank and Perry (1984) reported a 18% incidence of delirium in burn patients. Antoon et al. (1972) reported a 14% incidence of burn encephalopathy in children; however, these authors defined burn encephalopathy as "neurologic disturbances ranging from hallucination, personality changes, and delirium to seizures and coma" (p. 609), so the actual frequency of delirium in this study was much lower.

Rapid drug withdrawal in a patient with drug dependence, particularly rapid withdrawal from alcohol and benzodiazepines, is a risk factor for developing delirium. (Substance-induced delirium is discussed in detail in Chapter 19.)

According to DSM-IV, "Children may be more susceptible to delirium than adults, especially when it is related to febrile illness and certain medications (e.g., anticholinergics)" (American Psychiatric Association 1994, p. 126). However, little literature supports this statement. There is a dearth of published information on delirium in children and adolescents (Prugh et al. 1980). In Kornfeld et al.'s (1965) sample of 119 unselected open-heart patients that included 20 children, no child developed delirium, whereas 30% of the adults experienced delirium. Because of the lack of data, childhood is not listed as a risk factor for developing delirium in Table 18–3. However, children do experience delirium, as evidenced by reports of "encephalopathy," "confusion," or "posttraumatic amnesia" from a wide variety of etiologies, including AIDS; cancer chemotherapy; closed-head injury; emergence from anesthesia; organ failure; hypoxia due to status asthmaticus, near drowning, asphyxiation, or foreign body ingestion; CNS viral infections; fever; sepsis; seizures; alcohol dependence and withdrawal; anorexia nervosa; and inhalation syndromes (e.g., inhalation of typing correction fluid).

Sleep deprivation and perceptual (sensory) deprivation may facilitate the development of a delirium; however, Lipowski (1990), after a thorough review of the literature on the relation between sleep and delirium, stated that "experimental and clinical studies indicate a relationship between sleep disturbances and delirium but fail to clarify its exact nature" (p. 123). Without question, sleep-wake abnormalities are frequently an integral part of the symptomatology found in delirium. How critical sleep deprivation is to the development of the delirium remains unclear. Harrell and Othmer (1987) found that sleep disturbance developed after the score on the Mini-Mental State Exam (MMSE; Folstein et al. 1975) decreased (i.e., after the delirium developed) and not before. As Lipowski (1990) noted, "there is no evidence that sensory deprivation alone can cause delirium" (p. 128). The crucial issue may not be the quantity of stimuli but rather the quality. It is known, for example, that the EEG of a subject exposed to monotonous stimuli shows more slowing than the EEG of a sensory-deprived subject (Zubek and Welch 1963). Patients in an intensive care unit (ICU) do not lack stimulation; rather, they lack the kinds of stimuli that orient them to time and environment.

Despite investigations, no personality and psychological variables are associated with delirium. In their review of the postoperative literature, Dubin et al. (1979) indicated that no specific personality profile correlated with delirium. Lipowski (1980), concurring, reported that "it may be stated that so far not a single psychological variable has been conclusively shown to predispose one to delirium" (p. 115).

Clinical Features and Patient Assessment

Prodrome

The patient often manifests symptoms such as restlessness, anxiety, irritability, or sleep disruption immediately before the onset of a delirium. In children, developmental issues, particularly regressive behavior, may contribute to the clinical and subclinical manifestations of delirium (Prugh et al. 1980). Review of the patient's hospital medical chart, particularly the nursing notes, often reveals prodromal features.

Disorganized Thinking (Disturbance of Consciousness) and Impaired Speech

The delirious patient's thought patterns are disorganized and his or her reasoning is defective. In DSM-IV, this is described as a disturbance of consciousness or a reduced clarity of awareness of the environment. The presumptively delirious patient is asked to perform the following three tasks in sequence. The patient must perform each task correctly and return to normal posture before proceeding to the next task.

1. "Place your right hand on your left ear."
2. "Place your left hand on your right elbow."
3. "Place your right hand on your right elbow."

The last task challenges the patient's ability to reason clearly. A nondelirious patient typically will not even attempt the latter task and will look at the physician with a quizzical expression and state, "I can't do that!" The confused patient will either attempt the task, seemingly unaware that it is impossible; perseveratively repeat the first two tasks; or communicate in some other fashion that he or she does not understand. If the severity of the delirium increases, spontaneous speech can become "incoherent, rambling, and shifts from topic to topic" (Cummings 1985, p. 68).

Attention Deficits

The delirious patient has difficulty sustaining attention and is easily distracted by activities in the environment. If one were interviewing a delirious patient in the hospital and someone walked by, the patient would most likely attend to the distraction. Looking back, the patient may then say, "Did you ask me a question?" The patient's inability to sustain attention undoubtedly plays a key role in memory and orientation difficulties.

Acute Alterations in Cognitive Functioning

Impaired Memory

The short-term memory of a delirious patient is impaired. Whether because of attention deficits, perceptual disturbances, or malfunction of the brain, the patient fails tests of recent memory, such as orientation. After recovering from a delirium, some patients are amnestic for the entire episode; others have islands of memory for events during the episode. Whether these islands of memory correspond to "lucid intervals" is unknown.

Disorientation

The patient with a delirium is usually, except for lucid intervals, disoriented to time and often disoriented to place but very rarely, if ever, disoriented to person. It is not unusual for a delirious patient to feel that he or she is in a familiar place (e.g., a room at home) while nodding agreement that he or she is in a surgical ICU. The extent of the patient's disorientation fluctuates with the severity of the delirium.

Altered Perceptions

The delirious patient often experiences misperceptions (i.e., illusions, delusions, and hallucinations). Virtually all patients with a delirium have misperceptions. The patient may, for example, overhear people laughing in the hallway and believe a "wild party" is in progress. The patient, on hearing a postoperative patient moaning or a bedpan falling on the floor (i.e., "A shot?!"), typically weaves these events into a loosely knit paranoid system based on misperceptions; the patient may even attempt to leave the hospital to escape anticipated injury.

Visual hallucinations are common and can involve simple visual distortions or complex scenes. Vivid, detailed, complex visual hallucinations are often the product of substance-induced delirium. During a delirium, visual hallucinations occur more frequently than auditory hallucinations. Tactile hallucinations occur the least frequently. Auditory and tactile misperceptions that are called hallucinations are, in fact, illusions (e.g., an intravenous tubing brushes against the skin and is perceived as a snake crawling on the patient's arm).

Acute Onset and Rapidly Fluctuating Course

The clinical features of delirium are protean (Table 18–4). The symptoms develop abruptly and vary rapidly throughout the day. For example, the surgery team can find a friendly, noncomplaining patient on morning rounds; however, the psychiatric consultant, later that day, can find a grossly confused, paranoid, agitated, uncooperative, and visually hallucinating patient. It is difficult to convince the surgeon, who believes the patient is lucid, that the patient is delirious and requires immediate evaluation and treatment. Noting lucid intervals in the clinical course of a patient is an important observation and is a diagnostic feature of a delirium.

TABLE 18–4. Clinical features of delirium

Prodrome (restlessness, anxiety, sleep disturbance, irritability)
Disorganized thinking (disturbance of consciousness) **and impaired speech**
Attention deficits (easily distracted)
Acute alteration in cognitive functioning
Impaired memory (cannot register new information)
Disorientation (rarely, if ever, to person)
Altered perceptions (misperceptions, illusions, [poorly formed] delusions, hallucinations)
Acute onset and rapidly fluctuating course
Arousal disturbance and psychomotor abnormalities
Disturbance of the sleep-wake cycle
Affective lability
Neurological abnormalities
Constructional apraxia
Dysnomic aphasia
Dysgraphia
Motor abnormalities (tremor, asterixis, myoclonus, reflex, and tone changes)
Electroencephalographic abnormalities (usually global slowing on the electroencephalogram)
Other features (sadness, irritability, anger, or euphoria)

A few patients manifest delirium as a "reversible dementia" (Task Force Sponsored by the National Institute on Aging 1980). These patients lack the dramatic fluctuations that are so typical of delirium and, as a result, are often given the misdiagnosis of dementia.

Nocturnal agitation occurs in patients with Alzheimer's disease, Parkinson's disease, and other disorders (Lipowski 1980, 1989). A critical review of this agitation, also known as "sundowning," indicates that there are several differences between delirium and sundowning (Bliwise 1994; Bliwise et al. 1993). Patients with sundowning have agitation caused by, or at least strongly associated with, darkness and do not have fluctuations throughout the 24-hour period or the diurnal variation as do patients with delirium. Indeed, sundowning has been induced by bringing patients with dementia into a dark room during the daytime (Cameron 1941). Systematic observations of nursing home patients showed that sleep is less likely between 3:00 P.M. and 7:00 P.M., with adjustments made for potential disruption by dinner (Bliwise et al. 1990). Vocalizations and physically aggressive behaviors are more likely to occur between 4:30 P.M. and 11:00 P.M. relative to earlier in the day (Cohen-Mansfield et al. 1992), and wandering is most likely between 7:00 P.M. and

10:00 P.M. (Martino-Saltzman et al. 1991). Other factors that could affect agitation include staff-induced awakening, the patient-to-staff ratio, the shift change, the use of medication, the number and severity of medical conditions, and the physical environment. Circadian rhythmicity probably plays a part in sundowning; therefore, more information on the utility of bright-light exposure, melatonin, and other interventions is needed.

Arousal Disturbance and Psychomotor Abnormalities

Some delirious patients are hypoactive, in which case the patient appears apathetic, somnolent, and quietly confused. These patients commonly receive a diagnosis of "depression" from primary care providers and surgeons. According to a prospective study (Koponen and Riekkinen 1993), patients with the hypoactive, or "silent," form of delirium have the most severe cognitive disturbance, when compared with patients with the hyperactive or mixed variants. In hyperactive-type delirium, the patient is agitated and hypervigilant and has psychomotor hyperactivity. Some patients have a "mixed" picture, in which the level of activation vacillates between the hypoactive and the hyperactive states. According to Liptzin and Levkoff's study (1992) of elderly patients who developed delirium in a general hospital setting, 15% were "hyperactive," 19% were "hypoactive," 52% were "mixed," and 14% were classified as "neither."

Disturbance of the Sleep-Wake Cycle

Sleep-wake disturbance can be symptomatic of a delirium, with sleep deprivation likely exacerbating the confusion. The sleep-wake cycle of the patient with delirium is often reversed. The patient is often somnolent during the day and active during the night. Restoration of the normal diurnal sleep cycle is an important goal in treatment.

Affective Lability

Patients with delirium can have rapid fluctuations in their emotional state (e.g., from fear to incongruent crying to irritability) consistent with affective lability characteristic of "organicity." Emotional responses seen in patients with delirium include anxiety, panic, fear, anger, rage, sadness, apathy, and—rarely, except in steroid-induced delirium—euphoria. Medical and nursing staff often focus on the emotional or behavioral disturbance in the patient without recognizing the underlying delirium. This leads to inappropriate consultation for "depression" (Nicholas and Lindsey 1995) or "character problem." Prospective studies indicate that 23%–42% of the patients referred to a consultation-liaison service for depression by a staff-level physician were subsequently given a diagnosis of delirium by the psychiatrist (Farrell and Ganzini 1995; Valan and Hilty 1996).

Neurological Abnormalities

Neurological abnormalities appear frequently in patients with delirium. Testing for these signs at the bedside strengthens the clinician's confidence in the diagnosis and, when added to the chart, can help other physicians recognize the presence of cognitive dysfunction. An example of an easily performed bedside test—the clock face—is presented in Figure 18–1. The clinician draws a large circle on an unlined sheet of paper and asks the patient to draw a clock face. When the patient is about half finished with this task, the clinician asks the patient to "make the hands of the clock show 10 minutes before 11 o'clock when you fin-

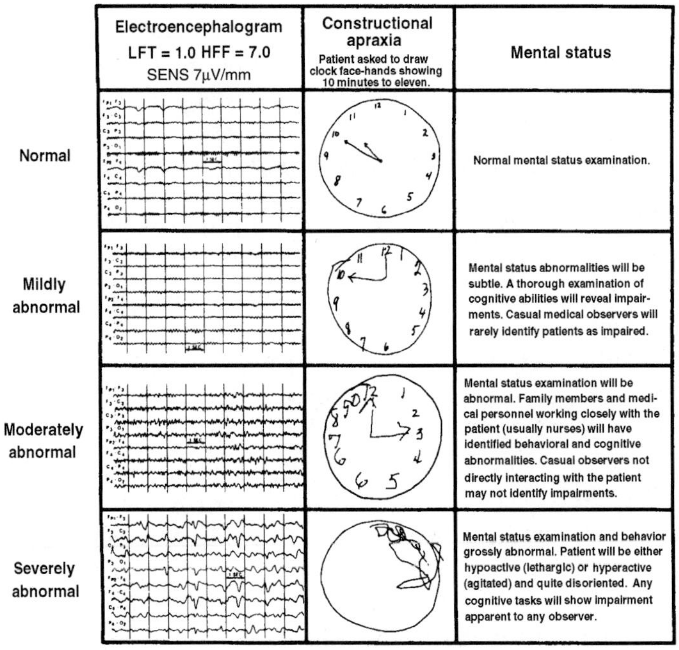

FIGURE 18–1. Comparison of electroencephalogram, constructional apraxia, and mental status in delirium.
Source. Reprinted from Wise MG: "Delirium," in *The American Psychiatric Press Textbook of Neuropsychiatry.* Edited by Hales RE, Yudofsky SC. Washington, DC, American Psychiatric Press. 1987, pp. 89–105. Copyright 1987, American Psychiatric Press. Used with permission.

ish." This and other constructional tasks (testing for constructional apraxia) are sensitive tests for the degree of confusion present. In addition, the patient is asked to name objects (testing for dysnomic aphasia) and to write a sentence (testing for dysgraphia). Dysgraphia is one of the most sensitive indicators of a delirium. In Chedru and Geschwind's (1972) study, 33 of 34 acutely confused patients had impaired writing. Writing shows motor impairment (from tremor to illegible scribble), spatial impairment (letter malalignment and line disorientation), misspelling, and linguistic errors. Dysgraphia is not specific to delirium and can occur with dementia and acute psychiatric disorders (Patten and Lamarre 1989), but dysgraphia in delirious patients is typically more severe.

Delirious patients can have motor abnormalities, such as tremor, myoclonus, asterixis, or reflex and muscle tone changes. The tremor associated with delirium, particularly toxic-metabolic delirium, is absent at rest but apparent during movement. Myoclonus and asterixis (so-called liver flap) occur in many toxic and metabolic conditions. Symmetric reflex and muscle tone changes can also occur. When symmetric hyperreflexia is found, one should suspect alcohol or sedative-hypnotic withdrawal.

Electroencephalographic Abnormalities

In their classic paper titled "Delirium, a Syndrome of Cerebral Insufficiency," Engel and Romano (1959) proposed that the basic etiology of delirium was a derangement in metabolism manifested at the clinical level by characteristic disturbances in cognitive functions and at the physiological level by characteristic slowing of the EEG. Pro and Wells (1977) reported that EEG changes virtually always accompany delirium. The EEG changes found in delirium are *not* always slowing, and the pattern can be low-voltage fast activity, as in DTs (Kennard et al. 1945). Low-voltage fast activity is usually found in hyperactive, agitated patients with heightened arousal (Pro and Wells 1977). EEG slowing is found in lethargic, anergic, abulic patients. The EEG slowing illustrated in Figure 18–1 is typical of deliriums with toxic-metabolic etiologies.

It is worth remembering that a patient's EEG can have significant slowing but is sometimes read as normal. For example, if a patient's normal background activity is 12 cycles per second and during a delirium (metabolic encephalopathy) the background slows to 8 cycles per second, significant slowing has occurred; however, 8 cycles per second still falls within the "normal" range, and the EEG could be read as normal. The encephalopathy might be documented only if the patient has a previous EEG on record or if a second EEG is obtained once the patient is cognitively normal. EEG abnormalities can also occur before, and linger after, the clinical manifestations of a delirium (Andreasen et al. 1977).

Making the Diagnosis

The diagnosis of delirium follows from an appreciation of the clinical features of the syndrome (Table 18–4) and a thorough evaluation of the patient's mental and physical status (Table 18–5). In addition to the usual mental status examination, the examiner should, at a minimum, test for constructional praxis (see Figure 18–1), writing ability, and the ability to name objects. If a delirium is present, every effort should be made to identify the specific etiology or etiologies. Francis et al. (1990) noted in their study that 56% of delirious patients had a single definite or probable etiology and that the remaining 44% had an average of 2.8 etiologies per patient. Although the etiology may not be apparent at the time of consultation, it will often become apparent within a few days.

The gold standard for diagnosis is the clinical evaluation, and the most useful diagnostic laboratory measure is the EEG. Several paper-and-pencil tests exist to aid the clinician in diagnosis. Folstein et al.'s (1975) MMSE provides a screening tool for organicity and is also used to follow the patient's clinical course. The major problem with the MMSE is its lack of sensitivity (i.e., high rate of false-negative results). For example, some patients who had slowed background activity on the EEG at the time of evaluation scored in the mid to upper 20s on the MMSE (M. G. Wise, unpublished data, December 1989). The Delirium Rating Scale (DRS; Trzepacz et al. 1988) and the Confusion Assessment Method (CAM; Inouye et al. 1990) are two more recently developed tests. Both of these tests translate the DSM diagnostic criteria for delirium into an assessment instrument. Some training is required for optimal use of the CAM. The DRS is the most widely used delirium assessment tool. In elderly patients, sensitivity and specificity improve if a cutpoint of 8 instead of the usual 10 is used (Rockwood et al. 1996).

The laboratory evaluation of a delirious patient has two levels: basic and additional tests. The basic laboratory battery is ordered in virtually every patient with delirium. Additional tests are available to the clinician and are ordered based on the specifics of a particular case. When information about the patient's mental and physical status is combined with the basic laboratory battery, the specific etiology (etiologies) is often apparent. If the etiology is not apparent, the clinician should review the case and consider ordering further diagnostic studies.

TABLE 18–5. Assessment of the delirious patient

Physical status

History

Physical examination (neurological examination important)

Review of vital signs (past and present, and [if postoperative] anesthesia record)

Review of medical records

Careful review of medications and correlation with behavioral changes

Mental status

Interview

Performance tests (e.g., clock face, Trails A and B)

Basic laboratory—needed in every delirious patient

Blood chemistries (electrolytes, glucose, Ca^{++}-albumin, BUN, NH_4^+, SGOT, bilirubin, alkaline phosphatase, Mg^{++}, PO_4^{--}, T_4, T_3RU, TSH, VDRL)

Blood count (hematocrit, white blood cell count and differential, MCV, sedimentation rate)

Drug levels (digoxin, theophylline, phenobarbital, etc.)

Arterial blood gases

Urinalysis

Electrocardiogram

Chest X ray

Laboratory—order as needed

Electroencephalogram

Lumbar puncture

CT or MRI

Blood chemistries (heavy metals, thiamine and folate levels, LE Prep, ANA, urinary porphyrins, HIV)

Neuropsychological testing

Note. BUN = blood urea nitrogen; SGOT = serum glutamic-oxaloacetic transaminase; T_4 = thyroxine; T_3RU = T_3 resin uptake; TSH = thyroid-stimulating hormone; VDRL = Venereal Disease Research Laboratory test; MCV = mean corpuscular volume; CT = computed tomography; MRI = magnetic resonance imaging; LE Prep = lupus erythematosus cell preparation; ANA = antinuclear antibodies; HIV = human immunodeficiency virus.

Differential Diagnosis

The differential diagnosis of delirium is extensive, so much so that a tendency to avoid the search for etiologies sometimes exists. It is important to realize that confusional states, particularly in elderly persons, can have multiple causes. For example, an elderly delirious patient might have a low hematocrit and multiple organ system disease (e.g., pulmonary insufficiency, cardiac failure, or dementia) and be taking multiple medications. The clinician must attempt to independently reverse each potential contributor to the delirium.

Pseudodiagnostic terms such as *ICU psychosis* are sometimes used as an explanation for delirium. When a term such as this is used, it usually means that no attempt at specific diagnosis has been made. Koponen et al. (1989) found clear organic etiologies in 87% of the delirious patients in their sample; they also found that the few patients who became confused because of psychological and environmental events had severe dementia. The task for the clinician is to organize the large number of potential causes for delirium into a usable differential diagnosis. The following two-tiered differential diagnostic system is an attempt to do that.

Emergent Items (WHHHHIMP)

The first level of this diagnostic system comprises the emergent diagnoses (mnemonic WHHHHIMP). The clinician must make these diagnoses early in the course of a delirium because failure to do so can result in irreversible injury to the patient.

W—Wernicke's Encephalopathy or Withdrawal

Patients with Wernicke's encephalopathy typically have the triad of confusion, ataxia, and ophthalmoplegia (usually lateral-gaze paralysis). If Wernicke's encephalopathy is not immediately treated with parenteral thiamine, the patient develops a permanent amnestic disorder called Korsakoff's psychosis, which is labeled alcohol-induced persisting amnestic disorder in DSM-IV. Findings that increase the suspicion of alcohol withdrawal/DTs are a history of alcohol-related arrests, alcoholic blackouts, medical complications associated with alcohol abuse, liver function abnormalities, and elevated red cell mean corpuscular volume. Hyperreflexia and increased sympathetic tone (e.g., tachycardia, tremor, sweating, hyperarousal) at the time of examination should lead the clinician to suspect a hyperadrenergic withdrawal state.

H, H, H, H—Hypoxemia, Hypertensive Encephalopathy, Hypoglycemia, or Hypoperfusion

Arterial blood gases and current and past vital signs should be checked to establish whether hypoxemia or hypertensive encephalopathy is present. The patient with hypoglycemia-induced delirium virtually always has a history of type 1 diabetes mellitus. Hypoglycemic delirium is also hyperadrenergic. Hypotension can result from multiple etiologies, such as decreased cardiac output from a myocardial infarction, cardiac failure or arrhythmias, and anemia. All medical conditions that cause hypotension can lead to a decrease in brain oxygenation.

I—Intracranial Bleeding or Infection

The patient who is confused may have had a subarachnoid bleed or another type of CNS hemorrhage. If the patient had a brief period of unconsciousness, with or without headache, and now has delirium or if the patient had or now has focal neurological signs, an intracranial bleed should be suspected. Immediate neurological/neurosurgical evaluation is needed. The clinician should look for signs of an infectious process (e.g., elevated white blood cell count, fever).

M—Meningitis or Encephalitis

Meningitis and encephalitis are typically acute febrile illnesses (vital signs should be checked for fever) and usually have either nonspecific localizing neurological signs (e.g., meningism with stiff neck) or more focal neurological signs.

P—Poisons or Medications

When a delirious patient is encountered in the emergency room, the clinician must consider a substance-induced reaction and order a toxic screen. The clinician should consider pesticides or solvent poisoning as well, although these agents are less likely to be the cause of the delirium. A very common cause of delirium is prescribed medications. The importance of taking a thorough medication history cannot be overemphasized. For the hospitalized patient who becomes delirious, the examiner must thoroughly review the patient's medication records. Attention must particularly be paid to drugs with anticholinergic activity, because they are quite deliriogenic (Tollefson et al. 1991; Tune et al. 1993). The doctor's order sheets are sometimes misleading because drugs are ordered but not given. Correlation of behavior with medication administration or discontinuation is often very helpful in sorting through a difficult case.

Critical Items (I WATCH DEATH)

Numerous insults can cause delirium, many of which are listed in Table 18–6 under the mnemonic I WATCH DEATH. Because the list is lengthy, it may be helpful for the clinician to carry a card containing the entire differential diagnosis of delirium. The mnemonic I WATCH DEATH may sound melodramatic, but this is not the case. The appearance of a delirium, which is equivalent to acute brain failure, should marshal the same medical forces as does failure of any other vital organ. The morbidity and mortality associated with delirium are substantial.

TABLE 18–6. Differential diagnosis for delirium—I WATCH DEATH

Infectious	Encephalitis, meningitis, and syphilis
Withdrawal	Alcohol, barbiturates, and sedative-hypnotics
Acute metabolic	Acidosis, alkalosis, electrolyte disturbance, hepatic failure, and renal failure
Trauma	Heat stroke, postoperative, and severe burns
CNS pathology	Abscesses, hemorrhage, normal pressure hydrocephalus, seizures, stroke, tumors, and vasculitis
Hypoxia	Anemia, carbon monoxide poisoning, hypotension, and pulmonary or cardiac failure
Deficiencies	Vitamin B_{12}, niacin, thiamine, and hypovitaminosis
Endocrinopathies	Hyper- or hypoadrenocorticism and hyper- or hypoglycemia
Acute vascular	Hypertensive encephalopathy and shock
Toxins or drugs	Medications, pesticides, and solvents
Heavy metals	Lead, manganese, and mercury

Prevention

Although research studies have described a variety of potential risk factors for developing delirium, until recently, little research existed about its prevention. Preoperative psychiatric interviews may reduce postoperative psychosis by 50% (Kornfeld et al. 1974; Layne and

Yudofsky 1971). In a factor analysis of 28 risk factors from 44 studies, Smith and Dimsdale (1989) found that only preoperative psychiatric intervention decreased the occurrence of postcardiotomy delirium. Recent reports describe potentially preventable problems that lead to delirium, including dehydration, immobilization, use of physical restraints, indwelling bladder catheters, sleep deprivation, and psychoactive medications (Inouye and Charpentier 1996; Inouye et al. 1999). In particular, medication-induced delirium commonly results from inappropriate use and overuse of sedative-hypnotic, narcotic, anticholinergic, and other psychoactive medications; specifically, the use of more than two psychoactive medications or the addition of three total medications to a regimen increases the risk for delirium (Inouye and Charpentier 1996). Finally, despite the acuity, number, and complexity of health problems among patients older than 65, physicians spend less time with them during medical encounters compared with younger patients (Keeler et al. 1982; Radecki et al. 1988).

Treatment

The treatment of delirium has two separate and important aspects. The first—the identification and reversal, when possible, of the reason(s) for the delirium—is critical and bears directly on the survival of the patient. The second aspect of treatment is to control the agitation that often accompanies the patient's confusion, paranoia, and misperceptions (see Table 18–7).

Reversal of Suspected Etiologies

The goal of diagnosis is to discover reversible causes for delirium. For example, a delirious patient found to have a blood pressure of 260/150 mm Hg and papilledema must immediately receive antihypertensive medications. The alcoholic patient having withdrawal symptoms must receive appropriate pharmacological intervention with drugs such as thiamine and oxazepam. In other words, the clinician must identify specific etiologies and apply appropriate treatment. Without this approach, one might, for example, attempt to treat the agitation and hallucinations of the patient who is septic with haloperidol and fail to treat the medical disorder that might rapidly result in the patient's death.

Research in patients who develop hepatic failure suggests that the γ-aminobutyric acid (GABA)ergic system is important in the development of hepatic encephalopathy (i.e., hypoactive delirium caused by liver dysfunction) (Basile et al. 1994). Specifically, endogenous benzodiazepine-like substances may play a role in delirium associated with hepatic failure; therefore, flumazenil, a benzodiazepine antagonist, might be used to treat these patients (Rothstein 1994). Unfortunately, 60% of the patients fail to respond to this treatment (Pomier-Layrargues et al. 1994).

Another potential cause of delirium is anticholinergic medications and substances. In severe cases of anticholinergic toxicity, physostigmine, administered at a rate of less than 1 mg/minute and at doses of 1–2 mg intravenously every 1 or 2 hours, is recommended (Liston 1989). Contraindications to the use of physostigmine include ulcerative colitis, asthma, diabetes mellitus, gangrene, mechanical obstruction of the urinary or gastrointestinal tract, and cardiovascular disease (especially conduction defects). Because of physostigmine's short duration of action (i.e., 1–2 hours), a continuous intravenous infusion at a rate of 1–3 mg/hour is possible; cardiac monitoring is recommended (Stern 1983).

TABLE 18–7. Medical management of delirium

Medical care
Monitor vital signs, fluid input and output, and oxygenation.
Discontinue nonessential medications.
Avoid addition of multiple medications at one time.
Identify sources of pain (may not be volunteered).
Avoid interruptions in sleep whenever possible.
Do regular laboratory evaluations as indicated.
Prevention and management of disruptive behaviors
Place the patient in a room near the nursing station.
If dangerous behaviors occur, consider a sitter.
Maintain bed in low position and use side rails only if patient insists on getting out of bed.
Use restraints only if necessary (for emergencies or if medication fails).
Avoid placement in a room with another delirious patient.
Avoid a room cluttered with equipment or furniture.
Use of medications
Use haloperidol for agitation; give intravenously whenever possible to avoid side effects and antagonizing the patient.
Avoid use of a benzodiazepine as a sole agent, except in alcohol or sedative-hypnotic withdrawal delirium.
Avoid use of narcotics unless significant pain is present.
Avoid anticholinergic medications.
Use low doses and increase slowly, except in emergencies.
Facilitation of reality
Encourage presence of family members.
Provide familiar clues (e.g., clock, calendar).
Provide adequate day and night lighting (e.g., use a night-light).
Minimize transfers (e.g., do procedures in room whenever possible).
Maximize staff continuity.
Reduce excessive environmental stimuli.
Orient the patient to staff, surroundings, and situations repetitively, particularly before procedures.
Make available hearing or vision assistive devices (e.g., hearing aid, eyeglasses).
Encourage use of personal belongings.
Reassure the patient.

Because of the high mortality and morbidity associated with delirium, proper medical management is important (Table 18–7). The patient is placed in a room near the nursing station, and vital signs are obtained frequently. The patient is observed closely for medical deterioration and for dangerous behaviors, such as trying to crawl over bed rails or pulling out intravenous lines. Fluid input and output are monitored, and good oxygenation must be ensured. All nonessential medications should be discontinued. The brain is a very sensitive forecaster of medical perils ahead. When an etiology for the confusional state is not immediately identified, daily laboratory examinations (e.g., blood count, blood chemistries, urinalysis) and physical examinations are recommended.

Treatment of Agitated Behavior

Pharmacological Interventions

A few studies have compared medications in the treatment of psychotic, disruptive behavior (Bick and Hannah 1986; Salzman et al. 1991). The applicability of these studies to delirium is unknown. Therefore, one must rely on clinical experience, known properties of drugs (particularly side effects), and anecdotal reports of various treatments. A drug used to control agitated psychotic behavior in an ICU should calm the patient without obtunding consciousness and stop hallucinations and paranoid ideation. A drug should not suppress respiratory drive, cause hypotension, or be deliriogenic (e.g., an anticholinergic). The drug should be available in a parenteral form.

A task force of more than 40 disciplines recently reviewed the literature with regard to practice parameters for intravenous sedation of adult patients in the intensive care setting (Shapiro et al. 1995). Literature was classified into one of three levels by a consensus process, according to the methodology of the research, from randomized, prospective, controlled investigations to non-peer-reviewed published opinions (e.g., textbook statements or official organizational publications):

1. Level 1—Use of sedatives is convincingly justifiable on scientific evidence alone.
2. Level 2—Use of sedatives is reasonably justifiable by available scientific evidence and strongly supported by expert critical care opinion.
3. Level 3—Adequate scientific evidence is lacking, but use of sedatives is widely supported by available data and expert critical care opinion.

Recommendations included haloperidol for delirium (level 1), lorazepam for anxiety (level 2), and midazolam or propofol for sedation of less than 24 hours (level 2).

Review of the literature and of clinical experience indicates that haloperidol is the drug of first choice for treatment of agitated behavior in a patient with delirium (American Psychiatric Association 1999; Lipowski 1980, 1990). Haloperidol, a potent antipsychotic with virtually no anticholinergic or hypotensive properties, can be given parenterally. In fact, intravenous haloperidol has been used in very high doses (e.g., 1,200 mg in a 24-hour period) for many years without harmful side effects in seriously ill patients (Sanders and Cassem 1993; Sos and Cassem 1980; Tesar et al. 1985). A continuous intravenous infusion of haloperidol also was used to control severe refractory agitation (Fernandez et al. 1988). (*Note:* Haloperidol is not approved by the U.S. Food and Drug Administration [FDA] for intravenous use.) Although extrapyramidal side effects are more likely with the higher-potency antipsychotic drugs, the actual rate of occurrence of such side effects in medically ill patients who receive haloperidol, particularly when intravenous administration is used, is strikingly low. When extrapyramidal symptoms of oral versus intravenous haloperidol were measured in a blind fashion, intravenous administration of haloperidol was associated with fewer severe extrapyramidal symptoms (Menza et al. 1987). In a few patients with a history of alcohol abuse or cardiomyopathy, intravenous haloperidol caused lengthening of the QT interval or torsades de pointes arrhythmia (Metzger and Friedman 1993). A recent review of 18 patients with arrhythmia associated with haloperidol suggested a pretreatment check of the

QTc interval and serum magnesium and potassium concentrations (Lawrence and Nasraway 1997). If the baseline QTc is 440 msec or longer and the patient is receiving other drugs that may prolong the QTc or has electrolyte disturbances, caution is recommended.

Other useful antipsychotic medications include thiothixene and droperidol. Droperidol is used by anesthesiologists as a preanesthetic agent and by other physicians for the control of nausea and vomiting. It is a butyrophenone, as is haloperidol, and has comparable antipsychotic potency. Droperidol is FDA-approved for intravenous use but is more sedating than haloperidol and has a slight risk of hypotension. In a double-blind study that compared intramuscular haloperidol with droperidol in actively agitated patients, droperidol appeared to give more rapid relief (Resnick and Burton 1984).

Other medications have been used for delirium with varying levels of success. Antipsychotic medications that are less potent, such as chlorpromazine and thioridazine, are more likely to cause hypotension and anticholinergic and quinidine-like side effects, and are not available in a parenteral form. Used in low doses (e.g., 10–100 mg), chlorpromazine appears efficacious and well tolerated (Breitbart et al. 1996), but it is not routinely recommended for delirium. Although risperidone and olanzapine are not available in parenteral formulation, open trials indicate that they may be clinically useful in treating delirium and may have fewer side effects than traditional antipsychotic medication (Sipahimalani and Masand 1997, 1998). Other medications, such as a combination of buspirone and carbamazepine, were reported to be beneficial in controlling agitation in several cases of traumatic brain injury (Pourcher et al. 1994).

A protocol for the use of haloperidol in delirious patients is given in Table 18–8. Regardless of the route of administration, the usual initial dose of haloperidol in the agitated younger patient is 2 mg for mild agitation, 5 mg for moderate agitation, and 10 mg for severe agitation. The initial dose for the elderly patient is 0.5 mg for mild agitation, 1 mg for moderate agitation, and 2 mg for severe agitation. The dose is repeated every 30 minutes until the patient is sedated and/or calm. After the confusion has cleared, the medications are continued for 3–5 days. Abrupt discontinuation of medication immediately following improvement may, within 24 hours, be followed by recurrence of the delirium. A more rational approach is to taper the medication over a 3- to 5-day period, administering the largest dose of the medication before bedtime to help normalize the sleep-wake cycle.

The use of benzodiazepines in delirium has its proponents. However, the sedation that accompanies benzodiazepines may further impair the delirious patient's sensorium. In addition, some patients are disinhibited when given benzodiazepines. Benzodiazepines are the drugs of choice in alcohol withdrawal and sedative-hypnotic withdrawal. Therefore, with the exception of drug-withdrawal states, benzodiazepines are not recommended as a sole agent in the treatment of delirium. Benzodiazepines are used as successful adjuncts to high-potency antipsychotics such as haloperidol (Adams 1984; Garza-Treviño et al. 1989). Small doses of intravenous lorazepam, particularly in patients who have not responded to haloperidol alone, often help decrease agitation. Regardless of what medications are used to control agitation, remember that delirium is defined by its variability; one assessment will evoke management and medical recommendations that are time-limited in efficacy. Only constant follow-up of the delirious patient will suffice.

Environmental Interventions

Environmental interventions are sometimes helpful but are not a primary treatment (Ribby and Cox 1996). Both nurses and family members can frequently reorient the patient to date

TABLE 18–8. Guidelines for haloperidol use in the treatment of agitated behavior

Level of agitation	Starting dose (mg)
Mild	0.5–2.0
Moderate	2.0–5.0
Severe	5.0–10.0

1. For frail elderly, use lower doses.
2. Allow 30 minutes between doses.
3. If agitation continues, double previous haloperidol dose.
4. After three doses of haloperidol, add 0.5–2.0 mg of intravenous lorazepam every 4 hours.
5. Once patient is calm, add the total mg of haloperidol and administer same number of mg in divided doses over the next 24 hours (give larger dose qhs to aid sleep).
6. After the patient remains calm, can reduce dose 50% every 24 hours.
7. Oral dose of haloperidol is twice the intravenous dose.

Note. If haloperidol is used intravenously, clear intravenous line with normal saline prior to bolus infusion. This is important, because heparin can precipitate intravenous haloperidol. Haloperidol is not approved by the U.S. Food and Drug Administration for intravenous use; however, its safety in critically ill patients is well established.

and surroundings. It may help to place a clock, calendar, and familiar objects in the room. Adequate light in the room during the night may decrease frightening illusions. A private room for the delirious patient is not recommended unless adequate supervision is provided. A room with a window helps to orient the patient to normal diurnal cues (Wilson 1972). If the patient normally wears eyeglasses or a hearing aid, returning these devices may improve the quality of sensory input and help the patient better understand his or her surroundings.

A common error on medical and surgical wards is to place more than one delirious patient in the same room. This makes reorientation of these patients impossible and often leads to confirmation, based on conversations with a paranoid roommate, that strange things are indeed happening in the hospital.

Psychosocial Interventions

The psychological support of a patient both during and after a delirium is important. A calm family member should, if possible, remain with the paranoid, agitated patient; this is reassuring and can stop mishaps (e.g., patient's pulling out arterial lines, falling out of bed). In lieu of a family member, close supervision by reassuring nursing staff is essential. After the delirium has cleared, it is therapeutic to help the patient understand the bizarre experience (Mackenzie and Popkin 1980). An explanation to the family about delirium also helps to reduce anxiety and calm fears. Many patients, if they remember the delirious period, are reluctant to discuss their experiences. The clinician should encourage the patient to talk about the delirium. Simple explanation and education are usually all that is required to reduce the likelihood of posttraumatic symptoms.

Course

The clinical outcome for a patient with delirium varies within a range of less than 1 week to 2 months, with a typical course of 10–12 days (American Psychiatric Association 1999).

The possibilities are full recovery; progression to stupor, coma, or death; seizures; chronic brain syndromes; and associated injuries (e.g., fracture or subdural hematomas resulting from falls). Most patients who have delirium may have a full recovery (Lipowski 1990), but only 4%–40% of patients have a full recovery by the time of hospital discharge, and the rate of recovery at discharge is closer to 15% for elderly patients (American Psychiatric Association 1999; Levkoff et al. 1992). Persistent cognitive deficits are common, particularly in AIDS patients, with only 27% having a full recovery of cognition (American Psychiatric Association 1999; Rockwood 1993). Cognitive deficits also may be caused by previously unrecognized dementia that was heralded by the delirium. Seizures can accompany delirium but are more likely to occur with drug withdrawal, particularly alcohol, and burn encephalopathy (Antoon et al. 1972).

Morbidity

Work with patients who are undergoing orthopedic surgery is a fertile ground for research in delirium. Rogers and colleagues (1989) reported that patients who had normal cognitive function when tested preoperatively showed no improvement in level of physical function at 6 months if they developed delirium. In other words, patients who became delirious gained no functional benefit from the surgery. Gustafson et al. (1988) found that delirium was the best predictor of outcome in patients who presented with femoral neck fractures. These authors reported that 37 of 111 patients were delirious preoperatively and that another 31 became delirious postoperatively. The group of delirious, nondemented patients had longer hospital stays (21.7 days vs. 13.5 for nondelirious patients) and were more likely to require walking aids, be bedridden, die, and require rehabilitation. The group of delirious patients spent four times as long in recuperation before discharge. Fernandez et al. (1989) found that only 37% of AIDS patients who became delirious had a complete recovery of cognitive function.

Clinicians who perform hospital consultations encounter patients like the one Moore (1977) described, who "became agitated, struck a nurse, and pulled out his nasogastric tube" (p. 1431). Delirious patients pull out intravenous lines, nasogastric tubes, arterial lines, nasopharyngeal tubes, and intra-aortic balloon pumps. Inouye et al. (1989) reported that the risk of complications, such as decubiti and aspiration pneumonia, was more than six times greater in the delirious patient compared with the nondelirious patient. Levkoff et al. (1986) projected a savings of $1–$2 billion if the hospital stay of each delirious patient was reduced by 1 day. Data on morbidity in children are not available.

Mortality

Most psychiatrists, and physicians in general, are unaware of the mortality associated with delirium. In one study, of the 77 patients who received a DSM-III (American Psychiatric Association 1980) diagnosis of delirium from a consultation psychiatrist, 19 (25%) died within 6 months (Trzepacz et al. 1985). In another study, 3 months following diagnosis, the mortality rate for delirium was 14 times greater (Weddington 1982) than the mortality rate for affective disorders. A patient who receives a diagnosis of delirium during a hospital admission has a 5.5 times greater hospital mortality rate than a patient who receives a diagnosis of dementia (Rabins and Folstein 1982). Furthermore, the elderly patient who develops a delirium in the hospital has a 22% (Rabins and Folstein 1982) to 76% (Flint and Richards 1956) chance of dying during that hospitalization. Cameron et al. (1987) reported that 13 of 20 (65%) delirious patients died during hospitalization. Patients who survive hospitalization have a very high death rate during the months immediately following discharge. Patients with a diagnosis of delirium followed up for several months showed a mortality rate equal to that for dementia patients followed up for several years (Roth 1955; Varsamis et al. 1972). Data on mortality in children are not available.

Conclusions

Delirium is a ubiquitous, underappreciated clinical syndrome that accompanies potentially life-threatening medical conditions. Delirium is especially common in elderly patients, patients with impaired cognitive functioning or structural brain injury, patients who are seriously burned, patients with HIV-related illness, and patients dependent on sedative-hypnotics or alcohol. Because these patients in many cases exhibit bizarre behavior when delirious, the psychiatrist is often consulted. The psychiatrist must be able to organize a systematic differential, make the correct diagnosis, help the primary physician identify the cause(s) of the delirium, and recommend and monitor treatment for agitation. Done properly, correct management and treatment of delirium are life-saving. Although the literature states that delirium is common in children, no epidemiological studies exist to support this. Other than early signs of delirium being mistaken for "normal" regression, delirium in children generally manifests like that in adults.

References

Aberg T, Ronquist G, Tyden H, et al: Release of adenylate kinase into cerebrospinal fluid during open-heart surgery and its relation to postoperative intellectual function. Lancet 1:1139–1141, 1982

Aberg T, Ronquist G, Tyden H, et al: Adverse effects on the brain in cardiac operations as assessed by biochemical, psychometric, and radiologic methods. J Thorac Cardiovasc Surg 87:99–105, 1984

Adams F: Neuropsychiatric evaluation and treatment of delirium in the critically ill cancer patient. Cancer Bulletin 36:156–160, 1984

Adams RD, Victor M: Principles of Neurology, 4th Edition. New York, McGraw-Hill, 1989

American Psychiatric Association: Diagnostic and Statistical Manual of Mental Disorders, 3rd Edition. Washington, DC, American Psychiatric Association, 1980

American Psychiatric Association: Diagnostic and Statistical Manual of Mental Disorders, 4th Edition. Washington, DC, American Psychiatric Association, 1994

American Psychiatric Association: Practice Guideline for the Treatment of Patients With Delirium. Washington, DC, American Psychiatric Association, 1999

Andreasen NC, Noyes R, Hartford C, et al: Management of emotional reactions in seriously burned adults. N Engl J Med 286:65–69, 1972

Andreasen NJC, Hartford CE, Knott JR, et al: EEG changes associated with burn delirium. Diseases of the Nervous System 38:27–31, 1977

Antoon AY, Volpe JJ, Crawford JD: Burn encephalopathy in children. Pediatrics 50:609–616, 1972

Basile AS, Harrison PM, Hughes RD, et al: Relationship between plasma benzodiazepine receptor ligand concentrations and severity of hepatic encephalopathy. Hepatology 19:112–121, 1994

Berrios GE: Delirium and confusion in the 19th century: a conceptual history. Br J Psychiatry 139:439–449, 1981

Bick PA, Hannah AL: Intramuscular lorazepam to restrain violent patients (letter). Lancet 1:206, 1986

Blachly PH, Kloster FE: Relation of cardiac output to postcardiotomy delirium. J Thorac Cardiovasc Surg 52:423–427, 1966

Blank K, Perry S: Relationship of psychological processes during delirium to outcome. Am J Psychiatry 141:843–847, 1984

Bliwise DL: What is sundowning? J Am Geriatr Soc 42:1009–1011, 1994

Bliwise DL, Bevier WC, Bliwise NG, et al: Systematic 24-hour behavioral observations of sleep and wakefulness in a skilled-care nursing facility. Psychol Aging 5:16–24, 1990

Bliwise DL, Carroll JS, Lee KA, et al: Sleep and "sundowning" in nursing home patients with dementia. Psychiatry Res 48:277–292, 1993

Breitbart W, Marotta R, Platt MM, et al: A double-blind trial of haloperidol, chlorpromazine, and lorazepam in the treatment of delirium in hospitalized AIDS patients. Am J Psychiatry 153:231–237, 1996

Cameron DE: Studies in senile nocturnal dementia. Psychiatr Q 5:47–53, 1941

Cameron D, Thomas R, Mulvihill M, et al: Delirium: a test of the Diagnostic and Statistical Manual III criteria on medical inpatients. J Am Geriatr Soc 35:1007–1010, 1987

Chedru F, Geschwind N: Writing disturbances in acute confusional states. Neuropsychologia 10:343–353, 1972

Chenoweth DE, Cooper SW, Hugli TE, et al: Complement activation during cardiopulmonary bypass. N Engl J Med 304:497–502, 1981

Cohen-Mansfield J, Marx MS, Werner P, et al: Temporal patterns of agitated nursing home residents. Int Psychogeriatr 4:197–206, 1992

Cole MG, Primeau FJ: Prognosis of delirium in elderly hospital patients. Can Med Assoc J 149:41–46, 1993

Cummings JL: Clinical Neuropsychiatry. Orlando, FL, Grune & Stratton, 1985

Dubin WR, Field NL, Gastfriend DR: Postcardiotomy delirium: a critical review. J Thorac Cardiovasc Surg 77:586–594, 1979

Engel GL: Delirium, in Comprehensive Textbook of Psychiatry. Edited by Freedman AM, Kaplan HI. Baltimore, MD, Williams & Wilkins, 1967, pp 711–716

Engel GL, Romano J: Delirium, a syndrome of cerebral insufficiency. Journal of Chronic Diseases 9:260–277, 1959

Farrell KR, Ganzini L: Misdiagnosing delirium as depression in medically ill elderly patients. Arch Intern Med 155:2459–2464, 1995

Fernandez F, Holmes VF, Adams F, et al: Treatment of severe, refractory agitation with a haloperidol drip. J Clin Psychiatry 49:239–241, 1988

Fernandez F, Levy JK, Mansell PWA: Management of delirium in terminally ill AIDS patients. Int J Psychiatry Med 19:165–172, 1989

Flint FJ, Richards SM: Organic basis of confusional states in the elderly. BMJ 2:1537–1539, 1956

Folstein MF, Folstein SE, McHugh PR: "Mini-Mental State": a practical method for grading the cognitive state of patients for the clinician. J Psychiatr Res 12:189–198, 1975

Folstein MF, Bassett SS, Romanoski AJ, et al: The epidemiology of delirium in the community: the Eastern Baltimore Mental Health Survey. Int Psychogeriatr 3:169–176, 1991

Francis J, Kapoor WN: Prognosis after hospital discharge of older medical patients with delirium. J Am Geriatr Soc 40:601–606, 1992

Francis J, Strong S, Martin D, et al: Delirium in elderly general medical patients: common but often unrecognized. Clin Res 36(3):711A, 1988

Francis J, Martin D, Kapoor WN: A prospective study of delirium in hospitalized elderly. JAMA 263:1097–1101, 1990

Garza-Treviño ES, Hollister LE, Overall JE, et al: Efficacy of combinations of intramuscular antipsychotics and sedative-hypnotics for control of psychotic agitation. Am J Psychiatry 146:1598–1601, 1989

Gustafson Y, Berggren D, Brannstrom B, et al: Acute confusional states in elderly patients treated for femoral neck fracture. J Am Geriatr Soc 36:525–530, 1988

Harrell RG, Othmer E: Postcardiotomy confusion and sleep loss. J Clin Psychiatry 48:445–446, 1987

Heller SS, Frank KA, Malm JR, et al: Psychiatric complications of open-heart surgery. N Engl J Med 283:1015–1020, 1970

Inouye SK, Charpentier PA: Precipitating factors for delirium in hospitalized elderly persons: predictive model and interrelationship with baseline vulnerability. JAMA 275:852–857, 1996

Inouye SK, Horwitz RI, Tinetti M, et al: Acute confusional states in the hospitalized elderly: incidence, factors, and complications. Clin Res 37(2):524A, 1989

Inouye SK, van Dyck CH, Alessi CA, et al: Clarifying confusion: the confusion assessment method: a new method for detection of delirium. Ann Intern Med 113:941–948, 1990

Inouye SK, Rushing J, Foreman M, et al: Does delirium contribute to poor hospital outcomes? A three-site epidemiologic study. J Gen Intern Med 13:234–242, 1998

Inouye SK, Schlesinger MJ, Lydon TJ: Delirium: a symptom of how hospital care is failing older persons and a window to improve quality of hospital care. Am J Med 106:565–573, 1999

Kane FJ, Remmell R, Moody S: Recognizing and treating delirium in patients admitted to general hospitals. South Med J 86:985–988, 1993

Keeler EB, Solomon DH, Beck JC, et al: Effect of patient age on duration of medical encounters with physicians. Med Care 20:1101–1108, 1982

Kennard MA, Bueding E, Wortis SB: Some biochemical and electroencephalographic changes in delirium tremens. Quarterly Journal of Studies on Alcohol 6:4–14, 1945

Kolbeinsson H, Jónsson A: Delirium and dementia in acute medical admissions of elderly patients in Iceland. Acta Psychiatr Scand 87:123–127, 1993

Koponen HJ, Riekkinen PJ: A prospective study of delirium in elderly patients admitted to a psychiatric hospital. Psychol Med 23:103–109, 1993

Koponen HJ, Stenbäck U, Mattila E, et al: Delirium among elderly persons admitted to a psychiatric hospital: clinical course during the acute stage and one-year follow-up. Acta Psychiatr Scand 79:579–585, 1989

Kornfeld DS, Zimberg S, Malm JR: Psychiatric complications of open-heart surgery. N Engl J Med 273:287–292, 1965

Kornfeld DS, Heller SS, Frank KA, et al: Personality and psychological factors in postcardiotomy delirium. Arch Gen Psychiatry 31:249–253, 1974

Lawrence K, Nasraway S: Conduction disturbances associated with administration of butyrophenone antipsychotics in the critically ill: a review of the literature. Pharmacotherapy 17:531–537, 1997

Layne OL, Yudofsky SC: Postoperative psychosis in cardiotomy patients: the role of organic and psychiatric factors. N Engl J Med 284:518–520, 1971

Levkoff SE, Besdine RW, Wetle T: Acute confusional states (delirium) in the hospitalized elderly. Annual Review of Gerontology & Geriatrics 6:1–26, 1986

Levkoff SE, Evans DA, Liptzin B, et al: Delirium: the occurrence and persistence of symptoms among elderly hospitalized patients. Arch Intern Med 152:334–340, 1992

Lewis LM, Miller DK, Morley JE, et al: Unrecognized delirium in ED geriatric patients. Am J Emerg Med 13:142–145, 1995

Lipowski ZJ: Delirium: Acute Brain Failure in Man. Springfield, IL, Charles C Thomas, 1980

Lipowski ZJ: Delirium in the elderly patient. N Engl J Med 320:378–382, 1989

Lipowski ZJ: Delirium: Acute Confusional States. New York, Oxford University Press, 1990

Liptzin B, Levkoff SE: An empirical study of delirium subtypes. Br J Psychiatry 161:843–845, 1992

Liston EH: Delirium, in Treatments of Psychiatric Disorders: A Task Force Report of the American Psychiatric Association, Vol 2. Washington, DC, American Psychiatric Association, 1989, pp 804–815

Mackenzie TB, Popkin MK: Stress response syndrome occurring after delirium. Am J Psychiatry 137:1433–1435, 1980

Maj M, Satz P, Janssen R, et al: WHO Neuropsychiatric AIDS Study, Cross-Sectional Phase II: neuropsychological and neurological findings. Arch Gen Psychiatry 51:51–61, 1994

Marcantonio ER, Goldman L, Mangione CM, et al: a clinical prediction rule for delirium after elective noncardiac surgery. JAMA 271:134–139, 1994

Martino-Saltzman D, Blasch BB, Morris RD, et al: Travel behavior of nursing home residents perceived as wanderers and nonwanderers. Gerontologist 31:666–672, 1991

Menza MA, Murray GB, Holmes VF, et al: Decreased extrapyramidal symptoms with intravenous haloperidol. J Clin Psychiatry 48:278–280, 1987

Mesulam M-M: Patterns in behavioral neuroanatomy: association areas, the limbic system, and hemispheric specialization, in Principles of Behavioral Neurology. Edited by Mesulam M-M. Philadelphia, PA, FA Davis, 1985, pp 1–70

Metzger E, Friedman R: Prolongation of the corrected QT and torsades de pointes cardiac arrhythmia associated with intravenous haloperidol in the medically ill. J Clin Psychopharmacol 13:128–132, 1993

Moore DP: Rapid treatment of delirium in critically ill patients. Am J Psychiatry 134:1431–1432, 1977

Mori E, Yamadori A: Acute confusional state and acute agitated delirium. Arch Neurol 44:1139–1143, 1987

Murray AM, Levkoff SE, Wetle TT, et al: Acute delirium and functional decline in the hospitalized elderly patient. J Gerontol 48:M181–M186, 1993

Naughton BJ, Moran MB, Kadah H, et al: Delirium and other cognitive impairment in older adults in an emergency room. Ann Emerg Med 25:751–755, 1995

Nicholas LM, Lindsey BA: Delirium presenting with symptoms of depression. Psychosomatics 36:471–479, 1995

Nussmeier N, Arlund C, Slogoff S: Neuropsychiatric complications after cardiopulmonary bypass: cerebral protection by a barbiturate. Anesthesiology 64:165–170, 1986

O'Keefe S, Lavan J: The prognostic significance of delirium in older hospital patients. J Am Geriatr Soc 45:174–178, 1997

Patten SB, Lamarre CJ: Dysgraphia (letter). Can J Psychiatry 34:746, 1989

Perry SW: Organic mental disorders caused by HIV: update on early diagnosis and treatment. Am J Psychiatry 147:696–710, 1990

Platt MM, Breitbart W, Smith M, et al: Efficacy of neuroleptics for hypoactive delirium (letter). J Neuropsychiatry Clin Neurosci 6:66–67, 1994

Pomier-Layrargues G, Giguere JF, Lavoie J, et al: Flumazenil in cirrhotic patients with hepatic coma: results of a randomized, double-blind, placebo-controlled crossover trial. Hepatology 19:32–37, 1994

Pourcher E, Filteau M-J, Bouchard RH, et al: Efficacy of the combination of buspirone and carbamazepine in early posttraumatic delirium (letter). Am J Psychiatry 151:150–151, 1994

Pro JD, Wells CE: The use of the electroencephalogram in the diagnosis of delirium. Diseases of the Nervous System 38:804–808, 1977

Prugh DG, Wagonfeld S, Metcalf D, et al: A clinical study of delirium in children and adolescents. Psychosom Med 42 (suppl):177–195, 1980

Rabins PV, Folstein MF: Delirium and dementia: diagnostic criteria and fatality rates. Br J Psychiatry 140:149–153, 1982

Radecki SE, Kane SL, Solomon DH, et al: Do physicians spend less time with older patients? J Am Geriatr Soc 36:713–718, 1988

Resnick M, Burton BT: Droperidol vs haloperidol in the initial management of acutely agitated patients. J Clin Psychiatry 45:298–299, 1984

Ribby KJ, Cox KR: Development, implementation, and evaluation of a confusion protocol. Clinical Nurse Specialist 10(5):241–247, 1996

Rockwood K: The occurrence and duration of symptoms in elderly patients with delirium. J Gerontol 48:M162–M166, 1993

Rockwood K, Goodman J, Flynn M, et al: Cross-validation of the delirium rating scale in older patients. J Am Geriatr Soc 44:839–842, 1996

Rogers MP, Liang MH, Daltroy LH, et al: Delirium after elective orthopedic surgery: risk factors and natural history. Int J Psychiatry Med 19:109–121, 1989

Ross CA, Peyser CE, Shapiro I, et al: Delirium: phenomenologic and etiologic subtypes. Int Psychogeriatr 3:135–147, 1991

Roth M: The natural history of mental disorder in old age. Journal of Mental Science 101:281–301, 1955

Rothstein JD: Benzodiazepine-receptor ligands and hepatic encephalopathy: a causal relationship? (editorial). Hepatology 19:248–250, 1994

Salzman C, Solomon D, Miyawaki E, et al: Parenteral lorazepam versus parenteral haloperidol for the control of psychotic disruptive behavior. J Clin Psychiatry 52:177–180, 1991

Sanders KM, Cassem EH: Psychiatric complications in the critically ill cardiac patient. Tex Heart Inst J 20:180–187, 1993

Shapiro BA, Warren J, Egol AB, et al: Practice parameters for intravenous analgesia and sedation for adult patients in the intensive care unit: an executive summary. Crit Care Med 23:1596–1600, 1995

Sipahimalani A, Masand PS: Use of risperidone in delirium: case reports. Ann Clin Psychiatry 9:105–107, 1997

Sipahimalani A, Masand PS: Olanzapine in the treatment of delirium. Psychosomatics 39:422–430, 1998

Smith LW, Dimsdale JE: Postcardiotomy delirium: conclusions after 25 years? Am J Psychiatry 146:452–458, 1989

Sos J, Cassem NH: Managing postoperative agitation. Drug Therapy 10(3):103–106, 1980

Stern TA: Continuous infusion of physostigmine in anticholinergic delirium: case report. J Clin Psychiatry 44:463–464, 1983

Task Force Sponsored by the National Institute on Aging: Senility reconsidered. JAMA 244:259–263, 1980

Tesar GE, Murray GB, Cassem NH: Use of high-dose intravenous haloperidol in the treatment of agitated cardiac patients. J Clin Psychopharmacol 5:344–347, 1985

Tollefson GD, Montague-Clouse J, Lancaster SP: The relationship of serum anticholinergic activity to mental status performance in an elderly nursing home population. J Neuropsychiatry Clin Neurosci 3:314–319, 1991

Trzepacz PT: The neuropathogenesis of delirium: a need to focus our research. Psychosomatics 35:374–391, 1994

Trzepacz PT, Teague GB, Lipowski ZJ: Delirium and other organic mental disorders in a general hospital. Gen Hosp Psychiatry 7:101–106, 1985

Trzepacz PT, Baker RW, Greenhouse J: A symptom rating scale for delirium. Psychiatry Res 23:89–97, 1988

Tune LE, Damlouh NF, Holland A, et al: Association of postoperative delirium with raised serum levels of anticholinergic drugs. Lancet 2:651–653, 1981

Tune L[E], Carr S, Cooper T, et al: Association of anticholinergic activity of prescribed medications with postoperative delirium. J Neuropsychiatry Clin Neurosci 5:208–210, 1993

Valan MN, Hilty DM: Incidence of delirium in patients referred for evaluation of depression. Psychosomatics 37:190–191, 1996

Varsamis J, Zuchowski T, Maini KK: Survival rates and causes of death in geriatric psychiatric patients: a six-year follow-up study. Canadian Psychiatric Association Journal 17:17–22, 1972

Weddington WW Jr: The mortality of delirium: an underappreciated problem? Psychosomatics 23:1232–1235, 1982

Wilson LM: Intensive care delirium. Arch Intern Med 130:225–226, 1972

Wise MG: Delirium, in The American Psychiatric Press Textbook of Neuropsychiatry. Edited by Hales RE, Yudofsky SC. Washington, DC, American Psychiatric Press, 1987, pp 89–105

Zubek JP, Welch G: Electroencephalographic changes after prolonged sensory and perceptual deprivation. Science 139:1209–1210, 1963

19

Substance-Induced Delirium and Related Encephalopathies

Thomas M. Brown, M.D.

Drugs may be the most common cause of delirium (Carter et al. 1996). Drugs are the cause of delirium in approximately 30% of elderly patients with the disorder (A.R. Moore and O'Keefe 1999). The fact that many drugs, with such varying actions on the human brain, can precipitate delirium speaks to the pathophysiology of delirium, as well as to the importance of recognizing and treating the disorder. A discussion of individual drugs and how they induce delirium can be found elsewhere (T.M. Brown and Stoudemire 1998c; Trzepacz et al. 1995). This chapter will review the basic mechanisms in the neuropathogenesis of drug-induced delirium (DID).

The Neuropathogenesis of Delirium

It appears that disruptions in certain brain structures and activities can induce delirium. Structures involved in the neuropathogenesis of delirium include presynaptic aminergic and cholinergic neurons, the circuits formed by the axons of these neurons, and the postsynaptic structures reached by these axons. Drugs that interfere with the function of any of these structures may precipitate delirium. The best-established correlations between drugs and delirium are those that involve dopaminergic drugs and muscarinic anticholinergic agents.

Neurotransmitter Imbalances

Current thinking about the chemical basis of delirium holds that a diffuse excess of brain dopaminergic activity, a diffuse deficit in brain muscarinic cholinergic activity, or both are essential to the induction of delirium (T. M. Brown 2000a; Trzepacz 1994). Antagonists of the muscarinic cholinergic receptor and agonists of central dopamine receptors are repeatedly identified as precipitants in cases of DID (Karlsson 1999). An important feature of DID is that drugs may have additive dopaminergic or anticholinergic toxicity; therefore, the clinician must consider the total burden of dopaminergic or anticholinergic activity rather than search for a single, most likely culprit. Table 19–1 lists the ways in which selected drugs may contribute to excessive activation of dopaminergic systems or to excessive inhibition of cholinergic systems (Banerjee et al. 1995; Chiu and Mishra 1980; Cott 1997; Furui et al. 1990; Giacomelli et al. 1998; Huber et al. 1999; Leshner and Koob 1999; Ota et al. 1991; Raffa 1998; Stone 1993; Tuxen and Hansen 1994; Unseld et al. 1990).

One of the striking features of this small selection of deliriogenic agents is its variety. Drugs of many otherwise distinct pharmacological and therapeutic classes may cause delirium. This means that if a patient who takes medication develops delirium, the medication—as well as any herbal remedies, other over-the-counter agents, and substances of abuse—must be considered potential contributors to the delirium. Furthermore, the deliriogenic effects of drugs may conspire in a pharmacodynamic manner, pharmacokinetic manner, or both.

The pharmacodynamic interactions by which drugs exacerbate delirium include additive anticholinergic activity, additive dopaminergic activity, a combination of these two actions, and the indirect potentiation of deliriogenic neurotransmitter imbalances (T. M. Brown 2000a). Other neurotransmitters may participate in the neuropathogenesis of delirium. For example, both elevations and reductions in central serotonin activity are associated with the development of delirium (van der Mast and Fekkes 2000). Other molecules that act as neurotransmitters in the brain, such as adenosine, eicosanoids, endorphins, and nitric oxide, may contribute to delirium, but their role is not well understood, and clinical manipulations based on altering the activities of these molecules is rarely attempted (T. M. Brown and Skop 1996). Of great relevance for the immediate future, though, are the potential roles of gamma-aminobutyric acid (GABA) and glutamate in the neuropathogenesis of delirium.

Aminergic and cholinergic neurons are critical modulators of the membrane potentials of postsynaptic neurons. However, most depolarizations and hyperpolarizations are triggered by the excitatory and inhibitory neurotransmitters of the brain. Currently, the main excitatory neurotransmitter that can be manipulated for clinical purposes is glutamate acting at the *N*-methyl-D-aspartate (NMDA) receptor; the main inhibitory neurotransmitter that can be manipulated is GABA acting at the various GABA receptors. Glutamate and GABA are the main neurotransmitters used by the brain structures thought to be affected by the hyperdopaminergic and hypocholinergic imbalances of delirium. Furthermore, these neurotransmitters may magnify the deliriogenic effects of dopamine and acetylcholine. For example, in rats, benzodiazepines inhibit acetylcholine release, whereas glutamate increases the release of brain-stem dopamine (H. Moore et al. 1995; Morare et al. 1993; Sarter et al. 1999). Although delineation of a role for GABA and glutamate in the neuropathogenesis of delirium seems inevitable, and the clinical utility of agents such as benzodiazepines in the management of some cases of delirium is recognized, how inhibitory and

TABLE 19–1. Dopaminergic and cholinergic deliriogenic effects of selected drugs

Drug	Effects
Amantadine	Stimulates dopamine, norepinephrine, and serotonin receptors; inhibits MAO_A
Amphetamine	Causes release of dopamine, blocks reuptake of dopamine, and inhibits MAO
Atropine	Acts as a potent antagonist at muscarinic cholinergic receptors
Caffeine	Acts as a nonspecific antagonist at adenosine receptors; stimulates the release of dopamine, norepinephrine, serotonin, glutamate, and acetylcholine
Cannabis	Stimulates dopaminergic neurons
Clozapine	Appears to act as a glutamate agonist at NMDA receptors and as an antagonist at $GABA_A$ receptors, which may potentiate the effects of excess dopamine; produces anticholinergic activity
Digoxin	Acts as an antagonist at muscarinic cholinergic receptors, but is about half as potent as atropine
Diphenhydramine	Acts as a potent inhibitor at muscarinic cholinergic receptors; blocks reuptake of dopamine
Lysergic acid diethylamide (LSD)	Acts as a nonspecific agonist at serotonin receptors and as a partial agonist at dopamine D_2 receptors; may act as an antagonist at muscarinic cholinergic receptors
Opiates	Increase release of dopamine
Prednisone	Acts as an antagonist at muscarinic cholinergic receptors, but is about half as potent as atropine; may increase the release, and decrease the reuptake, of dopamine
Procarbazine	Weakly inhibits MAO, which may increase dopamine levels; may inhibit formation of GABA, thereby tending to facilitate the central effects of excess dopamine
Quinolone antibiotics	Act as agonists at NMDA receptors and as antagonists at $GABA_A$ receptors; produce weak dopaminergic activity
St. John's wort	Has significant binding affinity for MAO_A and MAO_B receptors; produces activity at muscarinic cholinergic receptors
Vinca alkaloids	Disrupt axoplasmic flow, which affects the long, thin axons of aminergic and cholinergic neurons early; cause thrombocytosis and direct endothelial injury, which may cause local hypoxia, potentiating the effects of increased dopamine or decreased acetylcholine

Note. GABA = gamma-aminobutyric acid; MAO = monoamine oxidase; NMDA = *N*-methyl-D-aspartate.

excitatory neurotransmitters of the brain conspire to produce delirium is unknown.

Pharmacokinetic drug-drug interactions may contribute to the development of delirium. These interactions may be direct or indirect. Alteration of gut uptake or bioavailability, inhibition of hepatic enzymes, and displacement from albumin and other intravascular binding sites are examples of how one drug may directly alter the metabolism and action of another. Indirect effects on drug metabolism may occur when various organ systems are affected. For example, acute renal failure caused by an aminoglycoside may increase the anticholinergic effect of a tricyclic antidepressant. Other organs of metabolism, distribution, and elimination (e.g., the liver, the lungs, and the organs of the cardiovascular system) may also experience drug-induced impairments of function and thus magnify the deliriogenic potential of a drug. The neuron is another structure whose function may be disrupted in a delirium-inducing manner.

Neurons

The role of drugs in producing the hyperdopaminergic, hypocholinergic state of delirium has been examined. These examinations offer a postsynaptic explanation of the neuropathogenesis of DID. But drugs without obvious dopaminergic or muscarinic anticholinergic activity are also known to cause delirium. When these drugs cause delirium without causing structural damage, the deliriogenic effect may be exerted against the aminergic and cholinergic neurons themselves. The neurons that mediate arousal, including the aminergic and cholinergic neurons, have a morphology that places them at high risk for energetic stress. This increased risk results from at least three factors of these neurons—their large surface area–to–volume ratio (SAVR), their enormously branching and far-flung axonal processes, and their relationship with their glial supports.

The neuronal plasma membrane is an extremely active tissue. Approximately 40% of the brain's adenosine triphosphate (ATP) is consumed by neuronal Na^+-K^+-ATPase alone as this pump strives to maintain ion gradients across the plasma membrane (Park et al. 1992). The greater the SAVR of a neuron, the sooner it is likely to experience difficulty in maintaining ion gradients for any degree of energetic stress. Aminergic and cholinergic neurons are few in number and send slender axonal processes throughout the brain to modulate a variety of functions. These neurons may have one of the largest SAVRs of any neurons in the brain. This energetic risk is compounded by two other aspects of these neurons: the risk of conduction disturbance experienced by slender versus large axons and the susceptibility of oligodendrocytes to energetic stress.

Brain Circuits in Delirium and Drug-Induced Delirium

A recent development in neuropsychiatry is the recognition that dysfunction of certain regions or circuits within the brain are likely to be essential to the production of delirium. The fact that cortical regions generate the electroencephalographic slowing and executive dysfunctions of delirium has long been known. Lateralized dysfunction of executive function occurs in a variety of conditions (e.g., attention-deficit/hyperactivity disorder) in which "hypofrontality" is associated with a) a relative underperfusion of the right caudate nucleus and right mesial frontal territory and b) right parietal lesions, and it occurs in cases of severe head injury in which right-sided thalamic and frontal cortical hypometabolism is observed (Casey et al. 1997a, 1997b; Jagust et al. 1992; Robertson et al. 1995). The brain's alerting network is a system of connections between certain areas in the right frontal lobe, the right parietal lobe, and the locus coeruleus. Injury or dysfunction of these structures or their connecting fibers reduces a patient's ability to sustain attention, marshal appropriate levels of arousal, and organize behaviors appropriate to the immediate stimuli (Berger and Posner 2000; Posner and Petersen 1990). The executive dysfunction of delirium may also develop, at least initially, as a right-sided or bilateral brain dysfunction (Trzepacz 2000).

Some of the earliest evidence of lateralized dysfunction in delirium comes from clinical observations of stroke patients. Mesulam et al. (1979) reported the development of an acute confusional state after infarction in the right middle cerebral artery. Other reports of acute confusional states preceded by coma, liver failure, or postcardiotomy also describe localized reductions in cerebral blood flow or metabolism either to the right cerebral cortex and basal ganglia or globally (Deutsch and Eisenberg 1987; Doyle and Warden 1996; O'Carroll et al. 1982). Recent studies, both retrospective and prospective, link delirium to right-sided brain dysfunction (Henon et al. 1999). At this time, it is not certain which neural pathways are involved. But it is likely that aminergic and cholinergic nuclei; the projections of these nuclei to basal ganglia, to the thalamus, and to certain cortical areas; and these subcortical and cortical recipients of the aminergic and cholinergic projections create a neural pathway, the disturbance of which leads to delirium.

Oligodendrocytes and Astrocytes in Drug-Induced Delirium

In the brain, oligodendrocytes support neuronal function through myelin. Astrocytes serve as vital storage areas for potassium released by neuronal depolarization, a role termed "spatial buffering," and help regulate the activity and presence of neurotransmitters. These two types of glia may play important roles in the genesis and resolution of delirium.

Oligodendrocytes

The fact that axons of small diameter have a greater internal resistance to the conduction of electrochemical signals than large axons is well known. Less often recognized is the potential contribution of the brain's myelin-producing cells, the oligodendrocytes, to both transient and permanent signal propagation problems. In the brain, myelin is formed by oligodendrocytes to insulate neurons and thereby permit not just containment of electrochemical signaling, but also swifter propagation of waves of axonal depolarization. Small axons tend to be grouped together under the insulation of one oligodendrocyte. Because of their extreme sensitivity to oxidative insults and to changes in the extracellular potassium concentration (K_O), oligodendrocytes are susceptible to a variety of drug-induced impairments. Metabolically stressed oligodendrocytes do not reliably insulate axons. Axons shielded by a single malfunctioning oligodendrocyte tend to experience a synchronous disruption of plasma membrane function. The result is a heightening of the metabolic stress endured by the axons of aminergic and cholinergic neurons and a strong tendency toward synchronization of their activity. Table 19–2 describes how select drugs induce deliriogenic impairments to oligodendrocyte function (Hemachudha et al. 1987; Heurteaux et al. 1986; Krisanda 1993; Larocca et al. 1987; Murray and Steck 1984; Stambolic et al. 1996; Ulmer and Braun 1987).

Astrocytes

Astrocytes are critical to the regulation of the neuronal external milieu. Connected by gap junctions to each other, and in some cases to oligodendrocytes, astrocytes create a syncytium that retrieves potassium released by neuronal depolarization and distributes the potassium to areas of low internal potassium concentration. This stabilizes K_O for the neuron (Sontheimer 1994; Zahs 1998). In some encephalopathies, such as the postictal state of a generalized seizure and spreading depression, astrocytic potassium uptake is overwhelmed. In these cases, K_O rises and neuronal function is depressed. It has been noted that in the rat hippocampus, when the uptake of potassium by glia is overwhelmed or blocked, maintenance of the proper K_O level depends on the activity of Na^+-K^+-ATPase. This pump is likely to be found in the plasma membrane of the neurons that released the potassium (Xiong and Stringer 2000). Furthermore, the spatial buffering capacity of different brain regions may vary significantly. The rat spinal cord, for example, appears to

TABLE 19–2. Drug-induced deliriogenic impairments to oligodendrocyte function

Atropine	Blocks the generation of inositol monophosphates and biphosphates in myelin through antagonism of muscarinic cholinergic receptors found on myelin
Chloroform	Stimulates phosphorylation of myelin basic protein and therefore interferes with the regulation of neuronal activity by oligodendrocytes
Cyclosporine	Produces nephrotoxicity that may cause a deliriogenic elevation in K_O
Digoxin	Replicates the activity of the putative endogenous digitalis-like factor, inhibiting the activity of the plasma membrane's Na^+-K^+-ATPase; because oligodendrocytes respond primarily to K_O, changes in K_O caused by digoxin may interfere with oligodendrocyte function
Furosemide	Threatens oligodendrocyte metabolic stability by altering K_O
Heparin	Interferes with the production of aldosterone and thus indirectly interferes with oligodendrocyte function through elevation of K_O
IVIg	Precipitates an autoimmune response to myelin basic protein, which may cause an encephalitis similar to multiple sclerosis (called experimental autoimmune encephalitis [EAE] in animal models)
Lidocaine	Swiftly and frequently causes a variety of disorders of neuronal function by blocking the Na^+ channel; the dysfunction likely extends to oligodendrocytes
Lithium	Interferes with various second-messenger-mediated events in oligodendrocyte differentiation and function
Pentamidine	Indirectly impairs oligodendrocyte function through elevation of K_O by blocking the kaliuretic effect of aldosterone
Potassium	Replicates the toxicity of digoxin
Propranolol	May adversely affect oligodendrocyte function by interfering with redistribution of potassium
Semple rabies vaccine	Precipitates an autoimmune response to myelin basic protein, which causes EAE

Note. IVIg = intravenous immunoglobulin; K_O = extracellular potassium concentration.

have a vast spatial buffering capacity compared to that of the rat hippocampus (S. H. Lee et al. 1994). In delirium, the neurons most susceptible to energetic stress would probably be the least able to respond to reductions in the spatial buffering capacity of potassium by astrocytes. These synergistic limitations might exacerbate the deliriogenic process for susceptible neurons. Thus, the hippocampus and short-term memory might be affected in delirium before the spinal cord and its motor neuron reflexes. Another potential contributor to the neuropathophysiology of delirium may be the interaction of astrocytes with neurotransmitters.

The various interactions between neurotransmitters and glial cells has only just begun to be elucidated. However, animal models show that astrocytes regulate the amount of neurotransmitter in the synaptic cleft. Changes in the rate of glutamate uptake from the synaptic cleft by astrocytes occurs in a frequency-dependent manner and tends to depress synaptic activity when that activity is prolonged (Turecek and Trussell 2000). Also, the activity of the gap junctions between astrocytes increases as the release of glutamate as well as potassium increases (Enkvist and McCarthy 1994). Through the process of nonsynaptic diffusion neurotransmission, astrocytes can take up neurotransmitters that have traveled from remote synapses and that can affect diffuse brain processes such as arousal (Sykova and Chvatal 2000). Thus, the uptake of neurotransmitters by astrocytes is one important means of regulating synaptic activity. The sensitivity of astrocytes to modulation of their various activities opens the door to an astrocytic contribution to DID.

Drugs that alter the release or reuptake of a large number of neurotransmitters have the potential to alter the ability of astrocytes to protect the neuron's external milieu. The result may be an enhancement of deliriogenic processes. Included among the neurotransmitters bound by mammalian neuroglia are acetylcholine, dopamine, GABA, glutamate, histamine, norepinephrine, and serotonin (Muller et al. 2000; Zanassi et al. 1999). Peripheral benzodiazepine receptors (PBRs) are also located on oligodendrocytes (Serra et al. 1999).

The fact that psychoactive medications can precipitate or exacerbate delirium by affecting astrocytes or oligodendrocytes seems certain, but exactly how psychoactive drugs exert a deliriogenic effect on neuroglia is currently unknown. Conditions such as multiple sclerosis that favor delirium and involve prominent derangements of glial structure or function may provide clinical and research opportunities to explore the pathophysiological connections between glial dysfunction and delirium (Arias Bal et al. 1991; Mendez 1995; Rao 1995).

Vascular Contributions to Drug-Induced Delirium

DID may be exacerbated by agents that alter the function or structure of the blood-brain barrier or the vasculature. The vasculature of the brain may be affected by drugs in several deliriogenic ways. Drugs may cause hemodynamic abnormalities, such as hypoperfusion, that lead to delirium. Drugs may also lead the vasculature to synthesize chemotransmitters that ultimately cause or exacerbate delirium.

Perfusion of the brain can be disrupted by drugs. Drugs may cause at least two kinds of hypoperfusion. One is absolute hypoperfusion, or hypotension, in which a drug relaxes vascular smooth muscle excessively. Antihypertensive agents and tricyclic antidepressants often cause hypotensive hypoperfusion. When this occurs, the body's and brain's ability to coordinate and ensure the flow of blood to all regions of the brain is threatened. This is especially true for the nuclei and regions served by the smallest arterioles, such as the lenticulostriate arteries. Bound by physical laws of bulk flow, such as Bernoulli's law of flow, which states that flow is proportional to the fourth power of the radius of the vessel, the capacity of these vessels to autoregulate the flow of blood is severely challenged. There may occur not only a deliriogenic disruption of the supply of substrates for neuronal and glial aerobic metabolism, but a functional disconnection of important brain circuits as well.

This other type of hypoperfusion results when metabolic demand is not met with adequate perfusion. This may contribute significantly to delirium. The reason for the potentially important contribution of relative hypoperfusion to delirium is the fluctuating response of vascular tissue to sustained energy deficits. When 2-deoxyglucose, which blocks the metabolism of glucose, is given to human volunteers, the initial rise in cerebral blood flow declines throughout the brain back to baseline within an hour, despite ongoing hypoglycemia. Insulin and other hypoglycemic agents have similar effects (Elman et al. 1999). Hypoperfusion not only reduces the supply of energy substrates to the brain, it also functionally disconnects different brain regions from each other by interfering with their normal metabolic activity. Such metabolic disconnection may occur at a relatively low level of metabolic impairment and be of fluctuating severity. By disconnecting the brain circuits whose disruption results in delirium, hypoperfusion may itself induce delirium.

The blood-brain barrier carefully regulates the passage of molecules into and out of the brain. This limits the entry of potential neurotransmitters and neurotoxins into the brain and helps regulate the ionic and osmotic state of the brain's extracellular milieu. Drugs can disrupt blood-brain barrier integrity in both direct and indirect ways. Indirect disruption of blood-brain barrier function can result, for example, from amphotericin-induced renal failure or from penicillin-induced lipopolysaccharide release in the Jarisch-Herxheimer reaction (Patrick et al. 1992). When drugs impose a significant metabolic stress, such as hypoxia or hypoglycemia, the cerebral vasculature releases vascular endothelial growth factor (VEGF), which directly disrupts blood-brain barrier function. VEGF makes the blood-brain barrier hyperpermeable. Blood-brain barrier hyperpermeability results in vasogenic brain edema, which in turn is deliriogenic (Fischer et al. 1999). The vasculature may synthesize other deliriogenic molecules, such as nitric oxide, or it may help activate blood cells that subsequently release deliriogenic cytokines (del Zoppo et al. 2000). A cautious interpretation of the effects of drugs on the vasculature's interaction with the blood-brain barrier helps clarify the role of both the vasculature and the blood-brain barrier in the genesis of DID. The vasculature's ability to deliver the substrates of aerobic metabolism to the brain may also be affected by drugs.

Other Possible Deliriogenic Mechanisms

Many drugs can produce DID, but not always by the mechanisms described in this chapter. Drugs may simply lower the threshold for the induction of delirium. This may be especially true for drugs that act on the activity of GABA or glutamate or their receptors. For example, GABA acting at $GABA_A$ receptors inhibits the release of dopamine (Hauber 1998). $GABA_A$ antagonists may increase the risk of a hyperdopaminergic state. In turn, dopamine can enhance the action of glutamate at NMDA receptors by initiating depolarization (Cepeda and Levin 1998; Cepeda et al. 1998; Chase 1998; K. X. Huang et al. 1998). Agonists at the NMDA receptor may exacerbate the process of delirium or delay recovery from it. Barbiturates modulate chloride ion channel function through the $GABA_A$ receptor and may disrupt cerebral cortical modulation of arousal and attention. Such disruption could be deliriogenic by virtue of its impact on higher cortical function. When drugs interfere with higher cortical function, the likelihood of DID may increase.

Drug-Drug Interactions and Other Potentiators of Delirium

Pharmacokinetic Interactions

There are two ways in which two or more drugs may interact pharmacokinetically and increase the risk of DID. The first way is through drug-induced change in drug metabolism. Drug uptake, metabolism, distribution, and elimination are all susceptible to alteration by other drugs. For example, an anticholinergic agent such as amitriptyline may slow gut motility and subsequently increase the uptake (or bioavailability) of a dopaminergic drug such as levodopa. Displacement of one agent by another from serum albumin is another way in which the distribution, and thus the deliriogenic potential, of a drug may be altered by another drug.

A second, and indirect, mechanism of pharmacokinetic drug-drug interaction is through nonspecific organ injury. A drug may alter its own metabolism or that of another agent though injury to the gut, cardiovascular system, liver, or kidneys. In this case, the subsequent DID would likely be caused in part by toxins produced as a result of organ malfunction (T. M. Brown and Brown 1995).

Pharmacodynamic Interactions

Two drugs may interact by enhancing or inhibiting each other's deliriogenic effects. The total anticholinergic or dopaminergic burden of a drug regimen is likely to be an important determinant in the etiology of DID. Failure to recognize the ways in which drugs heighten their deliriogenic activity through pharmacodynamic interactions can contribute to the severity and refractoriness to treatment of some cases of DID. For example, rat studies show that estrogen stimulates the release of striatal dopamine; adenosine receptor antagonists such as caffeine increase the release of striatal glutamate; *m*-chlorophenylpiperazine (mCPP), a metabolite of trazodone, increases the release of acetylcholine within the hippocampus by about 100%; and benzodiazepines inhibit the release of GABA within the cerebral cortex. If these findings can be extrapolated to humans, the implication is that many drugs, drug-drug interactions, and drug-disease interactions can provoke delirium in unanticipated ways (Corsi et al. 1997; Exposito et al. 1999; Gobert et al. 1997; Grimaldi et al. 1999; Healy and Meador-Woodruff 1999; McDermott 1993; H. Moore et al. 1995; Morare et al. 1993; Popoli et al. 1998; Porras and Mora 1995; Porras et al. 1997; Sanz et al. 1997; Sarter 1994; Sarter et al. 1999; Segovia and Mora 1998; Segovia et al. 1997; Smolders et al. 1997; Steulet et al. 1989; Teoh et al. 1996; Zhelyazkova-Savova et al. 1999).

The Role of Aging

Elderly people have a greater risk of DID than young adults (Ritchie et al. 1996). Reasons for this include age-related changes in the absorption, metabolism, distribution, and elimination of drugs in elderly persons and their response to drugs (Lamy 1982). The aging body has less lean—or water—mass and more fat mass. Lipophilic agents are thus more likely to be distributed to the brain and to leave the brain more slowly. Age-related reductions in renal blood flow and in glomerular filtration rate, along with a decline in renal function, retard the elimination of drugs and therefore increase susceptibility to DID (Fliser et al. 1999; Muhlberg and Platt 1999). Reductions in hepatic blood flow and drug-elimination capacity also occur (Schmucker 1998). For example, the catalytic activities of enzymes such as cytochrome P450 1A2, 2C9, 2C19, 2D6, 2E1, and 3A3/4 decline with age (Tanaka 1998). The result of these changes in renal and hepatic function is an increase in the amount of drug available to act on the aging brain. The ability of the blood-brain barrier to regulate and impede the passage of drugs and other toxins into the brain also declines with age (Saija et al. 1992; Sankar et al. 1983; H. S. Sharma et al. 1995). Despite the importance of pharmacokinetic changes in aging, the most important factors in DID among elderly persons may be pharmacodynamic (Norman 1993).

Receptor function across various organs changes with age. These changes include an altered sensitivity of the brain to drug action (Klotz 1998). For example, a reduced response to adrenergic agonists and antagonists is common. This increases the susceptibility of elderly persons to drug-induced vascular problems such as orthostatic hypotension. Both the receptor changes and the subsequent effects on peripheral organ function may contribute to the reduced filtering effect of the blood-brain barrier (Mooradian 1994; Turnheim 1998). Therefore, many agents with the capacity to cause DID are likely to move into the brain and are better able to penetrate the blood-brain barrier in elderly persons. Reduced integrity of blood-brain barrier function is strongly associated with susceptibility to dementia; a similar association with susceptibility to delirium may exist (Skoog et al. 1998; van der Mast 1998).

Neurotransmitter changes in the aging brain include changes in neurotransmitter synthesis and elimination. As humans age, the rate at which the blood-brain barrier takes up choline declines (Shah and Mooradian 1997). This may limit the production of acetylcholine and therefore increase the risk of a central hypocholinergic state (Cohen et al. 1995). As the human brain ages, the availability of GABA appears to decline, the binding of GABA by $GABA_A$ and $GABA_B$ receptors decreases, and the availability of glutamate may increase (Milbrandt et al. 1996). The synthesis of dopamine also declines with age (Volkow et al. 1998). This may increase the risk of DID, because the brain responds with increased dopamine D_2 receptor sensitivity to dopamine agonists (Moy et al. 1997).

Elimination of potential neurotoxins declines with age. For example, the cerebrospinal circulatory system becomes less efficient, and its capacity to remove potential neurotoxins declines (Rubenstein 1998).

Other Deliriogenic Effects of Drugs

DID has thus far been presented as a constellation of abnormalities in neurotransmitter activity, neuronal and glial function, and brain circuits. Drugs may increase the risk of DID by reducing the brain's ability to resist the development or consequences of delirium. For example, anticholinergic agents and dopaminergic agents can impair thermoregulation, serotonergic agents can further reduce autonomic stability, and GABAergic agents can impair respiratory drive. Delirium, whether or not drug-induced, is rarely a static entity. Delirium tends to be associated with other pathological conditions that, if not recognized and dealt with, may aggravate or perpetuate the course of delirium (T. M. Brown 2000b; Ginsberg et al. 1992; Hayashi 1998; Sanna et al. 1999).

Concurrent Medical Problems

Medical problems can increase the risk of DID in two ways. First, medical problems can reduce a person's ability to sustain normal neuronal activity in the face of a pharmacological challenge. Table 19–3 describes how common medical problems contribute to DID (Freeman et al. 1962; Gibson and Blass 1976; Ginsberg et al. 1992; Hayashi 1998; Monda et al. 1998; Trzepacz and Francis 1990; Trzepacz et al. 1993; Zhao et al. 1998).

Second, medical disorders heighten susceptibility to DID by changing the baseline pattern of neurotransmitter release, reuptake, or postreceptor response. For example, acute febrile illness is associated with reduced serum anticholinergic activity among elderly individuals. Such a reduction in serum anticholinergic activity is associated with a higher incidence of delirium when fever is present (Flacker and Lipsitz 1999). Elderly patients are thus at greater risk of DID when they are febrile. Another, more familiar example of heightened risk of DID among elderly individuals is provided by Alzheimer's disease. The reduced neuronal cholinergic activity and reduced cerebral metabolism in Alzheimer's dementia heighten the risk of DID (Eikelenboom and Hoogendijk 1999; Wengel et al. 1998).

TABLE 19–3. Medical problems and their contribution to drug-induced delirium (DID)

Medical problem	Contribution to DID
Congestive heart failure	Decreased cardiac function may slow metabolism and excretion of deliriogenic agents and reduce oxygenation of the brain.
Fever	Hyperthermia causes the central release of Glu, NE, and DA. Studies in rats show a decreased reuptake of Glu accompanies the enhanced release of Glu in the hyperthermic brain.
Hepatic insufficiency	Reduces capacity to metabolize drugs, reduces the synthesis of albumin and related serum proteins, and decreases elimination of potential neurotoxins such as octopamine and ammonia.
Hypoalbuminemia	Decreased protein binding increases some drugs' activity.
Hypoglycemia	Hypoglycemia precipitates the release of neuronal dopamine and reduces central acetylcholine production and release.
Hyponatremia	Can alter the ability of neurons to signal properly.
Hypoxia	Same as for hypoglycemia.
Parkinson's disease	These patients require dopaminergic agents with or without muscarinic anticholinergic agents, and thus are at high risk for pharmacological induction of delirium.
Renal failure	May impair integrity of blood-brain barrier, or slow elimination, allowing more of a potentially toxic drug to reach the brain.

Note. DA = dopamine; Glu = glutamate; NE = norepinephrine.
Source. Reprinted from Brown TM: "Drug-Induced Delirium." *Seminars in Clinical Neuropsychiatry* 5:113–124, 2000. Copyright 2000. Used with permission.

Managing Drug-Induced Delirium

The diagnosis and treatment of DID depends on recognizing its hallmarks: confusion and abnormalities of arousal and attention. In some cases, such as in the quietly delirious and intubated patient in an intensive care unit, recognizing DID may be difficult. Thus, the possibility of DID must be considered for everyone who is at risk, because failure to diagnose and treat DID may prolong recovery and worsen outcome.

Once recognized, DID can be managed in several ways. The clinician must support and maintain basic vital functions; adequate oxygenation, hydration, nutrition, and normal temperature must be ensured. Specific pharmacological and physiological precipitants of DID must be identified and, when possible, removed. Active treatment of symptoms of delirium must also occur, even as precipitants are being identified and eliminated. The clinician must monitor for signs of recovery, as well as for side effects from any agents used to treat delirium. Finally, the clinician must taper and discontinue any pharmacological treatments for delirium as soon as possible to minimize the induction of other side effects, such as extrapyramidal side effects (EPS) from haloperidol. Agents commonly used to treat delirium include intravenous haloperidol and other high-potency antipsychotics, with adjunctive lorazepam for agitation and hydromorphone for pain (Adams 1989; American Psychiatric Association 1999; Wise 1995). Table 19–4 outlines a typical protocol for treating delirium at my institution (T. M. Brown 2000b; Hughes 1996).

Although haloperidol is not approved by the U.S. Food and Drug Administration for

TABLE 19–4. A general approach for using haloperidol to treat delirium

Time	Haloperidol use
Zero	Patient meets criteria for delirium. A baseline assessment of findings consistent with delirium and of extrapyramidal side effects (EPS: cogwheeling, tremor) is recorded. Signs and symptoms of delirium include the following: Disorientation Fluctuating level of arousal and disorientation Short-term memory impairment Generalized slowing on electroencephalogram Picking at bedsheets Autonomic instability Normal saline 10 cc is given to clear the iv line. (Normal saline prevents haloperidol from precipitating in the line with various agents, such as heparin.) Haloperidol 2 mg is given intravenously. Normal saline 10 cc is given to clear the iv line.
30 minutes	Reassessment of findings consistent with delirium and of EPS is made. If findings still present, the dose of haloperidol is doubled.
60 minutes	Reassessment of findings consistent with delirium and of EPS is made. If findings still present, the dose of haloperidol is doubled. Repeat the above step until the patient's delirium has resolved or unacceptable EPS develop. If patient's delirium resolves, dose haloperidol as follows: a. One-fourth of the total amount of haloperidol required to resolve delirium is given intravenously every 6 hours. b. The last dose required to achieve resolution of delirium is given intravenously PRN the return of delirium. The standing dose is reduced by 50% every day, until it is possible to remove haloperidol completely.

Source. Reprinted from Brown TM: "Drug-Induced Delirium." *Seminars in Clinical Neuropsychiatry* 5:113–124, 2000. Used with permission.

the treatment of delirium and case reports of torsades de pointes attributed to haloperidol make some physicians reluctant to use haloperidol in the management of delirium, it remains a very effective agent for the reversal of delirium (Hunt and Stern 1995; Lawrence and Nasraway 1997; N. D. Sharma et al. 1998). As basic neuroscience reveals more about the physiology and pharmacology of DID, a greater variety of agents for the treatment of delirium, with improved efficacy and safety, will likely be developed. It should remain for many years, however, the clinician's task to differentiate delirium from other drug-induced encephalopathies.

Other Substance-Induced Encephalopathies

The 1950s saw the emergence of rationally designed, laboratory-developed drugs for the relief of mental suffering. The impact of these drugs on human existence has been profound and largely beneficial. However, there have been problems. A devastating consequence of some of these drugs has been the unanticipated appearance of severe side effects. Entities such as the neuroleptic malignant syndrome (NMS) and the serotonin syndrome have joined ranks with established drug-induced encephalopathies such as anticholinergic toxicity and drug-induced seizures. One aspect of this problem has been the difficulty and the delays experienced by drug manufacturers, physicians, and patients in recognizing the role of medications in the genesis of severe side effects. In the following section I review the pathophysiology and treatment of some of the major drug-induced encephalopathies other than delirium.

The Varieties of Encephalopathy

In common clinical parlance, "delirium" means an acute confusional state. This definition has a telegraphic quality through which the importance of the clinical condition is captured, but any further clinical or pathophysiological meaning is lost. In this section, specific types of drug-induced acute confusional states are described. These descriptions are meant to serve as examples of how any acute confusional state may be first described as a constellation of findings and subsequently better understood as a particular set of physiological derangements. Ideally these descriptions will serve as models of, and a source of information on, the receptor mechanisms and neuroanatomic pathways involved in producing classic syndromes of drug-induced altered mental states. The syndromes discussed in this section are anticholinergic toxicity, inhibitotoxicity, NMS, seizures, and serotonin syndrome.

An important feature of these drug-induced encephalopathies is that they traditionally have been described as disorders of synaptic chemotransmission. Either too much or too little of a given neurotransmitter acting at one or more receptors has been offered as the cause of these encephalopathies. The assumption here is that neurotransmission may go awry in a point-to-point synaptic manner. Many useful—indeed, lifesaving—treatments have been developed using this disease model. But disease models are exploited only until their limitations point the way to more effective interventions. Where possible, these limitations will be highlighted and new directions in treatment explained. For instance, NMDA receptor antagonists are being deployed in the treatment of NMS, and nitric oxide may become a treatment for serotonin syndrome. The potential contributions of nonsynaptic diffusion neurotransmission, neuroglia, and non-neuronal brain connective tissue will not be discussed at length. Although these tissues are not likely to be mere bystanders in the evolution of a severe drug-induced encephalopathy, too little is known about their role in the initiation, maintenance, and resolution of these disorders to assist in their recognition and management. Yet the potential impact of basic neuroscience research, and the endless consumption of poorly characterized street and herbal agents, will ensure the emergence of new kinds of drug-induced encephalopathies, clarify the outlines of their distinct pathophysiologies, and suggest new treatments for decades to come.

The collection of drug-induced encephalopathies in this section is not exhaustive. Its purpose is to underscore the diversity of drug-induced encephalopathies and to suggest the importance of incorporating pathophysiological mechanisms in making treatment recommendations. This is especially important as the number and kinds of psychoactive drugs, ranging from new antitumor agents to herbal remedies obtained over the Internet, reveal their expected and their unexpected neuropsychiatric effects. The history of the diagnoses of the encephalopathies will be referred to occasionally to emphasize that the diagnostic outlines of these disorders are not static, but rather hypotheses in evolution.

Anticholinergic Toxicity

Diagnosis

Intoxication with anticholinergic agents is a well-described, and indeed ancient, form of psychotropic toxicity. "Red as a beet, dry as a bone, hot as a hare, blind as a bat, and mad as a hatter" describe the flushing, dryness, fever, pupillary dilation, and altered mentation of muscarinic anticholinergic toxicity (Mendez 1996). In doses used clinically, anticholinergic agents, particularly those with activity at the M_1 receptor, disrupt short-term memory (Bartus and Johnson 1976; Ghelardini et al. 1999). Recognition of the presence and persistence of the signs of anticholinergic intoxication is essential in differentiating it from delirium, which in this section is differentiated symptomatically from pure anticholinergic toxicity, although these two entities share pathophysiological features.

Table 19–5 lists selected agents with well-recognized and less-recognized muscarinic anticholinergic activity. The large number of agents with muscarinic anticholinergic activity speaks both to the importance of the muscarinic receptor in the clinical regulation of many diseases and to the risk of anticholinergic toxicity.

TABLE 19–5. Selected agents with antimuscarinic anticholinergic activity

Antidepressants	**Antispasmodics**
Amitriptyline	Various
Doxepin	**Over-the-counter agents**
Imipramine	Analgesics (e.g., Excedrin PM)
Nortriptyline	Cold remedies (e.g., Contac)
Paroxetine	Sedatives (e.g., Sominex)
Antihistamines	**Other**
Carbinoxamine	Cimetidine
Chlorpheniramine	Codeine
Cyclizine	Digoxin
Dimenhydrinate	Dipyridamole
Diphenhydramine	Furosemide
Promethazine	Isosorbide dinitrate
Tripelennamine	Nifedipine
Antipsychotic agents	Prednisolone
Clozapine	Ranitidine
Phenothiazines:	Theophylline
Chlorpromazine	Warfarin
Thioridazine	

Source. Reprinted from Brown TM, Stoudemire A: "Agents Used to Treat Movement Disorders," in *Psychiatric Side Effects of Prescription and Over-the-Counter Medications: Recognition and Management.* Washington, DC, American Psychiatric Press, 1998, pp. 35–52. Copyright 1998, American Psychiatric Press. Used with permission.

Pathophysiology of Antimuscarinic Agents

Knowing the location and function of the five muscarinic cholinergic receptor subtypes enables the clinician to interpret findings in cases of anticholinergic toxicity. Table 19–6 outlines the location and clinical significance of receptor antagonism of the muscarinic cholinergic receptor subtypes (P. J. Barnes 1993; Elhusseiny et al. 1999; Lechleiter et al. 1989; Linville and Hamel 1995; E. Perry et al. 1999; E. K. Perry and Perry 1995; Reever et al. 1997; Rodriguez-Puertas et al. 1997; V. K. Sharma et al. 1997).

In rat models of cortical pyramidal cell activity, ascending cholinergic fibers terminating at muscarinic receptors depolarize the pyramidal cells, upregulate glutamatergic NMDA receptors, and activate the phosphoinositide cascade (Jerusalinsky et al. 1997). The net effect of this muscarinic cholinergic activity is enhancement of attention, memory, and arousal, accompanied by desynchronization of the electroencephalogram (EEG). Acetylcholine has similar actions and effects within the hippocampus (Aigner 1995). Muscarinic receptor antagonists interfere with these processes, thereby impairing attention, memory, and arousal, and may give rise to visual hallucinations by impairing the ability of the cerebral cortex to filter "noise" from "signal."

An important feature of the muscarinic cholinergic system is its diffuse projection throughout the human brain. By diffusely and simultaneously regulating systems of attention, memory, and arousal, the muscarinic cholinergic system is susceptible to abrupt and widespread disruption by drugs. Metabolic stressors heighten the susceptibility of the muscarinic cholinergic system to drug side effects. This susceptibility is discussed in detail in the section on delirium.

Treatment

Recognizing anticholinergic toxicity is the first step in its management. Discontinuing or reducing the dosage of the offending drug or drugs is the next step. Because sedation, agitation, and hallucinations may presage convulsions, arrhythmias, cardiovascular collapse, and even death, swift consideration of the use of intravenous physostigmine is warranted (R. C. Hall et al. 1977). When reducing the burden of anticholinergic agents and using physostigmine, the clinician must monitor for the emergence of muscarinic cholinergic rebound (T. M. Brown and Stoudemire 1998a).

As is the case with inhibitotoxicity, which includes benzodiazepine intoxication, the many roles of the widely scattered muscarinic cholinergic receptors makes the use of any antidote a difficult procedure, and one that requires close monitoring.

Inhibitotoxicity

Diagnosis

Release from fear and anxiety is a desire that is probably as ancient as humankind. Not surprisingly, anxiolytic agents appear to have been among the first regularly used drugs to treat fear and anxiety. With these drugs there emerged the risk of a particular type of toxicity: excessive activation of neuronal inhibitory mechanisms. Such inhibitory toxicity, or inhibitotoxicity, can occur spontaneously, as in idiopathic recurring stupor (IRS). IRS is characterized by episodic stupor grading into coma, fast EEG activity in the range of 14–16 Hz with an unreactive background, elevated serum and cerebrospinal fluid levels of endozepine-4,

TABLE 19–6. Location and clinical significance of receptor antagonism of the muscarinic cholinergic receptor subtypes

Muscarinic cholinergic receptor subtype	Location	Clinical significance of receptor antagonism
M_1	Brain parenchyma Cerebral cortex Hippocampus	Impairs memory, possibly including memory mediated by long-term potentiation Impairs consciousness Causes hallucinations
	Brain connective tissue Astrocytes Vascular smooth muscle	May impair cerebral blood flow May dysregulate blood-brain barrier function
	Preganglionic neurons of airways	Inhibits ganglionic chemotransmission
	Cardiac myocytes	Increases heart rate
M_2	Brain parenchyma Cerebral cortex Hippocampus Striatum	Impairs memory Impairs consciousness Causes hallucinations
	Brain connective tissue Astrocytes Vascular endothelium Vascular smooth muscle	May impair cerebral blood flow May dysregulate blood-brain barrier function
	Postganglionic nerve terminals of airways	Disinhibits the release of acetylcholine in airways
	Cardiac myocytes	Increases heart rate
M_3	Brain parenchyma Cerebral cortex Hippocampus Striatum	Impairs memory, possibly including memory mediated by long-term potentiation Impairs consciousness Causes hallucinations
	Brain connective tissue Astrocytes Vascular smooth muscle	May impair cerebral blood flow May dysregulate blood-brain barrier function
	Airway Smooth muscle Submucosal glands	Causes bronchodilation Decreases mucus secretion
	Detrusor muscle of urinary bladder	Causes urinary hesitancy
	Gut Salivary glands	Decreases salivation, which causes dry mouth

TABLE 19–6. Location and clinical significance of receptor antagonism of the muscarinic cholinergic receptor subtypes *(continued)*

Muscarinic cholinergic receptor subtype	Location	Clinical significance of receptor antagonism
M_4	Brain parenchyma Cerebral cortex Hippocampus Striatum	Impairs memory Impairs consciousness Causes hallucinations
	Brain connective tissue Astrocytes	May impair cerebral blood flow May dysregulate blood-brain barrier function
M_5	Brain parenchyma Cerebral cortex Hippocampus Nucleus accumbens Striatum	Impairs memory Impairs consciousness Causes hallucinations
	Brain connective tissue Astrocytes Vascular endothelium Vascular smooth muscle	May impair cerebral blood flow May dysregulate blood-brain barrier function

and resolution of symptoms with administration of the $GABA_A$ antagonist flumazenil. There are no other structural or metabolic factors that account for the findings in IRS (Lugaresi et al. 1998; Rothstein et al. 1992; Soriani et al. 1997; Tinuper et al. 1992, 1994). By activating the endogenous inhibitory mechanisms of the brain, benzodiazepines and other $GABA_A$ agonists reproduce the distinct spectrum of findings in IRS. Figure 19–1 presents the evolution of findings in a case of benzodiazepine-induced inhibitotoxicity.

Two important questions are whether all benzodiazepines produce the same pattern of intoxication and whether nonbenzodiazepine $GABA_A$ agonists produce a similar state of intoxication. Although there is no definite answer to these questions yet, it seems that $GABA_A$ agonists produce a fairly typical syndrome of intoxication, as noted in Figure 19–1; however, it also seems that different agents have distinct forms of intoxication. The distinctions may take the form of a relapsing intoxication traditionally ascribed to barbiturates versus the sustained and gradually resolving intoxication of benzodiazepines (Plum and Posner 1980). The bottom line for the clinician is that profound benzodiazepine intoxication has a characteristic appearance and course that may culminate in death.

Many factors influence a person's risk of benzodiazepine intoxication. Table 19–7 lists some of these factors (Bell et al. 1987; Daderman and Lidberg 1999; MacDonald and Kapur 1999; Nagy et al. 1999; Ribeiro et al. 1999). When risk factors for benzodiazepine intoxication are identified, benzodiazepines should be used cautiously and their use should be monitored closely.

A variety of agents can exacerbate or replicate the toxicity of benzodiazepines. These include $GABA_A$ receptor agonists, such as barbiturates, kava kava, and progesterone; inhibitors of the metabolism of GABA, such as gabapentin and valerian; inhibitors of the neuronal reuptake of GABA, such as riluzole; and muscarinic cholinergic M_2 receptor antagonists, which tend to disinhibit the release of cortical GABA (Belelli et al. 1999; Ferraro et al. 1997;

Relaxation →	Sedation →	Disinhibition →	Coma
Reduction in anxiety without impairment in psychomotor performance	Drowsiness accompanied by a reduction in psychomotor activity level and performance	Impairment of coordinated activity of central and peripheral structures; may manifest as amnesia, agitation, and autonomic abnormalities such as atrioventricular conduction problems	Progression of severe depression of central nervous system from stupor to coma to death; abnormalities of autonomic function, including hypotension, bradycardia, and Cheyne-Stokes respiration, which can result from both central and peripheral disturbances

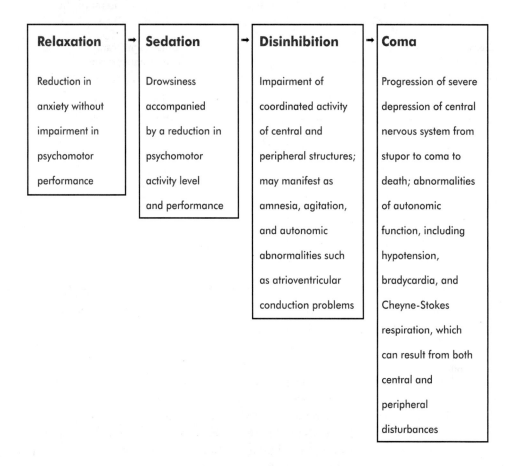

FIGURE 19–1. Evolution of findings in a case of benzodiazepine-induced inhibitotoxicity.

A. C. Hall et al. 1994; Kretschmer et al. 1998; Lovinger et al. 1993; Malatynska et al. 1999; Meldrum and Chapman 1999; Mihic et al. 1994; Rush et al. 1999; Roberge et al. 1998; Tunnicliff et al. 1999; Weight et al. 1992; Whiting 1999).

Pathophysiology

Two basic features of benzodiazepine intoxication are typically seen by clinicians: 1) stimulation of the intended $GABA_A$ receptors and 2) activation of other receptors, including the PBR. Agonist activity at the $GABA_A$ receptor is responsible for the traditional picture of benzodiazepine intoxication. Agonist activity at other receptors magnifies the toxicity of benzodiazepines and leads to their occasional refractoriness to flumazenil, a potent $GABA_A$ antagonist. Table 19–8 presents the main receptors activated by benzodiazepines and the consequences of such activation (T. M. Brown and Stoudemire 1998c).

The role of various GABA receptors in the modulation of both autonomic function and higher cortical activity is immense. Although labeled "peripheral," the PBR contributes to the toxicity of benzodiazepines by its widespread distribution and function.

The binding activities of benzodiazepines, and indeed of most $GABA_A$ receptor ago-

TABLE 19–7. Factors that influence risk of benzodiazepine intoxication

Factor	Influence
Age	Increasing age is strongly correlated with susceptibility to benzodiazepine intoxication: by age 70, patients are at very high risk for intoxication, including coma, even with low doses of benzodiazepines.
Personality disorders	Limited evidence suggests that persons with personality disorders characterized by impulsivity and aggressiveness may be at increased risk for benzodiazepine-induced disinhibition, aggressiveness, and amnesia.
Anxiety disorders	Rats identified as "anxious" have a higher density of hippocampal $GABA_A$ receptors than "nonanxious" rats, which may partly explain why some patients with anxiety disorders are sensitive to benzodiazepines and why these patients experience anxiety relief if treated with them.
Previous use of a benzodiazepine	Previous use of a benzodiazepine may reduce the extent to which a given dose of a $GABA_A$ agonist induces any stage of inhibitotoxicity.
Hepatic failure	Hepatic failure raises the risk of severe inhibitotoxicity, including coma.
Renal failure	Renal failure allows benzodiazepines to accumulate.
Status epilepticus	Status epilepticus may downregulate $GABA_A$ receptors in the hippocampus, making some patients less responsive to benzodiazepines.
Brain injury	Brain injury increases the risk of sedation, disinhibition, and coma.
Pregnancy	A marked decline in peripheral benzodiazepine receptors occurs in the third trimester of pregnancy, which may heighten sensitivity to many benzodiazepines.

Note. GABA = gamma-aminobutyric acid.

nists, to the receptors in Table 19–8 is not well described nor likely to be identical. This may help explain problems in the management of benzodiazepine overdose as well as in the differential utility of the benzodiazepines themselves in treating various syndromes. Different benzodiazepines have slightly different profiles of toxicity as well as utility. For example, although lorazepam appears to be effective in reversing serotonin syndrome, clonazepam does not reliably treat this disorder (T. M. Brown et al. 1996). Variations in the subunit composition of the $GABA_A$ receptor may be crucially important in determining sensitivity of $GABA_A$ receptors in different brain regions to different drugs. A $GABA_A$ receptor has five subunits, which tend to consist either of two alpha, two gamma, and one beta subunit or of two alpha, two beta, and one gamma subunit. For example, abecarnil is a full agonist at the $GABA_A$ receptor when the receptor is composed of $alpha_3beta_2gamma_3$ subunits, but abecarnil is only a partial agonist when the subunits of the $GABA_A$ receptor are $alpha_5beta_2gamma_2$. The subunit composition of $GABA_A$ receptors probably varies across brain regions (Mehta and Ticku 1999; Smith et al. 1998). The possibility of genetic and regional variations in the effect of benzodiazepines at the $GABA_A$ receptor alone is great.

TABLE 19–8. Benzodiazepine receptor subtypes

Type	Location	Activity	Effect
High-affinity A	Highest densities in superficial layers of cerebral cortex, thalamus, granule cell layer of cerebellum; low density in brain stem	GABA receptor–linked chloride ionophore	Regulates many functions, ranging from cellular polarization and endocrine and cardiovascular function to activation of preprogrammed behaviors
Low-affinity A	Widely dispersed: neocortex lamina VI, substantia nigra, amygdala, hippocampus, cerebellum	GABA receptor–linked chloride ionophore	Probably similar to high-affinity $GABA_A$ function
A: BZ1 *aka* omega1	High density in cerebellum; also in neocortex lamina VI and substantia nigra	Closely associated with the low-affinity $GABA_A$ receptor	Mediates sleep, anxiolytic, myorelaxant, and anticonvulsant effects
A: BZ2 *aka* omega2	Cerebral cortex, spinal cord, hippocampus	Likely similar to BZ1	Mediates aspects of memory and cognition
B	Cerebral cortex, hippocampus, spinal cord; may be found in lung	GABA receptor–linked G proteins and calcium ionophores	May regulate some aspects of memory, mood, and cognition
PBR	Cerebral cortex, hypothalamus, kidney, colon, blood cells, steroid-making endocrine organs	Involved in steroidogenesis	Uncertain at this time, but appears to be linked to endocrine and stress responses

Note. GABA = gamma-aminobutyric acid; PBR = peripheral benzodiazepine receptor.
Source. Reprinted from Brown TM, Stoudemire A: "Sedative-Hypnotic and Related Agents," in *Psychiatric Side Effects of Prescription and Over-the-Counter Medications: Recognition and Management.* Washington, DC, American Psychiatric Press, 1998, pp. 123–144. Copyright 1998, American Psychiatric Press. Used with permission.

Clinical manifestations of benzodiazepine intoxication probably result from the diffuse activation of various receptors that bind benzodiazepines as well the activation of various potential final common pathways of GABAergic intoxication. For example, diffuse activation of $GABA_B$ receptors in thalamic relay nuclei disinhibits low-threshold calcium currents. When activated, these calcium currents generate rhythmic activity within the thalamus that propagates to the cerebral cortex (Depaulis et al. 1997). Subsequent involvement of the substantia nigra results in the manifestations of the seizure. It appears that GABA receptors within the substantia nigra pars reticulata mediate the motor and autonomic features of benzodiazepine intoxication and withdrawal, whereas both GABA receptors and PBRs within the substantia nigra pars reticulata conspire to produce the electroencephalographic changes (Wala et al. 1999). Activation of thalamic $GABA_B$ receptors can enhance the effect of $GABA_A$ receptor activation on psychomotor activity level and cognition. The clinical picture may resemble an absence seizure, although the EEG would distinguish the spike-and-wave activity of an absence seizure from the enhanced beta activity of benzodiazepine intoxication (Z. C. Huang and Shen 1993, 1997; Pechadre et al. 1993). Indeed, the plasma level of the offending benzodiazepine and the quantitative extent of electroencephalographic changes appear directly correlated (Friedman et al. 1992).

Treatment

Treatment of benzodiazepine intoxication begins with recognition of the disorder, management of any acute medical disturbances, and, on occasion, use of flumazenil. More than 70% of patients with severe benzodiazepine intoxication respond to flumazenil. However, more than half of the responders will become re-sedated within 90 minutes of receiving flumazenil. Flumazenil's side effects include agitation, seizures, and rare disturbances of cardiac conduction (Flumazenil in Benzodiazepine Intoxication Multicenter Study Group 1992; Herd and Clarke 1991). Table 19–9 offers a simplified approach to the management of benzodiazepine intoxication. Although flumazenil may reverse many of the findings in benzodiazepine intoxication, such as profound psychomotor retardation and cardiovascular abnormalities, it may not reverse other findings attributed correctly to the offending benzodiazepine (Mullins 1999). For example, on occasion, flumazenil may not reverse benzodiazepine-induced amnesia (Hung et al. 1992). This is testimony to the diversity of $GABA_A$ receptor subtypes as well as to the many different types of receptors bound by benzodiazepines (Hevers and Luddens 1998).

Because of the potential for worsening as a result of autonomic impairment, patients at risk for airway compromise must be assumed to be at high risk for sudden decompensation. Seizures observed in benzodiazepine intoxication may suggest the presence of other intoxicants, including flumazenil, or of severe respiratory depression with secondary hypoxia. Cardiac arrhythmias may develop unpredictably, especially when other intoxicants are present. In such cases of extreme inhibitotoxicity, continuous cardiac and pulmonary monitoring by an intensivist are necessary.

Neuroleptic Malignant Syndrome

Diagnosis

One of the most spectacular, dangerous, and perhaps underrecognized drug-induced encephalopathies is NMS. NMS has been recognized as a complication of antipsychotic drug therapy since Delay and Deniker wrote about it in 1968, and the earliest case of NMS can be traced as far back as 1959 (Delay and Deniker 1968; Walker 1959). The classic findings in NMS are the quartet of fever, autonomic instability, altered mental status, and skeletal muscle rigidity. The incidence of NMS has been debated for decades. A low figure of 0.07% is sometimes offered, but the debated incidence has generally ranged from 0.1% to 2.5%. Pope et al. (1986) reviewed 500 patient records and found that 1.4% of patients developed "definite" or "probable" NMS. This correlated well with a figure of 0.5%–1.0% calculated for the development of NMS in a population of several hundred patients observed by Delay and Deniker (1968) (Addonizio et al. 1986; Caroff 1980; Pope et al. 1986). Although NMS is generally regarded as a rare complication of antipsychotic drug therapy, these percentages strongly suggest that underrecognition of NMS may play a role in the apparent infrequence of the disorder.

TABLE 19–9. A simplified approach to the management of benzodiazepine intoxication

Stage of intoxication	Management
Relaxation	May not reflect true intoxication, and usually does not require treatment.
Sedation	Depending on the degree of sedation, may or may not require intervention. Intervention may include 1) reduction in benzodiazepine dosage or 2) use of a stimulant.
Disinhibition	Disinhibition characterized by abnormal but directable behavior may require management of the environment only. When agitation accompanies disinhibition, interventions may include both physical and chemical restraints. Caution must be used when using either form of restraint: in both cases, autonomic function must be monitored and the risk of additive inhibitotoxicity with agents such as chlorpromazine must be considered.
Coma	If benzodiazepine intoxication has progressed to the point at which coma has occurred or is likely, protection of the airway becomes crucial. Intubation may be necessary. In these cases, flumazenil may be able to replace intubation or shorten its course. Monitoring of cardiovascular status is crucial.

The possibility of underrecognition of NMS is significant. Perhaps agents besides dopamine D_2 receptor antagonists contribute to the development of NMS. Drugs strongly associated with the development of NMS are listed in Table 19–10. Table 19–11 lists drugs implicated in at least one case of NMS (Ansseau et al. 1980; Bailly 1999; Boyarsky et al. 1999; Brazelton et al. 1997; C. S. Brown et al. 1999; Burke et al. 1981; Chan-Tack 1999; Corrigan et al. 1990; Cuesta Lopez et al. 1994; Duarte et al. 1996; Ehara et al. 1998; Fava and Galizia 1995; Gonner et al. 1999; Graber et al. 1994; Gradon 1991; Haggerty et al. 1987; Halman and Goldbloom 1990; Heinemann et al. 1997; June et al. 1999; Kern and Cernek 1996; Keyser and Rodnitzky 1991; Kiyatake et al. 1991; Koponen et al. 1993; Kornhuber et al. 1993; Kubota 1993; Larner et al. 1998; Lew and Tollefson 1983; Lin et al. 1999; Mateo et al. 1992; Miyaoka and Kamijima 1995; Nemecek et al. 1993; Nimmagadda et al. 2000; Nonino and Campomori 1999; Park-Matsumoto and Tazawa 1999; Portel et al. 1999; Reeves et al. 1998; Shintani et al. 1995; Spirt et al. 1992; Spivak et al. 1990, 1996; Stevens et al. 1998; Still et al. 1998; Swanson et al. 1995; Turjanski and Lees 1992; Wagner and Vause 1995; Young 1997).

Table 19–12 lists factors associated with the development of NMS and related parkinsonian states (Chopra et al. 1999; Fido 1999; James 1988; Portel et al. 1999; Ueda et al. 1999). This list is not exhaustive; as more is learned about NMS, more factors associated with its development are likely to be discovered.

The mortality rate of untreated NMS may exceed 10%. Severe residual injuries ranging from renal impairment to cerebral or cerebellar dysfunction may profoundly reduce the quality of a patient's life after an episode of NMS (T. M. Brown 1999; Pullicino et al. 1991; Slee et al. 1989). Clearly, the importance of recognizing an episode of NMS is high. Research criteria for the diagnosis of NMS are included in DSM-IV-TR (American Psychiatric Association 2000). Useful clinical diagnostic criteria for NMS were suggested by Pope et al.

TABLE 19–10. Drugs strongly associated with the development of neuroleptic malignant syndrome (NMS)

Dopamine D_2 antagonists	**Discontinuation of D_2 agonists**
Chlorpromazine[m]	Bromocriptine[c]
Domperidone[c]	Levodopa[m]
Droperidol[c]	Levodopa/carbidopa[m]
Fluphenazine[m]	**Atypical antipsychotic agents**
Haloperidol[m]	Clozapine[m]
Metoclopramide[m]	Olanzapine[m]
Molindone[c]	Quetiapine[r]
Nemonapride[c]	Remoxipride[c]
Pimozide[c]	Risperidone[m]
Promethazine[r]	Sulpiride (withdrawal)[r]
Dopamine-depleting agents	Tiapride[m]
Reserpine[r]	**Serotonergic agent**
Tetrabenazine[m]	Lithium[*m]

Note. c = occasional case reports; m = multiple case reports; r = rare case reports; * = likely had a mainly facilitatory, rather than directly causal, role in the development of NMS.

(1986). These emphasize an important difference between research criteria and clinical criteria when making a diagnosis of NMS. The American Psychiatric Association research criteria for NMS help ensure uniform and accurate diagnoses—even if some cases of NMS are excluded because they do not meet all criteria. In clinical settings, it is so important not to miss a diagnosis of NMS that the threshold for making the diagnosis is lowered. The risk here is that a clinician might make an incorrect diagnosis of NMS. However, the treatment for NMS is so benign compared to NMS itself that, in clinical practice, it often makes sense to err on the side of not missing the diagnosis.

A separate issue is whether there exists an atypical form of NMS that is unaccompanied by skeletal muscle rigidity. This issue has been raised with atypical antipsychotics, for which occasional cases of apparent NMS, but without skeletal muscle rigidity, have been reported. This is relevant, for example, with clozapine, for which typical cases of NMS involving all four findings and atypical cases without skeletal muscle rigidity exist (Amore et al. 1997; Goates and Escobar 1992; Nopoulos et al. 1990; Reddig et al. 1993; Sachdev et al. 1995). NMS without skeletal muscle rigidity has been observed with the typical antipsychotics (i.e., neuroleptics) as well (Rosebush and Stewart 1989). Some authors argue that "our understanding and diagnostic specificity for neuroleptic malignant syndrome is too rudimentary to advance the notion of a clinical spectrum, particularly in the context of atypical antipsychotics" (Buckley and Hasan 1998). This is probably the most reliable stance to take when distinguishing typical NMS from atypical NMS. In addition, this stance provides room for the inclusion of non-neuroleptic agents, such as fluoxetine, when these have been reported as having caused NMS (Halman and Goldbloom 1990). Of great interest to clinical researchers, this liberal stance toward the diagnosis of NMS has not undermined the immovable, important contributions of previous thinkers regarding the pathophysiology of NMS. On the contrary, the current understanding of this pathophysiology is founded on the older thinking.

TABLE 19–11. Drugs possibly associated with the development of neuroleptic malignant syndrome (NMS)

Adenosine antagonists

Diprophylline (7-(2,3-dihydroxy-propyl)theophylline)[r]

AMPA agonist

Basagran[r]

NMDA antagonists

The ability of NMDA antagonists such as amantadine and memantine to treat NMS suggests that their withdrawal may place some patients at risk for the development of NMS.

Dopamine-synthesis inhibitors

Alpha-methylparatyrosine[*r]

Discontinuation of D_2 antagonists

Chlorpromazine[r]

Haloperidol[r]

Metoclopramide[r]

Dopamine-reuptake inhibitor

Methylphenidate[r]

Monoamine oxidase inhibitor

Maprotiline (withdrawal)[*r]

Muscarinic cholinergic antagonists

Diphenhydramine (intoxication)[*r]

Trihexyphenidyl (withdrawal)[*r]

Noradrenergic-serotonergic agents

Amitriptyline[*r]

Clomipramine[*r]

Nortriptyline[r]

Serotonergic agents

Cisapride (potent 5-HT$_4$ agonist; weak 5-HT$_3$ antagonist)[c]

SSRIs: Fluoxetine[*r]; Fluvoxamine[r]; Paroxetine[*r]; Sertraline[*r]

MDMA ("Ecstasy")[r]

Mianserin (5-HT$_2$ and 5-HT$_3$ antagonist)[*r]

Nefazodone[r]

Trazodone[*r]

Venlafaxine[*r]

$GABA_A$ agonists

Lorazepam[*r]

Midazolam[r]

Zopiclone[r]

$GABA_A$ antagonists

$GABA_A$ antagonism may account for at least a portion of the capacity of some antipsychotic agents to cause NMS; for example, clozapine antagonizes GABA at the $GABA_A$ receptor.

TABLE 19–11. Drugs possibly associated with the development of neuroleptic malignant syndrome (NMS) *(continued)*

GABA transaminase inhibitor
Gamma vinyl GABA[r]
$GABA_B$ agonist withdrawal
Baclofen

Note. c = occasional case reports; m = multiple case reports; r = rare case reports; * = likely had a mainly facilitatory, rather than directly causal, role in the development of NMS; 5-HT = 5-hydroxytryptamine (serotonin); AMPA = alpha-amino-3-hydroxy-5-methyl-4-isoxazol propionic acid; GABA = gamma-aminobutyric acid; MDMA = methylenedioxymethamphetamine; NMDA = N-methyl-D-aspartate.

TABLE 19–12. Factors associated with the development of neuroleptic malignant syndrome (NMS)

Metabolic and pharmacological factors
Strongly associated with NMS development
Dehydration
Fever or other hyperthermic state
Higher dose of neuroleptic
Low serum iron
Low serum sodium
Mental retardation
Physical exertion
Preexisting parkinsonism or other extrapyramidal disorder
Weakly associated with NMS development
Low serum albumin
Low serum magnesium
Male gender
Malignant hyperthermia (prior to NMS)
Pregnancy
Premenstrual state
Postpartum period
Drug-drug interactions
Pharmacodynamic
Pharmacodynamic drug-drug interactions heighten the risk of NMS. Two types of pharmacodynamic interaction are relevant: 1) several drugs acting at the same site to cause NMS and 2) one or more drugs acting at several sites to cause NMS.
Pharmacokinetic
Pharmacokinetic drug-drug interactions may facilitate the development of NMS; for example, the interaction resulting from combining fluoxetine with a typical antipsychotic. In this case, fluoxetine would probably raise the serum level of the antipsychotic by inhibiting hepatic enzymes. Another example of a pharmacokinetic drug-drug interaction is an increase in the bioavailability of an antipsychotic as a result of anticholinergic-induced intestinal pseudo-obstruction.
Impaired excretion of offending agents may result from dehydration and renal injury in NMS. This is another vitally important pharmacokinetic factor that must be considered.

Pathophysiology

Blockade of brain dopamine D_2 receptors has long been recognized as a cause of NMS. Newer evidence suggests that dopamine D_2 receptor blockade may be only one path to induction of NMS. Much of this evidence has been sought and found since the discovery that clozapine, an antipsychotic agent with little activity at the dopamine D_2 receptor, causes NMS (Anderson and Powers 1991; DasGupta and Young 1991; Miller et al. 1991; Sachdev et al. 1995). At this time, NMS appears to occur when a drug, taken by a susceptible individual, disrupts coordinated central control of both centrally and peripherally mediated cognitive, motor, and autonomic function (Gurrera 1999). Starting with the effects of dopamine, GABA, glutamate, and serotonin on the production of extrapyramidal motor symptoms in humans, this section reviews the potential for agents acting through these neurotransmitters to cause the core findings in NMS.

Extrapyramidal Findings

Dopaminergic Agents

The role of dopamine D_2 receptor antagonism in NMS is well described and reviewed elsewhere (T. M. Brown and Stoudemire 1998b). What is perplexing is whether dopamine D_2 receptor antagonism is responsible for the induction of NMS when the responsible drug is clozapine, which exerts only a weak blockade of dopamine D_2 receptors, or fluoxetine, which does not directly antagonize dopamine D_2 receptors. In these cases, direct action at other receptors may be responsible for the appearance of NMS.

GABAergic Agents

Agents that alter activity at muscarinic cholinergic, dopamine D_1 and D_2, $GABA_A$, glutamate NMDA, and serotonin 5-hydroxytryptamine type 2 (5-HT_2) receptors may cause abnormal extrapyramidal motor findings. For example, Turjanski and Lees (1992) found that gamma vinyl GABA, an irreversible inhibitor of GABA transaminase, worsened parkinsonism in patients with Parkinson's disease. Although NMS is not typically thought of as a side effect of $GABA_A$ agonists, there are case reports of NMS resulting from their withdrawal or initiation (Kern and Cernek 1996; Larner et al. 1998). An imbalance between brain dopamine and GABA systems was suggested by Lew and Tollefson (1983) as a potential cause of NMS, given the response of a patient with NMS to diazepam. Diazepam-responsive NMS has been suggested as a subtype of NMS, given the possible association between good response and diazepam in patients with conditions such as low serum iron (J. W. Lee 1998; Miyaoka et al. 1997). Larner and colleagues reported that the addition of the cyclopyrrone zopiclone to benzodiazepine nitrazepam produced acute fever, autonomic instability, rigidity, and mental status changes in an elderly woman taking no other medication. Kern and Cernek (1996) attributed the induction of NMS to a delayed effect of risperidone. However, clonazepam had been withdrawn as well, and the temporal association between clonazepam withdrawal and the induction of NMS suggests that the withdrawal of clonazepam may have played a role in the emergence of NMS (Hasan and Buckley 1998). The development of probable NMS among patients exposed to, and withdrawn from, benzodiazepines and zopiclone suggests that profound underactivity or overactivity of the GABA system may be pathogenic for NMS (Bachli and Albani 1994; Ebadi et al. 1990). The neuroanatomy of central $GABA_A$

pathways helps explain the potential pharmacological association of $GABA_A$-active agents and EPS.

At least two major GABAergic pathways that mediate extrapyramidal motor function appear to run through the basal motor nuclei. One pathway, a direct GABAergic pathway that communicates between the internal segment of the globus pallidus and the pars reticulata of the substantia nigra, produces rigidity if overstimulated. The other, an indirect pathway from the external segment of the globus pallidus and subthalamic nucleus that runs to the precentral cortex, tends to cause rigidity if inhibited (DeLong 1990; Larner et al. 1998; Ridding et al. 1995). Abnormal modulation of either of these pathways may cause severe rigidity. In rats, GABAergic drugs have a biphasic effect on rigidity, with low doses of GABA agonists reducing rigidity and higher doses increasing it (Wardas et al. 1988; Worms and Lloyd 1980). Unfortunately, for a given patient, knowing what dose of, for example, a GABA agonist will precipitate EPS can be difficult to judge except empirically (Turjanski and Lees 1992). Figure 19–2 presents clinically relevant interactions among neurotransmitters that may produce rigidity associated with NMS, with emphasis on the direct and indirect systems of motor control (Gerfen and Engber 1992; Perlmutter et al. 1997; Watts and Mandir 1992). In addition to the actions of GABA mediated through these pathways, GABA agonists appear to inhibit the production of dopamine by tyrosine hydroxylase and to inhibit the postsynaptic response of striatal dopamine receptors to dopamine (Bartholini 1985). Among some patients, such as those with Parkinson's disease, these effects might produce a clinically profound consequence.

Figure 19–2 highlights the receptors thought to be involved in NMS and shows how these receptors (e.g., the dopamine D_2 receptor of the striatum and the NMDA receptor of the globus pallidus) are linked. In addition, it shows how other receptors may be involved in NMS and how other interventions for NMS may be developed.

Figure 19–2 cannot illustrate why some patients may be more susceptible to NMS with one agent versus another or why NMS recurs only about 50% of the time on rechallenge with the offending agent.

Glutamatergic Agents

Kornhuber and Weller (1994) have made a convincing argument that the release of glutamatergic systems from dopaminergic inhibition can cause profound skeletal muscle rigidity and may precipitate the full syndrome of NMS. There is little doubt that overactivity of basal motor glutamate circuits is involved in the pathogenesis of Parkinson's disease. Thus, either severe inhibition of dopaminergic neurotransmission or profound enhancement of glutamatergic neurotransmission may produce the severe skeletal muscle rigidity that typifies NMS. This theory is bolstered by several lines of evidence. First, haloperidol, clozapine, and olanzapine facilitate glutamatergic neurotransmission at the NMDA receptor (Banerjee et al. 1995; N. A. Moore et al. 1997). This means that even for haloperidol, antagonism of the dopamine D_2 receptor may not be the sole cause of either EPS or NMS. Second, Kornhuber and Weller (1994) support their idea that overactivity of glutamate may be responsible for NMS by referring to cases of NMS resulting from withdrawal of amantadine, an NMDA receptor antagonist. Figure 19–1 shows how glutamate excess may override counterregulatory dopaminergic activity. Again, overriding of an endogenous counterregulatory system is assumed to occur primarily among patients with an abnormality that predisposes them to NMS, and what these abnormalities are is unclear. But abnormalities of central glutamate activity may contribute to the development of schizophrenia, because persons

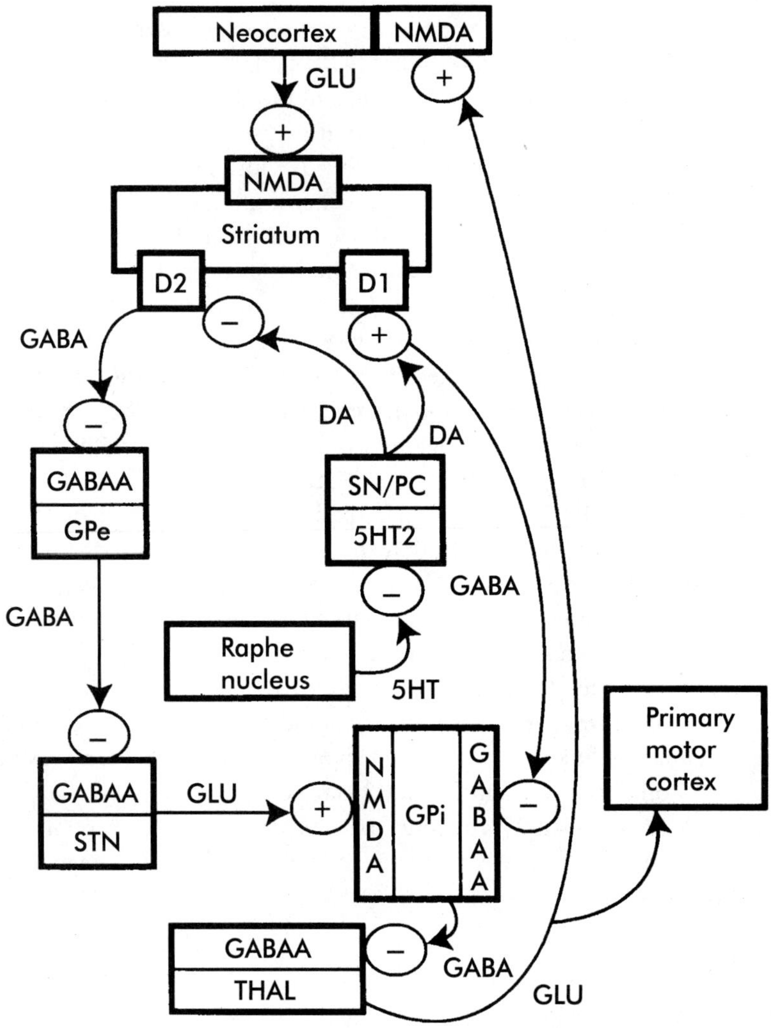

FIGURE 19–2. Interactions among neurotransmitters that may produce rigidity associated with neuroleptic malignant syndrome (NMS). Abbreviations: + = stimulates release of neurotransmitter; – = inhibits release of neurotransmitter; D1 = dopamine D_1 receptor; D2 = dopamine D_2 receptor; DA = dopamine; GABA = gamma-aminobutyric acid; GABAA = $GABA_A$ receptor; GLU = glutamate; GPe = external portion of the globus pallidus; GPi = internal portion of the globus pallidus; 5HT = 5-hydroxytryptamine (serotonin); 5HT2 = 5-HT_2 receptor; NMDA = *N*-methyl-D-aspartate; SN/PC = pars compacta of the substantia nigra; STN = subthalamic nucleus; THAL = thalamus.
Source. Adapted from Perlmutter JS, Tempel LW, Black KJ, et al: "MPTP Induces Dystonia and Parkinsonism: Clues to the Pathophysiology of Dystonia." *Neurology* 49:1432–1438, 1997.

with schizophrenia are also at risk for developing malignant catatonia (Banerjee et al. 1995; Riederer et al. 1991). Malignant catatonia resembles NMS except that it is not caused by medication.

Serotonergic Agents

Selective serotonin reuptake inhibitors have been noted to cause EPS (Coulter and Pillans 1995; Dave 1994; Schechter and Nunes 1997). A case of typical NMS precipitated by fluoxetine has been reported (Halman and Goldbloom 1990). Enhancement of central serotonergic activity has been implicated in the genesis of NMS (Heyland and Sauve 1991; Parsa et al. 1990). The severe skeletal muscle rigidity seen in the case reported by Halman and Goldbloom may have resulted from inhibition of dopamine release by serotonin acting on 5-HT_{2A} receptors located on striatal dopaminergic neurons (Arya 1994; Meltzer and Nash 1991). From this case, it appears that the risk of developing EPS or NMS stems from the indirect effects of serotonergic agents on striatal dopamine release (see Figure 19–2).

Fever

Body temperature appears to be regulated primarily by the hypothalamus, which coordinates peripheral heat-generating and heat-losing mechanisms (Berner and Heller 1998). Fever in NMS may reflect, at least in part, abnormal activation of heat-generating mechanisms. There are two ways in which the body generates heat. During skeletal muscle contraction, the incomplete use of energy substrates generates movement, which in turn produces heat. Heat is generated through normal activity and shivering and occurs in persons of abnormal heightened muscle tone. The other mechanism of heat generation, sometimes referred to as "nonshivering" thermogenesis, involves the dissipation of proton gradients in certain tissues. These tissues are primarily brown adipose tissue and secondarily skeletal muscle. Dissipation of proton gradients results when certain "uncoupling proteins" uncouple oxidative phosphorylation in mitochondria (Jezek et al. 1998; Palou et al. 1998; Vidal-Puig et al. 1997). Energy is once again converted into heat, although the heat produced is not a by-product of energy use. Heat-losing mechanisms include the elimination of heat through evaporation of sweat. The regulation of heat generation and loss involves multiple systems and neurotransmitters. Dysregulation of thermogenesis, and in particular the induction of fever in NMS, may result from disruption of this complex system at several points.

Fever in NMS has long been thought to be caused by dopamine D_2 receptor blockade. Such blockade in the striatum produces heat through muscle contraction, whereas the same blockade at the level of the hypothalamus impairs the dissipation of heat (Di Rosa et al. 1988; Figa-Talamanca et al. 1985; Henderson and Wooten 1981). Antagonism of the D_2 receptor on tuberoinfundibular neurons, for example, reduces the release of vasopressin, thus compromising the body's response to heat-induced fluid loss (Hennig et al. 1995). However, other neurotransmitters participate in thermogenesis and may also be responsible for the fever associated with NMS.

Stimulation of $GABA_B$ receptors in the ventral hypothalamus of the rat elevates body temperature at least in part by activating heat production in brown adipose tissue. This effect is antagonized by agonists of ventral hypothalamic $GABA_A$ receptors. However, although $GABA_A$ antagonists acting alone at the ventral hypothalamus can stimulate heat production, $GABA_A$ agonists acting alone have no effect on normal thermogenesis. It appears that GABA, acting at the ventral hypothalamus through $GABA_A$ receptors, tonically inhibits thermogenesis and, through $GABA_B$ receptors, activates thermogenesis in the rat (Amir 1990; Horton et al. 1988). In humans, benzodiazepines and inhibitors of GABA metabolism have long been recognized for their ability to inhibit increases in body temperature (Paredes and Agmo 1992; Vidal et al. 1983). An acute decrease in central $GABA_A$ activity, such as that resulting from benzodiazepine withdrawal, can cause hyperthermia (van Engelen et al. 1993). Conversely, diazepam appears to reverse the fever generated by the hypothalamus in response to exogenous pyrogens (Beattie and Smyth 1988). If GABAergic agents cause skeletal muscle rigidity, they are thermogenic. Finally, lethal catatonia, which resembles NMS except that it is not precipitated by antipsychotic use, is routinely managed with benzodiazepines, suggesting an underlying GABAergic deficit in hyperthermia (Tang et al. 1995).

Descending neocortical glutamatergic axons in the rat stimulate nonshivering thermogenesis (Monda et al. 1994, 1998; Shibata et al. 1984, 1985). At least three glutamatergic systems involving the hypothalamus or basal ganglia may stimulate thermogenesis. First, glutamate applied to the ventral hypothalamus in the rat activates brown adipose thermogenesis (Amir 1990; Halvorson et al. 1990). Second, glutamate acting at the hypothalamic supraoptic nucleus of the rat coordinates osmoregulatory effects on thermogenesis. It appears that osmotic stimulation of thermogenesis requires activation of the sympathetic nervous system to be effective (Amir and De Blasio 1991). Overactivity of the sympathetic nervous system may contribute to NMS (Gurrera 1999). Third, glutamatergic overactivity within the basal ganglia can cause hyperthermia through profound skeletal muscle rigidity. Kornhuber and Weller (1994) proposed that this thermogenesis stimulation occurs in humans and causes fever in NMS. Using clinical evidence from human patients, they noted, for example, that NMDA receptor antagonists can produce hypothermia. Basic neuroscience and clinical evidence suggest that overstimulation of central NMDA receptors may cause hyperthermia.

Serotonin acting centrally and peripherally may produce fever (Arancibia et al. 1996; Nimmo et al. 1993; Rothwell 1994). Activation of human brain 5-HT_2 receptors produces fever. Stimulation of human central 5-HT_{1A} receptors lowers body temperature and may cause frank hypothermia (Murphy et al. 1991). When human central 5-HT_2 receptors are stimulated, any skeletal muscle rigidity produced may become a peripheral means of elevating body temperature (T. M. Brown et al. 1996). In addition, serotonin acting on 5-HT_{2C} receptors in the adrenal medulla stimulates the release of glucocorticoids. Peripheral glucocorticoids stimulate thermogenesis (Schobitz et al. 1994).

Hyperthermia may have multiple disastrous consequences. Hyperthermia precipitates the release of glutamate and catecholamines, including norepinephrine and dopamine (Ginsberg et al. 1992; Hayashi 1998). This increase in dopamine may perpetuate the pathophysiology of NMS, particularly if the offending agent is a D_2 receptor blocker. The failure of dopamine to reverse the pathophysiology of NMS may stem from dopamine, acting at D_1 receptors, facilitating NMDA receptor activation and bypassing blocked D_2 receptors. Activated dopamine D_1 receptors facilitate the activation of NMDA receptors by glutamate in animal models and is thought to exert a similar effect in humans (Cepeda and Levin 1998; Cepeda et al. 1998; Chase 1998; K. X. Huang et al. 1998). The norepinephrine surge may also aggravate NMS by further stimulating activity of the sympathetic nervous system (Gurrera 1999).

Autonomic Instability

As is the case with fever, the autonomic instability observed in NMS may be caused by both central and peripheral components (Balzan 1995). Antagonism of peripheral dopamine D_2 receptors disinhibits the release of norepinephrine, which causes elevation of blood pressure (Frishman and Hotchkiss 1996; Olsen 1998). D_2 receptors on arterial endothelium and D_2-like D_3 receptors within the atria also modulate peripheral vascular tone (Amenta et al. 1995). Brain-stem dopamine D_2, D_3, and D_4 receptors of the nucleus of the solitary tract, all members of the D_2-like family of dopamine receptors, are intimately involved in the regulation of cardiovascular, gut, and pulmonary function (Hyde et al. 1996). The dopamine D_2 receptor is thus able to modulate a variety of autonomic functions and to dysregulate these functions in conditions of abnormal dopaminergic tone.

GABA is well known for its participation in autonomic function. It is well established that GABA, acting through $GABA_A$ receptors at multiple levels throughout the brain, including cortical, hypothalamic, and brain-stem sites, exerts a profound coordinating influence on autonomic function (Bernardis and Bellinger 1998; Daras et al. 1995; Gillis et al. 1987; Waldrop et al. 1988). In the rat it appears that GABA, probably acting through $GABA_A$ receptors of the posterior hypothalamus, tonically inhibits cardiorespiratory and locomotor activity. $GABA_A$ agonists usually suppresses such activity (Bonham 1995; Waldrop et al. 1988). Stimulation of either $GABA_A$ or $GABA_B$ receptors in the rat spinal cord causes hypotension (Garcia et al. 1998). GABAergic agents are thus able to exert the derangements of cardiovascular and respiratory function seen in NMS. Clinically, the effect of benzodiazepine withdrawal in humans provides dramatic evidence of the relative effect of GABA antagonism on cardiac and respiratory rate as well as blood pressure.

The role of glutamate in causing the autonomic instability of NMS is uncertain. In rats, NMDA receptor antagonists acting at the rostral ventrolateral medulla and paraventricular hypothalamic nucleus appear to inhibit tachycardia and hypertension that would normally be generated by peripheral stimuli acting through the carotid body, whereas NMDA injected into the rat paraventricular hypothalamic nucleus stimulates a pressor response (Berrino et al. 1996; Kubo et al. 1993, 1997). Similar effects, whose neuroanatomic causes are less certain, have been observed in humans. For example, NMDA receptor antagonists have been reported to cause hypertension and hypotension, depending on the agent used (Dextrorphan Study Group and Hoffmann–La Roche 1995; Muir et al. 1995, 1997). In humans, glutamate may act through both NMDA and non-NMDA receptors to generate respiratory drive (Bonham 1995). This suggests that glutamate acting through NMDA receptors plays a direct role in the autonomic instability of NMS.

Serotonin plays an important role in the modulation of human cardiovascular and respiratory activity (Bonham 1995). Platelet $5\text{-}HT_2$ receptors and endothelial $5\text{-}HT_1$ receptors coordinate vascular tone in a variety of mammals, including humans. Endogenous and iatrogenic dysfunction of these receptors can cause hypertension and ischemia. Serotonin exogenously introduced into the human cardiovascular system typically induces a triphasic physiological response. Mediated by central $5\text{-}HT_{1A}$ and peripheral $5\text{-}HT_3$ receptors, this response includes an initial von Bezold–Jarisch reflex, which is followed by a pressor phase and, finally, a hypotensive phase. The von Bezold–Jarisch reflex, which consists of bradycardia and secondary hypotension, is typically accompanied by rapid, shallow respiration. Tachycardia resulting from peripherally administered 5-HT is mediated at least in part by $5\text{-}HT_2$ receptors on the adrenal medulla. Stimulation of these receptors promotes release of adrenal catecholamines (Saxena and Villalon 1990, 1991). In humans, acute cardiovascular abnormalities may be induced by serotonergic agents. These effects, as well as the acute peripheral and central effects of serotonergic agents on human gut and respiratory function, are reviewed elsewhere (T. M. Brown et al. 1996; Skop et al. 1994). Serotonin-induced abnormalities of oxygenation in NMS may be caused by vasoconstriction, bronchoconstriction, or central abnormalities of cardiac or respiratory rhythm (Kalenda and Holzenspies 1981).

In peripheral sympathetic ganglia, there are small, intensely fluorescent cells that release biogenic amines, including dopamine, norepinephrine, and serotonin (Verhofstad et al. 1981). Dopamine, acting though D_2 receptors, inhibits sympathetic nervous system activity. Dopamine also participates in carotid body regulation of the baroreceptor reflex of many mammals, possibly acting through D_1 in addition to D_2 receptors (Bairam et al. 1998). The potential for D_2 antagonists to disinhibit sympathetic nervous system activity through peripheral mechanisms clearly exists.

Mental Status Changes

Mental status changes in NMS tend to be profound. Dopamine D_2 receptor blockade is known to induce a variety of severe changes in mentation and psychomotor activity, such as akathisia and parkinsonism. Glutamate agonists and antagonists acting at the NMDA receptor also cause mental status changes. For example, ketamine, phencyclidine, and MK-801, potent NMDA receptor antagonists, can cause psychosis and disrupt memory (Kornhuber and Weller 1997; Malhotra et al. 1997; Olney 1994). NMDA agonists such as glutamate may cause a variety of insults ranging from seizures to parkinsonism.

Similarly, acute deficits in GABAergic neurotransmission have adverse effects on mentation and psychomotor activity (Zalsman et al. 1998). Flumazenil, a $GABA_A$ antagonist, causes various adverse neuropsychiatric effects, including anxiety, confusion, and seizures (Brogden and Goa 1991). Withdrawal of benzodiazepines is a well-known cause of severe changes in mentation, resembling those resulting from flumazenil intoxication. Benzodiazepine intoxication produces a variety of mental status changes ranging from sedation and disinhibition to delirium and psychosis. Because of the close interaction between brain $GABA_A$ and glutamate systems, disruption of one is likely to affect the other and produce clinical symptoms (Ben-Ari et al. 1997; Mott and Lewis 1994).

Glutamate agonists and antagonists acting at the NMDA receptor are also known to cause mental status changes. For example, ketamine, phencyclidine, and MK-801, potent antagonists at the NMDA receptor, can precipitate psychosis and impair memory (Saxena and Villalon 1990, 1991; Skop et al. 1994). As noted previously, glutamate deficits are implicated in the pathogenesis of schizophrenia. NMDA agonists may also cause a variety of insults ranging from seizures to parkinsonism. The profound anxiety and confusion associated with NMS may be explained by excessive glutamate activity alone.

The effect of serotonin on human mentation is profound. Serotonin acting on human central $5\text{-}HT_{1A}$ or $5\text{-}HT_{2A}$ receptors may cause anxiety and confusion (T. M. Brown et al. 1996; Meltzer and Nash 1991). In this case, overstimulation of human central $5\text{-}HT_{2A}$ receptors might explain the mental status changes observed in NMS, as well as the fever, autonomic instability, and profound skeletal muscle rigidity. The localization of $5\text{-}HT_3$ and $5\text{-}HT_4$ receptors to the frontal cortex and hippocampus, and of $5\text{-}HT_4$ receptors to the basal ganglia, suggests a possible role for these serotonin receptor subtypes in the alteration of mental status (Hoyer et al. 1994). The $5\text{-}HT_4$ receptor is also found in the adrenal medulla, where its stimulation causes the release of cortisol (Lefebvre et al. 1998). Cortisol stimulates the release of serotonin from brain-stem raphe nuclei, which in turn acts on hypothalamic 5-HT_{1A} receptors to stimulate the release of corticotropin-releasing factor. This factor ultimately causes the release of cortisol; it also stimulates the brain-stem locus coeruleus (Valentino and Curtis 1991). The adrenal medullary 5-HT_4 receptor is thus able to stimulate both the serotonergic system directly and the sympathetic nervous system indirectly. It is possible that NMS is a condition in which normal endogenous counterregulatory mechanisms do not act effectively to limit such reverberating circuits. The possibility that other serotonin receptor subtypes, such as 5-HT_5, 5-HT_6, and 5-HT_7, may participate in causing abnormalities of psychomotor activity and mentation is under investigation.

Initiation

Much evidence suggests that multiple neurotransmitter systems participate in the genesis of NMS. Two possibilities can be gleaned from examining these neurotransmitter systems individually. The first is that a few brain structures seem to be central in the initiation of NMS. These are the hypothalamus, basal ganglia, and brain-stem nuclei involved in the regulation of the autonomic nervous system. The second, reviewed extensively by Gurrera (1999), is that peripheral systems, acting mainly through the sympathetic nervous system, may also participate in the initiation of NMS (T. M. Brown and Stoudemire 1998b). These possibilities are not intended to minimize the complexity of and uncertainty associated with the initiation of NMS. However, a clinically useful explanation of the role of several neurotransmitters in the initiation of NMS seems possible. Figure 19–3 illustrates the actions of various neurotransmitters on brain structures and functions and their relationship to NMS.

Figure 19–3 indicates that multiple neurotransmitters act together to produce NMS. This implies the possibility of multiple, simultaneous treatment interventions for refractory cases of NMS.

Many important aspects of NMS remain to be understood. These include the epidemiology of NMS, the factors that predispose certain individuals at certain times to NMS, and the roles of other neurotransmitters in the etiology of NMS. For example, although dehydration may be an important risk factor in the development of NMS, it has not been shown to be a risk factor in the development of serotonin syndrome. Serotonin syndrome is another clinically distinct state in which drug-related increases in serotonergic activity become pathologic. Similarly, even though chronic endothelial disease may be a marker, if not a risk factor, for the development of serotonin syndrome, it has not been observed to increase the risk of developing NMS (T. M. Brown and Stoudemire 1998b; Ginsberg et al. 1992).

Treatment

Recognizing that a spectrum of findings, rather than a fixed quartet, may characterize NMS, Pope et al. (1986) proposed an operationalized approach to diagnosis, and others have followed suit (Nierenberg et al. 1991). Three important points emerge from this research as well as later research on the management of NMS. First, *substituted findings* based on pathophysiology are valuable. The clinician may recognize autonomic abnormalities, for example, in the absence of an abnormal heart rate, or profound respiratory dysregulation may substitute for a cardiovascular abnormality (Delay and Deniker 1968). Substitute findings,

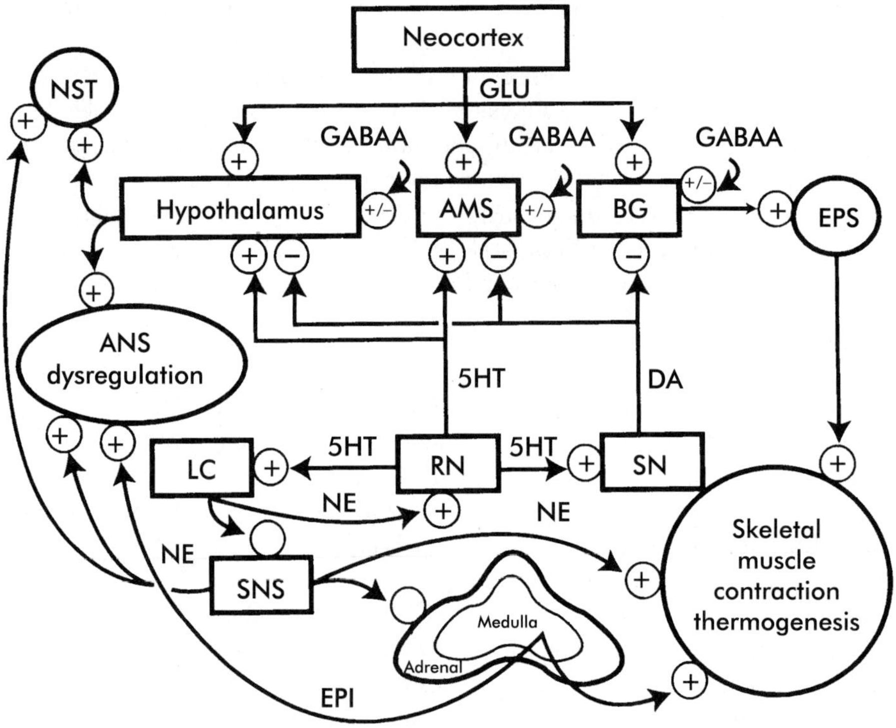

FIGURE 19–3. Actions of various neurotransmitters on brain structures and functions and their relationship to neuroleptic malignant syndrome (NMS). Abbreviations: + = stimulates release of neurotransmitter; – = inhibits release of neurotransmitter; AMS = altered mental status; ANS = autonomic nervous system; BG = basal ganglia; DA = dopamine; EPI = epinephrine; EPS = extrapyramidal side effects; GABA = gamma-aminobutyric acid; GABAA = $GABA_A$ receptor; GLU = glutamate; 5HT = 5-hydroxytryptamine (serotonin); LC = locus coeruleus; NE = norepinephrine; NST = nonshivering thermogenesis; RN = raphe nuclei; SN = substantia nigra; SNS = sympathetic nervous system.

as long as their pathophysiology reflects the dysfunction of NMS, expands the constellation of findings that characterize NMS, without reducing diagnostic validity.

Second, the insistence on the presence of altered mentation is important for a diagnosis of NMS. Because of the acute sensitivity of mental status to changes in neurotransmission, the likelihood of an agent causing NMS but not demonstrably affecting some aspect of mentation seems low.

Third, a cautious interpretation of the absence of classically associated findings in NMS is important. A normal creatinine phosphokinase level or a normal white blood cell level does not indicate the absence of NMS. If either level is elevated, as they usually are in NMS, they can help the clinician monitor treatment. However, if these levels are normal and all other evidence points to NMS, the clinician should seriously consider the diagnosis of NMS. The clinician must consider the fact that NMS is a potentially fatal syndrome for which treatments are relatively ineffective. If the patient's symptoms do not satisfy strict diagnostic criteria, but the clinician still believes that the correct diagnosis is NMS, the clinician should consider treating the patient for NMS and assess the possibility of other disorders in the differential diagnosis. These other disorders include malignant catatonia, malignant hyperthermia, akinetic hyperthermia of Parkinson's disease, status epilepticus, serotonin syndrome, tetanus, and basal motor nuclei infections or infarctions (Daras et al. 1995).

If a patient has NMS, all antipsychotics should be discontinued immediately. Special attention should be paid to other psychotropics and their potential role in the genesis of NMS. The clinician must also consider the acute consequences of stopping or starting any medication. For example, if a patient's benzodiazepine has recently been stopped, the clinician should consider whether resuming it may help reverse NMS. In another example, a patient who has taken chlorpromazine for years, and who has developed NMS after an increase in dosage, may develop cholinergic rebound after discontinuation of chlorpromazine.

While the clinician considers which agents are involved in causing NMS, the patient should be vigorously hydrated. Attention must be paid immediately to the risk of rhabdomyolysis and secondary renal failure. Urine studies for myoglobin and the search for evidence of renal injury are mandatory. Cooling the hyperthermic patient is important. Cooling blankets, fans, or chilled intravenous solutions may be helpful. In NMS, the reduction in skeletal muscle metabolism that accompanies cooling may directly facilitate resolution of the disorder (Ray 1997). In one case, pancuronium seems to have led to reduced temperature through muscle relaxation (Sangal and Dimitrijevic 1985). However, cooling measures usually raise the systemic metabolic rate; therefore, measures to cool the patient with NMS must be accompanied by monitoring for further derangements of autonomic function (Lenhardt et al. 1999). Once hydration and cooling begin, the clinician must decide whether to intervene further and whether to use medications or electroconvulsive therapy (ECT).

Treatment of NMS should be directed at what the clinician believes is the underlying insult. If the clinician suspects that a traditional dopamine D_2 receptor–blocking antipsychotic is responsible, a trial of bromocriptine is reasonable. Dantrolene is helpful in treating severe rigidity. If rigidity is lacking and the agent is an atypical antipsychotic or something other than an antipsychotic, or if benzodiazepine withdrawal is implicated in the etiology, a trial of a benzodiazepine may be warranted (Kontaxakis et al. 1988). If ECT is available and the patient's guardian or family have no objections to its use, a trial of ECT as a first-line intervention is reasonable. More theoretical interventions, such as a trial of an NMDA receptor partial agonist (e.g., amantadine), should probably be reserved for cases in which a very strong argument can be made for such a trial or if all other standard interventions are failing (Weller and Kornhuber 1992). Once effective therapy has been initiated, treatment for at least 10 days after resolution of the findings is often recommended. The cerebrospinal fluid observations of Nisijima and Ishigura (1995) support this recommendation. Table 19–13 outlines a treatment regimen for NMS (T. M. Brown and Stoudemire 1998b; Pelonero et al. 1998).

Seizures

Seizures reflect extreme overstimulation of the central nervous system (CNS). Restlessness and anxiety are the mildest forms of such stimulation, and anxiety may be an early warning sign of CNS stimulation. When drugs are responsible for CNS stimulation, other indications of abnormal brain arousal are often present, such as elevations of blood pressure and temperature, as well as acceleration of heart rate. Excitotoxicity, or abnormal excitation of the CNS occurring at the neuronal membrane, refers to a spectrum of findings ranging from

TABLE 19–13. A treatment regimen for neuroleptic malignant syndrome (NMS)

1. Discontinue all offending agents.
2. Initiate hydration and cooling.
3. Consider specific interventions:
   a. Electroconvulsive therapy (ECT), if available, for severe cases
   b. A dopamine agonist when dopamine D_2 receptor blockade is clearly implicated; especially useful as first-line agent if ECT is not available:

      Bromocriptine 5 mg by mouth three times a day; dosage can be escalated as tolerated and needed

      Dantrolene 60 mg iv every 6 hours can be added, but patient must be monitored for hepatotoxicity
   c. Ativan and diazepam are very safe and usually considered a second-line or adjunctive approach; consider as a first-line agent if NMS was precipitated by benzodiazepine withdrawal
   d. NMDA partial agonists usually considered a third-line approach; consider as adjunctive approach when discontinuation of an NMDA agonist is implicated in NMS
4. For 10 days after resolution of NMS, continue intervention that has been effective.
5. If it is necessary to resume an antipsychotic agent, wait until NMS has been resolved for *at least* 10 days, and select an agent considered least likely to replicate the suspected pathophysiology of NMS. If the agent that caused NMS must be resumed, resume agent in hospital and advise patient and significant others of risks and symptoms of NMS to facilitate monitoring for relapse.

Note. NMDA = N-methyl-D-aspartate.

anxiety with changes in vital signs to seizures. Figure 19–4 presents the evolution of findings in a case of excitotoxicity.

The challenge for the clinician is to recognize that a state of excitotoxicity exists before it has fully developed. For example, a patient may not be brought to a hospital until he or she has had a seizure, or a patient may move rapidly through the stages. Perhaps the most vexing problem is distinguishing excitotoxicity from conditions that partially mimic the signs and symptoms of excitotoxicity.

Excitotoxicity may develop in a susceptible region of the brain and spread. Regional susceptibility to drug side effects depends on the type of drug used, as well as the patient's underlying medical condition. Regional susceptibility to drug side effects thus helps determine why a drug may cause problems, as well as how the problems will develop. In excitotoxicity, a wave of abnormal neuronal activity may move across portions of the brain and declare itself as a recurring or relapsing dysfunction. This occurs in a variety of disorders, including epilepsy, migraine, and transient ischemic attacks, and possibly other conditions such as delirium.

Many drugs can cause excitotoxicity. Table 19–14 lists some of these drugs and their mechanisms of action (Farber et al. 1998; Jarrott 1999; Maksay et al. 1998; Smith et al. 1998; Wolf and Kirschbaum 1999). The clinician must also consider the possibility that an anticonvulsant may be responsible for deterioration of a patient's seizure control (Genton and McMenamin 1998).

The Physiology and Pharmacology of Drug-Induced Excitotoxicity

There are two main causes of drug-induced excitotoxicity: 1) excessive activation of the brain's stimulatory mechanisms and 2) disruption of the brain's normal inhibitory mechanisms.

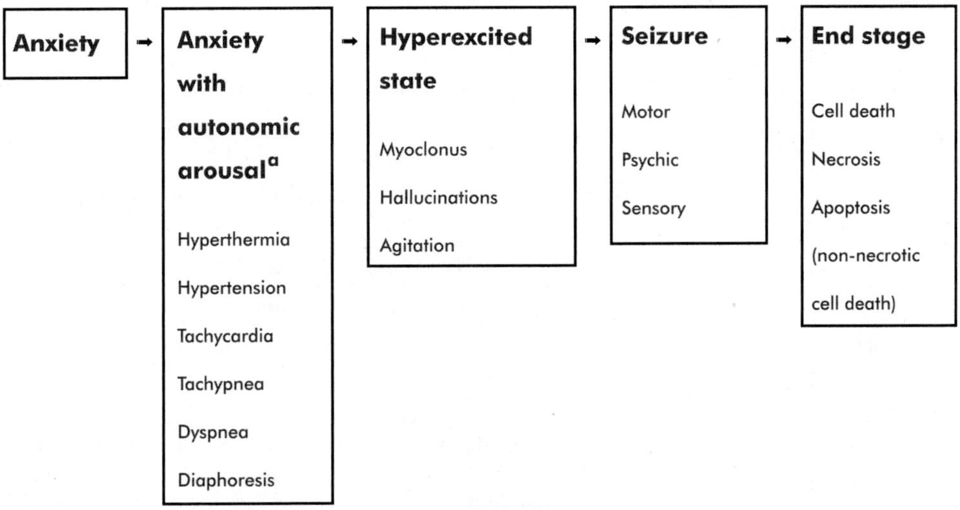

FIGURE 19–4. Evolution of findings in a case of excitotoxicity. [a]Not all findings may be present at any one time.

Drugs are particularly capable of causing excitotoxicity because of the diffuse way in which they are distributed to brain tissue. Once a susceptible brain structure is abnormally activated, neighboring tissue is more readily recruited into the wave of spreading excitation. Specific neuronal circuits may be abnormally activated and produce a seizure as a result. Beginning with the individual neuron, the sequence of tissues and events that lead to excitotoxicity can be explained.

The Neuron as the Basis of a Seizure

Neurons are the basic structural and functional units of the brain. They conduct signals by creating an electrochemical gradient and allowing it to collapse, which generates a wave of electrochemical activity. Such waves must occur only when needed; if neuronal activity occurs randomly, the signals that create thought, sensation, and movement would be reduced to a quagmire of random, meaningless nervous excitation. The work of electrochemical signaling is in creating these electrochemical gradients and preventing their collapse until the precise moment when such collapse will generate the desired signal. Because energy is required for the neuron to maintain these electrochemical gradients, anything that might hinder this maintenance increases the risk of excitotoxicity.

The neuron becomes susceptible to severe hyperexcitability and seizures when an action potential crosses into a region of depolarizing or depolarized neuronal membrane. In the presence of a shift toward depolarization, or depolarization shift, successive action potentials are able to propagate themselves repeatedly. The direct effects of the action potentials on the neuronal membrane, as well as the indirect effects of $K+$ ion accumulation in the extracellular space and depletion of neuronal energy reserves, enhances the state of depolarization (Selzer and Dichter 1992). The action potentials can be described in terms of the frequency, amplitude, and duration of each electrochemical wave. Each of these wave characteristics is modulated independently and can be disrupted by drugs independently. An agent may induce a convulsion by enhancing the frequency of neuronal discharge, the

TABLE 19–14. Selected excitotoxic drugs and their mechanisms of action

Drug	Mechanism of action
Aminophylline	Antagonizes inhibitory adenosine receptors
Amphetamine	Stimulates dopamine release, which facilitates glutamatergic activity at NMDA receptors
Atropine	Produces rebound cholinergic hyperactivity at muscarinic receptors
Baclofen	Acts as an NMDA agonist
Caffeine	Antagonizes inhibitory adenosine receptors
Chlorpromazine	Produces rebound cholinergic hyperactivity at muscarinic receptors
Cimetidine	Acts as an H_2 antagonist; causes excitotoxicity (other H_2 antagonists, however, are more excitotoxic: from most excitotoxic to least: famotidine, nizatidine, ranitidine, cimetidine)
Clozapine	Acts as an NMDA agonist and $GABA_A$ antagonist
Cocaine	Same as for amphetamine
Colchicine	Acts as a $GABA_A$ antagonist
Cyclosporine	Acts as a $GABA_A$ antagonist
Dehydroepiandrosterone	Acts as a $GABA_A$ antagonist and sigma receptor agonist, thereby potentiating NMDA receptor activity
Flumazenil	Acts an a $GABA_A$ antagonist
Fluoxetine	Increases serotonergic activity at 5-HT_3 receptors, depolarizing neurons
Furosemide	Acts as a $GABA_A$ antagonist
Ketamine	Acts as an NMDA antagonist; causes excitotoxicity during withdrawal
Lithium	Potentiates the effect of acetylcholine at muscarinic receptors
Penicillin	Acts as a $GABA_A$ antagonist
Phencyclidine	Acts as an NMDA antagonist; causes excitotoxicity during withdrawal
Pilocarpine	Facilitates NMDA receptor activity by stimulating muscarinic receptors
Progesterone metabolite (3alpha-OH-5alpha-pregnane-20-one)	Acts as a $GABA_A$ agonist; causes excitotoxicity during withdrawal
Tacrine	Inhibits breakdown of acetylcholine, which facilitates NMDA receptor activity by stimulating muscarinic receptors

Note. 5-HT = 5-hydroxytryptamine (serotonin); GABA = gamma-aminobutyric acid; NMDA = N-methyl-D-aspartate.

amplitude of the action potential, or the duration of the action potential. The abnormal generation and propagation of action potentials thus may be altered by drugs as well as by energetic stressors (Bikson et al. 1999). Drugs used to precipitate or terminate seizures may act on any part of the dissipation or the restoration of neuronal ion gradients. For example, diazepam increases the frequency of $GABA_A$ channel opening, whereas pentobarbital enhances primarily the duration of channel opening (Study and Baker 1981; Twyman et al. 1989). Pentylenetetrazol, a $GABA_A$ receptor antagonist, changes the frequency of channel opening (Madeja et al. 1996). Corticotropin-releasing hormone appears specifically to enhance the amplitude of neuronal discharges within the rat hippocampus (Hollrigel et al. 1998). Finally, abnormalities of the neuronal membrane's ability to create and maintain ion gradients can lead to abnormalities of neurotransmitter activity and cause a seizure. For example, ouabain inhibits Na^+-K^+-ATPase, which causes the release of GABA from hippocampal interneurons resulting from a reversal of neuronal GABA transporter function; the reversal of the transporter's function is replicated by other causes of energy impairment, such as glucose deprivation (Vizi and Sperlagh 1999).

Neuron-Neuron Interactions

The interactions of individual neurons are the "sites" of drug-induced excitotoxicity. Despite the complexity of neuronal interactions, and the many types of drugs and their various effects on electrochemical signaling, only two basic types of neuronal interaction initiate excitotoxicity. These are overexcitation of a neuron, such as the lowering of the seizure threshold caused by cocaine, and disinhibition of a neuron, such as the loss of the usual level of neuronal inhibition caused by abrupt withdrawal of chronic benzodiazepine treatment. The chemical messengers that neurons use to communicate include two that are significant from the standpoint of excitotoxicity and seizure regulation: the excitatory and inhibitory neurotransmitters. The primary excitatory neurotransmitters are glutamate and aspartate, and the main inhibitory neurotransmitters are GABA and glycine (MacDonald et al. 1998; Mihic 1999). The reader may note the proconvulsant activity of other endogenous neurotransmitters, such as acetylcholine and dopamine, and thus the proconvulsant actions of many important drugs. Scremin et al. (1998) offer a comprehensive discussion of the many agents that may alter the balance between excitatory and inhibitory neurotransmission.

Another issue in the development of a drug-induced seizure is whether a final common pathway for the generation of such a seizure exists. In generalized convulsion, this is likely to be the case. There are probably several final common pathways, which share several features. First, the neurons that initiate generalized seizures are usually arrayed in parallel bundles of the same polarity, which allows for the generation of large waves of synchronous electrical activity. The neurons of the hippocampus and neocortex contain such arrays. Second, the tissues that initiate drug-induced generalized seizures usually produce recurrent excitatory loops, which allows for signal amplification through positive feedback. Once again, the hippocampus and the neocortex, with their excitatory feedback loops, are able to unleash seizures (Selzer and Dichter 1992). For example, manipulation of $GABA_A$ receptors and PBRs in the substantia nigra pars reticulata generates a signal that is sent to the hippocampus and that produces a generalized convulsion (Depaulis et al. 1997; Wala et al. 1999). Application of an NMDA agonist or $GABA_A$ antagonist to the substantia nigra pars reticulata can initiate a generalized convulsion. The subthalamic nucleus sends glutamatergic input to the substantia nigra pars reticulata, which then relays a potentially convulsant signal to the hippocampus and amygdala (Deransart et al. 1998; Veliskova et al. 1998). Thalamic $GABA_B$ receptors inhibit the generation of rhythmic electrical activity; inhibition of these receptors can unleash a dangerous organizing influence on subcortical structures (e.g., the substantia nigra pars reticulata) that may ultimately produce a generalized convulsion (Dichter 1997). Activating this system at any point may induce a generalized seizure. Applying convulsant agents to the cerebral cortex can produce a wave of excitation that subsequently spreads throughout the cortex along cortico-cortical association fibers (Forti et al. 1997). Applying penicillin to the cerebral cortex is a well-known way to cause a focal epileptiform discharge that may subsequently generalize (Collins and Caston 1979). As in many cases of drug-induced derangements of brain function, there may be several distinct anatomic pathways to a given syndrome.

Factors that may lower the threshold for a drug-induced seizure include fever, estrogen (especially in patients with catamenial or perimenstrual susceptibility to seizures), extreme youth or age, acidemia, hypoxia, and hypoglycemia (Morrell 1999; Moshe 1997; Sperber et al. 1999; Velisek et al. 1998; Yuhas et al. 1999).

Once initiated, a seizure may beget another seizure in at least two ways. One way is through acute depletion of energy substrates. Increased neuronal activity and altered ion homeostasis demand energy. As neuronal energy stores are depleted, neurons are unable to restore ion gradients swiftly, which may contribute to propagation of a seizure. Reversal of energy deficits may be the mechanism by which the ketogenic diet is anticonvulsant (Janigro 1999).

The other, more chronic way in which seizures beget seizures is through *kindling*. In this pathological state, the balance of neurotransmission has been permanently altered in favor of excitation as a result of significantly increased basal levels of glutamate and simultaneously reduced levels of GABA (Jarrott 1999). These neurochemical changes are subsequently reflected in neuronal interactions; progressively smaller degrees of neurochemical stimulation are required to produce a seizure (Majkowski 1999). The deeper layers of the cerebral cortex appear to be especially susceptible to drug-induced kindling (Ekonomou and Angelatou 1999).

Drugs may contribute to the development of kindling, as evidenced by the effect of ethanol on the NMDA receptor. Acute ethanol consumption impairs the activity of the NMDA receptor. Chronic use of ethanol produces an upregulation of NMDA receptors as well as enhancement of NMDA receptor function (Wirkner et al. 1999). Chronic ethanol consumption also enhances the stimulatory activity of glutamate at alpha-amino-3-hydroxy-5-methyl-4-isoxazole propionic acid (AMPA) and kainate receptors and vasopressin at L-type calcium channels, and may enhance the activity of the N-type calcium channel (Netzeband et al. 1999; Walter and Messing 1999). Ethanol, acting through $GABA_A$ and glycine receptors, promotes convulsions upon withdrawal (Mihic 1999). Ethanol also potentiates function of the serotonin $5\text{-}HT_3$ receptor, which in turn enhances inhibitory neurotransmission in parts of the brain involved in the production of generalized seizures (Lovinger 1999). Chronic use of ethanol may downregulate the number or suppress the function of the $5\text{-}HT_3$ receptor, thereby enhancing the effect of ethanol in the production of seizures and the potentiation of kindling.

Treatment

Swift termination of a drug-induced seizure is important. A prolonged seizure not only may cause central and peripheral injury, but also may increase the patient's risk of further seizures. One brief seizure may not require intervention. However, if a patient has a prolonged or recurring seizure, the advice of a neurologist should be sought immediately.

Once a drug-induced seizure has been controlled, the clinician's next task is to determine its cause. The clinician must determine whether the drug caused the seizure or aggravated an underlying seizure disorder. If there is no underlying seizure disorder, the clinician must determine whether other patient-specific factors contributed to the development of the seizure or whether the drug's usual action on the brain accounted for the seizure. For example, if a penicillin is suspected of causing the seizure, determining how the drug was able to cross the blood-brain barrier may reveal an abnormality in blood-brain barrier integrity. Seizures that occur after a patient starts taking bupropion may suggest the presence of other problems, such as idiosyncrasies of bupropion metabolism or an eating disorder.

Serotonin Syndrome

Diagnosis

Sternbach (1991) provided the first set of operationalized diagnostic criteria for serotonin syndrome. These criteria improved recognition of and heightened interest in serotonin syndrome. Subsequent reports of death associated with the use of selective serotonin reuptake inhibitors (SSRIs) among patients with cardiovascular and respiratory disease challenged the idea that SSRIs could be safely prescribed regardless of a patient's cardiovascular or pulmonary status and inspired greater interest in the pathophysiology and management of serotonin syndrome (T. M. Brown and Skop 1996; T. M. Brown et al. 1996; Spier and Frontera 1991). Sternbach's criteria remain useful and accepted for the diagnosis of serotonin syndrome, and an understanding of what makes persons susceptible to the syndrome and how to treat it is evolving rapidly.

Pathophysiology

5-Hydroxytryptamine (5-HT), or serotonin, is found throughout the body. Erspamer and Asero (1952) identified 5-HT in the gut. 5-HT is most abundant in the gut, where more than 90% of the human body's 10-mg store of 5-HT is found. 5-HT was named "serotonin" when Rapport et al. (1948) discovered its seroactive effect on vascular smooth muscle tone. A debate ensued over what to name 5-HT when Erspamer and Asero (1952) named it "enteramine" to reflect its location and structure. However, the name "serotonin" remained. 5-HT was later identified in the brain. The role of 5-HT in mood disorders, such as major depression, is widely recognized. The role of psychoactive serotonergic agents in precipitating peripheral side effects, however, is not as recognized.

5-HT Function in the Gut

The role of 5-HT in gut function is increasingly being recognized (Gorard et al. 1994). Some recognized functions of 5-HT acting on receptors in the gut include the regulation of gastric and intestinal secretions as well as motility (Budhoo and Kellum 1994; Burleigh and Borman 1993; Maxton et al. 1996; Sanger 1996). Gut-derived 5-HT is important in understanding serotonin syndrome for three reasons. First, gut function may be locally deranged in hyperserotonergic states, including carcinoid syndrome and serotonin syndrome. Emesis and diarrhea are sometimes generated within the gut, rather than at the level of the brain. Second, the gut itself may produce nausea or anorexia sometimes seen in serotonin syndrome, depending on local 5-HT levels and activity (Coupland et al. 1997; Eberle-Wang et al. 1993). Finally, the gut is the source of vascular 5-HT, which is also implicated in the genesis of serotonin syndrome. Platelets, which cannot synthesize 5-HT, circulate through the gut, pick up 5-HT, and subsequently use the 5-HT. 5-HT does not cross the intact blood-brain barrier.

Cardiovascular Effects of 5-HT

As is the case with the gut, the cardiovascular system is regulated both centrally and peripherally by 5-HT. Thus, local effects of 5-HT on the cardiovascular system may contribute to the development of findings in serotonin syndrome. Peripheral vascular 5-HT receptors help regulate blood vessel tone, the tendency of platelets to form clots, and the contractility of cardiac myocytes (Bailey et al. 1996; Blauw et al. 1988; Saxena and Villalon 1990, 1991). For example, 5-HT exogenously introduced into the cardiovascular system typically induces a triphasic physiological response. Mediated by central 5-HT_{1A} and peripheral 5-HT_3 receptors, this response includes an initial von Bezold–Jarisch reflex, which is followed by a pressor phase and, finally, a hypotensive phase. The von Bezold–Jarisch reflex consists of bradycardia and secondary hypotension, and is typically accompanied by rapid, shallow respiration. Tachycardia resulting from peripherally administered 5-HT is mediated at least in part by 5-HT_2 receptors on the adrenal medulla. Stimulation of these receptors promotes the release of adrenal catecholamines (Saxena and Villalon 1990, 1991).

5-HT within the vascular system is derived from platelets. Circulating platelets release 5-HT, which produces a variety of normal effects. Platelet-derived 5-HT stimulates the intact blood vessel to dilate by binding to 5-HT_1-like receptors on endothelial cells. This stimulates endothelial cells to release nitric oxide, which diffuses toward underlying smooth muscle cells and relaxes them. Nitric oxide also diffuses toward platelets, inhibiting the further release of 5-HT. Simultaneously, 5-HT causes damaged vessels to contract by stimulating the underlying smooth muscle cells directly, bypassing the damaged endothelium. 5-HT also binds to 5-HT_{2A} receptors on platelets, stimulating the further release of 5-HT. 5-HT thus causes platelets to aggregate and plug damaged vessels, which contract around the platelet plug, while allowing blood to flow around the damaged portion of the vessel by causing vasodilation of the intact portion.

5-HT Function in the Central Nervous System

The CNS uses 5-HT for many purposes. Several 5-HT receptor subtypes have been identified, including 5-HT_5, 5-HT_6, and 5-HT_7. The physiology of 5-HT_5 and 5-HT_6 and behavioral effects of their activation are still under investigation (Adham et al. 1998; Hoyer et al. 1994; Jasper et al. 1997). Table 19–15 outlines some of the known functions of 5-HT in the CNS (N. M. Barnes and Sharp 1999). The behavioral consequences of receptor activation are derived primarily from animal (guinea pig, mouse, and rat) studies.

5-HT and Respiratory Function

5-HT is recognized as having a role in the modulation of respiration. The pulmonary role of 5-HT in humans, however, is unclear. In the guinea pig, peripheral 5-HT_2 receptors cause bronchoconstriction when stimulated (Selig et al. 1988). In the cat, stimulation of central 5-HT receptors increases respiratory rate (Gillis et al. 1989). The peripheral 5-HT_3 receptor also appears to be involved in the modulation of respiratory drive, producing rapid, shallow respirations in the rabbit when stimulated (Saxena and Villalon 1990). Pe-

TABLE 19–15. Serotonin function in the central nervous system (CNS)

Receptor subtype	Location	Physiology	Behavioral effects of receptor activation
$5\text{-}HT_{1A}$	Astrocytes Presynaptic neuronal membranes of axons from nucleus raphe magnus to substantia gelatinosus of spinal cord, hippocampus, midline thalamic nuclei, and frontal cortex Postsynaptic membrane in hippocampus and other forebrain areas	Regulates development of CNS Presynaptic $5\text{-}HT_{1A}$ receptors inhibit 5-HT release Postsynaptic $5\text{-}HT_{1A}$ receptors hyperpolarize by increasing K^+ conductance	Anxiolysis Hyperphagia Hypothermia Increased libido
$5\text{-}HT_{1B}$	Likely most concentrated in substantia nigra and basal ganglia; also likely in hippocampus and cortex	Inhibits release of 5-HT and possibly other neurotransmitters, including glutamate and acetylcholine	Hypophagia Hypothermia (effect is suspected but not proven) Increases in locomotor and rotational activity Myoclonus (effect is suspected, but not proven)
$5\text{-}HT_{1E}$	Concentrated in cortex (especially entorhinal), caudate, putamen, and claustrum; smaller amounts in hippocampus and amygdala	Little is known about the physiological significance of brain $5\text{-}HT_{1E}$ receptor activation	Little is known about the behavioral significance of brain $5\text{-}HT_{1E}$ receptor activation
$5\text{-}HT_{2A}$	Postsynaptic neuronal membranes, with highest concentrations in the neocortex, claustrum, anterior olfactory nucleus, and olfactory tubercle; lesser density in the basal ganglia; minimal in hippocampus, brain stem, and thalamus	Stimulation of central $5\text{-}HT_2$ receptors is linked to turnover of phosphatidylinositol	Hyperthermia Preprogrammed repetitive movements in various species, such as "wet dog shake"
$5\text{-}HT_{2C}$	Choroid plexus	Increases turnover of phosphatidylinositol	Anxiogenesis Hyperthermia Hypophagia Reduced locomotor activity Penile erections

TABLE 19–15. Serotonin function in the central nervous system (CNS) *(continued)*

Receptor subtype	Location	Physiology	Behavioral effects of receptor activation
5-HT_3	Postsynaptic neuronal membranes in area postrema Frontotemporal cortex and hippocampus	Regulation of emesis 5-HT_3 stimulation inhibits release of acetylcholine	Anxiogenesis Cognition Locomotor activity
5-HT_4	Frontal cortex, basal ganglia, hippocampus, substantia nigra, and superior and inferior colliculi	Reduces neuronal after-hyperpolarization and prolongs excitation via K^+ channels	Anxiogenesis Anxiolysis Cognition
5-HT_{5A}	Forebrain and cerebellum	Under investigation	Under investigation
5-HT_6	Striatum, olfactory tubercles, hippocampus, and nucleus accumbens	Under investigation	Under investigation
5-HT_7	Widely distributed in brain; probably highest density in thalamus, hypothalamus, and hippocampus	Activates adenylate cyclase	Circadian rhythms Epilepsy (effect is suspected but not proven)

Note. 5-HT = 5-hydroxytryptamine (serotonin).

ripheral 5-HT has a modest effect on pulmonary smooth muscle contractility. The intact lungs in turn provide a vast metabolic bed for clearance of 5-HT from the circulation (McIntyre et al. 1996). In some cases, acute respiratory distress syndrome (ARDS) may result from a hyperserotonergic state. The ability of the 5-HT_2 receptor antagonist ketanserin to relieve symptoms of ARDS supports a hyperserotonergic basis for the disorder (Frishman et al. 1995) and may help explain case reports of acute cardiorespiratory failure after initiation of serotonergic antidepressants (Spier and Frontera 1991).

Pathophysiology of Serotonin Syndrome

Background

An iatrogenic hyperserotonergic state was first described by Oates and Sjoerdsma (1960) in their report on the effects of combining tryptophan, the precursor of 5-HT, with a monoamine oxidase inhibitor. Three decades passed before such events were regarded as manifestations of a distinct syndrome. Sternbach (1991) hypothesized that excessive stimulation of central 5-HT_{1A} receptors produced the serotonin syndrome. Sternbach generated further interest in the serotonin syndrome by operationalizing its diagnosis. He proposed that the diagnosis could be made when there were three or more findings consistent with the disorder, in the absence of confounding entities such as adverse reactions to dopamine antagonists. It appears unlikely that central 5-HT_{1A} receptors alone participate in the genesis of the serotonin syndrome. Also, the existence of factors that may increase susceptibility to the serotonin syndrome has been proposed (Lane and Baldwin 1997; Sporer 1995). Subsequent proposals have been made regarding the temporal course of the syndrome, as well as the populations that may be at risk (T. M. Brown et al. 1996; Skop et al. 1994).

Unfortunately, it is not yet known what constellation of findings represents the core syndromal event of the serotonin syndrome. Whether there is just one distinct hyperserotonergic state or several is unknown. Prospective studies to address these concerns are being conducted. Current evidence indicates certain basic elements in the pathophysiology of the serotonin syndrome.

Acute Induction of Serotonin Syndrome

Serotonin syndrome may be induced by either of two possible pathophysiological scenarios. The first scenario is the acute introduction of a large amount of an exogenous 5-HT agonist. There are numerous 5-HT agonists, such as ergot derivatives, as well as illicit agents, such as LSD, mescaline, and psilocybin (Gravlin 1997). The second scenario is an impairment in the ability of the body to clear 5-HT, combined with an acute release of relatively large amounts of endogenous 5-HT. Factors leading to serotonin syndrome are presented in Table 19–16.

TABLE 19–16. Factors leading to serotonin syndrome[a]

Factor	Releasing agent or event
Endogenous	Adrenergic stimulus (e.g., pseudoephedrine)
Diabetes	
Hyperlipidemia	
Hypertension	
Smoking	
Iatrogenic	Stress (e.g., surgery)
SSRIs	
TCAs	
MAOIs	Other 5-HT releasers (e.g., alcohol)

Note. 5-HT = 5-hydroxytryptamine (serotonin); MAOIs = monoamine oxidase inhibitors; SSRIs = selective serotonin reuptake inhibitors; TCAs = tricyclic antidepressants.
[a]Findings in serotonin syndrome are gastrointestinal distress, hyperreflexia, hypertension, mental status changes, myoclonus, shivering, and tachycardia.

The second scenario may be replicated frequently, such as among depressed patients who take SSRIs, which block reuptake—an important endogenous mechanism of 5-HT clearance. This iatrogenic impairment of clearance is usually well tolerated. The next step in the genesis of serotonin syndrome among patients taking SSRIs is the release of large quantities of 5-HT. Table 19–17 lists potential 5-HT releasing agents and events and their mechanisms of action (Bel and Artigas 1992; Boadle-Biber 1993; Celada et al. 1992; Esler et al. 1991; Gimenez-Roldan et al. 1988; Gupta et al. 1992; Jarman et al. 1991; Kreiss et al. 1993; Mitrakou et al. 1991; Ortiz and Artigas 1992; Pattichis et al. 1994; Pope et al. 1985; Sandyk 1986; Schuldiner et al. 1993; Veith et al. 1994).

TABLE 19–17. Potential serotonin releasing agents and events and their mechanisms of action

Releasing agent or event	Mechanism of action
SSRI initiation or dosage increase	Increases the extent of 5-HT reuptake blockade, which causes a transient increase in extracellular 5-HT, until cells down-regulate 5-HT secretion
TCA use for more than 4 weeks	Increases sympathetic nervous system activity in patients with major depression; causes norepinephrine reuptake blockade, which increases extracellular norepinephrine
Sympathomimetics	Stimulate platelets and neurons to release 5-HT
Tryptophan	Causes the synthesis of serotonin (tryptophan hydroxylase activity is substrate-dependent)
Ethanol	Releases 5-HT from platelets and neurons
Acute psychosocial stress	May stimulate platelets and neurons to release 5-HT
Hypoxia, hypoglycemia	Cause significant release of catecholamines

Note. 5-HT = 5-hydroxytryptamine (serotonin); SSRI = selective serotonin reuptake inhibitor; TCA = tricyclic antidepressant.

Norepinephrine stimulates platelets and neurons to release 5-HT. The release of 5-HT may be aggravated in this case by the release of norepinephrine from the adrenal medulla in response to 5-HT (Saxena and Villalon 1990). Multiple cases of serotonin syndrome temporally linked to acute ingestion of a sympathomimetic suggest that this may be an important cause of the syndrome (Bostwick and Brown 1996; Sporer 1995). Table 19–18 lists adverse effects of central and peripheral 5-HT receptor stimulation (T. M. Brown et al. 1996; Hoyer et al. 1994; Pazos et al. 1987; Sastry et al. 1992).

Two motor events with a probable central etiology have resisted assignment to a specific 5-HT receptor subtype: 1) EPS associated with SSRI use and 2) repetitive motor behaviors. EPS, such as akathisia, are recognized, although infrequent, consequences of SSRI therapy (Coulter and Pillans 1995). Other agents with actions mediated by 5-HT have been associated with EPS, such as ondansetron (Finn 1992). The introduction of atypical antipsychotics that potently antagonize central 5-HT_2 receptors, and whose frequency of EPS is significantly lower than traditional antipsychotic agents, places the focus on the 5-HT_2 receptor. But a role for other 5-HT receptor subtypes, including 5-HT_1 and 5-HT_3, cannot be excluded (Arya 1994).

Repetitive motor behaviors seen in serotonin syndrome, such as hyperreflexia, myoclonus, shivering, and tremor, are probably linked to centrally acting 5-HT. 5-HT suppresses the afterhyperpolarization of spinal and cortical motor neurons, which permits ongoing activity of these neurons. As serotonergic input to these neurons increases, the frequency and duration of their discharges increase. This may induce hyperreflexia, myoclonus, and tremors. More complex repetitive behaviors, such as chewing and licking, may similarly be generated by serotonergic input to the facial nucleus (Gimenez-Roldan et al. 1988; Jacobs and Fornal 1993; Westheimer and Klawans 1974). Although these effects appear to be mediated by a 5-HT_1-like or a 5-HT_2 receptor, this is not yet established (Hoyer et al. 1994; Pranzatelli 1994).

TABLE 19–18. Serotonin receptor subtypes and adverse effects resulting from their activation

5-HT receptor subtype	Adverse effects resulting from activation
5-HT_{1A}	Shivering related to hypothermia Decreased heart rate and blood pressure Increased respiratory rate and decreased tidal volume Altered gut activity
$5\text{-HT}_{1B/D}$	Anxiety, hyperactivity, and acute confusional states
5-HT_2	Acute confusional states Incoordination mediated by cerebellar 5-HT_2 receptors Diaphoresis resulting from central 5-HT_2-mediated hyperthermia Elevated blood pressure and heart rate resulting from release of adrenal catecholamines, as well as activation of serovascular 5-HT_2 receptors
5-HT_3	Nausea, vomiting, and diarrhea Bradycardia and hypotension Rapid, shallow respiration
5-HT_4	Possible association with mood disturbances, psychosis, motor coordination, and arousal
5-HT_5	Unknown
5-HT_6	Unknown; however, this receptor has a high affinity for many typical and new antipsychotics and antidepressants
5-HT_7	Unknown

Note. 5-HT = 5-hydroxytryptamine (serotonin).

Treatment

Treatment of serotonin syndrome requires identification of populations that may be at risk, recognition of the syndrome when it occurs, and rational institution of treatments. As noted, populations at risk include patients with known abnormalities in serotonergic chemotransmission. Among these patients, those with cardiovascular disease have some of the better understood abnormalities and may be easier to monitor for side effects upon initiation of serotonergic agents. In addition to predicting and studying populations that may be at risk and recognizing serotonin syndrome when it occurs, there is the issue of rational management of acute cases of the syndrome.

Most authors agree that discontinuation of offending medications is an important first step in treating serotonin syndrome. The syndrome is generally short-lived, with most cases resolving spontaneously within 24–48 hours (Dike 1997; Gitlin 1997; LeJoyeux et al. 1995; Sternbach 1991). Mild cases of serotonin syndrome may resolve even if the serotonergic agents are continued (Edwards et al. 1994). Some cases of serotonin syndrome are of sufficient severity and duration that active measures are required to interrupt the process. Such measures usually fall into one of two categories: 1) drugs given to block the effects of 5-HT and 2) drugs given to halt the release of 5-HT.

Cyproheptadine antagonizes the postsynaptic action of 5-HT and is considered among the more effective nonspecific serotonergic antagonists for treating serotonin syndrome (George and Godleski 1996; Graudins et al. 1998; LeJoyeux et al. 1995). Other agents that block 5-HT include chlorpromazine, which blocks the $5\text{-}HT_2$ receptor, and propranolol, which antagonizes the action of 5-HT at the $5\text{-}HT_{1A}$ receptor (Gillman 1996; LeJoyeux et al. 1995; Oates and Sjoerdsma 1960). The use of specific $5\text{-}HT_2$ or $5\text{-}HT_3$ antagonists, which may be effective in other hyperserotonergic states, such as carcinoid syndrome, or putative hyperserotonergic states, such as ARDS, has not been adequately explored (Gillis et al. 1989; Greenshaw and Silverstone 1997). Agents that prevent the release of 5-HT may be equally effective for the treatment of serotonin syndrome.

Certain benzodiazepines, including lorazepam, have an excellent track record in managing serotonin syndrome (Baetz and Malcolm 1995; Nierenberg and Semprebon 1993). This may result from the ability of benzodiazepines to inhibit the release of 5-HT and subsequently permit the clearance of released 5-HT (Bonnafous et al. 1995). The receptor that mediates this effect is unclear because of the insufficient numbers of cases treated successfully or unsuccessfully with a variety of benzodiazepines. However, the PBR may be more important in mediating this effect than the $GABA_A$ receptor (Gavish et al. 1992). In a fulminant case of serotonin syndrome unresponsive to lorazepam, nitroglycerin was used to increase the release of nitric oxide, noted previously as an endogenous "off" signal for peripheral 5-HT release. The patient swiftly recovered (T. M. Brown and Skop 1996). I have repeated the use of nitroglycerin in another treatment-refractory case of serotonin syndrome, with equally swift, complete, and lasting effect. Note that many serotonergic drugs inhibit the nitric oxide synthase, including that found in brain and vascular tissue (Finkel et al. 1996; Marcoli et al. 1998; Yaron et al. 1999).

References

Adams F: Emergency intravenous sedation of the delirious, medically ill patient. J Clin Psychiatry 49 (suppl):22–26, 1989

Addonizio G, Susman VL, Roth SD: Symptoms of neuroleptic malignant syndrome in 82 consecutive inpatients. Am J Psychiatry 143:1587–1590, 1986

Adham N, Zgombick JM, Bard J, et al: Functional characterization of the recombinant human 5-hydroxytryptamine7(a) receptor isoform coupled to adenylate cyclase stimulation. J Pharmacol Exp Ther 287:508–514, 1998

Aigner TG: Pharmacology of memory: cholinergic-glutamatergic interactions. Curr Opin Neurobiol 5:155–160, 1995

Amenta F, Ferrante F, Ricci A: Pharmacological characterisation and autoradiographic localisation of dopamine receptor subtypes in the cardiovascular system and kidney. Hypertens Res 18 (suppl 1): S23–S27, 1995

American Psychiatric Association: Practice guideline for the treatment of patients with delirium. Am J Psychiatry 156 (5 suppl):1–20, 1999

American Psychiatric Association: Diagnostic and Statistical Manual of Mental Disorders, 4th Edition, Text Revision. Washington, DC, American Psychiatric Association, 2000

Amir S: Intra-ventromedial hypothalamic injection of glutamate stimulates brown adipose tissue thermogenesis in the rat. Brain Res 511:341–344, 1990

Amir S, De Blasio E: Activation of brown adipose tissue thermogenesis by chemical stimulation of the hypothalamic supraoptic nucleus. Brain Res 563:349–352, 1991

Amore M, Zazzeri N, Bernardi D: Atypical neuroleptic malignant syndrome associated with clozapine treatment. Neuropsychobiology 35:197–199, 1997

Anderson ES, Powers PS: Neuroleptic malignant syndrome associated with clozapine use. J Clin Psychiatry 52:102–104, 1991

Ansseau M, Diricq S, Grisar T, et al: Biochemical and neuroendocrine approaches to a malignant syndrome of neuroleptics. Acta Psychiatrica Belgica 80:600–606, 1980

Arancibia S, Rage F, Astier H, et al: Neuroendocrine and autonomous mechanisms underlying thermoregulation in cold environment. Neuroendocrinology 64:257–267, 1996

Arias Bal MA, Vazquez-Barquero JL, Pena C, et al: Psychiatric aspects of multiple sclerosis. Acta Psychiatr Scand 83:292–296, 1991

Arya DK: Extrapyramidal symptoms with selective serotonin reuptake inhibitors. Br J Psychiatry 165:728–733, 1994

Bachli E, Albani C: Akinetic crisis in Parkinson disease. Schweiz Med Wochenschr 124:1017–1023, 1994

Baetz M, Malcolm D: Serotonin syndrome from fluvoxamine and buspirone (letter). Can J Psychiatry 40:428–429, 1995

Bailey JE, Coupland NC, Potokar J, et al: A study of acute effects of an SSRI and a 5-HT_3 antagonist on autonomic reflexes (abstract). Clinical Autonomic Research Society Proceedings 6:52, 1996

Bailly D: Troubles neuropsychiatriques lies a la MDMA ("ecstasy"). Encephale 25:595–602, 1999

Bairam A, Frenette J, Dauphin C, et al: Expression of dopamine D_1-receptor mRNA in the carotid body of adult rabbits, cats and rats. Neurosci Res 31:147–154, 1998

Balzan MV: Paradoxical autonomic response to procyclidine in the neuroleptic malignant syndrome. Can J Neurol Sci 22:244–246, 1995

Banerjee SP, Zuck LG, Yablonsky-Alter E, et al: Glutamate agonist activity: implications for antipsychotic drug action and schizophrenia. Neuroreport 6:2500–2514, 1995

Barnes NM, Sharp T: A review of central 5-HT receptors and their function. Neuropharmacology 38:1083–1152, 1999

Barnes PJ: Muscarinic receptor subtypes: implications for therapy. Agents Actions Suppl 43:243–252, 1993

Bartholini G: GABA receptor agonists: pharmacological spectrum and therapeutic actions. Med Res Rev 5:55–75, 1985

Bartus RT, Johnson HR: Short-term memory in the rhesus monkey: disruption from the anti-cholinergic scopolamine. Pharmacol Biochem Behav 5:39–46, 1976

Beattie GJ, Smyth JF: Diazepam ablates the constitutional side-effects of gamma interferon. Medical Oncology and Tumor Pharmacotherapy 5:129–130, 1988

Bel N, Artigas F: Fluvoxamine preferentially increases extracellular 5-hydroxytryptamine in the raphe nuclei: an in vivo microdialysis study. Eur J Pharmacol 229:101–103, 1992

Belelli D, Pistis M, Peters JA, et al: The interaction of general anaesthetics and neurosteroids with $GABA_A$ and glycine receptors. Neurochem Int 34:447–452, 1999

Bell GD, Spickett GP, Reeve PA, et al: Intravenous midazolam for upper gastrointestinal endoscopy: a study of 800 consecutive cases relating dose to age and sex of patient. Br J Clin Pharmacol 23:241–243, 1987

Ben-Ari Y, Khazipov R, Leinekugel X, et al: $GABA_A$, NMDA and AMPA receptors: a developmentally regulated "menage a trois." Trends Neurosci 20:523–529, 1997

Berger A, Posner MI: Pathologies of brain attentional networks. Neurosci Biobehav Rev 24:3–5, 2000

Bernardis LL, Bellinger LL: The dorsomedial hypothalamic nucleus revisited: 1998 update. Proc Soc Exp Biol Med 218:284–306, 1998

Berner NJ, Heller HC: Does the preoptic anterior hypothalamus receive thermoafferent information? Am J Physiol 274:R9–R18, 1998

Berrino L, Pizzirusso A, Maione S, et al: Hypothalamic paraventricular nucleus involvement in the pressor response to *N*-methyl-D-aspartic acid in the periaqueductal grey matter. Naunyn Schmiedebergs Arch Pharmacol 353:157–160, 1996

Bikson M, Ghai RS, Baraban SC, et al: Modulation of burst frequency, duration, and amplitude in the zero-Ca(2+) model of epileptiform activity. J Neurophysiol 82:2262–2270, 1999

Blauw GJ, van Brummelen P, van Zwieten PA: Serotonin induced vasodilatation in the human forearm is antagonized by the selective 5-HT_3 receptor antagonist ICS 205–930. Life Sci 43:1441–1449, 1988

Boadle-Biber MC: Regulation of serotonin synthesis. Prog Biophys Mol Biol 60:1–15, 1993

Bonham AC: Neurotransmitters in the CNS control of breathing. Respir Physiol 101:219–230, 1995

Bonnafous C, Lefevre P, Bueno L: Benzodiazepine-withdrawal-induced gastric emptying disturbances in rats: evidence for serotonin receptor involvement. J Pharmacol Exp Ther 273:995–1000, 1995

Bostwick JM, Brown TM: Fluoxetine and phentermine interaction may produce the serotonin syndrome. J Clin Psychopharmacol 16:189–190, 1996

Boyarsky BK, Fuller M, Early T: Malignant catatonia-induced respiratory failure with response to ECT. J ECT 15:232–236, 1999

Brazelton T, Blanc PD, Olson KR: Toxic effects of nefazodone (letter). Ann Emerg Med 30:550–551, 1997

Brogden RN, Goa KL: Flumazenil: a reappraisal of its pharmacological properties and therapeutic efficacy as a benzodiazepine antagonist. Drugs 42:1061–1089, 1991

Brown CS, Markowitz JS, Moore TR, et al: Atypical antipsychotics, Part II: adverse effects, drug interactions, and costs. Ann Pharmacother 33:210–217, 1999

Brown TM: Clozapine, neuroleptic malignant syndrome, and pancerebellar syndrome. Psychosomatics 40:518–520, 1999

Brown TM: Basic mechanisms in the pathogenesis of delirium, and a proposed model for clinical assessment, in Psychiatric Care of the Medical Patient, 2nd Edition. Edited by Stoudemire A, Fogel B, Greenberg D. Oxford, Oxford University Press, 2000a, pp 571–580

Brown TM: Drug-induced delirium. Seminars in Clinical Neuropsychiatry 5:113–124, 2000b

Brown TM, Brown RL: The neuropsychiatric consequence of renal failure. Psychosomatics 36:244–253, 1995

Brown TM, Skop BP: Nitroglycerin in the treatment of the serotonin syndrome (letter). Ann Pharmacother 30:191–192, 1996

Brown TM, Stoudemire A: Agents used to treat movement disorders, in Psychiatric Side Effects of Prescription and Over-the-Counter Medications: Recognition and Management. Washington, DC, American Psychiatric Press, 1998a, pp 35–52

Brown TM, Stoudemire A: Antipsychotics, in Psychiatric Side Effects of Prescription and Over-the-Counter Medications: Recognition and Management. Washington, DC, American Psychiatric Press, 1998b, pp 3–33

Brown TM, Stoudemire A: Psychiatric Side Effects of Prescription and Over-the-Counter Medications: Recognition and Management. Washington, DC, American Psychiatric Press, 1998c

Brown TM, Stoudemire A: Sedative-hypnotic and related agents, in Psychiatric Side Effects of Prescription and Over-the-Counter Medications: Recognition and Management. Washington, DC, American Psychiatric Press, 1998d, pp 123–144

Brown TM, Skop BP, Mareth TR: Pathophysiology and management of the serotonin syndrome. Ann Pharmacother 30:527–533, 1996

Buckley PF, Hasan S: Atypical neuroleptic malignant syndrome and atypical antipsychotics (letter). Am J Psychiatry 155:1633, 1998

Budhoo MR, Kellum JM: The 5-HT receptor mediates 5-hydroxytryptamine-induced rise in short circuit current in the human jejunum in vitro. Surgery 116:396–400, 1994

Burke RE, Fahn S, Mayeux R, et al: Neuroleptic malignant syndrome caused by dopamine-depleting drugs in a patient with Huntington disease. Neurology 31:1022–1025, 1981

Burleigh DE, Borman RA: Short-circuit current responses to 5-hydroxytryptamine in human ileal mucosa are mediated by a 5-HT_4 receptor. Eur J Pharmacol 241:125–128, 1993

Caroff SN: The neuroleptic malignant syndrome. J Clin Psychiatry 41:79–83, 1980

Carter GL, Dawson AH, Lopert R: Drug-induced delirium. Incidence, management and prevention. Drug Saf 15:291–301, 1996

Casey BJ, Castellanos FX, Giedd JN, et al: Implication of right frontostriatal circuitry in response inhibition and attention deficit/hyperactivity disorder. J Am Acad Child Adolesc Psychiatry 36:374–383, 1997a

Casey BJ, Giedd J, Vauss Y, et al: The role of the anterior cingulate in automatic and controlled processes: a developmental neuroanatomical study. Dev Psychobiol 30:61–69, 1997b

Celada P, Dolera M, Alvarez E, et al: Effects of acute and chronic treatment with fluvoxamine on extracellular and platelet serotonin in the blood of major depressive patients. Relationship to clinical improvement. J Affect Disord 25:243–249, 1992

Cepeda C, Levin MS: Dopamine and *N*-methyl-D-aspartate receptor interactions in the neostriatum. Dev Neurosci 20:1–18, 1998

Cepeda C, Colwell CS, Itri JN, et al: Dopaminergic modulation of early signs of excitotoxicity in visualized rat neostriatal neurons. Eur J Neurosci 10:3491–3497, 1998

Chan-Tack KM: Neuroleptic malignant syndrome due to promethazine. South Med J 92:1017–1018, 1999

Chase TN: Levodopa therapy: consequences of the nonphysiologic replacement of dopamine. Neurology 50 (5 suppl 5):S17–S25, 1998

Chiu S, Mishra RK: Effects of dopaminergic and cholinergic drugs, naloxone and l-prolyl-leucyl-glycinamide on LSD-induced catalepsy. Naunyn Schmiedebergs Arch Pharmacol 313:45–50, 1980

Chopra MP, Prakash SS, Raguram R: The neuroleptic malignant syndrome: an Indian experience. Compr Psychiatry 40:19–23, 1999

Cohen BM, Renshaw PF, Stoll AL, et al: Decreased brain choline uptake in older adults. An in vivo magnetic resonance spectroscopic study. JAMA 274:902–907, 1995

Collins RC, Caston TV: Functional anatomy of occipital lobe seizures: an experimental study in rats. Neurology 29:705–716, 1979

Corrigan FM, Coulter F, Mackay AV: Neuroleptic malignant syndrome (NMS) on neuroleptic withdrawal (letter). Acta Psychiatr Scand 82:268–269, 1990

Corsi C, Pazzagli M, Bianchi L, et al: In vivo amino acid release from the striatum of aging rats: adenosine modulation. Neurobiol Aging 18:243–250, 1997

Cott JM: In vitro receptor binding and enzyme inhibition by Hypericum perforatum extract. Pharmacopsychiatry 30 (suppl 2):108–112, 1997

Coulter DM, Pillans PI: Fluoxetine and extrapyramidal side effects. Am J Psychiatry 152:122–125, 1995

Coupland NJ, Bailey JE, Potokar JP, et al: 5-HT receptors, nausea, and serotonin reuptake inhibition (letter). J Clin Psychopharmacol 17:142–143, 1997

Cuesta Lopez MJ, Moreno Brea MP, Munoz Malaga A: Sindrome neuroleptico maligno. Med Clin (Barc) 103:557–558, 1994

Daderman AM, Lidberg L: Flunitrazepam (Rohypnol) abuse in combination with alcohol causes premeditated, grievous violence in male juvenile offenders. J Am Acad Psychiatry Law 27:83–99, 1999

Daras M, Kakkouras L, Tuchman AJ, et al: Rhabdomyolysis and hyperthermia after cocaine abuse: a variant of the neuroleptic malignant syndrome. Acta Neurol Scand 92:161–165, 1995

DasGupta K, Young A: Clozapine-induced neuroleptic malignant syndrome. J Clin Psychiatry 52:105–107, 1991

Dave M: Fluoxetine-associated dystonia (letter). Am J Psychiatry 151:149, 1994

Delay J, Deniker P: Drug-induced extrapyramidal syndromes, in Handbook of Neurology: Diseases of the Basal Ganglia, Vol 6. Edited by Bruyn GW. Amsterdam, North-Holland, 1968, pp 248–266

DeLong MR: Primate models of movement disorders of basal ganglia origin. Trends Neurosci 13:281–285, 1990

del Zoppo G, Ginis I, Hallenbeck JM, et al: Inflammation and stroke: putative role for cytokines, adhesion molecules and iNOS in brain response to ischemia. Brain Pathol 10:95–112, 2000

Depaulis A, Deransart C, Vergnes M, et al: Mecanismes GABAergiques dans les epilepsies generalisees: la dimension neuronanatomique. Rev Neurol (Paris) 153 (suppl 1):S8–S13, 1997

Deransart C, Le BT, Marescaux C, et al: Role of the subthalamo-nigral input in the control of amygdala-kindled seizures in the rat. Brain Res 807:78–83, 1998

Deutsch G, Eisenberg HM: Frontal blood flow changes in recovery from coma. J Cereb Blood Flow Metab 7:29–34, 1987

Dextrorphan Study Group and Hoffmann-La Roche: Safety, tolerability and pharmacokinetics of the N-methyl-D-aspartate antagonist Ro-01-6794/706 in patients with acute ischemic stroke. Ann N Y Acad Sci 765:249–261, 1995

Dichter MA: Basic mechanisms of epilepsy: targets for therapeutic intervention. Epilepsia 38 (suppl 9): S2–S6, 1997

Dike GL: Triphasic waves in the serotonin syndrome (letter). J Neurol Neurosurg Psychiatry 62:200, 1997

Di Rosa AE, Morgante L, Coraci MA, et al: Functional hyperthermia due to central dopaminergic impairment. Funct Neurol 3:211–215, 1988

Doyle M, Warden D: Use of SPECT to evaluate postcardiotomy delirium. Am J Psychiatry 153:838–839, 1996

Duarte J, Campos JM, Cabezas C, et al: Neuroleptic malignant syndrome while on tiapride treatment (letter). Clin Neuropharmacol 19:539–540, 1996

Ebadi M, Pfeiffer RF, Murrin LC: Pathogenesis and treatment of neuroleptic malignant syndrome. Gen Pharmacol 21:367–386, 1990

Eberle-Wang K, Levitt P, Simansky KJ: Abdominal vagotomy dissociates the anorectic mechanisms for peripheral serotonin and cholecystokinin. Am J Physiol 265:R602–R608, 1993

Edwards JG, Inman WHW, Wilton L, et al: Prescription-event monitoring of 10,401 patients treated with fluvoxamine. Br J Psychiatry 164:387–395, 1994

Ehara H, Maegaki Y, Takeshita K: Neuroleptic malignant syndrome and methylphenidate. Pediatr Neurol 19:299–301, 1998

Eikelenboom P, Hoogendijk WJ: Do delirium and Alzheimer's dementia share specific pathogenetic mechanisms? Dement Geriatr Cogn Disord 10:319–324, 1999

Ekonomou A, Angelatou F: Upregulation of NMDA receptors in hippocampus and cortex in the pentylenetetrazol-induced "kindling" model of epilepsy. Neurochem Res 24:1515–1523, 1999

Elhusseiny A, Cohen Z, Olivier A, et al: Functional acetylcholine muscarinic receptor subtypes in human brain microcirculation: identification and cellular localization. J Cereb Blood Flow Metab 19:794–802, 1999

Elman I, Sokoloff L, Adler CM, et al: The effects of pharmacological doses of 2–deoxyglucose on cerebral blood flow in healthy volunteers. Brain Res 815:243–249, 1999

Enkvist MO, McCarthy KD: Astroglial gap junction communication is increased by treatment with either glutamate or high K^+ concentration. J Neurochem 62:489–495, 1994

Erspamer V, Asero B: Identification of enteramine, the specific hormone of the enterochromaffin cell system, as 5-hydroxytryptamine. Nature 169:800–801, 1952

Esler MD, Wallin G, Dorward PK, et al: Effects of desipramine on sympathetic nerve firing and norepinephrine spillover to plasma in humans. Am J Physiol 260:R817–R823, 1991

Exposito I, Del Arco A, Segovia G, et al: Endogenous dopamine increases extracellular concentrations of glutamate and GABA in striatum of the freely moving rat: involvement of D_1 and D_2 dopamine receptors. Neurochem Res 24:849–856, 1999

Farber NB, Newcomer JW, Olney JW: The glutamate synapse in neuropsychiatric disorders. Focus on schizophrenia and Alzheimer's disease. Prog Brain Res 116:421–437, 1998

Fava S, Galizia AC: Neuroleptic malignant syndrome and lithium carbonate. J Psychiatry Neurosci 20:305–306, 1995

Ferraro L, Beani L, Bianchi C, et al: Inhibitory cholinergic control of endogenous GABA release from electrically stimulated cortical slices and K(+)-depolarized synaptosomes. Neurochem Int 3:795–800, 1997

Fido AA: Postpartum period: a risk factor for neuroleptic malignant syndrome. Ann Clin Psychiatry 11:13–15, 1999

Figa-Talamanca L, Gualandi C, Di Meo L, et al: Hyperthermia after discontinuation of levodopa and bromocriptine therapy: impaired dopamine receptors a possible cause. Neurology 35:258–261, 1985

Finkel MS, Laghrissi-Thode F, Pollock BG, et al: Paroxetine is a novel nitric oxide synthase inhibitor. Psychopharmacol Bull 32:653–658, 1996

Finn AL: Toxicity and side effects of ondansetron. Semin Oncol 19 (suppl 10):53–60, 1992

Fischer S, Renz D, Wiesnet M, et al: Hypothermia abolishes hypoxia-induced hyperpermeability in brain microvessel endothelial cells. Brain Res Mol Brain Res 74:135–144, 1999

Flacker JM, Lipsitz LA: Serum anticholinergic activity changes with acute illness in elderly medical patients. J Gerontol A Biol Sci Med Sci 54:M12–M16, 1999

Fliser D, Bischoff I, Hanses A, et al: Renal handling of drugs in the elderly. Creatinine clearance underestimates renal function and pharmacokinetics remain virtually unchanged. Eur J Clin Pharmacol 55:205–211, 1999

Flumazenil in Benzodiazepine Intoxication Multicenter Study Group: Treatment of benzodiazepine overdose with flumazenil. Clin Ther 14:978–995, 1992

Forti M, Biella G, Caccia S, et al: Persistent excitability changes in the piriform cortex of the isolated guinea-pig brain after transient exposure to bicuculline. Eur J Neurosci 9:435–451, 1997

Freeman RB, Sheff MF, Matter JF, et al: The blood-cerebrospinal fluid barrier in uremia. Ann Intern Med 56:233–240, 1962

Friedman H, Greenblatt DJ, Peters GR, et al: Pharmacokinetics and pharmacodynamics of oral diazepam: effect of dose, plasma concentration, and time. Clin Pharmacol Ther 52:139–150, 1992

Frishman WH, Hotchkiss H: Selective and nonselective dopamine receptor agonists: an innovative approach to cardiovascular disease treatment. Am Heart J 132:861–870, 1996

Frishman WH, Huberfield S, Okin S, et al: Serotonin and serotonin antagonism in cardiovascular and non-cardiovascular disease. J Clin Pharmacol 35:541–572, 1995

Furui T, Tanaka I, Iwata K: Alterations in Na^+-K^+-ATPase activity and beta-endorphin content in acute ischemic brain with and without naloxone treatment. J Neurosurg 72:458–462, 1990

Garcia MC, Celuch SM, Adler-Graschinsky E: Involvement of GABA and glutamate receptors in the blood pressure responses to intrathecally injected sodium nitroprusside in anesthetized rats. Eur J Pharmacol 349:245–252, 1998

Gavish M, Katz Y, Bar-Ami S, et al: Biochemical, physiological, and pathological aspects of the peripheral benzodiazepine receptor. J Neurochem 58:1589–1601, 1992

Genton P, McMenamin J: Aggravation of seizures by antiepileptic drugs: what to do in clinical practice. Epilepsia 39 (suppl 3):S26–S29, 1998

George TP, Godleski LS: Possible serotonin syndrome with trazodone addition to fluoxetine (letter). Biol Psychiatry 39:384–385, 1996

Gerfen CR, Engber TM: Molecular anatomic mechanisms of Parkinson's disease: a proposed therapeutic approach. Neurol Clin 10:435–449, 1992

Ghelardini C, Galeotti N, Matucci R, et al: Antisense "knockdowns" of M1 receptors induces transient anterograde amnesia in mice. Neuropharmacology 38:339–348, 1999

Giacomelli S, Palmery M, Romanelli L, et al: Lysergic acid diethylamide (LSD) is a partial agonist of D_2 dopaminergic receptors and it potentiates dopamine-mediated prolactin secretion in lactotrophs in vitro. Life Sci 63:215–222, 1998

Gibson G, Blass J: Impaired synthesis of acetylcholine in brain accompanying mild hypoxia and hypoglycemia. J Neurochem 27:37–42, 1976

Gillis RA, Quest JA, DiMicco JA: Central regulation of autonomic function by GABA receptors, in GABA and Benzodiazepine Receptors, Vol 2. Edited by Squires RF. Boca Raton, FL, CRC, 1987, pp 47–61

Gillis RA, Hill KJ, Kirby JS, et al: Effect of activation of central nervous system serotonin 1A receptors on cardiorespiratory function. J Pharmacol Exp Ther 248:851–857, 1989

Gillman PK: Successful treatment of serotonin syndrome with chlorpromazine (letter). Med J Aust 165:345–346, 1996

Gimenez-Roldan S, Mateo D, Muradas V, et al: Clinical, biochemical, and pharmacological observation in a patient with postasphyxic myoclonus: association to serotonin hyperactivity. Clin Neuropharmacol 11:151–160, 1988

Ginsberg MD, Sternau LL, Globus MY, et al: Therapeutic modulation of brain temperature: relevance to brain injury. Cerebrovascular and Brain Metabolism Reviews 4:189–225, 1992

Gitlin MJ: Venlafaxine, monoamine oxidase inhibitors, and the serotonin syndrome (letter). J Clin Psychopharmacol 17:66–67, 1997

Goates MG, Escobar JI: An apparent neuroleptic malignant syndrome without extrapyramidal symptoms upon initiation of clozapine therapy: report of a case and results of a clozapine rechallenge. J Clin Psychopharmacol 12:139–140, 1992

Gobert A, Rivet JM, Cistarelli L, et al: Alpha$_2$-adrenergic receptor blockade markedly potentiates duloxetine- and fluoxetine-induced increases in noradrenaline, dopamine, and serotonin levels in the frontal cortex of freely moving rats. J Neurochem 69:2616–2619, 1997

Gonner F, Baumgartner R, Schupbach D, et al: Neuroleptic malignant syndrome during low dosed neuroleptic medication in first-episode psychosis: a case report. Psychopharmacology (Berl) 144: 416–418, 1999

Gorard AD, Libby GW, Farthing MJG: 5-Hydroxytryptamine and human small intestinal motility: effect of inhibiting 5-hydroxytryptamine reuptake. Gut 35:496–500, 1994

Graber MA, Hoehns TB, Perry PJ: Sertraline-phenelzine drug interaction: a serotonin syndrome reaction. Ann Pharmacother 28:732–735, 1994

Gradon JD: Neuroleptic malignant syndrome possibly caused by molindone hydrochloride. DICP. Ann Pharmacother 25:1071–1072, 1991

Graudins A, Stearman A, Chan B: Treatment of the serotonin syndrome with cyproheptadine. J Emerg Med 16:615–619, 1998

Gravlin MA: Serotonin syndrome: what causes it, how to recognize it, and ways to avoid it. Hospital Pharmacy 32:570–575, 1997

Greenshaw AJ, Silverstone PH: The non-antiemetic uses of serotonin 5-HT$_3$ receptor antagonists. Clinical pharmacology and therapeutic applications. Drugs 53:20–39, 1997

Grimaldi B, Bonnin A, Fillion MP, et al: 5-Hydroxytryptamine-moduline: a novel endogenous peptide involved in the control of anxiety. Neuroscience 93:1223–1225, 1999

Gupta G, Azam M, Baquer NZ: Effect of experimental diabetes on the catecholamine metabolism in rat brain. J Neurochem 58:95–100, 1992

Gurrera RJ: Sympathoadrenal hyperactivity and the etiology of neuroleptic malignant syndrome. Am J Psychiatry 156:169–180, 1999

Haggerty JJ Jr, Bentsen BS, Gillette GM: Neuroleptic malignant syndrome superimposed on tardive dyskinesia. Br J Psychiatry 150:104–105, 1987

Hall AC, Lieb WR, Franks NP: Stereoselective and non-stereoselective actions of isoflurane on the $GABA_A$ receptor. Br J Pharmacol 112:906–910, 1994

Hall RC, Popkin MK, McHenry LE: Angel's Trumpet psychosis: a central nervous system anticholinergic syndrome. Am J Psychiatry 134:312–314, 1977

Halman M, Goldbloom DS: Fluoxetine and neuroleptic malignant syndrome. Biol Psychiatry 28:518–521, 1990

Halvorson I, Gregor L, Thornhill JA: Brown adipose tissue thermogenesis is activated by electrical and chemical (L-glutamate) stimulation of the ventromedial hypothalamic nucleus in cold-acclimated rats. Brain Res 522:76–82, 1990

Hasan S, Buckley P: Novel antipsychotics and the neuroleptic malignant syndrome: a review and critique. Am J Psychiatry 155:1113–1115, 1998

Hauber W: Involvement of basal ganglia transmitter systems in movement initiation. Prog Neurobiol 56:507–540, 1998

Hayashi N: The control of brain tissue temperature and stimulation of dopamine-immune system to the severe brain injury patients. Nippon Rinsho 56:1627–1635, 1998

Healy DJ, Meador-Woodruff JH: Ionotropic glutamate receptor modulation of $5\text{-}HT_6$ and $5\text{-}HT_7$ mRNA expression in rat brain. Neuropsychopharmacology 21:341–345, 1999

Heinemann F, Assion HJ, Hermes G, et al: Paroxetin-induziertes malignes neuroleptisches Syndrom. Nervenarzt 68:664–666, 1997

Hemachudha T, Griffin DE, Giffels JJ, et al: Myelin basic protein as an encephalitogen in encephalomyelitis and polyneuritis following rabies vaccination. N Engl J Med 316:369–374, 1987

Henderson VW, Wooten GF: Neuroleptic malignant syndrome: a pathogenetic role for dopamine receptor blockade? Neurology 31:132–137, 1981

Hennig J, Rzepka U, Mai B, et al: Suppression of HPA-axis activity by haloperidol after experimentally induced heat stress. Prog Neuropsychopharmacol Biol Psychiatry 19:603–614, 1995

Henon H, Lebert F, Durieu I, et al: Confusional state in stroke. Relation to preexisting dementia, patient characteristics, and outcome. Stroke 30:773–779, 1999

Herd B, Clarke F: Complete heart block after flumazenil (letter). Hum Exp Toxicol 10:289, 1991

Heurteaux C, Baumaan N, Lachapelle F, et al: Lithium distribution in the brain of normal mice and of "quaking" dysmyelinating mutants. J Neurochem 46:1317–1321, 1986

Hevers W, Luddens H: The diversity of $GABA_A$ receptors. Pharmacological and electrophysiological properties of $GABA_A$ channel subtypes. Mol Neurobiol 18:35–86, 1998

Heyland D, Sauve M: Neuroleptic malignant syndrome without the use of neuroleptics. CMAJ 145:817–819, 1991

Hollrigel GS, Chen K, Baram TZ, et al: The pro-convulsant actions of corticotropin-releasing hormone in the hippocampus of infant rats. Neuroscience 84:71–79, 1998

Horton RW, LeFeuvre RA, Rothwell NJ, et al: Opposing effects of activation of central $GABA_A$ and $GABA_B$ receptors on brown fat thermogenesis in the rat. Neuropharmacology 27:363–368, 1988

Hoyer D, Clarke DE, Fozard JR, et al: International Union of Pharmacology classification of receptors for 5-hydroxytryptamine (serotonin). Pharmacol Rev 46:157–203, 1994

Huang KX, Bergstrom DA, Ruskin DN, et al: *N*-methyl-D-aspartate receptor blockade attenuates D_1 dopamine receptor modulation of neuronal activity in rat substantia nigra. Synapse 30:18–29, 1998

Huang ZC, Shen DL: The prognostic significance of diazepam-induced EEG changes in epilepsy: a follow-up study. Clin Electroencephalogr 24:179–187, 1993

Huang ZC, Shen DL: Studies on quantitative beat activity in EEG background changes produced by intravenous diazepam in epilepsy. Clin Electroencephalogr 28:172–178, 1997

Huber TJ, Dietrich DE, Emrich HM: Possible use of amantadine in depression. Pharmacopsychiatry 32:47–55, 1999

Hughes JR: A review of the usefulness of the standard EEG in psychiatry. Clin Electroencephalogr 27: 35–39, 1996

Hung DZ, Tsai WJ, Deng JF: Anterograde amnesia in triazolam overdose despite flumazenil treatment: a case report. Hum Exp Toxicol 11:289–290, 1992

Hunt N, Stern TA: The association between intravenous haloperidol and torsades de pointes. Three cases and a literature review. Psychosomatics 36:541–549, 1995

Hyde TM, Knable MB, Murray AM: Distribution of dopamine D_1–D_4 receptor subtypes in human dorsal vagal complex. Synapse 24:224–232, 1996

Jacobs BL, Fornal CA: 5-HT and motor control: a hypothesis. Trends Neurosci 16:346–352, 1993

Jagust WJ, Reed BR, Martin EM, et al: Cognitive function and regional cerebral blood flow in Parkinson's disease. Brain 115:521–537, 1992

James ME: Neuroleptic malignant syndrome in pregnancy. Psychosomatics 29:119–122, 1988

Janigro D: Blood-brain barrier, ion homeostasis and epilepsy: possible implications towards the understanding of ketogenic diet mechanisms. Epilepsy Res 37:223–232, 1999

Jarman J, Glover V, Sandler M: Release of ^{14}C 5-hydroxytryptamine from human platelets by red wine. Life Sci 48:2297–2300, 1991

Jarrott B: Epileptogenesis: biochemical aspects, in Antiepileptic Drugs: Pharmacology and Therapeutics. Edited by Eadie MJ, Vajda FJE. New York, Springer-Verlag, 1999, pp 87–121

Jasper JR, Kosaka A, To ZP, et al: Cloning, expression and pharmacology of a truncated splice variant of the human 5-HT_7 receptor (h5-HT7b). Br J Pharmacol 122:126–132, 1997

Jerusalinsky D, Kornisiuk E, Izquierdo I: Cholinergic neurotransmission and synaptic plasticity concerning memory processes. Neurochem Res 22:507–515, 1997

Jezek P, Engstova H, Zackova M, et al: Fatty acid cycling mechanism and mitochondrial uncoupling proteins. Biochim Biophys Acta 1365:319–327, 1998

June R, Yunus M, Gossman W: Neuroleptic malignant syndrome associated with nortriptyline (letter). Am J Emerg Med 17:736–737, 1999

Kalenda Z, Holzenspies AJ: Restoration of pulmonary perfusion by a serotonin antagonist. Angiology 32:463–475, 1981

Karlsson I: Drugs that induce delirium. Dement Geriatr Cogn Disord 10:412–415, 1999

Kern JL, Cernek PK: Delayed risperidone-induced neuroleptic malignant syndrome (letter). Ann Pharmacother 30:300, 1996

Keyser DL, Rodnitzky RL: Neuroleptic malignant syndrome in Parkinson's disease after withdrawal or alteration of dopaminergic therapy. Arch Intern Med 151:794–796, 1991

Kiyatake I, Yamaji K, Shirato I, et al: A case of neuroleptic malignant syndrome with acute renal failure after the discontinuation of sulpiride and maprotiline. Japanese Journal of Medicine 30:387–391, 1991

Klotz U: Effect of age on pharmacokinetics and pharmacodynamics in man. Int J Clin Pharmacol Ther 36:581–585, 1998

Kontaxakis VP, Christodoulou GN, Markidis MP, et al: Treatment of a mild form of neuroleptic malignant syndrome with diazepam. Acta Psychiatr Scand 78:396–398, 1988

Koponen HJ, Lepola UM, Leinonen EV: Neuroleptic malignant syndrome during remoxipride treatment. A case report. Eur Neuropsychopharmacol 3:517–519, 1993

Kornhuber J, Weller M: Neuroleptic malignant syndrome. Curr Opin Neurol 7:353–357, 1994

Kornhuber J, Weller M: Psychotogenicity and N-methyl-D-aspartate receptor antagonism: implications for neuroprotective pharmacotherapy. Biol Psychiatry 41:135–144, 1997

Kornhuber J, Weller M, Riederer P: Glutamate receptor antagonists for neuroleptic malignant syndrome and akinetic hyperthermic parkinsonian crisis. Journal of Neural Transmission: Parkinson's Disease and Dementia Section 6:63–72, 1993

Kreiss DS, Wieland S, Lucki I: The presence of a serotonin uptake inhibitor alters pharmacological manipulations of serotonin release. Neuroscience 52:295–301, 1993

Kretschmer BD, Kratzer U, Schmidt WJ: Riluzole, a glutamate release inhibitor, and motor behavior. Naunyn Schmiedebergs Arch Pharmacol 358:181–190, 1998

Krisanda TJ: Fab immunotherapy for digitalis toxicity. Topics in Emergency Medicine 15:41–49, 1993

Kubo T, Amano M, Asari T: *N*-methyl-D-aspartate receptors, but not non-*N*-methyl-D-aspartate receptors mediate hypertension induced by carotid body chemoreceptor stimulation in the rostral ventrolateral medulla of the rat. Neurosci Lett 164:113–116, 1993

Kubo T, Yanagihara Y, Yamaguchi H, et al: Excitatory amino acid receptors in the paraventricular hypothalamic nucleus mediate pressor response induced by carotid body chemoreceptor. Clin Exp Hypertens 19:1117–1134, 1997

Kubota T: Neuroleptic malignant syndrome induced by nemonapride. Acta Neurologica Napoli 15: 142–144, 1993

Lamy PP: Comparative pharmacokinetic changes and drug therapy in an older population. J Am Geriatr Soc 30 (11 suppl):S11–S19, 1982

Lane R, Baldwin D: Selective serotonin reuptake inhibitor–induced serotonin syndrome: review. J Clin Psychopharmacol 17:208–221, 1997

Larner AJ, Smith SC, Farmer SF: "Non-neuroleptic malignant" syndrome (letter). J Neurol Neurosurg Psychiatry 65:613, 1998

Larocca JN, Cervone A, Ledeen RW: Stimulation of phosphoinositide hydrolysis in myelin by muscarinic agonist and potassium. Brain Res 436:357–362, 1987

Lawrence KR, Nasraway SA: Conduction disturbances associated with administration of butyrophenone antipsychotics in the critically ill: a review of the literature. Pharmacotherapy 17:531–537, 1997

Lechleiter J, Peralta E, Clapham D: Diverse functions of muscarinic acetylcholine receptor subtypes. Trends Pharmacol Sci (suppl):34–38, 1989

Lee JW: Serum iron in catatonia and neuroleptic malignant syndrome. Biol Psychiatry 44:499–507, 1998

Lee SH, Kim WT, Cornell-Bell AH, et al: Astrocytes exhibit regional specificity in gap-junction coupling. Glia 11:315–325, 1994

Lefebvre H, Contesse V, Delarue C, et al: Serotonergic regulation of adrenocortical function. Horm Metab Res 30:398–403, 1998

LeJoyeux M, Rouillon F, Leon E, et al: Le syndrome serotonergique: revue de la litterateur et description d'une etude originale. Encephale 21:537–545, 1995

Lenhardt R, Negishi C, Sessler DI, et al: The effects of physical treatment on induced fever in humans. Am J Med 106:550–555, 1999

Leshner AI, Koob GF: Drugs of abuse and the brain. Proc Assoc Am Physicians 111:99–108, 1999

Lew TY, Tollefson G: Chlorpromazine-induced neuroleptic malignant syndrome and its response to diazepam. Biol Psychiatry 18:1441–1446, 1983

Lin TJ, Hung DZ, Hu WH, et al: Acute basagran poisoning mimicking neuroleptic malignant syndrome. Hum Exp Toxicol 18:493–494, 1999

Linville DG, Hamel E: Pharmacological characterization of muscarinic acetylcholine binding sites in human and bovine cerebral microvessels. Naunyn Schmiedebergs Arch Pharmacol 352:179–186, 1995

Lovinger DM: 5-HT_3 receptors and the neural actions of alcohols: an increasingly exciting topic. Neurochem Int 35:125–130, 1999

Lovinger DM, Zimmerman SA, Levitin M, et al: Trichloroethanol potentiates synaptic transmission mediated by gamma-aminobutyric acidA receptors in hippocampal neurons. J Pharmacol Exp Ther 264:1097–1103, 1993

Lugaresi E, Montagna P, Tinuper P, et al: Endozepine stupor. Recurring stupor linked to endozepine-4 accumulation. Brain 121:127–133, 1998

MacDonald JF, Xiong XG, Lu WY, et al: Modulation of NMDA receptors. Prog Brain Res 116:191–208, 1998

MacDonald RL, Kapur J: Pharmacological properties of recombinant and hippocampal dentate granule cell $GABA_A$ receptors. Adv Neurol 79:979–990, 1999

Madeja M, Musshoff U, Lorra C, et al: Mechanism of action of the epileptogenic drug pentylenetetrazol on a cloned neuronal potassium channel. Brain Res 722:59–70, 1996

Majkowski J: Kindling: clinical relevance for epileptogenicity in humans. Adv Neurol 81:105–113, 1999

Maksay G, Korpi ER, Uusi-Oukari M: Bimodal action of furosemide on convulsant $[^3H]$EBOB binding to cerebellar and cortical $GABA_A$ receptors. Neurochem Int 33:353–358, 1998

Malatynska E, Miller C, Schindler N, et al: Amitriptyline increases GABA-stimulated 36Cl-influx by recombinant ($alpha_1gamma_2$) $GABA_A$ receptors. Brain Res 851:277–280, 1999

Malhotra AK, Adler CM, Kennison SD, et al: Clozapine blunts N-methyl-D-aspartate antagonist-induced psychosis: a study with ketamine. Biol Psychiatry 42:664–668, 1997

Marcoli M, Maura G, Tortarolo M, et al: Trazodone is a potent agonist at 5-HT_{2C} receptors mediating inhibition of the *N*-methyl-D-aspartate/nitric oxide/cyclic GMP pathway in rat cerebellum. J Pharmacol Exp Ther 285:983–986, 1998

Mateo D, Munoz-Blanco JL, Gimenez-Roldan S: Neuroleptic malignant syndrome related to tetrabenazine introduction and haloperidol discontinuation in Huntington's disease. Clin Neuropharmacol 15:63–68, 1992

Maxton DG, Morris J, Whorwell PJ: Selective 5-hydroxytryptamine antagonism: a role in irritable bowel syndrome and functional dyspepsia? Aliment Pharmacol Ther 10:595–599, 1996

McDermott JL: Effects of estrogen upon dopamine release from the corpus striatum of young and aged female rats. Brain Res 606:118–125, 1993

McIntyre RC, Agrafojo J, Banerjee A, et al: Pulmonary vascular smooth muscle contraction. J Surg Res 61:170–174, 1996

Mehta AK, Ticku MK: An update on $GABA_A$ receptors. Brain Res Brain Res Rev 29:196–217, 1999

Meldrum BS, Chapman AG: Basic mechanisms of gabitril (tiagabine) and future potential developments. Epilepsia 40 (suppl 9):S2–S6, 1999

Meltzer HY, Nash JF: Effects of antipsychotic drugs on serotonin receptors. Pharmacol Rev 43:587–604, 1991

Mendez MF: The neuropsychiatry of multiple sclerosis. Int J Psychiatry Med 25:123–130, 1995

Mendez MF: Delirium, in Neurology in Clinical Practice: Principles of Diagnosis and Management, 2nd Edition, Vol 1. Edited by Bradley WG, Daroff RB, Fenichel GM, Marsden CD. Boston, MA, Butterworth-Heinemann, 1996, pp 29–38

Mesulam MM, Waxman SG, Geschwind N, et al: Acute confusional states with right middle cerebral artery infarction. J Neurol Neurosurg Psychiatry 39:84–89, 1979

Mihic SJ: Acute effects of ethanol on $GABA_A$ and glycine receptor function. Neurochem Int 35:115–123, 1999

Mihic SJ, McQuilkin SJ, Eger EI, et al: Potentiation of gamma-aminobutyric acid type A receptor-mediated chloride currents by novel halogenated compounds correlates with their abilities to induce general anesthesia. Mol Pharmacol 46:851–857, 1994

Milbrandt JC, Albin RL, Turgeon AM, et al: $GABA_A$ receptor binding in the aging rat inferior colliculus. Neuroscience 73:449–458, 1996

Miller DD, Sharafuddin MJA, Kathol RG: A case of clozapine-induced neuroleptic malignant syndrome. J Clin Psychiatry 52:99–101, 1991

Mitrakou A, Ryan C, Veneman T, et al: Hierarchy of thresholds for counterregulatory hormone secretion, symptoms, and cerebral dysfunction. Am J Physiol 260:E67–E74, 1991

Miyaoka H, Kamijima K: Encephalopathy during amitriptyline therapy: are neuroleptic malignant syndrome and serotonin syndrome spectrum disorders? Int Clin Psychopharmacol 10:265–267, 1995

Miyaoka H, Shishikura K, Otsubo T, et al: Diazepam-responsive neuroleptic malignant syndrome: a diagnostic subtype? (letter). Am J Psychiatry 154:882, 1997

Monda M, Amaro S, De Luca B: Non-shivering thermogenesis during prostaglandin E1 fever in rats: role of the cerebral cortex. Brain Res 651:148–154, 1994

Monda M, Viggiano A, Sullo A, et al: Aspartic and glutamic acids increase in the frontal cortex during prostaglandin E1 hyperthermia. Neuroscience 83:1239–1243, 1998

Mooradian AD: Potential mechanisms of the age-related changes in the blood-brain barrier. Neurobiol Aging 15:751–755, 761–762, 767, 1994

Moore AR, O'Keefe ST: Drug-induced cognitive impairment in the elderly. Drugs Aging 15:15–28, 1999

Moore H, Sarter M, Bruno JP: Bidirectional modulation of cortical acetylcholine efflux by infusion of benzodiazepine receptor ligands into the basal forebrain. Neurosci Lett 189:31–34, 1995

Moore NA, Leander JD, Benvenga MJ, et al: Behavioral pharmacology of olanzapine: a novel antipsychotic drug. J Clin Psychiatry 58 (suppl 10):37–44, 1997

Morare M, O'Connor WT, Ungerstedt U, et al: N-methyl-D-aspartic acid differentially regulates extracellular dopamine, GABA, and glutamate levels in the dorsolateral neostriatum of the halothane-anesthetized rat: an in vitro microdialysis study. J Neurochem 60:1884–1893, 1993

Morrell MJ: Epilepsy in women: the science of why it is special. Neurology 53 (4 suppl 1):S42–S48, 1999

Moshe SL: Sex and the substantia nigra: administration, teaching, patient care, and research. J Clin Neurophysiol 14:484–494, 1997

Mott DD, Lewis DV: The pharmacology and function of central $GABA_B$ receptors. Int Rev Neurobiol 36:97–223, 1994

Moy SS, Criswell HE, Breese GR: Differential effects of bilateral dopamine depletion in neonatal and adult rats. Neurosci Biobehav Rev 21:425–435, 1997

Muhlberg W, Platt D: Age-dependent changes in the kidney: pharmacological implications. Gerontology 45:243–253, 1999

Muir KW, Grosset DG, Lees KR: Clinical pharmacology of CNS 1102 in volunteers. Ann N Y Acad Sci 765:279–289, 1995

Muir KW, Grosset DG, Lees KR: Effects of prolonged infusion of the NMDA antagonist aptiganel hydrochloride (CNS 1102) in normal volunteers. Clin Neuropharmacol 20:311–321, 1997

Muller B, Qu H, Garseth M, et al: Amino acid metabolism in neurones and glia following kainate injection in rats. Neurosci Lett 279:169–172, 2000

Mullins ME: First-degree atrioventricular block in alprazolam overdose reversed by flumazenil. J Pharm Pharmacol 51:367–370, 1999

Murphy DL, Lesch KP, Aulakh CS, et al: Serotonin-selective arylpiperazines with neuroendocrine, behavioral, temperature, and cardiovascular effects in humans. Pharmacol Rev 43:527–552, 1991

Murray N, Steck AJ: Impulse conduction regulates myelin basic protein phosphorylation in rat optic nerve. J Neurochem 43:243–248, 1984

Nagy F, Chugani DC, Juhasz C, et al: Altered in vitro and in vivo flumazenil binding in human epileptogenic neocortex. J Cereb Blood Flow Metab 19:939–947, 1999

Nemecek D, Rastogi-Cruz D, Csernansky JG: Atropinism may precipitate neuroleptic malignant syndrome during treatment with clozapine (letter). Am J Psychiatry 150:1561, 1993

Netzeband JG, Trotter C, Caguioa JN, et al: Chronic ethanol exposure enhances AMPA-elicited $Ca2^{+}$ signals in the somatic and dendritic regions of cerebellar Purkinje cells. Neurochem Int 35:163–174, 1999

Nierenberg DW, Semprebon M: The central nervous system serotonin syndrome. Clin Pharmacol Ther 53:84–88, 1993

Nierenberg DW, Disch M, Manheimer E, et al: Facilitating prompt diagnosis and treatment of the neuroleptic malignant syndrome. Clin Pharmacol Ther 50:580–586, 1991

Nimmagadda SR, Ryan DH, Atkin SL: Neuroleptic malignant syndrome after venlafaxine (letter). Lancet 355:289–290, 2000

Nimmo SM, Kennedy BW, Tullett WM, et al: Drug-induced hyperthermia. Anaesthesia 48:892–895, 1993

Nisijima K, Ishigura T: Cerebrospinal fluid levels of monoamine metabolites and gamma-aminobutyric acid in neuroleptic malignant syndrome. J Psychiatr Res 29:233–244, 1995

Nonino F, Campomori A: Neuroleptic malignant syndrome associated with metoclopramide (letter). Ann Pharmacother 33:644–645, 1999

Nopoulos P, Flaum M, Miller DD: Atypical neuroleptic malignant syndrome (NMS) with an atypical neuroleptic: Clozapine-induced NMS without rigidity. Ann Clin Psychiatry 2:251–253, 1990

Norman TR: Pharmacokinetic aspects of antidepressant treatment in the elderly. Prog Neuropsychopharmacol Biol Psychiatry 17:329–344, 1993

Oates JA, Sjoerdsma A: Neurologic effects of tryptophan in patients receiving a monoamine oxidase inhibitor. Neurology 10:1076–1078, 1960

O'Carroll RE, Hayes PC, Ebmeier KP, et al: Regional cerebral blood flow and cognitive function in patients with chronic liver disease. Lancet 1:1250–1253, 1982

Olney JW: Neurotoxicity of NMDA receptor antagonists: an overview. Psychopharmacol Bull 30:533–540, 1994

Olsen NV: Effects of dopamine on renal haemodynamics tubular function and sodium excretion in normal humans. Dan Med Bull 45:282–297, 1998

Ortiz J, Artigas F: Effects of monoamine uptake inhibitors on extracellular and platelet 5-hydroxytryptamine in rat blood: different effects of clomipramine and fluoxetine. Br J Pharmacol 105:941–946, 1992

Ota M, Mefford IN, Naoi M, et al: Effects of morphine administration on catecholamine levels in rat brain: specific reduction of epinephrine concentration in hypothalamus. Neurosci Lett 121:129–132, 1991

Palou A, Pico C, Bonet ML, et al: The uncoupling protein, thermogenin. Int J Biochem Cell Biol 30:7–11, 1998

Paredes RG, Agmo A: GABA and behavior: the role of receptor subtypes. Neurosci Biobehav Rev 16: 145–170, 1992

Park HS, Kelly JM, Milligan LP: Energetics and cell membranes, in Energy Metabolism: Tissue Determinants and Cellular Corollaries. Edited by Kinney JM, Tucker HN. New York, Raven, 1992, pp 411–437

Park-Matsumoto YC, Tazawa T: Neuroleptic malignant syndrome associated with diphenhydramine and diprophyllin overdose in a depressed patient (letter). J Neurol Sci 162:108–109, 1999

Parsa MA, Rohr T, Ramirez LF, et al: Neuroleptic malignant syndrome without neuroleptics (letter). J Clin Psychopharmacol 10:437–438, 1990

Patrick D, Betts J, Frey EA, et al: Haemophilus influenzae lipopolysaccharide disrupts confluent monolayers of bovine brain endothelial cells via a serum-dependent cytotoxic pathway. J Infect Dis 165:865–872, 1992

Pattichis K, Louca LL, Jarman J, et al: Phenolic substances in red wine and release of 5-hydroxytryptamine (letter). Lancet 341:1104, 1994

Pazos A, Probst A, Palacios JM: Serotonin receptors in the human brain, IV: autoradiographic mapping of serotonin receptors. Neuroscience 2:123–139, 1987

Pechadre JC, Beudin P, Trolese JF, et al: A comparison of the electroencephalographic spectral modifications induced by diazepam and by hydroxyzine. J Int Med Res 21:234–242, 1993

Pelonero AL, Levenson JL, Pandurangi AK: Neuroleptic malignant syndrome: a review. Psychiatr Serv 49:1163–1172, 1998

Perlmutter JS, Tempel LW, Black KJ, et al: MPTP induces dystonia and parkinsonism: clues to the pathophysiology of dystonia. Neurology 49:1432–1438, 1997

Perry EK, Perry RH: Acetylcholine and hallucinations: disease-related compared to drug-induced alterations in human consciousness. Brain Cogn 28:240–258, 1995

Perry E, Walker M, Grace J, et al: Acetylcholine in mind: a neurotransmitter correlate of consciousness? Trends Neurosci 22:273–280, 1999

Plum F, Posner JB: Multifocal, diffuse, and metabolic brain diseases causing stupor or coma, in The Diagnosis of Stupor and Coma, 3rd Edition. Philadelphia, PA, FA Davis, 1980, pp 177–304

Pope HG Jr, Jonas M, Hudson JI, et al: Toxic reactions to the combination of monoamine oxidase inhibitors and tryptophan. Am J Psychiatry 142:491–492, 1985

Pope HG Jr, Keck PE Jr, McElroy SL: Frequency and presentation of neuroleptic malignant syndrome in a large psychiatric hospital. Am J Psychiatry 143:1227–1233, 1986

Popoli P, Betto P, Rimondini R, et al: Age-related alteration of the adenosine/dopamine balance in the rat striatum. Brain Res 795:297–300, 1998

Porras A, Mora F: Dopamine-glutamate-GABA interactions and ageing: studies in the striatum of the conscious rat. Eur J Neurosci 7:2183–2188, 1995

Porras A, Sanz B, Mora F: Dopamine-glutamate interactions in the prefrontal cortex of the conscious rat: studies on ageing. Mech Ageing Dev 99:9–17, 1997

Portel L, Hilbert G, Gruson D, et al: Malignant hyperthermia and neuroleptic malignant syndrome in a patient during treatment for acute asthma. Acta Anaesthesiol Scand 43:107–110, 1999

Posner MI, Petersen SE: The attention system of the human brain. Annu Rev Neurosci 13:25–42, 1990

Pranzatelli MR: Serotonin and human myoclonus: rationale for the use of serotonin receptor agonists and antagonists. Arch Neurol 51:605–617, 1994

Pullicino P, Galizia AC, Azzopardi C: Cerebral infarction in neuroleptic malignant syndrome. J Neuropsychiatry Clin Neurosci 3:75–77, 1991

Raffa RB: Screen of receptor and uptake-site activity of St. John's wort reveals sigma receptor binding. Life Sci 62:PL265–PL270, 1998

Rao SM: Neuropsychology of multiple sclerosis. Curr Opin Neurol 8:216–220, 1995

Rapport MM, Green AA, Page IH: Serum vasoconstrictor (serotonin) IV: isolation and characterization. J Biol Chem 176:1243–1251, 1948

Ray JG: Neuroleptic malignant syndrome associated with severe thrombocytopenia. J Intern Med 241:245–247, 1997

Reddig S, Minnema AM, Tandon R: Neuroleptic malignant syndrome and clozapine. Ann Clin Psychiatry 5:25–27, 1993

Reever CM, Ferrari-DiLeo G, Flynn DD: The M_5 (m5) receptor subtype: fact or fiction? Life Sci 60: 1105–1112, 1997

Reeves RK, Stolp-Smith KA, Christopherson MW: Hyperthermia, rhabdomyolysis, and disseminated intravascular coagulation associated with baclofen pump catheter failure. Arch Phys Med Rehabil 79:353–356, 1998

Ribeiro RL, Andreatini R, Wolfman C, et al: The "anxiety state" and its relation with rat models of memory and habituation. Neurobiol Learn Mem 72:78–94, 1999

Ridding MC, Inzelberg R, Rothwell JC: Changes in excitability of motor cortical circuitry in patients with Parkinson's disease. Ann Neurol 37:181–188, 1995

Riederer P, Lange KW, Kornhuber J, et al: Glutamate receptor antagonism: neurotoxicity, anti-akinetic effects, and psychosis. J Neural Transm Suppl 34:203–210, 1991

Ritchie J, Steiner W, Abrahamowicz M: Incidence of and risk factors for delirium among psychiatric inpatients. Psychiatr Serv 47:727–730, 1996

Roberge RJ, Atchley B, Ryan K, et al: Two chlorzoxazone (Parafon forte) overdoses and coma in one patient: reversal with flumazenil. Am J Emerg Med 16:393–395, 1998

Robertson IH, Tegner R, Tham K, et al: Sustained attention training for unilateral neglect: theoretical and rehabilitation implications. J Clin Exp Neuropsychol 17:416–430, 1995

Rodriguez-Puertas R, Pascual J, Vilaro T, et al: Autoradiographic distribution of M_1, M_2, M_3, and M_4 muscarinic receptor subtypes in Alzheimer's disease. Synapse 26:341–350, 1997

Rosebush P, Stewart T: A prospective analysis of 24 episodes of neuroleptic malignant syndrome. Am J Psychiatry 146:717–725, 1989

Rothstein JD, Guidotti A, Tinupe P, et al: Endogenous benzodiazepine receptor ligands in idiopathic recurring stupor. Lancet 340:1002–1004, 1992

Rothwell NJ: CNS regulation of thermogenesis. Crit Rev Neurobiol 8:1–10, 1994

Rubenstein E: Relationship of senescence of cerebrospinal fluid circulatory system to dementias of the aged. Lancet 351:283–285, 1998

Rush CR, Frey JM, Griffiths RR: Zaleplon and triazolam in humans: acute behavioral effects and abuse potential. Psychopharmacology (Berl) 145:39–51, 1999

Sachdev P, Kruk J, Kneebone M, et al: Clozapine-induced neuroleptic malignant syndrome: review and report of new cases. J Clin Psychopharmacol 15:365–371, 1995

Saija A, Princi P, Imperatore C, et al: Ageing influences haloperidol-induced changes in the permeability of the blood-brain barrier in the rat. J Pharm Pharmacol 44:450–452, 1992

Sandyk R: L-dopa induced "serotonin syndrome" in a Parkinsonian patient on bromocriptine (letter). J Clin Psychopharmacol 6:194–195, 1986

Sangal R, Dimitrijevic R: Neuroleptic malignant syndrome. Successful treatment with pancuronium. JAMA 254:2795–2796, 1985

Sanger GJ: 5-Hydroxytryptamine and functional bowel disorders. Neurogastroenterol Motil 8:319–331, 1996

Sankar R, Blossom E, Clemons K, et al: Age-associated changes in the effects of amphetamine on the blood-brain barrier of rats. Neurobiol Aging 4:65–68, 1983

Sanna E, Pau D, Tuveri F, et al: Molecular and neurochemical evaluation of the effects of etizolam on $GABA_A$ receptors under normal and stress conditions. Arzneimittelforschung 49:88–95, 1999

Sanz B, Exposito I, Mora F: M_1 acetylcholine receptor stimulation increases the extracellular concentrations of glutamate and GABA in the medial prefrontal cortex of the rat. Neurochem Res 22:281–286, 1997

Sarter M: Neuronal mechanisms of the attentional dysfunctions in senile dementia and schizophrenia: two sides of the same coin? Psychopharmacology (Berl) 114:539–550, 1994

Sarter M, Bruno JP, Turchi J: Basal forebrain afferent projections modulating acetylcholine, attention, and implications for neuropsychiatric disorders. Ann N Y Acad Sci 877:368–382, 1999

Sastry PS, Dixon JF, Hokin LE: Agonist-stimulated inositol polyphosphate formation in cerebellum. J Neurochem 58:1079–1086, 1992

Saxena PR, Villalon CM: Cardiovascular effects of serotonin agonists and antagonists. J Cardiovasc Pharmacol 15 (suppl 7):S17–S34, 1990

Saxena PR, Villalon CM: 5-Hydroxytryptamine: a chameleon in the heart. Trends Pharmacol Sci 12: 223–227, 1991

Schechter DS, Nunes EV: Reversible parkinsonism in a 90-year-old man taking sertraline (letter). J Clin Psychiatry 58:275, 1997

Schmucker DL: Aging and the liver: an update. J Gerontol A Biol Sci Med Sci 53:B315–B320, 1998

Schobitz B, Reul JM, Holsboer F: The role of the hypothalamic-pituitary-adrenocortical system during inflammatory conditions. Crit Rev Neurobiol 8:263–291, 1994

Schuldiner S, Steiner-Mordoch S, Yelin R, et al: Amphetamine derivatives interact with plasma membrane and secretory biogenic amine transporters. Mol Pharmacol 44:1227–1231, 1993

Scremin OU, Shih TM, Li MG, et al: Mapping of cerebral metabolic activation in three models of cholinergic convulsions. Brain Res Bull 45:167–174, 1998

Segovia G, Mora F: Role of nitric oxide in modulating the release of dopamine, glutamate, and GABA in striatum of the freely moving rat. Brain Res Bull 45:275–279, 1998

Segovia G, Del Arco A, Mora F: Endogenous glutamate increases extracellular concentrations of dopamine, GABA, and taurine through NMDA and AMPA/kainate receptors in striatum of the freely moving rat: a microdialysis study. J Neurochem 69:1476–1483, 1997

Selig WM, Bloomquist MA, Cohen ML, et al: Serotonin-induced pulmonary responses in the perfused guinea pig lung: evidence for 5-HT_2 receptor-mediated pulmonary vascular and airway smooth muscle constriction. Pulmonary Pharmacology 1:93–99, 1988

Selzer ME, Dichter MA: Cellular pathophysiology and pharmacology of epilepsy, in Diseases of the Nervous System: Clinical Neurobiology, 2nd Edition. Edited by Asbury AK, McKhann GM, McDonald WI. Philadelphia, PA, WB Saunders, 1992, pp 916–935

Serra M, Madau P, Chessa MF, et al: 2-Phenyl-imidazol[1,2-a]pyridine derivatives as ligands for peripheral benzodiazepine receptors: stimulation of neurosteroid synthesis and anticonflict action in rats. Br J Pharmacol 127:177–187, 1999

Shah GN, Mooradian AD: Age-related changes in the blood-brain barrier. Exp Gerontol 32:501–509, 1997

Sharma HS, Westman J, Navarro JC, et al: Probable involvement of serotonin in the increased permeability of the blood-brain barrier by forced swimming. An experimental study using Evans blue and ^{131}I-sodium tracers in the rat. Behav Brain Res 72:189–196, 1995

Sharma ND, Rosman HS, Padhi ID, et al: Torsades de pointes associated with intravenous haloperidol in critically ill patients. Am J Cardiol 81:238–240, 1998

Sharma VK, Colecraft HM, Rubin LE, et al: Does mammalian heart contain only the M_2 muscarinic receptor subtype? Life Sci 60:1023–1029, 1997

Shibata M, Hori T, Kiyohara T, et al: Activity of hypothalamic thermosensitive neurons during cortical spreading depression in the rat. Brain Res 308:255–262, 1984

Shibata M, Hori T, Nagasaka T: Effects of single cortical spreading depression on metabolic heat production in the rat. Physiol Behav 34:563–567, 1985

Shintani S, Murase H, Tsukagoshi H, et al: Glycyrrhizin (licorice)-induced hypokalemic myopathy. Report of two cases and review of the literature. Eur Neurol 32:44–51, 1995

Skoog I, Wallin A, Fredman P, et al: A population study on blood-brain barrier function in 85-year-olds: relation to Alzheimer's disease and vascular dementia. Neurology 50:966–971, 1998

Skop BP, Finkelstein J, Mareth TR, et al: The serotonin syndrome associated with paroxetine, an over-the-counter cold remedy, and vascular disease: a case report and review. Am J Emerg Med 12:642–644, 1994

Slee AM, Kim TS, Liebling M, et al: Cerebellar degeneration in neuroleptic malignant syndrome: neuropathologic findings and review of the literature concerning heat-related nervous system injury. J Neurol Neurosurg Psychiatry 52:387–391, 1989

Smith SS, Gong GH, Hsu FC, et al: GABA receptor $alpha_4$ subunit suppression prevents withdrawal properties of an endogenous steroid. Nature 392:926–930, 1998

Smolders I, Bogaert L, Ebinger G, et al: Muscarinic modulation of striatal dopamine, glutamate, and GABA release, as measured with in vivo microdialysis. J Neurochem 68:1942–1948, 1997

Sontheimer H: Voltage-dependent ion channels in glial cells. Glia 11:156–172, 1994

Soriani S, Carrozzi M, De Carlo L, et al: Endozepine stupor in children. Cephalalgia 17:658–661, 1997

Sperber EF, Veliskova J, Germano IM, et al: Age-dependent vulnerability to seizures. Adv Neurol 79: 161–169, 1999

Spier SA, Frontera MA: Unexpected deaths in depressed medical inpatients treated with fluoxetine. J Clin Psychiatry 52:377–382, 1991

Spirt MJ, Chan W, Thieberg M, et al: Neuroleptic malignant syndrome induced by domperidone. Dig Dis Sci 37:946–948, 1992

Spivak B, Weizman A, Wolvick L, et al: Neuroleptic malignant syndrome during abrupt reduction of neuroleptic treatment. Acta Psychiatr Scand 81:168–169, 1990

Spivak B, Gonen N, Mester R, et al: Neuroleptic malignant syndrome associated with abrupt withdrawal of anticholinergic agents. Int Clin Psychopharmacol 11:207–209, 1996

Sporer KA: The serotonin syndrome. Implicated drugs, pathophysiology and management. Drug Saf 13:94–104, 1995

Stambolic V, Ruel L, Woodgett JR: Lithium inhibits glycogen synthase kinase-3 activity and mimics wingless signalling in intact cells. Curr Biol 6:1664–1668, 1996

Sternbach H: The serotonin syndrome. Am J Psychiatry 148:705–713, 1991

Sternberg EM, Chrousos GP, Wilder RL, et al: The stress response and the regulation of inflammatory disease. Ann Intern Med 117:854–866, 1992

Steulet AF, Hauser K, Martin P, et al: Reversal by apomorphine of the gabaculine-induced GABA accumulation in mouse cortex. Eur J Pharmacol 174:161–170, 1989

Stevens E, Roman A, Houa M, et al: Severe hyperthermia during tetrabenazine therapy for tardive dyskinesia. Intensive Care Med 24:369–371, 1998

Still J, Friedman B, Law E, et al: Neuroleptic malignant syndrome in a burn patient. Burns 24:573–575, 1998

Stone TW: Neuropharmacology of quinolinic and kynurenic acids. Pharmacol Rev 45:309–379, 1993

Study RE, Baker JL: Diazepam and (-)-pentobarbital: fluctuation analysis reveals different mechanisms for potentiation of gamma-aminobutyric acid responses in cultured central neurons. Proc Natl Acad Sci U S A 78:7180–7184, 1981

Swanson CL Jr, Price WA, McEvoy JP: Effects of concomitant risperidone and lithium treatment (letter). Am J Psychiatry 152:1096, 1995

Sykova E, Chvatal A: Glial cells and volume transmission in the CNS. Neurochem Int 36:397–409, 2000

Tanaka E: In vivo age-related changes in hepatic drug-oxidizing capacity in humans. J Clin Pharm Ther 23:247–255, 1998

Tang CP, Leung CM, Ungvari GS, et al: The syndrome of lethal catatonia. Singapore Med J 36:400–402, 1995

Teoh H, Malcangio M, Bowery NG: GABA, glutamate and substance P-like immunoreactivity release: effects of novel $GABA_B$ antagonists. Br J Pharmacol 118:1153–1160, 1996

Tinuper P, Montagna P, Cortelli P, et al: Idiopathic recurring stupor: a case with possible involvement of the gamma-aminobutyric acid (GABA)ergic system. Ann Neurol 31:503–506, 1992

Tinuper P, Montagna P, Plazzi G, et al: Idiopathic recurring stupor. Neurology 44:621–625, 1994

Trzepacz PT: The neuropathogenesis of delirium: a need to focus our research. Psychosomatics 35:374–391, 1994

Trzepacz PT: Is there a final common neural pathway in delirium? Focus on acetylcholine and dopamine. Seminars in Clinical Neuropsychiatry 5:132–148, 2000

Trzepacz PT, Francis J: Low serum albumin levels and risk of delirium (letter). Am J Psychiatry 147:675, 1990

Trzepacz PT, DiMartini A, Tringali RA: Psychopharmacologic issues in organ transplantation. Part I: pharmacokinetics in organ failure and psychiatric aspects of immunosuppressants and anti-infectious agents. Psychosomatics 34:199–207, 1993

Trzepacz PT, Brown TM, Stoudemire A: Substance-induced delirium, in Treatments of Psychiatric Disorders, 2nd Edition, Vol 1. Edited by Gabbard GO. Washington, DC, American Psychiatric Press, 1995, pp 445–478

Tunnicliff G, Schindler NL, Crites GJ, et al: The $GABA_A$ receptor complex as a target for fluoxetine action. Neurochem Res 24:1271–1276, 1999

Turecek R, Trussell LO: Control of synaptic depression by glutamate transporters. J Neurosci 20:2054–2063, 2000

Turjanski N, Lees AJ: Gamma vinyl GABA in the treatment of levodopa-induced dyskinesias in Parkinson's disease (letter). J Neurol Neurosurg Psychiatry 55:413, 1992

Turnheim K: Drug dosage in the elderly. Is it rational? Drugs Aging 13:357–379, 1998

Tuxen MK, Hansen SW: Neurotoxicity secondary to antineoplastic drugs. Cancer Treat Rev 20:191–214, 1994

Twyman RE, Rogers CJ, MacDonald RL: Differential regulation of gamma-aminobutyric acid receptor channels by diazepam and pentobarbital. Ann Neurol 25:213–220, 1989

Ueda M, Hamamoto M, Nagayama H, et al: Susceptibility to neuroleptic malignant syndrome in Parkinson's disease. Neurology 52:777–781, 1999

Ulmer JB, Braun PE: Chloroform markedly stimulates the phosphorylation of myelin basic proteins. Biochem Biophys Res Commun 146:1084–1088, 1987

Unseld E, Ziegler G, Gemeinhardt A, et al: Possible interaction of fluoroquinolones with the benzodiazepine-$GABA_A$-receptor complex. Br J Clin Pharmacol 30:63–70, 1990

Valentino RJ, Curtis AL: Pharmacology of locus coeruleus spontaneous and sensory-evoked activity. Prog Brain Res 88:249–256, 1991

van der Mast RC: Pathophysiology of delirium. J Geriatr Psychiatry Neurol 11:138–145,157–158, 1998

van der Mast RC, Fekkes D: Serotonin and amino acids: partners in delirium pathophysiology? Seminars in Clinical Neuropsychiatry 5:125–131, 2000

van Engelen BG, Gimbrere JS, Booy LH: Benzodiazepine withdrawal reaction in two children following discontinuation of sedation with midazolam. Ann Pharmacother 27:579–581, 1993

Veith RC, Lewis N, Linares OQ, et al: Sympathetic nervous system activity in major depression. Arch Gen Psychiatry 51:411–422, 1994

Velisek L, Veliskova J, Moshe SL: Site-specific effects of local pH changes in the substantia nigra pars reticulata in flurothyl-induced seizures. Brain Res 782:310–313, 1998

Veliskova J, Loscher W, Moshe SL: Regional and age specific effects of zolpidem microinfusions in the substantia nigra on seizures. Epilepsy Res 30:107–114, 1998

Verhofstad AA, Steinbusch HW, Penke B, et al: Serotonin-immunoreactive cells in the superior cervical ganglion of the rat. Evidence for the existence of separate serotonin- and catecholamine-containing small ganglionic cells. Brain Res 212:39–49, 1981

Vidal C, Suaudeau C, Jacob J: Hyper- and hypothermia induced by non-noxious stress: effects of naloxone, diazepam and gamma-acetylenic GABA. Life Sci 33 (suppl 1):587–590, 1983

Vidal-Puig A, Solanes G, Grujic D, et al: UCP3: an uncoupling protein homologue expressed preferentially and abundantly in skeletal muscle and brown adipose tissue. Biochem Biophys Res Commun 235:79–82, 1997

Vizi ES, Sperlagh B: Separation of carrier mediated and vesicular release of GABA from rat brain slices. Neurochem Int 34:407–413, 1999

Volkow ND, Gur RC, Wang GJ, et al: Association between decline in brain dopamine activity with age and cognitive and motor impairment in healthy individuals. Am J Psychiatry 155:344–349, 1998

Wagner W, Vause EW: Fluvoxamine. A review of global drug-drug interaction data. Clin Pharmacokinet 29 (suppl 1):26–32, 1995

Wala EP, Sloan JW, Jing X: Substantia nigra: the involvement of central and peripheral benzodiazepine receptors in physical dependence on diazepam as evidenced by behavioral and EEG effects. Pharmacol Biochem Behav 64:611–623, 1999

Waldrop TG, Bauer RM, Iwamoto GA: Microinjection of GABA antagonists into the posterior hypothalamus elicits locomotor activity and a cardiorespiratory activation. Brain Res 444:84–94, 1988

Walker MFC: Simulation of tetanus by trifluoperazine overdosage. CMAJ 81:109–110, 1959

Walter HJ, Messing RO: Regulation of neuronal voltage-gated calcium channels by ethanol. Neurochem Int 35:95–101, 1999

Wardas J, Ossoska K, Wolfarth S: Evidence for the independent role of GABA synapses of the zona incerta-lateral hypothalamic region in haloperidol-induced catalepsy. Brain Res 462:378–382, 1988

Watts RL, Mandir AS: The role of motor cortex in the pathophysiology of voluntary movement deficits associated with parkinsonism. Neurol Clin 10:451–469, 1992

Weight FF, Aguayo LG, White G, et al: GABA- and glutamate-gated ion channels as molecular sites of alcohol and anesthetic action. Adv Biochem Psychopharmacol 47:335–347, 1992

Weller M, Kornhuber J: Pathophysiologie und therapie des malignen neuroleptischen syndroms. Nervenarzt 63:645–655, 1992

Wengel SP, Roccaforte WH, Burke WJ: Donepezil improves symptoms of delirium in dementia: implications for future research. J Geriatr Psychiatry Neurol 11:159–161, 1998

Westheimer R, Klawans HL: The role of serotonin in the pathophysiology of myoclonus seizures associated with acute imipramine toxicity. Neurology 24:1175–1177, 1974

Whiting PJ: The GABA-A receptor gene family: new targets for therapeutic intervention. Neurochem Int 34:387–390, 1999

Wirkner K, Poelchen W, Koles L, et al: Ethanol-induced inhibition of NMDA receptor channels. Neurochem Int 35:153–162, 1999

Wise MG: Delirium due to a general medical condition, delirium due to multiple etiologies, and delirium not otherwise specified, in Treatments of Psychiatric Disorders, 2nd Edition, Vol 1. Gabbard GO, Editor-in-Chief. Washington, DC, American Psychiatric Press, 1995, pp 423–443

Wolf OT, Kirschbaum C: Actions of dehydroepiandrosterone and its sulfate in the central nervous system: effects on cognition and emotion in animals and humans. Brain Res Brain Res Rev 30:264–288, 1999

Worms P, Lloyd KG: Biphasic effects of direct, but not indirect, GABA mimetics and antagonists on haloperidol-induced catalepsy. Naunyn Schmiedebergs Arch Pharmacol 311:179–184, 1980

Xiong ZQ, Stringer JL: Sodium pump activity, not glial spatial buffering, clears potassium after epileptiform activity in the dentate gyrus. J Neurophysiol 83:1443–1451, 2000

Yaron I, Shirazi I, Judovich R, et al: Fluoxetine and amitriptyline inhibit nitric oxide, prostaglandin E2, and hyaluronic acid production in human synovial cells and synovial tissue cultures. Arthritis Rheum 42:2561–2568, 1999

Young C: A case of neuroleptic malignant syndrome and serotonin disturbance (letter). J Clin Psychopharmacol 17:65–66, 1997

Yuhas Y, Shulman L, Weizman A, et al: Involvement of tumor necrosis factor alpha and interleukin-1-beta in enhancement of pentylenetetrazole-induced seizures caused by *Shigella dysenteriae*. Infect Immun 67:1455–1460, 1999

Zahs KR: Heterotypic coupling between glial cells of the mammalian central nervous system. Glia 24: 85–96, 1998

Zalsman G, Hermesh H, Munitz H: Alprazolam withdrawal delirium: a case report. Clin Neuropharmacol 21:201–202, 1998

Zanassi P, Paolillo M, Montecucco A, et al: Pharmacological and molecular evidence for dopamine (D_1) receptor expression by striatal astrocytes in culture. J Neurosci Res 58:544–552, 1999

Zhao H, Asai S, Kohno T, et al: Effects of brain temperature on CBF thresholds for extracellular glutamate release and reuptake in a rat model of graded global ischemia. Neuroreport 9:3183–3188, 1998

Zhelyazkova-Savova M, Giovannini MG, Pepeu G: Systemic chlorophenylpiperazine increases acetylcholine release from rat hippocampus—implication of 5-HT_{2C} receptors. Pharmacol Res 40:165–170, 1999

20

Alzheimer's Disease

Donna L. Masterman, M.D., M.S.
Jeffrey L. Cummings, M.D.

Alzheimer's disease (AD), a slowly progressive degenerative cortical dementia, is the most common dementing illness in elderly persons. The prevalence of AD has increased to become one of the most important diseases affecting society. Current estimates indicate that AD afflicts between 2 and 4 million persons in the United States (Evans 1990; Evans et al. 1989), a number that is expected to increase to 9 million by the year 2030 (U.S. Bureau of the Census 1992). It accounts for 40%–59% of nursing home admissions (Katzman et al. 1989) and imposes an expanding economic burden on patients, their families, and the nation. It is the third most expensive disease to treat in the United States behind heart disease and cancer, with an overall estimated annual cost between $80 and $100 billion. Effective treatments are urgently needed, and even seemingly small improvements can have a tremendous overall effect. For example, if treatments were identified that could delay the onset of symptoms by 5 years, the prevalence could be reduced by 50% in one generation. Moreover, effective symptomatic treatment would help delay nursing home placement and thereby reduce costs substantially.

Current research is actively focused on developing new drugs that not only will provide symptomatic improvement of cognitive function but also may slow disease progression, and, ultimately, researchers would like to find ways to prevent AD altogether.

This project was supported by the National Institute on Aging–Alzheimer's Disease Core Center Grant AG 10123.

In this chapter, we review a variety of treatment approaches under consideration for AD. We focus on pharmacological interventions aimed at treatment of both cognitive and behavioral symptoms of the disease and potential disease-modifying treatments. We also discuss nonpharmacological strategies for the management of neuropsychiatric symptoms frequently accompanying this illness.

Approaches to Therapy

Understanding of the pathological changes that occur in AD and their potential links to etiology and pathogenesis of the disease have major implications for the development and application of new therapeutic strategies. A complete and detailed discourse of the many research advances into potential disease pathogenesis is beyond the scope of this chapter, but pivotal findings and theories directly related to drug development are highlighted.

Current therapeutic strategies include symptomatic treatment directed at neurotransmitter and neuromodulator enhancement. Potential neuroprotective strategies and disease-modifying approaches have focused on the development of antiamyloidogenic compounds, free-radical scavengers, and anti-inflammatory agents; hormonal approaches; enhancement of cell growth or regeneration with compounds such as nerve growth factor (NGF); and the potential use of stem cell transplantation and genetically engineered tissue. Nootropics, nonspecific cerebral metabolic enhancers and herbal compounds, and other neutraceuticals are also areas of further investigation. The neuropsychiatric disturbances associated with AD are also a major source of disease morbidity and have been receiving increasing attention in AD research. Treatment approaches have been aimed largely at neurotransmitter manipulation. Effective disease management also must use nonpharmacological management strategies and continue to address the needs of the caregiver.

Moreover, as new therapies are rapidly being developed for AD, it becomes even more important to be able to accurately diagnose the underlying cause of the dementia and to recognize early cases of dementia that may benefit from these newer therapies. Delaying the time to onset of symptoms, slowing the progression of the disease, improving symptoms and reducing disease morbidity, modifying risk factors, and preventing the disease are all goals of current therapeutic research (Figure 20–1).

Pharmacological Interventions

Symptomatic Treatments

Cholinergic Augmentation

Since the acetylcholine (ACh) deficit associated with AD was recognized in the mid-1970s, there has been a systematic attempt to increase central cholinergic activity by pharmacological manipulation. Both animal and human studies indicate that the cholinergic system plays an important role in memory function, and cholinergic dysfunction resulting from loss of basal forebrain cholinergic neurons is the most marked and consistent neurotransmitter deficiency in AD. This stems from the loss of neurons that synthesize the choline acetyltransferase (ChAT) needed to catalyze the synthesis of ACh. Attempts to ameliorate the cognitive deterioration in AD through augmentation of the cholinergic system have included administering ACh precursors, increasing ACh release, inhibiting acetylcholin-

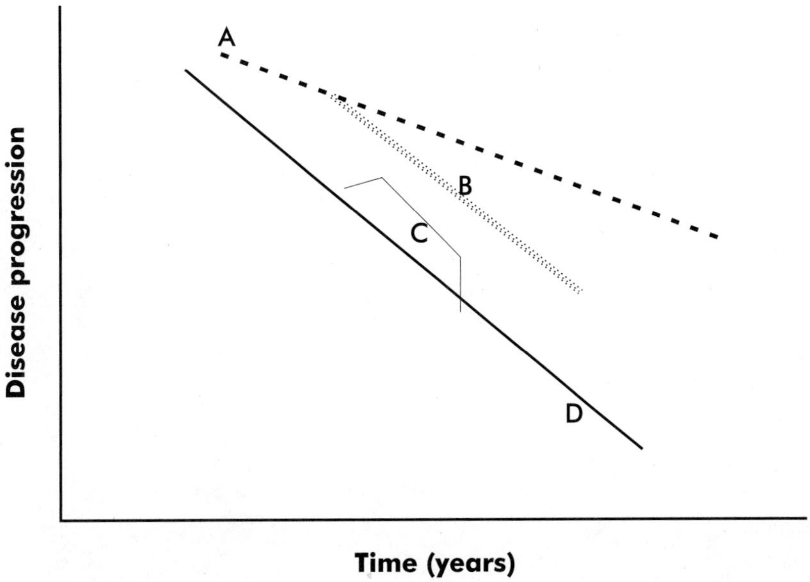

FIGURE 20–1. Therapeutic approaches to Alzheimer's disease include slowing the progression of the disease *(A)*, delaying the time to onset of symptoms *(B)*, and improving symptoms *(C)*. D = natural disease progression.

esterase (AChE) to slow synaptic degradation of ACh, directly stimulating muscarinic cholinergic receptors, and administering compounds that can retard cholinergic neuronal cell loss (Table 20–1).

Acetylcholine precursors. Use of the ACh precursors choline and phosphatidylcholine (lecithin) has been investigated as therapy for AD because these compounds have been shown to increase brain levels of ACh in rats (Heyman et al. 1987). Oral administration of choline results in elevated blood and cerebrospinal levels of choline. It was hoped that the effect of choline and phosphatidylcholine would be dramatic, comparable to the administration of dopamine precursors in the treatment of Parkinson's disease. However, results from several double-blind, placebo-controlled clinical trials were disappointing. Minimal improvement on a test of word recognition in one trial of choline was demonstrated, and only 10 of 43 clinical trials reported any positive effect (Becker and Giacobini 1988). The loss of ChAT in AD may prevent the formation of ACh from precursors, or the choline supply may not be the rate-limiting step in the formation of ACh (Galasko and Thal 1990).

Drugs enhancing acetylcholine release. 4-Aminopyridine, an agent that increases ACh release, has not been found to improve cognition in AD patients (Davidson et al. 1988; Galasko and Thal 1990). Linopridine, a novel phenylindolinone compound, increases ACh release. It appears to selectively enhance physiological ACh release and also enhances release of noradrenaline and serotonin, both of which are known to be decreased in AD (Cook et al. 1990). However, no clinical benefit was seen in a recent multicenter, randomized, double-blind, placebo-controlled trial with 382 patients (Rockwood et al. 1997).

TABLE 20–1. Cholinergic enhancers

Precursors/synthesis enhancers
Choline
Lecithin
Acetyl-L-carnitine (ALCAR)
Drugs enhancing acetylcholine release
4-Aminopyridine
Linopridine
Acetylcholinesterase inhibitors
Physostigmine
Tacrine
Donepezil
Rivastigmine
Galanthamine
Metrifonate
Eptastigmine
Huperazine A
Muscarinic agonists
Milameline
Xanomeline
Arecoline
Oxotremorine
Sabcomeline (SB-202026)
Talsaclidine

Acetylcholinesterase inhibitors. Investigation of cholinesterase inhibitors has been the predominant approach for the symptomatic treatment of AD. Synaptic ACh is hydrolized by a group of enzymes called cholinesterases, which can be classified into two groups: AChEs, found primarily in neuronal tissue, and butyrylcholinesterases (pseudocholinesterases), found primarily in peripheral tissue. The acetylcholinesterase inhibitors retard the breakdown of intrasynaptic ACh, thus prolonging the action of ACh at postsynaptic receptor sites. Furthermore, some recent evidence indicates that some cholinesterase inhibitors may also have direct effects on peptide processing, neurotransmitter receptors, and ion channels that are not yet fully understood. Early investigations with physostigmine, a very short-acting, reversible acetylcholinesterase inhibitor, showed modest improvement in subjects' memory and cognition (Becker and Giacobini 1988; Thal et al. 1996). This effect was enhanced in studies that used individualized dosing.

Tacrine. Tacrine (9-amino-1,2,3,4-tetrahydroacridine; THA), a longer-acting AChE agent, has been available in the United States since 1993 for the symptomatic treatment of mild to moderate AD. It is a reversible cholinesterase inhibitor and inhibits plasma and tissue cholinesterase with a higher affinity for butyrylcholinesterases and AChE. THA may also have direct effects on cholinergic receptors, synthesis and release of ACh and other neurotransmitters, sodium (Na^+) and potassium (K^+) ion channels, and other actions.

Early encouraging trials of THA (Summers et al. 1981, 1986) and the studies involving physostigmine suggested the importance of dosage individualization and led to the

National Institute on Aging/Mount Sinai Medical Center THA Study, a large-scale multicenter placebo-controlled trial with an enriched population design. This study included mildly to moderately impaired community-dwelling patients without significant medical illness. Small but statistically significant results favored THA over placebo (in THA responders) on the cognitive subscale of the Alzheimer's Disease Assessment Scale (ADAS) and on the Instrumental Activities of Daily Living (IADL) scale and the Progressive Deterioration Scale (PDS). However, no significant differences were found on the Clinicians' Global Impression of Change (CGIC), the behavioral subscale of the ADAS, or the Physical Self-Maintenance Scale (PSMS) (Davis et al. 1992).

Another large-scale multicenter trial (Farlow et al. 1992) with a 12-week two-stage double-blind, placebo-controlled, parallel-group design also found significant improvement on the cognitive subscale of the ADAS and on both physician- and caregiver-rated CGIC for 80 mg of THA compared with placebo and on the caregiver-rated CGIC for 40 mg/day. A French multisite study with a similar design demonstrated statistically significant results favoring THA only on the cognitive subscale of the ADAS (Schneider 1993). The treatment effects were again modest: about 4 points each on the 70-point ADAS cognitive subscale and the 115-point ADAS total scale. The ADAS total score has been found to deteriorate about 8 points per year in the natural history of AD. A parallel-group 30-week trial (Knapp et al. 1994) of THA at 80, 120, and 160 mg/day showed statistically significant dose-response trends favoring THA on the cognitive subscale of the ADAS, on the Clinician's Interview-Based Impression of Change (CIBIC), and on a global assessment instrument that included family member input (Clinician's Interview-Based Impression of Change with Caregiver Input [CIBIC-Plus]). Follow-up studies on THA have shown its use to delay the time to nursing home placement (Knopman et al. 1996).

The pharmacokinetics of THA are distinguished by dose nonlinearity with variability in elimination half-life, from 1.4 to 3.6 hours. Adverse effects of THA observed most commonly include peripheral cholinergic effects and reversible hepatotoxicity. Nausea, vomiting, diarrhea, dyspepsia, and anorexia appear to be dose-dependent and lead to patient withdrawal. In a combined analysis of five multicenter clinical trials involving 2,446 patients exposed to THA, the levels of alanine aminotransferase (ALT) were elevated in 49% of the exposed patients and were greater than three times the upper limit of normal in 25% of the patients. The average time to first ALT value greater than three times the upper limit of normal was 7 weeks, and 90% of such elevations occurred within the first 12 weeks of treatment. ALT levels returned to normal in all patients after drug discontinuation. Among 145 patients rechallenged with THA after discontinuation because of a rise in ALT to greater than three times the upper limit of normal, 128 (88%) were able to tolerate long-term therapy with THA.

THA is available in 10-, 20-, 30-, and 40-mg tablets and is to be initiated at 10 mg four times a day. This dose should be maintained for 6 weeks while ALT levels are monitored on a weekly basis. Dosage can be increased by 40 mg/day at 6-week intervals to a maximum dose of 160 mg, providing that no significant elevations of transaminase levels or other adverse reactions occur. THA has no effect on the underlying disease process, and deterioration in cognitive functions will recur as the number of functioning cholinergic neurons declines. Patients should be withdrawn from the drug when continuing functional decline is evident or when incapacity is severe.

A racemate of the primary metabolite, velnacrine, has also undergone clinical investigation as a possible treatment for AD but has been limited by hepatotoxicity.

Donepezil hydrochloride. Donepezil gained U.S. Food and Drug Administration (FDA) approval in 1996 for the treatment of mild to moderate AD. It was the first of the newer class of reversible cholinesterase inhibitors, the piperidines. It does not contain the acridine group, which has been linked to the hepatotoxicity. It has specificity for the neuronal form of AChE with little butyrylcholinesterase inhibition. In double-blind, placebo-controlled trials of donepezil in AD, treatment was associated with improvement in cognition and global function compared with placebo (S.L. Rogers et al. 1996, 1998). In the 30-week double-blind, placebo-controlled study of donepezil, clinical trial patients were randomized to 5 mg/day of donepezil, 10 mg/day of donepezil, or placebo followed by a 6-week single-blind washout period. The treatment benefit on the ADAS cognitive subscale and other global measures that was seen during the first 24 weeks was lost after a 6-week washout, which is what one might expect for a solely symptomatic therapy.

Donepezil has minimal hepatotoxic effects, and no laboratory monitoring is required by the FDA. The drug's half-life is approximately 70 hours, allowing for once-a-day dosing. Steady state is achieved usually by 15 days. It is highly protein-bound (94%) and is metabolized by the hepatic P450 system. No drug interactions were seen with warfarin, cimetidine, theophylline, or digoxin. The current recommendations are to start donepezil at a 5-mg oral dose in the evening, just before bedtime. This dosage should be maintained for at least 1 month before considering a dose increase to the maximum recommended, which is 10 mg once a day. This slow dose titration minimizes side effects. Patients should be followed up for 4 weeks after starting donepezil to determine tolerability and compliance. Most adverse effects are mild and transient, although they may require symptomatic management for a short period. The most common side effects of donepezil are diarrhea, muscle cramps, nausea, vomiting, fatigue, dizziness, and insomnia.

Most clinical trials with cholinesterase inhibitors have included only patients with Mini-Mental State Exam (MMSE; Folstein et al. 1975) scores of 10–26 at entry; therefore, particular thought and caution should be exercised in prescribing treatment to patients scoring above or below this range. Patients with very mild and early signs of cognitive failure that are insufficient to meet criteria for a dementia syndrome, usually will not be eligible for symptomatic treatment with donepezil. Requests by caregivers or families for treatment of patients with severe dementia should be dealt with sympathetically but realistically.

Patients whose condition has deteriorated significantly after 12 weeks of treatment usually should be advised to discontinue medication. Patients whose condition is unchanged at 3 months, or for whom uncertainty or disagreement about the response exists, should be reevaluated after a period of time (3–6 months). No information is currently available to guide prescribers as to when patients who have previously responded to donepezil should stop taking it. This judgment will need to be made in close consultation with the patient and caregiver and/or family. Patients should be closely observed after medication is stopped in case a precipitous decline occurs, which would justify rapid reinstatement.

A variety of postdiagnostic guidelines for treating patients with AD have been documented in the literature (American Medical Association 1999; American Psychiatric Association 1997; California Workgroup on Guidelines for Alzheimer's Disease Management 1999; Swanwick and Lawlor 1998; Small et al. 1997).

Other cholinesterase inhibitors. Three drugs—THA, donepezil, and rivastigmine—are currently approved in the United States for the treatment of AD, and a fourth drug—galanthamine (available in Europe)—is awaiting FDA approval. (The application for another drug—metrifonate—was recently withdrawn because of potential serious side effects.) Other similar compounds are under investigation (Table 20–2), and they differ somewhat with respect to their pharmacokinetic properties, their specificities for AChE and butyrylcholinesterase, and their reversibility.

Rivastigmine is a carbamate AChE inhibitor with selectivity for the central nervous system. It is pseudoirreversible, meaning that the drug has a prolonged duration of action, with AChE being inhibited for several hours after the drug has been metabolized and eliminated (Anand et al. 1996). Drug metabolism does not use the hepatic cytochrome P450 enzyme system. Several large-scale, multinational clinical trials have been conducted, and all showed efficacy in the symptomatic treatment of mild to moderate AD (Anand et al. 1996; Corey-Bloom et al. 1998; Rösler et al. 1999). In a large prospective, double-blind, placebo-controlled trial of 725 patients with mild to moderate AD in 45 centers across Europe and North America, significant improvement was seen in cognition, as measured by the ADAS cognitive subscale, and on global measures and in activities of daily living (Rösler et al. 1999). The dose was titrated up from 1–4 mg twice a day to a target dose of 6–12 mg/day. The drug was generally well tolerated, and the principal side effect was gastrointestinal symptoms, which were often transient and usually of mild to moderate severity.

Galanthamine, a phenanthrene alkaloid isolated from the European daffodil or common snowdrop, is a reversible inhibitor of AChE (Nordberg and Svensson 1998). It also exerts an effect on presynaptic nicotinic receptors. It is metabolized by the cytochrome P450 enzyme system and yields a potent metabolite, sanguinine, which is three times as powerful as the parent compound and accounts for 20% of the administered galanthamine. No liver toxicity has been reported, but as with the other acetylcholinesterase inhibitors, gastrointestinal symptoms are the most common side effect and occur in fewer than 4% of patients taking galanthamine (Rainer 1997a, 1997b). A recent multinational clinical trial with galantamine involving 653 patients with AD found galantamine to be more effective than placebo on the ADAS cognitive subscale, the CIBIC-Plus, and the Disability Assessment for Dementia over the 6 months of the trial (Wilcock et al. 2000). This finding is in keeping with results of a recent U.S. phase III clinical trial showing similar efficacy in patients with mild to moderate AD (Tariot et al. 2000).

Metrifonate is a prodrug that is converted nonenzymatically to the active metabolite 2,2-dichlorovinyl dimethyl phosphate (DDVP) (Hinz et al. 1996b). This metabolite forms a stable complex with the AChE enzyme, resulting in long-lasting inhibition (Hinz et al. 1996a), and can be given once a day. In a 6-month randomized, double-blind, placebo-controlled trial in patients with mild to moderate AD who received a single daily dose of 30–60 mg of metrifonate (based on the patient's weight), significant improvements were seen in cognition, as measured by the ADAS cognitive subscale; in global function; and in behavior, as measured by the Neuropsychiatric Inventory (NPI) (Cummings et al. 1998; Morris et al. 1998). In another prospective multicenter 26-week trial of 264 patients with mild to moderate AD receiving a fixed dosage of 50 mg/day of metrifonate, significant improvements also were seen in cognition, behavior, and daily functioning (Raskind et al. 1999). The new drug application for FDA approval of metrifonate was recently withdrawn because of serious potential side effects.

Eptastigmine is another AChE inhibitor that has been studied in phase III clinical trials. Although it has shown significant benefit, potential adverse hematological effects may limit its clinical utility (Imbimbo et al. 1999).

TABLE 20–2. Cholinesterase-inhibiting drugs approved or under investigation for the treatment of Alzheimer's disease

Drug	Trade name	Drug class	Relative degree of cholinesterase inhibition	Reversibility	Metabolism	Half-life (hours)	Dose (mg)	Frequency	Study duration (weeks)	ADAS-cog (placebo vs drug)
Tacrine	Cognex	Acridine	AChE = BChE	Reversible	Hepatic	1.3–7	10–40	qid	12–30	1.4–3.8
Donepezil	Aricept	Piperidine	AChE >> BChE	Reversible	Hepatic	70–80	5–10	qd	12–24	2.5–2.9
Rivastigmine	Exelon	Carbamate	AChE > BChE	Pseudo-irreversible	Nonhepatic	2	3–6	bid	26	1.9–3.8
Metrifonate	ProMem	Organophosphate	AChE = BChE	Irreversible	Enzymatic	2	50–80	qd	26	2.9
Galanthamine	Reminyl	Alkaloid	AChE > BChE	Reversible	Hepatic	5.7	10	tid	13	3.1
Physostigmine	Synapton	Tertiary amine	AChE > BChE	Reversible	Enzymatic	—	—	—	—	—

Note. AChE = acetylcholinesterase; BchE = butyrylcholinesterase; ADAS-cog = Alzheimer's Disease Assessment Scale cognitive subscale.

Direct receptor agonists. The fact that postsynaptic muscarinic receptors (the primary type of cholinergic receptor in the neocortex) are preserved in AD (Davies and Verth 1977) supports the use of direct agonists. The number of direct postsynaptic muscarinic receptor agonists is limited, and their use is curbed by prominent peripheral side effects on blood pressure, vision, and salivation. Trials of arecoline, RS-86, oxotremorine, and pilocarpine have not shown consistent benefit (Crook 1988). Arecoline, a muscarinic agonist that crosses the blood-brain barrier, was administered in 12 patients with AD under a 2-hour intravenous infusion compared with a placebo infusion. The infusions were well tolerated, but the treatment failed to show any significant improvement in cognitive performance (Tariot et al. 1988). Xanomeline, a muscarinic agonist, showed some modest benefit in clinical trials (Bodick et al. 1997). Other agonists such as sabcomeline (SB-202026), a functionally selective M_1-receptor partial agonist; RU35926; WAL 2014; and other novel muscarinic agonists have shown some promise in animal studies (Adamus et al. 1995; Hatcher et al. 1998; Sedman et al. 1995).

Trials of direct intraventricular therapy with bethanechol have shown modest improvement in behavior and mood (Penn et al. 1988) or memory (Read et al. 1990) in a subset of patients whose clinical diagnosis of probable AD was confirmed by senile plaque quantification in cortical biopsy specimens. Both a narrow therapeutic window for positive effects and substantial interindividual variation in optimum dose were observed. Significant neurosurgical morbidity was associated with the required intraventricular catheter placement.

Nicotinic receptors are also present in the neocortex, but these are thought to function as presynaptic receptors, and there is evidence of marked loss of cortical nicotinic receptors in AD brain at autopsy. In a pilot study, nicotine infusion decreased intrusion errors on memory testing but increased anxiety and depression (Newhouse et al. 1988). Positron-emission tomography (PET) studies also report losses of frontal and temporal nicotinic receptors in AD patients compared with control subjects, with a lower uptake of labeled nicotine. In one PET study, the cholinesterase inhibitor THA increased the uptake of nicotine, a finding that is compatible with a restoration of nicotinic cholinergic receptors, and normalized the ratio of the (R)(+)– and (S)(–D)-nicotinic enantiomers. These effects were associated with an increase in glucose metabolism, but not blood flow, and with improvement in neuropsychological test performance in some patients with early-onset AD (Nordberg 1993).

Acetyl-L-carnitine (ALCAR), developed with the aim of augmenting ACh synthesis, protects against excitotoxic injury in vitro and promotes membrane stability and energy production. It has shown only modest benefits in clinical trials (Rai et al. 1990; Spagnoli et al. 1991).

Drugs affecting other neurotransmitter systems. Certain populations of neurons are lost selectively in AD, namely, neurons of the association cortices, cholinergic neurons of the nucleus basalis of Meynert, and subcortical nuclei such as the serotonergic cells of the raphe and adrenergic cells in the locus coeruleus. Decreased cholinergic activity is well described in AD and has been discussed earlier in this chapter. Serotonergic neurons in the dorsal raphe nuclei contain many neuritic plaques and neurofibrillary tangles, and serotonin deficiencies are also documented in AD. Levels of γ-aminobutyric acid (GABA) are decreased, but dopaminergic neurons are relatively spared. Levels of somatostatin, neuropeptide Y, substance P, corticotropin-releasing hormone, and other neuropeptides are also characteristically decreased (for review, see Blass 1993). In one study in rats, performance on retention tests was enhanced when cholinomimetic therapy was combined with the noradrenergic receptor agonist clonidine (Davis and Haroutunian 1993). Combination pharmacotherapy with cholinergic and noradrenergic agents is currently being evaluated in AD patients.

Limited studies of the effects of selective serotonin reuptake inhibitors (SSRIs) in AD patients have failed to show significant effects on cognition (Cutler et al. 1985; Mody and Miller 1990). However, a trend toward a correlation between, on the one hand, cognitive improvement and, on the other, low pretreatment ratio of plasma tryptophan to other large neutral amino acids (indicative of low brain serotonin levels) was noted in a study of non-depressed dementia patients (Jorgenson et al. 1993). This suggestion of a subgroup of SSRI responders among dementia patients awaits confirmation.

Trials with GABA-agonist and dopaminergic compounds have had negative results, discouraging interventions directed at these neurotransmitter systems (Crook 1988). Memantine is a blocker of glutamate gated *N*-methyl-D-aspartate (NMDA) receptor channels, allowing physiological activation of the rapid, voltage-dependent gating mechanism, but blocking pathological activation (Kornhuber et al. 1989, Parsons et al. 1993). Placebo-controlled clinical trials of memantine in both patients with mild to moderate dementia and those with severe dementia have been evaluated (Görtelmeyer and Erbler 1992, Pantev et al. 1993; Winblad and Poritis 1999). The results have indicated mild improvements in function and reduced care dependence in severely demented patients.

Disease-Modifying Approaches

Antiamyloid and Tau Strategies

The cause and the mechanism by which neurons are triggered to die in AD are unknown. A key pathological feature of AD involves the extensive accumulation of neuritic plaques and neurofibrillary tangles in the brain. Amyloid plaques are extracellular, spherical, amorphous deposits composed of 6- to 10-nm fibrils of a protein known as β-amyloid with a surrounding cluster of dystrophic neuritic processes. The predominantly β-pleated sheet configuration of β-amyloid arises as a result of abnormal processing. It has 40–42 residues and is derived from a larger precursor known as amyloid precursor protein (APP). APP has either 695 or 770 residues and is found normally in neurons. The normal function of APP is not fully understood, but it is known that the longer extracellular domain is cleaved from the molecule as a soluble protein, which appears to have regulatory functions.

Several lines of evidence have implicated abnormal amyloid deposition as an important feature in the pathogenesis of AD (Hyman 1998). The reasons for abnormal APP processing are obscure, possibly related to abnormal protease activity. Evidence indicates that β-amyloid is directly neurotoxic by disrupting the function of membrane proteins involved in the neuron's calcium homeostasis (Mattson 1992). It has also been suggested that β-amyloid enhances the neurotoxicity of other agents, although this also may be caused by disturbed calcium regulation. There is also evidence that normal regulation of APP processing is controlled by a positive feedback system from cholinergic neurons. Treatment with cholinomimetic agents not only may enhance cognition in patients with AD but also may slow down neurodegeneration by inhibiting abnormal APP processing (Lahiri et al. 1998).

Therapeutic approaches to interfere with the accumulation and deposition of amyloid are under active investigation. Similarly, compounds such as protease inhibitors, which may interfere with amyloid processing, and calcium channel blockers, which are important in intracellular signaling, are also under investigation as potential targets for treatment. Recently, one of the enzymes believed to be involved in abnormal splicing of the APP gene was identified and isolated and has become a potential target for drug development (Vassar et al. 1999). β-Secretase cleavage of Alzheimer's APP by the transmembrane aspartic protease β-site APP cleaving enzyme (BACE) has been identified (Rai et al. 1999). Another recent report by Schenk et al. (1999) showed that immunization of a genetically engineered mouse model of AD could decrease the number of neuritic plaques that accumulated in the brains of these animals when treated early in life. The study went on to further report that when the animals were immunized later in life when a number of the neuritic plaques had clearly already formed, the number of neuritic plaques could actually be reduced. This has led to further studies in other species, and investigators anticipate that clinical trials in humans will begin in the very near future.

The second characteristic pathological change in AD is the neurofibrillary tangle, a collection of abnormally phosphorylated filamentous proteins that are a normal component of microtubules known as tau protein. The abnormal phosphorylation leads to the formation of intracellular paired helical filaments, which constitute the neurofibrillary tangle. Like β-amyloid, this abnormally phosphorylated tau protein is believed to be neurotoxic and aggregates into tangles after the death of neurons. Normal tau protein is located in the axons, where it binds to tubulin in the microtubules, thereby promoting microtubule assembly and stability. The presence of neurofibrillary tangles in the brain is not specific to AD but is also seen in many other neurological conditions. It remains a potential target for therapeutic intervention that has not yet been fully explored.

Antioxidants

α-Tocopherol (vitamin E). Vitamin E is a lipid-soluble vitamin within cell membranes that is capable of blocking hydrogen peroxide production and the resulting cytotoxicity in the form of lipid peroxidation. Vitamin E also reduces β-amyloid-induced cell death in rat hippocampal cell cultures (Goodman and Mattson 1994) and PC12 cells (Behl et al. 1992). Several lines of evidence suggest that free radical generation is an important step in the pathogenesis of the disease process.

Vitamin E and other antioxidants improve cognitive performance in aged animals and animal models of AD. Vitamin E and selegiline have been shown to slow the progression of AD (Sano et al. 1997). A double-blind, placebo-controlled study compared vitamin E, selegiline, vitamin E plus selegiline, and placebo. The treated groups progressed to the end points of death, nursing home placement, loss of activities of daily living, and severe dementia at a reduced rate compared with patients receiving placebo. No differences were found in the therapeutic efficacy of the three treatments, and all were superior to placebo. The rate of progression in those receiving treatment was approximately 25% less than the rate in the placebo group. The high dose of vitamin E (2,000 IU/day) was well tolerated. A few clinical studies have examined doses higher than this (3,000–3,200 IU/day) and noted gastrointestinal complaints of indigestion, gastric distress, severe cramps, and persistent diarrhea (Anderson and Reid 1974; Fahn 1992; Pappert et al. 1996). Another important potential side effect of high-dose vitamin E is reduced coagulation and possible clotting defects, so it should be used with caution in patients who have bleeding disorders or liver disease or who are receiving anticoagulation therapy. The dose of selegiline in this study was 5 mg twice a day. The side effects of selegiline include insomnia, confusion, orthostatic hypotension, and psychosis. The utility of vitamin E or selegiline in disease prophylaxis has not been established.

Other antioxidants. Many other antioxidants are currently under investigation. Idebenone, along with its parent compound coenzyme Q-10, is an antioxidant shown to inhibit lipid peroxidation in vitro and to improve behavior in aged and basal forebrain–lesioned rats. Clinical trials in patients with AD have suggested a mild benefit (Adkins and Noble 1998; Weyer et al. 1997). The free-radical-scavenging properties of ascorbic acid (vitamin C) have been well documented (Frei et al. 1989). One double-blind trial that compared the antioxidant vitamins C, B_1 (thiamine hydrochloride), B_2, (riboflavin), and B_6 (pyridoxine hydrochloride) in patients with AD and vascular dementia found that they had no effect (Burns et al. 1989).

Anti-Inflammatory Agents

Many lines of evidence point to an instrumental role of inflammatory mechanisms in AD. Several specific inflammatory and immune effector mechanisms are active in the brains of patients with AD. Acute-phase reactants are present in the neuritic plaques, and localized inflammatory reactions involving some elements of the classical complement pathway have been identified. Interaction between complement proteins and amyloid fragments may activate the complement cascade and may increase the toxicity of amyloid peptides (Oda et al. 1995; Schulz et al. 1994). Activated microglia also may be an important source of inflammatory cytokines and complement proteins.

Epidemiological studies show an inverse relationship between AD and rheumatoid arthritis; one study reported a prevalence rate of AD of 2% in patients with rheumatoid arthritis compared with 13% in control subjects (Jenkinson et al. 1989). In addition, epidemiological studies have suggested that nonsteroidal anti-inflammatory drugs (NSAIDs) reduce the risk of developing AD, with the magnitude of the effect approaching 50% in some studies (Breitner et al. 1994, 1995; Lucca et al. 1994; McGeer et al. 1996; Rich et al. 1995; Stewart et al. 1997). The effect of aspirin and acetaminophen was substantially less than that of NSAIDs. Patients received different agents in variable doses for varying lengths of time. The apparent protective effect of NSAIDs has been explained by the theory that they may limit destructive inflammation in the AD brain.

A study examining the effect of chronic use of low-dose prednisone (20 mg/day for 4 weeks followed by 10 mg/day over a 1-year period) in patients diagnosed with probable AD failed to show disease stabilization or any slowing of disease progression (Aisen et al. 2000).

A small, prospective, placebo-controlled clinical trial with 44 patients with early AD taking 100–150 mg/day of the potent NSAID indomethacin showed a clinical benefit in the treated group (J. Rogers et al. 1993). Indomethacin-treated subjects maintained constant MMSE scores over the 6-month period of the trial, whereas those taking placebo showed an expected 10%–12% decline. NSAIDs are not without significant potential side effects, however, and in the indomethacin trial, 42% of the patients in the active drug group dropped out. Another recent small study, in which diclofenac was given to AD patients, found similar results, suggesting a potential disease-modifying effect; however, a 40%–50% dropout rate was also seen, even though one treatment arm included the use of misoprostol for gastrointestinal protection (Scharf et al. 1999). Prospective controlled clinical treatment trials to define the potential role of these agents in the treatment of AD are in progress.

NSAIDS currently in use were developed to inhibit cyclooxygenase (COX-1); recently, a second isoform, COX-2, which is induced by inflammatory stimuli, has been identified. COX-2 is believed to be of primary importance in the inflammatory response. COX-2 is upregulated in the brains of AD subjects compared with control subjects (Pasinetti and Aisen 1998). Recent work suggests that COX-2 also may play a central role in neurodegeneration (Tocco et al. 1997). Currently, several treatment trials with these newer COX-2 inhibitors are under way in patients with AD. Other anti-inflammatory agents, such as colchicine and hydroxychloroquine, are also candidates for clinical trials in AD; both agents suppress the activity of mononuclear cells. Colchicine also has poorly understood antiamyloidogenic properties.

NSAIDS should not yet be considered as a preventive or therapeutic treatment for AD. Prospective clinical trials are under way to further clarify the potential role of these agents in preventing or delaying disease onset or in modifying the disease course. Similarly, cytokine inhibitors such as methotrexate recently have been shown to be beneficial in rodent models of neurodegeneration but have not yet been studied in patients with AD.

Hormones

Hormonal therapies have been a focus of research attention in AD. Estrogen promotes growth of cholinergic neurons, co-localizes with NGF receptors in the basal forebrain, promotes the survival of hippocampal neurons in vitro, and regulates the metabolism of APP. Several epidemiological studies provide evidence that estrogen replacement therapy (ERT) reduces the risk of AD in postmenopausal women and that ERT may reduce the severity of AD in postmenopausal women (Henderson 1997; Paganini-Hill and Henderson 1994). The effect size in these studies is similar to that of NSAIDs—approximately 50% (Birge 1994; Kawas et al. 1997; Ohkura et al. 1994; Yaffe et al. 1998). Moreover, the lack of ERT may contribute to the increased risk of AD among women compared with men. In some studies, postmenopausal women with AD receiving ERT performed at higher cognitive levels than those not receiving replacement hormones (Birge 1994; Ohkura et al. 1994). Women receiving ERT have been given various combinations of estrogen and progesterone for varying lengths of time, and specific dosage recommendations are not currently possible. Prospective studies are under way to examine the potential preventive role of ERT in AD.

ERT for the treatment of mild to moderate AD was recently studied in a large-scale randomized, placebo-controlled U.S. trial in hysterectomized women with AD. It was shown to be no better than placebo in altering disease progression in this 1-year trial (Mulnard et al. 2000). A smaller prospective, randomized placebo-controlled trial of estrogen replacement in postmenopausal women with AD revealed a similar lack of efficacy (Henderson et al. 2000). These studies do not address the issue of prevention of AD, and there remains a possibility that estrogen could have an important role in delaying onset of disease. Two large-scale prospective trials of ERT in postmenopausal women are currently under way. One of these, an ancillary study to the Women's Health Initiative, seeks to enroll 8,000 women to be followed over 5 years. Rates of dementia in the treated and nontreated groups will be compared (Shumakeer et al. 1998).

Androgens also may have an important effect on cognition. One study actually showed that higher levels of testosterone predicted better cognitive performance in women not receiving ERT (Barrett-Conner and Goodman-Gruen 1999). Although men do not undergo a sudden decline in sex hormones analogous to menopause in women, testosterone levels do decline throughout life. Testosterone is converted to estrogen by aromatases in the brain, and based on the emerging evidence that ERT enhances cognition in women, testosterone replacement in men with AD may have beneficial effects and is an area of current clinical research.

Calcium Channel Blockers

Calcium plays a critical role in overall physiological homeostasis. Alterations in calcium homeostasis have been implicated in brain aging and in AD (for a review, see Mattson et al. 1997). One mechanism postulated of β-amyloid toxicity involved calcium dysregulation. β-amyloid forms fibrils and induces membrane oxidation, leading to lipid peroxidation and impairment of the Na^+/K^+ adenosine triphosphatase (ATPase) and the Ca^{++} ATPase that can account for calcium dysregulation (Mattson et al. 1997; Pascale and Etcheberrigaray 1999). Current research indicates that most of the alterations in calcium regulation in AD arise from disturbances in the calcium release from stores and not from calcium influx through channels (Pascale and Etcheberrigaray 1999). It is therefore not surprising that agents such as nimodipine and related compounds have had a minimal effect in AD (Tollefson 1990). Nonetheless, aiming to restore proper calcium homeostasis and regulatory mechanisms remains an attractive therapeutic target in the effort to treat AD.

Nerve Growth Factor

Neurotrophic factors promote the maintenance and survival of neurons. The cholinergic neurons in the basal forebrain differ from other cholinergic neuron populations in the brain by possessing a high-density, low-affinity NGF receptor on their surface (Batchelor et al. 1989; Koh et al. 1989). Exogenously administered NGF does not cross the blood-brain barrier and must be delivered directly into the central nervous system. Intracerebroventricular (ICV) infusions of NGF are capable of preventing deterioration of nucleus basalis neurons but have been associated with undesirable effects. Cognitive benefits of NGF treatment have been reported in lesioned aged animals. However, NGF administered systemically does not cross the blood-brain barrier, and ICV administration requires surgical implantation of a device to administer the compound, which has some risks. Additionally, NGF has been associated with Schwann's cell hyperplasia (aberrant sprouting of sensory and sympathetic neurites) and weight loss (Winkler et al. 1995).

AIT-082, an oral agent that crosses the blood-brain barrier, stimulates the production of NGF and augments the effects of NGF on cells in culture (Middlemiss et al. 1995). A clinical trial with this agent is under way. Sabeluzole, a compound that potentiates the action of NGF, accelerates axonal transport, promotes neurite outgrowth, and prevents tangle formation, demonstrated only modest benefit in Alzheimer's patients in one study (Mohr et al. 1997).

Gene Therapy/Transplantation

Safety is a major concern in ex vivo gene therapy for the treatment of neurodegenerative disorders. Graft-induced tumor formation, inadvertent release of infectious viral particles into the host, and ineffective transgene levels are some of the potential risks associated with genetically engineered cells. Encapsulating cells within polymer membranes is one technique for restricting cellular growth and isolating certain cellularly released factors from the host. Exogenous manipulation of transduced cells undoubtedly will be necessary for directly controlling cells and/or transgene expression in vivo. Use of stem-cell transplantation is also under investigation in AD.

Nonspecific Cerebral Metabolic Enhancement (Nootropic Agents)

Nootropics (*noos*, mind; *tropein*, forward) are a novel class of agents that act through general metabolic enhancement independent of any direct neurotransmitter influence. Piracetam and analogs are nootropic agents that have been tested in clinical trials involving patients with AD. Piracetam is the prototypical drug of this group of pyrrolidinone agents developed to improve cognitive function. Although all agents in this group are GABA derivatives, they have no effects on GABA receptors. Agents clinically tested in dementia patients include piracetam and its analogs aniracetam, pramiracetam, and oxiracetam. Although there is evidence of a nonspecific arousal effect, no current evidence indicates that these agents enhance cognitive functioning in AD (Waters 1990). A recent high-dose (8 g/day) 1-year parallel-group, double-blind, placebo-controlled trial of piracetam in moderately impaired AD patients suggested a partial slowing of cognitive deterioration, as noted in performance on neuropsychological subtests involving memory and attention (Croisile et al. 1993). The authors suggested that previous trials of nootropic agents had involved drug doses that were too low and were too brief to demonstrate any effect. No significant adverse effects were observed in trials of piracetam.

Ergoloid Mesylates

Hydergine, a combination of ergoloid mesylates, was the only drug approved by the FDA for therapy of dementia before the approval and release of THA for AD in 1993. Despite researchers' extensive efforts, Hydergine's precise mode of pharmacological effect has not yet been delineated. Explanations of action include cerebral vasodilation, enhancement of cerebral metabolism, α-adrenergic receptor blockade, and dopaminergic and cyclic adenosine monophosphate (cAMP) effects. More recently, the cholinergic effects of Hydergine have been postulated via increase in receptor number or affinity, increased ACh synthesis due to general metabolic enhancement, or indirect stimulation of hippocampal cholinergic neurons through stimulation of locus coeruleus adrenergic projections (Yesavage 1990).

Only modest improvements in cognition have been reported with Hydergine in both mixed dementia and probable AD populations. These effects may be primarily the result of enhanced arousal (Gottlieb and Kumar 1993). Another double-blind, placebo-controlled, parallel-group 6-month trial of Hydergine (3 mg/day) in probable AD patients showed neither improvement in cognition or function nor a slowing of cognitive decline as had been reported in earlier studies (Thompson et al. 1990). Hydergine appears to be safe and well tolerated, and no significant adverse side effects were reported in this or other studies. At higher doses, Hydergine has antihypertensive effects and can cause mild slowing of heart rate (Yesavage 1990). Evidence is insufficient to support the use of Hydergine in AD patients.

Ginkgo Biloba and Huperazine A

Ginkgo biloba is derived from a Chinese herb and contains EGb 761, a mixture with free-radical-scavenging properties that appear to derive from the combined action of flavonoid and terpenoid fragments in conjunction with organic acids. In addition, it has platelet-activating-factor inhibitor properties (Packer et al. 1995). Ginkgo biloba has been approved for the treatment of dementia in Germany and has been under increasing investigation in clinical trials. In a recent double-blind, placebo-controlled randomized study in 309 dementia patients followed over a 1-year period, modest but statistically significant improvements in the ADAS cognitive subscale were seen in the Ginkgo-treated subjects compared with those receiving placebo (Le Bars et al. 1997).

Huperazine A is a Chinese herb that appears to have cholinesterase-inhibiting properties. It is currently being evaluated in controlled clinical trials (Cheng et al. 1996; Patocka 1998).

Therapies Found to Be Ineffective for Enhancement of Cognitive Function in Alzheimer's Disease

Of historical interest are multiple other therapies for which initial enthusiasm was later proven unfounded. These therapies included chelation therapy; high-potency vitamin preparations; RNA administration; anticoagulants; vasodilators; hemorrheological agents; combinations of the neurotransmitter precursors lecithin, tryptophan, and tyrosine; vasopressin; hyperbaric oxygen; thyrotropin-releasing hormone (TRH); adrenocorticotropic hormone (ACTH); psychostimulants; and narcotic antagonists (Gottlieb and Kumar 1993; Mody and Miller 1990).

Future Directions in Therapy

In addition to symptomatic therapies directed at the correction of neurotransmitter deficits, research is focusing on the development of drugs that may alter disease progression. Such approaches include drugs that regulate the expression and processing of β-APP, enhancing secretion of nontoxic β-APP fragments or blocking β-amyloid peptide production that is mediated by the endosomal-lysosomal system, which could decrease β-amyloid deposition and prevent neuronal degeneration (Growdon 1992). Other research is directed toward putative excitatory amino acid–mediated neuronal toxicity in AD. The use of neurotrophic factors such as NGF is also ongoing (Davis and Haroutunian 1993). Detection of upregulated levels of phagocytic receptors on reactive microglia and the fixation of complement proteins co-localized with neuritic plaques, dystrophic neurites, and some neurofibrillary tangles in AD brains suggest the possibility of autoimmune-mediated destruction (rather than passive phagocytosis) as a pathogenic component in AD (McGeer and Rogers 1992). The potential role of immunophyllins is being studied in Parkinson's disease, but there may be a role for their use in AD as well. Moreover, genetically engineered cell transplants and stem-cell research remain promising areas of study (Tuszynsky et al. 1996).

Importance of Behavioral Disturbances in Alzheimer's Disease

Cognitive impairment is a consistent clinical feature of AD, but psychiatric and behavioral disturbances and a progressive inability to perform instrumental and basic activities of daily living are also typical. Behavioral disturbances occur throughout the course of AD. Mega et al. (1996) reviewed the spectrum of behavioral changes seen in AD over the course of the disease. The spectrum included personality alterations, mood disturbances, perceptual disturbances such as delusions and hallucinations, vegetative symptoms, and motor disturbances. Their successful management can significantly improve the overall quality of life for patients and their caregivers, whereas persistent disruptive behavior is a common reason for institutionalization (Steele et al. 1990). Kaufer et al. (1998) recently reported on the interrelation between cognitive status as assessed by the MMSE, behavioral disturbances as measured by the NPI, and caregiver distress. The authors reported a strong correlation between the amount of neuropsychiatric disturbance and the degree of caregiver distress, which was statistically significant and emphasizes that the neuropsychiatric manifestations of this illness are a major source of disease morbidity. Little, if any, relation was found between the degree of impairment on the MMSE and caregiver distress. The neuropsychiatric disturbances are associated with increased costs for patient care because of greater medication use and more adverse side effects, more extensive institutional staffing needs, and earlier institutionalization of the AD patient. Rabins et al. (1990) found that both the severity of the neuropsychiatric symptomatology and caregiver distress are associated with nursing home placement. Improvement in the treatment and management of the noncognitive symptoms, therefore, could have significant relevant benefit.

Many studies have focused on the association between the cholinergic deficit and cognitive impairment; however, evidence is mounting that cholinergic abnormalities are related to the neuropsychiatric manifestations of AD as well. The neurobiology of these disturbances in AD is as yet inadequately understood. The known alterations in several neurotransmitter systems (i.e., noradrenergic, serotonergic, cholinergic, dopaminergic) that are implicated in the pathobiology of anxiety, mood disorders, and psychosis suggest that neurotransmitter changes in AD might contribute to behavioral disturbances in these patients.

Critical to the initial management of these disturbances is a search for any contributing medical, medication-related, or social/environmental factors. Superimposed delirium as a cause of behavioral deterioration should always be considered. Understanding the patient's underlying needs or motivation can lead to creative interventions that diminish disturbed behaviors without drugs (Gottlieb and Piotrowski 1990). If these approaches are not successful and behavioral disorders are severe enough to interfere with normal functioning, pharmacological therapy should be considered (Table 20–3).

Treatment of Behavioral Disturbances

Treatment of Psychosis and Agitation

Antipsychotics

Antipsychotics are the psychotropic medications most frequently prescribed for treatment of agitation associated with dementia (Salzman 1988). Antipsychotics are indicated for the treatment of specific target symptoms in AD: delusions, hallucinations, and severe aggression or agitation. Dementia patients often are unable to report symptoms of psychosis, and the presence of delusions and hallucinations must at times be inferred from behavioral alterations. Although the use of antipsychotics in the demented elderly patient has been widely studied, many investigations have been limited by methodological flaws (i.e., heterogeneous patient populations, inadequate definition and measurement of target symptoms, lack of randomization, inadequate controls, and lack of double-blind assessment methods). In a review of methodologically superior studies of the use of these agents in AD and other dementias (Wragg and Jeste 1988), three target symptoms—delusions, hallucinations, and agitation—were found to respond better to active drug than to placebo. Improvement was substantial in approximately one-third of the antipsychotic-treated patients. In general, de-

TABLE 20–3. Psychopharmacological treatments for behavioral disturbances in Alzheimer's disease

Drug	Trade name	Starting dosage (mg)	Frequency	Maximum dosage (mg/day)
Psychosis				
Haloperidol	Haldol	0.25–0.50	daily	2–4
Risperidone	Risperdal	0.5	daily	1–3
Olanzapine	Zyprexa	2.5	daily	5–10
Quetiapine	Seroquel	12.5–25.0	daily	50–150
Clozapine	Clozaril	6.25–12.5	daily	25–100
Agitation/aggression				
Antipsychotics (same as listed above under Psychosis)				
Trazodone	Desyrel	25–50	daily	200–300
Divalproex	Depakote	125	bid	1,500–2,000
Carbamazepine	Tegretol	50–100	daily	500–800
Buspirone	BuSpar	5	bid	45
Lorazepam	Ativan	0.5	daily	4–6
Propranolol	Inderal	10	bid	50–240
Depression				
Selective serotonin reuptake inhibitors				
Fluoxetine	Prozac	10	daily	20–40
Paroxetine	Paxil	5–10	daily	40
Sertraline	Zoloft	25–50	daily	150–200
Citalopram	Celexa	10–20	daily	40
Fluvoxamine	Luvox	50	daily	300
Tricyclic antidepressants				
Nortriptyline	Pamelor	10	daily	50–100
Desipramine	Norpramin	50	daily	150
Others				
Nefazodone	Serzone	150	bid	600
Venlafaxine	Effexor	75	daily	375
Anxiety				
Buspirone	BuSpar	5	daily	30–45
Lorazepam	Ativan	0.5	daily	2–6
Oxazepam	Serax	10	daily	30
Sleep disturbance				
Trazodone	Desyrel	50	daily	300
Zolpidem	Ambien	5–10	daily	10
Temazepam	Restoril	15	daily	30

gree of improvement was proportional to the initial severity of symptoms. Inappropriately repetitious nonaggressive behaviors and certain delusions (regarding theft or loss of previously discarded possessions, possibly related to amnesia) appear to be resistant to antipsychotic treatment (Raskind and Risse 1986). Overall responses are modest, and responses to placebo also occur. A modest benefit was also found in a statistical meta-analysis of controlled trials of antipsychotic treatment of agitation in patients with a primary diagnosis of dementia (Schneider et al. 1990); 18% of the dementia patients derived benefit from antipsychotic treatment beyond response attributable to placebo. The placebo response was significant in many studies, varying from 0% to 67%. The symptoms of agitation, uncooperativeness, and hallucinations responded to medication in the controlled studies reviewed. The authors concluded that, given the high nonresponse rate and the magnitude of the placebo response, many elderly dementia patients are being unnecessarily treated with antipsychotics.

No particular antipsychotic agent has emerged as therapeutically superior, and all have the potential to cause multiple side effects and to interact with other drugs in the AD patient, who is usually elderly and often has coexisting medical conditions. Antipsychotic agents can also contribute to cognitive deficits in AD patients (Devanand et al. 1989).

Selection of an antipsychotic agent in an individual patient should be made on the basis of the agent's side-effect profile. Potential side effects include sedation, orthostatic hypotension, central and peripheral anticholinergic effects, and extrapyramidal symptoms (EPS) (akathisia, parkinsonism, tardive dyskinesia, neuroleptic malignant syndrome) due to dopamine blockade. All of these side effects appear to occur with increased frequency and at lower dosage levels in elderly patients (Raskind et al. 1987). The one exception is neuroleptic malignant syndrome, which is more common among younger patients. The incidence and severity of tardive dyskinesia increase with advancing age (Salzman 1987). The lower incidence of parkinsonism and the increased occurrence of sedation, orthostatic hypotension, and anticholinergic effects with low-potency antipsychotics must be weighed against the converse side-effect profile of high-potency agents. Excessive sedation can potentially cause increased confusion and agitation. More serious consequences (e.g., hip fracture) can result from falls in elderly patients. Elderly patients are more likely to have preexisting medical conditions such as cardiac disease or prostatic hypertrophy, increasing the risk of adverse peripheral anticholinergic effects. AD patients may be more susceptible to central anticholinergic cognitive effects, given the widespread cortical cholinergic deficit present in AD. Decrements in MMSE scores have been observed with thioridazine at dosages greater than 75 mg/day (Steele et al. 1986) and also with haloperidol at dosages of 1–5 mg/day (Devanand et al. 1989). Most patients with AD experience severe EPS with dosages of haloperidol greater than approximately 4 mg/day. In a preliminary study, AD patients with psychosis or behavioral disturbance who responded to haloperidol therapy did so at plasma levels below the 4–18 ng/mL postulated to be therapeutic in schizophrenia (Devanand et al. 1992).

Because of the substantial risk of adverse side effects with only modest efficacy, antipsychotics should be used only in those agitated patients with psychotic symptomatology or those who require acute sedation. Antipsychotic therapy should be initiated with very small dosages (0.5 mg/day of haloperidol or 10–25 mg/day of thioridazine), and use of the newer atypical antipsychotics may be even better tolerated in this patient population. Titration upward should proceed slowly, with careful monitoring of outcome, both behavioral and functional. Patients should be followed up closely for orthostatic hypotension,

EPS, and anticholinergic side effects. Antipsychotic-induced akathisia may increase pacing and other repetitive nonaggressive behaviors (Wragg and Jeste 1988). Anticholinergic or antihistaminic drugs should not be prescribed prophylactically for EPS because they can affect behavior and cognition adversely. If significant EPS occur, antipsychotic dosage should be reduced. Behavioral disturbances in degenerative dementia may be transient or episodic, and periodic discontinuation of antipsychotic drugs is recommended given their potential morbidity (Risse and Barnes 1986).

Atypical Antipsychotics

The use of the atypical antipsychotics in the treatment of behavioral problems in dementia patients has been gaining more widespread approval. In a well-designed placebo-controlled trial comparing 0.5, 1.0, and 2.0 mg/day of risperidone with placebo in treating psychosis and aggressive behavior in 625 institutionalized elderly patients with dementia, the authors found significant reductions in these behaviors as measured by the Behavioral Pathology in Alzheimer's Disease rating scale (BEHAVE-AD; Reisberg et al. 1987). Seventy percent of the patients completed the study, and more side effects were seen with the 2-mg/day than with the 1-mg/day dose of risperidone (Katz et al. 1999). Another study in 344 nursing home patients found slightly less robust results, but efficacy was clearly demonstrated. In an open-label trial, patients with AD and other dementias showed some improvement with quetiapine fumarate, and olanzapine, another newer atypical antipsychotic agent, is also undergoing further investigation in clinical trials in dementia patients (Stoppe et al. 1999).

Clozapine was the first atypical antipsychotic agent approved by the FDA for the treatment of schizophrenia refractory to conventional antipsychotic drugs. Because of clozapine's relative freedom from EPS, its use has been advocated in patients who experience severe EPS at antipsychotic doses necessary to control psychosis or in those patients with severe tardive dyskinesia (Marder et al. 1993). Although not widely studied in the treatment of psychosis in AD, clozapine may prove useful when severe EPS occur at effective doses of typical antipsychotic agents. The risk of agranulocytosis (1%–2% during the first year of exposure) with clozapine therapy must be considered, and if clozapine therapy is initiated, hematological monitoring must be performed weekly. More common adverse effects include sedation, orthostatic hypotension, tachycardia, fever, weight gain, and gastrointestinal disturbance (Marder et al. 1993).

Benzodiazepines

Benzodiazepines are effective for reducing anxiety and agitation but not psychotic symptoms. Antipsychotics have been shown to have greater efficacy than benzodiazepines in controlled trials of treatment of agitation. This superiority was most evident with increasing severity of dementia and agitation (Wragg and Jeste 1988). Side effects of benzodiazepines include sedation, cognitive impairment, paradoxical disinhibition, amnestic effects, tolerance, and withdrawal syndromes. Short-acting agents such as lorazepam or oxazepam are preferred in elderly patients to minimize drug accumulation and drug interactions. Very small doses can be used intermittently for treatment of anxiety and mild agitation in mild AD with close monitoring of behavior and function. The literature does not support the use of benzodiazepines for agitation in patients with more severe dementia for whom antipsychotics, β-blockers, or possibly carbamazepine is more efficacious (Gottlieb and Kumar 1993; Stern et al. 1991).

Trazodone

Several case reports and small uncontrolled series have shown that trazodone, a serotonin reuptake inhibitor, can effectively control agitation in dementia. Daily dosage typically ranges from 200 to 400 mg (Schneider and Sobin 1992; Wragg and Jeste 1988). The mechanism of the antiagitation effect is unknown but appears to be unrelated to antidepressant or sedative properties and may be associated with calming effects observed in animal models after blockade of serotonin reuptake (Wragg and Jeste 1988). One group of investigators showed that serotonin deficiency was particularly severe in the frontal lobes in AD, and it was suggested that this neurotransmitter deficiency contributes significantly to aggressive behavior in AD patients (Palmer et al. 1988). Adverse effects of trazodone include sedation, hypotension, ventricular arrhythmias, and priapism.

Anticonvulsants

Divalproex sodium is an anticonvulsant that works by enhancing the release of the primarily inhibitory neurotransmitter GABA. It has been shown to be effective in managing agitation and aggression in dementia patients in a number of mostly open trials (Zayas and Grossberg 1996). In a small, controlled pilot study with 16 subjects, divalproex sodium was used for the treatment of agitation in dementia patients with good efficacy and tolerability (Herrmann 1998). The dosage was gradually titrated from 500 to 2,000 mg/day. It is well tolerated in the elderly but can cause gastrointestinal side effects as well as a benign tremor and sedation. Liver function tests also should be monitored periodically.

Carbamazepine, an anticonvulsant with psychotropic properties found to be effective in bipolar disorder, has also been reported to reduce emotional lability, aggression, and socially inappropriate behaviors in various brain disorders (Wragg and Jeste 1988). More recent controlled clinical trials in dementia patients have found it efficacious in reducing irritability, hostility, agitation, and combativeness in AD patients (Leibovici and Tariot 1988; Tariot et al. 1998). Carbamazepine can be started as low as 50 mg twice daily and slowly titrated upward to avoid oversedation and ataxia (Gleason and Schneider 1990; Leibovici and Tariot 1988). Daily dosages used in possible AD patients have ranged from 100 to 1,000 mg, and clinical improvement usually occurs within 2–4 weeks (Schneider and Sobin 1992). Central nervous system side effects of carbamazepine are dose-related and include sedation and ataxia. Baseline complete blood count and routine liver function tests should be obtained. Monthly measurements are recommended for the first 6 months, with measurements repeated at 3- to 12-month intervals thereafter.

Buspirone

Buspirone is a nonbenzodiazepine anxiolytic agent whose mechanism of action is unknown. A few case observations support the use of buspirone to treat agitation in AD. The binding of the drug to central dopamine receptors has raised concern about possible EPS. There have been a few open series and case reports of its effectiveness in dementia populations.

β-Adrenergic Receptor Blocking Agents

In a few small clinical series, propranolol at dosages ranging from 60 to 560 mg/day was successful in improving aggressive and agitated behavior in dementia patients (Gottlieb and Kumar 1993; Schneider and Sobin 1992). Other β-blockers have not been extensively studied. Cardiovascular side effects may limit the use of these agents in elderly patients. Concomitant conditions such as chronic obstructive lung disease and diabetes also can preclude use of these agents in some geriatric patients. Blood pressure and pulse should be monitored closely in any dementia patient receiving β-adrenergic blocking agents.

Lithium

Lithium carbonate is effective in reducing mania-associated agitation, aggressiveness, and irritability. The few case reports of its use in AD suggest that it may be ineffective except when symptoms of mania are present (pressured speech, sleeplessness, and motor hyperactivity). In view of its potential for adverse cognitive effects with advanced age and brain disease, lithium should probably be used only when there is clearly an affective component to the behavior (Leibovici and Tariot 1988; Wragg and Jeste 1988).

Cholinesterase Inhibitors

Anticholinergic toxicity is commonly accompanied by delirium with delusions and is reversible with physostigmine. In one study, physostigmine was compared with haloperidol in two pilot double-blind crossover trials involving patients with probable AD (Cummings et al. 1993; Gorman et al. 1993). Reductions in psychotic symptoms were similar with the two drugs. In an open-label study evaluating the effects of THA on behavioral symptoms in AD, the authors reported a significant reduction in behavioral symptoms, particularly apathy, in response to therapy (Kaufer et al. 1996). The effects of metrifonate on behavioral symptoms in AD were evaluated in a more recent randomized, placebo-controlled study. This acetylcholinesterase inhibitor significantly improved behavioral disturbances in AD as measured by the Neuropsychiatric Inventory (Cummings et al. 1998).

In summary, treatment of agitation in AD patients must be individualized. Agitation should be approached initially by investigation of potentially reversible causes. Acute management may include sedation with atypical and typical antipsychotics or short-acting benzodiazepines. Severe adverse effects and limited efficacy make these agents less useful for the management of chronic agitation. Low-dose antipsychotic therapy is, however, indicated for agitation related to psychotic symptomatology. The serotonergic agent trazodone is a reasonable first-line pharmacological agent in the management of agitation because it is well tolerated (Sultzer and Cummings 1993). Other antidepressants, such as the SSRIs, are generally well tolerated and may be helpful in treating both depressive symptoms and agitation in patients with dementia. Other available agents reported to be effective in some clinical studies are divalproex sodium and carbamazepine. Propranolol also may be helpful for aggressive, impulsive behaviors and is used frequently in patients with behavioral disturbances resulting from head trauma. These drugs must be used with care in the elderly because they are associated with common side effects. Lithium may be effective when manic symptoms are associated with agitation. Therapeutic approaches must be strongly influenced by consideration of potential side effects in the individual patient, and patients must be closely monitored for adverse effects. Periodic attempts should be made to reduce or discontinue any therapeutic agent.

Depressive Symptomatology

Depressive symptoms are common (40%–50%) in patients with AD and are more common than major depressive episodes (10%–20%). Depression may be difficult to identify in AD patients. The cognitive and vegetative symptoms of AD and depression often overlap. Persons with dementia may have difficulty describing subjective affective states. Little information exists about the relative frequency or course of depressive symptoms across the progressive stages of AD (Wragg and Jeste 1989). The etiology of depressive symptoms in AD is not clear. Reaction to cognitive and functional impairment is likely contributory. Degeneration of the noradrenergic and serotonergic projection systems also may be involved. Appropriate treatment of concomitant depression may improve the quality of life for the dementia patient and his or her family. Following successful treatment (with various antidepressants or electroconvulsive therapy [ECT]) of major depression in dementia (Alzheimer's disease or multi-infarct dementia) in one study, cognitive test performance improved (Greenwald et al. 1989). However, in a double-blind, placebo-controlled trial of imipramine in AD outpatients with and without depression, imipramine and placebo were equally effective in the treatment of depression; there was no concomitant cognitive improvement (Reifler et al. 1989).

Larger placebo-controlled trials of antidepressant therapy (both pharmacological and psychosocial) in depressed AD patients are needed. The best treatment for depression in AD remains to be determined. Cyclic agents, monoamine oxidase inhibitors, and ECT have all been beneficial in open clinical trials. Choice of a particular antidepressant agent should therefore be based primarily on the side-effect profile in an individual patient. Any agent used should be titrated upward from low starting doses with caution (Gottlieb and Kumar 1993; Salzman 1988). An electrocardiogram should be performed before tricyclic antidepressant therapy is initiated. The use of drug plasma levels is recommended in the event of adverse side effects or failure to respond.

The use of SSRIs in treating depressive symptoms in dementia has been evaluated in a few open trials. A randomized, double-blind, placebo-controlled trial of sertraline in treating behavioral symptoms, including depression, in patients with AD is currently being evaluated. In dementia patients in a European study, citalopram had significant efficacy in controlling problem behaviors and mood symptoms in subjects with AD (Pollock et al. 1997). The newer combination SSRI and noradrenergic reuptake inhibitors also may be of benefit in this patient population but remain to be systematically investigated.

Anxiety

Anxiety is common in patients with AD, reported in about 40% (Mendez et al. 1990). However, treatment of anxiety with standard benzodiazepine anxiolytic agents is problematic, as discussed earlier. Use of benzodiazepines must be accompanied by ongoing assessment of the risk-benefit ratio. Shorter-acting benzodiazepine agents (e.g., lorazepam, oxazepam) are preferable in elderly patients. Buspirone is a nonbenzodiazepine anxiolytic that is well tolerated and effective in the treatment of anxiety in nondemented elderly patients. It does not affect cognition adversely in young healthy persons. This agent holds promise for the treatment of anxiety in AD, but no results from well-designed trials in this population are yet available (Gottlieb and Kumar 1993).

Insomnia

Sleep disturbance is common in AD. The disturbance is characterized by reduced depth and efficiency as well as increased fragmentation of sleep. With progression of the disease, disruption of the normal circadian rhythm is observed, with multiple periods of sleeping and waking, daytime naps, and sundowning (nocturnal agitation, confusion, and wandering). This disruption of the normal sleep-wake cycle in AD patients may be related to degeneration of the suprachiasmatic nucleus. The cholinergic system is important in the generation of rapid eye movement sleep, and cholinergic dysfunction in AD is likely related to sleep disturbances (Culebras 1992). Poor nocturnal sleep may reduce daytime alertness, aggravating cognitive impairment in AD patients and further increasing caregiver stress.

Nonpharmacological management includes optimizing sleep hygiene by limiting time in bed to 6.5–7 hours per night, reducing daytime naps, establishing a consistent morning awakening time, and reducing evening fluids to prevent awakening for micturition (Reynolds et al. 1988). The use of light therapy has also been shown to be of some benefit in dementia patients (Lyketsos et al. 1999; Van Someren et al. 1997). Useful medications include trazodone, temazepam, chloral hydrate, zolpidem, and melatonin. Both temazepam and chloral hydrate are associated with tolerance and withdrawal syndromes.

Psychotherapy

A comprehensive approach to the management of psychiatric and behavioral disturbances in patients with AD is necessary. Given the rather modest effectiveness of the various pharmacological agents currently used for behavioral management, the importance of maximal use of all available treatment modalities is clear. Certain behavioral disturbances (e.g., wandering, verbal outbursts, hostility, repetitive questions, apathy, and disinhibition) are particularly resistant to medication (Sultzer and Cummings 1993).

Psychotherapeutic approaches include conventional insight-oriented, cognitive, group, family, supportive, reminiscent, directive, and reality therapies, as well as behavior modification and environmental manipulation (Maletta 1988). The approach to psychotherapeutic treatment should be flexible and appropriate to the patient's level of cognitive functioning, to the specific problem to be addressed, and to therapist availability. A close working alliance with both the patient and the primary caregiver is fundamental to effective psychotherapy. Psychodynamic and cognitive psychotherapy can be useful in the early stages of AD when the patient still has adequate insight and memory. Group therapy can also be beneficial and should involve small groups of patients at about the same cognitive level. Family therapy (with or without the patient present) can provide a nonjudgmental and safe forum for discussion of the complex emotional, financial, and legal issues involved in caring for the dementia patient. Supportive psychotherapy—reassurance, modulation of insecurity and anxiety, empathic listening, guidance in the selection of activities that bolster self-esteem, and assistance in accessing community resources—can be useful throughout the course of AD. As dementia becomes more severe, behavior modification and operant conditioning techniques are more appropriate (Maletta 1988).

Behavior modification treatment involves identification of the specific problem behavior and assessment of environmental factors that precipitate or reinforce the undesired behavior. The environment and actions of others are then modified to extinguish undesirable behaviors and increase desired behaviors. Operant techniques and environmental manipulation have been used to successfully reduce wandering behavior, verbal and physical aggression, and depressive behaviors and to increase self-care skills, appropriate ambulation, and socialization (McEvoy 1990).

Caregivers and family members benefit from education regarding the expected changes in memory, language skills, cognition, and behavior during the progressive course of AD.

A simple mnemonic (the three R's) can assist caregivers in decreasing distressing patient behaviors (Sultzer and Cummings 1993):

- Repetition: Frequent, clear reminders aid patients with mild to moderate memory loss.
- Reassurance: A short, calm conversation with a familiar person will often reduce a patient's anxiety, agitation, or verbal outbursts.
- Redirection: Distraction from the focus of frustration, preoccupation, or agitation is often beneficial (e.g., a brief walk or other activity enjoyed by the patient).

Other Nonpharmacological Management

Maintaining the maximal level of functioning for the individual patient with AD through attention to general measures such as good nutrition, regular exercise, attention to coexistent medical conditions, and regular dental care is extremely important. Patients with AD are susceptible to chronic age-related illnesses as well as to the specific medical complications of AD. Concurrent medical conditions sometimes go unrecognized and untreated in the person with dementia. Careful medical surveillance is critical to the identification and management of conditions such as drug toxicity, anemia, cardiovascular disease, arthritis, infection, chronic lung disease, and loss of hearing and vision, all of which can exacerbate functional impairment. Dementia patients are more likely than nondemented elderly patients to develop an acute confusional state with toxic or metabolic insults. There should be a high index of suspicion for the presence of delirium with any acute alteration in behavior, sleep patterns, or attention or with the onset of motor restlessness or increase in visual hallucinosis (Cummings and Benson 1992).

Urinary incontinence is common (occurring in 37%–57% of community-dwelling dementia patients), distressing, and often an important factor in the decision to place a patient in an extended-care facility. Moreover, 30%–50% of elderly patients with frequent urinary incontinence have episodic fecal incontinence. Reversible causes of incontinence include delirium, infection, restricted mobility, urinary retention with overflow, fecal impaction, atrophic vaginitis/urethritis, polyuria, and medication side effects (e.g., anticholinergic effects, sedation). These potentially treatable etiologies should be carefully considered before incontinence is attributed to dementia alone. Incontinence due to dementia can often be ameliorated by behavioral techniques such as implementing scheduled toileting, increasing the visibility and ease of use of toilet facilities, and instructing the patient to avoid evening fluid intake. Incontinence undergarments and pads and external urine collection devices can be helpful (Ouslander 1990).

In advanced stages of AD, patients are usually bedbound, incontinent, and dependent on being fed. Death is typically caused by the consequences of aspiration pneumonia, dehydration, malnutrition, or sepsis from urinary tract or decubitus infection, as well as by concomitant unrelated medical illness. At this stage of dementia, adequate nutrition and hydration must be provided, and frequent turning is necessary to avoid decubiti. Seizures often develop and require anticonvulsant therapy once metabolic etiologies have been excluded. Modifications in the physical environment to improve patient safety also should be considered. Such modifications include limiting access to exits, installing door locks and alarms, erecting outdoor fencing, improving lighting, and making stoves and automobiles inoperable by the patient. Patients with dementia should wear medical alert wrist bracelets or necklaces, and a recent photograph should be available to facilitate a search in the event the patient wanders away.

Psychosocial Management

Caregiver Support

Care for community-dwelling patients with AD is delivered primarily by family members. Experience with care of dementia patients has shown that the needs of the patient cannot be addressed in isolation from those of his or her family. Much research attention has been focused on the effect on family members of caring for persons with progressive dementia. Family caregivers are primarily women, usually the spouse or an adult daughter, and one-third of these women are older than 60 years. Often other family members supplement the service of these primary caregivers. The concept of caregiver burden has emerged to convey the adverse effect of caring for a demented relative in terms of the caregiver's physical and emotional health, economic resources, and social life (Mohide 1993). An inventory has been devised to assess the degree of caregiver stress (Zarit et al. 1980, 1986). Caregivers have been found to have poorer overall physical health, increased use of psychotropic medications, and more depressive symptomatology than age-matched control subjects (Levine and Lawlor 1991). The proportion of caregivers with clinically significant depression is not known, but one study found that 55% of family caregivers of AD patients had symptoms of depression (Cohen and Eisdorfer 1988). Caregivers should be assessed for depressive symptomatology and referred for individual therapy or medication if indicated. Participation in support groups, group therapy, or family therapy can ameliorate depressive symptoms. Evidence indicates that caregiver training directed at improving coping strategies and reducing psychological distress and isolation can delay nursing home placement of persons with dementia (Brodaty et al. 1993).

The clinician should educate the caregiver about AD so that he or she can better understand the disease and adjust to progressive changes in the patient's behavior and care needs. Several books are available to help family members understand the nature and course of Alzheimer's disease. These include *The 36-Hour Day* (Mace and Rabins 1981) and *Understanding Alzheimer's Disease* (Aronson 1988). Caregiver support groups are also an excellent source of information. They can increase informal support networks, enhance feelings of competence in the caregiver role, and improve psychological functioning (Toseland et al. 1989). Groups can be arranged through the local chapter of the Alzheimer's Disease and Related Disorders Association (ADRDA). (For information on local chapters and related services, call the national ADRDA at 1-800-272-3900.)

Alteration in sexual relationships can be a cause of distress for the caregiver, and these concerns should be frankly addressed. Variable changes in libido occur among AD patients, ranging from loss of interest in sexual activity to increased sexual drive and disinhibition in a minority of cases. Relational changes may also make continued sexual activities distasteful to the caregiver spouse. Suggestions for redirecting undesired sexual attention or encouraging desirable physical affection may be beneficial (Cummings and Benson 1992).

Community Resources

The need for community and family support changes during the progressive course of AD (Paveza 1993). A social worker, nurse, case manager, or family member can coordinate the continuum of required care. Local ADRDA chapters provide directories of available community resources and services, including home care services, day care programs, respite care for limited periods, extended-care institutions, and nursing home care. AD patients often qualify for other community senior citizen services (e.g., senior centers, meal services, and transportation programs).

Legal and Financial Considerations

Referral for legal and financial counseling should be made when AD is diagnosed. Planning for the future in regard to financial matters, advance medical directives, research participation, and autopsy should take place early in the course of AD, incorporating as clear an understanding of the patient's wishes as possible. The issues of competency, durable power of attorney, guardianship, inter vivos trusts, wills, living wills, financial planning, and protection of assets should be addressed with counsel from an experienced attorney and other professional advisers. Early attention to such matters can ease the burden of AD on the family by preserving economic stability and obviating complex legal dilemmas (Overman and Stoudemire 1988).

References

Adamus WS, Leonard JP, Tröger W: Phase I clinical trials with WAL 2014, a new muscarinic agonist for the treatment of Alzheimer's disease. Life Sci 56:883–890, 1995

Adkins JC, Noble S: Idebenone: a review of its use in mild to moderate Alzheimer's disease. CNS Drugs 9:403–419, 1998

Aisen PS, Davis KL, Berg JD, et al: A randomized controlled trial of prednisone in Alzheimer's disease. Alzheimer's Disease Cooperative Study. Neurology 54:588–593, 2000

American Medical Association: Diagnosis, Management and Treatment of Dementia: A Practical Guide for Primary Care Physicians. Chicago, IL, American Medical Association, Program on Aging and Community Health, 1999

American Psychiatric Association: Practice guideline for the treatment of patients with Alzheimer's disease and other dementias of late life. Am J Psychiatry 154(5 suppl):1–39, 1997

Anand R, Gharabawi G, Enz A: Efficacy and safety results of the early phase studies with Exelon (ENA-713) in Alzheimer's disease: an overview. Journal of Drug Development and Clinical Practice 8:1–14, 1996

Anderson DK, Reid DB: A double-blind trial of vitamin E in angina pectoris. Am J Clin Nutr 27:1174–1178, 1974

Aronson MK (ed): Understanding Alzheimer's Disease. New York, Scribners, 1988

Barrett-Connor E, Goodman-Gruen D: Cognitive function and endogenous sex hormones in older women. J Am Geriatr Soc 47:1289–1293, 1999

Batchelor PE, Armstrong DM, Blaker SN, et al: Nerve growth factor receptor and choline acetyltransferase colocalization in neurons within the rat forebrain: response to fimbria-fornix transection. J Comp Neurol 284:187–204, 1989

Becker RE, Giacobini E: Mechanisms of cholinesterase inhibition in senile dementia of the Alzheimer's type: clinical, pharmacological and therapeutic aspects. Drug Development Research 12:16–19, 1988

Behl C, Davis J, Cole GM, et al: Vitamin E protects nerve cells from amyloid beta protein toxicity. Biochem Biophys Res Commun 186:944-950, 1992

Birge SG: The role of estrogen deficiency in the aging central nervous system, in Treatment of the Postmenopausal Woman: Basic and Clinical Aspects. Edited by Lobo RA. New York, Raven, 1994, pp 153-157

Blass JP: Pathophysiology of the Alzheimer's syndrome. Neurology 43 (suppl 4):S25–S38, 1993

Bodick NC, Offen WW, Levey A, et al: Effects of xanomeline, a selective muscarinic receptor agonist, on cognitive function and behavioral symptoms in Alzheimer's disease. Arch Neurol 54:465–473, 1997

Breitner JC, Gau BA, Welsh KA, et al: Inverse association of anti-inflammatory treatments and Alzheimer's disease: initial results of a co-twin control study. Neurology 44:227–232, 1994

Breitner JC, Welsh KA, Helms MJ, et al: Delayed onset of Alzheimer's disease with nonsteroidal anti-inflammatory and histamine H2 blocking drugs. Neurobiol Aging 16:523–530, 1995

Brodaty H, McGilchrist C, Harris L, et al: Time until institutionalization and death in patients with dementia. Arch Neurol 50:643–650, 1993

Burns A, Marsh A, Bender D: A trial of vitamin supplementation in senile dementia. Int J Geriatr Psychiatry 4:333–338, 1989

California Workgroup on Guidelines for Alzheimer's Disease Management: Guidelines for Alzheimer's Disease Management. Sacramento, CA, California Department of Health Services, 1999

Cheng DH, Ren H, Tang XC: Huperzine A, a novel promising acetylcholinesterase inhibitor. Neuroreport 8:97–101, 1996

Cohen D, Eisdorfer C: Depression in family members caring for a relative with Alzheimer's disease. J Am Geriatr Soc 36:885–889, 1988

Cook L, Nickolson VJ, Steinfels GF, et al: Cognition enhancement by the acetylcholine releaser DUP 996. Drug Development Research 19:301–314, 1990

Corey-Bloom J, Anand R, Veach J for the ENA 713 B352 Study Group: A randomized trial evaluating the efficacy and safety of ENA 713 (rivastigmine tartrate), a new acetylcholinesterase inhibitor, in patients with mild to moderately severe Alzheimer's disease. International Journal of Geriatric Psychopharmacology 1:55–65, 1998

Croisile B, Trillet M, Fondari J, et al: Long-term and high-dose piracetam treatment of Alzheimer's disease. Neurology 43:301–305, 1993

Crook T: Pharmacotherapy of cognitive deficits in Alzheimer's disease and age-associated memory impairment. Psychopharmacol Bull 24:31–38, 1988

Culebras A: Update on disorders of sleep and the sleep-wake cycle. Psychiatr Clin North Am 15:467–486, 1992

Cummings JL, Benson DF: Dementia: A Clinical Approach, 2nd Edition. Boston, MA, Butterworth-Heinemann, 1992

Cummings JL, Gorman DG, Shapira J: Physostigmine ameliorates the delusions of Alzheimer's disease. Biol Psychiatry 33:536–541, 1993

Cummings JL, Cyrus PA, Bieger F, et al: Metrifonate treatment of the cognitive deficits of Alzheimer's disease. Neurology 50:1214–1221, 1998

Cutler NR, Lhaxby J, Kay AD, et al: Evaluation of zimelidine in Alzheimer's disease: cognitive and biochemical measures. Arch Neurol 42:744–748, 1985

Davidson M, Zemishlany Z, Mohs RC, et al: 4-Aminopyridine in the treatment of Alzheimer's disease. Biol Psychiatry 23:485–490, 1988

Davies P, Verth AH: Regional distribution of muscarinic acetylcholine receptor in normal and Alzheimer's type dementia brains. Brain Res 138:385–392, 1977

Davis KL, Haroutunian V: Strategies for the treatment of Alzheimer's disease. Neurology 43 (suppl 4): S52–S55, 1993

Davis KL, Thal LJ, Gamzu ER, et al: A double-blind, placebo-controlled multicenter study of tacrine for Alzheimer's disease: the Tacrine Collaborative Study Group. N Engl J Med 327:1253–1259, 1992

Devanand DP, Sackeim HA, Brown RP, et al: A pilot study of haloperidol treatment of psychosis and behavioral disturbance in Alzheimer's disease. Arch Neurol 46:854–857, 1989

Devanand DP, Cooper T, Sackeim HA, et al: Low dose oral haloperidol and blood levels in Alzheimer's disease: a preliminary study. Psychopharmacol Bull 28:169–173, 1992

Evans DA: Estimated prevalence of Alzheimer's disease in the United States. Milbank Q 68:267–289, 1990

Evans DA, Funkenstein H, Albert MS, et al: Prevalence of Alzheimer's disease in a community population of older persons: higher than previously reported. JAMA 262:2551–2556, 1989

Fahn S: A pilot trial of high-dose alpha-tocopherol and ascorbate in early Parkinson's disease. Ann Neurol 32 (suppl):S128–S132, 1992

Farlow M, Gracon SI, Hershey LA, et al: A controlled trial of tacrine in Alzheimer's disease. JAMA 268:2523–2529, 1992

Folstein MF, Folstein SE, McHugh PR: "Mini-Mental State": a practical method for grading the cognitive state of patients for the clinician. J Psychiatr Res 12:189–198, 1975

Frei B, England L, Ames BN: Ascorbate is an outstanding antioxidant in human blood plasma. Proc Natl Acad Sci U S A 86:6377–6381, 1989

Galasko DR, Thal LJ: Cholinomimetic agents, in Alzheimer's Disease: Treatment and Long-Term Management. Edited by Cummings JL, Miller BL. New York, Marcel Dekker, 1990, pp 23–36

Gleason RP, Schneider LS: Carbamazepine treatment of agitation in Alzheimer's outpatients refractory to neuroleptics. J Clin Psychiatry 51:115–118, 1990

Goodman Y, Mattson MP: Secreted forms of beta-amyloid precursor protein protect hippocampal neurons against amyloid beta-peptide-induced oxidative injury. Exp Neurol 128:1–12, 1994

Gorman DG, Read S, Cummings JL: Cholinergic therapy of behavioral disturbances in Alzheimer's disease. Neuropsychiatry Neuropsychol Behav Neurol 6:229–234, 1993

Görtelmeyer R, Erbler H: Memantine in treatment of mild to moderate dementia syndrome. Drug Research 42:904–913, 1992

Gottlieb GL, Kumar A: Conventional pharmacologic treatment for patients with Alzheimer's disease. Neurology 43 (suppl 4):S56–S63, 1993

Gottlieb GL, Piotrowski LS: Neuro are also typical, in Alzheimer's Disease: Treatment and Long-Term Management. Edited by Cummings JL, Miller BL. New York, Marcel Dekker; 1990, pp 89–108

Greenwald BS, Kramer-Ginsberg E, Marin DB, et al: Dementia with coexistent major depression. Am J Psychiatry 146:1472–1478, 1989

Growdon JH: Treatment for Alzheimer's disease? N Engl J Med 327:1306–1308, 1992

Hatcher JP, Looudon JM, Hagan JJ, et al: Sabcomeline (SB-202026), a functionally selective M1 receptor partial agonist, reverses delay-induced deficits in the T-maze. Psychopharmacology 138:275–282, 1998

Henderson VW: The epidemiology of estrogen replacement therapy and Alzheimer's disease. Neurology 48 (suppl):S27–S35, 1997

Henderson VW, Paganini-Hill A, Miller BL, et al: Estrogen for Alzheimer's disease in women: randomized, double-blind, placebo-controlled trial. Neurology 54:295–301, 2000

Herrmann N: Valproic acid treatment of agitation in dementia. Can J Psychiatry 43:69–72, 1998

Heyman A, Schmechel D, Wilkinson W, et al: Failure of long term high-dose lecithin to retard progression of early-onset Alzheimer's disease. J Neural Transm 24:279–286, 1987

Hinz V, Grewig S, Schmidt BH: Metrifonate and dichlorvos: effects of a single oral administration on cholinesterase activity in rat brain and blood. Neurochem Res 21:339–345, 1996a

Hinz V, Grewig S, Schmidt BH: Metrifonate induces cholinesterase inhibition exclusively via slow release of dichlorvos. Neurochem Res 21:331–337, 1996b

Hyman BT: New neuropathologic criteria for Alzheimer's disease. Arch Neurol 55:1174–1176, 1998

Imbimbo BP, Martelli P, Troetel WM, et al: Efficacy and safety of eptastigmine for the treatment of patients with Alzheimer's disease. Neurology 52:700–708, 1999

Jenkinson ML, Bliss MR, Brain AT, et al: Rheumatoid arthritis and senile dementia of the Alzheimer's type. Br J Rheumatol 28:86–88, 1989

Jorgenson J, Bile A, Anderson J, et al: Fluvoxamine treatment of dementia: tryptophan levels. Biol Psychiatry 34:587–588, 1993

Katz IR, Jeste DV, Mintzer JE, et al: Comparison of risperidone and placebo for psychosis and behavioral disturbances associated with dementia: a randomized, double-blind trial. J Clin Psychiatry 60: 107–115, 1999

Katzman R, Aronson M, Fuld PA, et al: Development of dementia in an 80-year-old volunteer cohort. Ann Neurol 25:317–324, 1989

Kaufer DI, Cummings JL, Christine D: Effect of tacrine on behavioral symptoms in Alzheimer's disease: an open-label study. J Geriatr Psychiatry Neurol 9:1–6, 1996

Kawas C, Resnick S, Morrison A, et al: A prospective study of estrogen replacement therapy and the risk of developing Alzheimer's disease: the Baltimore Longitudinal Study of Aging. Neurology 48:1517–1521, 1997

Knapp MJ, Knopman DS, Solomon PR, et al: A 30-week randomized controlled trial of high-dose tacrine in patients with Alzheimer's disease. The Tacrine Study Group. JAMA 271:985–991, 1994

Knopman D, Schneider L, Davis K, et al: Long-term tacrine (Cognex) treatment: effects on nursing home placement and mortality. Tacrine Study Group. Neurology 47:166–177, 1996

Koh S, Oyler GA, Higgins GA: Localization of nerve growth factor receptor messenger RNA and protein in the adult rat brain. Exp Neurol 106:209–221, 1989

Kornhuber J, Bormann J, Retz W, et al: Memantine displaces [3H]MK-801 at therapeutic concentrations in postmortem human frontal cortex. Eur J Pharmacol 166:589–590, 1989

Lahiri DK, Farlow MR, Sambamurti K: The secretion of amyloid β-peptides is inhibited in the tacrine-treated human neuroblastoma cells. Brain Res Mol Brain Res 62:131–140, 1998

Le Bars PL, Katz MM, Berman N, et al: A placebo-controlled, double-blind, randomized trial of an extract of Ginkgo biloba for dementia. North American EGb Study Group. JAMA 278:1327–1332, 1997

Leibovici A, Tariot PN: Carbamazepine treatment of agitation associated with dementia. J Geriatr Psychiatry Neurol 1:110–112, 1988

Levine I, Lawlor BA: Family counseling and legal issues in Alzheimer's disease. Psychiatr Clin North Am 14:385–396, 1991

Lucca U, Tettamanti M, Forloni G, et al: Nonsteroidal antiinflammatory drug use in Alzheimer's disease. Biol Psychiatry 36:854–856, 1994

Lyketsos CG, Lindell Veiel L, Baker A, et al: A randomized, controlled trial of bright light therapy for agitated behaviors in dementia patients residing in long-term care. Int J Geriatr Psychiatry 14:520–525, 1999

Mace NL, Rabins PV: The 36-Hour Day. Baltimore, MD, Johns Hopkins University Press, 1981

Maletta GJ: Management of behavior problems in elderly patients with Alzheimer's disease and other dementias. Clin Geriatr Med 4:719–747, 1988

Marder SR, Ames D, Wirshing WC, et al: Schizophrenia. Psychiatr Clin North Am 16:567–587, 1993

Mattson MP: Calcium as sculptor and destroyer of neuronal circuitry. Exp Gerontol 27:29–49, 1992

Mattson MP, Furukawa K, Bruce AJ, et al: Calcium homeostasis and free radical metabolism as convergence points in the pathophysiology of dementia, in Molecular Models of Dementia. Edited by Tanzi R, Wasco W. Clifton, NJ, Humana Press, 1997, p 103

McEvoy CL: Behavioral treatment, in Alzheimer's Disease: Treatment and Long-Term Management. Edited by Cummings JL, Miller BL. New York, Marcel Dekker, 1990, pp 207–244

McGeer PL, Rogers J: Anti-inflammatory agents as a therapeutic approach to Alzheimer's disease. Neurology 42:447–449, 1992

McGeer PL, Schulzer M, McGeer EG: Arthritis and anti-inflammatory agents and possible protective factors for Alzheimer's disease: a review of 17 epidemiologic studies. Neurology 47:425–432, 1996

Mega MS, Cummings JL, Fiorello T, et al: The spectrum of behavioral changes in Alzheimer's disease. Neurology 46:130–135, 1996

Mendez MF, Martin RJ, Smyth KA, et al: Psychiatric symptoms associated with Alzheimer's disease. J Neuropsychiatry Clin Neurosci 2:28–33, 1990

Middlemiss PJ, Glasky AJ, Rathbone MP, et al. AIT-082, a unique purine derivative, enhances nerve growth factor mediated neurite outgrowth from PC12 cells. Neurosci Lett 199:131–134, 1995

Mody CK, Miller BL: Unsuccessful treatments, in Alzheimer's Disease: Treatment and Long-Term Management. Edited by Cummings JL, Miller BL. New York, Marcel Dekker, 1990, pp 69–85

Mohide EA: Informal care of community-dwelling patients with Alzheimer's disease: focus on the family caregiver. Neurology 43 (suppl 4):S16–S19, 1993

Mohr E, Nair NP, Sampson M, et al: Treatment of Alzheimer's disease with sabeluzole: functional and structural correlates. Clin Neuropharmacol 20:338-345, 1997

Morris JC, Cyrus PA, Orazem J, et al: Metrifonate benefits cognitive, behavioral and global function in Alzheimer's disease patients. Neurology 50:1222–1230, 1998

Mulnard RA, Cotman CW, Kawas C, et al: Estrogen replacement therapy for treatment of mild to moderate Alzheimer disease: a randomized controlled trial. Alzheimer's Disease Cooperative Study. JAMA 283:1007–1015, 2000

Newhouse PA, Sunderland T, Tariot PN, et al: Intravenous nicotine in Alzheimer's disease: a pilot study. Psychopharmacology (Berl) 95:171–175, 1988

Nordberg A: In vivo detection of neurotransmitter changes in Alzheimer's disease. Ann N Y Acad Sci 695:27–33, 1993

Nordberg A, Svensson A-L: Cholinesterase inhibitors in the treatment of Alzheimer's disease: a comparison of tolerability and pharmacology. Drug Saf 19:465–480, 1998

Oda T, Lehrer-Graiwer J, Finch CE, et al: Complement and β-amyloid (Aβ) neurotoxicity in vitro: a model for Alzheimer's disease. Alzheimer's Research 1:29–34, 1995

Ohkura T, Isse K, Akazawa K, et al: Evaluation of estrogen treatment in female patients with dementia of the Alzheimer type. Endocr J 41:361–371, 1994

Ouslander JG: Incontinence, in Alzheimer's Disease: Treatment and Long-Term Management. Edited by Cummings JL, Miller BL. New York, Marcel Dekker, 1990, pp 177–206

Overman W Jr, Stoudemire A: Guidelines for legal and financial counseling of Alzheimer's disease patients and their families, Am J Psychiatry 145:1495–1500, 1988

Packer L, Haramaski N, Kawabata T, et al: Ginkgo biloba extract (EGb 761), in Effect of Ginkgo Biloba Extract (EGb 761) on Aging and Age-Related Disorders. Edited by Christen Y, Courtois Y, Droy-Lefaix MT. Paris, France, Editions Scientifiques Elsevier Paris, 1995, pp 23–47

Paganini-Hill A, Henderson VW: Estrogen deficiency and risk of Alzheimer's disease in women. Am J Epidemiol 140:256–261, 1994

Palmer AM, Stratmann GC, Procter AW, et al: Possible neurotransmitter basis of behavioral changes in Alzheimer's disease. Ann Neurol 23:616–620, 1988

Pantev M, Ritter R, Görtelmeyer R: Clinical and behavioural evaluation in long-term care patients with mild to moderate dementia under Memantine treatment. Zeitschrift für Gerontolpsychologie und Psychiatrie 6:103–117, 1993

Pappert EJ, Tangney CC, Goetz CG, et al: Alpha-tocopherol in the ventricular cerebrospinal fluid of Parkinson's disease patients: dose-response study and correlations with plasma levels. Neurology 47:1037–1042, 1996

Parsons CG, Gruner R, Rozental J, et al: Patch clamp studies on the kinetics and selectivity of N-methyl-D-aspartate receptor antagonism by Memantine (1-amino-3,5-dimethyl-adamantan). Neuropharmacology 32:1337–1350, 1993

Pascale A, Etcheberrigaray R: Calcium alterations in Alzheimer's disease: pathophysiology, models and therapeutic opportunities. Pharmacol Res 39(2):81–88, 1999

Pasinetti GM, Aisen PS: Cyclooxygenase-2 expression is increased in frontal cortex of Alzheimer's disease brain. Neuroscience 87:319–324, 1998

Patocka J: Huperzine A—an interesting anticholinesterase compound from the Chinese herbal medicine. Acta Medica 41:155–157, 1998

Paveza GJ: Social services and the Alzheimer's disease patient: an overview. Neurology 43 (suppl 4): S11–S15, 1993

Penn RD, Martin EM, Wilson RS, et al: Intraventricular bethanechol infusion for Alzheimer's disease: results of double-blind and escalating-dose trials. Neurology 38:219–222, 1988

Pollock BG, Mulsant BH, Sweet R, et al: An open pilot study of citalopram for behavioral disturbances of dementia: plasma levels and real-time observations. Am J Geriatr Psychiatry 5:70–78, 1997

Rabins PV, Fitting MD, Eastham J, et al: The emotional impact of caring for the chronically ill. Psychosomatics 31:331-336, 1990

Rai G, Wright G, Scott L, et al: Double-blind, placebo controlled study of acetyl-L-carnitine in patients with Alzheimer's dementia. Curr Med Res Opin 11:638–647, 1990

Rainer M: Clinical studies of galanthamine. Drugs Today 4:273–279, 1997a

Rainer M: Galanthamine in Alzheimer's disease: a new alternative to tacrine? CNS Drugs 7:89–97, 1997b

Raskind MA, Risse SC: Antipsychotic drugs and the elderly. J Clin Psychiatry 47 (no 5, suppl):17–22, 1986

Raskind MA, Risse SC, Lampe TH: Dementia and antipsychotic drugs. J Clin Psychiatry 48 (5 suppl): 16–18, 1987

Raskind MA, Cyrus PA, Ruzicka BB, et al for the Metrifonate Study Group: The effects of metrifonate on the cognitive, behavioral, and functional performance of Alzheimer's disease patients. J Clin Psychiatry 60:318–325, 1999

Read SL, Frazee J, Shapira J, et al: Intracerebroventricular bethanechol for Alzheimer's disease. Arch Neurol 47:1025–1030, 1990

Reifler BV, Teri L, Raskind M, et al: Double-blind trial of imipramine in Alzheimer's disease patients with and without depression. Am J Psychiatry 146:45–49, 1989

Reisberg B, Borenstein J, Salob SP, et al: Behavioral symptoms in Alzheimer's disease: phenomenology and treatment. J Clin Psychiatry 48 (suppl):9–15, 1987

Reynolds CF, Hoch CC, Stack J, et al: The nature and management of sleep/wake disturbance in Alzheimer's dementia. Psychopharmacol Bull 24:43–48, 1988

Rich JB, Rasmusson DX, Folstein MF, et al: Nonsteroidal anti-inflammatory drugs in Alzheimer's disease. Neurology 45:51–55, 1995

Risse SC, Barnes R: Pharmacologic treatment of agitation associated with dementia. J Am Geriatr Soc 34:368–376, 1986

Rockwood K, Beattie BL, Easwood MR, et al: A randomized, controlled trial of linopridine in the treatment of Alzheimer's disease. Can J Neurol Sci 24:140–145, 1997

Rogers J, Kirby LC, Hempelman SR, et al: Clinical trial of indomethacin in Alzheimer's disease. Neurology 43:1609–1611, 1993

Rogers SL, Friedhoff LT, and the Donepezil Study Group: The efficacy and safety of donepezil in patients with Alzheimer's disease: results of a US multicenter randomized double blind placebo controlled trial. Dementia 7:293–303, 1996

Rogers SL, Farlow MR, Doody RS, et al: A 24-week, double-blind, placebo-controlled trial of donepezil in patients with Alzheimer's disease. Donepezil Study Group. Neurology 50:136–145, 1998

Rösler M, Cicin-Sain A, Gautheir S, et al: Efficacy and safety of rivastigmine in patients with Alzheimer's disease: international randomised controlled trial. BMJ 318:633–638, 1999

Salzman C: Treatment of the elderly agitated patient. J Clin Psychiatry 48 (5 suppl):19–22, 1987

Salzman C: Treatment of agitation, anxiety, and depression in dementia. Psychopharmacol Bull 24:39–42, 1988

Sano M, Ernesto C, Thomas RG, et al: A controlled trial of selegiline, alpha-tocopherol, or both as treatment for Alzheimer's disease: the Alzheimer Disease Cooperative Study. N Engl J Med 336: 1216–1222, 1997

Scharf S, Mander A, Ugoni A, et al: A double-blind, placebo-controlled trial of diclofenac/misoprostol in Alzheimer's disease. Neurology 53:197–201, 1999

Schenk D, Barbour R, Dunn W, et al: Immunization with amyloid-β attenuates Alzheimer-disease-like pathology in the PDAPP mouse. Nature 400:173–177, 1999

Schneider LS: Clinical pharmacology of aminoacridines in Alzheimer's disease. Neurology 43 (suppl 4): S64–S79, 1993

Schneider LS, Sobin PB: Non-neuroleptic treatment of behavioral symptoms and agitation in Alzheimer's disease and other dementia. Psychopharmacol Bull 28:71–79, 1992

Schneider LS, Pollock VE, Lyness SA: A metaanalysis of controlled trials of neuroleptic treatment in dementia. J Am Geriatr Soc 38:553–563, 1990

Schultz J, Schaller J, McKinley M, et al: Enhanced cytotoxicity of amyloid beta-peptide by a complement dependent mechanism. Neurosci Lett 175:99–102, 1994

Sedman AJ, Bockbrader H, Schwarz RD: Preclinical and phase 1 clinical characterization of CI-979/RU35926, a novel muscarinic agonist for the treatment of Alzheimer's disease. Life Sci 56:877–882, 1995

Shumaker SA, Reboussin BA, Espeland MA, et al: The Women's Health Initiative Memory Study (WHIMS): a trial of the effect of estrogen therapy in preventing and slowing the progression of dementia. Control Clin Trials 19:604–621, 1998

Small GW, Rabins PV, Barry PP, et al: Diagnosis and treatment of Alzheimer disease and related disorders: consensus statement of the American Association for Geriatric Psychiatry, the Alzheimer's Association, and the American Geriatrics Society. JAMA 278:1363–1371, 1997

Spagnoli A, Lucca U, Menasce G, et al: Long-term acetyl-L-carnitine treatment in Alzheimer's disease. Neurology 41:1726–1732, 1991

Steele C, Lucas MJ, Tune L: Haloperidol versus thioridazine in the treatment of behavioral symptoms in senile dementia of the Alzheimer's type: preliminary findings. J Clin Psychiatry 47:310–312, 1986

Steele C, Rovner B, Chase GA, et al: Psychiatric symptoms and nursing home placement of patients with Alzheimer's disease. Am J Psychiatry 147:1049–1051, 1990

Stern RG, Duffelmeyer ME, Zemishlani Z, et al: The use of benzodiazepines in the management of behavioral symptoms in demented patients. Psychiatr Clin North Am 14:375–384, 1991

Stewart WF, Kawas C, Coron B, et al: Alzheimer's disease and duration of NSAID use. Neurology 48:626–632, 1997

Stoppe G, Brandt CA, Staedt JH: Behavioural problems associated with dementia: the role of newer antipsychotics. Drugs Aging 14:41–54, 1999

Sultzer DL, Cummings JL: Alzheimer's disease, in Conn's Current Therapy. Edited by Rakel RE. Philadelphia, PA, WB Saunders, 1993, pp 838–840

Sultzer DL, Gray KF, Gunay I, et al: A comparison of trazodone and haloperidol for treatment of agitation in dementia. Paper presented at the 148th annual meeting of the American Psychiatric Association, Miami, FL, May 1995

Summers WK, Viesselman JO, Marsh GM, et al: Use of THA in treatment of Alzheimer-like dementia; pilot study in twelve patients. Biol Psychiatry 16:145–153, 1981

Summers WK, Majovski LV, Marsh GM, et al: Oral tetrahydro-aminoacridine in long-term treatment of senile dementia, Alzheimer's type. N Engl J Med 315:1241–1245, 1986

Swanwick GR, Lawlor BA: Initiating and monitoring cholinesterase inhibitor treatment for Alzheimer's disease. Int J Geriatr Psychiatry 14:244–248, 1999

Tariot PN, Cohen RM, Welkowitz JA, et al: Multiple-dose arecoline infusions in Alzheimer's disease. Arch Gen Psychiatry 45:901–905, 1988

Tariot PN, Erb R, Podgorski DA, et al: Efficacy and tolerability of carbamazepine for agitation and aggression in dementia. Am J Psychiatry 155:54–61, 1998

Tariot PN, Solomon PR, Morris JC, et al: A 5-month, randomized, placebo-controlled trial of galantamine in AD. The Galantamine USA-10 Study Group. Neurology 54:2269–2276, 2000

Thal LJ, Schwartz G, Sano M: A multicenter double-blind study of controlled-release physostigmine for the treatment of symptoms secondary to Alzheimer's disease. Neurology 47:1389–1395, 1996

Thompson TL, Filley CM, Mitchell WD, et al: Lack of efficacy of Hydergine in patients with Alzheimer's disease. N Engl J Med 323:445–448, 1990

Tocco G, Freire-Moar J, Schreiber SS, et al: Maturational regulation and regional induction of cyclooxygenase-2 in rat brain: implications for Alzheimer's disease. Exp Neurol 144:339–349, 1997

Tollefson GD: Short-term effects of the calcium channel blocker nimodipine (Bay-e-9736) in the management of primary degenerative dementia. Biol Psychiatry 27:1133–1142, 1990

Toseland RW, Rossiter CM, Labreque MS: The effectiveness of peer-led and professionally led groups to support family caregivers. Gerontologist 29:465–471, 1989

Tuszynski MH, Roberts J, Senut M-C, et al: Gene therapy in the adult primate brain: intraparenchymal grafts of cells genetically modified to produce nerve growth factor prevent cholinergic neuronal degeneration. Gene Ther 3:305–314, 1996

Van Someren EJ, Kessler A, Mirmiran M, et al: Indirect bright light improves circadian rest-activity rhythm disturbances in demented patients. Biol Psychiatry 41:955–963, 1997

Vassar R, Bennett BD, Babu-Khan S, et al: Beta-secretase cleavage of Alzheimer's amyloid precursor protein by the transmembrane aspartic protease BACE. Science 286:735–741, 1999

Waters CH: Nootropics, in Alzheimer's Disease: Treatment and Long-Term Management. Edited by Cummings JL, Miller BL. New York, Marcel Dekker, 1990, pp 53–67

Weyer G, Babej-Dölle RM, Hadler D, et al: A controlled study of 2 doses of idebenone in the treatment of Alzheimer's disease. Neuropsychobiology 36:73–82, 1997

Wilcock GK, Lilienfeld S, Gaens E: Efficacy and safety of galantamine in patients with mild to moderate Alzheimer's disease: multicentre randomised controlled trial. BMJ 321:1445–1449, 2000

Winblad B, Poritis N: Memantine in severe dementia: results of the 9M-BEST Study (Benefit and Efficacy in Severely Demented Patients During Treatment With Memantine). Int J Geriatr Psychiatry 14:135–146, 1999

Winkler J, Fonten AN, Sung CM, et al: Induction of Schwann cell hyperplasia in vivo after intracerebroventricular administration of nerve growth factor. Soc Neurosci Abstr 21:278, 1995

Wragg RE, Jeste DV: Neuroleptics and alternative treatments: management of behavioral symptoms and psychosis in Alzheimer's disease and related conditions. Psychiatr Clin North Am 11:195–213, 1988

Wragg RE, Jeste DV: Overview of depression and psychosis in Alzheimer's disease. Am J Psychiatry 146:577–587, 1989

Yaffe K, Sawaya G, Lieberburg I, et al: Estrogen therapy in postmenopausal women: effects on cognitive function and dementia. JAMA 279:688–695, 1998

Yesavage I: Ergoloid mesylates (hydergine), in Alzheimer's Disease: Treatment and Long-Term Management. Edited by Cummings JL, Miller BL. New York, Marcel Dekker, 1990, pp 45–52

Zarit SH, Reever KE, Bach-Peterson I: Relatives of the impaired elderly: correlates of feelings of burden. Gerontologist 20:649–655, 1980

Zarit SH, Todd PA, Zarit JM: Subjective burden of husbands and wives as caregivers: a longitudinal study. Gerontologist 26:260–266, 1986

Zayas EM, Grossberg GT: Treating the agitated Alzheimer patient. J Clin Psychiatry 57 (suppl 7):46–51; discussion 52–54, 1996

21

Vascular Dementia

John W. Burruss, M.D.
Javier I. Travella, M.D.
Robert G. Robinson, M.D.

The term *vascular dementia* refers to a condition in which cerebrovascular disease has caused brain injury without a change in level of consciousness but with a global decline in cognitive functions. Until 25 years ago, elderly patients with focal neurological signs and dementia were classified as having *arteriosclerotic dementia.* In 1974, Hachinski and colleagues, based on their clinical investigations and neuropathological studies, suggested the term *multi-infarct dementia* for patients with cognitive impairments associated with multiple bilateral ischemic strokes. The authors emphasized that the vascular process was quantal and episodic rather than continuous and chronic. Since that time, multi-infarct dementia, defined as global decline of cognitive function produced by the cumulative effects of multiple cerebral strokes, is the best recognized form of vascular dementia, having been diagnosed in approximately 9% of the patients in a clinical series of dementia cases and 23% of autopsy brains from patients with dementia (Chui 1989).

Because advancing age is one of the most important risk factors for stroke, increases in life expectancy have been associated with increases in the prevalence of cerebrovascular disease and of vascular dementia. Thus, not only is stroke the third most common cause of death in the elderly population, but it has also become the second most common cause of dementia next to Alzheimer's disease. There is also a new emphasis on the so-called mixed dementia resulting from the complex interaction between vascular dementia and Alzheimer's disease. Identification of risk factors that predispose one to cerebrovascular disease may lead to improved prophylactic and therapeutic measures. The early diagnosis and prevention of further infarcts also may reduce morbidity and impairment (Meyer et al. 1988; Roberts et al. 1991).

Classification

The criteria used to define vascular dementia have included imprecise and sometimes confusing terminology. One of the problems is that there is considerable heterogeneity among the conditions that are included under the rubric of cerebrovascular disease. *Arteriosclerotic dementia,* which implies dementia associated with "hardening" of the arteries, is used to describe dementias that might be caused by thromboembolic cerebral vascular disease or by numerous brain regions of hypoperfusion resulting in neuronal death, cortical atrophy, and eventual dementia. On the other hand, the term *multi-infarct dementia* is sometimes considered to be synonymous with all types of dementias of vascular etiology, incorrectly implying that multiple brain infarcts are the only cause of vascular dementia.

Loeb and Meyer (1996) classified at least eight subtypes of vascular dementia based on clinical and neuropathological correlates. *Atherosclerotic dementia,* or the classic multi-infarct dementia, usually has been associated with one or more large areas of infarction with ischemic damage to the cortex and subcortical white matter of one or both hemispheres or with many lesions ranging from a few millimeters to several centimeters in diameter. The damage results from multiple emboli that often occur in the vascular territory of the major arteries. Neurological deficits are pronounced, and a physician can usually predict which vessel is occluded based on the clinical presentation of symptoms.

Arteriosclerotic dementia, by contrast, also has been associated with the presence of microinfarcts, white matter changes of various types, vascular changes, unidentified deposits in the lumen of small blood vessels, and decreased competence of the blood-brain barrier. Tomlinson and Henderson (1976) emphasized the large size of these areas of brain destruction and implied that arteriosclerotic dementia is not caused by simple pathological lesions. Other authors, however, have stressed the importance of lesion location as well as the vascular territory involved (Katz et al. 1987; Philips et al. 1987). These emphases led to a formulation of atherosclerotic dementia in which both the volume of infarcted brain and the distribution and strategic location of lesions are important in the development of this type of vascular dementia.

Multiple lacunar infarcts, originally described by Marie (1901) and later systematically investigated by Fisher (1968), are thought causative of another subtype of vascular dementia. They are small cerebral infarcts or lacunae (*état lacunaire*) that result from the occlusion of deeply penetrating arterioles. On computed tomography (CT) or magnetic resonance imaging (MRI), lesions appear as small lacunae or holes in the basal ganglia, thalamus, upper brain stem, and/or white matter. This regional specificity suggests the importance of subcortical involvement in dementia (Bamford et al. 1987).

Another category of vascular dementia could be identified based on the cumulative effects of *reductions in regional cerebral perfusion* (Howard et al. 1987; Samson et al. 1985). Patients with severe occlusive disease in carotid or vertebral arteries may develop vascular dementia as a result of the widespread area of reduced cerebral perfusion. This condition often can be diagnosed with arteriography or Doppler ultrasonography. Reduced cerebral perfusion also may be diagnosed by changes in blood flow detected by positron-emission tomography (PET) scanning (Hachinski et al. 1975; Samson et al. 1985).

In 1894, Binswanger described macroscopically a diffuse loss of white matter in patients with chronic hypertension and gradually progressive dementia. This clinicopathological entity has been referred to as *Binswanger's disease* or *subcortical arteriosclerotic encephalopathy.* The clinical picture of patients with Binswanger's disease is characterized by severe deep white matter changes, history of hypertension, gait disturbance, urinary incontinence, focal neurological symptoms, and a progressive decline in cognitive status. The relation between deep white matter pathological findings and dementia is difficult to establish because most patients with Binswanger's disease also have cerebral infarcts. Although some authors correlated the deep white matter changes with gait disturbance rather than with cognitive deficits (Loizou et al. 1981; Rao et al. 1989), others (Kertesz et al. 1990; Kluger et al. 1988) showed associations between deep white matter lesions and cognitive slowing, impaired comprehension, and attention deficits. Hachinski (1992), on the other hand, contended that deep white matter changes are attributed with unjustified frequency to Binswanger's disease because 40% of patients with Alzheimer's disease and more than 80% of patients with vascular dementia had such changes visualized on CT scan. Caplan (1995) went so far as to deny a single case of Binswanger's disease, instead attributing many diverse causes and pathophysiologies to the chronic ischemia that leads to periventricular and deep white matter changes, referred to as *leukoariosis.* Additional research is required to determine the importance of deep white matter lesions on the development of cognitive impairment.

Modern genetic technologies have established a new type of hereditary vascular dementia that was first described in Europe. *Cerebral autosomal dominant arteriopathy with subcortical infarcts and leukoencephalopathy (CADASIL)* is characterized by subcortical infarcts and dementia. This heritable dementing disorder can be mapped to the short arm of chromosome 19, but the gene has yet to be identified (Salloway and Hong 1998; Sondergaard et al. 1998). The discovery of CADASIL is particularly salient because it predicts the many potential variations on the common theme of vascular dementia that will likely occur in the coming years.

Finally, other types of vascular disease also could be used to classify subtypes of vascular dementia. Examples are inflammatory vasculitis associated with collagen vascular disease, ischemia of the brain secondary to shunting of blood into an arteriovenous malformation, and vasospasm due to subarachnoid hemorrhage or rupture of an intracranial aneurysm (Loeb 1985).

Thus, although the causal relation between the different sequelae of various vascular diseases and cognitive decline has yet to be established, numerous types of lesions that are produced by vascular insufficiency (e.g., white matter lesions of Binswanger's disease) are thought to be etiologically responsible for subsets of vascular dementia. Many investigators have used these pathological varieties to classify or subclassify the wide array of cognitive impairments (from verbal reasoning to visual construction) and vascular diseases (from large atherosclerotic infarcts to small lacunar infarcts) subsumed under the category of vascular dementia with varying degrees of success. Yet another classification scheme—based on genetic markers and more precise knowledge of the causative factors of cognitive impairment—will likely be presented in the near future.

Diagnostic Criteria

As discussed in the previous section, one of the major problems that has complicated the development of research studies of vascular dementia is the lack of consensus about the diagnosis and subclassification of this disorder. Advances in neuroimaging have been integral in earlier and more accurate diagnosis but have also hindered diagnostic clarity even further. Both CT and MRI scanning have enabled us to visualize infarcts that would otherwise be clinically silent. Some investigators have suggested that dementia might be overdiagnosed (Brust 1988) or underdiagnosed (O'Brien 1988) because of the lack of standardized diagnostic criteria for incorporating findings from imaging studies. Developers of the Hachinski Ischemia Score (HIS; Hachinski et al. 1974), which provided a useful guideline for the diagnosis of multi-infarct dementia, did not have the benefit of imaging criteria and based their instrument on the assumption that all vascular dementias are caused by infarcts. This instrument has proven helpful but imperfect, especially when Alzheimer's disease coexists with vascular dementia. The HIS also has been faulted for ignoring the occurrence of dementia caused by nonstroke ischemic mechanisms (Drachman 1993).

Criteria for vascular dementia have been developed by a group of Alzheimer's Disease Diagnostic and Treatment Centers (ADDTC) in California (Chui et al. 1992). To improve the sensitivity and specificity of clinical diagnosis, these new criteria were developed specifically to identify cognitive disturbances that result from ischemic, but not hemorrhagic or anoxic, injuries. Three categories of vascular dementia are described (definitive, probable, and possible) as well as a novel category of mixed dementia. Mixed dementia is a disorder in which other systemic or brain disorders, in addition to the primary disorder, may be causally related to the dementia (e.g., mixed dementia due to definitive vascular dementia or Alzheimer's disease and hypothyroidism). Histopathological examination of the brain is required to clarify the underlying etiology and to exclude the overlap with another disorder such as Alzheimer's disease.

With the same purpose, the Neuroepidemiology Branch of the National Institute of Neurological Disorders and Stroke (NINDS), with support from the Association Internationale pour la Recherche et l'Enseignement en Neurosciences (ARIEN), convened an international workshop to develop easily applicable criteria for reliable and valid diagnosis of vascular dementia (Roman et al. 1993). The guidelines developed by this workshop group emphasized, first, the heterogeneity of vascular dementia syndromes. The vascular pathological subtypes include ischemic and hemorrhagic strokes, cerebral hypoxyischemic events, and senile leukoencephalopathy. These guidelines also emphasized that the clinical course of vascular dementia may be static, remitting, or progressive. In an effort to distinguish vascular dementia from degenerative dementia, the workshop participants noted specific clinical findings early in the course of vascular dementia (e.g., incontinence, personality changes) that are more likely to be associated with vascular disease than with a degenerative cause. They also noted that there should be a close temporal relation between stroke onset and dementia onset. In addition, they recommended that brain imaging should support the clinical findings and highlighted the value of neuropsychological testing to address impairments in cognitive function. Finally, they proposed that there should be a protocol for neuropathological evaluations and an effort made to conduct correlative studies of clinical, radiological, and neuropsychological features. Gold et al. (1997) showed that each of these diagnostic criteria has its own limitations, particularly when faced with "mixed" cases of dementia.

A third set of diagnostic criteria was developed in DSM-IV (American Psychiatric Association 1994; Table 21–1). Although subject to the same criticisms as the NINDS-ARIEN and ADDTC criteria, the DSM-IV criteria take into account both the breadth of cognitive impairment and the importance of imaging studies to limit the diagnoses to patients with

TABLE 21–1. DSM-IV diagnostic criteria for vascular dementia

A. The development of multiple cognitive deficits manifested by both
   (1) memory impairment (impaired ability to learn new information or to recall previously learned information)
   (2) one (or more) of the following cognitive disturbances:
      (a) aphasia (language disturbance)
      (b) apraxia (impaired ability to carry out motor activities despite intact motor function)
      (c) agnosia (failure to recognize or identify objects despite intact sensory function)
      (d) disturbance in executive functioning (i.e., planning, organizing, sequencing, abstracting)

B. The cognitive deficits in criteria A1 and A2 each cause significant impairment in social or occupational functioning and represent a significant decline from a previous level of functioning.

C. Focal neurological signs and symptoms (e.g., exaggeration of deep tendon reflexes, extensor plantar response, pseudobulbar palsy, gait abnormalities, weakness of an extremity) or laboratory evidence indicative of cerebrovascular disease (e.g., multiple infarctions involving cortex and underlying white matter) that are judged to be etiologically related to the disturbance.

D. The deficits do not occur exclusively during the course of a delirium.

Code based on predominant features:

290.41 **With delirium:** if delirium is superimposed on the dementia

290.42 **With delusions:** if delusions are the predominant feature

290.43 **With depressed mood:** if depressed mood (including presentations that meet full symptom criteria for a major depressive episode) is the predominant feature. A separate diagnosis of mood disorder due to a general medical condition is not given.

290.40 **Uncomplicated:** if none of the above predominates in the current clinical presentation

Specify if:

With behavioral disturbance

Coding note: Also code cerebrovascular condition on Axis III.

evidence of widespread focal brain lesions caused by ischemia. This issue, however, is far from resolved, and until we know the mechanism by which ischemic lesions lead to the dementia syndrome, as we may soon with entities such as CADASIL, we cannot be certain what varieties of ischemic lesions constitute a vascular dementia.

Epidemiology

Vascular dementia is second to Alzheimer's disease as the most common cause of age-associated dementia in the Western world (Roman 1991). In Japan, vascular dementia is the most common type of dementia, representing up to 50% of all clinical cases and from 54% to 65% of all autopsy-confirmed dementia cases (Suzuki et al. 1991; Yamaguchi et al. 1992). Prevalence estimates from community samples indicate that, on average, 1%–4% of persons older than 65 have vascular dementia, resulting in 6–12 cases per 1,000 people older than 70 years (Hebert and Brayne 1995).

Clinicopathological studies have shown that Alzheimer's disease accounts for 50%–60%, and vascular disease (e.g., multi-infarct disease) about 10%–20%, of the cases of dementia in the United States (Loeb 1985). Furthermore, as many as 20% of patients have a mixture of both disorders. The remaining patients with dementia may have rare or reversible types of dementia. The annual incidence of vascular dementia ranges from 7 per 1,000 person-years in the general population to 16 per 1,000 person-years in subjects at risk for strokes, particularly those with high blood pressure (Forette et al. 1991).

The European Community Concerted Action on Epidemiology and Prevention of Dementia, in a review of population-based studies, found a consistent increase in the prevalence of vascular dementia with advancing age (Rocca et al. 1991). Prevalence rates ranged from 1.5 per 100 for women ages 75–79 years in the United States to 16.3 per 100 for men older than 80 years in Italy. In most age groups, men had a higher prevalence of vascular dementia than did women. This higher prevalence in men has also been confirmed by other authors (Meyer et al. 1989). In general, for patients with either stroke or vascular dementia, male-to-female ratios of between 1:5 and 2:1 have been reported in several studies (Roth 1978; Schoenberg et al. 1987).

In summary, cerebrovascular disease is the second leading cause of dementing illness in the United States and Scandinavia, whereas stroke is the leading cause of dementia in other countries such as Japan, Russia, and China. Incidence rates for vascular dementia rise significantly with age, and many investigations have reported slightly higher morbidity rates among men. Although projections of demographic trends toward a greater number of elderly individuals in the population might suggest that the prevalence of vascular dementia is likely to increase, the declining incidence of stroke over the past 20 years along with future efforts at stroke prevention may be important factors in ameliorating this major cause of dementing illness (Schoenberg et al. 1987).

Patient Assessment and Differential Diagnosis

Dementia is a syndrome that includes both deterioration of intellectual ability and alterations in the patient's emotional and personality functions (Cummings et al. 1980; McPherson and Cummings 1996). Multi-infarct dementia is characterized by an abrupt onset, by stepwise deterioration of intellectual function, and, clinically, by the gradual accumulation of neuropsychological deficits in which some cognitive functions are more impaired than others, resulting from ischemic injury in multiple brain regions (Hachinski et al. 1974). To make the diagnosis, these deficits must not be limited to a period of depression or delirium and must be of sufficient degree to impair work, usual social activities, or interpersonal relationships. Finally, there must be evidence of organic factors related to these disturbances, or, without evidence of an organic factor, an etiological organic factor can be presumed or another factor such as depression can be identified.

For the diagnosis of vascular dementia, cognitive decline should be demonstrated by loss of memory and at least one other deficit in domains including aphasia, apraxia, agnosia, or executive function (American Psychiatric Association 1994). Multifocal deficits are expected, and single defects in cognition, such as amnestic states, aphasias, and apraxias, do not fulfill the criteria. Therefore, although single cognitive deficits do not qualify as vascular dementia, single lesions may produce vascular dementia if they lead to loss of both memory and some other cognitive function of sufficient severity to produce impairment in daily living.

Impaired functioning in daily living as an inclusion criterion for epidemiological studies of vascular dementia is intended to ensure that changes are more than incidental and would increase the specificity of the criteria for detecting true dementia. The impairments in daily functioning, however, should be due to cognitive deficits and not to physical disabilities produced by stroke.

The clinical identification of vascular dementia requires a medical history, a neurological examination, and a thorough psychiatric interview. Often, psychometric testing with a dementia rating scale can help differentiate a complicated case. Testing that can be helpful to exclude less common and reversible causes of dementia includes blood chemistries (including B_{12}, folate, thyroid function), cerebrospinal fluid analysis, an electroencephalogram (EEG) and an EEG with evoked responses, CT, MRI, and, in certain cases, cerebral angiography. These test results will usually identify cases of potentially treatable forms of dementia caused by tumor, vascular malformation, cerebral hematoma, normal pressure hydrocephalus, infections, and metabolic, toxic, and drug-induced encephalopathy, as well as dementia due to vitamin or endocrine deficiencies.

The diagnosis of vascular dementia may be difficult at times. A particularly difficult differential diagnosis occurs in patients with cerebral infarction but without prominent (focal) neurological symptoms. This is frequently the case with thalamic or parietal lobe infarctions that present with confusion and drowsiness as the only clinical manifestations. Diagnostic problems also occur when nonvascular diseases present with focal neurological deficits of acute onset. Acute onset of focal neurological symptoms can occur in cases of intracranial neoplasms, subdural hematoma, cerebral abscess, subdural empyema, multiple sclerosis, Wernicke's encephalopathy, psychogenic disorders, or peripheral nervous system lesions. Distinguishing between embolism and thrombosis and between ischemia and hemorrhagic infarction also can be difficult.

In summary, the diagnosis of vascular dementia is based on a longitudinal history of symptoms of vascular disorder, focal neurological symptoms consistent with ischemia or infarction, demonstrated impairment in a wide range of neuropsychological functions, and laboratory testing consistent with vascular disease. The differential diagnosis should include other causes of dementia ranging from Alzheimer's disease to Huntington's disease. Vascular dementia is frequently misdiagnosed when there are no focal neurological findings or when neurological disorders mimic the temporal course and focal deficits of stroke.

Prevention

Prevention is crucial for patients who are most at risk for vascular dementia and appropriate for the remainder of the populace. The current state of treatment for any established dementing disorder leaves a great deal to be desired, making prevention the physician's most potent weapon. In general, prevention measures are centered on limiting the risk factors for cerebral vascular disease and stroke.

Both high and low blood pressure have been defined as risk factors for vascular dementia. Several studies (Gorelick 1997; Launer et al. 1995; Skoog et al. 1996) have developed sound epidemiological evidence that hypertension is a risk factor for dementia in late life. Similarly, a Japanese study has associated left ventricular hypertrophy, which is the direct result of hypertension, with preclinical, asymptomatic cerebrovascular damage, a harbinger of eventual dementing illness (Kohara et al. 1999). Perhaps most compelling is a double-blind, placebo-controlled study as part of the Systolic Hypertension in Europe trial that has reported a significant lowering in the incidence of dementia when elderly people (>60 years) were treated for isolated systolic hypertension (Forette et al. 1998). The treatment in this study was fairly aggressive, beginning with a calcium channel blocker as primary therapy but adding an angiotensin converting enzyme inhibitor or a diuretic if needed to reduce systolic blood pressure below 150 mm Hg.

Conversely, Meyer et al. (1988), in a longitudinal study of 173 patients, examined the frequency of risk factors for stroke and cerebral atherosclerosis among patients with vascular dementia. Although *hyper*tension is the single most potent risk factor for cerebral atherosclerosis and stroke, *hypo*tension was, by far, the most common risk factor for vascular dementia in this sample. Hypotension was present in 66% of the patients in these authors' series. Also, at least two studies have purported a protective and preventive effect of mildly elevated blood pressure once a patient has developed vascular dementia. Meyer et al. (1986) followed up 52 patients in a naturalistic study in which patients were divided into hypertensive and normotensive groups. The authors found that improved cognition was associated with systolic blood pressures in the upper normal range (135–150 mm Hg). Smoking cessation improved cognition in the normotensive group. Likewise, in a case-control study of demented compared with nondemented poststroke patients, Gorelick et al. (1993) reported improved cognition and clinical course when the hypertensive patients with dementia were managed with systolic blood pressures in the same range (135–150 mm Hg). The authors hypothesized that elevated blood pressures were necessary to maintain cerebral perfusion in the face of vascular distortion caused by chronic hypertension.

Heart disease of the atherosclerotic type, with or without cardiac arrhythmia, also was present in most of the cases of vascular dementia. This cardiac disease may have provided a source of cerebral emboli leading to vascular dementia (Flegel et al. 1987). Cigarette smoking of one or more packs per day was a risk factor in 21% of the patients. Hyperlipidemia of the type 4 form (hypertriglyceridemia) was present in 29% of the cases. Diabetes mellitus of sufficient clinical severity to require medical treatment was found in 20% of the cases, and symptomatic peripheral vascular disease with ischemic symptoms referable to the lower extremities was present in 6% of the cases.

Katzman and Saitho (1990) reported that low education is a risk factor for Alzheimer's disease. Although the explanation for this association is unknown, it has been hypothesized that education may lead to optimal cerebral neuronal plasticity and synaptic development. In a study comparing the risk factors for vascular dementia with those for Alzheimer's disease (Zhang et al. 1990), patients with vascular dementia had less education and a greater frequency of family history of cancer in women than did patients with Alzheimer's disease. The reason for the association of vascular dementia with a family history of cancer in women is unclear. However, high fibrinogen levels have been reported to be associated with both cancer and stroke (Miller and Heilmann 1989; Woimant et al. 1988). The association of vascular dementia with limited education suggests that education-related factors (perhaps neurobiological or social factors) place patients at greater risk for developing dementia from a vascular etiology. Finally, it should be remembered that although degenerative dementias are currently untreatable, the potential exists to prevent or to provide early treatment of cerebrovascular disease and to prevent some of the accompanying cognitive and physical impairments. Thus, identification of risk factors is an important goal of prevention in vascular dementia.

Treatment trials have endeavored to maximize cerebral blood flow in areas of reduced flow or in the "ischemic penumbra" (i.e., areas of partial ischemia surrounding the central area of infarction). Such areas occur immediately after acute stroke, and the resulting impairment may be ameliorated if cerebral blood flow in these areas is restored. The use of hemodilution therapy in combination with other therapies may play a significant role in preventing cognitive impairment due to extension of infarcts into areas of potentially reversible ischemia (Asplund 1987).

For patients who are in a "predementia" stage (i.e., history of transient ischemic attacks, stroke, previous cognitive impairment, or silent cerebral infarctions but without global cognitive impairment), prevention may include carotid endarterectomy (when carotid stenosis is from 70% to 99%), anticoagulants, aspirin, ticlopidine, agents that interfere with amyloid deposition in vessels (in the case of stroke secondary to lupus), and calcium channel blockers (as pretreatment to attenuate the effect of infarcts).

Thus, the identification of factors that place patients at risk for vascular dementia is the goal of prevention efforts. Patients with a history of stroke, hypertension or hypotension, smoking, diabetes mellitus, and atrial fibrillation or other cardiac disease, as well as those of advanced age and limited education, are at higher risk for vascular dementia. Controlling the risk factors in these persons is the key to prevention of vascular dementia.

Treatment

Some of the risk factors for stroke can be effectively treated, thus giving rise to the hope that the natural progression or even pathogenesis of vascular dementia might be treated. In the past decade, new agents have been identified that show promise in slowing or halting the progression of the cognitive loss itself. This predicts a future in which vascular dementia may be treated more directly and more effectively.

Successful management of a progressive dementing disorder requires multimodality treatment, beginning with psychotherapy and psychosocial interventions designed to maintain or improve functionality and safety. The 1997 American Psychiatric Association's "Practice Guideline for the Treatment of Patients with Alzheimer's Disease and Other Dementias of Late Life" recommends the following psychosocial management strategies: 1) establish and maintain an alliance with the patient and family; 2) perform a diagnostic evaluation, and refer the patient for any needed general medical care; 3) assess and monitor psychiatric status; 4) monitor safety and intervene when required; 5) intervene to decrease the hazards of wandering; 6) advise the patient and family about driving and other activities that put other people at risk; 7) educate the patient and family about the illness and available treatments; 8) advise the family about sources of care and support; and 9) guide the family in financial and legal issues.

An innovative and insightful study from New York (Mittelman et al. 1996) showed that addressing the considerable demands placed on the caregivers is crucial in the treatment of dementia. When support and counseling were provided for the spouses of demented patients, there was a statistically significant delay in time to nursing home placement compared with the control group. From a clinical standpoint, this delay was somewhat extraordinary, reaching almost 1 year (329 days, $P = 0.02$) of additional time with the family.

Psychotherapy for the dementia patient should be used if indicated, taking into account the remaining cognitive abilities of the patient and individualizing as necessary. Cognitive therapy, with or without behavioral strategies, supportive psychotherapy, and recreational therapy, can be helpful in maximizing functionality or addressing a concurrent mood or anxiety disorder in a patient with early, mild dementia.

Stroke of cardioembolic origin is responsible for about 15% of all ischemic strokes, and this percentage is even higher among younger patients. The most common disorders causing cardioembolic stroke are atrial fibrillation, with or without mitral stenosis; ischemic heart disease with mural thrombi; and prosthetic cardiac valves. Following cardioembolic stroke, anticoagulation is an effective treatment to reduce the risk of recurrence.

Treatment with antiplatelet aggregant drugs has reduced the number of repeated ischemic vascular episodes in patients with transient ischemic attacks (TIAs) (Fields et al. 1977). The efficacy of these drugs suggests that aspirin treatment also might modify the course of vascular dementia by curtailing the stepwise deterioration caused by each subsequent vascular event. Three large studies showed that acetylsalicylic acid (ASA) is effective in secondary prevention of stroke. The United Kingdom–TIA Aspirin Trial (UK-TIA Study Group 1988), Bousser et al. (1981), and Grotta (1987) all reported a reduction in the risk for stroke with daily ASA therapy. It is yet to be shown in controlled fashion whether this aspirin-mediated reduction in cerebral vascular events is protective against cognitive deterioration, but the results are very promising when combined with the presumed pathophysiology of this disorder.

One platelet aggregation inhibitor, pentoxifylline, has produced improvement in dementia rating scale scores when given in a dosage of 400 mg three times a day over 9 months. The European Pentoxifylline Multi-Infarct Dementia Study (1996) was a double-blind, placebo-controlled study of 289 patients. Those who completed the study showed a significant improvement on the Gottfries, Brane, Steen scale when compared with placebo. This is one of the first studies to show an actual benefit in the cognitive status of dementia patients treated with platelet aggregation inhibitors.

In another study, involving 73 patients with mild vascular dementia, a double-blind, randomized treatment was carried out for 90 days with 300 mg of buflomedil twice daily or placebo (Cucinotta et al. 1992). (Buflomedil is a vasodilator drug with hemorrheological and metabolic properties, capable of dilating collateral vessels and influencing microcirculation and red blood cell function.) At the end of the treatment period, all patients received buflomedil or no further treatment for another 90 days. The efficacy of buflomedil was monitored with rating scales and neuropsychological tests. Study findings indicated that buflomedil improved the symptoms of vascular dementia, with the greatest improvement found in patients who had received buflomedil for the longest time. Inadequacy of attention, poor cooperation, psychoaffective disorder, impaired self-care, and frequency of somatic complaints were all positively influenced by buflomedil. Treatment efficacy may have been the result of effects on platelet aggregation with improvement in blood flow and, ultimately, oxygenation of ischemic brain tissue.

Evidence to support the efficacy of other platelet aggregation inhibitors is scarce, although the European Stroke Prevention Study Group (1987) found that the risk of secondary ischemic lesions was significantly decreased when dipyridamole was added to ASA treatment. This study included 2,500 patients with either TIAs (defined as neurological deficits that resolve within 24 hours), reversible ischemic neurological deficits (defined as neurological deficits that resolve within 24 hours to 7 days), or completed strokes (defined as neurological deficits that persist for more than 7 days). The combination of 75 mg of dipyridamole and 330 mg of ASA daily, compared with placebo, significantly reduced the incidence of stroke or deaths by 33% in the TIA and completed-stroke subgroups. The reversible ischemic group, however, failed to show such improvement. The lack of statistical efficacy in this group may be attributed to the relatively small sample size.

Propentofylline, a neuroprotective glial cell modulator, also has now been shown to improve the cognitive status of patients with both Alzheimer's disease and vascular dementia (Mielke et al. 1998; Rother et al. 1998). In phase III trials, 359 patients with vascular dementia experienced an improvement in cognitive ability and functional level and a slowing of the progression of their disease when given 300 mg of propentofylline three times a day compared with placebo.

Perhaps the most intriguing new weapon in the armamentarium against vascular dementia is Ginkgo biloba, or more properly the active chemical EGb 761. Caution must be exercised in using this agent because it is marketed in the United States as a dietary supplement and therefore not subject to the stringent U.S Food and Drug Administration (FDA) controls applied to prescription medication. However, at least three double-blind, placebo-controlled, randomized studies now have established the safety and purported efficacy of EGb 761. The first study, by Kanowski et al. (1996), evaluated 156 patients with a mixture of Alzheimer's disease and vascular dementia who were given 240 mg/day of EGb 761 or placebo. They showed that EGb 761 led to significantly ($P < 0.005$) improved performance compared with placebo on tests of psychopathology, attention and memory, and activities of daily life. Haase et al. (1996), in a German study, gave intravenous EGb 761 or placebo to 40 patients with moderate severity Alzheimer's disease, vascular dementia, or both. The active treatment group showed significant ($P < 0.05$) improvement in behavior, psychopathology, and psychometric measures. Finally, in the largest and longest of the three trials (Le Bars et al. 1997), 202 patients received EGb 761 (120 mg/day) for 52 weeks. The results of this study showed that treatment could stabilize and, in many cases, improve cognitive performance and social function of demented patients as measured by the Alzheimer's Disease Assessment Scale—Cognitive subscale (ADAS-Cog) and the Geriatric Evaluation by Relatives Rating Instrument.

Other therapeutic measures that may be helpful in vascular dementia include smoking cessation, prevention or careful management of diabetes mellitus, potassium supplementation (because of its vascular protective effect), estrogen replacement (in postmenopausal women), antihypertensives (angiotensin-converting enzyme inhibitors and calcium channel blockers), lipid-lowering agents, anticoagulants (for cases in which emboli are likely), and aspirin. For patients who are in the "dementia stage" (i.e., patients with atherosclerosis of the extracranial arteries, cardiac embolism, or intracranial small vessel disease who have already shown evidence of cognitive decline in several areas of intellectual functioning), treatment measures may include antidepressants, antihypertensives, cholinergic agonists, nerve growth factor, aspirin, or ticlopidine (Hachinski 1992).

In summary, treatment studies have found that the risk of recurrence of cerebrovascular disease can be significantly reduced by the use of aspirin and perhaps dipyridamole. This preventive treatment would presumably reduce the risk of developing vascular dementia. In addition to aspirin/dipyridamole, there have been exciting recent findings regarding neuroprotective agents and EGb 761, which may offer much greater success when treating the dementia itself.

Dementia Related to Poststroke Depression

Comorbid depression deserves special attention as another clinical finding that appears to have a significant relation to dementia in stroke patients. Depression occurs in 25%–45% of patients who have had a stroke (Eastwood et al. 1989; Feibel and Springer 1982; Morris et al. 1990; Robinson et al. 1983). More specifically, one study (Newman 1999) showed a 21.2% prevalence of major depression with vascular dementia compared with a much lower 3.2% association with Alzheimer's disease. Evidence also indicates that major depression is more severe when associated with vascular disease (Ballard et al. 1996a, 1996b; Simpson et al. 1999).

Several studies have reported that patients with poststroke major depression have a greater degree of cognitive impairment than patients with comparable lesions but without major depression (Robinson et al. 1986; Starkstein and Robinson 1991). One study compared the severity of cognitive impairment in 13 pairs of stroke patients with major depression with that in nondepressed stroke patients who were matched for size and location of brain lesion (Starkstein et al. 1988). Patients with poststroke major depression had significantly lower Mini-Mental State Exam (MMSE; Folstein et al. 1975) scores (i.e., indicating more cognitive deficits) than did nondepressed patients with the same size and location of brain lesion (Starkstein et al. 1988) (Figure 21–1).

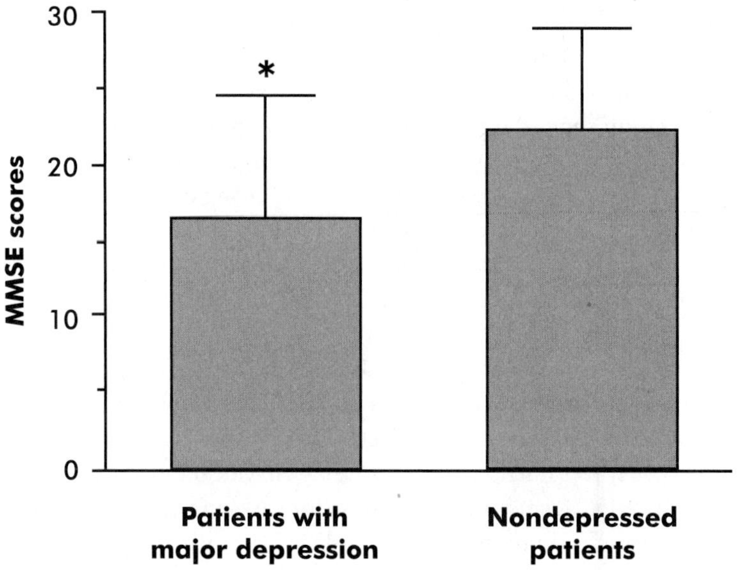

FIGURE 21–1. Severity of cognitive impairment in 13 pairs of stroke patients with major depression and nondepressed stroke patients who were matched for lesion volume and location. Patients with major depression were significantly more impaired in cognitive function as demonstrated by lower Mini-Mental State Exam (MMSE) scores than their lesion-matched nondepressed control subjects ($t = 3.21$, $df = 12$, $P = 0.15$). $^*P < 0.05$.
Source. Data obtained from Starkstein et al. 1988.

In another study, the variety of cognitive impairments associated with depression were examined by administering an extensive neuropsychological battery (Bolla-Wilson et al. 1989). The investigators found that among patients with left-hemisphere lesions, those with major depression were significantly more impaired in overall cognitive functions than were the nondepressed patients (Figure 21–2). In contrast, among patients with right-hemisphere lesions, overall severity of cognitive impairment did not differ significantly between nondepressed and major depression patients (see Figure 21–2).

In a follow-up study of poststroke depression and cognitive impairment, Downhill and Robinson (1994) found that stroke patients with major depression had more severe intellectual impairment than did nondepressed patients at 3, 6, and 12 months following stroke, but only among those patients with left-hemisphere lesions (Figure 21–3). The effect of depression on cognitive function was greatest during the acute poststroke period, but no

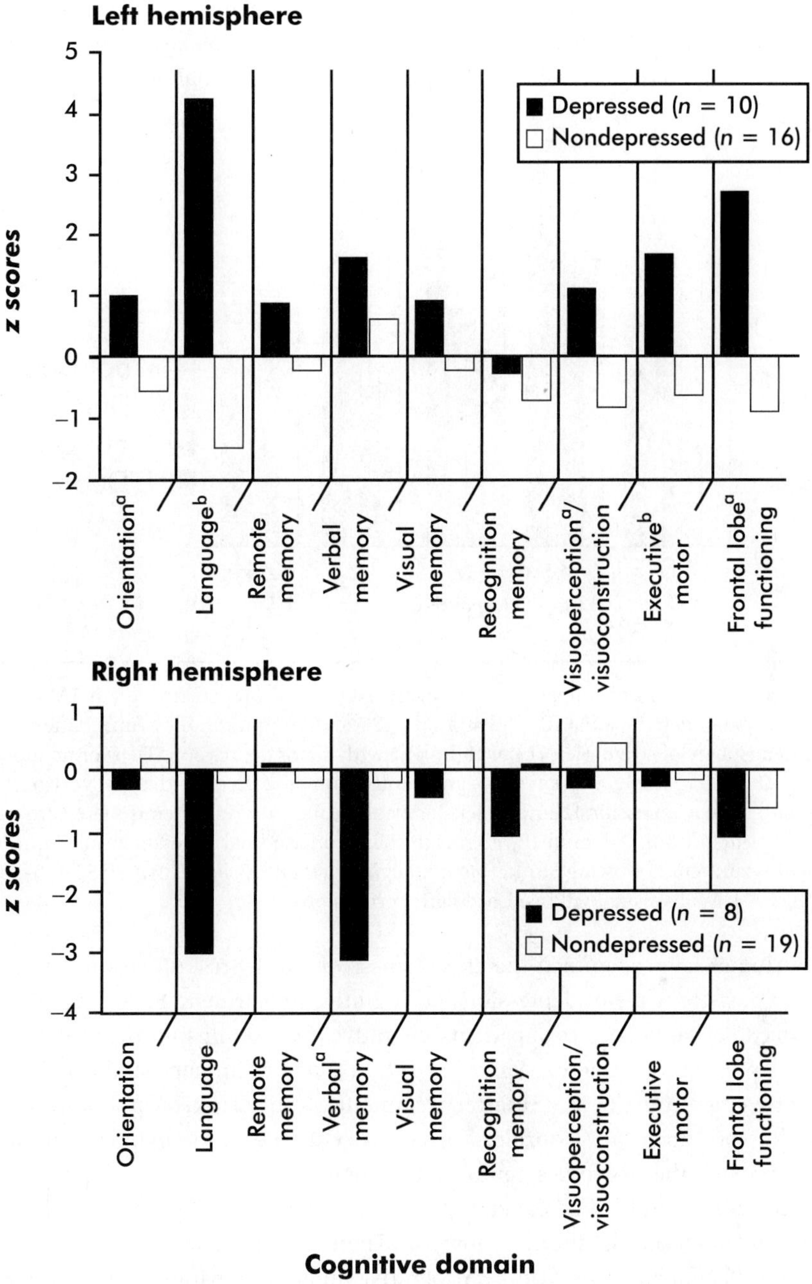

FIGURE 21–2. Performance in nine cognitive domains by depressed and nondepressed patients with left- or right-hemisphere stroke. $^{a}P < 0.05$ and $^{b}P < 0.01$ comparing depressed and nondepressed groups with one-way analysis of variance. Positive *z* scores indicate greater impairment. Note that only patients with major depression following left-hemisphere stroke showed general cognitive impairment compared with nondepressed patients.

Source. Reprinted from Bolla-Wilson K, Robinson RG, Starkstein SE, et al.: "Lateralization of Dementia of Depression in Stroke Patients." *American Journal of Psychiatry* 146:627–634, 1989. Copyright 1989, American Psychiatric Association. Used with permission.

effect could be shown even among patients with left-hemisphere lesions and major depression at 2 years poststroke. These findings suggest that left-hemisphere lesions (particularly lesions of the left frontal cortex or left basal ganglia) that lead to major depression may produce a different kind of depression and cognitive impairment that do not occur or are less severe in patients with right-hemisphere lesions.

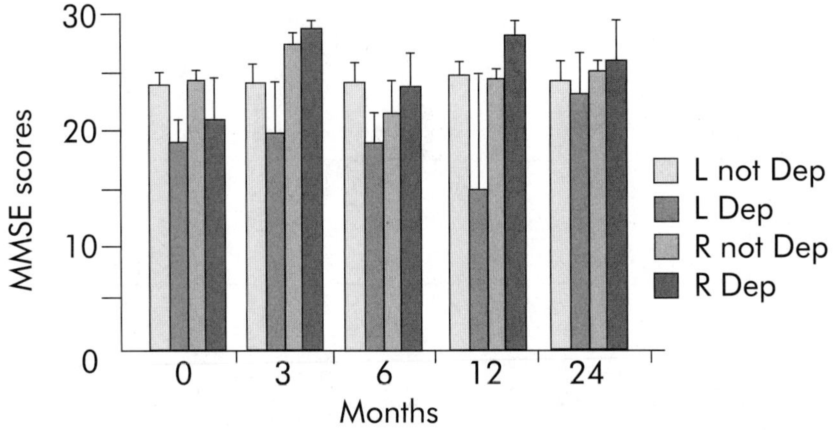

FIGURE 21–3. Cognitive impairment, as measured by Mini-Mental State Exam (MMSE) scores, in poststroke patients in hospital (0) and at 3-, 6-, 12-, and 24-month follow-up. Patients were divided by hemisphere of stroke (left [L] or right [R]) with major depression (Dep) or no mood disturbance (not Dep). Cognitive function was significantly more impaired for the first year poststroke in patients with major depression following left-hemisphere, but not right-hemisphere, stroke.
Source. Reprinted from Downhill JE, Robinson RG: "Longitudinal Assessment of Depression and Cognitive Impairment Following Stroke." *Journal of Nervous and Mental Disease* 182:425–431, 1994. Copyright 1994, Williams & Wilkins. Used with permission.

Few studies have examined the effectiveness of antidepressant treatment among patients with poststroke major depression and cognitive impairment. Several studies have reported anecdotal case histories of patients' cognitive functioning improving after treatment with antidepressants (Fogel and Sparadeo 1985). One preliminary study showed significant improvement on the MMSE after treatment of poststroke depression with either nortriptyline or fluoxetine (Gonzalez-Torrecillas et al. 1993). Methylphenidate was effective in improving the negative symptoms and cognitive scores of demented patients in a small uncontrolled study of 27 patients (Galynker et al. 1997). The stimulant's antidepressant effect did not reach significance, however. There have been no double-blind, controlled trials of the effect of antidepressants on cognitive function in patients with poststroke major depression.

However, three double-blind trials of an antidepressant in the treatment of poststroke depression have been published (Andersen et al. 1994; Lipsey et al. 1984; Reding et al. 1986). Lipsey et al. (1984) examined 14 patients who received nortriptyline and 20 control patients given placebo. The patients who received nortriptyline and completed the 6-week study ($n = 11$) showed significantly greater improvement in their Hamilton Rating Scale for Depression (Hamilton 1967) scores compared with the patients administered placebo. Serum nortriptyline levels in the 75- or 100-mg dose range were between 50 and 150 ng/mL.

Although cognitive function was not the principal outcome variable in this study, MMSE scores were examined before and after treatment. This study, however, failed to show a significant difference in MMSE scores between the actively treated patients and the patients administered placebo either before or after the study. The lack of an improvement in cognitive function after treatment of depression may have been because both major and minor depressions (only major depression is associated with cognitive impairment) and patients who were more than 6 months poststroke (the association with depression is strongest in the acute poststroke period) were included. In the other double-blind, placebo-controlled studies, conducted by Reding et al. (1986) and Andersen et al. (1994), patients were given trazodone, a serotonin reuptake inhibitor, at low dosage (50–100 mg) or citalopram (10–40 mg). In the Reding study, depressed patients who failed to suppress serum cortisol after dexamethasone administration (i.e., positive response on the dexamethasone suppression test [DST]) taking the active drug had significantly greater improvement in the Barthel activities of daily living scores than did comparable control patients who were administered placebo. In the Andersen study, significantly greater improvement was seen in depression scores among patients who received citalopram ($n = 33$) than among those who were given placebo ($n = 33$) based on either intention-to-treat analysis ($P < 0.05$) or efficacy analysis ($P < 0.005$). Cognitive function was not examined in either study.

Finally, in an uncontrolled study, Murray et al. (1986) reported that electroconvulsive therapy also was effective in the treatment of poststroke mood disorders. However, its influence on cognitive function remains to be determined.

In summary, many studies have found that depression may play an important role in cognitive impairment. More recent studies suggest that this may also be true even among patients with structural brain lesions. When the effect of the lesion on cognitive function is controlled, a significant effect of depression still can be seen. These findings indicate that the assessment of depression is an important element of the clinical examination of patients with possible vascular dementia. Because depression can influence a patient's cognitive performance and produce a severe and long-lasting emotional disorder, detection of depressive disorders is an important goal of clinical evaluation of patients with a history or clinical evidence of brain lesion. Some preliminary evidence suggests that treatment of poststroke depression may improve the cognitive function of patients at least during the acute poststroke period.

Conclusions

Vascular dementia is defined as a global decline in intellectual functioning, without a change in level of consciousness, produced by cerebrovascular disease. Vascular dementia can result from a wide variety of vascular diseases ranging from multiple infarcts to vascular insufficiency. Similarly, because of the focal nature of cerebral ischemia, the cognitive impairments may range from memory disturbance with predominantly language disorder to memory disturbance with predominantly visuospatial disorder.

The DSM-IV criteria for vascular dementia include multiple cognitive deficits with memory impairment; one or more deficits in aphasia, apraxia, agnosia, or executive function; and focal neurological signs and symptoms or laboratory evidence of cerebral vascular disease thought to be etiologically related to the dementia. In the United States, vascular dementia is second to Alzheimer's disease as the most common cause of dementia. A substantial number of patients (about 10%–20%) appear to have a mixture of both disorders.

Risk factors for vascular dementia include age, limited education, and accompanying medical disorders such as depression, prior stroke, hypertension or hypotension, diabetes mellitus, and cardiac disease. Prevention of vascular dementia is dependent on amelioration or control of one or more of these risk factors. Several studies have shown the efficacy of aspirin and perhaps dipyridamole in the prevention of stroke among patients with cerebrovascular disease. Control of other risk factors, as well as use of other anticoagulants, may limit the development or progression of vascular dementia. Recent advances have resulted in the use of neuroprotective agents, which show great promise in halting or even reversing the cognitive decline associated with vascular dementia.

Future research needs to clarify the clinical and etiological varieties of vascular dementia, which will lead to ever more focused and definitive treatments aimed at the precise etiology of the vascular compromise or dementing illness itself. Another area for future research is the effect of treatment on the progress of the cognitive decline associated with vascular dementia; for example, does the prevention of subsequent stroke in a patient with known vascular disease prevent or alter the course of dementia? Ultimately, however, only through an understanding of the relation of cerebral ischemia to cognitive function will we be able to specifically target treatments to ameliorate the dementia syndrome.

References

American Psychiatric Association: Diagnostic and Statistical Manual of Mental Disorders, 4th Edition. Washington, DC, American Psychiatric Association, 1994

American Psychiatric Association: Practice guideline for the treatment of patients with Alzheimer's disease and other dementias of late life. Am J Psychiatry 154 (suppl):1–39, 1997

Andersen G, Vestergaard K, Lauritzen L: Effective treatment of post-stroke depression with the selective serotonin reuptake inhibitor citalopram. Stroke 25:1099–1104, 1994

Asplund K: Scandinavian Stroke Study Group: multicenter trial of hemodilution in acute ischemic stroke, I: results from the total patient population. Stroke 18:691–699, 1987

Ballard C, Bannister C, Solis M, et al: The prevalence, associations and symptoms of depression amongst dementia sufferers. J Affect Disord 36:135–144, 1996a

Ballard CG, Patel A, Solis M, et al: A one-year follow-up study of depression in dementia sufferers. Br J Psychiatry 168:287–291, 1996b

Bamford J, Sandercock P, Jones L, et al: The natural history of lacunar infarction: the Oxfordshire Community Stroke Project. Stroke 18:545–551, 1987

Bolla-Wilson K, Robinson RG, Starkstein SE, et al: Lateralization of dementia of depression in stroke patients. Am J Psychiatry 146:627–634, 1989

Bousser MG, Eschewege E, Hagenau M, et al: Essai cooperatif controle "AICLA": prevention secondaire des accidents ischemiques cerebraux lies a l'atherosclerose par l'aspirine et le dipyridamole. Rev Neurol (Paris) 5:333–341, 1981

Brust JCM: Vascular dementia is overdiagnosed. Arch Neurol 45:799–800, 1988

Caplan LR: Binswanger's disease—revisited. Neurology 45:626–633, 1995

Chui HC: Dementia: a review emphasizing clinicopathologic correlation and brain-behavior relationship. Arch Neurol 46:806–814, 1989

Chui HC, Victoroff JI, Margolin D, et al: Criteria for the diagnosis of ischemic vascular dementia proposed by the State of California Alzheimer's Disease Diagnostic and Treatment Centers. Neurology 42:473–480, 1992

Cucinotta D, Aveni Casucci MA, Pedrazi F, et al: Multicentre clinical placebo-controlled study with buflomedil in the treatment of mild dementia of vascular origin. J Int Med Res 20:136–149, 1992

Cummings JL, Benson DF, LoVerme S: Reversible dementia. JAMA 243:2434–2439, 1980

Downhill JE, Robinson RG: Longitudinal assessment of depression and cognitive impairment following stroke. J Nerv Ment Dis 182:425–431, 1994

Drachman DA: New criteria for the diagnosis of vascular dementia: do we know enough yet? Neurology 43:243–245, 1993

Eastwood MR, Rifat SL, Nobbs H, et al: Mood disorder following cerebrovascular accident. Br J Psychiatry 154:195–200, 1989

European Pentoxifylline Multi-Infarct Dementia Study. Eur Neurol 36:315–321, 1996

European Stroke Prevention Study Group: The European Stroke Prevention Study: preliminary results. Lancet 2:1351–1354, 1987

Feibel JH, Springer CJ: Depression and failure to resume social activities after stroke. Arch Phys Med Rehabil 63:276–278, 1982

Fields WS, Lemak NA, Frankowski RF, et al: Controlled trial of aspirin in cerebral ischemia. Stroke 8:301–314, 1977

Fisher CM: Dementia in cerebrovascular disease, in Cerebral Vascular Disease: Sixth Princeton Conference. Edited by Toole JG, Siekert RG, Whisnant JP. New York, Grune & Stratton, 1968, pp 232–236

Flegel KM, Shipley MJ, Rose G: Risk of stroke in non-rheumatic atrial fibrillation. Lancet 1(8532):526–529, 1987 (Published erratum appears in Lancet 1(8537):878, 1987)

Fogel BS, Sparadeo FR: Focal cognitive deficits accentuated by depression. J Nerv Ment Dis 173:120–124, 1985

Folstein MF, Folstein SE, McHugh PR: "Mini-Mental State": a practical method for grading the cognitive state of patients for the clinician. J Psychiatr Res 12:189–198, 1975

Forette F, Amery A, Staessen J, et al: Is prevention of vascular dementia possible? The Syst-Eur Vascular Dementia Project. Aging 3:373–382, 1991

Forette F, Seux ML, Staessen JA, et al: Prevention of dementia in randomised double-blind placebo-controlled Systolic Hypertension in Europe (Syst-Eur) trial. Lancet 352:1347–1351, 1998

Galynker I, Ieronimo C, Miner C, et al: Methylphenidate treatment of negative symptoms in patients with dementia. J Neuropsychiatry Clin Neurosci 9:231–239, 1997

Gold G, Giannakopoulos P, Montes-Paixao C, et al: Sensitivity and specificity of newly proposed clinical criteria for possible vascular dementia. Neurology 49:690–694, 1997

Gonzalez-Torrecillas J-L, Mendlewicz J, Hildebrand J, et al: Early treatment of post-stroke depression: repercussion on neuropsychological rehabilitation. Paper presented at the 146th annual meeting of the American Psychiatric Association, San Francisco, CA, May 1993

Gorelick PB: Status of risk factors for dementia associated with stroke. Stroke 28:459–463, 1997

Gorelick PB, Brody J, Cohen D, et al: Risk factors for dementia associated with multiple cerebral infarcts. Arch Neurol 50:714–720, 1993

Grotta JC: Current medical and surgical therapy for cerebrovascular disease. N Engl J Med 317:1505–1516, 1987

Haase J, Halama P, Horr R: Effectiveness of brief infusions with ginkgo biloba special extract Egb 761 in dementia of the vascular and Alzheimer type. Z Gerontol Geriatr 29:302–309, 1996

Hachinski VC: Preventable senility: a call for action against the vascular dementias. Lancet 340:645–648, 1992

Hachinski VC, Lassen NA, Marshall J: Multi-infarct dementia: a cause of mental deterioration in the elderly. Lancet 2:207–209, 1974

Hachinski VC, Iliff L, Duboulay GH, et al: Cerebral blood flow in dementia. Arch Neurol 32:632–637, 1975

Hamilton M: Development of a rating scale for primary depressive illness. Br J Clin Psychol 6:278–296, 1967

Hebert R, Brayne C: Epidemiology of vascular dementia. Neuroepidemiology 14:240–257, 1995

Howard R, Trend PJ, Russell RWR: Clinical features of ischemic lesions in cerebral arterial border zones. Arch Neurol 44:934–939, 1987

Kanowski S, Herrmann WM, Stephan K, et al: Proof of efficacy of the ginkgo biloba special extract Egb 761 in outpatients suffering from mild to moderate primary degenerative dementia of the Alzheimer type or multi-infarct dementia. Pharmacopsychiatry 29:47–56, 1996

Katz DI, Alexander MP, Mandell AM: Dementia following strokes in the mesencephalon and diencephalon. Arch Neurol 44:1127–1133, 1987

Katzman R, Saitho T: Advance in Alzheimer's disease. FASEB J 5:278–286, 1990

Kertesz A, Polk M, Carr T: Cognition and white matter changes on magnetic resonance imaging in dementia. Arch Neurol 47:387–391, 1990

Kluger A, Gianutsos J, de Leon MJ, et al: Significance of age-related white matter lesions. Stroke 19:1054–1055, 1988

Kohara K, Zhao B, Jiang Y, et al: Relation of left ventricular hypertrophy and geometry to asymptomatic cerebrovascular damage in essential hypertension. Am J Cardiol 83:367–370, 1999

Launer LJ, Masaki K, Petrovich H, et al: The association between midlife blood pressure levels and late-life cognitive function. JAMA 274:1846–1851, 1995

Le Bars PL, Katz MM, Berman N, et al: A placebo-controlled, double-blind, randomized trial of an extract of ginkgo biloba for dementia. JAMA 278:1327–1332, 1997

Lipsey JR, Robinson RG, Pearlson GD, et al: Nortriptyline treatment of post-stroke depression: a double-blind treatment trial. Lancet 1:297–300, 1984

Loeb C: Vascular dementias, in Handbook of Clinical Neurology, Vol 2. Edited by Frederiks JAM. Amsterdam, Elsevier, 1985, pp 353–371

Loeb C, Meyer JS: Vascular dementia: still a debatable entity? J Neurol Sci 143:31–40, 1996

Loizou LA, Kendall BE, Marshall J: Subcortical arteriosclerotic encephalopathy: a clinical and radiological investigation. J Neurol Neurosurg Psychiatry 44:294–304, 1981

Marie P: Des foyers lacunaires de desintegration et de differents autres etats cavitaires du cerveau. Rev Med 21:281–298, 1901

McPherson SE, Cummings JL: Neuropsychological aspects of vascular dementia. Brain Cogn 31:269–282, 1996

Meyer JS, Judd BW, Tawaklna T, et al: Improved cognition after control of risk factors for multi-infarct dementia. JAMA 256:2203–2209, 1986

Meyer JS, McClintic KL, Rogers RL, et al: Aetiological considerations and risk factors for multi-infarct dementia. J Neurol Neurosurg Psychiatry 51:1489–1497, 1988

Meyer JS, Rogers RL, Mortel KF: Multi-infarct dementia: demography, risk factors, and therapy, in Cerebrovascular Diseases: Sixteenth Princeton Conference. Edited by Ginsberg MD, Dietrich WD. New York, Raven, 1989, pp 199–206

Mielke R, Moller HJ, Erkinjuntti T, et al: Propentofylline in the treatment of vascular dementia and Alzheimer-type dementia: overview of phase I and phase II clinical trials. Alzheimer Dis Assoc Disord 12 (suppl 2):S29–S35, 1998

Miller B, Heilmann L: Hemorheological parameters in patients with gynecological malignancies. Gynecol Oncol 33:177–181, 1989

Mittelman MS, Ferris SH, Shulman E, et al: A family intervention to delay nursing home placement of patients with Alzheimer's disease: a randomized controlled trial. JAMA 276:1725–1731, 1996

Morris PLP, Robinson RG, Raphael B: Prevalence and course of depressive disorders in hospitalized stroke patients. Int J Psychiatry Med 20:349–364, 1990

Murray GB, Shea V, Conn DK: Electroconvulsive therapy for poststroke depression. J Clin Psychiatry 47:258–260, 1986

Newman SC: The prevalence of depression in Alzheimer's disease and vascular dementia in a population sample. J Affect Disord 52:169–176, 1999

O'Brien MD: Vascular dementia is underdiagnosed. Arch Neurol 45:797–798, 1988

Philips S, Sangalang V, Sterns G: Basal forebrain infarction: a clinico-pathologic correlation. Arch Neurol 44:1134–1138, 1987

Rao SM, Mittenberg W, Bernardin L, et al: Neuropsychological test findings in subjects with leukoaraiosis. Arch Neurol 46:40–44, 1989

Reding JJ, Orto LA, Winter SW, et al: Antidepressant therapy after stroke: a double-blind trial. Arch Neurol 43:763–765, 1986

Roberts GW, Gentleman SM, Lynch A, et al: Beta A4 amyloid protein deposition in brain after head trauma. Lancet 338:1422–1433, 1991

Robinson RG, Starr LB, Kubos KL, et al: A two-year longitudinal study of poststroke mood disorders: findings during the initial evaluation. Stroke 14:736–744, 1983

Robinson RG, Bolla-Wilson K, Kaplan E, et al: Depression influences intellectual impairment in stroke patients. Br J Psychiatry 148:541–547, 1986

Rocca WA, Hofman A, Brayne C, et al: The prevalence of vascular dementia in Europe: facts and fragments from 1980–1990 studies. Ann Neurol 30:817–824, 1991

Roman GC: The epidemiology of vascular dementia, in Cerebral Ischemia and Dementia. Edited by Hartmann A, Kuschinsky W, Hoyer S. Berlin, Germany, Springer-Verlag, 1991, pp 9–15

Roman GC, Tatemichi TK, Erkinjuntti T, et al: Vascular dementia: diagnostic criteria for research studies. Report of the NINDS-AIREN International Workshop. Neurology 43:250–260, 1993

Roth M: Diagnosis of senile and related forms of dementia, in Alzheimer's Disease: Senile Dementia and Related Disorders (Aging, Vol 7). Edited by Katzman R, Terry RD, Bick KL. New York, Raven, 1978, pp 105–108

Rother M, Erkinjuntti T, Roessner M, et al: Propentofylline in the treatment of Alzheimer's disease and vascular dementia: a review of phase III trials. Dement Geriatr Cogn Disord 9 (suppl 1):36–43, 1998

Salloway S, Hong J: CADASIL syndrome: a genetic form of vascular dementia. J Geriatr Psychiatry Neurol 11:71–77, 1998

Samson Y, Baron JC, Bousser MG, et al: Effects of intracranial arterial bypass on cerebral blood flow and oxygen metabolism in humans. Stroke 16:609–616, 1985

Schoenberg BS, Kokmen E, Okazaki H: Alzheimer's disease and other dementing illness in a defined U.S. population: incidence rates and clinical features. Ann Neurol 22:724–729, 1987

Simpson S, Allen H, Tomenson B, et al: Neurological correlates of depressive symptoms in Alzheimer's disease and vascular dementia. J Affect Disord 53:129–136, 1999

Skoog I, Lernfelt B, Landahl S, et al: 15-year longitudinal study of blood pressure and dementia. Lancet 347:1141–1145, 1996

Sondergaard H, Jorgensen HS, Olsen TS: CADASIL—a newly discovered hereditary cerebrovascular disease. Ugeskr Laeger 160:1617–1620, 1998

Starkstein SE, Robinson RG: Dementia of depression in Parkinson's disease and stroke. J Nerv Ment Dis 179:593–601, 1991

Starkstein SE, Robinson RG, Price TR: Comparison of patients with and without poststroke major depression matched for size and location of lesion. Arch Gen Psychiatry 45:247–252, 1988

Suzuki K, Kutsuzawa T, Nakajinia K, et al: Epidemiology of vascular dementia and stroke in Akita, Japan, in Cerebral Ischemia and Dementia. Edited by Hartmann A, Kuschinsky W, Hoyer S. Berlin, Germany, Springer-Verlag, 1991, pp 16–24

Tomlinson BE, Henderson G: Some quantitative cerebral findings in normal and demented old people, in Neurobiology of Aging. Edited by Terry RD, Gershon S. New York, Raven, 1976, pp 183–204

UK–TIA Study Group: United Kingdom transient ischaemic attack (UK-TIA) aspirin trial: interim results. BMJ 296:316–320, 1988

Woimant F, Moulinier L, Lecoz P, et al: Cerebral ischemic accidents and chronic disseminated intravascular coagulation of cancerous origin. Rev Neurol (Paris) 144:120–124, 1988

Yamaguchi T, Ogata J, Yoshida F: Epidemiology of vascular dementia in Japan: proceedings of the NINDS-ARIEN International Workshop on Vascular Dementia. National Institutes of Health, Bethesda, MD, April 19–21, 1991. New Issues in Neurosciences 4:100–103, 1992

Zhang MY, Katzman R, Salmon D, et al: The prevalence of dementia and Alzheimer's disease in Shanghai, China: impact of age, sex and education. Ann Neurol 27:428–437, 1990

22

Dementia Due to Other General Medical Conditions and Dementia Due to Multiple Etiologies

David B. Arciniegas, M.D.
Steven L. Dubovsky, M.D.

Although Alzheimer's disease and vascular dementia are the most common causes of dementia, many other conditions can produce persistent impairment in cognition on their own and can contribute to vascular dementia and dementia from Alzheimer's disease. In this chapter, we review these additional dementing illnesses and their treatments. We then discuss the general pharmacological treatment of cognitive and behavioral problems that can complicate any dementing disorder.

Epidemiology

The current prevalence of dementia in persons ages 65 years or older is 6%–10%, and the prevalence rate doubles if milder cases of dementia are included (Hendrie 1997). About two-thirds of the cases of geriatric dementia are caused by Alzheimer's disease (Hendrie 1998). In a review of 32 studies of dementia in a total of 2,889 subjects, Alzheimer's disease was the diagnosis in 56.8% of cases, vascular dementia in 13.3%, and depression in 4.5%; other medical and neurological causes such as those reviewed in this chapter accounted for approximately 16.7% of cases (Clarfield 1988). The number of persons with dementia is expected to increase to at least 6.1 to 9.8 million by 2040, when the cost of care for dementia is predicted to be $92 to $149 billion annually (E. L. Schneider and Guralnik 1990).

Identification of Other Causes of Dementia

Causes of dementia to be considered in developing a treatment plan are summarized in Table 22–1 (Arnold and Kumar 1993; Mayeux et al. 1993). Cummings and Benson (1992) outlined a general approach to the differential diagnosis of these conditions. First, cortical dementias must be distinguished from subcortical or mixed dementias. Cortical dementia is generally characterized by impairment in specific domains of cognition, perception, and language associated with cortical function (e.g., aphasia, apraxia, agnosia, impaired new learning based on encoding problems, dysexecutive function). By contrast, subcortical and white matter dementias are more likely to be associated with dysarthria without aphasia, slowed cognition and movement, impaired retrieval of information, disturbance of mood, and diminished motivation. In all types of dementia, evidence of cerebrovascular disease, such as abrupt onset, stepwise deterioration, and focal neurological signs, should be sought, although such findings may be more common in patients with subcortical or mixed types (Cummings and Benson 1992). Within the group of subcortical dementias, those associated with extrapyramidal syndromes such as Huntington's disease or Parkinson's disease should be identified.

Cognitive impairment typical of subcortical dementia (depressive "pseudodementia") may occur in severe depression (Hill and Stoudemire 1993; Zapotoczky 1998). This syndrome of reversible dementia occurs in 18%–57% of depressed elderly patients (Alexopoulos et al. 1993). Mania, schizophrenia, obsessional ruminative states, severe anxiety disorders, and dissociative disorders may also present with apparent dementia. Cognitive changes in pseudodementia include forgetfulness, impaired attention, disorientation, decreased abstracting ability, and difficulty encoding (Hill and Stoudemire 1993) and retrieving (P. R. Martin and Welch 1993) new information. However, aphasia, agnosia, poor recognition, and other cognitive impairments seen in cortical dementias are not characteristic of pseudodementia (Cummings and Benson 1992). Slowed responses, diminished facial expression, stooped posture, and bradykinesia in pseudodementia can give a parkinsonian appearance to depressed patients, but lack of tremor helps to exclude Parkinson's disease (Yousef et al. 1998).

A careful history and examination can often identify a primary psychiatric illness that is producing symptoms of dementia. For example, depressed mood, expressions of guilt, neurovegetative signs, negative thinking, mood-congruent psychotic features, rapid progression, a history of depression, and a family history of mood disorders may help distinguish patients with pseudodementia from those with other dementias (Cummings and Benson 1992). However, improvement of dementia with a vigorous trial of an antidepressant or other appropriate treatment may be the only way to clarify the underlying psychiatric disorder. Impaired executive function (e.g., decreased initiation, perseveration, and psychomotor retardation) may predict a delayed and somewhat attenuated response to

TABLE 22–1. Medical causes of dementia

Degenerative disorders of the central nervous system
Frontotemporal dementia (including Pick's disease) and other focal cortical atrophies
Huntington's disease
Parkinson's disease
Diffuse Lewy body disease
Progressive supranuclear palsy
Hallervorden-Spatz syndrome
Spinocerebellar degenerations
Inherited disorders with dementia
Metachromatic leukodystrophy
Adrenoleukodystrophy
Membranous lipodystrophy
Cerebrotendinous xanthomatosis
Hereditary adult-onset leukodystrophy
G_{M1} and G_{M2} gangliosidoses
Gaucher's disease
Fabry's disease
Kufs' disease
Adult polyglucosan disease
Leigh's disease
Progressive myoclonic epilepsy
Mitochondrial encephalomyopathies
Mast syndrome
Sensory radicular neuropathy (Denny-Brown disease)
Homocystinuria
Acute intermittent porphyria
Myotonic dystrophy
Fahr's disease (idiopathic basal ganglia calcification)
Wilson's disease (hepatolenticular degeneration)
Endocrine and metabolic disorders
Thyroid disease
Parathyroid disease
Adrenal disease
Panhypopituitarism
Prolonged hypoglycemia
Pancreatitis
Chronic obstructive pulmonary disease
Congestive heart failure
Hypoxia
Hepatic encephalopathy
Hyponatremia
Hypernatremia
Uremia
Dialysis
Nutritional disorders
Thiamine (B_1) deficiency
B_{12} deficiency
Folate deficiency
Toxin- and drug-induced disorders
Alcohol-related syndromes
Drugs and toxins (see Table 22–2)
Infection-related disorders
Chronic meningitides (fungal, tuberculous, viral, bacterial)
Neurosyphilis
Neurobrucellosis
Lyme neuroborreliosis
Brain abscess
Human immunodeficiency virus
Arbovirus encephalitis
Progressive rubella panencephalitis
Progressive multifocal leukoencephalopathy
Subacute sclerosing panencephalitis
Creutzfeldt-Jakob disease
Gerstmann-Straussler disease
Postviral encephalitic syndromes
Kuru
Alpers' disease
Whipple's disease
Behçet's syndrome

TABLE 22–1. Medical causes of dementia *(continued)*

Collagen-vascular disorders	Miscellaneous disorders and conditions
Systemic lupus erythematosus	Multiple sclerosis
Temporal arteritis	Brain tumor
Rheumatoid vasculitis	Radiation-induced
Sarcoidosis	Limbic encephalitis
Thrombotic thrombocytopenic purpura	Subdural hematoma
Granulomatous angiitis	Hydrocephalus
Idiopathic hypereosinophilic syndrome	Sequelae of open and closed head injury
	Atrial myxoma

standard antidepressant therapy in late-life depression (Kalayam and Alexopoulos 1999).

On the other hand, the presence of a psychiatric disorder does not exclude a comorbid neurological condition or a primary neurological illness to which the psychiatric condition is a reaction (Cummings and Benson 1992). Ganser's syndrome, the syndrome of approximate answers, can occur in personality disorders and psychotic depression but also in left-hemisphere dysfunction, general paresis, head trauma, alcoholic dementia, and toxic and metabolic disorders (Cutting 1990). When a psychiatric illness such as depression coexists with a dementing illness, psychiatric treatment (e.g., an antidepressant) may not improve the underlying dementia (Hill and Stoudemire 1993), but it may reduce excess disability attributable to the mental disorder (Reifler et al. 1986; Tune 1998).

Once psychiatric conditions have been excluded, radiological evaluation for hydrocephalus is indicated (Cummings and Benson 1992). Further testing recommended by the 1985 National Institutes of Health Consensus Conference on Differential Diagnosis of Dementing Diseases (National Institutes of Health 1985) includes a complete blood count, electrolyte and metabolic screen, thyroid panel, vitamin B_{12} and folate levels, syphilis serology, urinalysis, chest radiograph (to help detect malignancy, cardiopulmonary disease, and sarcoidosis), electrocardiogram (ECG), and head computed tomography (CT) scan (to detect subdural hematomas, tumors, and evidence of vascular disease). Recent recommendations have changed little from these guidelines (Patternson et al. 1999), although magnetic resonance imaging (MRI) provides a more sensitive measure for the detection of white matter, posterior fossa, and brain-stem pathology and is probably a better neuroimaging study to order for the evaluation of dementia. However, as Frank (1998) noted in a comprehensive review of the literature on the laboratory evaluation of dementia, most recommendations are based on consensus rather than prospective trials, and clinical judgment remains the best measure by which to select the laboratory investigation in any given case.

Degenerative Disorders of the Central Nervous System

Pick's Disease and Other Frontal Lobe Disorders

Pick's disease, first described by Arnold Pick in 1892 (Pick 1892/1977), is the prototypic frontotemporal dementia, occurring at a frequency of 2%–10% of that of Alzheimer's disease (Civil et al. 1993). Pick's disease is inherited as an autosomal dominant in 20% of cases

(Cummings 1992b), and linkage to chromosome 17 (mutations of the *TAU* gene) has been reported in some families (Wilhelmsen et al. 1999). Onset usually occurs between ages 40 and 60, with death occurring within 2–15 years of disease onset (Cummings and Benson 1992). Psychiatric symptoms, including personality changes, impaired judgment, socially inappropriate behavior, and Klüver-Bucy syndrome–like symptoms, are often the first manifestations of this disease. Impairment of language and executive function becomes more apparent as the disease progresses, but memory loss occurs relatively late compared with Alzheimer's disease, a feature that most consistently distinguishes Pick's disease from Alzheimer's disease (Cummings and Benson 1992). In Pick's disease, in contrast to Alzheimer's disease, cortical choline acetyltransferase (ChAT) levels are normal, although activity of the basal ganglia cholinergic systems is variably diminished. Pick bodies and inflated cells are noted in the brains of most patients with Pick's disease (Civil et al. 1993). As in Alzheimer's disease, brain monoamine oxidase A (MAO-A) and B (MAO-B) activity may be increased (Civil et al. 1993). Treatment trials with monoamine oxidase inhibitors (MAOIs), agents that may improve cognitive functioning in Parkinson's disease and Alzheimer's disease (Lees 1991), may thus be appropriate in Pick's disease but have not yet been conducted.

Frontotemporal degeneration and frontal lobe atrophy (as opposed to the predominantly parietal lobe atrophy of Alzheimer's disease), which are present in a variety of conditions beyond the specific disease attributable to Pick, may be referred to as the frontotemporal dementias or Pick complex (Kertesz et al. 1999). These diseases include frontal lobe degeneration of the non-Alzheimer's type (clinically similar to Pick's disease but without the characteristic histological changes of that disorder), frontotemporal degeneration without Pick bodies, corticobasilar degeneration, primary progressive aphasia, semantic dementia, progressive subcortical gliosis, amyotrophic lateral sclerosis dementia syndrome, adult-onset neuronal intranuclear hyaline inclusion disease, and hereditary dysphasic dementia (Cummings and Benson 1992; Kertesz et al. 1999; Neary 1999). Primary progressive aphasia is an etiologically heterogeneous focal atrophy of the left hemisphere characterized by aphasia; dementia occurs late in the course of this disorder (Mesulam 1982). No specific treatment has been identified for any of these illnesses.

Huntington's Disease

Huntington's disease, first described by George Huntington in 1872, has its onset between ages 25 and 50; survival ranges from 10 to 17 years after onset (Harper 1991). The point prevalence among Caucasians is 5–7 cases per 100,000 (S.E. Folstein 1989). Huntington's disease is transmitted as an autosomal dominant with complete penetrance. Genetic linkage analysis indicates that the Huntington's disease gene (a trinucleotide CAG repeat sequence) is on the terminal short arm of chromosome 4 (Civil et al. 1993). Although chorea is the cardinal motor symptom in adult-onset Huntington's disease, rigidity, myoclonus, and dystonic movements are more characteristic of the 3%–9% of cases of Huntington's disease with juvenile onset (Whitehouse et al. 1992).

Psychiatric symptoms, particularly affective disorders, occur in 40%–50% of patients with Huntington's disease at some point in the course of the illness (Civil et al. 1993; Sano et al. 1996; Whitehouse et al. 1992). Chronic depression occurs in 20%–40% of patients and hypomania in about 10% (Caine and Shoulson 1983; Folstein 1989; Sano et al. 1996). Impulsive, irritable, and violent behavior may occur in nearly one-third of patients and alcoholism in 15% (Folstein 1989). Psychiatric symptoms may precede motor symptoms by several years (Folstein et al. 1983). Patients with Huntington's disease are also at a significantly increased risk for suicide, particularly early in the symptomatic stage of the disease (Sano et al. 1996).

Cognitive impairment appears relatively early in the course of Huntington's disease (Sano et al. 1996). Dementia in Huntington's disease follows a pattern consistent with disruption of frontal-subcortical circuitry that includes impairment of attention, concentration, executive function, cognitive flexibility and abstraction, visuospatial tasks, and verbal skills and delayed recall (Lange et al. 1995; Randolph et al. 1998; Zakzanis 1998). The cognitive impairments in Huntington's disease may also be attributable to impaired communication between frontal-subcortical and other information-processing networks (e.g., those involving the hippocampus and dorsal medial nucleus of the thalamus), resulting in memory impairment that is sometimes out of proportion to that predicted by IQ testing (Butters et al. 1978). Although the relative contribution of motor, psychiatric, and cognitive impairments to the degree of disability produced by Huntington's disease varies among individuals, the psychiatric and cognitive impairments generally produce significantly greater problems than do motor impairments over the entire course of the disease (Sano et al. 1996).

In the absence of controlled studies that could provide treatment guidelines for either the cognitive or the psychiatric symptoms of Huntington's disease (Leroi and Michalon 1998), treatment is informed by case reports and clinical experience. Antipsychotics such as perphenazine, haloperidol, and sulpiride have been shown to be effective in the treatment of chorea of Huntington's disease (Morris and Tyler 1991). Although lithium has not been found to reduce the motor manifestations of Huntington's disease, it has been used to treat aggression and irritability in Huntington's disease patients (Leonard et al. 1974; Morris and Tyler 1991). Tricyclic antidepressants (Folstein and Folstein 1981) and MAOIs (Ford 1986) have improved depression in Huntington's disease patients, and the antidopaminergic action of some of the serotonin reuptake inhibitors might make these antidepressants more specifically useful. Although depression in Huntington's disease is undertreated (Morris and Tyler 1991), antidepressants do not appear to improve the motor or cognitive deficits in nondepressed patients with Huntington's disease (Como et al. 1997). Inappropriate sexual behavior due to Huntington's disease may respond to leuprolide acetate, a gonadotropin-releasing hormone agonist that suppresses gonadotropin secretion when given in a continuous fashion (Rich and Ovsiew 1994).

The *N*-methyl-D-aspartate (NMDA) subgroup of glutamate receptors may mediate excitotoxic damage to the striatum (caudate) in Huntington's disease. Animal models suggest a possible role for NMDA antagonists (e.g., MK-801) in the treatment of Huntington's disease, and one such agent, remacemide hydrochloride, appears both well tolerated and promising with respect to reduction of choreiform movements (Kieburtz et al. 1996). Whether such agents might limit the progression of cognitive impairment attributable to striatal injury is not yet known. Antiexcitotoxins are discussed later in this chapter.

Parkinson's Disease

Parkinson's disease (paralysis agitans) is a degenerative disorder of unknown etiology involving the pigmented brain-stem nuclei and characterized by cogwheel rigidity, tremor, masked facies, bradykinesia, and postural instability. Because Parkinson's disease is further characterized neuropathologically by the presence of Lewy bodies, it is included in the family of Lewy body disorders with dementia (along with Parkinson's disease with Alzheimer's disease, cortical Lewy bodies and neuritic plaques, and cortical Lewy bodies and no concomitant Alzheimer's disease–

type pathology) (Cummings 1995). The average age at onset of Parkinson's disease is 50–65 years (Sano et al. 1997), and mean survival after disease onset is 8 years (Cummings and Benson 1992). The disease has a prevalence of approximately 1 in 1,000 in those older than 65 (Kessler 1972). Although Parkinson's disease is usually a sporadic disorder, familial cases have been reported (Pollock and Hornabrook 1966). The influenza pandemic of 1917 produced a substantial number of cases of parkinsonism, and poisoning (e.g., with carbon monoxide or heavy metals) also may be causative. In all of these cases, a complex interaction between genetic and environmental influences is likely contributory.

Although James Parkinson (1817) did not recognize the presence of mental changes in his original description of the disease that bears his name, subsequent experience has clearly shown that dementia is a feature of this illness. A relatively early review of more than 2,500 Parkinson's disease patients described in the literature (Brown and Marsden 1984) found an incidence of dementia of 15%. Other investigators report that delirium is present in 35%–55% of Parkinson's disease patients examined by standardized mental status examinations (Cummings and Benson 1992; Lieberman 1998). Advanced age, cerebrovascular disease, and family history of dementia may be risk factors for the development of dementia in Parkinson's disease (Civil et al. 1993).

The dementia of Parkinson's disease is of the subcortical type. Typical signs include failure to initiate behavior, visuospatial impairment, problem-solving difficulties, slowed memory, forgetfulness, poor word-list generation, and impaired spontaneous recall and procedural memory (Cummings and Benson 1992). Cortical features such as aphasia, agnosia, and severe amnesia are uncommon in Parkinson's disease but may occur when Alzheimer's disease is superimposed (Cummings et al. 1988). Depression, which occurs in 40%–60% of Parkinson's disease patients (Civil et al. 1993) and is probably an integral part of the basal ganglia disease rather than a psychological response to the disease itself (Cummings and Benson 1992; Mayeux et al. 1981), may complicate the dementia of Parkinson's disease.

In 60% of the patients who start taking L-dopa, symptomatic improvement of the movement disorder occurs, with akinesia responding better than tremor or rigidity (Cummings and Benson 1992). Cognitive impairment also improves with L-dopa treatment, with measurable enhancement of memory, visuospatial ability, perceptual organization, and sequencing (Cummings and Benson 1992). As the disease progresses, however, these gains are not maintained (Halgin et al. 1977). Although there are theoretical reasons to think that dopamine agonists should have an antidepressant effect (Jimerson 1987), and despite the transient improvement in mood of some patients receiving L-dopa therapy (Cantello et al. 1986) and methylphenidate (Cantello et al. 1989), dopaminergic agonists do not appear to treat depression reliably in Parkinson's disease (Cherington 1970; Marsh and Markham 1973; Mindham et al. 1976). On the other hand, tricyclic antidepressants are effective for depression in Parkinson's disease (Cummings and Benson 1992).

The selective MAO-B inhibitor selegiline (L-deprenyl) increases the average time that elapses before patients need L-dopa (Knoll 1992; Parkinson Study Group 1989; Tetrud and Langston 1989) and may improve life expectancy of Parkinson's disease patients (Birkmayer et al. 1985). Selegiline has been shown to improve cognitive and behavioral function in up to 50% of patients with Alzheimer's disease (Finali et al. 1991; Goad et al. 1991; Tariot et al. 1987). Selegiline also improves attention and episodic memory in nondemented Parkinson's disease patients (Lees 1991). One might predict that selegiline would be beneficial for the full dementia of Parkinson's disease, but, to our knowledge, trials have not yet been conducted to test this hypothesis. Although a parsimonious approach to the treatment of depression and cognitive impairment in Parkinson's disease might be to use an antidepressant dose of selegiline (e.g., 20–40 mg/day [Mann et al. 1989]), at these doses selegiline is no longer selective for the B form of MAO and may interact with L-dopa to produce cognitive impairment and possibly increased mortality (Ben-Shlomo et al. 1998). Depressed patients taking only selegiline for Parkinson's disease might benefit from an antidepressant dose of that drug.

The use of selective serotonin reuptake inhibitors (SSRIs) in Parkinson's disease is problematic for two reasons. First, even at low doses, MAOIs may produce a dangerous serotonin syndrome when combined with SSRIs (Valldeoriola et al. 1997). In addition, increased serotonergic input to striatal dopaminergic neurons leads to reduced dopamine release, which can aggravate parkinsonism. Because of its dopaminergic properties, bupropion improves parkinsonian symptoms in about one-third of patients (Cummings 1992a). However, aside from their capacity to reduce the dementia syndrome of depression, it is not known whether other antidepressant medications might primarily improve dementia in patients with Parkinson's disease.

Electroconvulsive therapy (ECT) improves not only depression but also the motor manifestations of Parkinson's disease, particularly in those patients with the on-off phenomenon (Kellner and Bernstein 1993; Moellentine et al. 1998). Repetitive transcranial magnetic stimulation (rTMS) also may improve the motor manifestations of Parkinson's disease, possibly by inducing changes in brain monoamine levels (Mally and Stone 1999). Whether rTMS may confer benefit for the cognitive or emotional disturbances of this disease is not yet known. Neurosurgical procedures such as bilateral pallidotomy (Ghika et al. 1999) or pallidal fetal tissue transplantation (Lopez-Lozano et al. 1997) can produce motor improvement in patients with severe Parkinson's disease, but it is not clear whether such procedures significantly improve mood or cognition.

L-Dopa and other dopaminergic medications cause psychosis in up to 12% of patients with Parkinson's disease (Celesia and Wanamaker 1972; Whitehouse et al. 1992), a problem that is more common in Parkinson's disease patients with dementia. Treatment with conventional antipsychotics or withdrawal of anti–Parkinson's disease agents may improve psychosis but worsen parkinsonism. Low doses of atypical antipsychotic medications (e.g., 6.25 mg/day of clozapine) have been reported to improve psychosis in Parkinson's disease without worsening parkinsonian symptoms (Musser and Akil 1996; Valldeoriola et al. 1997; Workman et al. 1997), but higher doses of the drug have resulted in poor compliance because of sedation and delirium (K. M. Jones and Stoukides 1992).

Progressive Supranuclear Palsy

Progressive supranuclear palsy, also known as Steele-Richardson-Olszewski syndrome (Steele et al. 1964), is characterized by paresis of vertical gaze, pseudobulbar palsy, axial rigidity, and dementia (Cummings and Benson 1992; Whitehouse et al. 1992). The median age at onset of progressive supranuclear palsy is 63 years, the median survival is 9.7 years, and the prevalence of this disorder is 1.39 in 100,000 (Golbe et al. 1988). Progressive supranuclear palsy appears to be a recessively inherited disorder involving a mutation of the *TAO* gene (Litvan and Hutton 1998); such familial types may be underrecognized as such (Rojo et al. 1999). Dopamine depletion and dopamine receptor loss in the striatum, reduced ChAT levels in the frontal cortex and basal ganglia, and reductions in subcortical levels of γ-aminobutyric acid (GABA) have been noted, as have neurofibrillary tangles structurally distinct from those seen in Alzheimer's disease (Civil et al. 1993). Frontal and temporal hypometabolism have been observed in positron-emission tomography (PET) studies (Whitehouse et al. 1992).

The dementia of progressive supranuclear palsy is of the subcortical type and is characterized by attentional impairment, rapid forgetting, apathy and depression, dramatically slowed mental processing and motor execution, impaired planning and conceptual shifting, and marked speech disturbances with hypophonia and dysarthria (Cummings and Benson 1992; Grafman et al. 1995; Salmon et al. 1997). Depression, anxiety, pathological laughing and crying (Menza et al. 1995), obsessive-compulsive behaviors (Destee et al. 1990), and schizophreniform psychoses (Aldrich et al. 1989) have been reported. Although early reports suggest variable benefit with L-dopa (Cummings and Benson 1992), when this syndrome is correctly distinguished from other subcortical dementias it appears that L-dopa is not beneficial (Litvan et al. 1997). Whether a similar result will pertain to treatment with amantadine, benztropine mesylate, methysergide (Newman 1985), amitriptyline (Engel 1996), and trazodone (L.S. Schneider et al. 1989) is not known, but to date none of these medications has been found to be consistently effective.

Hallervorden-Spatz Syndrome

Hallervorden-Spatz syndrome describes a group of etiologically distinct pallidal diseases that share a pathological triad of iron deposition, axonal spheroids, and gliosis (Halliday 1995). Several subgroups of this syndrome exist, including female patients with dementia, quadriparesis, and neurofibrillary tangles; patients with Lewy bodies; and patients without lipid abnormalities but with acanthocytosis and pigmentary retinal degeneration. Case-to-case variability in both presentation and neuropathological features is significant, but iron deposition in the pallidum appears to be the most consistent feature across these various subtypes. Hallervorden-Spatz syndrome is the designation reserved for the pediatric neurodegenerative form of these disorders and may occur as either a familial or a sporadic disorder. The familial form is an autosomal-recessive condition with onset between ages 7 and 9 years that may involve an enzymatic defect in the conversion of cysteine to taurine. Stiffness of gait, dysarthria, occasional dementia, and reddish-brown discoloration of the globus pallidus and substantia nigra due to iron and other metal deposition in those locations have been noted. There is no known treatment, and the disease relentlessly progresses to death (Cummings and Benson 1992).

Dementia Associated With Degeneration of the Cerebellum

The role of the cerebellum in cognitive function and behavior is not yet fully understood (Whitehouse et al. 1992), but it appears to be important for the initial learning of motor tasks, acquisition of cognitive information, and the efficient execution of previously learned sensorimotor responses (Hamilton et al. 1983; Heath et al. 1979; Hua and Houk 1997). Recent studies suggest that the cerebellum also may act in concert with the frontal lobes to facilitate efficient processing and retrieval of cognitive information (Allen et al. 1997; Berquin et al. 1998; Dormehl et al. 1999; Lesnik et al. 1998).

The olivopontocerebellar atrophies, accounting for 1.8% of the dementias in patients younger than 70 and 0.1% of the dementias in patients older than 70 (Feher et al. 1988), are a heterogeneous group of autosomal-dominant inherited disorders associated with progressive ataxia and neuronal degeneration of the cerebellum and brain stem (Gilman et al. 1981; Whitehouse et al. 1992), some subtypes of which are associated with dementia

(Schelhaas et al. 1997) and a decrease in ChAT activity (Civil et al. 1993). Congenital cerebellar atrophy is an autosomal-recessive disorder that may also produce cognitive impairment in affected individuals (Guzzetta et al. 1993).

Friedreich's ataxia, which is distinct from the olivopontocerebellar atrophies, is an autosomal-recessive illness with a prevalence of 1 in 100,000 and a gradual onset at puberty characterized by gait disturbance, clumsiness, and weakness of the lower extremities (Manyam 1993). Myocardial hypertrophy and dilatation, diabetes mellitus, and dysarthria are often associated with this disorder. More than half of Friedreich's ataxia patients require wheelchairs within 16 years of diagnosis, and the mean age at death is 38 years (Harding 1981). There have been some reports of preservation of intelligence, judgment, and other higher cortical functions (Hart et al. 1985), whereas other investigators have noted impaired visual construction, IQ, and nonverbal function; slowed information processing; and/or personality change (Fehrenbach et al. 1984). Treatment with physostigmine, choline, thyrotropin-releasing hormone, or amantadine has resulted in transient mild improvements in some patients (Manyam 1993).

Wilson's Disease

Wilson's disease, first described by Kennier Wilson in 1912, is an autosomal-recessive disease in which excessive amounts of copper are deposited in the brain, liver, kidney, and cornea because of lack of the copper-carrying globulin ceruloplasmin (Cummings and Benson 1992). Two variants are described: a juvenile type with rapid evolution and an adult variety with onset in the third or fourth decade and a more indolent course. Manifestations include dystonia, rigidity, drooling, incoordination, and dysarthria (Starosta-Rubinstein et al. 1987). The characteristic flapping tremor of the wrists and wing beating tremor of the shoulders seen in the adult type develop late, if at all, in the juvenile variant (Cummings and Benson 1992). Mood and personality changes are the most common psychiatric manifestations in both the juvenile and the adult types (Dening and Berrios 1989). A subcortical dementia becomes evident as the disease progresses (Lauterbach et al. 1998). Liver disease, thrombocytopenia and/or leukopenia, and Kayser-Fleischer rings caused by copper deposition in the cornea are observed; kidney involvement, including renal tubular acidosis and consequent osteomalacia, is rare (Cartwright 1978; Dobyns et al. 1979; Hoaglund and Goldstein 1978). Low serum ceruloplasmin concentration (<20 mg/dL), low serum copper (3–10 μM/L), and urinary copper excretion in excess of 100 μg Cu/24 hours strongly support the diagnosis in most cases. Because several patients with Wilson's disease have been reported to have normal serum ceruloplasmin, a urine copper assay is obtained in uncertain cases (Cummings and Benson 1992). Treatment consists of a low-copper diet, a cation exchange resin with each meal to limit intestinal absorption, and chelation of tissue copper with D-penicillamine (Cummings and Benson 1992). This protocol results in resolution of most manifestations of the disease including the dementia, although a transient worsening of neurological signs may occur with initiation of D-penicillamine therapy (Glass et al. 1990). Parkinsonian symptoms that do not resolve with penicillamine may respond to L-dopa (Barbeau and Friesen 1970).

Other Inherited Dementias

A variety of additional (usually recessively) inherited disorders that result in adult-onset dementia are listed in Table 22–1 (Cummings and Benson 1992). Metachromatic leukodystrophy may present as adult-onset psychosis (Waltz et al. 1987) or mania (Muller et al. 1969). Fahr's disease (idiopathic basal ganglia calcification) is an extrapyramidal syndrome accompanied by dementia inherited in an autosomal-dominant fashion that also may present as psychosis or mood disorder (Lauterbach et al. 1994; Whitehouse et al. 1992). Specific treatments exist for only Wilson's disease and adrenoleukodystrophy (Rizzo et al. 1989).

Endocrine and Metabolic Disorders

Thyroid dysfunction is second only to drug intoxication as a cause of reversible dementia (Feldmann and Plum 1993). Hyperthyroidism, which occurs most commonly in women younger than 40, may be associated with myopathy, peripheral neuropathy, chorea, seizures, hyperactivity, irritability, depression, euphoria, and psychosis (Cummings and Benson 1992; Goldman 1992). The dementia of hyperthyroidism may occur in up to 52% of elderly patients (F. I. Martin and Deam 1996), beginning as subtle impairment of attention, memory, and calculation, and in some patients may be the presenting feature of the disorder. Elderly thyrotoxic patients often have an apathetic dementia, with lethargy and psychomotor retardation (Reus 1993). Antithyroid treatment usually reverses the neuropsychiatric symptoms, including the dementia, although complete recovery may take up to a year (Bauer et al. 1987).

Hypothyroidism is common in the general population, with a prevalence of 4.4% among persons older than 60 (Reus 1993) and 10% in lithium-treated patients (Reus 1993). Cognitive symptoms and/or depression may be seen within weeks of the onset of hypothyroidism (Denicoff et al. 1990). Dementia, which may be the only apparent disturbance (Extein and Gold 1988), occurs in 5% of patients (Cummings and Benson 1992). Irritability, insomnia, and lability of mood occur more frequently. Dementia and milder neurocognitive impairment also may be seen in subclinical hypothyroidism with only modest elevations of serum thyrotropin (Ganguli et al. 1996), suggesting that thyroid replacement should be considered in patients presenting with mild cognitive impairment, elevated thyrotropin, but no other signs of hypothyroidism. Although hypothyroidism is generally considered among the most reversible dementias (Goldman 1992), cognitive function only partially recovers in many patients following hormone replacement therapy (Clarnette and Patterson 1994; Dugbartey 1998), especially in the presence of congenital hypothyroidism.

Hyperparathyroidism, myeloma, sarcoidosis, vitamin D intoxication, metastatic cancer, thiazide diuretics, and body immobilization can all result in hypercalcemia (Goldman 1992). Lithium induces mild increases in parathyroid hormone in 80% of patients within 1 month of treatment, and parathyroid adenomas may develop with prolonged treatment (Mallette and Eichhorn 1986). Chronic dementia occurs in 12% of hyperparathyroid patients in the absence of other signs (Feldmann and Plum 1993). This complication may be associated with psychosis (Rosenthal et al. 1997). In elderly patients, the dementia of hyperparathyroidism may occur in up to 40% (Ohrvall et al. 1994). Treatment is directed at the underlying cause of the hypercalcemia or hyperparathyroidism. Although other neuropsychiatric symptoms may respond well to treatment, the response of cognitive impairment is variable (Rosenthal et al. 1997). If a parathyroid adenoma is surgically resected within 2 years of illness onset, the dementia improves considerably within days postoperatively and appears to plateau after 3–6 months (Joborn et al. 1986). However, rapid decrements in serum calcium levels postoperatively can result in self-limited psychosis and an altered state of consciousness in some patients (Mikkelsen and Reider 1979).

Hypocalcemia is usually due to idiopathic or postoperative hypoparathyroidism, renal failure, vitamin D deficiency (occasionally related to anticonvulsants), hypomagnesemia (which occurs with chronic alcoholism or malabsorption), and pseudohypoparathyroidism (tissue unresponsiveness to parathyroid hormone) (Goldman 1992). Dementia, often accompanied by extrapyramidal symptoms produced by calcification of the basal ganglia, is common in hypoparathyroid patients (Cummings and Benson 1992). Normalization of serum calcium may improve the dementia (Slyter 1979), but in one series only 20 of 50 patients approached their former level of functioning after normalization of serum calcium (J. B. Martin and Reichlin 1987). Additionally, dementia may occur in hypoparathyroidism despite normal calcium levels, suggesting that hypocalcemia alone is not the sole determinant of dementia in this disorder (Stuerenburg et al. 1996).

The term *Cushing's disease* refers to corticotropin-producing nonmalignant pituitary tumors; other forms of hypercortisolism are called *Cushing's syndrome* (Goldman 1992). Cognitive changes, impaired concentration and memory, and visuospatial symptoms that may be associated with depression occur in about half of the patients with Cushing's syndrome (Starkman et al. 1986). The severity of neuropsychiatric symptoms correlates with the degree of cortisol elevation (Starkman and Schteingart 1981). Dementia improves with normalization of urinary free cortisol, although complete recovery may take months to years (Starkman et al. 1986). Even in the absence of Cushing's syndrome, milder chronic elevations of serum cortisol due to stress (Raber 1998) and depression (Mitchell and Dening 1996) have been associated with progressive cognitive impairment, particularly memory impairment. The extent to which cognitive impairment in these conditions responds to reduction of serum cortisol is not yet fully elucidated.

Adrenal insufficiency may be caused by adrenocortical destruction or failure (Addison's disease) or by pituitary failure. Memory impairment may occur and may be reversed by treatment with adrenal steroids (Cummings and Benson 1992). Persistence of symptoms despite treatment suggests the presence of other concurrent endocrinopathies (Johnstone et al. 1990).

Panhypopituitarism resulting in thyroid, adrenal, and gonadal insufficiency produces intellectual impairment in most patients (J.B. Martin and Reichlin 1987). Impaired concentration and memory may be accompanied by apathy, lethargy, delusions, hallucinations, and paranoia. Replacement therapy reverses the dementia within weeks; cortisone appears to be more important than thyroxine in this regard (Feldmann and Plum 1993; Hanna 1970; J.B. Martin and Reichlin 1987).

Prolonged or repeated hypoglycemia can result from insulinoma, postgastrectomy hypoglycemia, overadministration of insulin or oral hypoglycemic agents, cirrhosis, retroperitoneal and other large tumors, idiopathic postprandial hypoglycemia, various endocrine deficiencies, premature birth, and drugs (e.g., alcohol, propranolol) (Goldman 1992). Cognitive impairment is apparent with plasma glucose levels in the range of 45–70 mg/dL and becomes more severe as serum glucose levels decline further (Blackman et al. 1990). Pathological changes in the brain produced by hypoglycemia include patchy necrosis and loss of neurons in the cerebral cortex, basal ganglia, and cerebellum (Tom and Richardson 1951). Personality change, aggressive behavior, apathy, and emotional lability may accompany severe memory impairment. Identification and treatment of the underlying cause of hypoglycemia may halt progression of the dementia but may not reverse existing deficits (Cummings and Benson 1992).

Hypoxemia of various causes may produce dementia that is reversed by oxygen therapy (Krop et al. 1973). On the other hand, mountain climbers ascending summits greater than 6,500 meters without supplemental oxygen may experience persistent deficits in memory, naming, and concentration (Cummings and Benson 1992; Hornbein et al. 1989; Regard et al. 1989). Patients with chronic obstructive pulmonary disease (COPD) seldom develop dementia in the absence of hypercapnia, hypoxemia, congestive heart failure, or infection (Austen et al. 1967; W. J. Hall 1981; Feldmann and Plum 1993). However, hypoxemia in COPD may produce impairment in memory and attention related to insufficient oxygenation to limbic regions mediating memory and to diffuse brain areas required for attention (Stuss et al. 1997).

Sleep apnea may cause a reversible dementia due to chronic hypoxemia and sleep deprivation (Riley 1989) and may increase the risk of vascular dementia through associated hypertension and cardiac arrhythmias (Cummings and Benson 1992). Treatment includes weight loss, continuous positive airway pressure (CPAP), surgical correction of structural abnormalities, and tracheostomy for severe cases associated with cardiac arrhythmias and systemic hypertension (Arnold and Kumar 1993).

Chronic renal failure of any cause results in multiple metabolic perturbations that frequently lead to fatigue, apathy, poor concentration, memory impairment, disorientation, irritability, hallucinations, and paranoia (Cummings and Benson 1992; Ginn 1975; Kimmel et al. 1998; Raskin and Fishman 1976). Patients receiving hemodialysis may have significant reductions in frontal and thalamic cerebral blood flow and clinically important cognitive impairment without dementia (Fazekas et al. 1995, 1996), suggesting that these patients merit careful monitoring for changes in cognition and daily function before dementia becomes apparent. Dialysis dementia, which used to be caused by aluminum toxicity, is more common with hemodialysis than peritoneal dialysis (Mach et al. 1988). However, reduction of aluminum levels in dialysate has markedly diminished the incidence of dialysis dementia in areas where water supplies contain high levels of this element and has benefited some dialysis patients with dementia (Mach et al. 1988). Limiting use of aluminum-containing phosphate binders is also prudent. Deferoxamine, a chelating agent, has improved dialysis dementia in many patients (Ackrill et al. 1986; Milne et al. 1983).

A characteristic stuttering and speech hesitation are the most frequent presenting symptoms in dialysis dementia (Lederman and Henry 1978); personality changes also tend to occur early in its course (Mach et al. 1988). Agitation, paranoid delusions, hallucinations, and bizarre behavior are common (Chokroverty et al. 1976), and intellectual deterioration becomes apparent as the disease progresses (Cummings and Benson 1992). Even though clonazepam and diazepam can precipitate encephalopathy in dialysis patients (Mach et al. 1988), these benzodiazepines have been reported to temporarily ameliorate speech and cognitive disturbances in dialysis dementia (Snider et al. 1980; Trauner and Clayman 1979).

Nutritional Disorders: Vitamin B Deficiency

Vitamin B_{12} (cobalamin) and folate are required for the methylation of homocysteine to methionine, which is necessary for the synthesis of *S*-adenosylmethionine. This end product is needed for various methylation reactions in the brain, including neurotransmitter metabolism. When either vitamin B_{12} or folate is deficient, impairment of neurotransmitter (particularly monoamine) metabolism may ensue and produce neuropsychiatric symptoms such as dementia and depression (Bottiglieri 1996). Although such deficiencies have long been associated with dementia, recent studies suggest that hyperhomocysteinemia resulting from either vitamin B_{12} or folate deficiency may be the neurologically important factor because hyperhomocysteinemia is related to an increased risk of cerebrovascular problems, including stroke (Ebly et al. 1998).

Vitamin B_{12} deficiency results in peripheral neuropathy, myelopathy, optic atrophy, and dementia (Pallis and Lewis 1974). Although isolated vitamin B_{12} deficiency is a relatively rare cause of dementia, it may be a comorbid and possibly contributory factor in up to 27% of geriatric dementia (Nagga and Marcusson 1998). When the dementia is present, it tends to have a subcortical pattern with concurrent depressive symptoms that makes it difficult to distinguish from the dementia of depression (Saracaceanu et al. 1997). In 14%–25% of cases, the central nervous system (CNS) symptoms exist without anemia or macrocytosis (Lindenbaum et al. 1988; D. C. Martin 1988). Treatment with 100 μg of parenteral vitamin B_{12} for 1 week followed by every-other-day injections until 2,000 μg has been administered (Babior and Bunn 1987) in some cases may produce complete neurological recovery within 1 month (Zucker et al. 1981). If the deficiency is due to malabsorption, monthly 100-μg injections must be given for the rest of the patient's life (Cummings and Benson 1992). However, response to treatment is not universal, and although replacement therapy may arrest the progression of dementia, some patients do not recover lost cognitive function (Carmel et al. 1995; Crystal et al. 1994; Teunisse et al. 1996). Although this finding could argue against the etiological relevance of vitamin B_{12} deficiency to dementia (Crystal et al. 1994), it is also possible that downstream effects of vitamin B_{12} deficiency (e.g., cerebrovascular injury) may become permanent unless early replacement is instituted.

Low folate levels are associated with a significantly increased risk of stroke that, in turn, contributes to dementia (Clarke et al. 1998; Ebly et al. 1998). Low folate and vitamin B_{12} levels are associated with an increase in total serum homocysteine, which is itself a risk factor for stroke and may contribute to the development of Alzheimer's disease (Clarke et al. 1998). It is not clear whether low folate levels contribute to dementia or whether demented patients have an increased prevalence of low folate levels because cognitive impairment interferes with eating a proper diet. Most neurological symptoms are reversible with folate replacement (Feldmann and Plum 1993).

Niacin (vitamin B_6) deficiency results in pellagra, which is a triad of dermatitis, diarrhea, and dementia. Pellagra is rare in the United States because B_6 is supplied in wheat flour (Feldmann and Plum 1993). Confusion, disorientation, delusions, memory impairment, ataxia, rigidity, and peripheral neuropathy all improve within days to weeks of replacement with a normal diet and 300–500 mg of niacinamide daily for the first few days of treatment (Feldmann and Plum 1993).

Toxin- and Drug-Induced Disorders

Nearly any drug taken in excess can produce CNS toxicity, with impaired concentration, poor attention, memory disturbance, agitation, and stupor and coma at higher dosages (Cummings and Benson 1992). Table 22–2 summarizes some therapeutic and toxic agents associated with dementia at normal dosages.

Dementia caused by most therapeutic agents is reversible with discontinuation of the drug. However, oral contraceptives, ergot derivatives, and amphetamines may cause irreversible vascular dementia by inducing hypercoagulable states or cerebrovascular arteritis

TABLE 22–2. Drugs and toxic agents associated with dementia

Psychotropics	**Antineoplastic agents**	Ethanol
Benzodiazepines	Asparaginase	Hypoglycemic agents
Butyrophenones	Cisplatin	L-Dopa
Fluoxetine	Cytosine arabinoside	Opiates
Lithium	Interferon	Oral contraceptives
Phenothiazines	Methenamine	Ranitidine
Tricyclic antidepressants	Methotrexate	Steroids
	Vincristine	
Anticholinergics	X-radiation	**Heavy metals**
		Aluminum
Antihypertensives	**Antibiotics**	Bismuth
Clonidine	Chloramphenicol	Cadmium
Diuretics	Griseofulvin	Gold
Methyldopa	Metronidazole	Lead
Propranolol	Penicillin	Manganese
	Polymyxin B	Mercury
Anticonvulsants	Rifampin	Nickel
Barbiturates		Thallium
Carbamazepine	**Miscellaneous**	Tin
Ethosuximide	Amphetamines	
Mephenytoin	Aspirin	**Industrial agents/pollutants**
Phenytoin	Bromides	Carbon monoxide
Topiramate	Cimetidine	Carbon tetrachloride
Valproic acid	Digitalis	Ethylene glycol
	Disulfiram	Formaldehyde
	Ergot alkaloids	Jet fuels
		Organophosphate insecticides
		Toluene

Source. Adapted from Cummings and Benson 1992 and Dubovsky 1994.

(Cummings and Benson 1992). Hypoglycemic agents can cause irreversible CNS damage by depriving the brain of glucose. The combination of lithium and haloperidol was reported to produce irreversible neurotoxicity with dementia (Cohen and Cohen 1974), but the syndrome described may have represented neuroleptic malignant syndrome or lithium toxicity exacerbated by dehydration (Cummings and Benson 1992). Reports still emerge of irreversible neurological syndromes following lithium intoxication (Izzo and Brody 1985). Chronic barbiturate (Judd and Grant 1978) and solvent vapor (Hormes et al. 1986) abuse can produce dementia that does not reverse with abstinence. Methotrexate, cytosine arabinoside, and cerebral radiation may cause irreversible dementia, whereas other antineoplastics cause reversible syndromes (Cummings and Benson 1992). Heavy metals and industrial agents typically cause irreversible dementias. Partial resolution is noted with chelation therapy for some heavy metals. Cognitive impairment from organophosphates and carbon monoxide also is potentially reversible (Cummings and Benson 1992).

Human Immunodeficiency Virus Infection

Dementia is evident in 20%–40% of patients with human immunodeficiency virus (HIV) infection, and 90% of patients dying of acquired immunodeficiency syndrome (AIDS) show histological evidence of subacute encephalitis (McArthur et al. 1993). Microglia/monocyte and giant cells derived from fusion of monocytes appear to be the predominant cells in the CNS directly infected by HIV, and it has been suggested that cortical, subcortical, and white matter alterations seen in patients with HIV dementia result from the production of injurious soluble factors by these cells and by secondarily affected astrocytes (Dal Canto 1997). Independent replication of the virus in gray matter also may occur with some specific HIV strains in some patients (Cunningham et al. 1997). Infection of cortical and subcortical (especially basal ganglia) regions, deep hemispheric white matter (Cummings and Benson 1992), and the cerebellum can all contribute to HIV-related cognitive impairment (Tagliati et al. 1998).

HIV appears to induce a vacuolar myelopathy in both the central and the peripheral nervous systems, similar to that observed in vitamin B_{12} deficiency (Tan and Guiloff 1998; Tyor et al. 1995). This myelopathy may be the result of macrophage injury of myelin and oligodendrocytes and macrophage-derived products that interfere with the methyl transfer cycle, impairing repair mechanisms. Production of nitric oxide in the CNS of patients with HIV may further contribute to cell death and clinical symptoms of impaired cognition (Vincent et al. 1999).

HIV encephalopathy produces a subcortical dementia, with slowed mental processing, loss of initiative, poor short-term memory, apathy, and withdrawal from usual activities (Navia et al. 1986). Zidovudine treatment has been shown to improve cognitive function in patients with mild to moderate AIDS dementia (Sidtis et al. 1993), and zidovudine may offer time-limited neuroprotection against both AIDS dementia and opportunistic infection in AIDS patients (Baldeweg et al. 1995, 1998). In one report (Routy et al. 1993), 41% of the dementia patients who were intolerant of or derived no benefit from oral zidovudine responded to intrathecal zidovudine. The MAO-B inhibitor selegiline, which was discussed earlier in this chapter, has recently been shown to improve cognitive function in patients with HIV-related cognitive impairment (Dana Consortium on the Therapy of HIV Dementia and Related Cognitive Disorders 1998).

Collagen-Vascular Disorders

Many collagen-vascular disorders cause vascular dementia, which is discussed in Chapter 21. Systemic lupus erythematosus causes a variety of CNS symptoms, including seizures, depression, psychosis, chorea, delirium, and dementia (Cummings and Benson 1992; Miguel et al. 1994). Although many patients (up to 85%) with systemic lupus erythematosus report subjective symptoms of cognitive impairment, frank dementia is relatively uncommon (about 5%) (Miguel et al. 1994). The dementia of lupus may respond to corticosteroids (Manto et al. 1993), and ECT has occasionally produced dramatic improvement in delirium associated with lupus cerebritis unresponsive to immunosuppressive therapy (Abrams 1992).

Miscellaneous Disorders and Conditions

Up to half of all patients with multiple sclerosis (MS), an inflammatory demyelinating disease of unclear etiology that affects the white matter of the cerebral hemispheres, brain stem, optic nerves, cerebellum, and spinal cord, have measurable deficits on neuropsychological testing (Brassington and Marsh 1998; Peyser et al. 1980). Between 2% and 6.7% have impairment that is of sufficient severity to constitute dementia (Mendez 1993). Although cognitive impairment in MS has been described as subcortical (Rao 1986), more recent formulations suggest that MS may be a prototype for a pattern specific to white matter (white matter dementia) (Rao 1996). Indeed, cognitive impairment in MS appears to be a function of the extent of white matter injury rather than duration or other indices of illness severity (e.g., motor disturbance) (Patti et al. 1995). Examination of these findings suggests that extensively confluent white matter lesions extending from the periventricular regions toward the cortex (Patti et al. 1995) or subadjacent to the cortex (Damian et al. 1994) are most likely to produce cognitive impairments, such as decreased speed and efficiency of processing, inattention, decreased verbal and visuospatial memory, impaired retrieval of information, impaired judgment, perseveration, and difficulty shifting information sets (Rao et al. 1991; Troster et al. 1998; Tsolaki et al. 1994).

Although corticosteroids have been the mainstay of the treatment of MS (Francis 1993), interferon beta-1a and beta-1b (IFNB Multiple Sclerosis Study Group 1993), cladribine (Romine et al. 1999), glatiramer acetate (copolymer 1), and mizoribine with prednisolone (Saida et al. 1999) have been reported to reduce the risk of relapse (Tselis and Lisak 1999). Among these agents, interferon beta-1b (Paty and Li 1993), glatiramer acetate (Johnson et al. 1998; Mancardi et al. 1998), mizoribine with prednisolone (Saida et al. 1999), and azathioprine (Cavazzuti et al. 1997) may decrease relapse-associated demyelination as detected by MRI in patients with relapsing-remitting MS. No current evidence indicates that these approaches significantly decrease the incidence or severity of intellectual deficits produced by MS (Weinstein et al. 1999).

Brain tumors account for 1.5% of cases of dementia (Clarfield 1988), with an annual incidence of nonmetastatic primary brain tumors of 53.2 per 100,000 people older than 65 who present with dementia (Alexander et al. 1995). Tumors of the frontal lobes, temporal lobes, thalamus, basal ganglia, and hypothalamus can present with dementia, which occasionally is overlooked without neuroimaging (Cummings and Benson 1992; Sahadevan et al. 1997). Primary CNS lymphoma can produce a rapidly progressive dementia (Bakshi et al. 1999; Carlson 1996). Reduction of edema and intracranial pressure by corticosteroids can improve cognitive function. However, irradiation of brain neoplasms (usually with total doses in excess of 6,000 rads), especially in those who have also received chemotherapy, can result in a delayed degenerative white matter dementia that becomes apparent months or years after treatment (Asai et al. 1987; DeAngelis et al. 1989; Goldberg et al. 1982; So et al. 1987; Vigliani et al. 1999). This kind of tardive dementia is particularly troublesome for the fewer than 2% of long-term survivors of glioblastoma multiforme (Scott et al. 1998).

Subdural hematomas, which account for about 0.4% of dementias (Clarfield 1988), can produce mental status changes readily misdiagnosed as Alzheimer's disease or vascular dementia (Cummings and Benson 1992). The risk of subdural hematoma increases with age, largely as a result of falls, and is about three times as high in persons ages 75–85 years as in those ages 65–75 years (Alexander et al. 1995). Fluctuating arousal, poor attention, irritability, and memory impairment are common manifestations in elderly patients, and focal signs can mislead the clinician into diagnosing stroke or transient ischemic attacks. Although a history of trauma is often absent, a careful neurological examination may reveal deficits suggesting the presence of a focal mass lesion (Velasco et al. 1995). Although some lesions resolve spontaneously, surgical drainage is usually necessary to reverse cognitive deficits (Cummings and Benson 1992).

Hydrocephalus can be caused by congenital lesions, tumors, infections, hemorrhage, trauma, malignancies, aneurysms, and vascular malformations, or it may be idiopathic. Subacute hydrocephalus often causes dementia (Cummings and Benson 1992). Normal-pressure hydrocephalus, which accounts for 1.6% of dementias (Clarfield 1988), produces a triad of dementia, gait disturbance, and urinary incontinence, although only 12% of patients with this complex will prove to have normal-pressure hydrocephalus (Mulrow et al. 1987), and many patients with this condition will not have the entire triad (e.g., lack of urinary incontinence). The pattern of cognitive impairment of normal-pressure hydrocephalus is most consistent with that of a white matter disease dementia and is characterized by inattention, distractibility, psychomotor slowing, impaired initiation and frontal executive functions, poor judgment, and disinhibition, but not aphasia, agnosia, and apraxia (Filley et al. 1989; Gustafson and Hagberg 1978; Mendez 1993; Price and Tucker 1977). Enlarged ventricles are found on CT or MRI, but radioimmune serum albumin scanning may be necessary to distinguish normal-pressure hydrocephalus from hydrocephalus ex vacuo (i.e., ventricular enlargement due to loss of brain tissue). Radioisotope cisternography (Larsson et al. 1994), lumboventricular infusion techniques, intraventricular pressure monitoring, and the Fisher cerebrospinal fluid (CSF)–tap test help predict response to treatment (Mendez 1993). Measurement of CSF outflow resistance is also a useful predictor of response to surgical shunting, with values of 18 mL HG/mL/min or greater predicting the best cognitive and gait responses (Boon et al. 1998). Surgical shunting of the CSF results in acute reversal of all symptoms in 33%–80% of patients (Boon et al. 1998; Mendez 1993; St.-Laurent 1988). However, significant improvement is sustained in only 21% of all patients with normal-pressure hydrocephalus, and for every three or four successfully treated normal-pressure hydrocephalus patients, one serious complication arises (Vanneste et al. 1992). The best predictors of improvement or stabilization of neurological deficits following shunting are short duration of symptoms, onset without dementia, and only mild to moderate ventricular enlargement (Caruso et al. 1997).

More than 2 million Americans suffer traumatic brain injury (TBI) each year, most frequently from motor vehicle accidents, falls, and assaults (J.F. Kraus and Sorenson 1994; U.S. Department of Health and Human Services 1989). Three distinct neuropathological alterations may result from closed head injury: 1) diffuse axonal injury; 2) focal contusions, hemorrhages, and lacerations; and 3) hypoxic-ischemic insults (Cummings and Benson 1992). Poor functional outcome, including cognitive impairment, is more likely if either the period of anterograde posttraumatic amnesia or the duration of coma lasts more than 2 weeks (Bond 1986). Residual deficits are largely established within 6–9 months of the injury (Mendez 1993). Neuropsychiatric sequelae include problems with attention, concentration, and executive functioning; posttraumatic epilepsy; personality change; and a variety of secondary psychiatric disorders including depression, mania, anxiety, and psychosis (Arciniegas et al. 1999; Silver and Yudofsky 1994; Silver et al. 1992).

Cognitive impairment associated with mild to moderate TBI is usually relatively mild, with problems in selective and sustained attention, speed and efficiency of information processing, and delayed or impaired information retrieval. Alzheimer's disease is not caused by TBI. However, TBI may worsen Alzheimer's disease, especially in patients with one or more copies of the apolipoprotein E ε4 gene (Mayeux et al. 1995). Having one or more copies of the apolipoprotein E ε4 gene is associated with a poorer cognitive outcome following TBI (Friedman et al. 1999; Nicoll et al. 1995).

Antipsychotics (Feeney et al. 1982; Goldstein 1995a) and benzodiazepines (Goldstein 1995b) should be used sparingly in patients with TBI because these drugs may impede neuronal recovery following TBI. Methylphenidate (Cristomo et al. 1988; C.T. Gualtieri and Evans 1988; Plenger et al. 1996), amantadine (T. Gualtieri et al. 1989; M.F. Kraus and Maki 1997), bromocriptine (Powell et al. 1996), L-dopa (Lal et al. 1988), donepezil (Taverni et al. 1998), and naltrexone (Tennant and Wild 1987) may have salutary effects on cognitive function. Secondary mood disorders associated with TBI should be treated with medications with a low potential for cognitive impairment, such as bupropion, selegiline, and the calcium channel–blocking agents.

Mixed Dementias

Alzheimer's disease and vascular dementia frequently coexist (Lanska and Schoenberg 1993; Mölsä et al. 1985), constituting the most common mixed dementia. Parkinson's disease also may be comorbid with Alzheimer's disease, possibly because both diseases are more common with increasing age (Heston 1981).

One form of mixed dementia that poses a diagnostic challenge is comorbid depressive dementia and degenerative dementia, which can be difficult to differentiate from each other (Roth 1976). This is a common problem because 43%–89% of patients with depressive dementia eventually develop Alzheimer's disease or other primary degenerative dementias, even though the pseudodementia remits with improvement of depression (Alexopoulos et al. 1993; Gottfries and Hess 1990). One interpretation of this outcome is that depression increases the severity of subtle cognitive deficits, which eventually progress until they are evident even in the absence of conditions (e.g., depression) that lower the threshold for their expression. Because depression exacerbates cognitive and behavioral decline in dementia patients (Greenwald et al. 1989; Tune 1998), a trial of an antidepressant may be warranted in patients with dementia for which other reversible causes are not found (Hill and Stoudemire 1993; Katz 1998), even if a patient does not meet the formal criteria for major depressive disorder (Dubovsky 1994; Tune 1998).

Because sedating and anticholinergic antidepressants further impair cognitive function (Tariot 1992), the antidepressants of first choice for this indication are bupropion, venlafaxine, and the SSRIs (Tune 1998). The secondary amine tricyclic antidepressants are better tolerated than the tertiary amine preparations. Selegiline may slow neurological deterioration in some cases, but the dietary restrictions may be difficult for patients with dementia to remember. ECT is safe and effective for depressed patients with dementia (Benbow 1988; Kellner and Bernstein 1993; Stoudemire et al. 1995). ECT has a very high response rate in patients whose depression is accompanied by leukoencephalopathy on MRI (Coffey et al. 1988). Acute cognitive impairment with ECT is more common in patients with dementia than in other patients (Dubovsky 1995). However, ECT does not worsen preexisting brain damage (Coffey et al. 1991) and can be safely and effectively used as a maintenance treatment in elderly depressed patients with dementia (Rabheru and Persad 1997).

As is true of patients without dementia, attention to interactions with caregivers and the environment is an important component of treatment of depression in dementia patients. A study of a behavioral management program that included caregiver education found significant benefits on both depression and impaired cognition in patients with dementia living in a nursing home (Proctor et al. 1999) and on depression in their caregivers (Teri et al. 1997).

Treatment of Common Behavior Problems in Patients With Dementia

Patients with dementia often develop wandering, agitation, shouting, unexpected violent outbursts, and unprovoked hostility toward loved ones (Ross 1992). Most of these patients are given one or more psychotropic medications, which are considered essential by caregivers. However, reducing use of these agents does not increase the incidence of problem behaviors (Avorn et al. 1992). It is therefore important to consider withdrawing medications that could be aggravating confusion or causing delirium, especially benzodiazepines and anticholinergic drugs (Schor et al. 1992; Tariot 1999). Even aspirin can cause delirium in susceptible patients.

Because of the risk of oversedation, confusion, falls, paradoxical excitement, and further cognitive impairment, benzodiazepines are poor choices for treating behavioral disturbances in cognitively impaired patients (Goldstein 1995b; Risse and Barnes 1986). Antipsychotics are more effective than placebo in some studies of agitation, insomnia, irritability, and hostility in patients with dementia (Risse and Barnes 1986; Young and Meyers 1991), but the apparent benefit of these agents depends not on a primary antipsychotic action but on sedative side effects, which may aggravate cognitive impairment (Ahronheim 1992; Risse and Barnes 1986; Wragg and Jeste 1988). In addition, reports of positive effects are difficult to interpret because dementia in these reports has been diagnostically heterogeneous, and therapeutic trials are often brief (Risse and Barnes 1986). A careful reading of positive studies reveals that clinically meaningful improvement is usually modest and unsustained (Devanand and Levy 1995; Goldstein and Birnbom 1976; Smith et al. 1974).

The risk of motor side effects usually does not justify the benefit of the antipsychotics in treating agitation in dementia patients (Goldstein and Birnbom 1976; Smith et al. 1974) unless agitation is secondary to psychosis (Ross 1992). Indeed, in a double-blind study of institutionalized patients with dementia and physically aggressive behavior, withdrawal of antipsychotics was not associated with a significant increase in aggression, suggesting that many such patients are unnecessarily medicated (Bridges-Parlet et al. 1997). Atypical antipsychotic drugs, on the other hand, appear to have primary antiaggressive properties that are not linked to their antipsychotic effects and are better tolerated than the conventional antipsychotics by elderly patients with dementia (Collaborative Working Group on Clinical Trial Evaluations 1998).

In double-blind studies, propranolol in doses of 10–600 mg/day has been effective in reducing pacing, assaultiveness, and agitation in patients with dementia or brain damage (Lohr et al. 1992; Salzman 1990; L.S. Schneider and Sobin 1992; Shankle et al. 1995; Silver and Yudofsky 1988). Pindolol and nadolol have also been found to reduce impulsivity and assaultiveness in double-blind studies of dementia patients (L.S. Schneider and Sobin

1992). β-Blockers may take 4–6 weeks before ameliorating problem behaviors (Silver and Yudofsky 1985; Silver et al. 1992). Congestive heart failure, heart block, sinus bradycardia, insulin-dependent diabetes mellitus, asthma, and possibly COPD are contraindications (Lohr et al. 1992; Risse and Barnes 1986; Salzman 1990). High doses of β-blockers may cause hallucinations and aggravate aggression (L. S. Schneider and Sobin 1992). β-Blockers increase blood levels of antipsychotics and anticonvulsants.

Open trials and case series suggest additional potential treatments for agitation and aggression in dementia patients, including carbamazepine (Lemke 1995; Yudofsky et al. 1987), valproic acid (Giakas et al. 1990; Herrmann 1998), buspirone (Levine 1988), methylphenidate (Mooney and Haas 1993), selegiline (Goad et al. 1991), trazodone (L. S. Schneider and Sobin 1992), SSRIs (Greenwald et al. 1986), and estrogen (Kyomen et al. 1991; Shelton and Brooks 1999). Naltrexone decreases self-injurious behavior in some brain injury patients (Herman 1990), but it has not yet been studied in dementia patients. A recent study compared trazodone with haloperidol for the treatment of aggression and found both medications equally effective (Sultzer et al. 1997), although patients in this study with paranoia-related aggression appeared to respond somewhat better to haloperidol.

Behavioral interventions can be more effective than medications for managing many problem behaviors (Alessi 1991; Allen-Burge et al. 1999; Patterson et al. 1999). Wandering, for example, may be prevented by installing new locks that are difficult for the person with dementia to operate or that are located at an unusual place, such as the bottom of the door (Alessi 1991). Teaching caregivers to identify and lessen stressors that worsen the behavior of dementia patients, such as fatigue, change of routine, excess demands, overwhelming stimuli, and physical stressors such as acute illness or pain (G. R. Hall 1988), can decrease behavioral outbursts and the need for nursing home placement. Identifying antecedents and consequences of behavior can help caregivers devise behavioral treatment programs to modify maladaptive behavior (Alessi 1991; Allen-Burge et al. 1999). Patients with profound impairment of explicit memory may have preserved procedural (implicit) memory such that they can learn more appropriate behavior with positive reinforcement (Heinrichs 1990).

Treatment of Cognitive Impairment

Two kinds of primary treatment for dementia are under investigation. Correcting dysfunctional neurotransmitter activity can improve functions related to those transmitters and could slow the progression of the illness. Treatment of the underlying causes of neuronal death could have the potential to halt the disorder.

The finding of decreased cortical acetylcholine levels in Alzheimer's disease has given rise to 20 studies testing the effects of choline salts or phosphatidylcholine (precursors to acetylcholine) in Alzheimer's disease, of which only one study (Little et al. 1985) found significant benefit (Growdon 1993). Even though cholinergic muscarinic receptors are preserved in Alzheimer's disease, trials of the nonselective muscarinic agonists bethanechol and arecoline have not yielded positive results (Gauthier et al. 1991). Seven of 15 reports on physostigmine, a short-acting cholinesterase inhibitor, showed small and transient benefits of no clinical significance in most patients (Growdon 1993). A sustained-release form of physostigmine proved to be more effective, but it was poorly tolerated.

Tacrine (9-amino-1,2,3,4-tetrahydroacridine; THA) is a reversible cholinesterase inhibitor with a longer duration of action than physostigmine that was approved by the U.S.

Food and Drug Administration (1993) for the treatment of Alzheimer's disease in September 1993. Shortly after this medication became available in the United States, reports suggested that 40%–50% of patients who tolerate THA have some meaningful improvement in cognition and a reduction in the rate of progression over at least the first 3 months of treatment (Small 1992). A recent meta-analysis of all clinical trials of THA completed as of 1996 suggested that at least one-fourth of patients drop out of treatment because of intolerable side effects and that the cognitive benefit during the first 3 months of treatment for those who continue is modest at best (Qizilbash et al. 1998). The long-term benefit of THA is no greater than that of placebo, whereas the incidence of adverse effects is greater (Malaguarnera et al. 1998).

Donepezil, a more centrally selective acetylcholinesterase inhibitor that was approved for use in the United States in 1997, has been shown to improve cognition and clinical global functioning in patients with Alzheimer's disease with fewer systemic side effects than THA (Rogers et al. 1998). A large multicenter, multinational, double-blind, placebo-controlled study replicated this finding (Burns et al. 1999). It has also been suggested that donepezil may be useful for the treatment of dementia associated with Down's syndrome (trisomy 21) (Kishnani et al. 1999), persistent delirium superimposed on dementia (Wengel et al. 1998), and TBI (Taverni et al. 1998), although controlled trials of donepezil in these disorders have not yet been conducted.

Other drugs recently have been found to selectively inhibit acetylcholinesterase in neurofibrillary tangles and plaques, although the clinical significance of this finding is unclear (Wright et al. 1993). Because cortical levels of ChAT are decreased in Parkinson's disease, Lewy body dementia, Gerstmann-Straussler syndrome, progressive supranuclear palsy, olivopontocerebellar atrophy, and Creutzfeldt-Jakob disease and basal ganglia levels of ChAT are decreased in Huntington's disease and Pick's disease (Court and Perry 1991), it is reasonable to speculate that cholinesterase inhibitors may eventually have a role in the treatment of these disorders as well. Because cholinesterase inhibitors prolong the availability of acetylcholine from neurons that produce it, long-term benefits would be expected to be limited by continued degeneration of cholinergic neurons (Ahronheim 1992).

A purified Ginkgo biloba extract (Egb 761) has recently received attention as a possible treatment for uncomplicated dementia (Curtis-Prior et al. 1999). In a meta-analysis of all articles examining the effect of this agent on cognitive function in dementia, a small but significant effect was apparent over 3–6 months of treatment with 120–240 mg/day of Ginkgo biloba extract (Oken et al. 1998). Although the mechanism of action by which the effect occurs is not known, current hypotheses include vasoregulatory, "cognition-enhancing," stress-alleviating, and gene-regulatory mechanisms (Curtis-Prior et al. 1999).

Another approach to normalizing neurotransmitter function in dementia grew out of the observation that monoamine oxidase levels are increased in the brains of Alzheimer's disease patients. Selegiline, the selective MAO-B inhibitor discussed earlier in this chapter, may improve cognitive function in some Alzheimer's patients (Finali et al. 1991; Tariot et al. 1987), although earlier studies varied in their ability to detect clear improvements (Burke et al. 1993). More recent double-blind, placebo-controlled studies of patients with Alzheimer's disease have found a significant benefit of selegiline over placebo on cognitive performance (Filip and Kolibas 1999; Lawlor et al. 1997), and in another study, selegiline (alone or in combination with vitamin E) significantly delayed institutionalization, functional disability, and/or death in Alzheimer's patients with moderately severe cognitive impairment (Sano et al. 1997). However, this finding continues to be inconsistent even in relatively large and well-controlled studies (Freedman et al. 1998; Tariot et al. 1998), suggesting that selegiline does not benefit all patients with Alzheimer's disease. Moclobemide, a reversible inhibitor of MAO-A, also may improve cognition in these patients (Amrein et al. 1999). However, at present, too few trials of moclobemide in patients with dementia have been done to determine whether it will prove more consistently effective than selegiline. Because monoamine oxidase levels are increased in Pick's disease, trials of MAOIs in this disease also may be warranted.

Another line of investigation that may have more promise involves the role of the intracellular calcium ion (Ca^{2+}) in neuronal degeneration (Branconnier et al. 1992; Choi 1988). All known cytotoxic processes, including ischemia, toxins, immune mechanisms, and genetically programmed cell death, increase free intracellular Ca^{2+} concentration. Although Ca^{2+} stimulates many crucial cellular actions including learning and gene activation, excessive elevation of free intracellular Ca^{2+} activates enzymes such as proteases, which degrade structural proteins, and phospholipases, which break down the cell membrane, leading to free-radical formation.

Sustained increases in free intracellular Ca^{2+} can be produced by excitatory amino acids such as glutamate (Choi 1988; Garthwaite 1991). In moderate concentrations, excitatory amino acids facilitate learning and neuronal development; however, excessive excitatory amino acid release and decreased uptake inhibition have been implicated in various forms of brain damage, including Alzheimer's disease (Court and Perry 1991). Through their interaction with specific receptors, the best studied of which is the NMDA receptor (Shaw 1993), glutamate and other excitatory amino acids produce sustained influx of Ca^{2+} through a receptor-operated calcium channel that persists after the excitatory amino acid is withdrawn.

One approach to reducing excitotoxicity involves the noncompetitive NMDA antagonists such as MK-801, ketamine, and dextromethorphan. These drugs bind to a phencyclidine receptor linked to the NMDA complex to attenuate Ca^{2+} influx. In animals with ligated cerebral arteries, MK-801 improved learning and reduced neuronal death in regions such as the hippocampus and neocortex, where high concentrations of NMDA receptors are found and vulnerability to glutamate toxicity seems greatest (Albers et al. 1989). Like all drugs that bind to the phencyclidine receptor, however, noncompetitive NMDA receptor antagonists could have psychotomimetic effects. D-Cycloserine, an antitubercular drug that modulates the NMDA receptor, has shown promise in scopolamine-induced memory impairment in healthy volunteers (R. W. Jones et al. 1991). As discussed earlier in this chapter, remacemide hydrochloride, an NMDA receptor antagonist, reduced choreiform movements and appeared well tolerated in a preliminary trial (Kieburtz et al. 1996). Whether such agents might limit neurodegeneration related to the progression of cognitive impairments is not yet known.

Another approach to reducing excitotoxicity and Ca^{2+}-stimulated neurotoxicity (and therefore perhaps decreasing the rate of cognitive decline) is to attenuate elevations of free intracellular Ca^{2+} by reducing calcium influx through potential dependent channels. Nimodipine, a lipid-soluble dihydropyridine calcium channel blocker, has antidepressant benefits in elderly patients and may have importance in the treatment of depression and dementia (De Vry et al. 1997). Some studies have reported a benefit of nimodipine on slowing progression of memory impairment in double-blind, placebo-controlled trials (Ban et al. 1990; Tollefson 1990), although questions have been raised about the clinical relevance of these findings (Fritze and Walden 1995; Jarvik 1991). More recently, a large study of cognitive function in elderly persons taking calcium channel blockers or other antihypertensive agents showed a significant adverse effect of the calcium channel blockers on cognitive performance over time that was not accounted for by factors other than medication type (Maxwell et al. 1999).

Other antioxidant therapies, including α-tocopherol (vitamin E), have been (Sano et al. 1997) and are being investigated as yet another mechanism by which to limit cellular injury and progression of cognitive impairment. Whether such therapies will consistently confer protection in the neurodegenerative dementias is not yet clear.

Conclusions

Dementia is a feature of many degenerative, metabolic, endocrine, and toxin-induced disorders. Patterns of dementia in these conditions may be cortical or subcortical and may affect gray matter or white matter. Depression produces a dementia syndrome that can be indistinguishable from neurological causes of subcortical dementia. Because depressive dementia often complicates neurological dementia and aggravates both cognitive decline and behavioral symptoms, addition of antidepressants to the regimens of patients newly diagnosed with dementia can provide substantial relief even if the underlying illness eventually progresses.

Treatment of behavioral disorders in depression involves both pharmacological and nonpharmacological interventions. The former include β-adrenergic–blocking agents, antidepressants, buspirone, anticonvulsants, and atypical antipsychotic medications. Antipsychotics should be reserved for the treatment of agitation secondary to psychosis. Promising treatments that may be useful in a variety of dementia syndromes include drugs that modify the NMDA receptor, calcium influx, and excitotoxicity.

References

Abrams R: Electroconvulsive Therapy, 2nd Edition. New York, Oxford University Press, 1992

Ackrill P, Ralston AJ, Day JP: Role of desferrioxamine in the treatment of dialysis encephalopathy. Kidney Int 29 (suppl 18):S104–S107, 1986

Ahronheim JC: Handbook of Prescribing Medications for Geriatric Patients. Boston, MA, Little, Brown, 1992

Albers GW, Goldberg MP, Choi DW: N-methyl-D-aspartate antagonists: ready for clinical trial in brain ischemia? Ann Neurol 25:398–403, 1989

Aldrich MS, Foster NL, White RF, et al: Sleep abnormalities in progressive supranuclear palsy. Ann Neurol 25:577–581, 1989

Alessi CA: Managing the behavioral problems of dementia in the home. Clin Geriatr Med 7:787–801, 1991

Alexander EM, Wagner EH, Buchner DM, et al: Do surgical brain lesions present as isolated dementia? A population-based study. J Am Geriatr Soc 43:138–143, 1995

Alexopoulos GS, Meyers BS, Young RC, et al: The course of geriatric depression with reversible dementia: a controlled study. Am J Psychiatry 150:1693–1699, 1993

Allen G, Buxton RB, Wong EC, et al: Attentional activation of the cerebellum independent of motor involvement. Science 275(5308):1940–1943, 1997

Allen-Burge R, Stevens AB, Burgio LD: Effective behavioral interventions for decreasing dementia-related challenging behavior in nursing homes. Int J Geriatr Psychiatry 14:213–228, 1999

Amrein R, Martin JR, Cameron AM: Moclobemide in patients with dementia and depression. Adv Neurol 80:509–519, 1999

Arciniegas DB, Adler LE, Topkoff J, et al: Attention and memory dysfunction after traumatic brain injury: cholinergic mechanisms, sensory gating, and a hypothesis for further investigation. Brain Inj 13:1–13, 1999

Arnold SE, Kumar A: Reversible dementias. Med Clin North Am 77:215–230, 1993

Asai A, Matsutani M, Takakura K: Subacute brain atrophy induced by radiation therapy of malignant brain tumors. Gan No Rinsho [Japanese Journal of Cancer Clinics] 33:753–761, 1987

Austen FK, Carmichael MW, Adams RD: Neurologic abnormalities of chronic pulmonary insufficiency. N Engl J Med 257:579–590, 1967

Avorn J, Soumerai SB, Everitt DE, et al: A randomized trial of program to reduce the use of psychoactive drugs in nursing homes. N Engl J Med 327:168–173, 1992

Babior BM, Bunn HF: Megaloblastic anemias, in Harrison's Principles of Internal Medicine, 11th Edition. Edited by Braunwald E, Isselbacher KJ, Petersdorf RG, et al. New York, McGraw-Hill, 1987, pp 1498–1504

Bakshi R, Mazziotta JC, Mischel PS, et al: Lymphomatosis cerebri presenting as a rapidly progressive dementia: clinical, neuroimaging and pathologic findings. Dement Geriatr Cogn Disord 10:152–157, 1999

Baldeweg T, Catalan J, Lovett E, et al: Long-term zidovudine reduces neurocognitive deficits in HIV-1 infection. AIDS 9:589–596, 1995

Baldeweg T, Catalan J, Gazzard BG: Risk of HIV dementia and opportunistic brain disease in AIDS and zidovudine therapy. J Neurol Neurosurg Psychiatry 65:34–41, 1998

Ban TA, Morey L, Aguglia E, et al: Nimodipine in the treatment of old age dementias. Prog Neuro-psychopharmacol Biol Psychiatry 14:525–551, 1990

Barbeau A, Friesen H: Treatment of Wilson's disease with L-dopa after failure with penicillamine. Lancet 1:1180–1181, 1970

Bauer MS, Droba M, Whybrow PC: Disorders of the thyroid and parathyroid, in Handbook of Clinical Psychoneuroendocrinology. Edited by Nemeroff CB, Loosen PT. New York, Guilford, 1987, pp 41–70

Benbow SM: ECT for depression in dementia (letter). Br J Psychiatry 152:859, 1988

Ben-Shlomo Y, Churchyard A, Head J, et al: Investigation by Parkinson's Disease Research Group of United Kingdom into excess mortality seen with combined levodopa and selegiline treatment in patients with early, mild Parkinson's disease: further results of randomised trial and confidential inquiry. BMJ 316(7139):1191–1196, 1998

Berquin PC, Giedd JN, Jacobsen LK, et al: Cerebellum in attention-deficit hyperactivity disorder: a morphometric MRI study. Neurology 50:1087–1093, 1998

Birkmayer W, Knoll J, Riederer R, et al: Increased life expectancy resulting from addition of L-deprenyl to Madopar treatment in Parkinson's disease: a long-term study. J Neural Transm 64:113–127, 1985

Blackman JD, Towle VL, Lewis GF, et al: Hypoglycemic thresholds for cognitive dysfunction in humans. Diabetes 39:828–835, 1990

Bond MR: Neurobehavioral sequelae of closed head injury, in Neuropsychological Assessment of Neuropsychiatric Disorders. Edited by Grant I, Adams KM. New York, Oxford University Press, 1986, pp 347–373

Boon AJ, Tans JT, Delwel EJ, et al: Does CSF outflow resistance predict the response to shunting in patients with normal pressure hydrocephalus? Acta Neurochir Suppl (Wien) 71:331–333, 1998

Bottiglieri T: Folate, vitamin B_{12}, and neuropsychiatric disorders. Nutr Rev 54:382–390, 1996

Branconnier RJ, Branconnier ME, Walshe TM, et al: Blocking the Ca^{2+}-activated cytotoxic mechanisms of cholinergic neuronal death: a novel treatment strategy for Alzheimer's disease. Psychopharmacol Bull 28:175–181, 1992

Brassington JC, Marsh NV: Neuropsychological aspects of multiple sclerosis. Neuropsychol Rev 8:43–77, 1998

Bridges-Parlet S, Knopman D, Steffes S: Withdrawal of neuroleptic medications from institutionalized dementia patients: results of a double-blind, baseline-treatment-controlled pilot study. J Geriatr Psychiatry Neurol 10:119–126, 1997

Brown RG, Marsden CD: How common is dementia in Parkinson's disease? Lancet 2:1262–1265, 1984

Burke WJ, Ranno AE, Roccaforte WH, et al: L-Deprenyl in the treatment of mild dementia of the Alzheimer type: preliminary results. J Am Geriatr Soc 41:367–370, 1993

Burns A, Rossor M, Hecker J, et al: The effects of donepezil in Alzheimer's disease—results from a multinational trial. Dement Geriatr Cogn Disord 10:237–244, 1999

Butters N, Sax D, Montgomery K, et al: Comparison of the neuropsychological deficits associated with early and advanced Huntington's disease. Arch Neurol 35:585–589, 1978

Caine ED, Shoulson I: Psychiatric syndromes in Huntington's disease. Am J Psychiatry 140:728–733, 1983

Cantello R, Gilli M, Riccio A, et al: Mood changes associated with "end-of-dose deterioration" in Parkinson's disease: a controlled study. J Neurol Neurosurg Psychiatry 49:1182–1192, 1986

Cantello R, Aguggia M, Gilli M, et al: Depression in Parkinson's disease: a quantitative and qualitative analysis. J Neurol Neurosurg Psychiatry 52:724–731, 1989

Carlson BA: Rapidly progressive dementia caused by nonenhancing primary lymphoma of the central nervous system. AJNR Am J Neuroradiol 17:1695–1697, 1996

Carmel R, Gott PS, Waters CH, et al: The frequently low cobalamin levels in dementia usually signify treatable metabolic, neurologic and electrophysiologic abnormalities. Eur J Haematol 54:245–253, 1995

Cartwright GE: Diagnosis of treatable Wilson's disease. N Engl J Med 298:1347–1350, 1978

Caruso R, Cervoni L, Vitale AM, et al: Idiopathic normal-pressure hydrocephalus in adults: result of shunting correlated with clinical findings in 18 patients and review of the literature. Neurosurg Rev 20:104–107, 1997

Cavazzuti M, Merelli E, Tassone G, et al: Lesion load quantification in serial MR of early relapsing multiple sclerosis patients in azathioprine treatment: a retrospective study. Eur Neurol 38:284–290, 1997

Celesia GG, Wanamaker WM: Psychiatric disturbances in Parkinson's disease. Diseases of the Nervous System 33:577–583, 1972

Cherington M: Parkinsonism, L-dopa, and mental depression. J Am Geriatr Soc 18:513–516, 1970

Choi DW: Glutamate neurotoxicity and diseases of the nervous system. Neuron 1:623–634, 1988

Chokroverty S, Bruetman ME, Berger V, et al: Progressive dialytic encephalopathy. J Neurol Neurosurg Psychiatry 39:411–419, 1976

Civil RH, Whitehouse PJ, Lanska DJ, et al: Degenerative dementias, in Dementia. Edited by Whitehouse PJ. Philadelphia, PA, FA Davis, 1993, pp 167–214

Clarfield AM: The reversible dementias: do they reverse? Ann Intern Med 109:476–486, 1988

Clarke R, Smith AD, Jobst KA, et al: Folate, vitamin B_{12}, and serum total homocysteine levels in confirmed Alzheimer disease. Arch Neurol 55:1449–1455, 1998

Clarnette RM, Patterson CJ: Hypothyroidism: does treatment cure dementia? J Geriatr Psychiatry Neurol 7:23–27, 1994

Coffey CE, Figiel GS, Djang WT, et al: Leukoencephalopathy in elderly depressed patients referred for ECT. Biol Psychiatry 24:143–161, 1988

Coffey CE, Weiner RD, Djang WT, et al: Brain anatomic effects of electroconvulsive therapy: a prospective magnetic resonance imaging study. Arch Gen Psychiatry 48:1013–1021, 1991

Cohen WJ, Cohen NH: Lithium carbonate, haloperidol, and irreversible brain damage. JAMA 230: 1283–1287, 1974

Collaborative Working Group on Clinical Trial Evaluations: Treatment of special populations with the atypical antipsychotics. J Clin Psychiatry 59 (suppl 12):46–52, 1998

Como PG, Rubin AJ, O'Brien CF, et al: A controlled trial of fluoxetine in nondepressed patients with Huntington's disease. Mov Disord 12:397–401, 1997

Court JA, Perry EK: Dementia: the neurochemical basis of putative transmitter oriented therapy. Pharmacol Ther 52:423–443, 1991

Cristomo EA, Duncan PW, Propst M, et al: Evidence that amphetamine with physical therapy promotes recovery of motor function in stroke patients. Ann Neurol 23:94–97, 1988

Crystal HA, Ortof E, Frishman WH, et al: Serum vitamin B12 levels and incidence of dementia in a healthy elderly population: a report from the Bronx Longitudinal Aging Study. J Am Geriatr Soc 42:933–936, 1994

Cummings JL: Depression and Parkinson's disease: a review. Am J Psychiatry 149:443–454, 1992a

Cummings JL: Neuropsychiatric aspects of Alzheimer's disease and other dementing illnesses, in The American Psychiatric Press Textbook of Neuropsychiatry, 2nd Edition. Edited by Yudofsky SC, Hales RE. Washington, DC, American Psychiatric Press, 1992b, pp 605–620

Cummings JL: Lewy body diseases with dementia: pathophysiology and treatment. Brain Cogn 28:266–280, 1995

Cummings JL, Benson DF: Dementia: A Clinical Approach, 2nd Edition. Boston, MA, Butterworth-Heinemann, 1992

Cummings JL, Darkins A, Mendez M, et al: Alzheimer's disease and Parkinson's disease: comparison of speech and language alterations. Neurology 38:680–684, 1988

Cunningham AL, Naif H, Saksena N, et al: HIV infection of macrophages and pathogenesis of AIDS dementia complex: interaction of the host cell and viral genotype. J Leukoc Biol 62:117–125, 1997

Curtis-Prior P, Vere D, Fray P: Therapeutic value of Ginkgo biloba in reducing symptoms of decline in mental function. J Pharm Pharmacol 51:535–541, 1999

Cutting J: The Right Cerebral Hemisphere and Psychiatric Disorders. Oxford, UK, Oxford University Press, 1990

Dal Canto MC: Mechanisms of HIV infection of the central nervous system and pathogenesis of AIDS-dementia complex. Neuroimaging Clin N Am 7:231–241, 1997

Damian MS, Schilling G, Bachmann G, et al: White matter lesions and cognitive deficits: relevance of lesion pattern? Acta Neurol Scand 90:430–436, 1994

Dana Consortium on the Therapy of HIV Dementia and Related Cognitive Disorders: A randomized, double-blind, placebo-controlled trial of deprenyl and thioctic acid in human immunodeficiency virus-associated cognitive impairment. Neurology 50:645–651, 1998

DeAngelis L, Delattre J-Y, Posner JB: Radiation-induced dementia in patients cured of brain metastases. Neurology 39:789–796, 1989

Denicoff KD, Joffe RT, Lakshmanan MC, et al: Neuropsychiatric manifestations of altered thyroid state. Am J Psychiatry 147:94–99, 1990

Dening TR, Berrios GE: Wilson's disease: psychiatric symptoms in 195 cases. Arch Gen Psychiatry 46: 1126–1134, 1989

Destee A, Gray F, Parent M, et al: Obsessive-compulsive behavior and progressive supranuclear palsy. Rev Neurol (Paris) 146:12–18, 1990

Devanand DP, Levy SR: Neuroleptic treatment of agitation and psychosis in dementia. J Geriatr Psychiatry Neurol 8 (suppl 1):S18–S27, 1995

De Vry J, Fritze J, Post RM: The management of coexisting depression in patients with dementia: potential of calcium channel antagonists. Clin Neuropharmacol 20:22–35, 1997

Dobyns WB, Goldstein NP, Gordon H: Clinical spectrum of Wilson's disease (hepatolenticular degeneration). Mayo Clin Proc 54:35–42, 1979

Dormehl IC, Jordaan B, Oliver DW, et al: SPECT monitoring of improved cerebral blood flow during long-term treatment of elderly patients with nootropic drugs. Clin Nucl Med 24:29–34, 1999

Dubovsky SL: Geriatric neuropsychopharmacology, in The American Psychiatric Press Textbook of Geriatric Neuropsychiatry. Edited by Coffey CE, Cummings JL. Washington, DC, American Psychiatric Press, 1994, pp 595–631

Dubovsky SL: Electroconvulsive therapy, in Comprehensive Textbook of Psychiatry/VI, 6th Edition. Edited by Kaplan HI, Sadock BJ. Baltimore, MD, Williams & Wilkins, 1995, pp 2129–2140

Dugbartey AT: Neurocognitive aspects of hypothyroidism. Arch Intern Med 158:1413–1418, 1998

Ebly EM, Schaefer JP, Campbell NR, et al: Folate status, vascular disease and cognition in elderly Canadians. Age Ageing 27:485–491, 1998

Engel PA: Treatment of progressive supranuclear palsy with amitriptyline: therapeutic and toxic effects. J Am Geriatr Soc 44:1072–1074, 1996

Extein IL, Gold MS: Thyroid hormone potentiation of tricyclics. Psychosomatics 29:166–174, 1988

Fazekas G, Fazekas F, Schmidt R, et al: Brain MRI findings and cognitive impairment in patients undergoing chronic hemodialysis treatment. J Neurol Sci 134(1–2):83–88, 1995

Fazekas G, Fazekas F, Schmidt R, et al: Pattern of cerebral blood flow and cognition in patients undergoing chronic haemodialysis treatment. Nucl Med Commun 17:603–608, 1996

Feeney DM, Gonzalez A, Law WA: Amphetamine, haloperidol, and experience interact to affect rate of recovery after motor cortex injury. Science 217:855–857, 1982

Feher EP, Inbody SB, Nolan B, et al: Other neurologic disease with dementia as a sequela. Clin Geriatr Med 4:799–814, 1988

Fehrenbach RA, Wallesch W, Claus D: Neuropsychologic findings in Friedreich's ataxia. Arch Neurol 41:306–308, 1984

Feldmann E, Plum F: Metabolic dementia, in Dementia. Edited by Whitehouse PJ. Philadelphia, PA, FA Davis, 1993, pp 307–336

Filip V, Kolibas E: Selegiline in the treatment of Alzheimer's disease: a long-term randomized placebo-controlled trial: Czech and Slovak Senile Dementia of Alzheimer Type Study Group. J Psychiatry Neurosci 24:234–243, 1999

Filley CM, Franklin GM, Heaton RK, et al: White matter dementia: clinical disorders and implications. Neuropsychiatry Neuropsychol Behav Neurol 1:239–254, 1989

Finali G, Piccirilli M, Oliani C, et al: L-Deprenyl therapy improves verbal memory in amnesic Alzheimer patients. Clin Neuropharmacol 14:523–536, 1991

Folstein SE: Huntington's Disease: A Disorder of Families. Baltimore, MD, Johns Hopkins University Press, 1989

Folstein SE, Folstein M: Diagnosis and treatment of Huntington's disease. Compr Ther 7:60–66, 1981

Folstein SE, Abbott MH, Chase GA, et al: The association of affective disorder with Huntington's disease in a case series and in families. Psychol Med 12:537–542, 1983

Ford MF: Treatment of depression in Huntington's disease with monoamine oxidase inhibitors. Br J Psychiatry 149:654–656, 1986

Francis DA: The current therapy of multiple sclerosis. J Clin Pharm Ther 18:77–84, 1993

Frank C: Dementia workup: deciding on laboratory testing for the elderly. Can Fam Physician 44:1489–1495, 1998

Freedman M, Rewilak D, Xerri T, et al: L-deprenyl in Alzheimer's disease: cognitive and behavioral effects. Neurology 50:660–668, 1998

Friedman G, Froom P, Sazbon L, et al: Apolipoprotein E-epsilon4 genotype predicts a poor outcome in survivors of traumatic brain injury. Neurology 52:244–248, 1999

Fritze J, Walden J: Clinical findings with nimodipine in dementia: test of the calcium hypothesis. J Neural Transm Suppl 46:439–453, 1995

Ganguli M, Burmeister LA, Seaberg EC, et al: Association between dementia and elevated TSH: a community-based study. Biol Psychiatry 40:714–725, 1996

Garthwaite J: Glutamate, nitric oxide and cell-cell signaling in the nervous system. Trends in Neurological Science 14:60–67, 1991

Gauthier S, Gauthier L, Bouchard R, et al: Treatment of Alzheimer's disease: hopes and reality. Can J Neurol Sci 18:394–397, 1991

Ghika J, Ghika-Schmid F, Fankhauser H, et al: Bilateral contemporaneous posteroventral pallidotomy for the treatment of Parkinson's disease: neuropsychological and neurological side effects: report of four cases and review of the literature. J Neurosurg 91:313–321, 1999

Giakas WJ, Seibyl JP, Mazure CM: Valproate in the treatment of temper outbursts (letter). J Clin Psychiatry 51:525, 1990

Gilman S, Bloedel JR, Lechtenberg R: Disorders of the Cerebellum. Philadelphia, PA, FA Davis, 1981

Ginn HE: Neurobehavioral dysfunction in uremia. Kidney Int 217 (suppl 2):S217–S221, 1975

Glass JD, Reich SG, DeLong MR: Wilson's disease: development of neurological disease after beginning penicillamine therapy. Arch Neurol 47:595–596, 1990

Goad DL, Davis CM, Liem P, et al: The use of selegiline in Alzheimer's patients with behavior problems. J Clin Psychiatry 52:342–345, 1991

Golbe LI, Davis PH, Schoenberg BS, et al: Prevalence and natural history of progressive supranuclear palsy. Neurology 38:1031–1034, 1988

Goldberg ID, Bloomer WD, Dawson DM: Nervous system toxic effects of cancer therapy. JAMA 247: 1437–1441, 1982

Goldman MB: Neuropsychiatric features of endocrine disorders, in The American Psychiatric Press Textbook of Neuropsychiatry, 2nd Edition. Edited by Yudofsky SC, Hales RE. Washington, DC, American Psychiatric Press, 1992, pp 519–540

Goldstein LB: Basic and clinical studies of pharmacologic effects on recovery from brain injury. J Neural Transplant Plast 4:175–192, 1995a

Goldstein LB: Prescribing of potentially harmful drugs to patients admitted to hospital after head injury. J Neurol Neurosurg Psychiatry 58:753–755, 1995b

Goldstein SE, Birnbom F: Piperacetazine versus thioridazine in the treatment of organic brain disease: a controlled double-blind study. J Am Geriatr Soc 24:355–359, 1976

Gottfries CG, Hess C: Pharmacotherapy in psychogeriatrics: an update, in Clinical and Scientific Psychogeriatrics, Vol 2: The Interface of Psychiatry and Neurology. Edited by Bergner M, Finkel SI. New York, Springer, 1990, pp 288–313

Grafman J, Litvan I, Stark M: Neuropsychological features of progressive supranuclear palsy. Brain Cogn 28:311–320, 1995

Greenwald BS, Marin DB, Silverman SM: Serotoninergic treatment of screaming and banging in dementia. Lancet 2:1464–1465, 1986

Greenwald BS, Kramer-Ginsberg E, Marin DB, et al: Dementia with coexistent major depression. Am J Psychiatry 146:1472–1478, 1989

Growdon JH: Biologic therapies for Alzheimer's disease, in Dementia. Edited by Whitehouse PJ. Philadelphia, PA, FA Davis, 1993, pp 375–399

Gualtieri CT, Evans RW: Stimulant treatment for the neurobehavioral sequelae of traumatic brain injury. Brain Inj 2:273–290, 1988

Gualtieri T, Chandler M, Coons TB, et al: Amantadine: a new clinical profile for traumatic brain injury. Clin Neuropharmacol 12:258–270, 1989

Gustafson L, Hagberg B: Recovery in hydrocephalic dementia after shunt operation. J Neurol Neurosurg Psychiatry 41:940–947, 1978

Guzzetta F, Mercuri E, Bonanno S, et al: Autosomal recessive congenital cerebellar atrophy: a clinical and neuropsychological study. Brain Dev 15:439–445, 1993

Halgin R, Riklan M, Misiak H: Levodopa, parkinsonism, and recent memory. J Nerv Ment Dis 164:268–272, 1977

Hall GR: Care of the patient with Alzheimer's disease living at home. Nurs Clin North Am 23:31–46, 1988

Hall WJ: Psychiatric problems in the elderly related to organic pulmonary disease, in Neuropsychiatric Manifestations of Physical Disease in the Elderly. Edited by Levinson AJ, Hall RCW. New York, Raven, 1981, pp 41–46

Halliday W: The nosology of Hallervorden-Spatz disease. J Neurol Sci 134 (suppl):84–91, 1995

Hamilton NG, Frick RB, Takahashi T, et al: Psychiatric symptoms and cerebellar pathology. Am J Psychiatry 140:1322–1326, 1983

Hanna SM: Hypopituitarism (Sheehan's syndrome) presenting with organic psychosis. J Neurol Neurosurg Psychiatry 33:192–193, 1970

Harding AE: Friedreich's ataxia: a clinical and genetic study of 90 families with an analysis of early diagnostic criteria and interfamilial clustering of clinical features. Brain 1041:589–620, 1981

Harper P: The natural history of Huntington's disease, in Huntington's Disease. Edited by Harper PS. Philadelphia, PA, WB Saunders, 1991, pp 127–139

Hart RP, Kwentus JA, Leshner RT, et al: Information processing speed in Friedreich's ataxia. Ann Neurol 17:612–614, 1985

Heath RG, Franklin DE, Shraberg D: Gross pathology of the cerebellum in patients diagnosed and treated as functional psychiatric disorders. J Nerv Ment Dis 167:585–592, 1979

Heinrichs RW: Relationship between neuropsychological data and response to behavioral treatment in a case of carbon monoxide poisoning. Brain Cogn 14:213–219, 1990

Hendrie HC: Epidemiology of Alzheimer's disease. Geriatrics 52 (suppl 2):S4–S8, 1997

Hendrie HC: Epidemiology of dementia and Alzheimer's disease. Am J Geriatr Psychiatry 6 (2 suppl 1): S3–S18, 1998

Herman BH: A possible role of proopiomelanocortin peptides in self-injurious behavior. Prog Neuropsychopharmacol Biol Psychiatry 14 (suppl):109–139, 1990

Herrmann N: Valproic acid treatment of agitation in dementia. Can J Psychiatry 43:69–72, 1998

Heston LL: Genetic studies of dementia: with emphasis on Parkinson's disease and Alzheimer's neuropathology, in The Epidemiology of Dementia. Edited by Mortimer JA, Schuman LM. New York, Oxford University Press, 1981, pp 101–114

Hill CD, Stoudemire A: Diagnostic and treatment implications of memory dysfunction in mood disorders, in American Psychiatric Press Review of Psychiatry, Vol 12. Edited by Oldham JM, Riba MB, Tasman A. Washington, DC, American Psychiatric Press, 1993, pp 783–804

Hoaglund HC, Goldstein NP: Hematologic (cytopenic) manifestations of Wilson's disease (hepatolenticular degeneration). Mayo Clin Proc 53:498–500, 1978

Hormes JT, Filley CM, Rosenberg NL: Neurologic sequelae of chronic solvent vapor abuse. Neurology 36:698–702, 1986

Hornbein TF, Townes BD, Schoene RB, et al: The cost to the central nervous system of climbing to extremely high altitude. N Engl J Med 321:1714–1719, 1989

Hua SE, Houk JC: Cerebellar guidance of premotor network development and sensorimotor learning. Learning and Memory 4(1):63–76, 1997

IFNB Multiple Sclerosis Study Group: Interferon beta-1b is effective in relapsing-remitting multiple sclerosis, I: clinical results of a multicenter, randomized, double-blind, placebo-controlled trial. Neurology 43:655–661, 1993

Izzo KL, Brody R: Rehabilitation in lithium toxicity. Arch Phys Med Rehabil 66:779–782, 1985

Jarvik LF: Calcium channel blocker nimodipine for primary degenerative dementia (letter). Biol Psychiatry 30:1171, 1991

Jimerson DC: Role of dopamine mechanisms in the affective disorders, in Psychopharmacology: The Third Generation of Progress. Edited by Meltzer HY. New York, Raven, 1987, pp 505–511

Joborn C, Hetta J, Frisk P, et al: Primary hyperparathyroidism in patients with organic brain syndrome. Acta Medica Scandinavica 219:91–98, 1986

Johnson KP, Brooks BR, Cohen JA, et al: Extended use of glatiramer acetate (Copaxone) is well tolerated and maintains its clinical effect on multiple sclerosis relapse rate and degree of disability: Copolymer 1 Multiple Sclerosis Study Group. Neurology 50:701–708, 1998

Johnstone PAS, Rundell JR, Esposito M: Mental status changes of Addison's disease. Psychosomatics 31:103–107, 1990

Jones KM, Stoukides CA: Clozapine in treatment of Parkinson's disease. Ann Pharmacother 26:1386–1387, 1992

Jones RW, Wesnes KA, Kirby J: Effects of NMDA modulation in scopolamine dementia. Ann N Y Acad Sci 640:241–244, 1991

Judd LL, Grant I: Intermediate duration organic mental disorder among polydrug abusing patients. Psychiatr Clin North Am 1:153–167, 1978

Kalayam B, Alexopoulos GS: Prefrontal dysfunction and treatment response in geriatric depression. Arch Gen Psychiatry 56:713–718, 1999

Katz IR: Diagnosis and treatment of depression in patients with Alzheimer's disease and other dementias. J Clin Psychiatry 59 (suppl 9):38–44, 1998

Kellner CH, Bernstein HJ: ECT as a treatment for neurologic illness, in The Clinical Science of Electroconvulsive Therapy. Edited by Coffey CE. Washington, DC, American Psychiatric Press, 1993, pp 183–210

Kertesz A, Davidson W, Munoz DG: Clinical and pathological overlap between frontotemporal dementia, primary progressive aphasia and corticobasal degeneration: the Pick complex. Dement Geriatr Cogn Disord 10 (suppl 1):46–49, 1999

Kessler H: Epidemiological studies of Parkinson's disease, III: a community based study. Am J Epidemiol 96:242–254, 1972

Kieburtz K, Feigin A, McDermott M, et al: A controlled trial of remacemide hydrochloride in Huntington's disease. Mov Disord 11:273–277, 1996

Kimmel PL, Thamer M, Richard CM, et al: Psychiatric illness in patients with end-stage renal disease. Am J Med 105:214–221, 1998

Kishnani PS, Sullivan JA, Walter BK, et al: Cholinergic therapy for Down's syndrome (letter). Lancet 353(9158):1064–1065, 1999

Knoll J: L-Deprenyl-medication: a strategy to modulate the age-related decline of the striatal dopaminergic system. J Am Geriatr Soc 40:839–847, 1992

Kraus JF, Sorenson SB: Epidemiology, in The Neuropsychiatry of Traumatic Brain Injury. Edited by Silver JM, Yudofsky SC, Hales RE. Washington, DC, American Psychiatric Press, 1994, pp 3–41

Kraus MF, Maki PM: Effect of amantadine hydrochloride on symptoms of frontal lobe dysfunction in brain injury: case studies and review. J Neuropsychiatry Clin Neurosci 9:222–230, 1997

Krop HD, Block AJ, Cohen E: Neuropsychologic effects of continuous oxygen therapy in chronic obstructive pulmonary disease. Chest 64:317–322, 1973

Kyomen HH, Nobel KW, Wei JY: The use of estrogen to decrease aggressive physical behavior in elderly men with dementia. J Am Geriatr Soc 39:1110–1112, 1991

Lal S, Merbtiz CP, Grip JC: Modification of function in head-injured patients with Sinemet. Brain Inj 2:225–233, 1988

Lange KW, Sahakian BJ, Quinn NP, et al: Comparison of executive and visuospatial memory function in Huntington's disease and dementia of Alzheimer type matched for degree of dementia. J Neurol Neurosurg Psychiatry 58:598–606, 1995

Lanska DJ, Schoenberg BS: The epidemiology of dementia: methodologic issues and approaches, in Dementia. Edited by Whitehouse PJ. Philadelphia, PA, FA Davis, 1993, pp 3–33

Larsson A, Arlig A, Bergh AC, et al: Quantitative SPECT cisternography in normal pressure hydrocephalus. Acta Neurol Scand 90:190–196, 1994

Lauterbach EC, Spears TE, Prewett MJ, et al: Neuropsychiatric disorders, myoclonus, and dystonia in calcification of basal ganglia pathways. Biol Psychiatry 35:345–351, 1994

Lauterbach EC, Cummings JL, Duffy J, et al: Neuropsychiatric correlates and treatment of lenticulostriatal diseases: a review of the literature and overview of research opportunities in Huntington's, Wilson's, and Fahr's diseases: a report of the ANPA Committee on Research: American Neuropsychiatric Association. J Neuropsychiatry Clin Neurosci 10:249–266, 1998

Lawlor BA, Aisen PS, Green C, et al: Selegiline in the treatment of behavioural disturbance in Alzheimer's disease. Int J Geriatr Psychiatry 12:319–322, 1997

Lederman RJ, Henry CE: Progressive dialysis encephalopathy. Ann Neurol 4:199–204, 1978

Lees AJ: Selegiline hydrochloride and cognition. Acta Neurol Scand Suppl 136:91–94, 1991

Lemke MR: Effect of carbamazepine on agitation in Alzheimer's inpatients refractory to neuroleptics. J Clin Psychiatry 56:354–357, 1995

Leonard DP, Kidson MA, Shannon PJ, et al: Double-blind trial of lithium carbonate and haloperidol in Huntington's chorea. Lancet 2:1208–1209, 1974

Leroi I, Michalon M: Treatment of the psychiatric manifestations of Huntington's disease: a review of the literature. Can J Psychiatry 43:933–940, 1998

Lesnik PG, Ciesielski KT, Hart BL, et al: Evidence for cerebellar-frontal subsystem changes in children treated with intrathecal chemotherapy for leukemia: enhanced data analysis using an effect size model. Arch Neurol 55:1561–1568, 1998

Levine AM: Buspirone and agitation in head injury. Brain Inj 2:165–167, 1988

Lieberman A: Managing the neuropsychiatric symptoms of Parkinson's disease. Neurology 50 (suppl 6): S33–S38, 1998

Lindenbaum J, Healton EB, Savage DG, et al: Neuropsychiatric disorders caused by cobalamin deficiency in the absence of anemia or macrocytosis. N Engl J Med 318:1720–1728, 1988

Little A, Levy R, Chuaqui-Kidd P, et al: A double-blind, placebo controlled trial of high-dose lecithin in Alzheimer's disease. J Neurol Neurosurg Psychiatry 48:736–742, 1985

Litvan I, Hutton M: Clinical and genetic aspects of progressive supranuclear palsy. J Geriatr Psychiatry Neurol 11:107–114, 1998

Litvan I, Campbell G, Mangone CA, et al: Which clinical features differentiate progressive supranuclear palsy (Steele-Richardson-Olszewski syndrome) from related disorders? A clinicopathological study. Brain 120 (Pt 1):65–74, 1997

Lohr JB, Jeste DV, Harris MJ, et al: Treatment of disordered behavior, in Clinical Geriatric Psychopharmacology, 2nd Edition. Edited by Salzman C. Baltimore, MD, Williams & Wilkins, 1992, pp 80–113

Lopez-Lozano JJ, Bravo G, Brera B, et al: Long-term improvement in patients with severe Parkinson's disease after implantation of fetal ventral mesencephalic tissue in a cavity of the caudate nucleus: 5-year follow up in 10 patients: Clinica Puerta de Hierro Neural Transplantation Group. J Neurosurg 86:931–942, 1997

Mach JR, Korchik WP, Mahowald MW: Dialysis dementia. Clin Geriatr Med 4:858–867, 1988

Malaguarnera M, Pistone G, Vinci M, et al: Tacrine treatment of Alzheimer's disease: many expectations, few certainties. Neuropsychobiology 38:226–231, 1998

Mallette LE, Eichhorn E: Effects of lithium carbonate on human calcium metabolism. Arch Intern Med 146:770–776, 1986

Mally J, Stone TW: Improvement in Parkinsonian symptoms after repetitive transcranial magnetic stimulation. J Neurol Sci 162:179–184, 1999

Mancardi GL, Sardanelli F, Parodi RC, et al: Effect of copolymer-1 on serial gadolinium-enhanced MRI in relapsing remitting multiple sclerosis. Neurology 50:1127–1133, 1998

Mann JJ, Aarons SF, Wilner PJ, et al: A controlled study of the antidepressant efficacy and side effects of L-deprenyl: a selective monoamine oxidase inhibitor. Arch Gen Psychiatry 46:45–50, 1989

Manto M, Badot V, Koulischer C: Reversible dementia and polyneuritis in an elderly woman: a case of late-onset disseminated lupus erythematosus. Acta Neurol Belg 93:139–145, 1993

Manyam BV: Friedreich's disease, in Handbook of Cerebellar Diseases. Edited by Lechtenberg R. New York, Marcel Dekker, 1993, pp 431–452

Marsh GG, Markham CH: Does levodopa alter depression and psychopathology in parkinsonism patients? J Neurol Neurosurg Psychiatry 36:925–935, 1973

Martin DC: B_{12} and folate deficiency dementia. Clin Geriatr Med 4:841–852, 1988

Martin FI, Deam DR: Hyperthyroidism in elderly hospitalised patients: clinical features and treatment outcomes. Med J Aust 164:200–203, 1996

Martin JB, Reichlin S: Clinical Neuroendocrinology, 2nd Edition. Philadelphia, PA, FA Davis, 1987

Martin PR, Welch LW: Psychopharmacologic treatment of memory disorders, in American Psychiatric Press Review of Psychiatry, Vol 12. Edited by Oldham JM, Riba MB, Tasman A. Washington, DC, American Psychiatric Press, 1993, pp 805–830

Maxwell CJ, Hogan DB, Ebly EM: Calcium-channel blockers and cognitive function in elderly people: results from the Canadian Study of Health and Aging. CMAJ 161:501–506, 1999

Mayeux R, Stern Y, Rosen J, et al: Depression, intellectual impairment, and Parkinson's disease. Neurology 31:645–650, 1981

Mayeux R, Foster NL, Rossor M, et al: The clinical evaluation of patients with dementia, in Dementia. Edited by Whitehouse PJ. Philadelphia, PA, FA Davis, 1993, pp 92–129

Mayeux R, Ottman R, Maestre G, et al: Synergistic effects of traumatic head injury and apolipoprotein-epsilon 4 in patients with Alzheimer's disease. Neurology 45 (3 pt 1):555–557, 1995

McArthur JC, Roos RP, Johnson RT: Viral dementias, in Dementia. Edited by Whitehouse PJ. Philadelphia, PA, FA Davis, 1993, pp 237–275

Mendez MF: Miscellaneous causes of dementia, in Dementia. Edited by Whitehouse PJ. Philadelphia, PA, FA Davis, 1993, pp 337–358

Menza MA, Cocchiola J, Golbe LI: Psychiatric symptoms in progressive supranuclear palsy. Psychosomatics 36:550–554, 1995

Mesulam M-M: Slowly progressive aphasia without generalized dementia. Ann Neurol 11:592–598, 1982

Miguel EC, Pereira RM, Pereira CA, et al: Psychiatric manifestations of systemic lupus erythematosus: clinical features, symptoms, and signs of central nervous system activity in 43 patients. Medicine 73:224–232, 1994

Mikkelsen EJ, Reider AA: Post-parathyroidectomy psychosis: clinical and research implications. J Clin Psychiatry 40:352–358, 1979

Milne FJ, Sharf B, Bell P, et al: The effect of low aluminum water and desferrioxamine on the outcome of dialysis encephalopathy. Clin Nephrol 20:202–207, 1983

Mindham RHS, Marsden CD, Parkes JD: Psychiatric symptoms during L-dopa therapy for Parkinson's disease and their relationship to physical disability. Psychol Med 6:23–33, 1976

Mitchell AJ, Dening TR: Depression-related cognitive impairment: possibilities for its pharmacological treatment. J Affect Disord 36(3–4):79–87, 1996

Moellentine C, Rummans T, Ahlskog JE, et al: Effectiveness of ECT in patients with parkinsonism. J Neuropsychiatry Clin Neurosci 10:187–193, 1998

Mölsä PK, Paljärvi L, Rinne JO, et al: Validity of clinical diagnosis in dementia: a prospective clinicopathological study. J Neurol Neurosurg Psychiatry 48:1085–1090, 1985

Mooney GF, Haas LJ: Effect of methylphenidate on brain injury-related anger. Arch Phys Med Rehabil 74:153–160, 1993

Morris M, Tyler A: Management and therapy, in Huntington's Disease. Edited by Harper PS. Philadelphia, PA, WB Saunders, 1991, pp 205–250

Muller D, Pilz H, TerMeulen V: Studies on adult metachromatic leukodystrophy, I: clinical, morphological, and histochemical observations in two cases. J Neurol Sci 9:567–584, 1969

Mulrow CD, Feussner JR, Williams BC, et al: The value of clinical findings in the detection of normal pressure hydrocephalus. J Gerontol 42:277–279, 1987

Musser WS, Akil M: Clozapine as a treatment for psychosis in Parkinson's disease: a review. J Neuropsychiatry Clin Neurosci 8:1–9, 1996

Nagga AK, Marcusson J: Associated physical disease in a demented population. Aging 10:440–444, 1998

National Institutes of Health: Consensus Conference on Differential Diagnosis of Dementing Diseases. JAMA 258:3411–3416, 1985

Navia BA, Jordan BD, Price RW: The AIDS dementia complex, I: clinical features. Ann Neurol 19:517–524, 1986

Neary D: Overview of frontotemporal dementias and the consensus applied. Dement Geriatr Cogn Disord 10 (suppl 1):6–9, 1999

Newman GC: Treatment of progressive supranuclear palsy with tricyclic antidepressants. Neurology 35:1189–1193, 1985

Nicoll JA, Roberts GW, Graham DI: Apolipoprotein E ε4 allele is associated with deposition of amyloid β-protein following head injury. Nat Med 1:135–137, 1995

Ohrvall U, Akerstrom G, Ljunghall S, et al: Surgery for sporadic primary hyperparathyroidism in the elderly. World J Surg 18:612–618, 1994

Oken BS, Storzbach DM, Kaye JA: The efficacy of Ginkgo biloba on cognitive function in Alzheimer disease. Arch Neurol 55:1409–1415, 1998

Pallis CA, Lewis PD: The Neurology of Gastrointestinal Disease. Philadelphia, PA, WB Saunders, 1974

Parkinson J: An Essay on the Shaking Palsy. London, UK, Sherwood, Neely, & Jones, 1817

Parkinson Study Group: Effect of L-deprenyl in the progression of disability in early Parkinson's disease. N Engl J Med 321:1364–1371, 1989

Patterson CJ, Gauthier S, Bergman H, et al: Canadian Consensus Conference on Dementia: a physician's guide to using the recommendations. CMAJ 160:1738–1742, 1999

Patti F, Di Stefano M, De Pascalis D, et al: May there exist specific MRI findings predictive of dementia in multiple sclerosis patients? Funct Neurol 10:83–90, 1995

Paty DW, Li DK: Interferon beta-1b is effective in relapsing-remitting multiple sclerosis, II: MRI analysis results of a multicenter, randomized, double-blind, placebo-controlled trial. Neurology 43:662–667, 1993

Peyser JM, Edwards KR, Poser CM, et al: Cognitive deficits in patients with multiple sclerosis. Arch Neurol 37:577–579, 1980

Pick A: On the relation between aphasia and senile atrophy of the brain (1892), in Neurological Classics in Modern Translation. Translated by Schoene WC. Edited by Rottenberg DA, Hochberg FH. New York, Hafner, 1977, pp 35–40

Plenger PM, Dixon CE, Castillo RM, et al: Subacute methylphenidate treatment for moderate to moderately severe traumatic brain injury: a preliminary double-blind placebo-controlled study. Arch Phys Med Rehabil 77:536–540, 1996

Pollock M, Hornabrook RW: The prevalence, natural history, and dementia of Parkinson's disease. Brain 89:429–448, 1966

Powell JH, al-Adawi S, Morgan J, et al: Motivational deficits after brain injury: effects of bromocriptine in 11 patients. J Neurol Neurosurg Psychiatry 60:416–421, 1996

Price TRP, Tucker GJ: Psychiatric and behavioral manifestations of normal pressure hydrocephalus. J Nerv Ment Dis 164:51–55, 1977

Proctor R, Burns A, Powell HS, et al: Behavioural management in nursing and residential homes: a randomised controlled trial. Lancet 354(9172):26–29, 1999

Qizilbash N, Whitehead A, Higgins J, et al: Cholinesterase inhibition for Alzheimer disease: a meta-analysis of the tacrine trials. Dementia Trialists' Collaboration. JAMA 280:1777–1782, 1998

Raber J: Detrimental effects of chronic hypothalamic-pituitary-adrenal axis activation: from obesity to memory deficits. Mol Neurobiol 18:1–22, 1998

Rabheru K, Persad E: A review of continuation and maintenance electroconvulsive therapy. Can J Psychiatry 42:476–484, 1997

Randolph C, Tierney MC, Mohr E, et al: The Repeatable Battery for the Assessment of Neuropsychological Status (RBANS): preliminary clinical validity. J Clin Exp Neuropsychol 20:310–319, 1998

Rao SM: Neuropsychology of multiple sclerosis: a critical review. J Clin Exp Neuropsychol 8:503–542, 1986

Rao SM: White matter disease and dementia. Brain Cogn 31:250–268, 1996

Rao SM, Leo GJ, Bernandin L, et al: Cognitive dysfunction in multiple sclerosis, I: frequency, patterns, and prediction. Neurology 41:685–691, 1991

Raskin NH, Fishman RA: Neurologic disorders in renal failure. N Engl J Med 294:143–148, 204–210, 1976

Regard M, Oelz O, Brugger P, et al: Persistent cognitive impairment in climbers after repeated exposure to extreme altitude. Neurology 39:210–213, 1989

Reifler BV, Larson E, Teri L, et al: Dementia of the Alzheimer's type and depression. J Am Geriatr Soc 34:855–859, 1986

Reus VI: Psychiatric aspects of thyroid disease, in The Thyroid Axis and Psychiatric Illness. Edited by Joffe RT, Levitt AJ. Washington, DC, American Psychiatric Press, 1993, pp 171–194

Rich SS, Ovsiew F: Leuprolide acetate for exhibitionism in Huntington's disease. Mov Disord 9:353–357, 1994

Riley T: Neurological aspects of sleep, in Neurology and General Medicine. Edited by Aminoff MJ. New York, Churchill Livingstone, 1989, pp 431–447

Risse SC, Barnes R: Pharmacologic treatment of agitation associated with dementia. J Am Geriatr Soc 34:368–376, 1986

Rizzo WB, Leshner RT, Odone A, et al: Dietary erucic therapy for X-linked adrenoleukodystrophy. Neurology 39:1415–1422, 1989

Rogers SL, Farlow MR, Doody RS, et al: A 24-week, double-blind, placebo-controlled trial of donepezil in patients with Alzheimer's disease: Donepezil Study Group. Neurology 50:136–145, 1998

Rojo A, Pernaute RS, Fontan A, et al: Clinical genetics of familial progressive supranuclear palsy. Brain 122 (pt 7):1233–1245, 1999

Romine JS, Sipe JC, Koziol JA, et al: A double-blind, placebo-controlled, randomized trial of cladribine in relapsing-remitting multiple sclerosis. Proc Assoc Am Physicians 111:35–44, 1999

Rosenthal M, Gil I, Habot B: Primary hyperparathyroidism: neuropsychiatric manifestations and case report. Isr J Psychiatry Relat Sci 34:122–125, 1997

Ross CA: Alzheimer's disease and other neuropsychiatric disorders. Current Opinion in Psychiatry 5: 561–566, 1992

Roth M: The psychiatric disorders of later life. Psychiatric Annals 6:417–445, 1976

Routy JP, Allegre T, Toma E, et al: Intrathecal (IT) zidovudine for AIDS dementia complex (ADC). Ninth International Conference on AIDS 9:61 (Abstract No WS-B18-6), June 1993

Sahadevan S, Pang WS, Tan NJ, et al: Neuroimaging guidelines in cognitive impairment: lessons from 3 cases of meningiomas presenting as isolated dementia. Singapore Med J 38:339–343, 1997

Saida K, Zhigang Z, Ozawa K, et al: Long-term open-trial of mizoribine with prednisolone in 24 patients with multiple sclerosis: safety, clinical and magnetic resonance imaging outcome. Intern Med 38:636–642, 1999

Salmon E, Van der Linden MV, Franck G: Anterior cingulate and motor network metabolic impairment in progressive supranuclear palsy. Neuroimage 5:173–178, 1997

Salzman C: Principles of psychopharmacology, in Verwoerdt's Clinical Geropsychiatry, 3rd Edition. Edited by Bienenfeld D. Baltimore, MD, Williams & Wilkins, 1990, pp 234–249

Sano M, Marder K, Dooneief G: Basal ganglia diseases, in Neuropsychiatry. Edited by Fogel BS, Schiffer RB, Rao SM. Baltimore, MD, Williams & Wilkins, 1996, pp 805–826

Sano M, Ernesto C, Thomas RG, et al: A controlled trial of selegiline, alpha-tocopherol, or both as treatment for Alzheimer's disease. The Alzheimer's Disease Cooperative Study. N Engl J Med 336: 1216–1222, 1997

Saracaceanu E, Tramoni AV, Henry JM: An association between subcortical dementia and pernicious anemia—a psychiatric mask. Compr Psychiatry 38:349–351, 1997

Schelhaas HJ, Hageman G, Post JG: Cerebellar ataxia, dementia, pyramidal signs, cortical cataract of the posterior pole and a raised IgG index in a patient with a sporadic form of olivopontocerebellar atrophy. Clin Neurol Neurosurg 99:99–101, 1997

Schneider EL, Guralnik JM: The aging of America: impact on health care costs. JAMA 263:2335–2340, 1990

Schneider LS, Sobin PB: Non-neuroleptic treatment of behavioral symptoms and agitation in Alzheimer's disease and other dementia. Psychopharmacol Bull 28:71–79, 1992

Schneider LS, Gleason RP, Chui HC: Progressive supranuclear palsy with agitation: response to trazodone but not to thiothixine or carbamazepine. J Geriatr Psychiatry Neurol 2:109–112, 1989

Schor JD, Levkoff SE, Lipsitz LA, et al: Risk factors for delirium in hospitalized elderly. JAMA 267:827–831, 1992

Scott JN, Rewcastle NB, Brasher PM, et al: Long-term glioblastoma multiforme survivors: a population-based study. Can J Neurol Sci 25:197–201, 1998

Shankle WR, Nielson KA, Cotman CW: Low-dose propranolol reduces aggression and agitation resembling that associated with orbitofrontal dysfunction in elderly demented patients. Alzheimer Dis Assoc Disord 9:233–237, 1995

Shaw PJ: Excitatory amino acid receptors, excitotoxicity, and the human nervous system. Curr Opin Neurol Neurosurg 6:414–422, 1993

Shelton PS, Brooks VG: Estrogen for dementia-related aggression in elderly men. Ann Pharmacother 33(7–8):808–812, 1999

Sidtis JJ, Gatsonis C, Price RW, et al: Zidovudine treatment of the AIDS dementia complex: results of a placebo-controlled trial. Ann Neurol 33:343–349, 1993

Silver JM, Yudofsky SC: Propranolol for aggression: literature review and clinical guidelines. International Drug Therapy Newsletter 20:9–12, 1985

Silver JM, Yudofsky SC: Psychopharmacology and electroconvulsive therapy, in The American Psychiatric Press Textbook of Psychiatry. Edited by Talbott JA, Hales RE, Yudofsky SC. Washington, DC, American Psychiatric Press, 1988, pp 767–853

Silver JM, Yudofsky SC: Psychopharmacology, in Neuropsychiatry of Traumatic Brain Injury. Edited by Silver JM, Yudofsky SC, Hales RE. Washington, DC, American Psychiatric Press, 1994, pp 631–670

Silver JM, Hales RE, Yudofsky SC: Neuropsychiatric aspects of traumatic brain injury, in The American Psychiatric Press Textbook of Neuropsychiatry, 2nd Edition. Edited by Yudofsky SC, Hales RE. Washington, DC, American Psychiatric Press, 1992, pp 363–395

Slyter H: Idiopathic hypoparathyroidism presenting as dementia. Neurology 29:393–394, 1979

Small GW: Tacrine for treating Alzheimer's disease. JAMA 268:2564–2565, 1992

Smith GR, Taylor CW, Linkous P: Haloperidol versus thioridazine for the treatment of psychogeriatric patients: a double-blind clinical trial. Psychosomatics 15:134–138, 1974

Snider WD, DeMaria AA, Mann JD: Diazepam and dialysis encephalopathy. Neurology 29:414–415, 1980

So NK, O'Neill BP, Frytak S, et al: Delayed leukoencephalopathy in survivors with small cell lung cancer. Neurology 37:1198–1201, 1987

Starkman MN, Schteingart DE: Neuropsychiatric manifestations of patients with Cushing's syndrome. Arch Intern Med 141:215–219, 1981

Starkman MN, Schteingart DE, Schork MA: Correlation of bedside cognitive and neuropsychological tests in patients with Cushing's syndrome. Psychosomatics 27:508–511, 1986

Starosta-Rubinstein S, Young AB, Kluin K, et al: Clinical assessment of 31 patients with Wilson's disease: correlations with structural changes on magnetic resonance imaging. Arch Neurol 44:365–370, 1987

Steele JC, Richardson JC, Olszewski J: Progressive supranuclear palsy. Arch Neurol 10:333–359, 1964

St.-Laurent M: Normal pressure hydrocephalus in geriatric medicine: a challenge. J Geriatr Psychiatry Neurol 1:163–168, 1988

Stoudemire A, Hill CD, Morris R, et al: Improvement in depression-related cognitive dysfunction following ECT. J Neuropsychiatry Clin Neurosci 7:31–34, 1995

Stuerenburg HJ, Hansen HC, Thie A, et al: Reversible dementia in idiopathic hypoparathyroidism associated with normocalcemia. Neurology 47:474–476, 1996

Stuss DT, Peterkin I, Guzman DA, et al: Chronic obstructive pulmonary disease: effects of hypoxia on neurological and neuropsychological measures. J Clin Exp Neuropsychol 19:515–524, 1997

Sultzer DL, Gray KF, Gunay I, et al: A double-blind comparison of trazodone and haloperidol for treatment of agitation in patients with dementia. Am J Geriatr Psychiatry 5:60–69, 1997

Tagliati M, Simpson D, Morgello S, et al: Cerebellar degeneration associated with human immunodeficiency virus infection. Neurology 50:244–251, 1998

Tan SV, Guiloff RJ: Hypothesis on the pathogenesis of vacuolar myelopathy, dementia, and peripheral neuropathy in AIDS. J Neurol Neurosurg Psychiatry 65:23–28, 1998

Tariot PN: Neurobiology and treatment of dementia, in Clinical Geriatric Psychopharmacology, 2nd Edition. Edited by Salzman C. Baltimore, MD, Williams & Wilkins, 1992, pp 277–299

Tariot PN: Treatment of agitation in dementia. J Clin Psychiatry 60 (suppl 8):11–20, 1999

Tariot PN, Cohen RM, Sunderland T, et al: L-Deprenyl in Alzheimer's disease: preliminary evidence for behavioral change with monoamine oxidase B inhibition. Arch Gen Psychiatry 44:427–433, 1987

Tariot PN, Goldstein B, Podgorski CA, et al: Short-term administration of selegiline for mild-to-moderate dementia of the Alzheimer's type. Am J Geriatr Psychiatry 6:145–154, 1998

Taverni JP, Seliger G, Lichtman SW: Donepezil mediated memory improvement in traumatic brain injury during post acute rehabilitation. Brain Inj 12:77–80, 1998

Tennant FS Jr, Wild J: Naltrexone treatment for postconcussional syndrome. Am J Psychiatry 144:813–814, 1987

Teri L, Logsdon RG, Uomoto J, et al: Behavioral treatment of depression in dementia patients: a controlled clinical trial. J Gerontol B Psychol Sci Soc Sci 52:P159–P166, 1997

Tetrud JW, Langston JW: The effect of L-deprenyl (selegiline) on the natural history of Parkinson's disease. Science 245:519–522, 1989

Teunisse S, Bollen AE, van Gool WA, et al: Dementia and subnormal levels of vitamin B_{12}: effects of replacement therapy on dementia. J Neurol 243:522–529, 1996

Tollefson GD: Short-term effects of the calcium channel blocker nimodipine (Bay-e-9736) in the management of primary degenerative dementia. Biol Psychiatry 27:1133–1142, 1990

Tom MI, Richardson JC: Hypoglycemia from islet cell tumor of pancreas with amyotrophy and cerebrospinal nerve cell changes. J Neuropathol Exp Neurol 10:57–66, 1951

Trauner DA, Clayman M: Dialysis encephalopathy treated with clonazepam. Ann Neurol 6:555–556, 1979

Troster AI, Fields JA, Testa JA, et al: Cortical and subcortical influences on clustering and switching in the performance of verbal fluency tasks. Neuropsychologia 36:295–304, 1998

Tselis AC, Lisak RP: Multiple sclerosis: therapeutic update. Arch Neurol 56:277–280, 1999

Tsolaki M, Drevelegas A, Karachristianou S, et al: Correlation of dementia, neuropsychological and MRI findings in multiple sclerosis. Dementia 5:48–52, 1994

Tune LE: Depression and Alzheimer's disease. Depress Anxiety 8 (suppl 1):91–95, 1998

Tyor WR, Wesselingh SL, Griffin JW, et al: Unifying hypothesis for the pathogenesis of HIV-associated dementia complex, vacuolar myelopathy, and sensory neuropathy. Journal of Acquired Immune Deficiency Syndromes 9:379–388, 1995

U.S. Department of Health and Human Services: Interagency Head Injury Task Force Report. Washington, DC, U.S. Government Printing Office, 1989

U.S. Food and Drug Administration: First Alzheimer's drug. FDA Medical Bulletin 23(3):5–6, 1993

Valldeoriola F, Nobbe FA, Tolosa E: Treatment of behavioural disturbances in Parkinson's disease. J Neural Transm Suppl 51:175–204, 1997

Vanneste J, Augustijn P, Dirven C, et al: Shunting normal-pressure hydrocephalus: do the benefits outweigh the risks? A multicenter study and literature review. Neurology 42:54–59, 1992

Velasco J, Head M, Farlin E, et al: Unsuspected subdural hematoma as a differential diagnosis in elderly patients. South Med J 88:977–979, 1995

Vigliani MC, Duyckaerts C, Hauw JJ, et al: Dementia following treatment of brain tumors with radiotherapy administered alone or in combination with nitrosourea-based chemotherapy: a clinical and pathological study. J Neurooncol 41:137–149, 1999

Vincent VA, De Groot CJ, Lucassen PJ, et al: Nitric oxide synthase expression and apoptotic cell death in brains of AIDS and AIDS dementia patients. AIDS 13:317–326, 1999

Waltz G, Harik SI, Kaufman B: Adult metachromatic leukodystrophy: value of computed tomographic scanning and magnetic resonance imaging of the brain. Arch Neurol 44:225–227, 1987

Weinstein A, Schwid SI, Schiffer RB, et al: Neuropsychologic status in multiple sclerosis after treatment with glatiramer. Arch Neurol 56:319–324, 1999

Wengel SP, Roccaforte WH, Burke WJ: Donepezil improves symptoms of delirium in dementia: implications for future research. J Geriatr Psychiatry Neurol 11:159–161, 1998

Whitehouse PJ, Friedland RP, Strauss ME: Neuropsychiatric aspects of degenerative dementias associated with motor dysfunction, in The American Psychiatric Press Textbook of Neuropsychiatry, 2nd Edition. Edited by Yudofsky SC, Hales RE. Washington, DC, American Psychiatric Press, 1992, pp 585–604

Wilhelmsen KC, Clark LN, Miller BL, et al: Tau mutations in frontotemporal dementia. Dement Geriatr Cogn Disord 10 (suppl 1):88–92, 1999

Wilson SAK: Progressive lenticular degeneration: a familial nervous disease associated with cirrhosis of the liver. Brain 34:295–299, 1912

Workman RH Jr, Orengo CA, Bakey AA, et al: The use of risperidone for psychosis and agitation in demented patients with Parkinson's disease. J Neuropsychiatry Clin Neurosci 9:594–597, 1997

Wragg RE, Jeste DV: Neuroleptics and alternative treatments: management of behavioral symptoms and psychosis in Alzheimer's disease and related conditions. Psychiatr Clin North Am 11:195–213, 1988

Wright CI, Geula C, Mesulam M-M: Protease inhibitors and indoleamines selectively inhibit cholinesterases in the histopathologic structures of Alzheimer disease. Proc Natl Acad Sci U S A 90:683–686, 1993

Young RC, Meyers BS: Psychopharmacology, in Comprehensive Review of Geriatric Psychiatry. Edited by Sadavoy J, Lazarus LW, Jarvik LF. Washington, DC, American Psychiatric Press, 1991, pp 435–467

Yousef G, Ryan WJ, Lambert T, et al: A preliminary report: a new scale to identify the pseudodementia syndrome. Int J Geriatr Psychiatry 13:389–399, 1998

Yudofsky SC, Silver JM, Schneider SE: Pharmacologic treatment of aggression. Psychiatric Annals 17: 397–404, 406–407, 1987

Zakzanis KK: The subcortical dementia of Huntington's disease. J Clin Exp Neuropsychol 20:565–578, 1998

Zapotoczky HG: Problems of differential diagnosis between depressive pseudodementia and Alzheimer's disease. J Neural Transm Suppl 53:91–95, 1998

Zucker DK, Livingston RL, Nakra R, et al: B_{12} deficiency and psychiatric disorders: case report and literature review. Biol Psychiatry 16:197–205, 1981

23

Substance-Induced Persisting Dementia and Substance-Induced Persisting Amnestic Disorder

Edward V. Nunes, M.D.
Michael Y. Hwang, M.D.
Pantelis G. Lazaridis, M.D.

Dementia is a broadly defined clinical syndrome characterized by general deterioration of intellectual abilities accompanied by behavioral changes. A growing geriatric population and the widespread use of both licit and illicit drugs, as well as increasing environmental exposure to neurotoxic chemicals, have contributed to a rising prevalence of substance-induced persisting dementia (SIPD) and substance-induced persisting amnestic disorder (SIPAD). In SIPD, unlike in substance-induced delirium, in which acute disturbance of mental status is caused by overwhelming exposure to a neurotoxic chemical, a gradual and prolonged exposure can cause more insidious cognitive dysfunction with progressive development of the dementia. In addition, neurotoxic agents may further exacerbate symptoms in patients with other forms of dementia. SIPD and SIPAD may mimic various functional psychiatric disorders with diverse clinical manifestations, thus challenging clinicians in terms of diagnosis and treatment. Yet, these disorders are among the few dementia syndromes in which early assessment and treatment can prevent further deterioration and even bring about improvements in intellectual and functional abilities. Because of the wide overlap in diagnosis and treatment of SIPD and SIPAD, we review these disorders here in a single chapter.

Definition and Diagnostic Criteria

SIPD refers to a clinical syndrome manifested by prominent impairments in neurocognitive processes including memory and other intellectual abilities as a result of exposure to a neurotoxic substance. The hallmark of *SIPAD* is impairment of both short- and long-term memory without immediate memory or the ability to repeat items being significantly affected. In SIPAD, in contrast to SIPD, the impairment is confined to memory function, with other cognitive abilities (e.g., judgment, abstraction, language, executive functioning) being spared. For the diagnosis of both SIPD and SIPAD, several criteria must be present: 1) onset of the symptoms temporally related to persistent exposure to medication, drugs of abuse, or neurotoxic chemicals; 2) memory loss and/or loss of other intellectual ability; 3) deterioration in cognitive ability resulting in impairment of social or occupational activities and representing decline from a previous level of functioning; and 4) absence of delirium. The DSM-IV (American Psychiatric Association 1994) diagnostic criteria for SIPD and SIPAD are presented in Tables 23–1 and 23–2, respectively.

TABLE 23–1. DSM-IV diagnostic criteria for substance-induced persisting dementia (SIPD)

A. The development of multiple cognitive deficits manifested by both
   (1) memory impairment (impaired ability to learn new information or to recall previously learned information)
   (2) one (or more) of the following cognitive disturbances:
      (a) aphasia (language disturbance)
      (b) apraxia (impaired ability to carry out motor activities despite intact motor function)
      (c) agnosia (failure to recognize or identify objects despite intact sensory function)
      (d) disturbance in executive functioning (i.e., planning, organizing, sequencing, abstracting)

B. The cognitive deficits in criteria A1 and A2 each cause significant impairment in social or occupational functioning and represent a significant decline from a previous level of functioning.

C. The deficits do not occur exclusively during the course of a delirium and persist beyond the usual duration of substance intoxication or withdrawal.

D. There is evidence from the history, physical examination, or laboratory findings that the deficits are etiologically related to the persisting effects of substance use (e.g., a drug of abuse, a medication).

Code [Specific substance]–induced persisting dementia:
   (291.2 alcohol; 292.82 inhalant; 292.82 sedative, hypnotic, or anxiolytic; 292.82 other [or unknown] substance)

TABLE 23–2. DSM-IV diagnostic criteria for substance-induced persisting amnestic disorder (SIPAD)

A. The development of memory impairment as manifested by impairment in the ability to learn new information or the inability to recall previously learned information.

B. The memory disturbance causes significant impairment in social or occupational functioning and represents a significant decline from a previous level of functioning.

C. The memory disturbance does not occur exclusively during the course of a delirium or a dementia and persists beyond the usual duration of substance intoxication or withdrawal.

D. There is evidence from the history, physical examination, or laboratory findings that the memory disturbance is etiologically related to the persisting effects of substance use (e.g., a drug of abuse, a medication).

Code [Specific substance]–induced persisting amnestic disorder:

(291.1 alcohol; 292.83 sedative, hypnotic, or anxiolytic; 292.83 other [or unknown] substance)

Epidemiology

The prevalence of dementia in subjects age 65 years and older in North America is approximately 6%–10%; if milder cases are included, the prevalence rates almost double. The prevalence of dementia doubles approximately every 5 years after age 65 (Hofman et al. 1991; Jorm et al. 1987). Although the prevalence of SIPD and SIPAD has not been well established, review of earlier studies among elderly populations suggests that a significant proportion of dementia is caused by persistent exposure to alcohol, drugs, or other neurotoxic chemicals. Most of those earlier studies indicated that about half of dementias result from Alzheimer's disease, whereas 5%–15% are due to prolonged exposure to alcohol, drugs, or other neurotoxic chemicals (F.R. Freeman 1976; Grant and Judd 1976; Hutton 1981; Maletta et al. 1982; Marsden and Harrison 1972; N.S. Miller et al. 1991; J.S. Smith and Kiloh 1981). Yet, this may be an underestimate of the prevalence of SIPD and SIPAD, in part because Alzheimer's disease is a clinical diagnosis of exclusion and in part because the role of drugs or other neurotoxic chemicals may be poorly explored as an etiological factor in dementia. Recent advances in the diagnosis of Alzheimer's disease and increasing awareness of neurotoxic effects of various drugs and chemicals are likely to enhance the significance of SIPD in the differential diagnosis and management of dementia. If the occupational risk factor is taken into consideration, excess mortality is observed in neurodegenerative diseases, including presenile dementia and Alzheimer's disease, in occupations involving pesticides, solvents, heavy metals, and other chemicals (Schulte et al. 1996). Recent studies indicate that "heavy alcohol use" is a contributing factor in 21%–24% of cases of dementia. Research difficulties include a lack of well-established positive diagnostic criteria for alcohol-related dementia, except those that are based almost exclusively on clinical judgment, and few postmortem studies. Moreover, no guidelines are available to assist the clinician or the researcher in distinguishing alcohol-related dementia from other causes of dementia such as Alzheimer's disease (Oslin et al. 1998; D.M. Smith and Atkinson 1995).

The prevalence of pure amnestic syndromes has not been well studied. SIPAD is most commonly associated with the use of medications and with thiamine deficiency in chronic alcohol abuse. Although reports have implicated short-acting benzodiazepines in SIPAD, all benzodiazepines can cause amnesia, probably as a result of reduced attention and sedation (King 1992). A variety of other sedative-hypnotics may also cause transient amnesia as a part of their side effects. Acute onset of oculomotor disturbance, cerebellar ataxia, and memory impairment is often a presenting feature of thiamine deficiency, known as Wernicke's encephalopathy (Reuler et al. 1985). Wernicke's encephalopathy is diagnosed in 0.05% of general hospital admissions but is detected in 1% at autopsy (Nakada and Knight 1984).

Clinical Syndromes

SIPD is characterized clinically by variable onset of impairment of memory, perception, language, and other intellectual functions. Affective and personality changes often accompany the cognitive disturbances. These presentations are often difficult to distinguish from other forms of dementia such as Alzheimer's disease. However, unlike Alzheimer's disease, which is characterized by a gradual onset and steady deterioration of cognition and functioning abilities, SIPD often manifests with varied onset and progression that are usually determined by the nature and extent of exposure to the neurotoxic agents. Furthermore, with cessation of exposure to the offending agent, most SIPD patients undergo variable degrees of recovery. On the other hand, continued exposure to the neurotoxic substance will invariably cause further deteriorations in intellectual and functional abilities.

SIPAD is characterized by relatively well-circumscribed impairments in both short- and long-term memory without widespread cognitive dysfunction.

The principal clinical features of SIPD and SIPAD are reviewed in the following subsections.

Memory Dysfunction

Impairment in registration and retrieval of information is one of the most sensitive indicators of underlying brain damage and an important clinical symptom in both SIPD and SIPAD. Evidence suggests the registration, storage, and retrieval processes of memory involve two important sites in the brain: the hypothalamic-diencephalic and the hippocampal formation, which is necessary for the correct function of recent and declarative memory for facts and events. In addition to these two sites, the memory involves wide areas of the brain, because memory is extensively linked with diverse sensory, motor, and emotional processes.

Neurotransmitters also play a critical role in the brain circuits involved in various aspects of memory. The importance of acetylcholine is outlined by the pathophysiology of Alzheimer's disease. Cholinergic replacement therapy is now available for treating the cognitive decline associated with this form of degenerative disease. Dopamine in the prefrontal cortex also contributes to information storage, particularly working memory (Iversen 1998). Glutamic acid is the principal excitatory neurotransmitter in the mammalian central nervous system (CNS). Glutamic acid binds to a variety of excitatory amino acid receptors, which are ligand-gated ion channels. Activation of these receptors, such as *N*-methyl-D-aspartate (NMDA) receptors, leads to depolarization and neuronal excitation. Normal functioning of the NMDA receptor is essential to thought, movement, and perception. Antagonists to NMDA receptors or low availability of glutamate impairs learning and memory. Excess glutamate results in overexcitation of the NMDA receptor, allowing excess calcium to enter the neurons. These neurons may then swell and rupture, releasing more glutamate into the surrounding area, which in turn overexcites NMDA receptors on adjacent neurons.

This cascade of neuronal injury, referred to as *excitotoxicity,* is probably another cause of neuronal death, leading to neurodegeneration and dementia.

Hormones and neuropeptides are also very important in the process of memory and learning. Neuropeptides are peptides derived from large precursor proteins. These are converted to neurohormones, neuropeptides of the "first generation," which can be further converted to neuropeptides of the "second generation." Sex hormones, oxytocin, vasopressin, cholecystokinin, endogenous opioids, corticotropin-releasing factor, cortisol, and thyroid hormones are well known to contribute to learning and memory process.

Organically induced memory impairment must be differentiated from functional psychogenic amnesia or psychogenic fugue. Functional amnestic disorders tend to present as a dense amnesia for events and may be limited to certain well-circumscribed themes. In addition, general intellect is relatively well preserved, and the ability to retain new information is generally normal.

Language Dysfunction

Aphasia may occur as part of SIPD and is often a clinically important localizing sign for underlying neurological deficits, but it also may reflect diffuse cerebral dysfunction.

Apraxia

Apraxia, an inability to carry out purposeful voluntary movements in the absence of paralysis, incoordination, sensory loss, or involuntary movements, is commonly seen in patients with dementia. Apraxia is often accompanied by dysphasia and agnosia, which may further hinder the patient from carrying out purposeful movements.

Agnosia

Agnosia is the failure to recognize an object by sight in the presence of intact primary sensory functions. In addition to visual agnosia, auditory and tactile agnosias have been reported. The fact that primary sensory pathways are intact suggests that these disturbances reside at the higher level of sensory information processing.

Intellectual Functioning

Intellectual functioning refers broadly to the ability to learn and apply knowledge in varying circumstances. Cognitive functions involved in intellectual functioning include organizing, reasoning, planning, and abstract thinking, as well as insight and judgment. Some degree of cognitive impairment is associated with aging; when one looks at average performance, great variability is found among individuals, with many showing little or no deleterious effects of aging on intellectual abilities. Significant loss or decline of these abilities is an important clinical finding in dementia. These functions are thought to be modulated by the prefrontal areas of the brain. The prefrontal lobe is also known to regulate initiation and integration of complex motor activities and to inhibit emotional impulses in response to the environment. Thus, in addition to intellectual impairment, emotional outbursts and poor impulse control are frequently found among patients with dementia, including those with SIPD, and may account for personality changes or exacerbation of premorbid personality traits often observed at the early stage of dementia.

Other associated clinical features in patients with dementia include depression, anxiety, disturbed levels of consciousness, delusional thoughts, and hallucinations. These symptoms often appear in response to perceived or real physical and psychosocial stressors in the environment. Patients with SIPD or SIPAD also may show variable neurological signs during the course of the illness.

Differential Diagnosis

The differential diagnosis of SIPD and SIPAD is broadly categorized into normal aging processes, organic mental disorder, and functional psychiatric disorder (pseudodementia). Organic causes of dementia include Alzheimer's disease, vascular dementia, and a wide variety of neurological and systemic disorders, including infections, developmental anomalies, trauma, neoplasm, degenerative processes, atherosclerosis, diabetes, emphysema, high blood pressure, obesity, thyroid dysfunction, and other endocrine and metabolic disorders that contribute to or are the direct cause of a dementia syndrome. Such multiple etiologies are especially important in elderly patients, who are at increased risk to develop various medical and psychiatric disorders.

Major diagnostic categories and etiological factors associated with the dementia syndrome are reviewed in the following subsections.

Normal Aging

The integrity of the hippocampal formation is necessary for the correct function of declarative memory for facts and events. Cortical areas relevant in memory function, and anatomically linked to the hippocampus, present a small degree of atrophy with aging (Insausti et al. 1998). Changes in mental functioning are commonly observed as a part of the aging process. A slowing of mental processes and a diminishing of psychomotor agility, as well as difficulties in recalling names and events, often occur. Such memory disturbances are, however, usually due to difficulties with recall rather than to impaired registration. These changes do not significantly interfere with the person's social or occupational functioning.

Primary Degenerative Dementia

Primary degenerative dementia of the Alzheimer's type is the most important single cause of dementia. It constitutes approximately half of all dementias in elderly patients, and the risk of developing this form of dementia increases steadily throughout adult life (Heston and Mastri 1982; Tomlinson et al. 1970). The clinical presentation of Alzheimer's disease includes insidious onset and pervasive deterioration of intellectual abilities often accompanied by behavioral changes and neurological signs. These symptoms are difficult to differentiate from symptoms of other types of dementia such as SIPD. However, because Alzheimer's disease is a diagnosis of exclusion, definitive diagnosis being possible only by pathological examination of brain tissue, the prevalence of Alzheimer's disease may have been overestimated. On more careful assessment, some apparent cases of Alzheimer's disease may actually be SIPD, or substance exposure may contribute to the greater intellectual decline. The value of morphological imaging (computed tomography [CT], magnetic resonance imaging [MRI]) in the diagnosis of dementias is clear although usually not specific for the underlying causes. Volumetric measurements of certain brain structures at onset, and even before the first clinical signs appear, might be a useful diagnostic approach for early detection. Furthermore, functional brain imaging methods (positron-emission tomography

[PET], functional MRI, and single photon emission computed tomography [SPECT]) appear particularly suited to the diagnosis of degenerative dementias. The presence of functional abnormalities is clearly valuable, particularly in early stages. Further discussion of Alzheimer's disease may be found in Chapter 20.

Vascular Dementia

Dementia as a result of multiple cerebrovascular occlusions depends on the extent and location of brain tissue involvement. Vascular dementia is usually associated with various underlying medical disorders such as diabetes, hypertension, or other cardiovascular diseases (myocardial infarction, arrhythmias). Involvement of the hippocampus, mammillary bodies, thalamus, or base of the frontal lobes is known to cause severe memory deficits (Scheinberg 1988). Most cases of vascular dementia, however, appear to be related to posterior cerebral vessel infarct and may involve cortex or subcortex, or both. Clinically, vascular dementia is characterized by stepwise deteriorations usually accompanied by episodes of confusion and localizing neurological signs. Patients with vascular dementia also may have patchy patterns of cognitive deficits and more labile emotions. These clinical presentations in vascular dementia, however, are again often difficult to distinguish from those in Alzheimer's disease, SIPD, and other forms of dementia. Diagnostic neuroimaging with CT and MRI may reveal characteristic wedge-shaped areas of infarction in the brain.

Treatment of vascular dementia consists primarily of efforts to prevent cerebral infarct by controlling underlying medical disorders or of use of aspirin and other drugs to reduce clotting. Anticoagulant therapy may be instituted with evidence of active embolic episodes or repeated transient ischemic attacks. Concurrent depression may contribute to intellectual decline in poststroke patients and should be identified and treated. Detailed discussion of vascular dementia may be found in Chapter 21.

Functional Psychiatric Disorders (Pseudodementias)

Intellectual impairments have been observed in association with various functional psychiatric disorders. Besides major depression, whose association with dementia has been better recognized, other disorders such as mania, schizophrenia, and anxiety disorders are associated with dementia syndrome. Pseudodementia accounts for approximately 10% of all dementia syndromes (Hutton 1981; Maletta et al. 1982; Marsden and Harrison 1972; J.S. Smith and Kiloh 1981). Rabins (1981) found that up to 30% of depressed patients have cognitive impairment. Clinical presentation of depressive pseudodementia is frequently characterized by psychomotor retardation and neurovegetative signs. Patients with pseudodementia, in contrast to patients with organic dementia, are usually acutely aware of their memory deficits and complain of recent cognitive and functional difficulties. Signs of cortical deficits seen in organic dementia, such as aphasia, agnosia, apraxia, and focal neurological signs, are also absent. The cognitive impairment in pseudodementia is often fully reversed with appropriate treatment of the underlying functional disorders.

Delirium

Delirium and dementia may coexist, or dementia could follow delirium if the underlying pathology persists through time or is extremely severe, leading to permanent brain damage. However, delirium is characterized by severe cognitive and sensorium disturbances, usually of acute onset and fluctuating course and of brief duration. Patients with delirium typically have underlying systemic disorders or acutely evolving neurological processes and may recover when these are corrected. Electroencephalographic findings in delirium are characterized by generalized slowing. Further discussion of delirium may be found in Chapters 18 and 19.

Psychogenic Amnestic Disorder

The primary manifestation of psychogenic amnestic disorder is memory impairment in the absence of other cognitive disturbances. The impairment is characterized by sudden and usually brief loss of personal information, often with significant or symbolic psychological content. Such loss may be focal or systematized, covering an extensive period of the person's life history. Psychogenic amnesia affects both short- and long-term memory without clouding consciousness or resulting in any general loss of intellectual abilities. Psychiatric history or histrionic personality traits also may help in differential diagnosis.

Neurological Disorders

Any disorders that can damage the diencephalic and medial temporal structures of the brain can result in an amnestic syndrome. Common causes include head trauma, degenerative disorders (e.g., Huntington's disease, Parkinson's disease), encephalitis, anoxia, and brain tumors.

Systemic Medical Disorders

Various medical conditions, including endocrine, metabolic, cardiovascular, hepatic, pulmonary, neoplastic, renal insufficiency, and nutritional deficiency states (e.g., thiamine, nicotinic acid, cyanocobalamin), may cause brain tissue damage or functional derangement and manifest as dementia. Further discussion of dementia caused by medical disorders may be found in Chapter 22.

Substance-Induced Dementia and Amnestic Disorders

Numerous prescription, nonprescription, and illicit drugs and toxic chemicals can adversely affect brain functioning and cause dementia and amnestic syndromes. Chronic use of alcohol impairs memory, often through thiamine deficiency. Examples of other drugs implicated are cocaine, toluene-based solvents, amphetamine, and steroids (Lishman 1990; O'Malley et al. 1992; Ron 1986). Amnestic episodes have been observed with benzodiazepines such as triazolam (Bixler et al. 1991; Kalynchuk and Beck 1992; King 1992) and drugs with anticholinergic effects, including many antidepressants (Sakulsripong et al. 1991). Acute and excessive exposure and chronic exposure to industrial toxins or pollutants have been associated with intellectual deterioration (Allen 1979; Feldman and Cummings 1981; Hartman 1988; Prockop 1979). Common drugs and chemicals associated with dementia or amnesia are listed in Table 23–3 and are reviewed below.

Alcohol

Chronic, excessive use of alcohol is one of the most frequent causes of dementia (Carlen et al. 1981; Charness 1993; Cutting 1982; Thal 1988). Major forms of alcohol-induced intellectual impairments include alcoholic dementia, subacute and chronic alcohol-induced encephalopathies, Marchiafava-Bignami disease, and dietary deficiency syndromes. Dementia

TABLE 23–3. Etiological agents associated with dementia

Prescription medications	Antibiotics	*Toxic chemicals*
Psychotropics	Antihypertensives	Acrylamide
Antipsychotics (phenothiazines)	Antineoplastics	Arsenic
Antidepressants (tricyclics)	Cardiac glycosides	Carbon monoxide
Antimanic agents (lithium)	Calcium channel blockers	Carbon tetrachloride
Antihistamines	Diuretics	Formaldehyde
Antiparkinsonian drugs	Oral contraceptives	Hydrogen sulfide
Barbiturates	Steroids	Lead
Benzodiazepines		Methyl alcohol
Sedative-hypnotics	**Illicit or toxic substances**	Methyl chloride
	Drugs of abuse	Mercury
Nonpsychotropics	Alcohol	Organophosphates
Analgesics	Amphetamine	Perchloroethylene
Anticonvulsants	Cocaine	Toluene
Antiarrhythmics	Ergot alkaloids	Trichloroethylene

Source. Adapted from Cummings and Benson 1992.

related to alcoholism is responsible for approximately 6%–10% of dementia cases (Hutton 1981; Marsden and Harrison 1972) and is more common among elderly alcoholic persons than among younger persons who have been drinking for a similar period of time (Finlayson et al. 1988).

Alcoholic dementia. Chronic use of alcohol may result in deterioration of cognitive ability with general decline in self-care and occupational and social functions, mimicking early signs of Alzheimer's disease. However, in alcoholic dementia, unlike in Alzheimer's disease, the progression of cognitive and functional deterioration may slow with cessation of drinking alcohol, although full return to premorbid functioning is unusual (Brandt et al. 1983; Grant et al. 1984; Martin et al. 1989; Page and Linden 1974). As many as half of chronic alcoholic patients have been found to have some intellectual deterioration (Carlen et al. 1981; Cutting 1982), and such deterioration is more likely to occur if drinking has been continuous. The clinical presentation of alcoholic dementia is usually mild and either nonprogressive or only slowly progressive and may include forgetfulness, circumstantiality, psychomotor retardation, perseveration, and disorientation (Lee et al. 1979; Lishman 1981). This functional and intellectual deterioration may be accompanied by neuroanatomic and neurophysiological changes (Carlen et al. 1978; Newman 1978; Sachs et al. 1987). These changes may be at least partially reversible if identified early and if the patient remains abstinent (Brandt et al. 1983; Carlen et al. 1978; Grant et al. 1984).

Marchiafava-Bignami disease. Marchiafava-Bignami disease occurs almost exclusively in alcoholic individuals and is associated with demyelination of the corpus callosum and other midline white matter structures. Although numerous etiological hypotheses have been proposed, the pathophysiology of Marchiafava-Bignami disease remains unknown. A few cases have been described in nonalcoholic persons, demonstrating that ethanol alone is not responsible for the lesions (Navarro and Noriega 1999). Recent studies of regional cerebral glucose metabolism obtained by PET showed diffusely reduced whole brain metabolism and strongly decreased metabolism in the frontal and parietal lobes, orbital gyrus, and thalamus. Cerebral perfusion images showed a pattern with decreased radioactivity similar to that in the metabolic images (Ishii et al. 1999). The clinical course of Marchiafava-Bignami disease is varied, and it may be acute, subacute, or chronic. Clinical symptoms include personality changes, amnesia, aphasia, disorientation, and occasionally coma. In addition, progressive dementia occurs over weeks to months, with signs of callosal disconnection such as left-side apraxia, left-hand agraphia, and left-hand tactile anomia (Ironside et al. 1961; Lechevalier et al. 1977; Lhermitte et al. 1977). Magnetic resonance imaging shows that corpus callosum thinning is present in persons with chronic alcoholism without clinical manifestations of Marchiafava-Bignami disease, severe liver disease, amnesia, or alcoholic dementia. These data suggest that chronic alcoholism can be characterized by a continuum of brain toxicity rather than classical alcoholic-related subsyndromes, such as Marchiafava-Bignami disease (Pfefferbaum et al. 1996).

Alcohol-related encephalopathies. In addition to the direct toxic neurological effects of alcohol, chronic alcoholic persons are susceptible to deficiency syndromes such as Wernicke's encephalopathy, Korsakoff's syndrome, and pellagra (Tomlinson et al. 1976). Wernicke's encephalopathy may present with abrupt onset of sensorial disturbances, inattentiveness, confusion, apathy, ophthalmoplegia, nystagmus, and ataxia and should be considered as a possible diagnosis in comatose and hypothermic patients because the history of alcohol abuse or other causes of thiamine deficiency may be unknown, and the classic triad of confusion, ophthalmoplegia (or nystagmus), and ataxia may be absent. Left untreated, acute Wernicke's encephalopathy has a 17% mortality rate (Lindberg and Oyler 1990). Drinking alcohol, even in relatively small quantities, could precipitate the development of Wernicke's encephalopathy in gastrectomized individuals because they already have low thiamine absorption.

Korsakoff's syndrome (alcohol amnestic disorder) often accompanies Wernicke's encephalopathy and is characterized by confabulation with severe short- and long-term memory impairments. Immediate memory, however, may be fairly well preserved. Impaired abstraction and perseveration are also commonly observed. Symmetrical lesions in the mammillary bodies, in the periventricular regions of the thalamus and hypothalamus, and in the periaqueductal midbrain are present in both Wernicke's and Korsakoff's syndromes. PET with oxygen 15 isotope inhalation in Korsakoff's syndrome shows decreased regional cerebral blood flow and decreased regional cerebral metabolic ratio for oxygen in the bilateral frontotemporal areas and in the left thalamus, suggesting that dysfunction of the frontal-thalamic neural network plays a role in the pathophysiology of this syndrome (Matsuda et al. 1997). Levels of plasma oxytocin, vasopressin, estrone, and β-endorphin are also altered in chronic alcoholic persons, contributing to learning and memory disturbances (Marchesi et al. 1997). Fluvoxamine (100–200 mg/day) was found to improve memory consolidation and retrieval in patients with alcohol amnestic disorder. These improvements in memory were significantly correlated with reduced cerebrospinal fluid (CSF) 5-hydroxyindoleacetic acid (5-HIAA) levels and high fluvoxamine plasma concentrations, suggesting that facilitation of serotonergic neurotransmission may ameliorate the episodic memory failure in patients with alcohol amnestic disorder (Martin et al. 1995).

Because thiamine deficiency plays a key role in Wernicke's encephalopathy and Korsakoff's syndrome, parenteral administration of thiamine, 100 mg/day in divided doses, may rapidly alleviate the symptoms. Reports of rare anaphylactoid reactions have led to a reduction in the use of parenteral thiamine, and this change in treatment may have led, or will lead, to an increase in morbidity and mortality (Thomson and Cook 1997). Once the patient can eat again, thiamine, 100 mg/day, can be given orally, which provides effective prophylaxis. Thiamine treatment is efficient in the early stages, and a delay often causes permanent damage. It is recommended that routine management of alcohol-related disease should include oral thiamine at 50–100 mg/day even if neurological or cognitive signs are absent or unclear.

Deficiency in nicotinic acid associated with malnutrition among persons with chronic alcoholism may result in pellagra. This condition is characterized by dermatitis, diarrhea, and dementia with thickened sun-exposed areas of the skin and, occasionally, spastic leg weakness. Vitamin supplementation, including B_{12}, folic acid, and pyridoxine, and improved general nutrition may alleviate the symptoms.

Finally, alcoholic persons are more susceptible to various CNS infections (e.g., meningitis), hepatic encephalopathies, head trauma, and cerebral hemorrhage, all of which may produce dementia or amnesia.

Sedative-Hypnotics

A variety of sedative-hypnotics, including barbiturates and nonbarbiturates such as meprobamate and benzodiazepines, are commonly used in the general population. These agents are available through prescription by physicians, although some sedatives are available as over-the-counter products. There is significant cross-tolerance between these drugs and a tendency associated with these drugs for the user to develop both psychological and physiological dependence. Grant and colleagues reported significant neuropsychological impairments such as abstraction, perceptual-motor integration, and memory deficits among subjects dependent primarily on sedative-hypnotics. These impairments persisted several months into drug abstinence, and their severity correlated with the amount of drug used (Grant and Judd 1976; Grant et al. 1976; R.M. Murray et al. 1971). More recently, significant amnestic effects have been observed among persons who chronically use benzodiazepines; these effects also appeared to correlate with the dosage of the benzodiazepines (Curran 1992; King 1992).

Treatment should include an attempt at dose reduction and discontinuation of sedative drugs. This reduction should proceed gradually over 2–3 weeks to prevent the risks of sedative withdrawal, which include seizures and delirium. The maximum daily dose reduction should be less than 10% of the initial established dosage. The offending agent itself may be tapered, or a long-acting sedative such as chlordiazepoxide or clonazepam may be substituted and then tapered. Buspirone, a serotonin type 1A (5-HT_{1A}) receptor but not γ-aminobutyric acid (GABA)-ergic anxiolytic drug without implications in learning and memory process and without abuse potential, also should be considered as an alternative therapeutic approach. Further discussion of techniques for sedative-hypnotic withdrawal may be found in Chapter 26.

Psychotropic Drugs

Various psychotropic medications have been associated with cognitive disturbances. Lithium carbonate, even at therapeutic levels, can occasionally produce a dementia syndrome with disorientation, poor attention and concentration, and impaired comprehension (Shopsin et al. 1970). Lithium has a greater neuropsychological effect in younger, less depressed patients with higher lithium concentrations in plasma (Kocsis et al. 1993). Cognitive impairment also may result from lithium-induced hypothyroidism (Fieve and Platman 1968). Preliminary study results suggest the use of thyroid hormone (triiodothyronine [T_3]) to diminish the cognitive side effects of psychiatric treatment with lithium (Tremont and Stern 1997).

The CNS toxicity of tricyclic antidepressants is attributable to their anticholinergic activity. As many as 10%–15% of all patients and 35% of elderly patients receiving tricyclics may experience some degree of cognitive impairment (Hollister 1979). Newer selective serotonergic or noradrenergic antidepressants should be considered in case of cognitive impairment with tricyclics, although subtle memory impairment can also result from treatment with these agents.

Conventional antipsychotics can further reduce cognitive function, which is already impaired in most patients with schizophrenia. It has been suggested that the origins of negative symptoms in schizophrenia may be related to a reduction in dopamine activity in the prefrontal cortex. If this is the case, dopamine D_2 blockade would be expected to impair some aspects of neurocognitive function further (Borison 1996). In addition, long-term use of antiparkinsonian medications (e.g., trihexyphenidyl), often used in conjunction with antipsychotics for treatment of extrapyramidal symptoms, can have additive, cognitive function–impairing effects (Kajimura et al. 1993). Atypical antipsychotics, with their weak dopamine affinity and rather strong 5-HT_2 blockage, have a better effect on cognitive function than conventional antidopaminergic antipsychotics and usually require fewer or no anticholinergic drugs because of their low incidence of extrapyramidal symptoms. Antipsychotic medications are also widely used to treat behavioral disorders, especially among elderly patients with Alzheimer's and Parkinson's dementia. Both phenothiazine and butyrophenone antipsychotics have been associated with chronic confusional states and cognitive impairment (Petrie et al. 1982; Thornton 1976; Van Putten et al. 1974).

In general, the CNS effects of any prescribed medications should be carefully evaluated in elderly patients presenting with recent onset or worsening of cognitive disturbances (Blazer et al. 1983).

The treatment of psychotropic medication–induced dementia includes dose reduction, elimination of the causative drugs, or substitution with other agents. Anticholinergic cognitive dysfunction may be reversed acutely by administration of physostigmine (Granacher and Baldessarini 1975).

Nonpsychotropic Drugs

Numerous nonpsychotropic medications have been associated with the dementia syndrome. Corticosteroid treatment may produce Cushing's syndrome, which is associated with excitation, depression, and psychosis, but may also produce deficits in declarative episodic, spatial-constructional, and contextual memory performance (Brown et al. 1999; Whelan et al. 1980). Cushing's syndrome is infrequent with short-term low-dose corticosteroid treatment. With long-term or high-dose treatment, however, the incidence may be quite high. In diseases such as lupus cerebritis and multiple sclerosis, the differentiation between cognitive difficulties secondary to the underlying illness, which might warrant more aggressive corticosteroid treatment, and those secondary to corticosteroid treatment itself, which might warrant dosage reduction, may be problematic (Wolkowitz et al. 1997). Corticosteroids increase hippocampal neuronal cell death in the CA3 region under conditions of metabolic stress, and it has been hypothesized that this effect might contribute to chronic memory deficits (Lupien et al. 1998; Meaney et al. 1991; Tombaugh and Sapolsky 1993).

Other medications that may produce memory impairment, dementia, or delirium include digoxin (Sagel and Matisonn 1972), antihypertensives (Solomon et al. 1983), diuretics (Moses and Miller 1974), anticonvulsants (Trimble and Reynolds 1976), antibiotics (Goetz et al. 1981), contraceptives (Shafey and Scheinberg 1966), and analgesics (e.g., aspirin, phenacetin) when used chronically and in large amounts (Murray et al. 1971).

Medication-induced CNS toxic effects may constitute an idiosyncratic response at normal therapeutic doses, or they may occur in conjunction with excessive blood levels either because of pharmacokinetic interactions between several medications or because of excessive dosage. Elderly patients and patients with physical illness or incipient dementia may be at highest risk. The clinician should always be alert to whether a patient is taking prescribed medications correctly, and careful review of the patient's current medications is recommended.

HIV-Associated Dementia and SIPD-SIPAD

Significant progress was made in recent years in the treatment of human immunodeficiency virus (HIV)-1-associated dementia and in unraveling the pathophysiology that follows viral invasion of the CNS. It is now known that CNS damage induced by HIV-1 infection occurs mainly indirectly. Neuron death is mediated through immune activation and viral infection of brain macrophages and microglia. It appears that viral growth in the brain is necessary, but not sufficient, to produce cognitive and motor impairments in affected individuals. Indeed, the best predictor of neurological impairment following HIV-1 infection is the absolute number of immune-competent macrophages, not the level of virus production in affected brain tissue. Cellular and viral factors secreted by brain macrophages and microglia produce, over time, neuronal damage and dropout (Swindells et al. 1999).

Psychoactive drugs are commonly abused by acquired immunodeficiency syndrome (AIDS) patients, and a growing body of evidence indicates that this population is more vulnerable to developing HIV-1-associated dementia than are homosexuals, hemophiliacs, or other groups of HIV-infected patients who are not drug abusers (Fein et al. 1995; Goodkin et al. 1998; Starace et al. 1998; Tyor and Middaugh 1999).

Alcohol and especially cocaine are the best-studied drugs in HIV-infected patients and probably have the greater toxic effects on the brain in patients with HIV-1-associated dementia. The "cerebral reserve" model was introduced to highlight the neurotoxic effects of those drugs so that HIV-infected subjects become more vulnerable to direct and indirect neurotoxic effects of HIV.

Chronic alcohol consumption and HIV infection have at least additive effects on memory and cognitive deficits. Both alcohol and HIV infection have been shown to produce CNS morbidity in frontal brain regions. Auditory P3A evoked potentials provide a sensitive index of frontal lobe functionality. HIV-positive persons with alcoholism show delayed P3A latency compared with HIV-positive persons without alcoholism or HIV-negative persons with alcoholism (Fein et al. 1995). According to Meyerhoff et al. (1995), chronic alcohol abuse and HIV infection have cumulative effects on phospholipid and energy metabolism in the white matter, leading to further neuropsychological deterioration.

Many recent studies indicate that cocaine abuse has profound effects on the immune system that, in many respects, are enhanced by retroviral infection contributing to HIV-1-associated dementia pathogenesis. Cocaine is well known to stimulate the hypothalamic-pituitary-adrenal axis to increase both anti- and proinflammatory hormonal secretion, which has wide-ranging effects on the immune and neuroendocrine systems (Fiala et al. 1996), resembling an inflammatory "stress" response with upregulation of proinflammatory cytokines (Gan et al. 1999). Recent data suggest that mononuclear cells from cocaine-addicted persons are sensitized to in vitro cocaine challenge with hypersecretion of inflammatory cytokines. Cocaine's in vivo manifestations are compatible with these in vitro effects (Fiala et al. 1998). Chronic cocaine abuse also has been associated with vascular disorders, including cerebral vasculitis and vasospasm, and evidence indicates that cocaine perturbs the function of endothelial cells, including the blood-brain barrier, facilitating the entrance of the retrovirus, immune cells, and cytokines into the CNS (Goodkin et al. 1998; Shapshak et al. 1996). Collectively, these results suggest that the effects of cocaine on endothelial, immune, and neuroendocrine cells impair the function of the blood-brain barrier, increase cell emigration from the blood vessels into the brain, and may cause wide toxic and inflammatory effects in the brain of HIV-infected patients. Although SPECT images are a sensitive indicator of HIV-1-associated dementia brain perfusion patterns, they cannot be distinguished from chronic cocaine use, demonstrating cortical defects most frequently in the frontal, temporal, and parietal lobes in both cases. Caution is therefore needed before entertaining a specific diagnosis and therapeutic approach (Holman et al. 1992).

Intravenous drug use is also correlated with HIV-1-associated dementia, suggesting that differences in the route of transmission may play a role in the manifestation of HIV-related brain toxicity.

HIV replication in and outside of the CNS was significantly reduced by new potent combined antiretroviral therapies. This has resulted in partial repair of cellular immune function with improvement in, and the prevention of, neurological deficits associated with progressive HIV-1 disease. Nonetheless, adjunctive anti-inflammatory and neuroprotective therapies are being developed, and immediate efforts should be made in treating comorbid disorders such as cocaine and alcohol abuse, which contribute to or trigger the manifestation of HIV-1-associated dementia neuropathogenesis (Swindells et al. 1999).

Substance Abuse

Chronic use of illicit drugs has been associated with intellectual impairment, although this remains an area of considerable controversy. Substance-induced cognitive impairment may involve memory, attention, or abstraction and problem-solving abilities (L. Miller 1985). The persistence and severity of cognitive and electroencephalogram (EEG) abnormalities appear to correlate with the extent of drug exposure (Judd and Grant 1978).

Among chronic opiate-dependent patients, Rounsaville and colleagues (1981) found a substantial prevalence of cognitive impairment. Although opiates themselves are not thought to be neurotoxic, persons with chronic opiate addiction often have substantial exposures to other, more toxic substances such as alcohol and are at high risk for debilitating medical illnesses that can contribute to cognitive impairment, such as AIDS.

Chronic use of cocaine (Herning et al. 1990; Manschreck et al. 1990) and phencyclidine (PCP) (Cosgrove and Newell 1991) is associated with cognitive impairment. Cocaine abuse has been associated with brain vasculitis and stroke. Recent neuroimaging studies found significant reduction in blood flow and metabolic activity in diverse brain regions among patients with chronic cocaine dependence (London et al. 1990; Pearlson et al. 1993; Volkow et al. 1988). Cerebral perfusion deficits also were detected in methamphetamine abusers even after a long abstinence period, suggesting that vascular changes were irreversible to some degree. Those pathophysiological changes may lead to severe cognitive and memory disturbances, which usually persist long after abstinence is achieved.

The toxic effects of marijuana have been underestimated for a long time; recent studies found delta-9-tetrahydrocannabinol-induced cell death with shrinkage of neurons and DNA fragmentation in the hippocampus. Two subtypes of cannabinoid receptors, CB1 and CB2, have been described to date, although future investigations may elucidate other receptors. The CB1 receptor and its splice variant CB1A are found predominantly in the brain, with highest densities in the hippocampus, cerebellum, and striatum (Ameri 1999). Long-term abuse of marijuana by humans can induce profound behavioral deficits characterized by cognitive and memory impairments. In particular, deficits in tasks dependent on frontal lobe function have been reported in cannabis abusers. Cognitive deficits in heavy abusers of cannabis may be related to drug-induced alterations in frontal cortical dopamine transmission (Jentsch et al. 1998). However, whether this impairment is caused by a residue of drug in the brain, a withdrawal effect from the drug, a frank neurotoxic effect of the drug, or preexisting deficits is unknown. Recent data suggest that beginning cannabis use during early adolescence may lead to enduring effects on specific attention functions in adulthood. Apparently, vulnerable periods during brain development are subject to persistent alterations by interfering exogenous cannabinoids (Ehrenreich et al. 1999).

Methylenedioxymethamphetamine (MDMA, or "Ecstasy") is a recreational drug of abuse with growing popularity that is well known to damage brain serotonergic neurons in animals, and recent data suggest that this may occur in humans as well. Repeated administration of MDMA produces lasting decreases in serotonergic activity in various brain areas, including the hippocampus, resulting in deficits in a variety of psychological processes involving learning and memory. MDMA users also had significant selective decreases in CSF 5-HIAA. Abstinent MDMA users had persisting impairment in verbal and visual memory correlating with the degree of MDMA exposure and the reduction in brain serotonin, as indexed by CSF 5-HIAA. Preclinical data suggest that treatment with selective serotonin reuptake inhibitors (SSRIs) could prevent or attenuate damage to brain serotonergic neurons (Bolla et al. 1998; Morgan 1999; McCann et al. 1999; Parrott and Lasky 1998).

The treatment of substance-induced dementia includes medically supervised withdrawal from drugs of abuse, treatment of associated medical and psychiatric disorders, and psychosocial or pharmacological intervention to prevent further drug dependence. For an in-depth discussion of the treatment of substance abuse, see Section 4 of this volume.

Solvent Vapor Exposure and Abuse

Chronic inhalation of the vapors of various volatile organic solvents has been associated with the dementia syndrome. Offending agents include toluene-containing products such as model airplane glue; acetone; xylene; halogenated hydrocarbons such as trichloroethylene, carbon tetrachloride, and trichloroethane found in paints, varnishes, and cleaning fluids; methyl alcohol (wood alcohol); methyl chloride; ethylene glycol (Sterno); acrylamide; and gasoline, which contains various hydrocarbons in addition to lead in some countries. Exposure occurs mainly in two types of patients: 1) industrial workers exposed to fumes at the workplace and 2) substance-abusing persons who inhale the fumes for their euphorigenic properties. Persons who abuse these substances are most commonly individuals living in remote communities, those whose occupations give ready access to abusable substances, and adolescents for whom solvents, which are cheap and available through various household products, are often a first drug of abuse and a point of entry into a lifelong pattern of substance abuse (Westermeyer 1987). Thus, with any alcoholic or drug-abusing patient with cognitive impairment, it is worthwhile to inquire about a past or early history of solvent abuse.

Chronic solvent exposure can result in multiple organ system damage, including bone marrow suppression, glomerulonephritis, respiratory tract irritation, and CNS effects (Westermeyer 1987). CNS effects can include encephalopathy or dementia, pyramidal and cerebellar dysfunction, brain-stem and cranial-nerve signs, ataxia, motor and sensory disturbances, and hallucinations (Hormes et al. 1986). Higher doses may produce life-threatening effects, such as convulsions and coma. Death may occur after inhalation of vomit or from direct cardiac or CNS toxicity. Cross-sectional studies support the hypothesis that occupational, low-level, long-term solvent exposure may cause adverse CNS effects. The cumulative findings suggest that occupational solvent exposure may cause mental and cognitive impairment that may become chronic and disabling (Mikkelsen 1997). Neuroimaging findings in chronic solvent vapor abuse have shown diffuse white matter abnormalities (Hormes et al. 1986; Rosenberg et al. 1988). Filley et al. (1990) reported that the extent of white matter abnormality correlated with the severity of the dementia. SPECT, using technetium 99m ethyl cysteinate dimer, may detect early CNS injury from toluene inhalation even when neurological examination and neuroanatomic imaging such as MRI are normal (Ryu et al. 1998). Electrophysiological data show markedly lower P300 amplitudes in patients with solvent-induced toxic encephalopathy under event-related potentials (Lindgren et al. 1997).

The cornerstone of treatment for solvent-induced cognitive dysfunction is elimination of exposure. Patients who abuse these substances will likely require drug abuse treatment (see Section 4 of this volume). Family evaluation and treatment are particularly important because many solvent-abusing patients are adolescents (Westermeyer 1987).

Heavy Metals

Numerous metallic compounds used in industry are potentially toxic to the CNS. Some of these compounds are aluminum, cadmium, lead, mercury, manganese, arsenic, thallium, and bismuth (Hartman 1988; Namba et al. 1971).

Aluminum. A link between exposure to aluminum or aluminum compounds and Alzheimer's disease has been suggested because severe neurological effects similar to those of Alzheimer's disease have been observed in patients receiving dialysis treatment (with dialysis fluids containing aluminum); also, aluminum levels are elevated in the brains of patients with Alzheimer's disease. At present, whether this association is a true effect is controversial, and findings are inconsistent. Recent reviewers have concluded that the evidence is inadequate to establish a link between occupational exposure to aluminum and specific effects on the nervous system or Alzheimer's disease in healthy subjects.

The dialysis encephalopathy syndrome is a progressive neurological disease with severe cognitive decline, deafness, tremor, and ataxia that usually causes death in 6–8 months and has a geographical distribution related to the aluminum content of the dialysis water supply. A close relation exists between concentrations of water aluminum and serum aluminum, and patients with dialysis encephalopathy have serum aluminum concentrations greater than 400 μg/L. High serum aluminum is also associated with osteomalacic bone disease and anemia. In dialysis encephalopathy, concentrations of aluminum are elevated in both CSF and gray matter, and a total aluminum load of 2–8 g is calculated from whole-body in vivo analysis (Elliott and Macdougall 1978).

Cadmium. Occupational cadmium exposure occurs mainly to workers in battery and coil manufacturing plants. Workers with high urinary cadmium levels perform less well than those with low urinary cadmium levels on measures of attention, psychomotor speed, and memory. In addition, cadmium body burden has previously been related to intelligence and school achievement of children (Hart et al. 1989). Cadmium interferes with several important nervous system functions, but the mechanisms of neurotoxicity are uncertain. Other toxic effects of cadmium are Fanconi's syndrome and osteomalacic bone disease (Marumo and Li 1996). Treatment with humic acid–based complex microelement preparation (potassium, magnesium, iron, zinc, manganese, copper, vanadium, cobalt, molybdenum, and selenium bound to humic acids) for 6 weeks (10 mL/day) decreases cadmium load, which leads to reduced neurotoxicity (Hudak et al. 1997). Also, preliminary evidence suggests that glycine, one of the major inhibitory neurotransmitters in the mammalian CNS and a modulator of excitatory amino acid transmission mediated by NMDA receptors, appears to protect against chronic cadmium toxicity by reducing oxidative stress (Shaikh and Tang 1999).

Lead. Lead poisoning in association with the domestic water supply, although less prevalent than in previous eras, still may occur. Children who eat lead-containing paint chips or dust are also susceptible. Tetraethyl lead, a gasoline additive, also may be a source of exposure (Boyd et al. 1957). Blood lead levels are often used as a general indicator of recent exposure to lead. Average blood lead levels of adults with no occupational exposure vary widely depending on factors such as smoking habits, nutritional status, and geographic area. In most industrialized countries, blood lead levels in adults without occupational exposure are typically less than 20–30 μg/dL. Blood lead levels below 50 μg/dL are considered to reflect relatively low lead exposure; blood lead levels of 51–100 μg/dL reflect moderate lead exposure, and blood lead levels greater than 100 μg/dL would reflect high lead exposure. Chronic lead encephalopathy patients may present with anorexia, constipation, intestinal colic attacks, and joint pains and headache, in addition to CNS effects such as dullness, poor concentration, impaired memory, deafness, transitory episodes of aphasia and hemianopsia, delirium, and peripheral neuropathy. More severe effects, including convulsions, paralysis, coma, and death, occur at very high exposures. Encephalopathic episodes may be precipitated by infections or dehydration, resulting in acidosis with subsequent mobilization of lead compounds in the body (Byers 1959). However, lead poisoning, particularly at lower levels, may present simply with intellectual impairment (Gellert et al. 1993; Ruff et al. 1993).

Diagnosis of lead poisoning includes basophilic stippling of the erythrocytes, elevated lead content on repeat blood and urine examinations, and dense bands of condensation in the lines of calcification on the X rays of long bones of young children. Treatment includes use of chelating agents that promote the urinary excretion of lead and treatment of any associated iron deficiency. One such agent is ethylene diaminetetraacetic acid (EDTA), and in severe cases dimercaprol or D-penicillamine may be given as well. Symptoms of acute lead encephalopathy can be rapidly relieved, although residual cognitive deficits are common (Gordon et al. 1998; Perlstein and Attala 1966). It has come to be generally accepted that low levels of lead exposure may result in mental deficits and retardation in young children, and it has been shown in young children that reduction in blood lead levels is associated with improvement in cognitive functioning over the long term (Ruff et al. 1993). Controversially, according to De Silva and Christophers (1997), mental retardation may lead to pica, which causes lead exposure (i.e., to support the theory of reverse causation).

Mercury. The harmful effects of long-term exposure to elemental mercury are generally thought to be caused by inhalation. However, mercury liquid and vapor are absorbed through the skin in small amounts, and this route of exposure can contribute to the overall exposure. Effects after absorption through the skin are expected to be similar to those reported for long-term inhalation exposure. Chronic mercury poisoning usually occurs among industrial workers and photoengravers. Sources of nonoccupational exposure include new dental fillings. Mercury levels in urine are often used as a general indicator of exposure and are reported in micrograms/gram of creatinine. Urine mercury levels in adults without occupational exposure are typically less than 3 μg/g of creatinine. Levels below 25 μg/g of creatinine are considered to reflect relatively low exposure, levels between 25 and 50 μg/g reflect moderate exposure, and levels greater than 100 μg/g are considered high exposure. Clinical manifestations may include paresthesias, narrowing of the visual field, ataxia, dysarthria, deafness, and dementia (Marsh 1979; Vroom and Greer 1972). Insomnia, agitation, depression, hallucinations, and short-term memory deficits also may occur. The CNS effects of mercury toxicity are sometimes referred to as "mad hatter's disease" because mercurous nitrate was used in making felt hats.

EEG findings are often abnormal in cases of mercury poisoning (Brenner and Snyder 1980). Chelation with penicillamine facilitates the excretion of mercury and may effect at least partial improvement of the symptoms (Kark 1979; Marsh 1979).

Manganese. Manganese is an essential mineral but is toxic when taken in excess. Because manganese is primarily cleared by the liver, patients with chronic liver disease have higher and sometimes toxic manganese concentrations, and it has been suggested that manganese contributes to the manifestation of and may be the pathogenesis of hepatic encephalopathy. Manganese toxicity of the brain occurs also in industrial workers involved with manganese ore and steel manufacturing, as well as in those involved with bleach, paint, enamel, and dry battery manufacturing. However, manganese poisoning is relatively rare and may require exposure to large quantities over a long time. Neurological symptoms include extrapyramidal signs, ataxia, dysarthria, tremor, bradykinesia, and increased muscle tone. If extrapyramidal findings are present, they are likely to be irreversible and even progress after termination of the exposure to manganese. Clinical features are usually sufficient to distinguish these patients from those with Parkinson's disease. The neurological syndrome does not respond to L-dopa. Imaging of the brain may reveal MRI signal changes in the globus pallidus, striatum, and midbrain (Pal et al. 1999). Neuropsychological features may include memory impairments, irritability, poor concentration, euphoria, hallucinations, and aggressiveness (Abd el Naby and Hassanein 1965; Mena 1979; Saric et al. 1977). The mechanisms of manganese neurotoxicity are still speculative, but evidence suggests that manganese deposition in the striatum, hypothalamus, and pallidum may lead to dopaminergic dysfunction. The cellular and molecular mechanisms underlying manganese-mineral interactions in the brain are still poorly defined and merit further investigation. Chelation with EDTA may alleviate psychiatric symptoms in some patients but is minimally effective for the extrapyramidal symptoms (Cook et al. 1974; Mena 1979).

Arsenic. Chronic arsenic exposure may occur in the manufacturing of paints, prints, and enamels (J.W. Freeman and Couch 1978; Goetz et al. 1981). The arsenic-induced dementia syndrome is characterized by somnolence, poor attention, disorientation, and memory disturbances (Hartman 1988). Myelopathy, peripheral and optic neuropathy, hyperpigmentation of skin, diabetes mellitus, transverse lines on the nails, and gastrointestinal, respiratory, and cardiac symptoms also may accompany the mental status changes. Diagnosis is made by identifying arsenic levels above 0.01 mg per 100 mL of blood or 0.1 mg per 100 g in the hair or nails (Goetz et al. 1981; Jenkins 1966). In addition to elimination of exposure, dimercaprol therapy may be helpful in some patients (Jenkins 1966).

Thallium. Thallium that is used in rodent poison and pesticides is sometimes ingested accidentally, causing headache, vomiting, abdominal pain, salivation, and tachycardia. The toxic effects of thallium on the kidney can produce hypertension. Neurological symptoms include ataxia, tremor, seizures, and visual disturbances (Reed et al. 1963). Thallium's effects on mental status include anxiety, somnolence, hallucinations, memory impairment, and confabulation (Prick 1979). The treatment should be directed at removing the offending agent.

Other metals and chemicals. Gold-induced encephalopathy may occur in the treatment of arthritic conditions and may manifest with apathy, disorientation, and memory disturbances (McAuley et al. 1977). Chronic exposure to bismuth may result in depression, anxiety, hallucinations, delusions, and intellectual impairments (Goetz and Klawans 1979). Tin poisoning may produce poor attention and memory in addition to apathy, headache, and pseudotumor cerebri (Foncin and Gruner 1979). Chronic exposure to nickel (Hartman 1988), methyl bromide (Baker and Tichy 1953), or carbon disulfide (Braceland 1942) has been implicated in causing the dementia syndrome.

Diagnostic Assessment

The cornerstone of diagnostic assessment of SIPD and SIPAD is a thorough clinical history and careful inquiry into potential exposures to toxic substances. Alcohol abuse, drug abuse, use of prescription and over-the-counter medications, and environmental or occupational exposures should be elicited. Past and current exposures should be sought, because permanent damage from a past episode of exposure could contribute to a current dementia syndrome. Collateral informants such as family members, caregivers, co-workers, or other physicians may be helpful in detecting sources of exposure.

A general dementia workup to identify other neurological or medical disorders that may cause dementia is of course essential. Such a workup includes standard history, physical and neurological examinations, and laboratory studies. In addition, lumbar puncture may be important if an infectious etiology or an inflammatory or demyelinating disorder such as multiple sclerosis is suspected. CT scans or MRIs are often performed to rule out space-occupying lesions or to detect infarcts or patterns associated with specific diseases such as atrophy of bilateral frontal or temporal lobe in Pick's disease (Cummings and Duchen 1981), atrophy of the caudate nucleus in Huntington's disease (Hayden et al. 1986), and enlarged ventricles in obstructive or normal-pressure hydrocephalus. Cerebral blood flow or metabolic studies (SPECT, PET, or functional MRI) may be useful in identifying vascular lesions. Electroencephalography is usually not useful, because various forms of dementia, including those that are substance induced, generally produce only nonspecific slow-wave activity. The EEG can, however, be diagnostic in certain conditions such as Creutzfeldt-Jakob disease, hepatic encephalopathy, and seizure disorders. Detailed discussion of the general dementia workup can be found in Chapter 20.

The physical, neurological, and laboratory examinations should be conducted with particular attention to findings indicative of substance exposure. Examples include the physical stigmata of alcoholism; elevated liver function tests that could indicate alcohol, other drug, or solvent exposure; red cell abnormalities such as macrocytosis in alcoholism or basophilic stippling in lead poisoning; and those neurological signs, discussed earlier in this section, that may be associated with specific substances. Measurement of blood levels of lead and other toxic chemicals should be considered. A urine toxicology screen is important for detecting drugs of abuse.

A structured mental status examination such as the Mini-Mental State Exam (Folstein et al. 1975) is often useful in documenting the initial degree of impairment and establishing a baseline against which clinical progress can be followed after removal of the offending agent(s). Neuropsychological testing usually reveals nonspecific impairment in dementia, although, again, such testing may be useful in designing rehabilitative or intervention strategies or in documenting progress with treatment.

Treatment

Management of SIPD and SIPAD requires integration of knowledge of medicine; neurology; pharmacology; cognitive, behavioral, and psychological treatments; and family dynamics. Removal of the offending agent is clearly the cornerstone of treatment for SIPD and SIPAD, and methods specific to various substances have already been alluded to in previous sections of this chapter. However, removal of the offending agent does not always bring about complete recovery. Treatment of the residual cognitive deficits is similar to the symptomatic or palliative treatment of other forms of dementia. The treatment plan may be organized according to the following outline, each step of which is discussed in the remainder of this chapter:

1. Cessation or reduction of exposure to the offending agent
2. Identification and treatment of comorbid medical, neurological, or psychiatric disorders
3. Alleviation of associated symptoms such as agitation, depression, and psychosis
4. Consideration of nootropic (cognition-enhancing) medications
5. Use of psychosocial and family interventions

Cessation or Reduction of Exposure to the Offending Agent

Addictive drugs and alcohol require detoxification to establish abstinence, followed by rehabilitative treatment to prevent relapse or, at least, to minimize subsequent use. Most alcoholic persons can cease alcohol use without undergoing significant withdrawal that would require medical treatment. However, the complications of frank alcohol withdrawal, mainly seizures and delirium tremens, are serious. The risk of serious withdrawal probably increases with duration and severity of alcohol use, and patients with SIPD or SIPAD are more likely to have histories of prolonged, heavy use. Such patients may have more difficulty giving up alcohol, and their cognitive deficits may make it harder for them to engage in the treatment effort. Finally, it has been suggested that the large quantities of cortisol released during alcohol withdrawal could have neurotoxic effects that are damaging to memory and cognition (Adinoff et al. 1991). These factors suggest that medically supervised inpatient detoxification should be considered more strongly for alcoholic patients with SIPD or SIPAD. Essential features include close monitoring for signs and symptoms of alcohol withdrawal; administration of thiamine, vitamin B_{12}, folate, and magnesium (if the latter is depleted or if there is concern about seizure risk); and substitution and tapering with cross-tolerant, long-acting sedative-hypnotics such as chlordiazepoxide, diazepam, or phenobarbital. A complete discussion of alcohol detoxification treatment may be found in Chapter 26.

Similar considerations are required for other drugs of abuse implicated in SIPD and SIPAD. Sedative-hypnotics and solvents have withdrawal syndromes resembling alcohol withdrawal, including risks of seizures and delirium, and management of withdrawal of these agents is similar to that for alcohol. Persons who abuse sedative-hypnotics may have great difficulty giving up the drugs, and inpatient treatment may be required simply to achieve compliance with detoxification. A complete discussion of sedative-hypnotic detoxification treatment may be found in Chapter 26. Cocaine withdrawal is medically benign. However, the craving, anergy, and depression of cocaine withdrawal may lead to further use, and for patients who are severely addicted, cocaine is difficult to give up. Again, inpatient treatment may be necessary to achieve initial compliance with detoxification (see Chapter 32).

Prescribed or over-the-counter drugs may be discontinued as long as either they are not essential or another effective agent can be substituted. Alternatively, a reduction in dosage may be sufficient to reverse cognitive deficits in some instances. It must be borne in mind, however, that many drugs, both psychotropic and nonpsychotropic, have withdrawal syndromes, so when the clinician is in doubt, a gradual taper, or cross-taper to another agent, is prudent.

For heavy metals and other industrial or environmental toxins, attention to the patient's environment is required to eliminate exposure to the offending agent(s). Chelation strategies are useful for heavy metal poisoning, and specific agents have been discussed earlier in this chapter in the subsections describing the heavy metals and their effects.

Identification and Treatment of Comorbid Medical, Neurological, or Psychiatric Disorders

As previously emphasized, patients with SIPD or SIPAD, particularly those who are elderly, may have other medical or neurological disorders that contribute to cognitive impairment. Some of these disorders may be treatable. Thus, a thorough dementia workup and general medical workup are essential to ensure optimum outcome. In addition to the CNS, particular attention should be paid to other organ systems that may be damaged by a particular toxin. For example, in alcoholic patients, nutritional status, vitamin deficiencies, and hepatic and cardiac status should all be evaluated. Many alcohol- and drug-abusing persons also smoke chronically and may have significant pulmonary disease. A careful review of all prescribed and over-the-counter medications is important to ensure that none of these agents is contributing to cognitive impairment.

Alleviation of Associated Symptoms

The cognitive impairment of dementia may be accompanied by other troublesome mental status changes, including agitation, insomnia, psychosis with paranoid delusions and hallucinations, and depression. There are few data on the treatment of these complications specifically in patients with alcohol- or other substance-induced dementias, and thus we are guided mainly by studies in populations with other dementing disorders (Martin et al. 1989).

Antipsychotics are commonly used to treat agitation, irritability, and psychotic symptoms (e.g., hallucinations, paranoia) accompanying dementia. Various antipsychotics have been found to be helpful, generally at doses that are low in comparison with the doses used to treat functional psychosis (Barnes et al. 1982; Rada and Kellner 1976; Raskind et al. 1987). Selection of a specific antipsychotic agent and determination of dosage are based mainly on the side-effect profile. Low doses of high-potency agents (e.g., haloperidol 0.5–2.0 mg) can be given in divided doses several times a day. Early-evening doses may lessen daytime sedation and decrease "sundowning" (i.e., insomnia with increased agitation and confusion at night). High-potency antipsychotics are also less often associated with anticholinergic and hypotensive side effects. This is important because cholinergic blockade is likely to further impair memory and cognitive functioning, and postural hypotension may be harmful when the dementia has a vascular component. The main disadvantage of high-potency antipsychotics is the increased risk of extrapyramidal side effects (i.e., dystonia, parkinsonism, neuroleptic malignant syndrome, and tardive dyskinesia). This risk is, however, moderated by the low antipsychotic doses generally sufficient to treat dementia. Low-potency antipsychotics may be useful in patients who require more sedation or in patients who are susceptible to extrapyramidal side effects. Atypical antipsychotics such as risperidone at low dosages (0.5–2.0 mg/day) seem to be especially useful for the treatment of behavioral symptoms in dementia because of their negligible anticholinergic adverse effects. The use of clozapine is limited by its anticholinergic activity, at least in dementia of the Alzheimer's and Lewy body types. However, in patients with psychosis arising from Parkinson's disease, it seems to be the drug of choice, and similar activity is likely for olanzapine. There are no published data on other newer drugs, such as sertindole, quetiapine, or ziprasidone (Stoppe et al. 1999).

Depression is a frequent clinical complication of dementia (Lazarus et al. 1987). Moreover, psychomotor retardation and pseudodementia of depression may worsen the clinical presentation of a dementia patient. Therefore, a thorough review of the psychiatric history is warranted, because depression is readily treatable and successful treatment should result in resolution of that component of cognitive impairment that is due to the pseudodementia. Antidepressant medications have been found to be effective in patients with Alzheimer's disease and vascular dementia (Greenwald et al. 1989; Reifler et al. 1989; Reynolds et al. 1987). The choice of antidepressant is based mainly on relative side-effect profiles. Patients with depression accompanied by agitation or insomnia may benefit from sedating medications such as a tricyclic antidepressant (imipramine, desipramine, or nortriptyline) or trazodone. The more anticholinergic tricyclics (e.g., amitriptyline) should be avoided because they are likely to worsen cognitive functioning (Sakulsripong et al. 1991; Thienhaus et al. 1990), although the less anticholinergic agents in the class (desipramine and nortriptyline) can also impair memory and cognition.

Preliminary findings suggest that fluoxetine may be as effective as tricylics in elderly depressed patients while producing fewer adverse effects and less cognitive impairment (Altamura and Mauri 1991; Montgomery 1989). However, its long elimination half-life suggests caution in patients with liver disease. Further, fluoxetine markedly impairs hepatic metabolism of drugs at cytochrome P450; drugs whose metabolism is impaired include prescribed and abused drugs that may cause cognitive deficits, such as tricyclic antidepressants and some benzodiazepines (Preskorn et al. 1990, 1993). Sertraline has a relatively short half-life and little tendency to impair P450 and may be preferable in patients with SIPD and SIPAD (Preskorn et al. 1990, 1993). Citalopram is another SSRI with an attractive pharmacokinetic profile for elderly patients (i.e., few side effects and a low potential for interaction with other drugs). Citalopram has shown efficacy in improving dementia-related behavioral symptoms, and preliminary evidence indicates reduction of irritability in these disorders (Flint and van Reekum 1998). Finally, the potential of SSRIs such as fluoxetine and sertraline to cause an akathisia-like syndrome with agitation must be borne in mind.

Agitation, anxiety, and sleep disturbances occur frequently in patients with dementia, and early reports suggested that benzodiazepines were useful for these symptoms (Chesrow et al. 1965; DeLamos et al. 1965). However, as reviewed earlier in this chapter, sedative-hypnotics are themselves implicated in the etiology of SIPD and SIPAD, and their adverse effects include clouding of sensorium, impairment of memory, and a disinhibition syndrome (Bixler et al. 1991; Ghoneim and Mewaldt 1990; King 1992; Rothschild 1992). Use of the benzodiazepines should therefore be limited to small doses in patients with poor tolerance of antipsychotic side effects. Patients' medications should be reviewed to identify agents that may interfere with sleep. Attention to sleep hygiene, including decreasing daytime sleep, avoiding caffeine in the afternoon and evening, and providing an environment conducive to sleep, also should be attempted by the patient before pharmacological intervention.

Consideration of Nootropic Medications

In recent years, cognition-enhancing medications (nootropics) have been extensively investigated, although their therapeutic efficacy has yet to be determined. These medications are intended to improve learning and other cognitive abilities through effects on central cholinergic and other neurotransmitter systems (Nicholson 1990). Piracetam, a cyclic GABA derivative, and several chemically related drugs (e.g., oxiracetam, anaracetam) are hypothesized to improve memory by supplementing the central cholinergic system (Ferris et al. 1982). However, Vernon and Sorkin (1991), in their review, found no clear evidence of cognition-improving effects from these agents. Studies with combined piracetam and cholinergic precursors (e.g., piracetam-lecithin, piracetam-choline) have not demonstrated cognition-enhancing effects in Alzheimer's disease patients (Davidson et al. 1987; Friedman et al. 1981). Recent studies support the use of very high dosages—up to 30 g/day—based on the benign safety profile and lack of organ toxicity shown by piracetam during its 25 years of clinical use. These studies have shown that piracetam might have a positive cytoprotective effect in brain tissue (De Reuck and Van Vleymen 1999; Goscinski et al. 1999).

NMDA receptor antagonists have therapeutic potential in many CNS disorders ranging from acute neurodegeneration (e.g., stroke and trauma) to chronic neurodegeneration (e.g., Parkinson's disease, Alzheimer's disease, Huntington's disease, amyotrophic lateral sclerosis [Lou Gehrig's disease]) to symptomatic treatment (e.g., epilepsy, Parkinson's disease, cocaine and heroin dependence, and chronic pain). However, many NMDA receptor antagonists (PCP, ketamine, dextromethorphan) also produce highly undesirable psychotomimetic side effects at doses within their putative therapeutic range. Memantine, a noncompetitive NMDA antagonist, is essentially devoid of such side effects at doses within the therapeutic range. This has been attributed to memantine's moderate potency and associated rapid, strongly voltage-dependent blocking kinetics. It stays in the channel long enough to reduce the calcium influx, preventing excitotoxicity, but not so long that it blocks calcium flow completely, interfering with normal functioning of the receptor (Parsons et al. 1999). Two double-blind studies in Europe (Ditzler 1991; Gortelmeyer and Erbler 1992) reported clinical and statistically relevant improvements with memantine in mild to moderate Alzheimer's disease with a low side-effect profile. Another placebo-controlled multicenter study (Schneider et al. 1984) with memantine, used either as monotherapy or as an adjuvant, in milder and initial forms of Parkinson's disease showed a positive statistically significant influence on tremor and on neurological overall symptomatology.

The long-acting central cholinesterase inhibitor tacrine (9-amino-1,2,3,4-tetrahydroacridine; THA) has been widely used outside the United States for its nootropic effects. Evidence suggests that THA produces a small and temporary improvement early in the course of Alzheimer's disease (Davis et al. 1992; Growdon 1992; Summers et al. 1986). The efficacy of nootropic medications in SIPD and SIPAD, however, has not been systematically studied.

Use of Psychosocial and Family Interventions

Involvement of family members is to be encouraged in the long-term management of dementia. Education and counseling about the nature of the illness should begin at the time of diagnosis. Goals include maintaining the patient's well-being and preventing further exposure to the offending neurotoxic agent. Moreover, both patient and family may benefit from supportive psychotherapy focusing on the nature of the illness; associated feelings of anger, shame, frustration, and helplessness; and ways to cope with intellectual impairment. Group therapy for family members may be located through national organizations such as the Alzheimer's Disease and Related Disorders Association.

For patients whose SIPD or SIPAD stems from substance abuse, psychosocial treatment of the alcohol or drug use disorder(s) is essential to maintain abstinence, prevent relapses, and contain relapses when they do occur so that exposure to the offending substance is at least reduced, if not eliminated. Participation in standard inpatient or outpatient rehabilitation programs and self-help groups such as Alcoholics Anonymous should be attempted. However, the cognitive impairments of SIPD or SIPAD may interfere with participation, because such programs rely heavily on psychoeducational and cognitive-behavioral techniques that require learning and memory. A more individualized treatment plan, again involving family members, may therefore be required. Treatment of substance abuse is covered in detail in Section 4 of this volume.

Conclusions

A wide array of drugs, medications, and neurotoxic chemicals can cause SIPD and SIPAD. Although most cases of SIPD and SIPAD are related to alcoholism, sedative-hypnotics, other psychotropic drugs, various nonpsychotropic drugs, drugs of abuse, solvent vapor inhalation, heavy metals, and other industrial chemicals have been implicated as well. Clinicians should be vigilant in the pursuit of substance-induced etiologies, because these represent a treatable form of dementia. In addition to the standard medical and neurological workup of dementia, thorough history taking and pursuit of clues regarding possible substance exposures are required. Prompt elimination of the offending neurotoxic agent(s) and alleviation of associated medical and psychiatric symptoms should prevent further deterioration and may improve cognitive functioning and overall well-being. This process may involve medical detoxification from alcohol and other drugs of abuse or use of chelation agents in the case of various heavy metal poisonings. As in the management of other dementia syndromes, clinicians should intervene pharmacologically, when indicated, to relieve associated symptoms. Psychosocial treatment should aim at environmental management and support of the patient's family. Appropriate rehabilitation and relapse prevention efforts are essential when SIPD or SIPAD is related to alcohol or other substance abuse.

References

Abd el Naby S, Hassanein M: Neuropsychiatric manifestations of chronic manganese poisoning. J Neurol Neurosurg Psychiatry 28:282–288, 1965

Adinoff B, Risher-Flowers D, DeJong J, et al: Disturbances of hypothalamic-pituitary-adrenal axis functioning during ethanol withdrawal in six men. Am J Psychiatry 148:1023–1025, 1991

Allen N: Solvents and other industrial organic compounds, in Handbook of Clinical Neurology, Part I, Vol 36: Intoxication of the Nervous System. Edited by Vinken PJ, Bruyn GW. New York, North-Holland, 1979, pp 361–389

Altamura AC, Mauri MC: Aspects of treatment of elderly depression: the fluoxetine experience, in The Use of Fluoxetine in Clinical Practice (International Congress and Symposium Series No 183). Edited by Freeman HL. London, Royal Society of Medicine Services, 1991, pp 53–59

Ameri A: The effects of cannabinoids on the brain. Prog Neurobiol 58:315–348, 1999

American Psychiatric Association: Diagnostic and Statistical Manual of Mental Disorders, 4th Edition. Washington, DC, American Psychiatric Association, 1994

Baker AB, Tichy FY: The effects of the organic solvents and industrial poisonings on the central nervous system, in Metabolic and Toxic Diseases of the Nervous System (Association for Research in Nervous and Mental Disease, Vol 32). Baltimore, MD, William & Wilkins, 1953, pp 475–505

Barnes R, Veith R, Okimoto J, et al: Efficacy of antipsychotic medications in behaviorally disturbed dementia patients. Am J Psychiatry 139:1170–1174, 1982

Bixler EO, Kales A, Manfredi RL, et al: Next-day memory impairment with triazolam use. Lancet 337(8745):827–831, 1991

Blazer DG, Federspiel CF, Ray WA, et al: The risk of anticholinergic toxicity in the elderly: a study of prescribing practice in two populations. J Gerontol 38:31–35, 1983

Bolla KI, McCann UD, Ricaurte GA: Memory impairment in abstinent MDMA ("Ecstasy") users. Neurology 51:1532–1537, 1998

Borison RL: The role of cognition in the risk-benefit and safety analysis of antipsychotic medication. Acta Psychiatr Scand Suppl 389:5–11, 1996

Boyd PR, Walker G, Henderson IN: The treatment of tetraethyl lead poisoning. Lancet 1:181–185, 1957

Braceland FJ: Mental symptoms following carbon disulfide absorption and intoxication. Ann Intern Med 16:246–261, 1942

Brandt J, Butters N, Ryan C, et al: Cognitive loss and recovery in long-term alcohol abusers. Arch Gen Psychiatry 40:435–442, 1983

Brenner RP, Snyder RD: Late EEG findings and clinical status after organic mercurial poisoning. Arch Neurol 37:282–284, 1980

Brown ES, Rush AJ, McEwen BS: Hippocampal remodeling and damage by corticosteroids: implications for mood disorders. Neuropsychopharmacology 21:474–484, 1999

Byers RK: Lead poisoning: review of the literature and report on 45 cases. Pediatrics 23:585–603, 1959

Carlen PL, Wortzman G, Holgate RC, et al: Reversible atrophy in recently abstinent chronic alcoholics measured by computed tomography scans. Science 200:1076–1078, 1978

Carlen PL, Wilkinson A, Wortzman G, et al: Cerebral atrophy and functional deficits in alcoholics without clinically apparent liver disease. Neurology 31:377–385, 1981

Charness ME: Brain lesions in alcoholics. Alcohol Clin Exp Res 17:2–11, 1993

Chesrow EJ, Kaplitz SE, Vetra H, et al: Double-blind study of oxazepam in the management of geriatric patients with behavioral problems. Clin Med 72:1001–1005, 1965

Cook DJ, Fahn S, Brait KA: Chronic manganese intoxication. Arch Neurol 30:59–64, 1974

Cosgrove J, Newell TG: Recovery of neuropsychological functions during reduction in use of phencyclidine. J Clin Psychol 47:159–169, 1991

Cummings JL, Benson DF: Dementia: A Clinical Approach, 2nd Edition. Boston, MA, Butterworth-Heinemann, 1992

Cummings JL, Duchen LW: Kluver-Bucy syndrome in Pick disease: clinical and pathologic correlations. Neurology 31:1415–1422, 1981

Curran HV: Memory functions, alertness and mood of long-term benzodiazepine users: a preliminary investigation of the effects of a normal daily dose. J Psychopharmacol 6:69–75, 1992

Cutting J: Alcoholic dementia, in Psychiatric Aspects of Neurologic Disease, Vol 2. Edited by Benson DF, Blumer D. New York, Grune & Stratton, 1982, pp 149–164

Davidson M, Mohs RC, Hollander E, et al: Lecithin and piracetam in patients with Alzheimer's disease. Biol Psychiatry 22:112–114, 1987

Davis KL, Thal LJ, Gamzu ER, et al: A double blind, placebo-controlled multicenter study of tacrine for Alzheimer's disease: the Tacrine Collaborative Study Group. N Engl J Med 327:1253–1259, 1992

DeLamos GP, Clements WR, Nickels E: Effects of diazepam suspension in geriatric patients hospitalized for psychiatric illness. Am J Geriatr Soc 13:355–359, 1965

De Reuck J, Van Vleymen B: The clinical safety of high-dose piracetam—its use in the treatment of acute stroke. Pharmacopsychiatry 32 (suppl 1):33–37, 1999

De Silva PE, Christophers AJ: Lead exposure and children's intelligence: do low levels of lead in blood cause mental deficit? J Paediatr Child Health 33:12–17, 1997

Ditzler K: Efficacy and tolerability of memantine in patients with dementia syndrome: a double-blind, placebo controlled trial. Arzneimittelforschung 41:773–780, 1991

Ehrenreich H, Rinn T, Kunert HJ, et al: Specific attentional dysfunction in adults following early start of cannabis use. Psychopharmacology (Berl) 142:295–301, 1999

Elliott HL, Macdougall AI: Aluminum studies in dialysis encephalopathy. Proceedings of the European Dialysis and Transplant Association 15:157–163, 1978

Fein G, Biggins CA, MacKay S: Alcohol abuse and HIV infection have additive effects on frontal cortex function as measured by auditory evoked potential P3A latency. Biol Psychiatry 37:183–195, 1995

Feldman RG, Cummings JL: Treatable dementia, in Geriatric Neurology. Edited by Slade WR Jr. New York, Futura, 1981, pp 173–197

Ferris SH, Reisberg B, Crook T, et al: Pharmacologic treatment of senile dementia: cholin, L-DOPA, piracetam, and cholin plus piracetam, in Alzheimer's Disease: A Report of Progress in Research. Edited by Corkin S, Davis KL, Growdon JH, et al. New York, Raven, 1982, pp 475–481

Fiala AM, Gan XH, Newton T, et al: Divergent effects of cocaine on cytokine production by lymphocytes and monocyte/macrophages: HIV-1 enhancement by cocaine within the blood-brain barrier. Adv Exp Med Biol 402:145–156, 1996

Fiala M, Gan XH, Zhang L, et al: Cocaine enhances monocyte migration across the blood-brain barrier: cocaine's connection to AIDS dementia and vasculitis. Adv Exp Med Biol 437:199–205, 1998

Fieve RR, Platman S: Lithium and thyroid function in manic-depressive psychosis. Am J Psychiatry 125:527–530, 1968

Filley CM, Heaton RK, Rosenberg NL: White matter dementia in chronic toluene abuse. Neurology 40:532–534, 1990

Finlayson RE, Hurt RD, Davis LJ Jr, et al: Alcoholism in elderly persons: a study of psychiatric and psychosocial features of 216 inpatients. Mayo Clin Proc 63:761–768, 1988

Flint AJ, van Reekum R: The pharmacologic treatment of Alzheimer's disease: a guide for the general psychiatrist. Can J Psychiatry 43:689–697, 1998

Folstein MF, Folstein SE, McHugh PR: "Mini-Mental State": a practical method for grading the cognitive state of patients for the clinician. J Psychiatr Res 12:189–198, 1975

Foncin JF, Gruner JE: Tin toxicity, in Handbook of Clinical Neurology, Part I, Vol 36: Intoxication of the Nervous System. Edited by Vinken PJ, Bruyn GW. New York, North-Holland, 1979, pp 279–290

Freeman FR: Evaluation of patients with progressive intellectual deterioration. Arch Neurol 33:658–659, 1976

Freeman JW, Couch JR: Prolonged encephalopathy with arsenic poisoning. Neurology 28:853–855, 1978

Friedman E, Sherman KA, Ferris SH, et al: Clinical response to choline plus piracetam in senile dementia: relation to red-cell choline level. N Engl J Med 304:1490–1491, 1981

Gan X, Zhang L, Berger O, et al: Cocaine enhances brain endothelial adhesion molecules and leukocyte migration. Clin Immunol 91:68–76, 1999

Gellert GA, Wagner GA, Maxwell RM, et al: Lead poisoning among low-income children in Orange County, California. JAMA 270:69–71, 1993

Ghoneim MM, Mewaldt SP: Benzodiazepines and human memory: a review. Anesthesiology 72:926–938, 1990

Goetz CG, Klawans HL: Neurologic aspects of other metals, in Handbook of Clinical Neurology, Part I, Vol 36: Intoxication of the Nervous System. Edited by Vinken PJ, Bruyn GW. New York, North-Holland, 1979, pp 319–345

Goetz CG, Klawans HL, Cohen MM: Neurotoxic agents, in Clinical Neurology. Edited by Baker AB, Baker LH. New York, Harper & Row, 1981, pp 1–84

Goodkin K, Shapshak P, Metsch LR, et al: Cocaine abuse and HIV-1 infection: epidemiology and neuropathogenesis. J Neuroimmunol 83(1–2):88–101, 1998

Gordon RA, Roberts G, Amin Z, et al: Aggressive approach in the treatment of acute lead encephalopathy with an extraordinarily high concentration of lead. Arch Pediatr Adolesc Med 152:1100–1104, 1998

Gortelmeyer R, Erbler H: Memantine in the treatment of mild to moderate dementia syndrome: a double-blind placebo-controlled study. Arzneimittelforschung 42:904–913, 1992

Goscinski I, Moskala M, Cichonski J: Clinical observations concerning piracetam treatment of patients after craniocerebral injury. Przegl Lek 56(2):119–120, 1999

Granacher RP, Baldessarini RJ: Physostigmine: its use in acute anticholinergic syndrome with antidepressant and antiparkinson drugs. Arch Gen Psychiatry 32:375–380, 1975

Grant I, Judd LL: Neuropsychological and EEG disturbances in poly drug users. Am J Psychiatry 133: 1039–1042, 1976

Grant I, Mohns L, Miller M, et al: A neuropsychological study of polydrug users. Arch Gen Psychiatry 33:973–978, 1976

Grant I, Adams KM, Reed R: Aging, abstinence, and medical risk factors in the prediction of neuropsychologic deficit among long term alcoholics. Arch Gen Psychiatry 41:710–718, 1984

Greenwald BS, Kramer-Ginsberg E, Marin DB, et al: Dementia with coexistent major depression. Am J Psychiatry 146:1472–1478, 1989

Growdon JH: Treatment for Alzheimer's disease? N Engl J Med 327:1306–1308, 1992

Hart RP, Rose CS, Hamer RM: Neuropsychological effects of occupational exposure to cadmium. J Clin Exp Neuropsychol 11:933–943, 1989

Hartman DE: Neuropsychological Toxicology. New York, Pergamon, 1988

Hayden MR, Martin AJ, Stoessl AJ, et al: Positron emission tomography in the early diagnosis of Huntington's disease. Neurology 36:888–894, 1986

Herning RI, Glover BJ, Koeppl B: Cognitive deficits in abstaining cocaine abusers (NIDA Research Monograph 101). Rockville, MD, National Institute on Drug Abuse, 1990, pp 167–178

Heston LL, Mastri AR: Age of onset of Pick's and Alzheimer's dementia: implications for diagnosis and research. J Gerontol 37:422–424, 1982

Hofman A, Rocca WA, Brayne C, et al: The prevalence of dementia in Europe: a collaborative study of 1980–1990 findings. Eurodem Prevalence Research Group. Int J Epidemiol 20:736–748, 1991

Hollister LE: Psychotherapeutic drugs, in Neuropsychiatric Side Effects of Drugs in the Elderly. Edited by Levenson AJ. New York, Raven, 1979, pp 79–88

Holman BL, Garada B, Johnson KA, et al: A comparison of brain perfusion SPECT in cocaine abuse and AIDS dementia complex. J Nucl Med 33:1312–1315, 1992

Hormes JT, Filley CM, Rosenberg NL: Neurologic sequelae of chronic solvent vapor abuse. Neurology 36:698–702, 1986

Hudak A, Naray M, Nagy I, et al: The favorable effect of humic acid based complex micro-element in cadmium exposure. Orv Hetil 138(22):1411–1416, 1997

Hutton JT: Results of clinical assessment for the dementia syndrome: implications for epidemiologic studies, in The Epidemiology of Dementia. Edited by Mortimer JA, Schuman LM. New York, Oxford University Press, 1981, pp 62–69

Insausti R, Insausti AM, Sobreviela MT, et al: Human medial temporal lobe in aging: anatomical basis of memory preservation. Microsc Res Tech 43:8–15, 1998

Ironside R, Bosanquet FD, McMenemy WH: Central demyelination of the corpus callosum (Marchiafava-Bignami disease). Brain 84:212–230, 1961

Ishii K, Ikerjiri Y, Sasaki M, et al: Regional cerebral glucose metabolism and blood flow in Marchiafava-Bignami disease. AJNR Am J Neuroradiol 20:1249–1251, 1999

Iversen SD: The pharmacology of memory. C R Acad Sci III 321(2–3):209–215, 1998

Jenkins RB: Inorganic arsenic and nervous system. Brain 89:479–498, 1966

Jentsch JD, Verrico CD, Le D, et al: Repeated exposure to delta 9-tetrahydrocannabinol reduces prefrontal cortical dopamine metabolism in the rat. Neurosci Lett 246:169–172, 1998

Jorm AF, Korten AE, Henderson AS: The prevalence of dementia: a quantitative integration of the literature. Acta Psychiatr Scand 76:465–479, 1987

Judd LL, Grant I: Intermediate duration organic mental disorder among poly drug abusing patients. Psychiatr Clin North Am 1:153–167, 1978

Kalynchuk LE, Beck CH: Behavioral analysis of diazepam-induced memory deficits: evidence for sedation-like effects. Psychopharmacology (Berl) 106:297–302, 1992

Kark RAP: Clinical and neurochemical aspects of inorganic mercury intoxication, in Handbook of Clinical Neurology, Part I, Vol 36: Intoxication of the Nervous System. Edited by Vinken PJ, Bruyn GW. New York, North-Holland, 1979, pp 147–197

Kajimura N, Mizuki Y, Kai S, et al: Memory and cognitive impairments in a case of long-term trihexyphenidyl abuse. Pharmacopsychiatry 26:59–62, 1993

King DJ: Benzodiazepines, amnesia and sedation: theoretical and clinical issues and controversies. Human Psychopharmacology: Clinical and Experimental 7(2):79–87, 1992

Kocsis JH, Shaw ED, Stokes PE, et al: Neuropsychologic effects of lithium discontinuation. J Clin Psychopharmacol 13:268–275, 1993

Lazarus LW, Newton N, Cohler B, et al: Frequency and presentation of depressive symptoms in patients with primary degenerative dementia. Am J Psychiatry 144:41–45, 1987

Lechevalier B, Andersson JC, Morin P: Hemispheric disconnection syndrome with a "crossed-avoiding" reaction in a case of Marchiafava-Bignami disease. J Neurol Neurosurg Psychiatry 40:483–497, 1977

Lee K, Moller L, Hardt F, et al: Alcohol induced brain damage and liver damage in young males. Lancet 2:759–761, 1979

Lhermitte F, Marteau R, Serdaru M, et al: Signs of interhemispheric disconnection in Marchiafava-Bignami disease. Arch Neurol 34:254, 1977

Lindberg MC, Oyler RA: Wernicke's encephalopathy. Am Fam Physician 41:1205–1209, 1990

Lindgren M, Osterberg K, Orbaek P, et al: Solvent-induced toxic encephalopathy: electrophysiological data in relation to neuropsychological findings. J Clin Exp Neuropsychol 19:772–783, 1997

Lishman WA: Cerebral disorder in alcoholism: syndrome of impairment. Brain 104:1–20, 1981

Lishman WA: Alcohol and the brain. Br J Psychiatry 156:635–644, 1990

London ED, Cascella NG, Wong DF, et al: Cocaine-induced reduction of glucose utilization in human brain. Arch Gen Psychiatry 47:567–574, 1990

Lupien SJ, de Leon M, de Santi S, et al: Cortisol levels during human aging predict hippocampal atrophy and memory deficits. Nature Neuroscience 1(1):69–73, 1998

Maletta GJ, Pirozzolo FT, Thompson G, et al: Organic mental disorders in geriatric outpatient population. Am J Psychiatry 139:521–523, 1982

Manschreck TC, Schneyer ML, Weisstein CC, et al: Freebase cocaine and memory. Compr Psychiatry 31:369–375, 1990

Marchesi C, Chiodera P, Brusamonti E: Abnormal plasma oxytocin and beta-endorphin levels in alcoholics after short and long term abstinence. Prog Neuropsychopharmacol Biol Psychiatry 21: 797–807, 1997

Marsden CD, Harrison MJG: Outcome of investigation of patients with presenile dementia. BMJ 2:249–252, 1972

Marsh DO: Organic mercury: methyl mercury compounds, in Handbook of Clinical Neurology, Part I, Vol 36: Intoxication of the Nervous System. Edited by Vinken PJ, Bruyn GW. New York, North-Holland, 1979, pp 73–81

Martin PR, Eckardt MJ, Linnoila M: Treatment of chronic organic mental disorders associated with alcoholism. Recent Dev Alcohol 7:329–350, 1989

Martin PR, Adinoff B, Lane E, et al: Fluvoxamine treatment of alcoholic amnestic disorder. Eur Neuropsychopharmacol 5:27–33, 1995

Marumo F, Li JP: Renal disease and trace elements. Nippon Rinsho 54:93–98, 1996

Matsuda K, Yamaji S, Ishii K: Regional cerebral blood flow and oxygen metabolism in a patient with Korsakoff syndrome. Ann Nucl Med 11:33–35, 1997

McAuley DLF, Lecky BRF, Earl CJ: Gold encephalopathy. J Neurol Neurosurg Psychiatry 40:1021–1022, 1977

McCann UD, Mertl M, Eligulashvili V, et al: Cognitive performance in (+/-) 3,4-methylenedioxymethamphetamine (MDMA, "Ecstasy") users: a controlled study. Psychopharmacology (Berl) 143: 417–425, 1999

Meaney MJ, Aitken DH, Bhatnagar S, et al: Postnatal handling attenuates certain neuroendocrine, anatomical, and cognitive dysfunctions associated with aging in female rats. Neurobiol Aging 12: 31–38, 1991

Mena I: Manganese poisoning, in Handbook of Clinical Neurology, Part I, Vol 36: Intoxication of the Nervous System. Edited by Vinken PJ, Bruyn GW. New York, North-Holland, 1979, pp 217–237

Meyerhoff DJ, MacKay S, Sappey-Marinier D, et al: Effects of chronic alcohol abuse and HIV infection on brain phosphorus metabolites. Alcohol Clin Exp Res 19:685–692, 1995

Mikkelsen S: Epidemiological update on solvent neurotoxicity. Environ Res 73:101–112, 1997

Miller L: Neuropsychological assessment of substance abusers: review and recommendations. J Subst Abuse Treat 2:5–17, 1985

Miller NS, Belkin BM, Gold MS: Alcohol and drug dependence among the elderly: epidemiology, diagnosis, and treatment. Compr Psychiatry 32:153–165, 1991

Montgomery SA: The efficacy of fluoxetine as an antidepressant in the short and long term. Int Clin Psychopharmacol 4 (suppl 1):113–119, 1989

Morgan MJ: Memory deficits associated with recreational use of "ecstasy" (MDMA). Psychopharmacology (Berl) 141:30–36, 1999

Moses AM, Miller M: Drug-induced dilutional hyponatremia. N Engl J Med 291:1234–1238, 1974

Murray RM, Greene JG, Adams JH: Analgesic abuse and dementia. Lancet 2:242–245, 1971

Nakada T, Knight RT: Alcohol and central nervous system. Med Clin North Am 68:121–131, 1984

Namba T, Nolte CT, Jackrel J, et al: Poisoning due to organophosphate insecticides. Am J Med 50:475–492, 1971

Navarro JF, Noriega S: Marchiafava-Bignami disease. Rev Neurol 28:519–523, 1999

Newman SE: The EEG manifestations of chronic ethanol abuse: relation to cerebral cortical atrophy. Ann Neurol 3:299–304, 1978

Nicholson CD: Pharmacology of nootropics and metabolically active compounds in relation to their use in dementia. Psychopharmacology (Berl) 101:147–159, 1990

O'Malley S, Adamse M, Heaton RK, et al: Neuropsychological impairment in chronic cocaine abusers. Am J Drug Alcohol Abuse 18:131–144, 1992

Oslin D, Smith DM, Atkinson RM: Alcohol related dementia: proposed clinical criteria. Int J Geriatr Psychiatry 13:203–212, 1998

Page RD, Linden JD: "Reversible" organic brain syndrome in alcoholics. J Stud Alcohol 35:98–107, 1974

Pal PK, Samii A, Calne DB: Manganese neurotoxicity: a review of clinical features, imaging and pathology. Neurotoxicology 20:227–238, 1999

Parrott AC, Lasky J: Ecstasy (MDMA) effects upon mood and cognition: before, during and after a Saturday night dance. Psychopharmacology (Berl) 139:261–268, 1998

Parsons CG, Danysz W, Quack G: Memantine is a clinically well tolerated N-methyl-D-aspartate (NMDA) receptor antagonist—a review of preclinical data. Neuropharmacology 38:735–767, 1999

Pearlson GD, Jeffery PJ, Harris GJ, et al: Correlation of acute cocaine-induced changes in local cerebral blood flow with subjective effects. Am J Psychiatry 150:495–497, 1993

Perlstein MA, Attala R: Neurologic sequelae of plumbism in children. Clin Pediatr 5:292–298, 1966

Petrie W, Ban T, Berncy S, et al: Loxapine in psychogeriatrics: a placebo and standard controlled clinical investigation. J Clin Psychopharmacol 2:122–126, 1982

Pfefferbaum A, Lim KO, Desmond JE: Thinning of the corpus callosum in older alcoholic men: a magnetic resonance imaging study. Alcohol Clin Exp Res 20:752–757, 1996

Preskorn SH, Beber JH, Faul JC, et al: Serious adverse effects of combining fluoxetine and tricyclic antidepressants (letter). Am J Psychiatry 147:532, 1990

Preskorn SH, von Moltke L, Alderman J, et al: In vitro and in vivo evaluations of the potential for desipramine interaction with fluoxetine or sertraline (NR673), in 1993 New Research Program and Abstracts, 146th annual meeting of the American Psychiatric Association, San Francisco, CA, May 1993, p 229

Prick JJG: Thallium poisoning, in Handbook of Clinical Neurology, Part I, Vol 36: Intoxication of the Nervous System. Edited by Vinken PJ, Bruyn GW. New York, North-Holland, 1979, pp 239–278

Prockop L: Neurotoxic volatile substances. Neurology 29:862–865, 1979

Rabins PV: The prevalence of reversible dementia in psychiatric hospital. Hospital and Community Psychiatry 32:490–492, 1981

Rada RT, Kellner R: Thiothixene in the treatment of geriatric patients with chronic organic brain syndrome. J Am Geriatr Soc 24:105–107, 1976

Raskind MA, Risse SC, Lampe TH: Dementia and antipsychotic drugs. J Clin Psychiatry 48 (suppl 5):16–18, 1987

Reed D, Crawley J, Faro SN, et al: Thallotoxicosis. JAMA 183:516–522, 1963

Reifler BV, Teri L, Raskind M, et al: Double-blind trial of imipramine in Alzheimer's disease patients with and without depression. Am J Psychiatry 146:45–49, 1989

Reuler JB, Girard DE, Cooney TG: Wernicke's encephalopathy. N Engl J Med 312:1035–1039, 1985

Reynolds CF, Perel JM, Kupfer DJ, et al: Open-trial response to antidepressant treatment in elderly patients with mixed depression and cognitive impairment. Psychiatry Res 21:111–122, 1987

Ron MA: Volatile substance abuse: a review of possible long-term neurological, intellectual and psychiatric sequelae. Br J Psychiatry 148:235–246, 1986

Rosenberg NL, Kleinschmidt-DeMasters BK, Davis KA, et al: Toluene abuse causes diffuse central nervous system white matter changes. Ann Neurol 23:611–614, 1988

Rothschild AJ: Disinhibition, amnestic reactions, and adverse reactions secondary to triazolam: a review of the literature. J Clin Psychiatry 53 (suppl):69–79, 1992

Rounsaville BJ, Novelly RA, Kleber HD: Neuropsychological impairment in opiate addicts: risk factors. Ann N Y Acad Sci 362:79–90, 1981

Ruff HA, Bijur PE, Markowitz M, et al: Declining blood lead levels and cognitive changes in moderately lead-poisoned children. JAMA 269:1641–1646, 1993

Ryu YH, Lee JD, Yoon PH, et al: Cerebral perfusion impairment in a patient with toluene abuse. J Nucl Med 39:632–633, 1998

Sachs H, Russell JAG, Christman DR, et al: Alteration of regional cerebral glucose metabolic rate in non-Kosakoff chronic alcoholism. Arch Neurol 44:1242–1251, 1987

Sagel J, Matisonn R: Neuropsychiatric disturbance as the initial manifestation of digitalis toxicity. S Afr Med J 46:512–514, 1972

Sakulsripong M, Curran HV, Lader M: Does tolerance develop to the sedative and amnestic effects of antidepressants? A comparison of amitriptyline, trazodone and placebo. Eur J Clin Pharmacol 40:43–48, 1991

Saric M, Markicevic A, Hrustic O: Occupational exposure to manganese. Br J Ind Med 34:114–118, 1977

Scheinberg P: Dementia due to vascular disease: a multifactorial disorder. Stroke 19:1291–1298, 1988

Schneider E, Fischer PA, Clemens R, et al: Effects of oral memantine administration on Parkinson symptoms: results of a placebo-controlled multicenter study. Dtsch Med Wochenschr 109:987–990, 1984

Schulte PA, Burnett CA, Boeniger MF, et al: Neurodegenerative diseases: occupational occurrence and potential risk factors, 1982 through 1991. Am J Public Health 86:1281–1288, 1996

Shafey S, Scheinberg P: Neurological syndromes occurring in patients receiving synthetic steroids (oral contraceptives). Neurology 16:205–211, 1966

Shaikh ZA, Tang W: Protection against chronic cadmium toxicity by glycine. Toxicology 132:139–146, 1999

Shapshak P, Crandall KA, Xin KQ, et al: HIV-1 neuropathogenesis and abused drugs: current reviews, problems, and solutions. Adv Exp Med Biol 402:171–186, 1996

Shopsin B, Johnson G, Gershon S: Neurotoxicity with lithium: differential drug responsiveness. Int Pharmacopsychiatry 5:170–182, 1970

Smith DM, Atkinson RM: Alcoholism and dementia. Int J Addict 30:1843–1869, 1995

Smith JS, Kiloh LG: The investigation of dementia: result of 200 consecutive admissions. Lancet 1:824–827, 1981

Solomon S, Hotchkiss E, Saravay SM, et al: Impairment of memory function by antihypertensive medication. Arch Gen Psychiatry 40:1109–1112, 1983

Starace F, Baldassarre C, Biancolilli V, et al: Early neuropsychological impairment in HIV-seropositive intravenous drug users: evidence from the Italian Multicentre Neuropsychological HIV Study. Acta Psychiatr Scand 97:132–138, 1998

Stoppe G, Brandt CA, Staedt JH: Behavioural problems associated with dementia: the role of newer antipsychotics. Drugs Aging 14:41–54, 1999

Summers WK, Majovski LV, Marsh GM, et al: Oral tetrahydro-aminoacridine in long term treatment of senile dementia, Alzheimer's type. N Engl J Med 315:1241–1245, 1986

Swindells S, Zheng J, Gendelman HE: HIV-associated dementia: new insights into disease pathogenesis and therapeutic interventions. Aids Patient Care STDS 13:153–163, 1999

Thal LJ: Dementia update: diagnosis and neuropsychiatric aspects. J Clin Psychiatry 49 (suppl 5):5–7, 1988

Thienhaus OJ, Allen A, Bennett JA, et al: Anticholinergic serum levels and cognitive performance. European Archives of Psychiatry and Neurological Sciences 240:28–33, 1990

Thomson AD, Cook CC: Parenteral thiamine and Wernicke's encephalopathy: the balance of risks and perception of concern. Alcohol Alcohol 32:207–209, 1997

Thornton WE: Dementia induced by methyldopa and haloperidol. N Engl J Med 294:1222, 1976

Tombaugh GC, Sapolsky RM: Endocrine features of glucocorticoid endangerment in hippocampal astrocytes. Neuroendocrinology 57:7–13, 1993

Tomlinson BE, Blessed G, Roth M: Observations on the brains of demented old people. J Neurol Sci 11:205–242, 1970

Tomlinson BE, Pierides AM, Bradley WG: Central pontine myelinolysis. Q J Med 45:373–386, 1976

Tremont G, Stern RA: Use of thyroid hormone to diminish the cognitive side effects of psychiatric treatment. Psychopharmacol Bull 33:273–280, 1997

Trimble MR, Reynolds EH: Anticonvulsant drugs and mental symptoms: a review. Psychol Med 6:169–178, 1976

Tyor WR, Middaugh LD: Do alcohol and cocaine abuse alter the course of HIV-associated dementia complex? J Leukoc Biol 65:475–481, 1999

Van Putten T, Mutalipassi LR, Malkin MD: Phenothiazine-induced decompensation. Arch Gen Psychiatry 30:102–105, 1974

Vernon MW, Sorkin EM: Piracetam: an overview of its pharmacological properties and a review of its therapeutic use in senile cognitive disorders. Drugs Aging 1:17–35, 1991

Volkow ND, Mullani N, Gould KL, et al: Cerebral blood flow in chronic cocaine users: a study with PET. Br J Psychiatry 152:641–648, 1988

Vroom FQ, Greer M: Mercury vapor intoxication. Brain 95:305–318, 1972

Westermeyer J: The psychiatrist and solvent-inhalant abuse: recognition, assessment, and treatment. Am J Psychiatry 144:903–907, 1987

Whelan TB, Schteingart DE, Starkman MN, et al: Neuropsychological deficits in Cushing's syndrome. J Nerv Ment Dis 168:753–757, 1980

Wolkowitz OM, Reus VI, Canick J, et al: Glucocorticoid medication, memory and steroid psychosis in medical illness. Ann N Y Acad Sci 823:81–96, 1997

24

Amnestic Disorder Due to a General Medical Condition and Amnestic Disorder Not Otherwise Specified

William J. Burke, M.D.
Daryl L. Bohac, Ph.D.

The amnestic disorders are not frequently encountered clinically.[1] When amnestic disorders do occur, however, they assume great clinical importance because of their effect on the individual. Persons with deficits in memory are typically disabled by their condition and may spend years of their life in a dependent role. One of the most famous patients with an amnestic disorder is "H.M.," who underwent bilateral medial temporal lobe resection for the treatment of severe epilepsy (Milner 1959; Milner et al. 1968). As a result of his operation, H.M. developed difficulty recalling some events of the past but an

[1]The study of amnestic disorders has provided crucial insights into the organization and functioning of memory. Investigation of patients with selective deficits in memory has led to the recognition of the diencephalon and the medial temporal lobe as critical areas for the processing and storage of those internal and external events called *memories*.

even more severe inability to make new memories. Because of his severe amnesia, he was said to have felt as if he were continuously waking from a dream. He would feel the events of the preceding moments slipping away from him even as he attempted to grasp at them. The case of H.M. also highlights the relatedness of the concepts of memory and learning. Learning can be seen as the process of acquiring new information, whereas memory is the persistence of learning in such a way that it can be used at a later time. As Squire (1987) noted, "memory is the usual consequence of learning" (p. 3).

The attempt to arrive at suitable, effective treatment for the amnestic disorders has been a slow and arduous journey. In this chapter, some of these efforts are reviewed. First, however, an overview of the diagnostic criteria for the amnestic disorders and discussion of some of the medical conditions that can produce amnesia are presented.

Definitions and Diagnostic Criteria

The essence of the amnestic disorders is an acquired memory deficit. This memory deficit is not the result of a developmental process but rather the result of some insult to the central nervous system (CNS). For a diagnosis of amnestic disorder to be made, the amnesia must have functional relevance and thus must cause a loss in social or occupational abilities.

The amnestic disorders, deliriums, and dementias all involve a deficit in memory. The dementias, however, feature impaired ability to learn new information *and* reduced ability to freely recall previously learned information, whereas the amnestic disorders can be diagnosed on the basis of a deficit in either realm. Also, the amnestic disorders, unlike the dementias, are not characterized by signs of impairment of other cognitive faculties, such as language, visuospatial abilities, attention, or reasoning ability. A person with an amnestic disorder typically is alert, has a normal level of consciousness, and is able to focus, maintain, and shift attention. This last feature distinguishes the amnestic disorders from the deliriums, in which the key feature is a disturbance in consciousness that tends to develop over a short time and to fluctuate throughout the course of the day.

When a general medical condition is judged to be etiologically linked to the amnesia, the category of *amnestic disorder due to a general medical condition* is used. The duration of the disturbance in memory is specified as *transient* (i.e., lasting 1 month or less) or *chronic* (i.e., lasting longer than 1 month). The DSM-IV (American Psychiatric Association 1994) criteria for amnestic disorder due to a general medical condition are given in Table 24–1. When no definite etiology can be imputed, the category of *amnestic disorder not otherwise specified* (NOS) is selected. DSM-IV specifies that "this category should be used to diagnose an amnestic disorder that does not meet criteria for any of the specific types [of amnestic disorders]" (American Psychiatric Association 1994, p. 163). When the etiology is thought to be secondary to the use of a substance, *substance-induced persisting amnestic disorder* is diagnosed. (For discussion of this disorder, see Chapter 23.) When the amnesia is thought to have a dissociative etiology, the diagnosis of *dissociative amnesia* should be used.

Epidemiology

Amnestic disorder due to a general medical condition is uncommon, and, as such, little is known about the incidence and prevalence of this condition.

TABLE 24–1. DSM-IV diagnostic criteria for amnestic disorder due to a general medical condition

A. The development of memory impairment as manifested by impairment in the ability to learn new information or the inability to recall previously learned information.

B. The memory disturbance causes significant impairment in social or occupational functioning and represents a significant decline from a previous level of functioning.

C. The memory disturbance does not occur exclusively during the course of a delirium or a dementia.

D. There is evidence from the history, physical examination, or laboratory findings that the disturbance is the direct physiological consequence of a general medical condition (including physical trauma).

Specify if:

Transient: if memory impairment lasts for 1 month or less

Chronic: if memory impairment lasts for more than 1 month

Coding note: Include the name of the general medical condition on Axis I, e.g., 294.0 amnestic disorder due to head trauma; also code the general medical condition on Axis III (see Appendix G for codes).

Etiology

Amnestic disorder, implying a complete loss of memory, is a misnomer. The person with an amnestic disorder instead has *dysmnesia,* that is, a difficulty recalling certain kinds of memories. To appreciate this difference, the organization of memory first must be discussed. Among the many possible ways to categorize the various processes lumped under the rubric of "memory," one of the most useful is to begin with the distinction between memory that is accessible to consciousness and that which is not. These types of memory have been referred to as *declarative (explicit) memory,* which can be brought to conscious recollection, and *nondeclarative (implicit) memory,* which is expressed and detected through performance rather than conscious recall (Zola-Morgan and Squire 1990a). Declarative memory includes memory for facts (semantic memory) and events (episodic memory), whereas nondeclarative memory includes a number of abilities such as priming, simple classical conditioning, nonassociative learning, and certain skills and habits (Squire and Zola-Morgan 1991) (Figure 24–1).

A further useful way to categorize memory is based on the recency of that which is remembered. Thus, *short-term (immediate) memory* refers to recall of material immediately after it is presented (Delis 1993). This system is finite in capacity and generally is tested by asking the person to recall a series of digits. The model of immediate memory was further expanded by Baddeley (1986) when he introduced the concept of *working memory.* Working memory generally refers to the ability to temporarily hold and manipulate information, in contrast to the more passive concept of simple short-term storage. For example, looking up the name and telephone number of a bookstore, dialing that number, and remembering why one is calling the bookstore is a case in which working memory is activated. This is different from passive short-term memory, in which a series of digits is read to the patient and then he or she is asked to immediately repeat the digits. This distinction is important in that it may have neuroanatomical implications. *Long-term memory* includes information that is recalled after a delay period. It is believed to have a very large capacity (Delis 1993). It is important to note that "short-term" memory means very different things in various classifications, with many schemes counting information recalled after a few minutes as "short-term" memory.

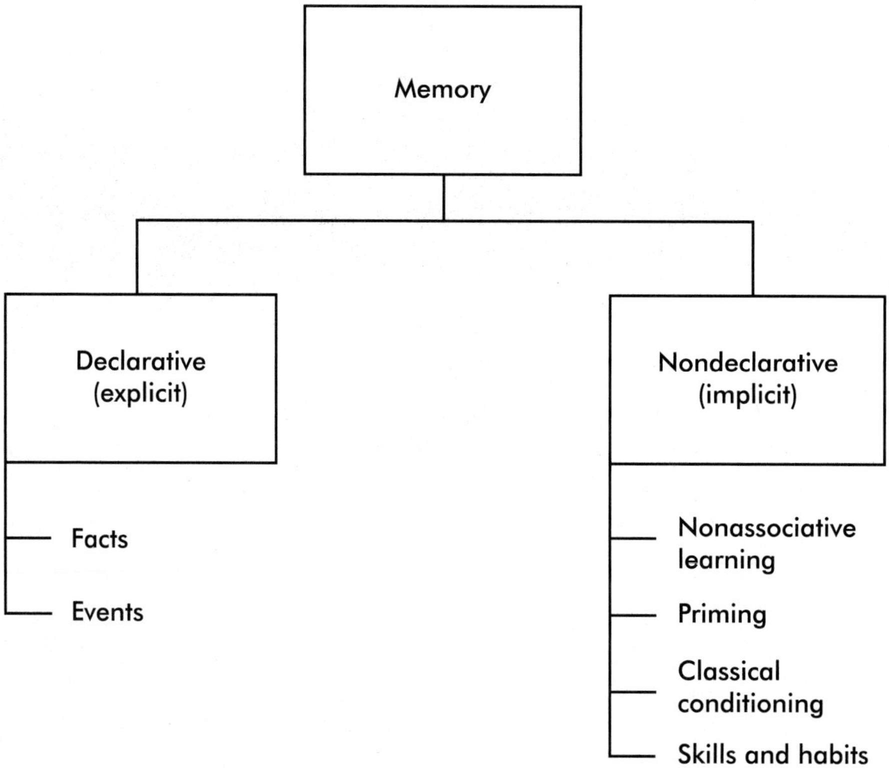

FIGURE 24–1. Classification of memory.
Source. After Squire and Zola-Morgan 1991.

These distinctions have developed as experimental work has focused on the selective deficits shown by patients with amnestic disorders (Cermak 1976; Parkin 1984; Squire and Zola-Morgan 1991; Zola-Morgan and Squire 1990a). From this work, it has been shown that memory is composed of many systems, only one of which is impaired in amnestic disorder patients. The key deficit in the patient with an amnestic disorder is in declarative memory, whereas nondeclarative memory is spared. Such patients manifest difficulty recalling information from the past (retrograde amnesia) and/or difficulty in making new memories (anterograde amnesia). Yet, these patients can have intact short-term memory and perform normally on some tests of learned motor skills, such as the Porteus maze, jigsaw puzzle assembly, and pursuit rotor task (Brooks and Baddeley 1976). In the latter circumstance, learning of a motor skill can be demonstrated even though the individual may have no conscious recollection of ever having performed the task before.

Studies of patients with an amnestic disorder, followed by the development of elegantly detailed animal models, have focused attention on two primary areas of the brain that seem to be affected in amnestic disorder. These two regions, the medial temporal lobe and the hypothalamic-diencephalic system, appear to be the essential sites associated with amnestic disorders. The medial temporal lobe memory system, as described by Squire and Zola-Morgan (1991), includes the hippocampus and the adjacent perirhinal, entorhinal, and parahippocampal cortices. These structures are essential for declarative memory. The role of this system seems to be that of a temporary "way station." Information that will eventually become a memory must first spend some time in the hippocampus before consolidation into long-term memory. The hippocampus-based system thus has a time-limited role in memory, eventually supplanted by a more permanent memory system (which at our current state of knowledge is assumed to be anatomically widely distributed) (Squire and Zola-Morgan 1991; Zola-Morgan and Squire 1990b). Squire and Zola-Morgan (1991) proposed that "the capacity for later retrieval is achieved because the hippocampal system has 'bound together' the relevant cortical sites that together represent memory for a whole event" (p. 1384). Other features of this system are its speed and its limited capacity. Injury produces anterograde amnesia as well as a retrograde amnesia that shows a temporal gradient. Memories of the distant past are recalled more readily than those memories more recently acquired, a phenomenon known as Ribot's law (Ribot 1881).

The components of the hypothalamic-diencephalic system have been less clearly identified but may include areas around the third ventricle, the periaqueductal gray matter, the upper brain stem, selected thalamic nuclei, the posterior hypothalamus, and the mammillary bodies (Lishman 1987). Isolated lesions to a single one of these areas may be sufficient to produce an amnestic disorder. Damage to the mammillary bodies or to the dorsomedial nucleus of the thalamus has been proposed as underlying Korsakoff's syndrome (see Chapter 23).

In addition to the above systems, the lateral surface of the frontal lobe has been suggested to have a role in working memory performance (Petrides 1989). Baddeley (1986) proposed two components to working memory: the subarticulatory loop system for verbal information and the visuospatial sketch pad for visual information. Petrides (1994) described these two processing systems as involving the lateral frontal cortex, which mediates the different aspects of working memory through connections to modality-specific posterior association areas of the cortex. For example, connections between the hippocampal formation and the frontal cortex have been described by Goldman-Rakic (1990), who speculated that these connections imply a reciprocal relationship in working memory. Thus, lesions of the lateral aspects of the frontal lobes may lead to the expression of working memory deficits in the amnesic patient. Much like the patient with hippocampal lesions whose ability to acquire new information for consolidation to long-term memory is significantly disrupted, patients with lesions of the lateral frontal cortex also may be prevented from acquiring new information for consolidation to long-term memory because they cannot effectively use and manipulate the information.

In general, for a medical condition to cause an amnestic disorder, it must do so by affecting one or more of these areas of the brain. The medical conditions that can selectively damage these areas are relatively few (see Table 24–2).

A variety of vascular insults, including interruption of blood flow to—with subsequent infarction of—the hippocampus (posterior cerebral artery occlusion) and the medial thalamus (von Cramon et al. 1985; Winocur et al. 1984), can result in an amnestic disorder. Amnestic disorders also have been reported after subarachnoid hemorrhage typically affecting the anterior circulation, particularly the anterior communicating artery (Cummings 1993). Transient global amnesia is seen in middle-aged and older adults who repetitively ask questions while exhibiting a time-limited anterograde and retrograde amnesia. Transient global amnesia has been widely attributed to a vascular etiology (Cummings 1993; Gorelick et al. 1988; Kushner and Hauser 1985), although in some patients a relationship

TABLE 24–2. Structures or regions of the brain affected in medical conditions causing amnestic disorders

Structure	General medical condition affecting the structure or region
Medial temporal lobe	Posterior cerebral artery occlusion
	Herpes simplex encephalitis
	Hypoxia
	Trauma
	Hypoglycemia
	Neurosarcoidosis
	Temporal lobectomy
Hypothalamic-diencephalic system	Thalamoperforant artery occlusion
	Thiamine deficiency (Wernicke-Korsakoff syndrome, malnutrition, pregnancy, severe vomiting)
	Tumors
	Trauma
Uncertain or diffuse region	Subarachnoid hemorrhage, aneurysm of anterior communicating artery
	Transient global amnesia
	Electroconvulsive therapy
	Closed brain injury

to migraine and epilepsy has been suggested (Hodges and Warlow 1990).

The amnestic disorders induced by substances, including Korsakoff's syndrome, are discussed in Chapter 23. As mentioned there, the underlying etiology of Korsakoff's syndrome is a deficiency of thiamine. Thiamine deficiency can occur in a variety of other medical presentations, such as stomach carcinoma, pregnancy, severe malnutrition, and persistent vomiting, and produces a Korsakoff-like syndrome (Lishman 1987). A Korsakoff-like syndrome also can be produced by other lesions of the diencephalon, such as tumors and tuberculous meningitis (Lishman 1987).

Discrete trauma to the region of the dorsomedial nucleus of the thalamus, although unusual, can occur, as in the famous case of N.A., who developed severe amnesia after a stab wound with a miniature fencing foil. The damage on computed tomography (CT) scan was found to be restricted to the left dorsal thalamus (Squire and Moore 1979).

Damage to the temporal lobes either by surgical ablation or as a result of herpes simplex encephalitis (which is particularly likely to affect the temporal lobes) can result in a severe amnesia. Herpes encephalitis is caused by the type I herpes simplex virus and can be accompanied to a variable extent by other symptoms reflecting temporal lobe damage, including elements of the Klüver-Bucy syndrome. This syndrome, seen experimentally in monkeys after ablation of the temporal lobe, includes a variety of behavioral disturbances, including visual agnosia, hyperorality, altered sexual behavior, and hypermetamorphosis. In humans, the syndrome is usually only partially expressed.

Another clinical setting in which amnestic disorders can be encountered is following traumatic brain injury. In this setting, amnesia is the result of a more diffuse cerebral insult in which the amnesia may simply be, or become, the most intrusive symptom. Other diffuse insults that can produce an amnestic syndrome include hypoxia and hypoglycemia. The cells of the hippocampus are particularly sensitive to hypoxic insult (Cummings et al.

1984). Neurosarcoidosis also has been reported as a very rare cause of an amnesia syndrome (Willigers and Koehler 1993).

An amnestic disorder may result from electroconvulsive therapy (ECT). At one time, the production of an amnestic disorder was considered by some to be necessary for the therapeutic efficacy of ECT, but this has been shown not to be the case (Squire 1984). Currently, the disturbance in memory function that can occur with ECT should be considered a complication rather than a necessary end point of the treatment. During and after the course of ECT, the patient may show retrograde and anterograde amnesia. The severity of the disorder has been reported to vary according to the number of treatments administered and to various aspects of technique, including the laterality and the waveform of the stimulus (Calev et al. 1993). The effect of ECT on memory has a strong temporal component, with memory of events occurring just before and just after ECT being the most affected.

The issue of whether any lasting deficits are associated with ECT remains open. Several studies have been unable to show any objective evidence of deficits lasting beyond 6 months after ECT. However, some patients will have subjective memory complaints beyond this time. A 3-year follow-up of patients who had received ECT reported that approximately one-half of the persons who had received bilateral ECT reported poor memory at follow-up (Squire and Slater 1983). The authors found that these complaints were associated with three circumstances. First, some patients had a recurrence or persistence of the original clinical reason for which they had received ECT. Second, other persons recalled the experience of amnesia after ECT and thereafter tended to question if their memory ever completely recovered. Third, the disturbance in memory was focused in the period representing 6 months preceding and 2 months following ECT. Thus, the focus of complaints in these patients 3 years after receiving ECT was not in new learning or in recent memories but instead centered on memory of events around the time of the treatment. This pattern would be consistent with the picture of a discrete temporal lobe amnestic disorder (Squire and Slater 1983).

In older populations, there has been a great deal of interest in the boundary area between normal aging and dementia, particularly of the Alzheimer's type. Persons in this boundary area have been labeled with terms such as *mild cognitive impairment, isolated memory impairment, age-associated memory impairment,* and *late-life forgetfulness,* although mild cognitive impairment has become the most prevalent clinical label. Mild cognitive impairment has been operationally defined by Petersen et al. (1995) with the following criteria: 1) memory complaints, 2) normal activities of daily living, 3) normal general cognitive functioning, 4) abnormal memory for age, and 5) no dementia. Patients whose symptoms meet these criteria may have had long-standing memory impairment or may be at risk for developing Alzheimer's disease. Petersen et al. (1999) followed up 76 patients with mild cognitive impairment for 4 years and found that the conversion rate from mild cognitive impairment to Alzheimer's disease was 12% per year, suggesting that patients with mild cognitive impairment are at risk for developing dementia (see Chapter 20).

Assessment and Differential Diagnosis

As with all diagnostic endeavors, the road to accurate diagnosis begins with the history and physical, which must include information from a collateral source whenever possible. On mental status examination, the patient is alert and attends to tasks as best as his or her memory deficits allow. The patient's immediate memory is preserved, and thus, he or she should have a normal ability to recite a series of digits. The fundamental problem experienced by these patients is in consolidating information held in short-term memory for later use. Because of the enduring nature of this anterograde amnesia, patients gradually develop a retrograde amnesia of continuously increasing duration (Lishman 1987). The patient will have a retrograde amnesia of variable length beyond which distant memory should be relatively intact. This amnesia tends to be most severe closest to the time of its onset and becomes gradually less severe for more remote events. Sense of time may be disturbed, and the patient may have difficulty correctly placing events in time. Tests of orientation may have abnormal results. Confabulatory responses may occur but are by no means universal. Postencephalitic patients and patients with other temporal lobe amnestic disorders are typically concerned, show insight about their memory loss, and have little evidence of confabulation. Lack of insight and confabulation do occur in diencephalic amnesia, but they tend to be relatively short-lived (Parkin 1984). Other cognitive functions are typically preserved. There is no evidence of aphasia, apraxia, or agnosia. Patients can acquire new motor skills.

Neuropsychological evaluation can be invaluable. Testing should establish both the severity and the selectivity of the memory deficit (Squire and Shimamura 1986). Through testing, subtle memory impairments can be detected, the degree of impairment can be estimated by comparison with normative data, and the relative integrity of components of the memory system can be ascertained (Delis 1993). To fully characterize the amnesic patient, a broad spectrum of tests assessing the domains of intelligence, memory and learning, language, attention and concentration, academic skills, motor ability, concept formation and reasoning skills, and emotional status should be used. Although a full discussion of memory assessment is beyond the scope of this chapter, two important caveats are worth noting about neuropsychological assessment of the amnesic patient. First, age has been shown to influence performance on measures of learning and memory. That is, as the patient becomes older, changes are likely because of reduced information-processing efficiency, which in turn influences working memory capabilities, suggesting that older patients will have greater difficulty with explicit memory tasks (Smith 1996). Therefore, it is important to use tests that have a representative normative base with which the patient's performance can be compared. Second, assessment of both learning and memory is important in the neuropsychological evaluation. For example, simply assessing a patient's ability to immediately recall a paragraph-length story and then later recall it can only provide information about single trial learning and rate of forgetting. Incorporating a measure of word-list learning such as the Rey Auditory-Verbal Learning Test (Lezak 1983) allows for examination of the patient's ability to benefit from rehearsal of information, or to learn the list, and its effect on later recall.

Neuropsychological evaluation also can be very helpful in distinguishing dissociative amnesia. In this condition, the patient has one or more episodes of an inability to recall important personal information that is too extensive to be explained by ordinary forgetfulness. The person may state that he or she has lost *all* of his or her past memories. More typically, the memories that cannot be recalled are of a personal nature, whereas memories for general information are preserved. A profound inability to recall past events coupled with a normal ability to retain new information is suggestive of a dissociative amnestic disorder and should prompt further investigation.

Another group of patients presenting with memory complaints may be malingering patients. With these persons, testing may show some helpful inconsistencies. These patients may claim a total inability to retain new information, including a normal digit span. In turn, they may insist that certain events could not have occurred despite having no basis on which to refute their occurrence (Lishman 1987). On word-list memory tests, truly amnesic patients tend to recall words from the end of the list (the so-called recency effect), whereas malingering patients tend to recall more items from the early part of the list (Delis 1993). Forced-choice recognition testing has become a standard assessment technique for patients suspected of malingering memory deficits. In this strategy, the neuropsychologist presents a word or numerical string to the patient followed by a pair of words or numbers, one of which is the previously presented item, and asks him or her to indicate which one he or she had just seen. Patients who perform below chance level are suspected to have deliberately performed poorly.

Prevention

The medical conditions causing amnestic disorders are for the most part preventable only in the most general sense. Some of these amnesias are the results of accidents, and others reflect the cerebral manifestation of a more systemic illness or disease diathesis. The only general recommendation for most of these disorders can be attention to good general preventive health measures.

One cause of amnestic disorder that is to some extent preventable, or at least can be minimized, involves ECT administration. Some clinical variables are known or suspected to be important factors influencing this amnestic disorder. It is clearly established that amnesia will generally be more severe after a course of ECT that uses a bilateral stimulus technique rather than a unilateral electrode placement (Calev et al. 1993). Bifrontal application of the stimulus has been reported to cause fewer cognitive effects than either unilateral or bilateral ECT while also having superior therapeutic efficacy (Letemendia et al. 1993).

Treatment

Because the amnestic disorders produced by most of the medical conditions discussed in an earlier section are relatively uncommon, there is very little extant treatment literature. It has been observed that the natural history of many of the amnestic disorders, regardless of cause, entails a gradual lessening of the severity of the retrograde and anterograde amnesia with time. The bulk of the treatment literature addressing rehabilitation of amnestic disorders concerns a group of individuals with a condition that, unfortunately, is not all that uncommon—traumatic brain injury. Persons with traumatic brain injury typically present with amnesia as one of an array of cognitive deficits, but memory problems are often the most persistent problem experienced by these patients. In theory, much of this cognitive rehabilitation literature on traumatic brain injury can be applied to individuals with an isolated amnestic disorder. A review of this literature is also essential to grasp what techniques have been applied to this population and with what success. Following this discussion, the even more modest psychopharmacological treatment literature is reviewed.

Psychological and Behavioral Treatments: Memory Rehabilitation

The literature on memory rehabilitation is relatively sparse and of limited scope. Many of the reports are single cases or uncontrolled series of cases. The approaches taken in the studies generally can be categorized as involving either *restoration* or *compensation* (Franzen and Haut 1991). Restorative therapies attempt to bring back normal function by repeated training on a skill such as memory. Thus, the subject with impaired memory might be taught to remember a list of words by repeated exposure to that list. Compensatory approaches, on the other hand, acknowledge the deficit but attempt to help the person master a task by the use of other intact or preserved cognitive abilities. Thus, attempts might be made to have the person use visual imagery as a substitute for verbal intake of information. A variation of the compensatory approach, so-called behavioral prosthetics, teaches the use of other behaviors to compensate for the deficit. An example is the use of a memory book that a person is taught to consult and that serves as an "external memory bank." Each approach has been used with varying degrees of success.

Performing practice and exercise drills has been metaphorically likened to training a "mental muscle." Repetition of certain mental activities is hoped to strengthen the brain, just as repeated exertions will strengthen a muscle. These drills are also similar to certain techniques that teach children basic math and language skills by rote memorization (Franzen and Haut 1991). Such training is commonly used in rehabilitation programs, and many such programs are now available on computer (Matthews et al. 1991). The person with a memory difficulty will be presented repeatedly with a list of words, letters, or numbers, and by repeated exposure it is hoped that he or she will gradually become more adept at recalling stimuli. Importantly, the material that is repeatedly presented has no practical relevance and does not apply to any real-world situation. The intent of the exercise is to strengthen the ability to remember in a nonspecific fashion in the hope that this ability will generalize to everyday life.

Two objections have been made to this process. Simple repetition has not been shown to circumvent this basic defect for encoding information and an inability to learn (Franzen and Haut 1991). Although very minor increases in the ability to recall lists of items have been seen in a few patients, ample evidence indicates that this increased ability is very specific to the artificial task and shows no generalization to other tasks or situations. This lack of generalization is a serious limitation of many cognitive rehabilitative efforts. Also, it is clear that improving the ability to recall lists of items, even if successful, would not be a great deal of help to most persons with memory disorders because in everyday life, little information confronts people in the form of lists.

If the "mental muscle" technique has been found lacking, what are the alternatives? One of the compensatory approaches that has been used involves the use of visual imagery as a mnemonic strategy. As described by Patten (1972), the "ancient art of memory" was invented by Simonides of Ceos in 477 B.C. Simonides had recited a lyric poem at a banquet. After he left the room, the ceiling collapsed and crushed the guests beyond all recognition. Simonides was able to correctly identify all of the corpses by recalling the visual image of the banquet room and associating the image with each guest. Through the years, this technique has served as a reliable method for persons with intact memories who want to increase their ability to recall lists of items. The basic mnemonic strategy involves creating a series of memory "pegs" on which to "hang" the items to be recalled. For example, the peg for the first item on a list might be a candle. The first word to be recalled might be an airplane. The mnemonic technique would be to associate the peg with the word to be recalled through a visual image, such as an airplane flying through the flame of a candle. It should be obvious that the first task in successfully employing this technique is to master the recall of the pegs. This process can be facilitated by tricks such as using a characteristic of the peg to help recall the order of the pegs. For example, the shape of the candle helps the person associate it with the number 1 and the silhouette of a swan makes it a useful cue for the second peg. As a general rule, the more concrete the image to be remembered, and the more ridiculous the mental image associated with the item, the more easily the subject remembers (Patten 1972).

This technique has been an attractive one to persons trying to remediate memory problems. The appeal is not only that it is relatively easy to show improvement in cognitively normal adults but also that the technique presents information in a manner that invites encoding in a visual form rather than a verbal form. In theory, this may avoid an obstruction in encoding by using other residual cognitive abilities. In practice, however, the technique has a major limitation. The technique requires that the person be able to encode and recall a set of pegs. This, in and of itself, is a formidable task analogous to the practice and exercise drills mentioned above. The person must somehow be taught a list of concrete objects that in turn must be linked to a numerical sequence so that the items ultimately to be recalled can be indexed. Because it is precisely this ability that many patients with amnestic disorders lack, the peg mnemonic technique often proves problematic with these patients.

Visual imagery need not incorporate a "peg" system. Amnesic patients can be taught to learn pairs of words by simply imagining some interaction between the words (Gasparrini and Satz 1979). "Ridiculously imaged stories" is another imaging technique that has been shown to increase the recall of a word list by incorporating it into a humorous story line (Kovner and Mattis 1983). Yet another method requires the person to elaborate a story using a list of words to be recalled and then to rehearse the story. The process of elaboration and rehearsal can improve recall of the list (Gianutsos 1981; Gianutsos and Gianutsos 1979).

A critical limitation of using visual imagery as a mnemonic strategy is that a limited number of real-life situations present the opportunity to use paired associates in a meaningful way. Thus, if the initial hurdle can be overcome and the patient masters the technique, it may still be of very little practical value. Attempts at linking visual imagery to practical consequences have met with mixed success (Wilson 1982, 1987). The hard-won skills that may be learned by cognitively disabled persons are frequently "hyperspecific" (Franzen and Haut 1991) and do not generalize to the tasks of the everyday world. This hyperspecificity seems to be a characteristic of such analog techniques. Although in some persons, gains can be made on the specific task, it is unclear whether the person in each of these cases in the end has achieved anything that is helpful in gaining functional independence.

Rather than attempting to strengthen the "mental muscle" or teaching a visual memory mnemonic technique, some investigators focus on alternative approaches that take a more real-life, problem-oriented approach. These techniques use external aids to solve the problems of everyday life. An example of such an aid is a memory book. A memory book is a notebook that contains information that the amnesic person can use as a "memory extender." In theory, this obviates the need for the person to recall the reams of information necessary to live in the external world. Sohlberg and Mateer (1989) described the contents of a typical notebook containing sections such as "Orientation," "Calendar," "Things to Do," "Transportation," "Names," "Today at Work," "Memory Log," and "Feelings Log." The latter two logs are places for persons to chart information about what they have done on an hourly basis and how they felt at the time of the event.

The training that goes into the use of a memory book is extensive. Three training phases, borrowed from learning theory, are recognized: acquisition, application, and adaptation (Sohlberg and Mateer 1989). During *acquisition,* the person is taught the purpose and use of each notebook section. Extensive role-playing is the teaching tool during *application,* at which time the person learns the appropriate methods of recording in the notebook. During *adaptation,* the person must demonstrate the appropriate use of the notebook in naturalistic settings in the community.

The theory behind the memory book goes back to the classification of memory into declarative and nondeclarative forms. Because the amnesic patient can be shown to retain nondeclarative memory skills such as perceptual motor skills, memory for overlearned behavior, and repetition priming effects (see Figure 24–1), these skills are recruited as much as possible in memory book training (Sohlberg and Mateer 1989). In particular, the emphasis in training is on constant repetition of certain skills, such as consulting the schedule, writing in the log, and marking a calendar section. The ability to perform the motor skills aspects of such behaviors is hoped to increase, even though the person may have no conscious recollection of having performed the tasks. Indeed, for some severely amnesic persons, the skills developed by using a memory book have led to an increase in functional independence.

The acquisition stage of the three-part memory book training process is dependent on some residual declarative memory skill. The patient must be able to consciously recall the purpose of the book and the nature of its sections and to select the appropriate section for use in particular situations. Guided repetition seems to be able to accomplish this goal. Even though this repetition bears similarity to the "mental muscle" approach, which, as noted earlier, is of very limited benefit, the crucial difference seems to be that the memory book process focuses repetition on a practical skill rather than on an analog skill such as memorizing lists of words. Even the severely amnesic person retains some degree of declarative memory, and the goal is to maximize use of declarative memory in complementing nondeclarative memory.

Resource use can be very intense with the memory book technique (i.e., it can require many resources, such as time, money, clinicians). In the case described by Sohlberg and Mateer (1989), it took the person 6 months of intensive notebook use to achieve independence in the system. At the conclusion of the training, repeated testing showed that the person had improved attention and delayed recall after distraction but continued to have persistent, profound limitations in memory and new learning. Nevertheless, this patient was able to live with only minimal daily assistance and was working in a sheltered environment. No mention was made of the economics of this approach.

An important concept that techniques such as the memory book raise is the notion of *prospective memory* (Sohlberg and Mateer 1989; Sohlberg et al. 1992). For a memory book to be useful, the person must remember to use it. This act of "remembering to remember" has been called prospective memory. It is the process by which a person lays down a memory trace and then initiates scanning for that memory or intention at some future time. Prospective memory is not about *what* the person recalls but about *whether* the person recalls a task. Prospective memory is demonstrated by the execution of an action and is usually cued by the person himself or herself (Sohlberg et al. 1992; Winograd 1988). Thus, the successful use of a memory book relies not only on being trained in the use of the book but also on actually remembering to use the book. The emphasis during memory book training on recording information and following it up is intended to facilitate the prospective recall of the amnesic person. Unfortunately, very little is known about the process of prospective memory, and it has been the experience of some investigators that patients with memory books rarely consult their books (Glisky and Schacter 1986). On the other hand, Zencius et al. (1990), in reviewing memory rehabilitative strategies, found that only memory books were of significant help to patients with traumatic brain injury.

Another way to exploit nondeclarative memory in the amnesic patient is the method of *vanishing clues*. This method is based on amnesic patients' ability, as noted above, to retain some ability to learn. If presented with a particular word such as "drawer" to recall, the amnesic patient is unlikely to spontaneously produce it. However, if presented with the letters "dra__," he or she is more likely to come up with the target word despite having no conscious recollection of its presentation. This is an example of *visual priming*. The vanishing-clues method makes use of this residual skill by then gradually withdrawing parts of the clues until the patient is able to produce the targeted response spontaneously. This technique has been used to teach amnesic persons to operate a computer and, in one case, enabled a 32-year-old who was amnesic after contracting herpes simplex encephalitis to hold a data entry job (Glisky and Schacter 1989).

Psychopharmacological Approaches

The literature addressing psychopharmacological interventions in the amnestic disorders is quite sparse. Whereas a tremendous amount of clinical attention has been devoted to developing pharmacological treatments for dementia, very little attention has been focused on the amnestic disorders. As was true for the memory rehabilitative approaches, almost all of the data on amnestic disorders are in the form of single case reports. Treatment efforts have certainly been hampered by the fact that discrete amnestic disorders are infrequently found or diagnosed because they are rare and by a lack of basic biochemical and physiological information on the nature of the underlying deficits in these disorders.

Several attempts have been made to pharmacologically alter the memory impairment associated with ECT. There have been negative trials of naloxone (Nasrallah et al. 1986), ergoloid mesylates (Sachs et al. 1989), and vasopressin (Mattes et al. 1990) to reduce the memory deficits associated with ECT. One positive trial found that physostigmine reversed the impairment of verbal and visual short- and long-term memory that had resulted from ECT (Levin et al. 1987).

Another series of cases examined the utility of a variety of drugs in amnestic disorders of different etiologies. Clonidine (McIntyre and Gasquoine 1990), vasopressin (Jenkins et al. 1981; Koch-Henriksen and Nielsen 1981), and nimodipine (Bailey et al. 1991) have been used in patients with head injury with no demonstrable benefit. Goldberg et al. (1982) reported on a patient with posttraumatic amnesia treated with physostigmine and lecithin who showed a selective improvement in verbal recall but not verbal recognition, visual memory, or conceptual reasoning. Both storage and retrieval of words in verbal memory were facilitated. Physostigmine also was helpful in two cases involving patients with an amnestic disorder due to herpes simplex encephalitis (Catsman-Berrevoets et al. 1986; Peters and Levin 1977). However, Gianutsos (1981) described a case of a college professor with an encephalitic amnesia whose condition was not improved by physostigmine. Vasopressin also has been used in a postencephalitic case with minimal results (Koizumi et al. 1981). In a recent report of the use of donepezil in the treatment of traumatic brain injury in two patients (Taverni et al. 1998), improvement in subjective and objective memory performance was noted.

Dobkin and Hanlon (1993) reported the case of a woman with a persistent anterograde amnesia after her brain had been surgically impaled. The injury left a 1-cm-wide mediobasal tract of encephalomalacia that extended anterior to the septal nuclei and medial to the nucleus accumbens. The patient's verbal learning, functional memory, and daily recall improved after she was given bromocriptine.

Conclusions

As in many arenas in the neurosciences, the rate of acquisition of new information about the memory systems of the brain has been breathtaking. Yet the treatment of amnestic disorders remains in its infancy. Important basic science research is under way that for the first time will allow us the opportunity to examine the roots of what a memory is and how it is made. With these theories in hand, we hope the time will come when an unequivocally effective treatment for the amnestic disorders is available. In the meantime, the effort to help our patients using the tools of today must continue. We must live by the words of Ambroise Paré (1510–1590), the father of French surgery, who said that the mission of the physician is "to cure occasionally, to relieve often, to comfort always."

References

American Psychiatric Association: Diagnostic and Statistical Manual of Mental Disorders, 4th Edition, Washington, DC, American Psychiatric Association, 1994

Baddeley AD: Working Memory. New York, Oxford University Press, 1986

Bailey I, Bell A, Gray J, et al: A trial of the effect of nimodipine on outcome after head injury. Acta Neurochir (Wein) 110:97–105, 1991

Brooks DN, Baddeley AD: What can amnesic patients learn? Neuropsychologia 14:111–122, 1976

Calev A, Pass HL, Sapira B, et al: ECT and memory, in The Clinical Science of Electroconvulsive Therapy. Edited by Coffey CE. Washington, DC, American Psychiatric Press, 1993, pp 125–142

Catsman-Berrevoets CE, Van Harskamp F, Applehof A: Beneficial effect of physostigmine on clinical amnesic behavior and neuropsychological test results in a patient with a post-encephalitis amnesic syndrome. J Neurol Neurosurg Psychiatry 49:1088–1090, 1986

Cermak LS: The encoding capacity of a patient with amnesia due to encephalitis. Neuropsychologia 14:311–326, 1976

Cummings JL: Amnesia and memory disturbances in neurological disorders, in American Psychiatric Press Review of Psychiatry, Vol 12. Edited by Oldham JM, Riba MB, Tasman A. Washington, DC, American Psychiatric Press, 1993, pp 727–745

Cummings JL, Tomiyasu U, Read S, et al: Amnesia with hippocampal lesions after cardiopulmonary arrest. Neurology 34:679–681, 1984

Delis DC: Neuropsychological assessment of memory disorders, in American Psychiatric Press Review of Psychiatry, Vol 12. Edited by Oldham JM, Riba MB, Tasman A. Washington, DC, American Psychiatric Press, 1993, pp 689–723

Dobkin BH, Hanlon R: Dopamine agonist treatment of anterograde amnesia from a mediobasal forebrain injury. Ann Neurol 33:313–316, 1993

Franzen MD, Haut MW: The psychological treatment of memory impairment: a review of empirical studies. Neuropsychol Rev 2:29–63, 1991

Gasparrini B, Satz P: A treatment for memory problems in left hemisphere CVA patients. Journal of Clinical Neuropsychology 1:137–150, 1979

Gianutsos R: Training the short- and long-term verbal recall of a postencephalitic amnesic. Journal of Clinical Neuropsychology 3:143–153, 1981

Gianutsos R, Gianutsos J: Rehabilitating the verbal recall of brain-injured patients by mnemonic training: an experimental demonstration using single-case methodology. Journal of Clinical Neuropsychology 1:117–135, 1979

Glisky EL, Schacter DL: Remediation of organic memory disorders: current status and future prospects. J Head Trauma Rehabil 1:54–63, 1986

Glisky EL, Schacter DL: Extending the limits of complex learning in organic amnesia: computer training in a vocational domain. Neuropsychologia 27:107–120, 1989

Goldberg E, Gerstman LJ, Mattis S, et al: Selective effects of cholinergic treatment on verbal memory in posttraumatic amnesia. Journal of Clinical Neuropsychology 4:219–234, 1982

Goldman-Rakic PS: Cellular and circuit basis of working memory in prefrontal cortex of nonhuman primates, in Progress in Brain Research, Vol 85. Edited by Uylings HBM, Van Eden CG, De Bruin JPC, et al. Amsterdam, Elsevier, 1990, pp 325–336

Gorelick PG, Amico LL, Ganellen R, et al: Transient global amnesia and thalamic infarction. Neurology 38:496–499, 1988

Hodges JR, Warlow CP: The aetiology of transient global amnesia. Brain 113:639–657, 1990

Jenkins JS, Mather HM, Coughlan AK, et al: Desmopressin and desglycinamide vasopressin in post-traumatic amnesia (letter). Lancet 1(8210):39, 1981

Koch-Henriksen N, Nielsen H: Vasopressin in post-traumatic amnesia. Lancet 1(8210):38–39, 1981

Koizumi HM, Rowe M, Clark R: Vasopressin (anti-diuretic hormone) for post encephalitis memory loss: a pilot study (letter). J Clin Psychiatry 42:217, 1981

Kovner R, Mattis S: A technique for promoting robust free recall in chronic organic amnesia. Journal of Clinical Neuropsychology 5:65–71, 1983

Kushner MJ, Hauser WA: Transient global amnesia: a case-control study. Ann Neurol 18:684–691, 1985

Letemendia FJJ, Delva NJ, Rodenburg M, et al: Therapeutic advantages of bifrontal electrode placement in ECT. Psychol Med 23:349–360, 1993

Levin Y, Elizur A. Korczyn AD: Physostigmine improves ECT-induced memory disturbances. Neurology 37:871–875, 1987

Lezak MD: Neuropsychological Assessment, 2nd Edition. New York, Oxford University Press, 1983

Lishman WA: Organic Psychiatry: The Psychological Consequences of Cerebral Disorder, 2nd Edition. Oxford, UK, Blackwell Scientific, 1987

Mattes JA, Pettinati HM, Stephens S, et al: A placebo-controlled evaluation of vasopressin for ECT-induced memory impairment. Biol Psychiatry 27:289–303, 1990

Matthews CG, Harley JP, Malec JF: Guidelines for computer-assisted neuropsychological rehabilitation and cognitive remediation. The Clinical Neuropsychologist 5:3–19, 1991

McIntyre FL, Gasquoine P: Effect of clonidine on post-traumatic memory deficits. Brain Inj 4:209–211, 1990

Milner B: The memory defect in bilateral hippocampal lesions. Psychiatric Research Reports 11:43–52, 1959

Milner B, Corkin S, Teuber H-L: Further analyses of the hippocampal amnestic syndrome: 14-year follow-up study of H.M. Neuropsychologia 6:215–234, 1968

Nasrallah HA, Varney N, Coffman JA, et al: Opiate antagonism fails to reverse post-ECT cognitive deficits. J Clin Psychiatry 47:555–556, 1986

Parkin AJ: Amnesic syndrome: a lesion-specific disorder? Cortex 20:479–508, 1984

Patten BM: The ancient art of memory: usefulness in treatment. Arch Neurol 26:25–31, 1972

Peters BH, Levin HS: Memory enhancement after physostigmine treatment in the amnesic syndrome. Arch Neurol 34:215–219, 1977

Petersen RC, Smith GE, Ivnik RJ, et al: Apolipoprotein E status as a predictor of the development of Alzheimer's disease in memory impaired individuals. JAMA 273:1274–1278, 1995

Petersen RC, Smith GE, Waring SC, et al: Mild cognitive impairment: clinical characterization and outcome. Arch Neurol 56:303–308, 1999

Petrides M: Frontal lobes and memory, in Handbook of Neuropsychology, Vol 3. Edited by Boller F, Grafman J. Amsterdam, Elsevier, 1989, pp 75–90

Petrides M: Frontal lobes and working memory: evidence from investigations of the effects of cortical excisions in nonhuman primates, in Handbook of Neuropsychology, Vol 9. Edited by Boller F, Grafman J. Amsterdam, Elsevier, 1994, pp 59–82

Ribot T: Les Maladies de la Memoire. Paris, Germer Baillere, 1881

Sachs GS, Gelenberg AJ, Bellinghausen B, et al: Ergoloid mesylates and ECT. J Clin Psychiatry 50:87–90, 1989

Smith AD: Memory, in Handbook of the Psychology of Aging, 4th Edition. Edited by Birren JE, Warner Schaie K. San Diego, CA, Academic Press, 1996, pp 236–250

Sohlberg MM, Mateer CA: Training use of compensatory memory books: a three-stage behavioral approach. J Clin Exp Neuropsychol 11:871–891, 1989

Sohlberg MM, White O, Evans E, et al: Background and initial case studies into the effect of prospective memory training. Brain Inj 6:129–138, 1992

Squire LR: ECT and memory dysfunction, in ECT: Basic Mechanisms. Edited by Lerer B, Weiner RD, Belmaker RH. London, John Libbey, 1984, pp 156–163

Squire LR: Memory and Brain. New York, Oxford University Press, 1987

Squire LR, Moore RY: Dorsal thalamic lesion in a noted case of human memory dysfunction. Ann Neurol 6:503–506, 1979

Squire LR, Shimamura AP: Characterizing amnesic patients for neurobehavioral study. Behav Neurosci 100:866–877, 1986

Squire LR, Slater PC: Electroconvulsive therapy and complaints of memory dysfunction: a prospective three-year follow-up study. Br J Psychiatry 142:1–8, 1983

Squire LR, Zola-Morgan S: The medial temporal lobe memory system. Science 253:1380–1386, 1991

Taverni JP, Seliger G, Lichtman SW: Donepezil medicated memory improvement in traumatic brain injury during post acute rehabilitation. Brain Inj 12:77–80, 1998

von Cramon DY, Hebel N, Schuri U: A contribution to the anatomical basis of thalamic amnesia. Brain 108:993–1008, 1985

Willigers H, Koehler PJ: Amnesic syndrome caused by neurosarcoidosis. Clin Neurol Neurosurg 95: 131–135, 1993

Wilson B: Success and failure in memory training following a cerebrovascular accident. Cortex 18:581–594, 1982

Wilson B: Identification and remediation of everyday problems in memory-impaired patients, in Neuropsychology of Alcoholism: Implications for Diagnosis and Treatment. Edited by Parson OA, Butters N, Nathan PE. New York, Guilford, 1987, pp 322–338

Winocur G, Oxbury S, Roberts R, et al: Amnesia in a patient with bilateral lesions to the thalamus. Neuropsychologia 22:122–143, 1984

Winograd E: Some observations on prospective remembering, in Practical Aspects of Memory: Current Research and Issues, Vol 1. Edited by Gruneber MM, Morris PE, Sykes RN. London, Wiley, 1988, pp 348–353

Zencius A, Wesolowski MD, Burke WH: A comparison of four memory strategies with traumatically brain-injured clients. Brain Inj 4:33–38, 1990

Zola-Morgan S, Squire LR: The neuropsychology of memory: parallel findings in humans and nonhuman primates. Ann N Y Acad Sci 608:4343–4356, 1990a

Zola-Morgan S, Squire LR: The primate hippocampal formation: evidence for a time-limited role in memory storage. Science 250:288–298, 1990b

SECTION 4

Substance-Related Disorders

Section Editors

Herbert D. Kleber, M.D.

Marc Galanter, M.D.

Introduction

In spite of progress on a number of fronts, the major public health problem facing the United States today remains that of substance abuse and dependence. This section on substance abuse disorders is organized so that problems with individual drugs and certain common treatment modalities are given separate chapters. Within each chapter are sections written by separate authors who are experts on that particular topic. We have been fortunate in obtaining for this section the contributions of some of the country's leading researchers and practitioners in the field of substance abuse. The emphasis throughout is on useful clinical practices rather than on research or academic concerns.

Staggering health care costs, crime, domestic violence, acquired immunodeficiency syndrome (AIDS), homelessness, and education and welfare problems all are related to our failure to adequately deal with substance abuse and dependence. The number of persons addicted to or in trouble with various substances is enormous: more than 60 million people addicted to tobacco; more than 15 million alcoholic persons, or "problem drinkers"; in excess of 5 million people using marijuana more than once a week; more than 2 million people addicted to cocaine; 800,000 or more people addicted to heroin; and up to half a million people who regularly use hallucinogens such as lysergic acid diethylamide (LSD), phencyclidine (PCP), and methylenedioxymethamphetamine (MDMA; also known as "Ecstasy"). The extent of the national experiment that has endured in the United States over the past three decades is often not fully recognized. In 1962, only about 4 million Americans had ever used an illicit drug; by 1992, that number had climbed to almost 80 million. Although every physician will see a substantial number of persons whose substance abuse either leads to or complicates their reasons for seeking treatment, psychiatrists in particular see large numbers of such patients, either for primary substance abuse or for substance abuse comorbid with other psychiatric disorders.

Marc Schuckit, Richard Schottenfeld, and Michael Pantalon begin the section by reviewing the overall goals and principles of treatment and how to evaluate patients when they present for treatment. Maintaining abstinence, although an obvious goal, usually needs to be supplemented by activities aimed at improving multiple aspects of life functioning and training in relapse prevention. Clinicians will not be surprised to learn that diagnosis can sometimes be difficult and that it will often be necessary to supplement information gathered from the patient with laboratory data that reveal the presence of drugs whose use is denied, and with information from interviews with family members who reveal material the patient has been reluctant to disclose. Because substance abuse disorders can be life-threatening, and because denial and deception so often accompany them, the clinician must begin with a high index of suspicion regarding the presence of substance abuse in addition to or instead of other psychiatric disorders. Robert DuPont, in a subsection added since the last edition, reviews the strengths and weaknesses of the various laboratory tests designed to detect drug use.

The most common substance of abuse/dependence in patients presenting for treatment is alcohol. In Chapter 26, Don Gallant reviews what is known about the pharmacological treatment of this disorder in all of its phases, from detoxification to abstinence/maintenance. Pharmacotherapy for alcoholism is advancing, and the future looks even more promising for adding new medications to existing nonpharmacological approaches. Although both use of and dependence on benzodiazepine and other sedative-hypnotic medications have diminished, a large problem remains, and David Smith and Donald Wesson cogently summarize the diagnosis and treatment of these disorders.

There has been a resurgence in the use of hallucinogens, both old favorites such as LSD and psilocybin, and new ones such as MDMA, in high schools and colleges. Robert Pechnick and Thomas Ungerleider, in Chapter 27, provide a succinct overview of interventions for adverse reactions involving these agents. The most common illicit drug of abuse is cannabis. Although cannabis is often viewed in the lay press as a benign substance, its use by more than 5 million persons a week is associated with thousands of cases a year coming to emergency rooms for problems secondary to marijuana use and numerous cases of abuse and dependence that require psychiatric intervention. Mark Gold, Michelle Tullis, and Kimberly Frost-Pineda review what is known about the diagnosis and treatment of cannabis abuse and dependence. Resurgence of marijuana use in the 1990s by the young suggests that many clinicians will have occasion to see the "casualties" of such use in their practices. Studies suggest that marijuana may be much more difficult to stop than commonly thought.

The major drug epidemic in the 1980s was cocaine. That decade also witnessed the sharp decline in nonaddictive use of cocaine and the transition from snorting cocaine hydrochloride to smoking the rapidly absorbed base form, often known as "crack." The decline in nonaddictive use has not been paralleled by a decline in cocaine dependence, and treatment of patients with cocaine dependency remains a difficult and at times intractable problem. In Chapter 28, Tom Kosten and Amrita Singha review the phases of cocaine abuse, the problem of finding an adequate treatment medication, and the current knowledge base on pharmacological and psychological treatments of cocaine abuse and dependence. Phencyclidine abuse is experiencing a revival among certain subgroups in selected cities (unlike the more universal abuse of cocaine). Michael Weaver and Sidney Schnoll offer guidelines for diagnosing patients with phencyclidine or ketamine abuse when they present, often in an emergency fashion, and for treating the toxic consequences; they also address the even more difficult task of bringing about long-term abstinence. A new subsection by David McDowell addresses the "club drugs"—MDMA, gamma-hydroxybutyrate (GHB), and ketamine (which is covered in more detail by Schnoll and Weaver)—that are becoming increasingly popular in our urban areas. Finally, Lori Pbert, Sarah Reiff, and Judith Ockene tackle the treatment of tobacco withdrawal and tobacco dependence, a timely subject in view of the controversy about nicotine's addicting nature and smoking's association with more than 400,000 deaths a year in the United States as well as enormous health care costs. Practitioners often ignore their patients' smoking out of a belief that other problems are of more pressing concern. Successful interventions for nicotine addiction, however, do not need to be time-consuming and can be of great help to the person's overall health. Pbert and colleagues provide the tools for clinicians to be of such assistance.

Although cocaine use has been declining, heroin use has been on the rise, and the first decade of the new millennium may well be the decade of opiate abuse. Effective medications are available that can improve outcome. In Chapter 29, Herbert Kleber addresses detoxification from opiate addiction, discussing the standard technique of gradual methadone reduction as well as the newer approaches involving clonidine, the ultrarapid clonidine-naltrexone method, and experimental approaches such as acupuncture, buprenorphine, and rapid detoxification under anesthesia. Buprenorphine, a partial agonist, may be the most exciting advance in treatment of heroin addiction since methadone. Used in office-based prescribing, it has the potential to revolutionize delivery of opiate addiction treatment. Edward Senay outlines the strengths and weaknesses of methadone maintenance, the most commonly used treatment for opiate addiction as well as the most successful and most controversial. The narcotic antagonist naltrexone is both less controversial and less acceptable to most addicted persons. Charles O'Brien offers guidance on how to use antagonists in ways that may make them more acceptable and successful.

Regardless of what medications are developed for treatment of substance use disorders, psychotherapy will continue to be necessary to foster compliance with the medications and, more important, to help addicted persons to learn they can have lives beyond substance dependence. In Chapter 30, on individual treatment, a number of different approaches are reviewed. Richard Frances, Avram Mack, Lisa Borg, and John Franklin review psychodynamic therapy; Sheldon Zimberg, individual therapy for alcoholism; and George Woody and Delinda Mercer, individual therapy for treatment of other drugs of abuse. Relapse prevention training has become an essential ingredient in any rehabilitation program. Alan Marlatt, one of the pioneers in the field, and Kimberly Barrett describe the background and methods. Marc Galanter uses the insights of psychiatry along with family and peer support techniques in a combination called "network therapy."

Many clinicians believe that substance use disorders are better treated in group and family settings than in individual ones. In Chapter 31, Edward Khantzian, Sarah Golden, and William McAuliffe review group therapy for psychoactive substance use disorders. Peter Steinglass discusses family therapy for alcoholism, and Edward Kaufman, family therapy in the treatment of other substance abuse.

The final chapter deals with programs and populations that are not easily characterized and yet are of vital importance in the overall treatment of a substance use disorder. Chad Emrick discusses the widely used Alcoholics Anonymous (AA) and other 12-Step approaches and provides guidelines for integrating these programs with professional treatment. He reviews both the strengths and weaknesses of the 12-Step approach, offers recommendations for how physicians can best refer patients to AA, and outlines what is known about AA's effectiveness. Many patients will need an inpatient stay as part of their continuum of care, and Roger Weiss describes current inpatient approaches to these patients. Jonathan Ritvo and James Shore provide an overview of community-based treatment. George De Leon discusses the residential therapeutic community. There are fewer than 12,000 beds for such long-term therapeutic communities in the United States, and retention has been difficult. It has been recognized, however, especially because of the research done by De Leon, that graduates of such programs, as well as those who stay in the program any appreciable length of time, do quite well as far as later use of addicting substances. Finally, a new subsection by Kathleen Brady and Robert Malcolm provides insight into treating the large percentage of substance abusers with comorbid disorders.

While noncompliance and relapse rates are found among patients with chronic medical disorders such as diabetes and hypertension as well as among substance abusers, patients with these former disorders are not usually stigmatized for relapse. Substance-using patients who relapse are, in contrast, judged much more harshly. There is no one effective treatment for substance abuse. The substance abuse population is heterogeneous, and patients may need different approaches at different stages in their drug-using careers. What emerges from reviewing all of the chapters in this section is that, all in all, there are effective treatments for these patients. A variety of useful pharmacological and nonpharmacological approaches exist and can provide either temporary or long-term help. Clinicians need to take into account patient heterogeneity when confronted with the individual patient and deciding how to treat the patient or, if referring, what kind of treatment might be most suitable. This section attempts to bring together the knowledge that can help the clinician in making these decisions.

25

Overview of Treatment

Marc A. Schuckit, M.D.
Richard S. Schottenfeld, M.D.
Michael V. Pantalon, Ph.D.
Robert L. DuPont, M.D.

Goals of Treatment

Marc A. Schuckit, M.D.

At first glance, the appropriate goals of treatment for substance use disorders appear obvious. We all strive to help our patients and clients achieve their optimal levels of functioning for as long as possible (Schuckit 2000). However, we function in a complex world where health care deliverers must share scarce resources while reaching out to a pool of persons with impairment who, at least theoretically, have many more needs than we can possibly meet. Thus, we have to make decisions about which of the possible treatment tools we should use, which patients are most appropriate for care, and which treatment setting is most relevant.

In the first portion of this chapter subpart, I focus on how clinicians in the field of substance use disorders need to make important decisions about specific treatment goals to be applied in the day-to-day situations in which we function. In the first section I examine the components incorporated in our desire to help our patients function at an optimal level. In the next section I discuss the administrative and programmatic objectives that must be considered in our efforts to meet our patients' needs. This discussion is followed by an overview of some of the goals that may be less appropriate (and at times quite inappropriate) in substance use disorders treatment programs. Finally, I pull these thoughts together into a clinically oriented summary.

Patient- and Client-Oriented Goals

Several decades ago, treatment programs focused mostly on the achievement and maintenance of abstinence. However, increasing levels of sophistication have helped us to realize that being substance-free, although an essential step in the right direction, does not by itself guarantee optimal life functioning (McLellan et al. 1996). Thus, we can, somewhat arbi-

---

This work was supported by Veterans Affairs Research Service and National Institute on Alcohol Abuse and Alcoholism grants 05226, 08401, and 08403.

This chapter subpart is a revised version of my chapter "Goals of Treatment," which appeared in Galanter MA, Kleber HD (eds): *The American Psychiatric Press Textbook of Substance Abuse Treatment,* 2nd Edition. Washington, DC, American Psychiatric Press, 1999, pp. 89–95.

trarily, conceive of our patient-oriented goals as involving 1) helping the patient achieve a substance-free life, 2) maximizing multiple aspects of life functioning, and 3) preventing relapse. Today, it is difficult to envision a successful treatment program that ignores any of these domains.

Achieving a Substance-Free Lifestyle

There are at least two components to the important goal of achieving a substance-free lifestyle (Schuckit 2000). The first involves maximizing patients' motivation for abstinence, and the second relates to teaching our patients how to rebuild their lives after redirecting the focus of their activities away from the use of substances.

Maximizing Motivation for Abstinence

Substance dependence is, essentially, a condition in which the use of alcohol or other drugs has become such a central part of the person's life that he or she is willing to give up important activities in order to continue to use the substance or to resume substance intake. Prior to treatment, the usual clinical course of substance-related problems often involves temporary periods of controlled substance intake established through rules regarding particular situations, times of day, or other conditions during which substances will be taken but "kept under control" (Schuckit et al. 1997c; Vaillant 1996). Unfortunately, persons with a history of severe substance-related life impairment are very likely to discover that rules can be bent, which often leads to escalation of intake and development of a crisis. This discovery is followed by a new intense level of resolve to stop taking the drug, at least for a period of time, after which use begins again, efforts of control are instituted, and new crises develop.

In recognition of this pattern of repeated efforts at "controlled substance use," with the high likelihood (some would say almost certainty) of progression to the point of problems once use resumes, most programs dealing with substance-dependent persons have chosen to make abstinence a clear goal. However, some persons with substance dependence at least initially refuse a goal of abstinence. In the alcohol field, some clinicians and researchers have thus attempted to develop experimental programs aimed at teaching dependent persons "controlled use," but there are few data to support use of this approach once dependence has developed (Helzer et al. 1985). Some researchers have reported promising results regarding teaching control of alcohol use to persons who have not met criteria for dependence but have expressed concerns over their occasional heavy intake of alcohol, yet have refused to abstain totally.

Various maneuvers are appropriate for attempting to maximize substance-dependent persons' motivation for abstinence (Schuckit 2000). These include lectures, counseling sessions, and self-help groups. The goals are to educate the individual and his or her family about the dangers involved with substance use and the usual clinical course of substance use disorders, and to emphasize that each person is responsible for his or her own actions. Thus, any return to substance use is likely to set off a series of events leading to a fairly predictable group of severe life problems (Schuckit et al. 1998). On the other hand, abstinence is achievable, life patterns can change, and there is a high level of hope for success.

In summary, abstinence is accepted as the only clinically relevant goal for treatment programs focusing on persons who meet criteria for dependence on any substance, including tobacco and illegal drugs.

Helping the Patient/Client Rebuild a Lifestyle Free of Substances

Most programs admit to their patients that giving up all substance use is far from easy. Patients are likely to have experienced years of heavy substance intake and to have developed a life pattern in which a good deal of their time and the majority of their friends are involved with heavy, repeated substance intake. Even substance-free relatives and friends are likely to have developed expectations about the individual's behaviors and subtly, or sometimes more blatantly, communicated these probabilities to the individual, sometimes producing an almost "scripted" style of interaction. Thus, important elements in developing a substance-free lifestyle include helping the person to discover ways of dealing with free time; to develop friendships, independent of the context of drug use, with persons who themselves do not use substances; to adjust to the more "mundane" aspects of day-to-day living in the absence of the crisis-upon-crisis lifestyle associated with substance use; and to reestablish rewarding relationships with family members.

Maximizing Multiple Aspects of Life Functioning

As briefly discussed earlier in this section, becoming substance-free is an essential first step in rebuilding one's life. However, by itself, it is rarely sufficient to optimize functioning. Thus, most treatment programs attempt to address essential elements of day-to-day living. Although not all programs incorporate efforts directly aimed at each area of functioning, almost all recognize the need to deal with the majority of these domains.

Optimizing Medical Functioning

The heavy use of alcohol and other drugs is likely to damage body systems, increase the risk for physical trauma through accidents, and (for depressants, stimulants, and opiates) produce clinically relevant levels of physical dependence (Schuckit et al. 1999). Therefore, it is hard to conceive of an effective program that would ignore the importance of a careful physical examination, neglect emergent physical difficulties, fail to deal with the appropriate treatment of withdrawal when needed, and make no effort to prevent future medical difficulties. These steps not only are essential parts of the responsibility assumed by a treatment program but also are important for optimizing the patient's ability to participate fully in rehabilitation efforts.

Identifying and Treating Psychiatric Symptoms and Disorders

During intoxication and withdrawal from substances, as many as 80% of substance-dependent persons demonstrate psychiatric symptoms (Schuckit et al. 1997a). For example, perhaps as many as two-thirds of alcohol-dependent persons experience social phobia–like symptoms or panic attacks during withdrawal, and a similar proportion of actively drinking alcoholic persons and persons undergoing withdrawal from stimulants such as cocaine or amphetamines demonstrate serious depressive symptoms that can last 2–4 weeks or longer (Gawin and Ellinwood 1988; Schuckit et al. 1997a, 1997b). Treatment programs must be aware of these temporary conditions, carefully evaluate their patients for the possibility of independent psychiatric disorders, and take appropriate steps to address the clinical symptoms, even when these are only temporary and part of the substance use pattern. In this latter instance, education, reassurance, and evaluations for the potential temporary need for suicide precautions, along with cognitive, supportive, or behavioral counseling techniques, should be instituted on a temporary basis when appropriate. The intense depression and anxiety related to intoxication or withdrawal improve fairly quickly, although some low-grade symptoms can linger for several months as part of a protracted abstinence syndrome (Satel et al. 1993).

In addition to these fairly common substance-related temporary conditions, persons with substance use disorders have at least as high a risk for independent psychiatric disorders as does the general population. Therefore, at least 5% of men and 10% of women might have major depressive disorders, and as many as 10% of both sexes could by chance alone be expected to have one of the anxiety disorders (Regier et al. 1990). However, men and women with bipolar disorder, schizophrenia, or antisocial personality disorder have higher risks for subsequent substance-related problems than does the general population (Holdcraft et al. 1998). Therefore, most treatment programs incorporate a careful history-gathering procedure, obtaining information from both the patient and at least one knowledgeable friend or relative, to determine whether psychiatric syndromes actually meeting criteria for severe disorders were apparent either before the onset of severe life problems from substance use or during a period of perhaps several months or more when the person was totally abstinent (Schuckit et al. 1997c). Programs also are likely to incorporate procedures for observing the persistence of intense psychiatric symptomatology remaining 4 weeks or so after abstinence, documenting these as indicative of potentially important independent disorders.

When an independent psychiatric syndrome has been established through this careful history taking or through observation of the patient over time following abstinence, appropriate treatments must be instituted. Thus, the relatively small proportion of patients who have both substance dependence and an independent major depressive disorder are candidates for intense cognitive therapy and/or antidepressant medications; the 1%–2% of substance-dependent men and women who actually have bipolar illness may well require lithium, and the 1%–2% of patients who have both substance dependence and schizophrenia are almost certain to require antipsychotic medications (Schuckit 2000). Recognizing and appropriately treating these independent psychiatric disorders in the minority of our patients are as important a part of our goals for substance-related treatment as is carrying out steps to optimize medical functioning.

Dealing With Marital and Other Family Issues

Reestablishing and maintaining close relationships with one's spouse, one's children, and other family members are demanding tasks for our patients. As difficult as these issues are to deal with for anyone, the nature of the behaviors likely to be observed in the course of substance use problems is likely to jeopardize these relationships even further. Thus, most treatment programs in the substance use field have incorporated efforts that reach out to family members by establishing couples- and family-counseling sessions and including as many family members and friends as appropriate into relevant aspects of rehabilitation efforts. These steps not only make good sense but also increase the probability of long-term abstinence in our patients (Epstein et al. 1997).

Enriching Job Functioning and Financial Management

Most men and women who come to alcohol- and other substance-related programs have multiple financial problems. Although they might function quite well and hold good jobs, they still spend far too much money on the use of their substance, and they have developed a pattern of responding to financial crises rather than planning ahead. Obviously, an important part of helping persons to optimize their life functioning involves vocational rehabilitation—helping them to find jobs that are not as closely intertwined in their minds with substance use—and development of patterns of financial planning that will keep food on the table. Thus, financial management along with vocational education efforts is an important part of therapeutic interventions.

Addressing Relevant Spiritual Issues

Many treatment programs have developed from the basis of the Alcoholics Anonymous (AA) tradition and teach the tenet of reconstituting one's life while recognizing the importance of the care and nurturing of one's soul (Longabaugh et al. 1998). Although there is a debate about whether spirituality is an *essential* aspect of treatment, most clinicians in the field agree that issues of spirituality are worth exploring with patients who are attempting to rebuild their lives free of substance-related problems.

Dealing With Homelessness

Homelessness as a factor in treatment used to be a topic that only applied to central-city, skid-row programs. It is an unfortunate sign of our times that now most treatment programs attempting to optimize functioning of their patients have to take the time to determine the stability of their patients' current living situation. An important part of treatment is determining appropriate placement. Thus, it is worth the time and effort to assess not only present living situations but also the likelihood of the need for help in the near future.

Preventing Relapse

Many of the programmatic goals discussed in the next section emphasize the necessity of recognizing the limitation of financial resources. In part reflecting this reality, the period of time allowed for the intensive intervention phase in either an inpatient or an outpatient mode has been considerably shortened in recent years. This limitation underscores the importance of efforts aimed at helping to prevent relapse.

An integral part of helping persons to function is to raise their awareness of the need to develop high levels of vigilance regarding potential relapse, and to help them produce a plan of action for those occasions when they find themselves in a situation where relapse is highly likely or even when a "slip," or temporary resumption of substance use, has occurred (Allsop et al. 1997). Most treatment programs use the intensive phase of care to teach about relapse prevention, a subject that is emphasized even more fully through aftercare groups. Ways to minimize the risk of returning to substance use are taught through lectures, group discussions, and individual counseling sessions. Topics likely to be covered include the recognition of situations in which craving is likely to increase, the person's responsibility for avoiding "accidental" exposure to stressful situations in which substances are freely available, the development of a scenario of what to do and whom to contact if problems begin, and how to avoid allowing a temporary resumption of substance intake to be used as an excuse for escalating intake even further.

Programmatic Goals

The pragmatics of the need for resources in order to develop a treatment program require that clinicians recognize that the goals for patients outlined in the previous section are not enough to develop and maintain a program. The "institution" formed by people attempting to reach out to men and women with substance-related problems must itself function in relationship to a number of goals. These goals can be summarized as steps that are required to develop an atmosphere that is optimally conducive to helping patients and clients with substance-related problems.

1. **It is important to consider fiscal and political realities.** The amount of monies available in comparison with the number of patients seeking care establishes some realities of day-to-day life. This ratio helps to determine the type of facility that will be used (e.g., inpatient vs. outpatient; freestanding facility vs. one affiliated with a medical institution), the therapeutic regimen (e.g., more vs. less emphasis on physician care), the number of staff, the length of contact with patients, the number of hours that the facility will be open, and so on. The source of funding also dictates some political realities that have an impact on treatment goals. For instance, for a city-funded skid-row facility, the probable low 1-year rate of absolute abstinence for homeless drug- and alcohol-dependent persons entering rehabilitation makes it unwise to judge the program solely on the number of men and women who abstain over long periods of time (Schuckit 2000). The funding agencies (including insurers) might consider that a more appropriate immediate goal is to deal with severe medical problems that require active treatment, because efforts in this area can be lifesaving and outcomes more easily documented. This goal can, of course, be achieved in the context of efforts to help patients and clients achieve and maintain abstinence.
2. **Financial and staff resources must be used carefully.** In general, such management requires that treatment approaches be kept as simple as possible, with potentially expensive or potentially dangerous additions to a standard regimen being avoided until controlled studies have demonstrated that these more costly approaches are justified.
3. **The philosophy of the staff must be clearly stated.** In the substance use disorders field, it is not clear that one theoretical approach is likely to be more effective than another. Thus, after taking into account the realities of financial and staff resources, different programs are likely to demonstrate different theoretical biases, without one being apparently superior to any other. The specific theoretical bent chosen by a program probably rests as much with chance and the training of the director as with any solid literature review. In any event, staff who hope to function optimally while reaching out to patients must develop a level of comfort with one another. Achieving such rapport, in turn, often requires that the philosophy of the program (be it eclectic or committed to any specific model) be clearly stated and understood.
4. **It is wise to remember that no treatment is totally safe.** Patients can have adverse reactions to medications, develop complications of diagnostic procedures, act on bad advice, and run the risk of exhausting their scarce resources of time and money. Therefore, all programs should attempt to conform with the goal of doing the most good possible while exposing their patients to the least possible risks (Goodwin and Guze 1996). This cost-benefit ratio depends on knowledge of the usual course of alcohol- and drug-related problems in order for the clinician to be certain that the intervention poses less risk to the patient than does the clinical course likely to be observed in the subsequent months. Thus, isolated alcohol and drug problems, although certainly cause for concern, do not necessarily justify full-scale intervention.

One way to predict the probable course of problems likely to be observed over time with or without treatment is to carefully establish the diagnosis of abuse or dependence (Goodwin and Guze 1996; Schuckit 2000). Once one is certain that actual dependence has developed, the risks and costs of most of the usual substance-related rehabilitation efforts are likely to be outweighed by the benefits of such treatments. At the same time, documenting isolated problems or showing that a patient fulfills criteria for substance abuse (in the absence of dependence) indicates that a confrontation is likely to be beneficial and that some form of intervention is justified (Schuckit 2000). However, the lower level of intensity of the future course (assuming dependence does not subsequently develop) might not be sufficient to justify admitting the patient into a multiple-week inpatient rehabilitation program or assigning a patient to a long-term halfway or recovery home.

5. **It is important to determine that the treatment approaches being considered are more effective than chance alone.** Substance misuse problems fluctuate in intensity (Vaillant 1996). Patients and clients are likely to come to a treatment program for care at the time of their most intense problems. Therefore, it should not be surprising that with the passage of time alone and in the absence of intensive treatment, persons are likely to continue to experience a waxing and waning of symptom intensity. The fact that a patient shows improvement in functioning 6 months after intervention X was used does not prove that it was the intervention that was responsible for the improvement. Only through careful studies can we be sure that any particular intervention is actually useful.

Ideally, this requirement for careful studies that document that an intervention be superior to the passage of time alone should be applied to all treatment efforts in medicine and in the behavioral sciences. Because of the costs involved in such studies, however, most clinicians in most programs have a basic treatment approach that they accept as potentially beneficial and that is rarely tested. This basic approach often includes the efforts described above for increasing motivation for abstinence and helping persons to rebuild their lives without the substance. On the other hand, the addition of any intervention beyond the basic program should require documentation through carefully controlled research that the additional approach adds significantly to the outcome. Therefore, it is not wise to add a medication or additional therapy time, or to change the length of treatment, without carefully considering whether our patients benefit adequately from the altered approach.

Some Potentially Inappropriate Goals

As is true of most things in life, sometimes the things we do not do are as important as the things we do. Once a treatment program accepts the caveat of "Do no harm," it is important to recognize goals that are potentially inappropriate in dealing with substance-related problems.

For example, while attempting to help a patient achieve and maintain abstinence as well as develop a lifestyle free of substance use, it is unwise to use medications to treat insomnia, anxiety, or depression observed during intoxication or withdrawal (Schuckit 1996, 2000). For the physically addicting drugs (i.e., depressants, stimulants, and opiates), withdrawal-related psychological symptoms can be expected to be most intense during the first several weeks, with a great deal of improvement over the subsequent weeks (Raimo and

Schuckit 1998; Schuckit et al. 1997a). However, it is likely that the body will not reach its optimal level of functioning in a substance-free environment for perhaps 3–6 months following abstinence (Satel et al. 1993). For patients in this position, counseling, cognitive therapy, and behavioral approaches can help them deal with their temporary but troubling problems (e.g., insomnia, mood swings, nervousness) that are likely to plague their existence in an on-again, off-again fashion during the early months of recovery. Of course, there are two exceptions to this general prohibition against medications for substance-related anxiety or depression. The first exception is that medications may be necessary to treat acute withdrawal, especially from depressant- and opiate-type drugs. The second exception is that those patients who have been documented to have an independent major psychiatric disorder may require an appropriate medication (e.g., lithium for bipolar disorder, antidepressant medication(s) for severe major depressive disorder, or antipsychotic drugs for schizophrenia).

A related concern is the need to distinguish between treatments that *might enhance* recovery rates and those that have been demonstrated through careful study to be worth the risks involved. Using this approach, one finds that there are few medications that are justified for use among persons with substance use problems. The exceptions include methadone for severely impaired opiate-dependent persons (Marsch 1998), and possibly naltrexone, acamprosate, or disulfiram (Antabuse) for alcohol-dependent persons (Carroll et al. 1998). Although many other drugs are being evaluated for their potential in treating substance use disorders, few, if any, of these have been subject to enough carefully controlled studies to justify their routine use.

Another potentially inappropriate goal is any attempt to change long-standing personality characteristics as a routine part of substance-dependence rehabilitation. There are few convincing data that a specific personality profile, other than the antisocial personality disorder, is an important cause of substance dependence (Holdcraft et al. 1998). Even if such data existed, it is likely to be far beyond the financial and staff resources of the usual treatment program to offer intensive efforts at altering personality styles as an integral part of treatment.

Conclusions

The goals of treatment for substance use disorders appear, at first glance, obvious. Few would argue with the appropriateness of stating that abstinence and the development of a substance-free lifestyle over an extended period of time are the central goals in almost all treatment efforts with substance-dependent persons.

Implementation of these general goals requires the recognition of many realities regarding our patients and the political and fiscal environments in which we work. Thus, it is the manner in which we go about attempting to achieve our more global objectives that is likely to have a marked influence on the survival both of our patients and of our programs.

The general goals of treatment, however, should be placed into proper perspective. Being general in nature, some individual goals will not apply to specific programs. Nonetheless, it is hoped that the thoughts offered in the preceding discussion will help interested clinicians reading this text to develop a framework through which many of the subsequent chapters in Section 4 may be viewed. Perhaps some of these thoughts might also be of use in developing new programs and in optimizing existing ones.

References

Allsop S, Saunders B, Phillips M, et al: A trial of relapse prevention with severely dependent male problem drinkers. Addiction 92:61–74, 1997

Carroll KM, Nich C, Ball SA, et al: Treatment of cocaine and alcohol dependence with psychotherapy and disulfiram. Addiction 93:713–728, 1998

Epstein EE, McCrady BS, Hirsch LS: Marital functioning in early versus late-onset alcoholic couples. Alcohol Clin Exp Res 21:547–556, 1997

Gawin FH, Ellinwood EH Jr: Cocaine and other stimulants. N Engl J Med 318:1173–1182, 1988

Goodwin DW, Guze SB: Psychiatric Diagnosis, 5th Edition. New York, Oxford University Press, 1996

Helzer JE, Robins LN, Taylor JR, et al: The extent of long-term moderate drinking among alcoholics discharged from medical and psychiatric treatment facilities. N Engl J Med 312:1678–1682, 1985

Holdcraft LC, Iacono WG, McGue MK: Antisocial personality disorder and depression in relation to alcoholism: a community-based sample. J Stud Alcohol 59:222–226, 1998

Longabaugh R, Wirtz PW, Zweben A, et al: Network support for drinking, Alcoholics Anonymous and long-term matching effects. Addiction 93:1313–1333, 1998

Marsch LA: The efficacy of methadone maintenance interventions in reducing illicit opiate use, HIV risk behavior and criminality: a meta-analysis. Addiction 93:515–532, 1998

McLellan AT, Woody GF, Metzger D: Evaluating the effectiveness of addiction treatments: reasonable expectations, appropriate comparisons. Milbank Q 74:51–83, 1996

Raimo EB, Schuckit MA: Alcohol dependence and mood disorders. Addict Behav 23:933–946, 1998

Regier DA, Farmer ME, Rae DS, et al: Comorbidity of mental disorders with alcohol and other drug abuse. JAMA 264:2511–2518, 1990

Satel SL, Kosten TR, Schuckit MA, et al: Should protracted withdrawal from drugs be included in DSM-IV? Am J Psychiatry 150:695–704, 1993

Schuckit MA: Drug and Alcohol Abuse: A Clinical Guide to Diagnosis and Treatment, 5th Edition. J Consult Clin Psychol 64:669–676, 1996

Schuckit MA: Recent developments in pharmacotherapy of alcohol dependence. New York, Kluwer Academic, 2000

Schuckit MA, Tipp JE, Bergman M, et al: Comparison of induced and independent major depressive disorders in 2,945 alcoholics. Am J Psychiatry 154:948–957, 1997a

Schuckit MA, Tipp JE, Bucholz KK, et al: The life-time rates of three major mood disorders and four major anxiety disorders in alcoholics and controls. Addiction 92:1289–1304, 1997b

Schuckit MA, Tipp JE, Smith TL, et al: Periods of abstinence following the onset of alcohol dependence in 1,853 men and women. J Stud Alcohol 58:581–589, 1997c

Schuckit MA, Daeppen JB, Tipp JE, et al: The clinical course of alcohol-related problems in alcohol dependent and nonalcohol dependent drinking women and men. J Stud Alcohol 59:581–590, 1998

Schuckit MA, Daeppen JB, Danko GP, et al: Clinical implications for four drugs of the DSM-IV distinction between substance dependence with and without a physiological component. Am J Psychiatry 156:41–49, 1999

Vaillant GE: A long-term follow-up of male alcohol abuse. Arch Gen Psychiatry 53:243–249, 1996

Assessment of Patients

Richard S. Schottenfeld, M.D.
Michael V. Pantalon, Ph.D.

The primary goals of the substance abuse clinical evaluation are 1) to make an accurate diagnostic assessment of substance abuse or dependence and of the relationship of substance use to other psychiatric and medical disorders, 2) to plan and initiate effective interventions and treatment where indicated, and 3) to enhance the patient's motivation for treatment.

The failure to assess substance use patterns and problems related to use as a routine part of the medical or psychiatric history has resulted in unacceptably low rates of routine detection of substance use disorders in medical and psychiatric practice in many studies. Physicians most often miss the diagnosis of substance abuse or dependence in patients who are employed, married, white, insured, or female (Clark 1981; Cleary et al. 1988; Moore et al. 1989; Wolf et al. 1965), suggesting that mistaken stereotypes about alcoholic and addicted persons continue to affect clinical practice adversely. Needless to say, the failure to diagnose substance abuse or dependence precludes effective intervention or treatment and contributes to continued and more severe problems.

The characteristic defenses of patients with substance use disorders (minimization, denial, projection [i.e., blaming others for their problems], and grandiosity), as well as the reluctance of patients' family, friends, or co-workers to confront patients or to disclose information to physicians about these sensitive issues, contribute to the failure to diagnose these disorders (Nace 1987). Covert and overt attitudes of physicians about drug and alco-

---

This chapter subpart is a revised version of our chapter "Assessment of the Patient," which appeared in Galanter MA, Kleber HD (eds): *The American Psychiatric Press Textbook of Substance Abuse Treatment*, 2nd Edition. Washington, DC, American Psychiatric Press, 1999, pp. 109–119.

hol dependence may also interfere with timely diagnosis and treatment (Clark 1981; Lisansky 1975). These attitudes often include a reluctance to recognize the harmful effects of a patient's substance use because of the physician's own pattern of alcohol or drug use, a tendency to view addictive disorders as moral shortcomings of the patient rather than valid psychiatric disorders, or concerns about "labeling" a patient and about the patient's potentially angry response. Far from stigmatizing the patient, however, accurately diagnosing a substance use disorder and clearly labeling the patient's problems as resulting from alcohol or drug use are critical steps in motivating behavioral change and commitment to treatment.

In the remaining sections of this chapter subpart, we first review the concept of the dependence syndrome and the diagnostic features of substance use disorders and then discuss ways of eliciting an accurate history, observing signs of substance use disorders during the psychiatric examination, and assessing the relationship between substance use and other comorbid psychiatric disorders. In addition to the diagnostic interview with the patient and the mental status examination, a complete evaluation must be performed, consisting of reviewing the patient's medical records and the results of physical examination and laboratory studies; utilizing reports from family members, friends, co-workers, or supervisors; and monitoring the patient's breath alcohol concentration and urine for toxicological evidence of drug use. The utility of commonly used screening questionnaires and structured interviews is also considered. Finally, we review methods for assessing the patient's motivation for changing substance use and discuss the application of motivational interventions to substance-involved patients.

Dependence Syndrome and Diagnosis of Substance Use Disorders

DSM-IV criteria (American Psychiatric Association 1994) for substance use disorders continue to reflect the consensus that dependence is best conceptualized as a biobehavioral construct characterized by compulsive use of a substance rather than as a purely or primarily physical state (Rounsaville and Kranzler 1989). Viewed in this fashion, the concept of dependence can be applied to the pathological use of any of a variety of psychoactive substances, including some highly addicting drugs, such as cocaine, that do not produce significant signs of physical dependence. The DSM-IV criteria for substance dependence (Table 25–1) stress the importance of impaired control of psychoactive substance use and the increasing salience of continued use, in addition to physiological measures of dependence (tolerance and withdrawal), as the diagnostic hallmarks of dependence.

In DSM-IV, 11 specific classes of psychoactive substances are identified, including nicotine (cigarettes, cigars, chewing tobacco), caffeine (coffee, tea, and other caffeinated beverages; food products; medications), alcohol (beer, wine, and distilled spirits such as whiskey, vodka, gin), cannabinoids (marijuana, hashish), cocaine, amphetamines, opioids (heroin, morphine, Dilaudid, methadone, oxycodone, etc.), sedative-hypnotics and anxiolytics (barbiturates, benzodiazepines), psychotomimetics (e.g., phencyclidine [PCP]), hallucinogens (e.g., lysergic acid diethylamide [LSD]), and inhalants (glue, paint thinners, solvents). Organic mental syndromes can be associated with use of, intoxication from, or withdrawal from any of the 11 classes; caffeine is not considered to cause either abuse or dependence, and nicotine is considered to lead to dependence but not abuse.

TABLE 25–1. DSM-IV diagnostic criteria for substance dependence

A maladaptive pattern of substance use, leading to clinically significant impairment or distress, as manifested by three (or more) of the following, occurring at any time in the same 12-month period:

(1) tolerance, as defined by either of the following:

- (a) a need for markedly increased amounts of the substance to achieve intoxication or desired effect
- (b) markedly diminished effect with continued use of the same amount of the substance

(2) withdrawal, as manifested by either of the following:

- (a) the characteristic withdrawal syndrome for the substance (refer to criteria A and B of the criteria sets for withdrawal from the specific substances)
- (b) the same (or a closely related) substance is taken to relieve or avoid withdrawal symptoms

(3) the substance is often taken in larger amounts or over a longer period than was intended

(4) there is a persistent desire or unsuccessful efforts to cut down or control substance use

(5) a great deal of time is spent in activities necessary to obtain the substance (e.g., visiting multiple doctors or driving long distances), use the substance (e.g., chain-smoking), or recover from its effects

(6) important social, occupational, or recreational activities are given up or reduced because of substance use

(7) the substance use is continued despite knowledge of having a persistent or recurrent physical or psychological problem that is likely to have been caused or exacerbated by the substance (e.g., current cocaine use despite recognition of cocaine-induced depression, or continued drinking despite recognition that an ulcer was made worse by alcohol consumption)

Specify if:

With physiological dependence: evidence of tolerance or withdrawal (i.e., either item 1 or item 2 is present)

Without physiological dependence: no evidence of tolerance or withdrawal (i.e., neither item 1 nor item 2 is present)

Course specifiers (see text for definitions):

Early full remission
Early partial remission
Sustained full remission
Sustained partial remission
On agonist therapy
In a controlled environment

In DSM-IV, a diagnosis of psychoactive substance dependence requires the occurrence of at least three symptoms from a list of seven during the same 12-month period. *Remission*, defined by the absence of all of the symptoms for more than 1 month, may be classified as either early (less than 12 months) or sustained and may be either partial (intermittent or occasional symptoms) or full (no symptoms). Remissions associated with being on agonist therapy (e.g., methadone maintenance) or with living in a controlled environment (where access to the substance is restricted) should be classified as "on agonist therapy" or "in a controlled environment."

Symptoms of the dependence syndrome can be viewed as forming three clusters. The first two symptoms listed in DSM-IV (see Table 25–1) indicate *neurophysiological adaptations*. These symptoms include tolerance, as defined by a need for markedly increased amounts to obtain desired effects or markedly diminished effects with continued use of the same amount, and withdrawal, as manifested by either characteristic withdrawal symptoms following discontinuation of use or use of the substance to relieve or avoid withdrawal symptoms. The next two symptoms indicate *impaired control* of substance use: taking of the drug in larger amounts or over longer periods than originally intended, and persistent desire or one or more efforts to cut down or control substance use. The last three symptoms indicate that use of the substance has become increasingly important to the person. The *salience* of substance use to the person is indicated by spending a great deal of time acquiring, using, or recovering from substance use; reduction in or discontinuation of important social, occupational, or recreational activities because of substance use; and continued use despite knowledge of having a persistent or recurrent psychological or physical problem that is likely to be caused or exacerbated by the use of the substance.

In DSM-IV, psychoactive substance abuse is defined as a maladaptive pattern of substance use that leads to clinically significant impairment or distress over a 12-month period, but has never met the criteria for dependence (Table 25–2). Abuse is indicated by any one of the following four symptoms: 1) failure to fulfill major role occupations at work, school, or home as a result of substance use; 2) recurrent use in situations in which use is physically hazardous; 3) occurrence of recurrent legal problems related to substance use; and 4) continued use despite having persistent or recurrent social or interpersonal problems caused or exacerbated by the use.

TABLE 25–2. DSM-IV diagnostic criteria for substance abuse

A. A maladaptive pattern of substance use leading to clinically significant impairment or distress, as manifested by one (or more) of the following, occurring within a 12-month period:
   (1) recurrent substance use resulting in a failure to fulfill major role obligations at work, school, or home (e.g., repeated absences or poor work performance related to substance use; substance-related absences, suspensions, or expulsions from school; neglect of children or household)
   (2) recurrent substance use in situations in which it is physically hazardous (e.g., driving an automobile or operating a machine when impaired by substance use)
   (3) recurrent substance-related legal problems (e.g., arrests for substance-related disorderly conduct)
   (4) continued substance use despite having persistent or recurrent social or interpersonal problems caused or exacerbated by the effects of the substance (e.g., arguments with spouse about consequences of intoxication, physical fights)

B. The symptoms have never met the criteria for substance dependence for this class of substance.

Diagnostic features of organic mental syndromes associated with psychoactive substances are also detailed in DSM-IV. Included among these disorders are intoxication, withdrawal, delirium, withdrawal delirium, psychotic disorders, mood disorders, and other syndromes (e.g., sleep or sexual dysfunctions associated with substance use; amnestic disorders and dementias).

Patient's History

Pattison (1986) identified components of an alcohol history that serve as a useful summary of the areas that need to be addressed in the patient's substance use history. These components include assessment of quantity and frequency of intake and of symptoms of tolerance and withdrawal, as well as assessment of adverse medical, interpersonal, vocational, social, and legal consequences. Additional components include assessment of the behaviors engaged in when the patient is drinking alcohol or using drugs, personality changes associated with drinking or drug use, and emotional consequences (such as shame, diminished self-esteem, paranoid ideation, anxiety, and dissociative states).

As in all aspects of the psychiatric interview, a straightforward, nonjudgmental approach is most likely to elicit accurate information. Psychiatrists need to take into consideration the characteristic defenses of patients with substance use disorders and to take note of what the patient is trying to hide. It goes without saying, however, that patients who are intoxicated or delirious at the time of assessment cannot give an accurate history.

When the clinician is eliciting the history, the patient's concerns about disclosure of information to family members, employers, legal authorities, or licensing boards also need to be addressed directly. Sometimes the patient's reluctance to disclose sensitive information is lessened by a frank discussion about why this information is important, how the information will be used, and what measures can and will be taken to safeguard the patient's confidentiality. Confidentiality regulations are set by both federal and state authorities and may differ according to whether the patient is an adult or a minor. Consequently, physicians need to be informed about the specific reporting requirements and confidentiality statutes affecting their practice (Senay 1992).

One general strategy for eliciting the history is to begin by reviewing the patient's life history, including successes and problems experienced in work, school, family, and friendships, as well as medical, legal, and psychological and emotional problems, without linking any of these problems to the patient's use of alcohol or other drugs. Following this overview, a parallel chronology of the patient's use of alcohol and drugs can be obtained, and, finally, specific inquiry can be directed to the relationship between alcohol or drug use and the patient's life problems. This strategy may reveal a correlation not previously recognized by the patient between substance use and his or her life problems.

Although sensitivity to the patient's defensiveness is necessary, it is essential to obtain a complete alcohol and drug history. Specific questions need to be addressed to all categories of psychoactive substances. Inquiry should be directed to a history of lifetime and recent use of substances from each of the categories. For drugs that can be prescribed for medical purposes, it is also essential to determine whether these drugs were taken only for the prescribed purpose and whether use ever exceeded the prescribed dose or duration. It may be useful to ask about the general category and then name specific substances, using generic, brand, and street names as examples—for example, "Have you ever used any opioid or opiate-like drugs, such as morphine, Demerol, Dilaudid, methadone, or Percodan? What about heroin, P-dope, smack, or horse?"

For each of the drug categories, patients should be asked about lifetime use, recent or current use, periods of heaviest use, and pattern of use during each period. Pattern of use refers to quantity used per occasion (average and maximum), frequency (how often used), duration of episodes of use, route of administration, and expense. Age at and circumstances of first use, how the person reacted initially, who was with the person at the time of first use, and how soon the person used it again are often of diagnostic and therapeutic import (Kaufman and Reoux 1988).

Clinicians need to be alert to early and subtle indications of problematic use. With regard to alcohol, for example, indications may include relief drinking, surreptitious drinking, anticipatory drinking, and gulping drinks. Rationalizing drinking, protecting the supply, making geographic escapes to facilitate drinking, and drinking regularly in the morning are later occurrences and indicate greater problem severity (Pokorny and Kansas 1980). Changes in the pattern of alcohol or other drug use, including narrowing of the patient's alcohol or drug-taking repertoire, may also be a clue to a diagnosis of dependence. Some patient comments, such as "I never drink before five o'clock," "I never drink alone," or "I never drink spirits, only beer," may indicate a struggle over controlling use.

Finally, attention needs to be directed to any medical, psychological or emotional, and social complications of substance use. Early signs of problematic alcohol or drug use may include occurrence of blackouts, accidental overdoses, behavior changes, driving or other dangerous or aggressive activities while intoxicated, or guilt about behaviors engaged in while using. Later sequelae include loss of nonusing friends; loss of interest in non-drug-related activities; impaired relationships with family, friends, and co-workers; disruptions of occupational or social functioning; and occurrence of medical or legal problems.

Physical and Mental Status Examinations

The physical examination and mental status examination provide critical information regarding diagnosis, management, and treatment of substance abuse and dependence and of their medical and psychiatric sequelae. They should also be directed at detecting signs of acute intoxication, withdrawal, or delirium. Some potentially life-threatening complications such as impending drug overdose, sepsis, or severe nutritional deficiency may be evident on physical examination.

Slurred speech, incoordination, unsteady gait, nystagmus, impairment in attention or memory, or a flushed face may be signs of alcohol, sedative, or anxiolytic intoxication. Pupillary dilatation, diaphoresis, restlessness, nervousness, excitement, flushed face, muscle twitching, psychomotor agitation, or pressured or rambling speech may result from stimulant intoxication (including caffeine intoxication). Evidence of opioid intoxication includes pupillary constriction, drowsiness, slurred speech, and impairment in attention or memory. Cannabinoid intoxication may be indicated by conjunctival injection (i.e., bloodshot eyes), increased appetite, dry mouth, and tachycardia.

On physical examination, signs of opioid withdrawal include fever, lacrimation, rhinorrhea, dilated pupils, diaphoresis, and piloerection. Tachycardia, elevated blood pressure, and tremulousness are consistent with withdrawal from alcohol, sedatives, or anxiolytics. Delirium, which may result from intoxication with stimulants or withdrawal from alcohol, for example, is characterized by disorganized thinking, disorientation, perceptual disturbances, reduced attention to external stimuli, psychomotor agitation or retardation, and a reduced level of consciousness.

A careful mental status examination, including assessment of cognitive functioning, is also essential to detect other major sequelae of substance use disorders, such as transient or persistent hallucinatory phenomena, delirium, mood and affective disturbances (panic, anxiety, depression, guilt, shame, diminished self-esteem), and paranoid, suicidal, or violent ideation or behavior. Delirium may result from intoxication with stimulants, cannabis, and hallucinogens or from withdrawal from alcohol, sedatives, or anxiolytics. Assessment of cognitive functioning should include evaluation of attention and concentration, recent and remote memory, abstract reasoning, and problem-solving ability. All of these functions may be impaired by recent alcohol, sedative, anxiolytic, stimulant, or polydrug use. At least in the case of alcohol, and, as documented more recently, cocaine, memory deficits and other cognitive impairments may be persistent or permanent (Grant 1987; O'Malley et al. 1992).

Sleep and appetite disturbances, mood lability, irritability, anxiety, and depressed mood all can be symptoms of current substance abuse or dependence. Patients may be completely unaware that these problems result from or are exacerbated by substance use, but these symptoms should be considered presumptive evidence of problematic substance use in patients who otherwise report "controlled" use. Frank discussion with the patient about the relationship between these symptoms and his or her substance use will lead the patient without a substance use disorder to abstain and may help to overcome a substance-dependent patient's denial and to increase recognition of the need to abstain.

Finally, the mental status examination is critical to ascertain the presence of any comorbid psychiatric disorders, such as schizophrenia, bipolar disorder, major depression, and anxiety disorders. These comorbid disorders occur frequently, affect prognosis, and have important treatment implications.

Screening Instruments and Structured Interviews

A number of short self-report questionnaires are available to aid in the routine detection of alcohol abuse and dependence. The four-question CAGE—"Have you ever 1) attempted to *C*ut back on alcohol, 2) been *A*nnoyed by comments made about your drinking, 3) felt *G*uilty about drinking, 4) had an *E*ye-opener first thing in the morning to steady your nerves?" (Mayfield et al. 1974)—has been found to improve routine detection rates in primary care and medical settings (Bradley et al. 1998b; Lawner et al. 1997). Modified versions of the CAGE—including the four-item T-ACE (*T*olerance, *A*nnoyed, *C*ut back, *E*ye-opener; Sokol et al. 1989) or the five-item TWEAK (*T*olerance, *W*orried, *E*ye-opener, *A*nnoyed, *K*ut back; Russell et al. 1991), which contain items assessing alcohol tolerance—appear to have even greater sensitivity and specificity than the CAGE for assessing lifetime alcohol abuse or dependence (Chan et al. 1993; O'Connor and Schottenfeld 1998), especially among women (Bradley et al. 1998a). To improve their sensitivity in detecting current disorders, these questionnaires can be supplemented with standardized questions regarding quantity and frequency of drinking, such as those included in the Alcohol Use Disorders Identification Test (AUDIT; Saunders et al. 1993) (Bradley et al. 1998b; Bush et al. 1998; Volk et al. 1997), or more detailed questionnaires, such as the Michigan Alcoholism Screening Test (MAST; Selzer 1971) (Wetterling et al. 1998).

Utilization of structured interviews provides a reliable way to elicit diagnostic information and decrease omission of questioning about significant signs or symptoms. Two of these merit special attention. The Structured Clinical Interview for DSM-IV (SCID; First et al. 1995) is a clinically based interview that facilitates definitive diagnosis of DSM-IV substance-related and other psychiatric disorders. The Addiction Severity Index (ASI; McLellan et al. 1992) facilitates a multidimensional assessment of patients with substance use disorders by evaluating alcohol and drug problem severity and the severity of medical, psychiatric, social, legal, and occupational problems experienced by the patient. Initial ASI ratings of problem severity are highly correlated with treatment outcome and can be used to determine the need for specialized psychiatric, vocational, or medical interventions. The ASI can also be used to monitor the effects of treatment and changes in the patient's functioning.

Interviews With Significant Others

Whenever possible, evaluation should include an interview with family members or others who are in contact with the patient and do not themselves have alcohol or drug problems. Use of multiple informants can substantially increase the validity of the evaluation and reliability of patient self-reports. Family members may be able to provide critical information regarding the patient's behavioral changes or problems experienced as a direct result of alcohol or other drug use even while knowing little about how much or often the patient is using. Involvement of family members in the initial stages of the evaluation will also facilitate family-based interventions, including limit setting and long-term family support of treatment goals.

Laboratory Examination

Urine toxicology testing for drugs of abuse is an essential component of the substance abuse evaluation. Such testing is critical in cases of suspected drug overdose or when there are acute changes in mental status. Patients with any indication of alcohol or drug problems should be asked to give voluntary consent to urine toxicology testing as a routine part of the evaluation. In situations where there are no adverse consequences to a positive test, most patients, including most drug users, will consent to testing. With the exception of medical emergencies, it is unethical to test a person for drugs without the person's consent. Refusal to be tested in a medical setting, however, is often indicative of a problem. For some patients, toxicology testing may be the only way to document the problem and confront the patient about drug use. Even for patients who acknowledge drug problems, urine toxicology testing often reveals surprising results. Many patients openly admit to using one substance that has become a problem for them while continuing to deny their other drug use.

The clinical utility of drug abuse testing is enhanced by a thorough understanding of the methodologies that are used in the testing procedures, the sensitivity and specificity of the assays used, and the substances that can be detected and their duration in urine (Cone 1997). Because metabolites of heroin and cocaine can be detected reliably for only a few days following use, a weekend binge may not be detected in a urine sample collected on a Friday morning. Hair testing may increase the detection period following last use, but it is less useful as a means of monitoring relapse. Use of a breathalyzer is a convenient, reliable, and inexpensive method of determining current alcohol intoxication or alcohol consumption within the last 6–8 hours.

A variety of biochemical tests have been used as markers of harmful alcohol use, but their value is limited by problems with sensitivity and specificity. Sensitivity and specificity of these markers may be increased by using combinations of measures (e.g., serum gamma-glutamyltransferase [GGT] or aspartate aminotransferase [AST]), especially in conjunction with measures of increased red blood cell size (mean corpuscular volume [MCV]). Carbohydrate-deficient transferrin is currently the most sensitive and specific marker of heavy drinking (Wetterling et al. 1998) and may be particularly useful in monitoring abstinence during treatment (Allen et al. 1994).

To detect adverse medical consequences of alcohol and other drug use, initial evaluation of a patient with a substance use disorder should include a urinalysis (to detect kidney damage), a complete blood count, blood chemistry and liver enzymes, serology (venereal disease research laboratory [VDRL] test or fluorescent treponemal antibody absorption

[FTS-ABS] and hepatitis antibody and antigen), and testing for tuberculosis (purified protein derivative [PPD]). After appropriate counseling, testing for human immunodeficiency virus (HIV) infection is also indicated.

Assessment of Comorbid Psychiatric Disorders

Acute and chronic use of psychoactive substances can have profound effects on cognitive functioning, mood, thought processes, and personality functioning. In the absence of a history of substance use, many of these effects may be indistinguishable, on the basis of signs and symptoms alone, from primary Axis I or Axis II psychiatric disorders. Although these substance-induced syndromes are classified as organic mental disorders, accurate diagnosis is made problematic because patients with substance use disorders also experience high rates of psychiatric disorders independent of substance use.

Guidelines for distinguishing primary psychiatric disorders from substance abuse–related disorders are still evolving. In alcohol-dependent patients a diagnosis of an independent psychiatric disorder can only be made if onset of the disorder either preceded the initial onset of alcoholism, persisted during past periods of abstinence, or continues after 4 weeks of abstinence (Schuckit 1985). This approach avoids diagnosing a primary mood disorder in the majority of alcoholic patients whose mood will recover spontaneously during the first 4 weeks of abstinence. With other drugs that may be less likely to cause mood disorders, however, it may be prudent to shorten the period of abstinence required both to make a presumptive diagnosis and to begin pharmacological treatment.

Regardless of the diagnostic criteria utilized to diagnose comorbid psychiatric disorders and the exact timing of implementation of treatment for underlying psychiatric disorders, a diagnosis of comorbid psychiatric disorders has important prognostic and clinical implications. With the exception of depression among alcoholic women, the occurrence of comorbid psychiatric disorders usually confers a poorer treatment prognosis (Rounsaville et al. 1986, 1987). Psychiatric treatment of underlying psychiatric disorders, however, has been shown to improve treatment outcome for both opioid-dependent patients and alcoholic patients (Rounsaville et al. 1986, 1987). Matching of patients to treatments on the basis of an assessment of comorbid psychiatric disorders may also improve treatment outcome (McLellan et al. 1983, 1997). In a comparison of interactional group therapy and coping skills training in a structured group setting, Kadden et al. (1989) and Litt et al. (1992) documented that the structured group treatment was associated with improved treatment outcomes for sociopathic alcoholic patients, whereas the interactional group therapy was more effective for less sociopathic alcoholic patients. More recently, in Project MATCH (Matching Alcoholism Treatment to Client Heterogeneity) it was found that alcohol-dependent patients with low psychiatric severity (as measured by the ASI) who were treated with 12-Step facilitation had a significantly greater number of days abstinent and fewer drinks per drinking day at posttreatment than when treated with cognitive-behavioral therapy (Project MATCH Research Group 1997). However, no such differences were observed for patients with high psychiatric severity.

Enhancement of Motivation

The assessment also affords a unique opportunity to enhance the patient's motivation for treatment, if any treatment is indicated. Motivational strategies are critical, because resistance and ambivalence are often at their highest at the time of initial assessment, and patients may not be ready even to talk about or acknowledge their problems, much less agree to treatment recommendations.

Assessing the patient's motivation for change involves gaining an understanding of the patient's goals and reasons for seeking consultation at this particular point in time. The patient's stage of change may be classified along a continuum from *precontemplation* (patient does not think he/she has a problem), to *contemplation* (patient is considering that he/she might have a problem but is not taking steps to change), to *determination* (patient has made a decision to change but has yet to act on it), to *action* (patient is actively taking steps to change), and finally to *maintenance* (patient is trying to maintain a current level of successful change by preventing relapse). Although assessment of the patient's stage of change can often be made on the basis of the information received during the assessment, standardized questionnaires are also available (Beiner and Abrams 1991; DiClemente et al. 1991; McConnaughy et al. 1989).

Once the assessment is completed, motivational enhancement techniques can be selected based on the patient's stage of change. For a patient in the precontemplation stage, noting discrepancies between the patient's current life situation or emotional state and the patient's ideal or desired situation may engender less resistance than directly confronting denial (Miller and Rollnick 1991). The assessment provides an opportunity to identify these discrepancies and to elicit from the patient self-motivating statements that point to the patient's ambivalence about and interest in change (Samet et al. 1996). Thus, for example, the clinician might comment, on the basis of the patient's statements, that it appears that although the patient experiences most of his or her best times (e.g., times when the patient feels the happiest, most energetic) when using, the patient is also concerned that his or her job may be in jeopardy because of frequent absences after binge drinking. Once a patient begins to identify some negative consequences of use and to contemplate curtailing use, identifying the impediments to change experienced by the patient and supporting the patient's perceived ability to make a change can be beneficial. Exploration of the patient's history of attempts to curtail or control use may also afford an opportunity for identifying appropriate treatment options and suggesting reasons that the patient might now be successful in making and sustaining a change.

Summary

In this chapter subpart, we have discussed methods for conducting an assessment of substance abuse so as to make an accurate diagnosis, delineate the effect of substance use on other medical and psychiatric disorders, plan treatment interventions, and increase the patient's motivation or readiness for initiating such treatment. The information obtained during the assessment will enable the clinician to determine whether the patient needs to make changes with regard to substance use and to recommend or plan appropriate treatment based on current practice guidelines (e.g., American Psychiatric Association 1995). A carefully conducted assessment will also increase the patient's interest in and capability for initiating and maintaining change.

References

Allen JP, Litten RZ, Anton RF, et al: Carbohydrate-deficient transferrin as a measure of immoderate drinking: remaining issues. Alcohol Clin Exp Res 18:799–812, 1994

American Psychiatric Association: Diagnostic and Statistical Manual of Mental Disorders, 4th Edition. Washington, DC, American Psychiatric Association, 1994

American Psychiatric Association: Practice guideline for the treatment of patients with substance use disorders: alcohol, cocaine, opioids. Am J Psychiatry 152 (11 suppl):1–59, 1995

Beiner L, Abrams DB: The contemplation ladder: validation of a measure of readiness to consider smoking cessation. Health Psychol 10:360–365, 1991

Bradley KA, Boyd-Wickizer J, Powell SH, et al: Alcohol screening questionnaires in women: a critical review (comment). JAMA 280:1904–1905, 1998a

Bradley KA, Bush KR, McDonell MB, et al: Screening for problem drinking: comparison of CAGE and AUDIT, Ambulatory Care Quality Improvement Project (ACQUIP). J Gen Intern Med 13:379–388, 1998b

Bush K, Kivlahan DR, McDonell MB, et al: The AUDIT alcohol consumption questions: an effective brief screening test for problem drinking, Ambulatory Care Quality Improvement Project (ACQUIP). Arch Intern Med 158:1789–1795, 1998

Chan AWK, Pristach EA, Welte JW, et al: Use of the TWEAK test in screening for alcoholism/heavy drinking in three populations. Alcohol Clin Exp Res 17:1188–1192, 1993

Clark WD: Alcoholism: blocks to diagnosis and treatment. Am J Med 71:275–285, 1981

Cleary PD, Miller M, Bush BT, et al: Prevalence and recognition of alcohol abuse in a primary care population. Am J Med 85:466–471, 1988

Cone EJ. New developments in biological measures of drug prevalence, in Validity of Self-Reported Drug Use: Improving the Accuracy of Survey Estimates. NIDA Research Monograph 167 (NTIS 97-175889). Edited by Harrison L, Hughes A. Rockville, MD, Department of Health and Human Services, 1997, pp 108–129

DiClemente CC, Prochaska JO, Fairhurst SK, et al: The process of smoking cessation: an analysis of precontemplation, contemplation, and preparation stages of change. J Consult Clin Psychol 59: 295–304, 1991

First MB, Spitzer RL, Gibbon M, et al: Structured Clinical Interview for DSM-IV Axis I Disorders—Patient Version 2.0 (SCID-I/P). New York, New York State Psychiatric Institute, 1995

Grant I: Alcohol and the brain: neuropsychological correlates. J Consult Clin Psychol 55:310–314, 1987

Kadden RM, Getter H, Cooney NL, et al: Matching alcoholics to coping skills or interactional therapies: posttreatment results. J Consult Clin Psychol 57:698–704, 1989

Kaufman E, Reoux J: Guidelines for the successful psychotherapy of substance abusers. Am J Drug Alcohol Abuse 14:199–209, 1988

Lawner K, Doot M, Gausas J, et al: Implementation of CAGE alcohol screening in a primary care practice. Fam Med 29:332–335, 1997

Lisansky ET: Why physicians avoid early diagnosis of alcoholism. N Y State J Med 75:1788–1792, 1975

Litt MD, Babor TF, DelBoca FK, et al: Types of alcoholics, II: application of an empirically derived typology to treatment matching. Arch Gen Psychiatry 49:609–614, 1992

Mayfield DG, McLeon G, Hall P: The CAGE Questionnaire: validation of a new alcoholism screening instrument. Am J Psychiatry 131:1121–1123, 1974

McConnaughy EA, DiClemente CC, Prochaska JO, et al: Stages of change in psychotherapy: a follow-up report. Psychotherapy: Theory, Research and Practice 26:494–503, 1989

McLellan AT, Woody GE, Luborsky L, et al: Increased effectiveness of substance abuse treatment: a prospective study of patient-treatment "matching." J Nerv Ment Dis 171:597–605, 1983

McLellan AT, Kushner H, Metzger D, et al: The fifth edition of the Addiction Severity Index. J Subst Abuse Treat 9:199–212, 1992

McLellan AT, Grissom GR, Zanis D, et al: Problem-service "matching" in addiction treatment: a prospective study in 4 programs. Arch Gen Psychiatry 54:730–735, 1997

Miller WR, Rollnick S: Motivational Interviewing: Preparing People to Change Addictive Behavior. New York, Guilford, 1991

Moore RD, Bone LR, Geller G, et al: Prevalence, detection, and treatment of alcoholism in hospitalized patients. JAMA 261:403–407, 1989

Nace EP: The Treatment of Alcoholism. New York, Brunner/Mazel, 1987

O'Connor PG, Schottenfeld RS: Patients with alcohol problems. N Engl J Med 338:592–602, 1998

O'Malley SS, Adamse M, Heaton RK, et al: Neuropsychological impairment in chronic cocaine abusers. Am J Drug Alcohol Abuse 18:131–144, 1992

Pattison ME: Clinical approaches to the alcoholic patient. Psychosomatics 27:762–767, 770, 1986

Pokorny AD, Kansas TE: Stages in the development of alcoholism, in Phenomenology and Treatment of Alcoholism. Edited by Fann WE, Karcan I, Pokorny AD, et al. New York, SP Medical & Scientific, 1980, p 62

Project MATCH Research Group: Matching alcoholism treatment to client heterogeneity: Project MATCH posttreatment drinking outcomes. J Stud Alcohol 58:7–29, 1997

Rounsaville BJ, Kranzler HR: The DSM-II-R diagnosis of alcoholism, in American Psychiatric Press Review of Psychiatry, Vol 8. Edited by Tasman A, Hales RE, Frances AJ. Washington, DC, American Psychiatric Press, 1989, pp 323–340

Rounsaville BJ, Kosten TR, Weissman MM, et al: Prognostic significance of psychiatric disorders in treated opiate addicts: a 2.5-year follow-up study. Arch Gen Psychiatry 43:739–745, 1986

Rounsaville BJ, Dolinsky ZS, Babor TF, et al: Psychopathology as a predictor of treatment outcome in alcoholics. Arch Gen Psychiatry 44:505–513, 1987

Russell M, Martier SS, Sokol RJ, et al. Screening for pregnancy risk drinking: tweaking the tests. Alcohol Clin Exp Res 15:368, 1991

Samet JH, Rollnick S, Barnes H: Beyond CAGE: a brief clinical approach after detection of substance abuse. Arch Intern Med 156:2287–2293, 1996

Saunders JB, Aasland OG, Babor TF, et al: Development of the Alcohol Use Disorders Identification Test (AUDIT): WHO Collaborative Project on Early Detection of Persons With Harmful Alcohol Consumption—II. Addiction 88:791–804, 1993

Schuckit MA: The clinical implications of primary diagnostic groups among alcoholics. Arch Gen Psychiatry 42:1043–1049, 1985

Selzer ML: The Michigan Alcoholism Screening Test: the quest for a new diagnostic instrument. Am J Psychiatry 127:1653–1658, 1971

Senay EC: Diagnostic interview and mental status examination, in Substance Abuse: A Comprehensive Textbook. Baltimore, MD, Williams & Wilkins, 1992, pp 416–424

Sokol RJ, Martier SS, Ager JW: The T-ACE questions: practical prenatal detection of risk drinking. Am J Obstet Gynecol 160:863–870, 1989

Volk RJ, Steinbauer JR, Cantor SB, et al: The Alcohol Use Disorders Identification Test (AUDIT) as a screen for at-risk drinking in primary care patients of different racial/ethnic backgrounds. Addiction 92:197–206, 1997

Wetterling T, Kanitz RD, Rumpf HJ, et al: Comparison of CAGE and MAST with the alcohol markers CDT, gamma-GT, ALAT, ASAT and MCV. Alcohol Alcohol 33:424–430, 1998

Wolf I, Chafetz ME, Blane HT, et al: Social factors in the diagnosis of alcoholism, II: attitudes of physicians. Quarterly Journal of Studies on Alcohol 26:72–79, 1965

Laboratory and Psychological Testing in Addiction Medicine

Robert L. DuPont, M.D.

While the diagnosis of substance use disorders remains primarily clinical, laboratory and psychological testing are important in screening, in identifying comorbid disorders, in assessing addiction severity, and in performing case management (Brostoff 1994; DuPont 1994).

Laboratory Testing

Identifying Recent Drug Use

Because ethyl alcohol is volatilized in the lungs, it is the only abused drug easily identified in breath, but drugs and their metabolites are identifiable in virtually all fluids and in all body tissues—for example, urine, blood, sweat, saliva, hair, and fingernails (DuPont 1997; Schwartz 1988). Ease of access, cost of the test, and the most appropriate detection window affect the type of sample selected for drug testing. Organ samples (such as liver biopsies) are the most difficult to obtain. Blood is more difficult to obtain than urine in most settings. Breath, saliva, and hair samples are the most easily collected.

Costs of analysis are similar among the sample types, although hair, sweat, and blood testing are somewhat more expensive than urine testing. Sweat and hair testing are done only at a few specialized laboratories, but urine testing for drugs of abuse is done at most clinical laboratories. Urine testing kits produce reliable results within a few minutes of collec-

---

This chapter subpart is a revised version of my chapter "Diagnostic Testing—Laboratory and Psychological," which appeared in Galanter MA, Kleber HD (eds): *The American Psychiatric Press Textbook of Substance Abuse Treatment,* 2nd Edition. Washington, DC, American Psychiatric Press, 1999, pp. 521–527.

tion. If alcohol and other drug testing occur in the workplace, legal regulations, including secure collection with forensic standards of specimen handling and laboratory confirmation (U.S. Department of Health and Human Services 1988; Vogl and Bush 1997), are important considerations.

Blood has the shortest detection window; most drugs are cleared from the blood at measurable levels in 12 hours or less. Urine has a detection window of about 1–3 days, because most drugs are cleared rapidly after the most use of the drug. This is true even for marijuana, unless the tested individual was a chronic heavy user, in which case the urine results may remain positive for a month or longer after marijuana use stops. After smoking 1 or 2 joints of marijuana, many subjects without prior heavy chronic marijuana use will have negative urine results within 24 hours, and all will have negative results at the 100-nanogram cutoff within 3 days. After smoking 1 or 2 joints, all subjects—chronic heavy smokers and light users alike—will have negative urine testing results at the more sensitive 20-nanogram cutoff within 5 days (Schwartz 1988; Vogl and Bush 1997).

Head hair grows about 0.5 inch (or a bit more than 1 cm) a month. Drugs are laid down in the hair matrix when it is created in the follicle. It takes about a week for hair to grow long enough to be sampled in routine clipping of head hair. A standard 1.5-inch sample of head hair contains drug residuals from the prior 90 days minus the week immediately before sample collection. Hair testing is particularly useful when a longer detection window is important (DuPont and Baumgartner 1995). Because preemployment drug testing is scheduled, a drug user must refrain from nonmedical drug use for only 3–5 days to test negative in a urine sample, whereas the drug user must refrain for 90 days to test negative in a hair sample. Most drug abusers find it more difficult to refrain from use for 90 days.

Unlike urine samples, hair samples cannot be substituted, adulterated, or diluted. However, hair treatments such as perming, bleaching, and straightening may slightly reduce drug levels in hair so that borderline positives can become negative results. Substantial drug use in the 90 days prior to sample collection is required to create a positive hair test result (Cone et al. 1995; Kintz 1996). This higher threshold for a positive hair test means that eating poppy seeds or consuming hemp oil will not produce a positive test for opiates or marijuana, as commonly occurs with urine tests. Medical review officers routinely reverse the results of urine tests that are positive for opiates, making these tests all but worthless.

Sweat patch testing is the newest of the commonly used drug tests. The person wears a patch similar to the nicotine patch used by people attempting to quit smoking. If the patch is removed, it cannot be replaced without noticeable puckering of the edges. Sweat is continuously absorbed into the patch, with the water in the sweat evaporating through the outer patch membrane while drugs and drug metabolites are affixed to the absorbent patch. Because skin normally desquamates, patches can be worn for only 2–4 weeks before they fall off. However, during the time they are worn (which can range from a few hours to a few weeks), drug detection sweat patches reliably identify any substantial drug use. Once removed, the patches are tested by a laboratory.

Patches are commercially available for the detection of cocaine, opiates, marijuana, phencyclidine (PCP), and amphetamine/methamphetamine. Though not yet commercially available, sweat patches for alcohol detection are expected to become available soon. Sweat patch testing is especially useful for follow-up monitoring, such as return-to-work drug testing when daily urine testing and virtually hourly breath alcohol testing are impractical.

Hair testing and sweat patches offer important advantages over urine testing in some settings. Both are more resistant to cheating, both offer rough quantitative analysis (enabling the separation of heavy users from light users), and neither produces positive tests for opiates after poppy seed ingestion. Table 25–3 presents a comparison of blood, urine, hair, and sweat patch testing for abused drugs.

TABLE 25–3. Blood, urine, hair, and sweat patch testing for drugs of abuse

	Blood	Urine	Hair	Sweat patch
Surveillance window	3–12 hours	1–3 days	7–90 days	1–21 days
Intrusiveness of collection	Severe	Moderate	None	Slight
Retest of same sample	Yes	Yes	Yes	Yes
Retest of new sample if original test disputed	No	No	Yes	No
Number of drugs screened	Unlimited[a]	Unlimited	5[b]	5[c]
Cost/sample (HHS-5)	About $200	About $15–$30	About $40–$65	About $20
Permits distinction between light, moderate, and heavy use	Yes, acutely	No	Yes	Yes
Resistance to cheating	High	Low	High	High
Best applications	Postaccident and overdose testing for alcohol and other drugs Alcohol Blood alcohol level	Reasonable-cause and random testing Frequent testing of high-risk groups such as posttreatment follow-up and criminal justice system	Random and periodic testing Preemployment and survey testing	Abstinence maintenance

Note. Blood, urine, hair, and sweat patch tests all are done with an immunoassay screen with a gas chromatography/mass spectrometry (GC/MS) confirmation option. HHS-5 drugs = U.S. Department of Health and Human Services–regulated drug classes (cocaine, opiates [morphine/heroin/codeine], marijuana, amphetamine/methamphetamine, and phencyclidine).

[a]Blood testing for alcohol is routine, costing about $25 per sample, but blood testing for drugs is done by only a few laboratories in the country. Blood testing for drugs is relatively expensive, costing about $60 for each drug detected.

[b]Currently, hair testing is available only for the HHS-5 drugs.

[c]HHS-5 drugs only. Additional sweat patch tests may become available for alcohol.

The insurance industry now commonly uses saliva testing to detect use of nicotine (cotinine), cocaine, and other drugs. This approach is coming to the workplace and other settings. Saliva testing for alcohol is now available. Saliva is in equilibrium with blood; therefore, saliva testing can detect only recent drug use (i.e., within the prior 6–12 hours). Because saliva is easily obtained (unlike urine and blood), it is especially useful in postaccident tests, highway testing, and other settings where immediate results and easy collection are important.

Identifying Common Correlates of Alcohol and Other Drug Use

Because chronic heavy drinking produces a wide range of adverse biological effects, clinical chemistry tests can track the effects of heavy alcohol use (Allen and Litten 1994). Laboratory tests are neither as specific nor as sensitive as clinical assessment for diagnosing alcoholism (DuPont 1994). It is helpful to have a familiarity with the laboratory results typically seen after heavy drinking. Abnormal laboratory results are more common in older drinkers, reflecting years of alcohol's negative health effects. Younger people, even if they are heavy drinkers, are less likely to have abnormal laboratory results.

Gamma-glutamyltransferase (GGT) is elevated in about two-thirds of chronic heavy drinkers. GGT sensitively but nonspecifically reflects alcohol and, to a lesser extent, drug damage to the liver as well as infiltrative liver disorders and biliary obstruction. GGT elevation results from both liver damage and enzyme induction secondary to heavy drinking over extended periods of time. GGT levels return to normal after about 3 weeks of abstinence from alcohol use. GGT is induced not only by alcohol but also by phenobarbital, dilantin, and many other drugs.

Mean corpuscular volume (MCV) is elevated in about one-quarter of alcoholic patients. Elevation of the MCV is a relatively late manifestation of alcoholism and can result both from direct toxic effects of alcohol on the bone marrow and from disruptions in folate metabolism. Unlike GGT elevations, MCV elevations persist for several months after abstinence from alcohol. The specificity of GGT elevation in identifying alcoholism is enhanced when such elevation occurs in conjunction with MCV elevation, because the nonalcohol factors that raise GGT levels do not raise MCV levels.

Alanine aminotransferase (ALT) and aspartate aminotransferase (AST) are elevated in about one-half of chronic heavy drinkers. Elevations of these transaminase levels are nonspecific signs of liver damage. ALT (formerly called serum glutamic-pyruvic transaminase [SGPT]) and AST (formerly called serum glutamic-oxaloacetic transaminase [SGOT]) are elevated in many conditions, including liver disorders such as cirrhosis, fatty liver, and alcoholic hepatitis; myocardial infarction; circulatory dysfunction; muscle injury; central nervous system disorders; and other diseases unrelated to the liver. The ratio of mitochondrial AST to total AST is more specific to alcoholic liver damage than is the AST level itself. AST levels may be greater than ALT levels in alcoholism because of the toxic effects of alcohol on ALT synthesis. Although ALT is equally sensitive and possibly more specific to liver damage than is AST, it adds little of clinical value to AST levels alone.

Carbohydrate-deficient transferrin (CDT) is elevated in about 80% of people who drink heavily every day for 1 week or longer. CDT returns to normal during periods of abstinence from alcohol consumption, with values falling by about 50% after 2 weeks of abstinence. Unlike transaminase levels, CDT is not commonly elevated in liver diseases unrelated to heavy alcohol consumption. CDT may be elevated in severe hepatic failure unrelated to heavy drinking and in individuals with rare genetic variants of transferrin, a β-globulin that transports iron. CDT can be a useful marker of heavy drinking in follow-up studies and in the clinical management of recovering alcoholic patients.

Uric acid is elevated in about one-tenth of alcoholic patients, because alcohol produces an excessive amount of lactic acid, which competes with uric acid in the kidney, causing elevations in serum uric acid levels. Additional abnormal laboratory findings in alcoholism include lowered potassium, magnesium, calcium, phosphate, and zinc levels; lowered red and white blood cell counts; and lowered platelet levels. Amylase is elevated in alcoholic pancreatitis. Triglycerides, bilirubin, and alkaline phosphatase may be elevated in heavy drinkers, whereas glucose levels may be depressed.

Psychological Testing

Screening Tests

Psychological tests can augment clinical interviews and help clinicians recognize addiction. The simplest psychological screening test, and still one of the best, is the CAGE test (Mayfield et al. 1974). The interviewer asks patients if they have attempted to Cut down on drinking, if they have been Annoyed by people's comments about their drinking, whether they have felt Guilty about any aspect of their drinking, and whether they have used alcohol early in the day as an Eye-opener to get going. This simple test is remarkably effective in identifying drinking problems. Even a single positive answer is ample reason to explore drinking and its consequences more fully.

Another commonly used psychological test is the Michigan Alcoholism Screening Test (MAST; Selzer 1971), which has several versions. The original MAST test is a 25-item, self-administered questionnaire. The Short MAST (SMAST; Selzer et al. 1975) has 13 items, while the Brief MAST (BMAST; Pokorny et al. 1972) has only 10 items. Both CAGE and MAST screen for drinking but not drug use, because neither is designed to identify problems related to nonmedical drug use. Three other screening tests enjoy wide support: the Alcohol Use Disorders Identification Test (AUDIT; Saunders et al. 1993), the Self-Administered Alcoholism Screening Test (SAAST; Swenson and Morse 1975), and the Adolescent Drinking Inventory (ADI; Harrell and Wirtz 1989) (Allen and Litten 1994).

Assessment Tests

Because third-party payers want clinicians to reduce costs and raise health care quality, the 1990s saw a new movement to establish systematic approaches to diagnosis and treatment of addictive disorders. Controversies over the use of inpatient addiction treatment, which were especially intense in the 1980s when such treatment represented one of the most rapidly growing health-care costs, have encouraged structured assessment of patients' addiction problems and efforts to match these problems to specific levels of addiction treatment. Psychological instruments can provide standardization and credibility for treatment selection and can facilitate the study of treatment outcomes (Gastfriend et al. 1994).

Patient Placement Criteria, published by the American Society of Addiction Medicine (ASAM) in 1991, was one of the earliest and most influential of the efforts to standardize data collection related to treatment. Since their initial publication (American Society of Addiction Medicine 1991), these criteria have had a major impact on treatment decisions. The ASAM criteria divide addiction treatment into four levels of care defined by treatment setting: 1) hospital, 2) nonhospital inpatient, 3) day treatment, and 4) outpatient. The criteria were expanded in 1996 (American Society of Addiction Medicine 1996) to include a broader range of addiction treatments within each of the four major levels of care. ASAM criteria assess six patient-related dimensions: 1) acute intoxication and/or withdrawal, 2) medical diagnoses or complications, 3) emotional/behavioral disorders or complications, 4) treatment acceptance or resistance, 5) relapse or continuing use, and 6) recovery/living environment.

Diagnosis of Substance Use Disorder

The Structured Clinical Interview for DSM-IV (SCID; First et al. 1996) is suitable for both clinical and research use. It is the most highly developed of the assessment instruments currently used to establish the diagnosis of alcohol or drug abuse or dependence. The SCID is designed to be administered by trained clinical evaluators from the master's to the doctorate level. However, it is not easily administered by clinicians. It is labor intensive and is not compatible with the more intuitive, subjective way that clinicians usually approach patients.

Detailing both Axis I and Axis II diagnoses, the entire SCID requires more than 2 hours to administer, whereas the Psychoactive Use Disorders module of the SCID can be administered alone in about 30–60 minutes, depending on the extent of the subject's substance use history and the current intensity of substance use and related problems. This module, like the total SCID, now has questions specifically related to each item in the DSM-IV (American Psychiatric Association 1994) diagnostic criteria. Data are collected to establish lifetime and current diagnoses, age at onset of first abuse, and first dependence for each category of drug.

SCID diagnoses have shown good interrater reliability for substance use disorders but only moderate reliability for comorbid conditions such as anxiety and depression (Skre et al. 1991). The SCID is systematic and comprehensive in gathering the information required to fit the DSM-IV diagnostic criteria.

Substance Abuse and Dependence Severity

The Addiction Severity Index (ASI; McLellan et al. 1992) is the most widely used instrument for assessing substance use disorder severity. Through administration of a 30-minute semistructured interview, the ASI assesses seven areas typically affected by substance use: medical problems, employment/support, drug/alcohol use, legal status, family history, family/social relationships, and psychiatric problems. Information is obtained about lifetime drug and alcohol use as well as use in the prior 30 days. The ASI can be administered by a trained technician (not necessarily a licensed clinician, as is required for the SCID) and has been used widely for clinical, administrative, and research purposes. A smaller subset of ASI items has been used in follow-up studies.

The ASI is based on patient report without independent verification or review of collateral material (workplace, criminal justice, or family sources). The rater uses a 10-point scale to assess the severity of the patient's overall substance use disorder and the reliability of the patient's self-reports. Thus, the ASI is not totally dependent on what the patient says about his or her own problem. Although the ASI was developed for and initially used in the methadone treatment of heroin addiction, it is now employed in a wide variety of settings, including drug-free treatment, homeless shelters, and inpatient psychiatric hospitals (McLellan et al. 1980). Reflecting its origins, the ASI reliably identifies severe alcohol- and other drug-related impairments but is not as good at characterizing less severely impaired patients, including those commonly seen in outpatient alcohol treatment programs and in many drug-free outpatient programs.

Motivation for Recovery and Treatment Readiness

The Recovery Attitude and Treatment Evaluator Clinical Evaluation (RAATE-CE; Mee-Lee 1992) is the most promising of the new instruments for assessing treatment readiness. The RAATE-CE systematically and quantifiably assesses the patient's resistance and impediments to addiction treatment. This clinician-rated structured interview (like the SCID) assesses five dimensions related to substance treatment planning: 1) resistance to treatment; 2) resistance to continuing care; 3) severity of medical problems; 4) severity of psychiatric problems; and 5) extent of unsupportive family, social, and environmental factors. The RAATE-CE has 35 items scored from 1 to 4; higher scores indicate greater resistance and impediments to recovery.

Conclusions

While clinical judgment remains the foundation of addiction medicine, laboratory testing in recent years has provided important new opportunities to identify alcohol and other drug use and to study the effects of alcohol and other drug use on the physiology of alcohol and drug abusers. Psychological testing now provides an objective and quantifiable basis for the identification of alcohol and other drug problems and a more scientific way to follow the progress of treated individuals over time. Wise clinicians have learned to use these new laboratory and psychological tests in ways that enhance the effectiveness of patient care and provide powerful evidence that addiction treatment often works to produce cost-effective outcomes.

References

Allen JP, Litten RZ: Biochemical and psychometric tests, in Principles of Addiction Medicine. Edited by Miller NS. Chevy Chase, MD, American Society of Addiction Medicine, 1994, pp 1–8

American Psychiatric Association: Diagnostic and Statistical Manual of Mental Disorders, 4th Edition. Washington, DC, American Psychiatric Association, 1994

American Society of Addiction Medicine: Patient Placement Criteria. Washington, DC, American Society of Addiction Medicine, 1991

American Society of Addiction Medicine: Patient Placement Criteria, 2nd Edition. Chevy Chase, MD, American Society of Addiction Medicine, 1996

Brostoff WS: Clinical diagnosis, in Principles of Addiction Medicine. Edited by Miller NS. Chevy Chase, MD, American Society of Addiction Medicine, 1994, pp 1–5

Cone EJ, Welch, MJ, Babecki MB (eds): Hair Testing for Drugs of Abuse: International Research on Standards and Technology. Rockville, MD, National Institute on Drug Abuse, 1995

DuPont RL: Laboratory diagnosis, in Principles of Addiction Medicine. Edited by Miller NS. Chevy Chase, MD, American Society of Addiction Medicine, 1994, pp 1–8

DuPont RL: Drug testing, in Manual of Therapeutics for Addictions. Edited by Miller NS, Gold MS, Smith DE. New York, Wiley-Liss, 1997, pp 86–94

DuPont RL, Baumgartner WA: Drug testing by urine and hair analysis: complementary features and scientific issues. Forensic Sci Int 70:63–76, 1995

First M, Gibbon M, Spitzer R, et al: Users Guide for the Structured Clinical Interview for DSM-IV Axis I Disorders—Research Version (SCID I, Version 2.0, February 1996). New York, New York State Psychiatric Institute, Biometrics Research Department, 1996

Gastfriend DR, Najavits LM, Reif S: Assessment instruments, in Principles of Addiction Medicine. Edited by Miller NS. Chevy Chase, MD, American Society of Addiction Medicine, 1994, pp 1–8

Harrell AV, Wirtz PW: Screening for adolescent problem drinking: validation of a multidimensional instrument for case identification. Psychological Assessment 1:61–63, 1989

Kintz P (ed): Drug Testing in Hair. Boca Raton, FL, CRC Press, 1996

Mayfield DG, McLeon G, Hall P: The CAGE Questionnaire: validation of a new alcoholism screening instrument. Am J Psychiatry 131:1121–1123, 1974

McLellan AT, Luborsky L, Woody GE: An improved diagnostic evaluation instrument for substance abuse patients: the Addiction Severity Index. J Nerv Ment Dis 168:26–33, 1980

McLellan AT, Kushner H, Metzger D, et al: The fifth edition of the Addiction Severity Index. J Subst Abuse Treat 9:199–213, 1992

Mee-Lee D: An instrument for treatment progress and matching: the Recovery Attitude and Treatment Evaluator (RAATE). J Subst Abuse Treat 5:183–186, 1992

Pokorny AD, Miller BA, Kaplan HB: The brief MAST: a shortened version of the Michigan Alcoholism Screening Test. Am J Psychiatry 129:342–345, 1972

Schwartz RH: Urine testing in the detection of drugs of abuse. Arch Intern Med 148:2407–2412, 1988

Selzer ML: The Michigan Alcoholism Screening Test: the quest for a new diagnostic instrument. Am J Psychiatry 127:1653–1658, 1971

Selzer ML, Vinokur A, van Rooijen L: A self-administered Short Michigan Alcoholism Screening Test (SMAST). J Stud Alcohol 36:117–126, 1975

Skre I, Onstad S, Torgersen S, et al: High interrater reliability for the Structured Clinical Interview for DSM-III-R Axis I. Acta Psychiatr Scand 84:167–173, 1991

Swenson WM, Morse RM: The use of a self-administered alcoholism screening test (SAAST) in a medical center. Mayo Clin Proc 50:204–208, 1975

U.S. Department of Health and Human Services: Mandatory guidelines for federal workplace drug testing programs. Federal Register, pp 11979–11989, April 11, 1988

Vogl WF, Bush DM: Medical Review Officer Manual for Federal Workplace Programs. Rockville, MD, Center for Substance Abuse Prevention, 1997

26

Alcohol and Other Depressant Drugs

Don Gallant, M.D.

David E. Smith, M.D.

Donald R. Wesson, M.D.

Alcoholism

Don Gallant, M.D.

Detoxification

Recent findings on treatment of the alcohol withdrawal syndromes and pharmacotherapy and behavioral therapy of the abstinence phase, including the treatment of comorbid conditions, will be presented in this chapter subpart. These findings should influence the ways we treat alcoholic individuals at each stage of illness. However, important problems, such as selection of the most appropriate treatment modality for a specific subtype of alcoholic patient, need to be solved.

Promising data for treatment matching do exist (Litt et al. 1992). In a 2-year study, a group of alcoholic patients labeled Type B (resembling Cloninger's Type II early-onset alcoholism with antisocial traits) showed better treatment outcomes with coping skills treatment and worse outcomes with interactional psychotherapy, whereas the converse was true for the Type A group (resembling Cloninger's mild, late-onset form of alcoholism [Type I]) (Cloninger et al. 1996). Because other research attempts at treatment matching of patient subgroups for specific treatment modalities have been unsuccessful, it is important that these study results by Litt and colleagues be replicated (Project MATCH Research Group 1997). Interestingly, the antisocial characteristics of the Type II alcoholic patients described by Cloninger et al. and the Type B alcoholism patients described by Litt et al. resemble

I would like to thank W. W. Norton & Co. for permission to publish several excerpts from my book *Alcoholism: A Guide to Diagnosis, Intervention, and Treatment*; and Williams & Wilkins for permission to publish excerpts from several review articles that I wrote for their journal *Alcoholism: Clinical and Experimental Research*.

This chapter subpart is a revised version of my chapter "Alcohol," which appeared in Galanter MA, Kleber HD (eds): *The American Psychiatric Press Textbook of Substance Abuse Treatment*, 2nd Edition. Washington, DC, American Psychiatric Press, 1999, pp. 151–164.

those of the "underarousal criminal types" studied in a 9-year *prospective* neurophysiological evaluation of central and autonomic measures of arousal in 101 Caucasian male schoolchildren that was initiated when the children were 14–16 years of age (Raine et al. 1990).

The continued increase in patients with combined alcohol and cocaine addiction not only requires modification of treatment procedures originally devised for the "pure" alcoholic or drug-addicted patient but also presents more complicated hepatotoxicity problems (Boyer and Petersen 1990).

It should be stressed that quantitative criteria measures are a necessary part of the clinical management of detoxification. The revised Clinical Institute Withdrawal Assessment for Alcohol (CIWA-A) Scale (Sullivan et al. 1991), a 10-item scale, and the Alcohol Withdrawal Scale (AWS; Cushman et al. 1985), a 6-item scale, contain both objective and subjective criteria that enable the clinician to make a decision about the use of pharmacological medication. One of these short-form scales should be administered routinely to all patients admitted to detoxification units.

The CIWA-A Scale is a practical clinical instrument that offers the benefit of good acceptance by ward personnel in addition to being clinically valid and reliable. The 10 items on the scale are sweating, anxiety, tremor, auditory disturbances, visual disturbances, agitation, nausea, tactile disturbances, headache, and orientation. All of the items except orientation (0–4) are weighted equally on a scale of 0–7. If the patient scores less than 10 on the scale, pharmacological treatment is usually not indicated, and the patient may be managed with supportive care alone. In one study in which the guideline of instituting psychopharmacological medication only if the score was greater than 10 was used, the results showed that patients scoring high on the scale (i.e., those with a greater degree of physical dependence) appropriately received higher doses of benzodiazepines, whereas those scoring lower on the scale appropriately received lower doses of benzodiazepines (Sullivan et al. 1991). Thus, use of the CIWA-A Scale both minimized inadequate dosing of benzodiazepines for patients in moderate to severe withdrawal and reduced overmedication with benzodiazepines in alcoholic patients experiencing only mild withdrawal. However, it should be emphasized that the clinician must be extremely careful not to undertreat those alcoholic patients who have experienced repeated withdrawal, because some investigators believe that repeated inadequately treated withdrawal episodes could produce future withdrawal syndromes of increased severity with possible permanent central nervous system (CNS) changes (Ballenger and Post 1978).

The treatment of alcohol withdrawal syndromes has two primary goals: to help a patient achieve detoxification in as safe and as comfortable a way as possible, and to foster the patient's motivation to enter rehabilitation therapy. Recent advances in the treatment of alcohol withdrawal syndromes promise improvements in our ability to realize both goals.

Uncomplicated Alcohol Withdrawal

Outpatient treatment may be sufficient for a significant number of patients displaying the syndrome of alcohol withdrawal. In addition to the CIWA-A Scale or the AWS, the blood alcohol level can be used as a guideline for making a decision to place the patient in a social detoxification unit, to refer him or her to a medical ward for more intensive treatment of severe withdrawal symptoms, or to follow the patient at home with proper supervision. For example, if the alcohol level is 250–300 mg% and the patient appears to be alert and not dysarthric, the physician should be on guard for possible moderate to severe withdrawal symptoms as the blood alcohol level decreases. In this situation, the tolerance for alcohol is too high and the patient may have a predisposition to develop marked withdrawal symptoms upon cessation of alcohol use.

Successful outpatient treatment of patients with mild to moderate alcohol withdrawal symptoms has been described in a number of studies (Hyashida et al. 1989; Pattison 1977; Whitfield 1980; Wiseman et al. 1997). The clinician may feel relatively safe in treating an outpatient with alcohol withdrawal symptoms if the CIWA-A Scale score is less than 10 and if the patient has no previous history of alcohol-related convulsions or delirium. Such patients may be helped to decrease the intake of alcohol with family support and the use of a short-acting hypnotic for sleep in association with moderate dosages of benzodiazepines for daytime anxiety. The use of a short-acting benzodiazepine (e.g., oxazepam 30 mg qid or lorazepam 1 mg tid or qid) in association with a short-acting hypnotic (e.g., chloral hydrate) will enable the patient to withdraw from alcohol comfortably over a period of 4–7 days.

Clonidine, an α-adrenergic agonist, as well as guanabenz, also an α-adrenergic agonist, has also been found to be effective in suppressing the symptoms and signs of alcohol withdrawal (Manhem et al. 1985). In one study comparing clonidine (doses as high as 0.2 mg tid) with chlordiazepoxide (doses as high as 50 mg tid), the results showed clonidine to be more effective than chlordiazepoxide in lowering AWS scores, especially during the first 24 hours after cessation of alcohol use (Baumgartner and Rowen 1988). The use of these α-adrenergic agonists, as well as the use of β-blockers, has resulted in relatively nonsedative treatment approaches that enable the patient to participate in rehabilitation therapy within several days after admission to a detoxification unit or in treatment as an outpatient. Unfortunately, the β-blockers and the α-adrenergic agonists *do not* have anticonvulsant and antihallucinogenic effects in human subjects (Liskow and Goodwin 1987). Thus, a benzodiazepine would be indicated for patients with a previous history of alcohol-induced or postalcohol withdrawal seizures.

Complicated Alcohol Withdrawal

Patients with alcohol withdrawal delirium usually score higher than 20 on the CIWA-A Scale. Symptoms of alcohol withdrawal delirium occur within the first week after cessation or reduction of heavy alcohol ingestion. With adequate treatment, the symptoms should disappear by the end of the first week or by no later than the beginning of the second week (Gallant 1987). The diagnosis of alcohol withdrawal delirium warrants immediate hospitalization, because it implies that the patient is unable to care for him- or herself and is seriously ill. The use of a benzodiazepine may be of considerable help in alcoholic patients who have experienced recent alcohol withdrawal convulsions, because these compounds possess anticonvulsant activity. If the patient is suspected of having a moderate amount of liver damage, the most appropriate benzodiazepine may be oxazepam or lorazepam, because these agents do not require metabolism by the liver. The dosage range for the benzodiazepine should be based on the quantity of alcohol consumed before withdrawal, the weight of the patient, and the severity of the presenting symptomatology (e.g., a very high score on the CIWA-A Scale). Although patients who present with high blood alcohol levels usually experience more severe withdrawal symptoms than do patients with relatively low blood alcohol levels, this is not always the case. Exceptions may include patients who have experienced severe withdrawal symptoms following previous drinking episodes or those who have developed intercurrent illnesses during the present withdrawal stage. In severe cases of alcohol withdrawal syndrome with delirium, oxazepam dosages as high as 60 mg four times a day, lorazepam dosages as high as 1–2 mg four times a day, or diazepam dosages up to 20 mg four times a day may be required. Diazepam loading regimens (e.g., dosages of 40 mg hs) have also been successfully used (Romach and Sellers 1991).

In a recent paper summarizing a meta-analysis of English-language medical articles on treatment of ethanol withdrawal published before July 1, 1995, benzodiazepines were reported to be the most suitable agents for this purpose (Mayo-Smith 1997). If a patient is vomiting profusely and is unable to tolerate oral medication, the use of intramuscular lorazepam would be indicated, because this compound is absorbed quite readily after intramuscular administration. Prochlorperazine 25 mg as a suppository can be used temporarily to inhibit the emesis. It should be stressed that intravenous infusions should be used only in patients who are definitely dehydrated from excessive vomiting or diarrhea. Even in these cases, the clinician must be cautious with glycogen-depleted patients who may have a thiamine deficiency, because these patients may develop Wernicke's encephalopathy if a glucose infusion is administered without additional thiamine. These patients should be weighed daily in order to evaluate their hydration state.

During the past several years, encouraging results in the treatment of severe alcohol withdrawal syndromes have been reported. One double-blind, controlled evaluation of carbamazepine and oxazepam for the treatment of alcohol withdrawal confirmed the results of previous evaluations of the efficacy of carbamazepine (Malcolm et al. 1989). To be included in this trial, patients had to meet the DSM-III (American Psychiatric Association 1980) criteria for alcohol dependence and had to score 20 or higher on the CIWA-A Scale. Eighty-six subjects were randomly assigned to either the carbamazepine (200 mg qid) or the oxazepam (30 mg qid) group. The CIWA-A Scale, physiological measures, and neurological examinations were administered twice daily. The clinical measures in both treatment groups showed that maximal reduction of symptoms was achieved between days 4 and 5. There were no significant differences between groups on the CIWA-A Scale or on the other measures. More recent studies have confirmed the value of carbamazepine for the treatment of alcohol withdrawal (Stuppaeck et al. 1992). Stuppaeck et al. (1992) included in their report a detailed reference section on the use of carbamazepine for alcohol withdrawal.

Alcoholic patients who have made multiple attempts at alcohol withdrawal may be more likely to experience seizures and to develop long-term neurological and psychiatric disabilities. If these sequelae are associated with "kindling-like" changes in the limbic areas, the "antikindling" effects of carbamazepine may offer future protection against this type of CNS damage as well as ameliorate the acute phase of the withdrawal syndrome (Adinoff et al. 1988). It should be noted that thrombocytopenia secondary to carbamazepine treatment is rare, but when it does occur, it is usually within the first 3 weeks of treatment (Tohen et al. 1991). However, the hematological abnormalities apparently are rapidly corrected by discontinuing medication; in a review of the literature on the use of carbamazepine, I was unable to find any reports of irreversible hematological side effects occurring with a 1-week administration of carbamazepine for alcohol withdrawal syndrome.

The anticonvulsant agent sodium valproate, which is associated with more gastric distress but fewer and less severe CNS side effects than is carbamazepine, and the calcium channel blockers such as verapamil show some promise of therapeutic efficacy for the severe alcohol withdrawal states, but they have not yet been adequately evaluated in double-blind trials in the United States (Brady et al. 1996). Data on the use of these compounds have been summarized in a published symposium by the National Institute on Alcohol Abuse and Alcoholism (NIAAA) (Linnoila et al. 1987) and in a review article by investigators from NIAAA (Adinoff et al. 1988).

For patients with a recent history of alcohol withdrawal seizures, the use of phenytoin or magnesium has not been well established. In one double-blind, controlled study of 100 alcoholic patients displaying withdrawal symptomatology, the addition of magnesium to the chlordiazepoxide regimen did not result in additional therapeutic efficacy compared with placebo, even in those patients with low magnesium levels (Wilson and Vulcano 1986). Intramuscular magnesium administration does cause discomfort to the patient and is not indicated for the management of alcohol withdrawal unless the patient develops low magnesium levels in association with cardiac arrhythmias or neurological symptoms. Many authors recommend elimination of the use of phenytoin for the prophylactic treatment of withdrawal seizures (Adinoff et al. 1988; Alldredge et al. 1989). In animal and human research related to alcohol withdrawal seizures, diazepam has been shown to be a very effective anticonvulsant (Guerrero-Figueroa et al. 1970). If seizures are present on admission to the hospital, diazepam may be given intravenously at a dosage of 10 mg for a period of 1–2 minutes and then repeated until seizures stop, but no more than a total of 30 mg should be administered over a period of 15–20 minutes. Diazepam should be administered slowly to avoid laryngospasm.

European journals contain reports of other compounds, such as gamma-hydroxybutyric acid (GHB) and chlormethiazole, that have shown promise in controlled studies for the treatment of moderate to severe alcohol withdrawal symptoms (Schuckit 1991).

In the treatment of alcohol withdrawal, it is important to consider the increasing numbers of primary alcoholism patients who abuse habituating drugs in association with their intake of alcohol. The patient with an addiction to both alcohol and benzodiazepines presents an additional medical problem in the treatment of withdrawal because he or she is more likely to have seizures (Gallant 1987). The combined alcohol-benzodiazepine withdrawal syndrome appears to be different from the classical alcohol withdrawal syndrome. Combined alcohol-benzodiazepine withdrawal symptoms can start anywhere from 2 to 10 days after abrupt discontinuation of drugs and are characterized by more psychomotor and autonomic nervous system signs than are usually seen in alcohol withdrawal (Benzer and Cushman 1980). Carbamazepine should be effective for combined alcohol-benzodiazepine addictions, particularly since carbamazepine has been shown to be effective for both alcohol and benzodiazepine withdrawal (Ries et al. 1989).

Pharmacotherapy During the Abstinence Phase

Disulfiram

The efficacy of disulfiram in promoting abstinence has been demonstrated in a number of studies by different authors (Fuller and Williford 1981; Gerrein et al. 1973; Sereny et al. 1986). In one well-designed, controlled evaluation of disulfiram in a Department of Veterans Affairs (VA) hospital (Fuller and Williford 1981), a life-table analysis showed that the group of patients who were administered this compound had a significantly increased number of *abstinent months* compared with a placebo group, despite the fact that both groups of patients had requested disulfiram at the outset of the study, thus negating the variable of motivation for taking the medication. Although at the 12-month endpoint of the study no significant differences in total abstinence rates were found between the groups, evaluation of the effect of disulfiram on abstinence over time provided information about the number of additional months of abstinence before the 12-month endpoint; these additional months of abstinence may delay or possibly prevent the occurrence of alcohol-induced tissue damage to various organs (Fuller and Williford 1981). Perhaps even more important than these results are the studies that show supervised disulfiram maintenance to be significantly superior to voluntary disulfiram therapy in keeping patients in treatment (Gerrein et al. 1973; Sereny et al. 1986). In fact, patients administered disulfiram by spouses or cohabitants who had received positive reinforcement therapy with social skills training for administering the disulfiram showed more therapeutic gains than did patients receiving disulfiram on a routine basis from cohabitants who had not been given such training (Azrin et al. 1982). All of the aforementioned studies have shown that disulfiram as an adjunct to other treatment modalities helps to increase the abstinence rate and is only rarely associated with serious side effects (Gallant 1987). Disulfiram compliance can be determined by testing the urine for diethylamine, a metabolite of disulfiram (Fuller and Niederhiser 1980).

Because disulfiram inhibits dopamine-β-hydroxylase activity, it should be used only in small doses (125 mg) in alcoholic patients with a comorbid diagnosis of schizophrenia. For such patients, it may be advisable to prescribe an adequate dopamine-blocking agent such as a high-potency antipsychotic while disulfiram is being administered. Other side effects of disulfiram (e.g., peripheral nerve damage, including optic neuritis) have been described but are quite rare and are usually observed in association with daily disulfiram dosages of more than 250 mg (Gallant 1987). Published reports indicate that disulfiram-induced hepatotoxicity is a definite possibility (Berlin 1989). Despite the fact that only approximately 30 cases of disulfiram-induced permanent liver damage have been reported in the world medical literature, the physician is obligated to monitor hepatic transaminases and to warn the patient that if any clinical symptoms of hepatitis occur, the patient should immediately contact a physician and discontinue the disulfiram.

At times it may be difficult for the clinician to evaluate patients' reports of side effects. In one placebo-disulfiram double-blind, controlled study in alcoholic patients, the evaluation of side effects in 158 patients completing the study showed no statistically significant differences between the two groups except for a larger number of complaints of sexual problems in the placebo group (Christensen et al. 1984). Skin reactions, itching, fatigue or lethargy, and unpleasant taste were no more common in the disulfiram group than in the placebo group. Complaints of "bad breath" tended to be more frequent in the disulfiram group. The dosage of disulfiram in this study was 250 mg dissolved in plain soda water and administered daily for 6 weeks under staff supervision.

Other Pharmacological Approaches to Reducing Alcohol Intake

Another interesting and potentially valuable pharmacological approach incorporates the use of the long-acting oral narcotic antagonist naltrexone. Volpicelli et al. (1992) conducted a 12-week, double-blind, placebo-controlled evaluation of naltrexone at 50 mg/day in 70 alcoholism patients receiving outpatient group therapy. The naltrexone group had a significantly lower relapse rate and showed a decrease in subsequent drinking in those subjects who had at least one drink. In the evaluation of these patients who had "sampled" alcohol, 95% of the placebo subjects and only 40% of the naltrexone patients lost control of their drinking and met the criteria for relapse. Volpicelli and colleagues raised the possibility that the initial drink stimulates alcohol craving in some subjects by increasing the activity of the opioid system and that the blocking of this system by naltrexone dampens the alcohol craving. In another 12-week controlled study of naltrexone at 50 mg/day and psychotherapy with specific guidelines, 97 alcoholic patients were divided into four treatment groups: naltrexone with coping skills therapy, naltrexone with supportive therapy, placebo with coping skills therapy, and placebo with supportive therapy (O'Malley et al. 1992). The naltrexone group had a higher abstention rate, a lower severity of alcohol-related problems, fewer drinking days, and fewer relapses than did the placebo subjects. Although the overall rate of abstinence was highest in the patient group receiving naltrexone with supportive therapy, the investigators observed that those patients who received naltrexone and coping skills therapy were the least likely to relapse to heavy drinking after an initial lapse or drinking episode. There appeared to be a significant correlation between degree of craving and abstinence success in the naltrexone group, and this finding offers a possible guide for determining which subgroup of alcoholic patients (e.g., binge drinkers) might be more likely to profit from treatment. Naltrexone appears to be a relatively safe compound without serious long-term side effects.

In controlled trials, acamprosate (calcium acetyl homotaurinate) at oral dosages of 2,000 mg/day was significantly superior to placebo in increasing abstinence (Sass et al. 1996). The value of these studies is increased because of the length of the trials, which were of 1 and 2 years' duration. Acamprosate resembles L-glutamate and may indirectly block the reinforcing effects of alcohol. This compound has not yet been approved for clinical use by the U.S. Food and Drug Administration, although it is available in Europe. It must be emphasized that medications for the abstinence phase, such as disulfiram, naltrexone, GHB, and acamprosate, should be used only as part of a psychosocial-behavioral treatment program. If these drugs are used alone without such a program, the dropout rate is likely to be extremely high and the potential value of these medications will not be realized.

Medications for Comorbid Disorders Associated With Alcoholism

Incidence Reports of Comorbidity With Alcohol

In a study of lifetime and 12-month prevalence of psychiatric disorders in the noninstitutionalized civilian population, 48.0% of the respondents reported at least one lifetime disorder and 29.5% reported at least one 12-month disorder; alcohol abuse and dependence were reported as a lifetime illness by 23.5% and as a 12-month prevalence by 9.7% of the 8,098 persons interviewed (Kessler et al. 1994). In the Epidemiologic Catchment Area (ECA) survey conducted by the National Institute of Mental Health (NIMH), patients with an alcohol use disorder had seven times the chance of having another addictive disorder compared with the rest of the population, and 37% of these patients had a comorbid mental disorder (Regier et al. 1990). Of the mental disorders in persons with alcohol diagnoses, anxiety disorders were most frequent (19.4%), followed by antisocial personality disorders

(14.3%) and affective disorders (13.4%), with some overlapping of more than one comorbid diagnosis for certain persons. These data are extremely important, because psychiatric diagnoses generally predict poor treatment outcome for alcoholic patients (Rounsaville et al. 1987). Given the high incidence of major psychiatric diagnoses in alcoholic patients, which has important therapeutic and prognostic implications, it becomes apparent that skilled interviewing or screening techniques associated with diagnostic abilities and the appropriate use of psychopharmacological compounds are essential for any clinician treating alcoholic patients.

Use of Antidepressant Agents

Delineation of primary versus secondary mood disorder in patients presenting with alcoholism may be one of the most difficult diagnostic problems in psychiatry. A number of patients have a history of alcoholism and mood disorder that began at approximately the same age, and it is often quite difficult to decide whether the excessive use of alcohol resulted in depression or whether the patient was self-medicating the depression with alcohol. Certain biographical and clinical data are helpful to the clinician in making the diagnosis of a primary major depression (or bipolar disorder): 1) mood disorder preceding the onset of alcoholism or a history of mood disorder occurring during sustained periods of abstinence; 2) early childhood history of separation anxiety, phobic behavior, or neurasthenia; 3) a hypomanic or manic reaction to antidepressant medication; 4) family history of bipolar illness; 5) family history of affective illness in two or more consecutive generations; and 6) a positive dexamethasone suppression test (DST) after the patient has been abstinent for 4 or more weeks (Gallant 1987). If the affective symptomatology is secondary to excessive alcohol intake and the accompanying life failures, the mood disorder should resolve within a period of several weeks as abstinence continues. Patients for whom this occurs usually do not require specific psychopharmacological intervention for their affective symptomatology. However, if the affective illness persists for more than 1–2 months despite psychotherapeutic attempts to alleviate the discomfort, it may then be worthwhile to initiate psychopharmacological therapy to avoid a relapse of alcohol use or a suicide attempt secondary to painful affective symptomatology.

The serotonergic system has been implicated in a number of studies in both animals and humans, not only in relation to the onset of depression but also in relation to the decrease of alcohol intake (Gatto et al. 1990; Naranjo et al. 1986; Pietraszek et al. 1991). It has been suggested that fluoxetine increases "the physiologically active pool of 5-HT [serotonin] in neuronal circuits mediating the aversive properties of ethanol" (Gatto et al. 1990, p. 532). Thus, selective serotonin reuptake inhibitors do look promising, but additional long-term studies are needed with larger numbers of patients who have definitive diagnoses of alcohol dependence as defined by ICD-10 (World Health Organization 1992) or DSM-IV (American Psychiatric Association 1994) criteria.

Some of the antidepressants that are capable of producing sedative side effects, such as doxepin, amitriptyline, and trazodone, can be used for hypnotic purposes in alcoholic patients without fear of habituation. A controlled trial of trazodone 50–100 mg at bedtime versus placebo was conducted with 10 alcoholic inpatients who were receiving nonsedating antidepressants and experiencing persistent insomnia. In a 4-day crossover study of this group, all of the trazodone patients showed significant improvement on the sleep measures compared with the placebo patients. The patients receiving trazodone were able to distinguish the active drug from the placebo and wanted to continue treatment with trazodone (Nirenberg et al. 1991). These medications, which are not habit forming, are easily discontinued after the patient has developed adequate sleep habits.

Use of Anxiolytic Agents

The use of a benzodiazepine for anxiety reduction in alcoholic patients during the maintenance phase of abstinence is somewhat controversial. Benzodiazepines such as diazepam and alprazolam have been shown in placebo-controlled studies to cause a significant increase in symptoms of euphoria, not only in male alcoholic patients but also in the adult male offspring of male alcoholic patients who had not yet developed alcoholism (Ciraulo et al. 1989). If the clinician finds it necessary to use a benzodiazepine in an alcoholic patient with a comorbid diagnosis of social phobia (social anxiety disorder), a good rule of thumb is to plan the duration of therapy for no more than 4–6 weeks, using that period to instruct the patient in the use of cognitive and behavior therapies to reduce anxiety. If the alcoholic patient has a history of abusing other drugs, the use of mild to moderate dosages of some antidepressant medications (e.g., venlafaxine or doxepin) may be of help (Gallant et al. 1969). In one controlled evaluation of doxepin versus diazepam in 100 abstinent chronic alcoholic inpatients exhibiting the target symptomatology of anxiety and tension, an average doxepin dosage of 100–150 mg/day appeared to be just as effective as 15–30 mg/day of diazepam (Gallant et al. 1969). In addition to the potential habituation problems that benzodiazepines pose for the alcoholic patient, the side effects of performance decrements in cognitive tasks, reduced manual dexterity, and anterograde amnesia may interfere with the alcoholic patient's recovery phase (Gallant et al. 1969).

Buspirone is a compound that does not appear to be addicting or to cause significant impairment of the cognitive processes, but its practical utility for alcoholic patients with anxiety is still in question.

In posttraumatic stress disorder patients with substance abuse, we have found the α-adrenergic agonists to have a significant effect both in reducing the intensity and, in many cases, in eliminating the horrible nightmares that these patients experience. For those patients who first develop nightmares during the latter phase of sleep, we use guanfacine, which has a longer half-life than clonidine and causes less sedation and hypotension side effects. However, we do caution patients using both types of agents to sit up slowly and stand up slowly the morning after taking a nighttime dose of medication.

Use of Antipsychotic Medications

Before making a definitive diagnosis of schizophrenia, the clinician must rule out alcohol-induced psychotic disorder with hallucinations and/or delusions, a syndrome that can occur within a month of alcohol withdrawal (American Psychiatric Association 1994). Patients with this syndrome present with delusional thought processes and/or hallucinations accompanied by clear sensoriums. Exclusion criteria of other diagnoses include no history of a primary major psychiatric disorder prior to the development of the alcoholism or during sustained periods of abstinence. In one study, alcohol-induced psychotic disorder was reported by approximately 10% of 220 patients consecutively admitted to an inpatient alcohol treatment center, although the psychotic symptoms cleared within several weeks (Schuckit 1982). A review of the literature indicated that alcohol-induced psychosis appears to be a separate illness and may not be linked to the risk of schizophrenia (Schuckit 1982).

The clinician must exercise caution in the dosage regimen for alcoholic patients with a comorbid diagnosis of schizophrenia. It may be that some of the schizophrenic patients who are abusing alcohol are actually self-medicating one of their antipsychotic-induced side effects, such as akathisia. Therefore, the clinician must seek the minimal optimal dosage of the antipsychotic that alleviates the psychotic symptomatology but induces minimal or no extrapyramidal side effects, particularly akathisia.

The clinician should be aware that antipsychotic-induced tardive dyskinesia may be more frequent in psychiatric patients with comorbid alcoholism. In one sample of 284 psychiatric patients who chronically abused street drugs and had received antipsychotic treatment for an average duration of 10.5 ± 5.8 years, the overall incidence of tardive dyskinesia was 15.9% (Olivera et al. 1990). Those groups of psychiatric patients who abused alcohol, either alone or in combination with cannabis, had the *highest* incidences of tardive dyskinesia (25.4% and 26.7%, respectively). The possibility exists that chronic alcohol intake may be associated with structural or chemical changes that provide a substrate for development of tardive dyskinesia when antipsychotic drugs are administered over a relatively long period. Therefore, the atypical antipsychotics are preferred as the initial pharmacological therapy for schizophrenic patients with a comorbid diagnosis of alcohol dependence.

A comment should be made about alcoholic patients who have an accompanying drug dependence problem that requires methadone maintenance. Alcoholic patients who were formerly addicted to heroin should usually be treated for alcoholism without being withdrawn from methadone (Gordis 1988). Although the prevalence of alcoholism among patients on methadone maintenance is as high as 50%, rates of relapse to heroin use may be as high as 70%–80% if methadone maintenance is discontinued (Gordis 1988). Although these patients are difficult to treat, treatment is more likely to be successful if the patients are maintained on methadone throughout the duration of the alcoholism rehabilitation program. Maintaining a rigid guideline against continuing methadone in these patients prior to alcoholism rehabilitation not only will result in an increase in hepatitis and possible human immunodeficiency virus (HIV) infections but also will subsequently cause a spread of these infections to the patients' sexual partners. Gordis (1988), in the *NIAAA Alcohol Alert*, concluded that "requiring individuals to terminate methadone maintenance as a condition of acceptance into alcoholism treatment should be rejected as a standard practice by alcohol treatment service providers" (p. 3).

Use of Vitamins

It is not unusual for an alcoholic patient to have one or more nutritional deficiencies of, for example, magnesium, zinc, and/or various vitamins. It is generally agreed that supplemental thiamine should be administered to all patients who have a history of chronic alcoholism. Thiamine administration is the recommended treatment for Wernicke's encephalopathy, a rapidly degenerative organic mental syndrome that may be difficult to diagnose (Gallant 1987). Another disease whose treatment may benefit from supplemental thiamine therapy is alcoholic amblyopia, which is characterized by blurring of vision due to central scotomas and can develop into optic atrophy if left untreated (Edmondson 1980). Improvement of alcoholic amblyopia has been reported in association with vitamin B supplements, but there are no controlled studies in this area; controlled data are similarly lacking in most of the other areas involving vitamin therapy of alcohol-related diseases. A significant percentage of alcoholic patients have peripheral neuropathies; it may be that chronic thiamine deficiency, as well as pantothenic acid and pyridoxine deficiency, is responsible for the development of this syndrome (Gallant 1987). However, it is not known whether one or several of these vitamin deficiencies are specific causes of peripheral neuropathy; it is also uncertain what part direct alcohol toxicity plays in producing the condition. Multiple mega–B vitamin therapy is recommended for patients with neuropathies. Thiamine therapy, vitamin A, and zinc supplements have been recommended by some clinicians for alcoholic patients who complain about night blindness. If the patient does not show any significant neurological or hematological problems secondary to chronic excessive alcohol intake, routine orders should include only thiamine 100 mg daily and a multivitamin supplement.

Pharmacotherapy of Organ Damage Secondary to Chronic Excessive Ethanol Intake

Based on the available data on prophylactic therapy for large esophageal varices and recurrent bleeding from severe portal hypertensive gastropathy in men with chronic liver disease, propranolol administration appears to be the safest and most effective treatment at this time (Gallant 1992). In fact, a meta-analysis of all of the controlled clinical trials of β-adrenoreceptor–blocking drugs showed that these agents have significantly reduced the occurrence of variceal bleeding deaths (Hayes et al. 1990). These results indicate the value of β-adrenergic–blocking drugs in the prevention of hemorrhage from large esophageal varices.

Other encouraging results in patients with chronic alcoholic liver disease have been reported with the use of propylthiouracil (Orrego et al. 1987). In a long-term, double-blind, randomized clinical trial involving 310 alcoholic patients with mild to severe liver disease, the group receiving propylthiouracil at 300 mg/day had a mortality rate at the end of the 2-year study that was half the mortality rate in the group receiving placebo ($P < 0.05$) and less than half of that in the placebo subgroup of severely ill patients. The criteria for admission to the study included clinical or laboratory evidence of liver disease; the severity of each case was determined with the use of a clinical and laboratory index. The authors itemized the graded score for severity of liver disease using the clinical and laboratory abnormalities (Orrego et al. 1987). It should be emphasized that protective effect of propylthiouracil was not observed in patients who continued to drink during the study. Despite the fact that propylthiouracil can cause hepatitis in rare instances, administration of this drug is definitely recommended to reduce mortality secondary to alcoholic liver disease (Orrego et al. 1987, 1988).

Conclusions

In summary, we now see serious efforts devoted not only to the treatment of alcoholism before permanent liver and CNS damage develop but also to the maintenance of patients who have already developed permanent organ damage.

References

Adinoff B, Bone GHA, Linnoila M: Acute ethanol poisoning and the ethanol withdrawal syndrome. Med Toxicol Adverse Drug Exp 3:172–196, 1988

Alldredge BK, Lowenstein DH, Simon RP: Placebo-controlled trial of intravenous dyphenylhydantoin for short-term treatment of alcohol withdrawal seizures. Am J Med 87:645–648, 1989

American Psychiatric Association: Diagnostic and Statistical Manual of Mental Disorders, 3rd Edition. Washington, DC, American Psychiatric Association, 1980

American Psychiatric Association: Diagnostic and Statistical Manual of Mental Disorders, 4th Edition. Washington, DC, American Psychiatric Association, 1994

Azrin WH, Sisson RW, Meyers R, et al: Alcoholism treatment by disulfiram and community reinforcement therapy. J Behav Ther Exp Psychiatry 13:105–112, 1982

Ballenger JC, Post RM: Kindling as a model for alcohol withdrawal syndromes. Br J Psychiatry 133:1–14, 1978

Baumgartner GR, Rowen RC: Follow-up crossover comparison of clonidine with chlordiazepoxide in alcohol withdrawal management. J Psych Neurol 1:5–6, 1988

Benzer D, Cushman P Jr: Alcohol and benzodiazepines: withdrawal syndromes. Alcohol Clin Exp Res 4:243–247, 1980

Berlin RG: Disulfiram toxicity: a consideration of biochemical mechanism and clinical spectrum. Alcohol Alcohol 24:241–246, 1989

Boyer CS, Petersen DR: Potentiation of cocaine-induced hepatotoxicity by acute and chronic ethanol administration. Alcohol Clin Exp Res 14:28–31, 1990

Brady KT, Malcolm R, Ballenger JC: Anticonvulsants in substance use disorders. Psychiatr Ann 26:5488–5491, 1996

Christensen JK, Ronstead P, Vaag UH: Side effects after disulfiram. Acta Psychiatr Scand 69:265–273, 1984

Ciraulo DA, Barnhill JG, Ciraulo AM, et al: Parental alcoholism as a risk factor in benzodiazepine abuse: a pilot study. Am J Psychiatry 146:1333–1335, 1989

Cloninger CR, Sigvardsson S, Bohman M: Type I and type II alcoholism: an update. Alcohol Health Res World 20:18–23, 1996

Cushman P, Forbes R, Lerner W, et al: Alcohol withdrawal syndromes: clinical management with lofexidine. Alcohol Clin Exp Res 9:103–108, 1985

Edmondson HA: Pathology of alcoholism. Am J Clin Pathol 74:725–742, 1980

Fuller RK, Niederhiser DH: Evaluation and application of urinary diethylamine method to measure compliance with disulfiram therapy. J Stud Alcohol 42:202–207, 1980

Fuller RK, Williford WO: Life-table analysis of abstinence in a study evaluating the efficacy of disulfiram. Alcohol Clin Exp Res 4:298–301, 1981

Gallant DM: Alcoholism: A Guide to Diagnosis, Intervention and Treatment. New York, WW Norton, 1987

Gallant DM: Prophylactic therapy of first-episode bleeding in esophageal varices. Alcohol Clin Exp Res 16:139–140, 1992

Gallant DM, Biship MP, Guerrero-Figueroa R: Doxepin versus diazepam. A controlled evaluation in 100 chronic alcoholic patients. J Clin Pharmacol 9:57–61, 1969

Gatto GJ, Murphy JM, McBride WJ, et al: Effects of fluoxetine and desipramine on palatability-induced ethanol consumption in the alcohol-nonpreferring (NP) line of rats. Alcohol 7:531–536, 1990

Gerrein JR, Rosenberg C, Manohar V: Disulfiram maintenance in outpatient treatment of alcoholism. Arch Gen Psychiatry 28:798–802, 1973

Gordis E: Methadone maintenance and patients in alcoholism treatment. NIAAA Alcohol Alert, No. 1, August 1988

Guerrero-Figueroa R, Rye MM, Gallant DM, et al: Electrographic and behavioral effects of diazepam during alcohol withdrawal stage in cats. Neuropharmacology 9:143–150, 1970

Hayes PC, Davis JM, Lewis JA, et al: Meta-analysis of propranolol in prevention of variceal haemorrhage. Lancet 336:153–156, 1990

Hyashida M, Alterman AI, McClellan AT, et al: Comparative effectiveness and costs of inpatient and outpatient detoxification of patients with mild to moderate withdrawal syndrome. N Eng J Med 320:358–365, 1989

Kessler RC, McGonagle KA, Zhao S, et al: Lifetime and 12-month prevalence of DSM-III-R psychiatric disorders in the United States. Arch Gen Psychiatry 51:8–19, 1994

Linnoila M, Mefford I, Nutt D, et al: Alcohol withdrawal and noradrenergic function. Ann Intern Med 107:875–889, 1987

Liskow BI, Goodwin DW: Pharmacological treatment of alcohol intoxication, withdrawal, and dependence: a critical review. J Stud Alcohol 48:356–370, 1987

Litt MD, Babor TF, DelBoca FK, et al: Types of alcoholics, II: application of an empirically derived typology to treatment-matching. Arch Gen Psychiatry 49:609–614, 1992

Malcolm R, Ballenger JC, Sturgis ET, et al: Double-blind controlled trial comparing carbamazepine to oxazepam treatment of alcohol withdrawal. Am J Psychiatry 146:617–621, 1989

Manhem P, Nilsson LH, Moberg A, et al: Alcohol withdrawal: effects of clonidine treatment on sympathetic activity, the renin-aldosterone system, and clinical symptoms. Alcohol Clin Exp Res 9:238–243, 1985

Mayo-Smith MF: Pharmacological management of alcohol withdrawal. JAMA 278:144–151, 1997

Naranjo CA, Sellers EM, Lawrin MO: Modulation of ethanol intake by serotonin uptake inhibitors. J Clin Psychiatry 47:16–22, 1986

Nirenberg AA, Adler LA, Peselow E, et al: A controlled trial of trazodone in antidepressant-associated insomnia. Abstract presented at American College of Neuropsychopharmacology Annual Meeting, December 1991

Olivera AA, Kiefer MW, Manley NK: Tardive dyskinesia in psychiatric patients with substance use disorders. Am J Drug Alcohol Abuse 16:57–66, 1990

O'Malley SS, Jaffe A, Chang G, et al: Naltrexone and coping skills therapy for alcohol dependence: a controlled study. Arch Gen Psychiatry 49:881–887, 1992

Orrego H, Blake JE, Blendis LM, et al: Long-term treatment of alcoholic liver disease with propylthiouracil. N Engl J Med 317:1421–1427, 1987

Orrego H, Blake KE, Blendis LM, et al: Long-term treatment of alcoholic liver disease with propylthiouracil (letter). Lancet 1(8590):892, 1988

Pattison ME: Management of alcoholism in medical practice. Med Clin North Am 61:797–809, 1977

Pietraszek MH, Urano T, Sumioshi K, et al: Alcohol-induced depression: involvement of serotonin. Alcohol Alcohol 26:155–159, 1991

Project MATCH Research Group: Matching alcoholism treatments to client heterogeneity: Project MATCH post-treatment outcome. J Stud Alcohol 58:7–29, 1997

Raine A, Venables PH, Williams M: Relationship between central and autonomic measures of arousal at 15 years and criminality at age of 24 years. Arch Gen Psychiatry 47:1003–1007, 1990

Regier DA, Farmer ME, Rae DS, et al: Comorbidity of mental disorders with alcohol and other drug abuse. JAMA 264:2511–2518, 1990

Ries RK, Roy-Byrne PP, Ward NG, et al: Carbamazepine treatment for benzodiazepine withdrawal. Am J Psychiatry 146:536–537, 1989

Romach MK, Sellers EM: Management of the alcohol withdrawal syndrome, in Annual Review of Medicine. Edited by Creger WP, Coggins CH, Hancock EW. Palo Alto, CA, Annual Reviews, 1991, pp 323–339

Rounsaville BJ, Dolinsky ZS, Babor TF: Psychopathology as a predictor of treatment outcome in alcoholics. Arch Gen Psychiatry 44:505–513, 1987

Sass H, Soyka M, Mann K, et al: Relapse prevention by acamprosate: results from a placebo-controlled study on alcohol dependence. Arch Gen Psychiatry 53:673–680, 1996

Schuckit MA: The history of psychotic symptoms in alcoholism. J Clin Psychiatry 43:53–57, 1982

Schuckit MA: Chlormethiozole (Hemmerrin): a drug for alcohol withdrawal? Drug Abuse Alcohol News 19:1–3, 1991

Sereny G, Sharma V, Holt J, et al: Mandatory supervised Antabuse therapy in an outpatient alcoholism program: a pilot study. Alcohol Clin Exp Res 10:290–292, 1986

Stuppaeck CH, Pycha R, Miller C, et al: Carbamazepine versus oxazepam in the treatment of alcohol withdrawal: a double-blind study. Alcohol 27:153–158, 1992

Sullivan JT, Swift RM, Lewis DC: Benzodiazepine requirements during alcohol withdrawal syndrome: clinical implications of using a standardized withdrawal scale. J Clin Psychopharmacol 11:291–295, 1991

Tohen M, Castillo J, Cole JO: Thrombocytopenia associated with carbamazepine: a case series. J Clin Psychiatry 52:496–498, 1991

Volpicelli JR, Alterman AI, Hyashida M, et al: Naltrexone in the treatment of alcohol dependence. Arch Gen Psychiatry 49:876–880, 1992

Whitfield CL: Nondrug detoxification, in Phenomenology and Treatment of Alcoholism. Edited by Whitfield C. New York, Spectrum, 1980, pp 112–127

Wiseman EJ, Henderson KL, Briggs MJ: Outcomes of patients in a VA ambulatory detoxification program. Psychiatr Serv 48:200–203, 1997

Wilson A, Vulcano B: A double-blind, placebo-controlled trial of magnesium sulfate in the ethanol withdrawal syndrome. Alcohol Clin Exp Res 8:542–545, 1986

World Health Organization: International Classification of Diseases, 10th Revision. Geneva, World Health Organization, 1992

Benzodiazepine and Other Sedative-Hypnotic Dependence

David E. Smith, M.D.
Donald R. Wesson, M.D.

Chronic use of benzodiazepines or sedative-hypnotics *at dosages exceeding the usual therapeutic range* can produce physiological dependence and is often associated with a DSM-IV (American Psychiatric Association 1994) substance use disorder. Chronic use of *therapeutic doses* of benzodiazepines may also produce physiological dependence. Often, physiological dependence develops in the context of pharmacotherapy and is not necessarily associated with a substance use disorder.

High-Dose Benzodiazepine Withdrawal Syndrome

Studies in humans have established that large doses of chlordiazepoxide (Hollister et al. 1961) or diazepam (Hollister et al. 1963) taken for a month or more produce a withdrawal syndrome that is clinically similar to the withdrawal syndrome produced by high doses of barbiturates (Isbell 1950). Numerous case reports leave no doubt that other benzodiazepines, although not studied under such precise conditions, also produce a similar withdrawal syndrome.

Signs and symptoms of sedative-hypnotic withdrawal include anxiety, tremors, nightmares, insomnia, anorexia, nausea, vomiting, postural hypotension, seizures, delirium, and hyperpyrexia. The syndrome is qualitatively similar for all sedative-hypnotics; however, the time course of symptoms depends on the particular drug. With the short-acting sedative-hypnotics (e.g., pentobarbital, secobarbital, meprobamate, methaqualone) and the short-acting benzodiazepines (e.g., oxazepam, alprazolam, triazolam), withdrawal symptoms typically begin 12–24 hours after the last dose and peak in intensity at between 24 and 72 hours. (Symptoms may develop more slowly in patients with liver disease or in elderly patients because of decreased drug metabolism.) With the long-acting agents (e.g., phenobarbital, diazepam, chlordiazepoxide), withdrawal symptoms peak on the fifth to eighth day.

During untreated sedative-hypnotic withdrawal, the electroencephalogram (EEG) may show paroxysmal bursts of high-voltage, slow-frequency activity that precede the development of seizures. The withdrawal delirium may include confusion and visual and auditory hallucinations. The delirium generally follows a period of insomnia. Some patients may have only delirium, others may have only seizures, and still others may have both delirium and convulsions.

Low-Dose Benzodiazepine Withdrawal Syndrome

In addiction medicine literature, the low-dose benzodiazepine withdrawal syndrome is also referred to as *therapeutic-dose withdrawal*, *normal-dose withdrawal*, or *benzodiazepine-discontinuation syndrome*. During the 1980s, clinical studies and case reports established that therapeutic doses of benzodiazepines could produce physiological dependency. Many patients experienced a transient increase in symptoms for 1–2 weeks postwithdrawal. A few patients experienced a severe, protracted withdrawal syndrome that included symptoms (e.g., paresthesias and psychosis) that had not been present before. It is this latter withdrawal syndrome that has generated much of the concern about the long-term safety of the benzodiazepines.

Because of psychiatrists' concerns about the serious side effects and the associated dependency of benzodiazepines, the American Psychiatric Association formed a task force to review the issues. In its published report (American Psychiatric Association 1990), the task force's conclusions about therapeutic dose dependency were unambiguous:

> Physiological dependence on benzodiazepines, as indicated by the appearance of discontinuance symptoms, can develop with therapeutic doses. Duration of treatment determines the onset of dependence when typical therapeutic anxiolytic doses are used; clinically significant dependence indicated by the appearance of discontinuance symptoms usually does not appear before four months of such daily dosing. Dependence may develop sooner when higher antipanic doses are taken daily. (p. 56)

Many persons who have taken benzodiazepines in therapeutic doses for months to years can abruptly discontinue the current drug without developing symptoms. But others, taking similar amounts of a benzodiazepine, develop mild to severe symptoms when the benzodiazepine is stopped or the dosage is substantially reduced. Characteristically, patients tolerate a gradual tapering of the benzodiazepine until they are at 10%–20% of their peak dose. Further reduction in benzodiazepine dose causes patients to become increasingly symptomatic.

There are at least three categories of symptoms that emerge following benzodiazepine cessation: symptom rebound, protracted withdrawal syndrome, and symptom reemergence (or recrudescence). Symptom rebound and the protracted withdrawal syndrome are the result of physiological dependence, whereas symptom reemergence is not.

Symptom rebound is an intensified return of the symptoms for which the benzodiazepine was prescribed (e.g., insomnia or anxiety). The term comes from sleep research, in which it was observed that "rebound" insomnia may occur following long-term, daily sedative-hypnotic use. Symptom rebound lasts from a few days to weeks following discontinuation of the benzodiazepine (American Psychiatric Association 1990). Symptom rebound is the most common withdrawal consequence of prolonged benzodiazepine use.

Protracted withdrawal syndrome for benzodiazepines should be distinguished from the protracted withdrawal syndrome that has been described for most other drugs, including alcohol (Geller 1991). The symptoms attributed to protracted withdrawal syndromes for other drugs consist of relatively mild symptoms, such as irritability, anxiety, insomnia, and mood instability. The protracted withdrawal syndrome for benzodiazepines can be severe and disabling and lasts many months.

Some symptoms—increased sensitivity to sound, light, and touch; paresthesias—are particularly suggestive of low-dose withdrawal.

The protracted benzodiazepine withdrawal syndrome has no pathognomonic signs or symptoms. Many symptoms are nonspecific and often mimic obsessive-compulsive disorder with psychotic features. Protracted withdrawal-like symptoms that appear could also be attributable to the reemergence of agitated depression, generalized anxiety disorder, panic disorder, partial complex seizures, or schizophrenia. The time course of symptom resolution is the primary feature differentiating symptoms generated by withdrawal and symptoms produced by reemergence of psychopathology. Symptoms of withdrawal gradually subside with continued abstinence, whereas symptom reemergence does not.

The low-dose protracted benzodiazepine withdrawal syndrome is characterized in part by a waxing and waning intensity of symptoms (Figure 26–1). Patients are sometimes asymptomatic for several days, and then, without apparent psychological reason, they become acutely anxious. There may be concomitant physiological signs (e.g., dilated pupils, increased resting heart rate and blood pressure). The intense waxing and waning of symptoms is important in distinguishing low-dose withdrawal symptoms from symptom reemergence.

Patients' symptoms of anxiety, insomnia, or muscle tension abate during benzodiazepine treatment. *Symptom reemergence* (or *recrudescence*) occurs when the benzodiazepine is stopped and symptoms return to the same level as before benzodiazepine therapy. Distinguishing between symptom reemergence and symptom rebound has important treatment implications in that symptom reemergence suggests that the original symptoms have not been adequately treated, whereas symptom rebound suggests that a transient withdrawal syndrome is present.

Benzodiazepine Receptor Hypothesis of Low-Dose Withdrawal

From a clinical perspective, we have postulated that the low-dose benzodiazepine withdrawal syndrome is caused by alteration in gamma-aminobutyric acid (GABA) receptor function (D. E. Smith and Wesson 1983, 1985). A receptor site–mediated withdrawal syndrome would explain why benzodiazepine withdrawal symptoms develop at low doses and why symptoms develop when tapering patients from the last few milligrams of the benzodiazepine. These characteristics are consistent with those of withdrawals mediated by other receptors.

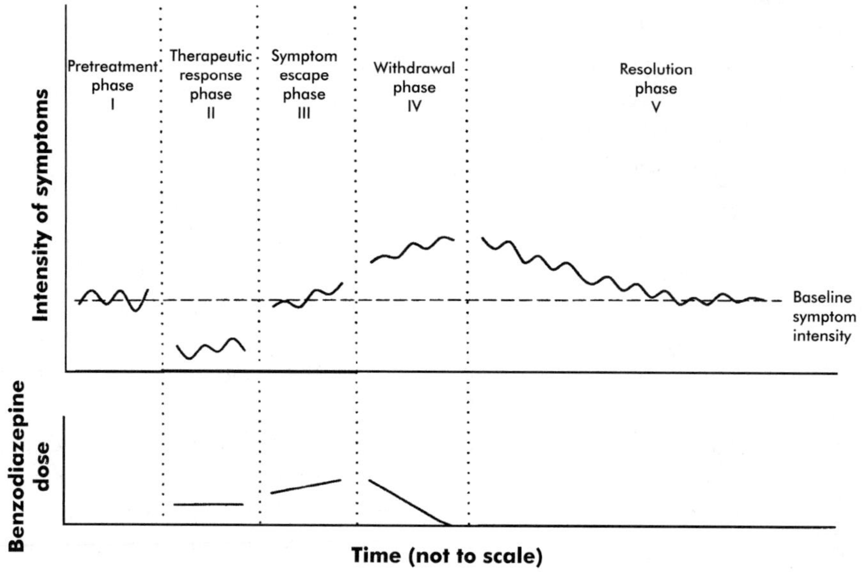

FIGURE 26–1. The dependence/withdrawal cycle for benzodiazepines. The symptom intensity before treatment (I) is reduced as part of the initial therapeutic response (II). Symptom amelioration may last months to many years. Some patients then enter a phase in which benzodiazepines no longer ameliorate the patients' symptoms. With intensifying symptoms, patients commonly increase their daily intake of the benzodiazepine and may develop cognitive impairment from the accumulation of the benzodiazepine (III). Withdrawal of the benzodiazepine initially increases symptoms still further (IV). If, however, patients remain off benzodiazepines, symptoms will eventually return to the level that the patients were experiencing before taking benzodiazepines (V). This resolution phase may take a few weeks or many months. The dotted line represents patients' average severity of symptoms before treatment with benzodiazepine.

Risk Factors for Low-Dose Withdrawal

Some drugs or medications may facilitate neuroadaptation by increasing the affinity of benzodiazepines for their receptors. Phenobarbital, for example, increases the affinity of diazepam to benzodiazepine receptors (Olsen and Loeb-Lundberg 1981; Skolnick et al. 1981), and prior treatment with phenobarbital has been found to increase the intensity of chlordiazepoxide (45 mg/day) withdrawal symptoms (Covi et al. 1973). Patients at increased risk for development of the low-dose withdrawal syndrome are those with a family or personal history of alcoholism, those who use alcohol daily, or those who concomitantly use other sedatives. Case-control studies suggest that patients with a history of addiction, particularly to other sedative-hypnotics, are at high risk for low-dose benzodiazepine dependence. The short-acting, high-milligram-potency benzodiazepines appear to produce a more intense low-dose withdrawal syndrome (Rickels et al. 1990).

Dependence/Withdrawal Cycle

When benzodiazepine dependence arises during therapeutic treatment, it often follows a sequence of phases, as illustrated in Figure 26–1. The clinical course described below most often occurs during long-term treatment of generalized anxiety disorder, panic disorder, or severe insomnia.

Pretreatment Phase

Before being treated with a benzodiazepine, patients have symptoms that generally vary in intensity from day to day depending on life stresses and the waxing and waning of their underlying disorder.

Therapeutic Response Phase

When treatment with a benzodiazepine is started, patients often have initial side effects such as drowsiness or psychomotor impairment. Tolerance to these side effects usually develops within a few days, and the patient's overall level of symptoms decreases. The therapeutic phase may last months to years.

Symptom Escape and Dosage Escalation Phase

When used daily for long-term treatment, benzodiazepines may suddenly lose their effectiveness in controlling symptoms. For some patients, the "symptom escape" coincides with a period of increased life stress; for others, no unusual psychological stressor is apparent. Patients often say that "the medication no longer works."

As the usual dosage of benzodiazepine loses effectiveness, patients may increase their benzodiazepine consumption in the hope that symptoms will again be controlled. As the daily dosage of benzodiazepine increases, they may develop subtle cognitive impairment that is difficult to diagnose without psychometric assessment. Such benzodiazepine-induced cognitive impairment may be a common clinical problem that is unrecognized. Patients may not be aware that their impairment is benzodiazepine-induced. Coping skills that were previously bolstered by the benzodiazepine become compromised. Some patients make suicide attempts or participate in self-defeating behavior that is out of character for them. Our evidence for this assertion is clinical observation of patients; research evidence is scanty and indirect. Many studies have demonstrated that acute doses of benzodiazepines impair cognitive function; however, there has been little systematic study of long-term cognitive effects. One psychometric study of nonrandomized patients compared long-term benzodiazepine users with patients who were benzodiazepine abstinent. Long-term benzodiazepine users performed poorly on tasks involving visuospatial ability and sustained attention (Golombok et al. 1988).

The symptom escape and dosage escalation phase is not an invariable consequence of long-term benzodiazepine treatment. Patients who have experienced symptom escape and dosage escalation may also be the most likely to have a protracted withdrawal syndrome.

Withdrawal Phase

When patients stop taking the benzodiazepine or the daily dose falls below 25% of the peak maintenance dose, patients become increasingly symptomatic. This increase in symptoms may be the result of symptom rebound or symptom reemergence, or the beginning of a protracted withdrawal syndrome. The symptoms that occur during this phase may be a mixture of symptoms that were present during the pretreatment phase and *new* symptoms.

During the first few weeks, it is not possible to know exactly what is producing the symptoms or to estimate how long they will last. Symptoms of the same type that occurred during the pretreatment phase suggest symptom rebound or symptom reemergence. New symptoms, particularly alterations in sensory perception, suggest the beginning of a protracted withdrawal syndrome. The response to increasing benzodiazepine dose is not useful in discrimination. Increasing the benzodiazepine dose will reduce both kinds of symptoms because either benzodiazepines have not completely lost effectiveness or the withdrawal syndrome is reversed.

Resolution Phase

Most patients will have symptom rebound lasting only a few weeks; a few patients will have a severe, protracted abstinence syndrome lasting months to over a year. During early abstinence, the patient's symptoms will generally vary in intensity from day to day. If abstinence from benzodiazepines is maintained, symptoms will gradually return to their baseline level. An encouraging finding of one discontinuation study was that "patients who were able to remain free of benzodiazepines for at least 5 weeks obtained lower levels of anxiety than before benzodiazepine discontinuation" (Rickels et al. 1990, p. 899).

Pharmacological Treatment of Benzodiazepine Withdrawal

Physicians' response during the withdrawal phase is critical to achieving a resolution. Some physicians interpret patients' escalating symptoms as evidence of these patients' "need" for benzodiazepine treatment and reinstitute higher doses of benzodiazepines or switch to another benzodiazepine. Reinstitution of any benzodiazepine agonist usually does not achieve satisfactory symptom control and may prolong the recovery process. Benzodiazepine withdrawal, using one of the strategies described in the following subsections, generally achieves the best long-term outcome.

Another common response is to declare patients "addicted to benzodiazepines" and refer them to primary chemical dependency treatment. Referral to a chemical dependency program is not appropriate unless the patient's benzodiazepine use meets the criteria for substance abuse or dependence.

Benzodiazepines and their phenobarbital withdrawal equivalents are summarized in Table 26–1.

Benzodiazepine withdrawal strategies must be tailored to suit three possible dependence situations:

1. A high-dose withdrawal (i.e., doses greater than the recommended therapeutic doses for more than 1 month)
2. A low-dose withdrawal (i.e., doses below those in the upper therapeutic range shown in Table 26–1)
3. A combined high-dose and low-dose withdrawal (i.e., the occurrence, following daily high doses for more than 6 months, of both a high-dose sedative-hypnotic withdrawal syndrome and a low-dose benzodiazepine withdrawal syndrome)

TABLE 26–1. Benzodiazepines and their phenobarbital withdrawal equivalents

Generic name	Trade name	Therapeutic dosage range (mg/day)	Dose equal to 30 mg of phenobarbital for withdrawal (mg)[a]	Phenobarbital conversion constant
Alprazolam	Xanax	0.75–6	1	30
Chlordiazepoxide	Librium	15–100	25	1.2
Clonazepam	Klonopin	0.5–4	2	15
Clorazepate	Tranxène	15–60	7.5	4
Diazepam	Valium	4–40	10	3
Estazolam	ProSom	1–2	1	30
Flumazenil	Mazicon	NA[b]	NA	NA
Flurazepam	Dalmane	15–30[c]	15	2
Halazepam	Paxipam	60–160	40	0.75
Lorazepam	Ativan	1–12	2	15
Midazolam	Versed	NA	NA	NA
Oxazepam	Serax	10–120	10	3
Prazepam	Centrax	20–60	10	3
Quazepam	Doral	15[c]	15	2
Temazepam	Restoril	15–30[c]	15	2
Triazolam	Halcion	0.125–0.50[c]	0.25	120

[a]Phenobarbital withdrawal conversion equivalence is not the same as therapeutic dose equivalency. Withdrawal equivalence is the amount of the drug that 30 mg of phenobarbital will substitute for and prevent serious high-dose withdrawal signs and symptoms.
[b]Not applicable.
[c]Usual hypnotic dose.

High-Dose Benzodiazepine Withdrawal

Abrupt discontinuation of a sedative-hypnotic agent in patients who are severely physiologically dependent on the agent can result in serious medical complications and even death. There are three general strategies for withdrawing patients from sedative-hypnotics, including benzodiazepines. The first is to use decreasing doses of the agent of dependence. The second is to substitute phenobarbital or some other long-acting barbiturate for the addicting agent and then gradually withdraw the substitute medication (D. E. Smith and Wesson 1970, 1971, 1983, 1985). The third, used for patients with a dependence on both alcohol and a benzodiazepine, is to substitute a long-acting benzodiazepine, such as chlordiazepoxide, and then taper it over 1–2 weeks.

The pharmacological rationale for phenobarbital substitution is that phenobarbital is long-acting, and little change in blood levels of phenobarbital occurs between doses. This allows the safe use of a progressively smaller daily dose. Phenobarbital is safer than the shorter-acting barbiturates; lethal doses of phenobarbital are manyfold higher than toxic doses, and the signs of toxicity (e.g., sustained nystagmus, slurred speech, and ataxia) are easy to observe. Finally, phenobarbital intoxication usually does not produce disinhibition, so most patients view it as a medication, not as a drug of abuse.

The method selected will depend on the particular benzodiazepine, the involvement of other drugs of dependence, and the clinical setting in which the detoxification program takes place.

The gradual reduction of the benzodiazepine of dependence is used primarily in medical settings for dependence arising from treatment of an underlying condition. The patient must be cooperative and able to adhere to dosing regimens and must not be abusing alcohol or other drugs.

Substitution of phenobarbital can also be used to withdraw patients who have lost control of their benzodiazepine use or who are polydrug dependent. Phenobarbital substitution has the broadest use for all sedative-hypnotic drug dependencies and is widely used in drug treatment programs.

Stabilization Phase

The patient's history of drug use during the month before treatment is used to compute the stabilization dose of phenobarbital. Although many addicted persons exaggerate the number of pills they are taking, patients' history is the best *guide* to initiating pharmacotherapy for withdrawal. Patients who have overstated the amount of drug they were taking will become intoxicated during the first day or two of treatment. Intoxication is easily managed by omitting one or more doses of phenobarbital and recalculating the daily dose.

The patient's average daily sedative-hypnotic dose is converted to phenobarbital equivalents and the daily amount divided into three doses. The conversion equivalents for various benzodiazepines are listed in Table 26–1 and for other sedative-hypnotics, in Table 26–2.

The computed phenobarbital equivalence dosage is given in three or four doses daily. If the patient is using significant amounts of other sedative-hypnotics (including alcohol), the amounts of all the drugs are converted to phenobarbital equivalents and *added together*. (For example, 30 cc of 100-proof alcohol is equivalent to 30 mg of phenobarbital for withdrawal purposes.) The maximum starting phenobarbital dosage is 500 mg/day.

Before receiving each dose of phenobarbital, the patient is checked for signs of phenobarbital toxicity: sustained nystagmus, slurred speech, or ataxia. Of these, sustained nystagmus is the most reliable indicator. If nystagmus is present, the scheduled dose of phenobarbital is withheld. If all three signs are present, the next two doses of phenobarbital are withheld and the daily dosage of phenobarbital for the following day is halved.

If the patient is in acute withdrawal and has had or is in danger of having withdrawal seizures, the initial dose of phenobarbital is administered by intramuscular injection. If nystagmus and other signs of intoxication develop after 1–2 hours following the intramuscular dosage, the patient is in no immediate danger from barbiturate withdrawal. Patients are maintained on the initial dosing schedule of phenobarbital for 2 days. If the patient has neither signs of withdrawal nor signs of phenobarbital toxicity (e.g., slurred speech, nystagmus, unsteady gait), then phenobarbital withdrawal is begun.

Withdrawal Phase

Unless the patient develops signs and symptoms of phenobarbital toxicity or sedative-hypnotic withdrawal, phenobarbital is decreased by 30 mg/day. Should signs of phenobarbital toxicity develop during withdrawal, the daily phenobarbital dose is decreased by 50% and the 30-mg-per-day withdrawal continued from the reduced phenobarbital dose. Should the patient have objective signs of sedative-hypnotic withdrawal, the daily dose is increased by 50% and the patient restabilized before continuing the withdrawal.

TABLE 26–2. Sedative-hypnotic agents and their phenobarbital withdrawal equivalents

Generic name	Trade name	Common therapeutic indication	Therapeutic dosage range (mg/day)	Dose equal to 30 mg of phenobarbital for withdrawal (mg)[a]	Phenobarbital conversion constant
Barbiturates					
Amobarbital	Amytal	Sedative	50–150	100	0.33
Butabarbital	Butisol	Sedative	45–120	100	0.33
Butalbital	Fiorinal Sedapap	Sedative/ analgesic[b]	100–300	100	0.33
Pentobarbital	Nembutal	Hypnotic	50–100	100	0.33
Secobarbital	Seconal	Hypnotic	50–100	100	0.33
Other sedative-hypnotics					
Buspirone	BuSpar	Sedative	15–60	—[c]	—[c]
Chloral hydrate	Noctec Somnos	Hypnotic	250–1,000	500	0.06
Ethchlorvynol	Placidyl	Hypnotic	500–1,000	500	0.06
Glutethimide	Doriden	Hypnotic	250–500	250	0.12
Meprobamate	Miltown Equagesic	Sedative	1,200–1,600	1,200	0.025
Methyprylon	Noludar	Hypnotic	200–400	200	0.15

[a]Phenobarbital withdrawal conversion equivalence is not the same as therapeutic dose equivalency. Withdrawal equivalence is the amount of the drug that 30 mg of phenobarbital will substitute for and prevent serious high-dose withdrawal signs and symptoms.
[b]Butalbital is usually available in combination with opiate or nonopiate analgesics.
[c]Not cross-tolerant with barbiturates.

Low-Dose Benzodiazepine Withdrawal

Most patients experience only mild to moderate symptom rebound that disappears after a few days to weeks. Patients may need much reassurance that rebound symptoms are common and that, with continued abstinence, the symptoms will likely subside.

Patients may experience severe symptoms that are quite different from their preexisting symptoms. The phenobarbital regimen described in the previous subsection will not be adequate to suppress symptoms to tolerable levels. Several pharmacological options are available.

One strategy is to increase the phenobarbital to 200 mg/day and slowly taper the phenobarbital over several months. Another strategy is to use propranolol to block somatic symptoms such as tachycardia. A propranolol dose of 20 mg every 6 hours can be administered, either alone or in combination with phenobarbital (Tyrer et al. 1981). The propranolol is continued for 2 weeks and then stopped. Even after phenobarbital withdrawal is complete, propranolol can be used episodically if needed to control tachycardia, increased blood pressure, and anxiety. *Continuous* propranolol therapy for more than 2 weeks is not recommended, however, because propranolol use may itself result in symptom rebound when the agent is discontinued after prolonged therapy (Glaubiger and Lefkowitz 1977).

Valproate and Carbamazepine

A final strategy in treating low-dose withdrawal is use of mood stabilizers, such as valproate or carbamazepine. This strategy has been particularly clinically useful in the management of patients with a comorbid physiological dependence and anxiety and alcohol dependence (Brady et al. 1994). The medications most studied have been carbamazepine (Tegretol) and valproate (Depakene, Depakote, Epilim EC), although gabapentin (Neurontin) and lamotrigine (Lamictal) have also received scrutiny. Carbamazepine and valproate enhance GABA function, seemingly by a different mechanism than the benzodiazepines. Neither carbamazepine nor valproate produces subjective effects that sedative-hypnotic abusers find desirable.

Valproate was first proposed for benzodiazepine withdrawal in the late 1980s (Roy-Byrne et al. 1989). Subsequently, clinical case reports of its use in benzodiazepine withdrawal have appeared (Apelt and Emrich 1990; McElroy et al. 1991). When valproate is employed for low-dose benzodiazepine withdrawal, dosages in the range of 500–1,500 mg/day are used. The most common side effect of valproate is gastrointestinal upset.

Case reports suggest the utility of carbamazepine in treating benzodiazepine withdrawal (Klein et al. 1986; Lawlor 1987; Neppe 1988; Rickels et al. 1990; Ries et al. 1989, 1991; Roy-Byrne et al. 1993; Schweizer et al. 1991). Withdrawal protocols use carbamazepine daily dosages in the range of 400–800 mg/day.

In both clinical experience with treatment of benzodiazepine withdrawal and controlled clinical trials with treatment of epilepsy, valproate appears to be better tolerated than carbamazepine (Richens et al. 1994).

Outpatient Treatment of Withdrawal

Withdrawal from high doses of barbiturates and other sedative-hypnotics should be done in a hospital when possible. Outpatient barbiturate withdrawal is not generally successful unless the patient is unusually motivated to stop using drugs. Patients must be evaluated daily, and withdrawal medication must be dispensed daily.

With patients who are withdrawing from therapeutic doses of benzodiazepines, a slow taper on an outpatient basis is generally a reasonable strategy and should be continued as long as the patient can tolerate withdrawal symptoms.

Postwithdrawal Treatment

Withdrawal is usually successful when the patient cooperates, but many patients do not remain abstinent. Detoxification is not in itself an adequate treatment of sedative-hypnotic dependency but rather constitutes the first step in the recovery process. Patients must learn alternative methods of coping with anxiety (e.g., biofeedback, exercise, cognitive psychotherapy).

Supportive individual psychotherapy or a self-help recovery group is virtually always needed. The goal of psychotherapy is to enable the patient to remain abstinent. Psychotherapy techniques that mobilize anxiety should not be used during early recovery.

Conclusions

Benzodiazepines have many therapeutic uses, and in treatment of some conditions, such as panic disorder, chronic treatment is an appropriate strategy for patients who do not respond to selective serotonin reuptake inhibitors. Physiological dependency is not always an avoidable complication of long-term benzodiazepine therapy. Before initiating a course of prolonged therapy, physicians should discuss with patients the possibility of their developing new or intensified symptoms when the benzodiazepines are discontinued.

Knowledge about low-dose dependency developed from clinical observations is still sketchy and controversial. The U.S. Food and Drug Administration has been remarkably silent about low-dose dependency, and benzodiazepine package inserts give physicians little practical guidance.

The American Psychiatric Association has played a leadership role in reframing dependency that develops during pharmacotherapy. Currently, DSM-IV includes substance-induced diagnoses in numerous categories, such as anxiety disorders and sleep disorders. For patients whose benzodiazepine dependency develops during pharmacotherapy, benzodiazepine dependency does not necessarily constitute a substance use disorder. To label it as such unnecessarily stigmatizes patients.

References

American Psychiatric Association: Benzodiazepine Dependence, Toxicity, and Abuse: A Task Force Report of the American Psychiatric Association. Washington, DC, American Psychiatric Association, 1990

American Psychiatric Association: Diagnostic and Statistical Manual of Mental Disorders, 4th Edition. Washington, DC, American Psychiatric Association, 1994

Apelt S, Emrich HM: Sodium valproate in benzodiazepine withdrawal (letter). Am J Psychiatry 147:950–951, 1990

Brady KT, Sonne S, Lydiard RB: Valproate treatment of comorbid panic disorder and affective disorders in two alcoholic patients (letter). J Clin Psychopharmacol 14:81–82, 1994

Covi L, Lipman RS, Pattison JH, et al: Length of treatment with anxiolytic sedatives and response to their sudden withdrawal. Acta Psychiatr Scand 49:51–64, 1973

Geller A: Protracted abstinence, in Comprehensive Handbook of Drug and Alcohol Addiction. Edited by Miller N. New York, Marcel Dekker, 1991, pp 905–913

Glaubiger G, Lefkowitz RJ: Elevated beta-adrenergic receptor number after chronic propranolol treatment. Biochem Biophys Res Commun 78:720–725, 1977

Golombok S, Moodley P, Lader M: Cognitive impairment in long-term benzodiazepine users. Psychol Med 18:365–374, 1988

Hollister LE, Motzenbecker FP, Degan RO: Withdrawal reactions from chlordiazepoxide (Librium). Psychopharmacology 2:63–68, 1961

Hollister LE, Bennett JL, Kimbell I Jr, et al: Diazepam in newly admitted schizophrenics. Diseases of the Nervous System 24:746–750, 1963

Isbell H: Addiction to barbiturates and the barbiturate abstinence syndrome. Ann Intern Med 33:108–120, 1950

Klein E, Uhde TW, Post RM: Preliminary evidence for the utility of carbamazepine in alprazolam withdrawal. Am J Psychiatry 143:235–236, 1986

Lawlor BA: Carbamazepine, alprazolam withdrawal, and panic disorder (letter). Am J Psychiatry 144:265–266, 1987

McElroy SL, Keck PE Jr, Lawrence JM: Treatment of panic disorder and benzodiazepine withdrawal with valproate (letter). J Neuropsychiatry Clin Neurosci 3:232–233, 1991

Neppe VM: Carbamazepine for withdrawal pseudohallucinations (letter). Am J Psychiatry 145:1605–1606, 1988

Olsen RW, Loeb-Lundberg F: Convulsant and anti-convulsant drug binding sites related to GABA-regulated chloride ion channels, in GABA and Benzodiazepine Receptors. Edited by Costa E, DiChiara G, Gessa GL. New York, Raven, 1981, pp 93–102

Richens A, Davidson DL, Cartlidge NE, et al: A multicentre comparative trial of sodium valproate and carbamazepine in adult onset epilepsy. J Neurol Neurosurg Psychiatry 57:682–687, 1994

Rickels K, Case WG, Schweizer E, et al: Benzodiazepine dependence: management of discontinuation. Psychopharmacol Bull 26:63–68, 1990

Ries RK, Roy-Byrne PP, Ward NG, et al: Carbamazepine treatment for benzodiazepine withdrawal. Am J Psychiatry 146:536–537, 1989

Ries R, Cullison S, Horn R, et al: Benzodiazepine withdrawal: clinicians' ratings of carbamazepine treatment versus traditional taper methods. J Psychoactive Drugs 23:73–76, 1991

Roy-Byrne PP, Ward NG, Donnelly PJ: Valproate in anxiety and withdrawal syndromes. J Clin Psychiatry 50 (suppl):44–48, 1989

Roy-Byrne PP, Sullivan MD, Cowley DS, et al: Adjunctive treatment of benzodiazepine discontinuation syndromes: a review. J Psychiatr Res 27 (suppl 1):143–153, 1993

Schweizer E, Rickels K, Case WG, Greenblatt DJ: Carbamazepine treatment in patients discontinuing long-term benzodiazepine therapy. Effects on withdrawal severity and outcome. Arch Gen Psychiatry 48:448–452, 1991

Skolnick P, Concada V, Barker JL, et al: Pentobarbital: dual action to increase brain benzodiazepine receptor affinity. Science 211:1448–1450, 1981

Smith DE, Wesson DR: A new method for treatment of barbiturate dependence. JAMA 213:294–295, 1970

Smith DE, Wesson DR: Phenobarbital technique for treatment of barbiturate dependence. Arch Gen Psychiatry 24:56–60, 1971

Smith DE, Wesson DR: Benzodiazepine dependency syndromes. J Psychoactive Drugs 15:85–95, 1983

Smith DE, Wesson DR: Benzodiazepine dependency syndromes, in The Benzodiazepines: Current Standards for Medical Practice. Edited by Smith DE, Wesson DR. Hingham, MA, MTP Press, 1985, pp 235–248

Tyrer P, Rutherford D, Huggett T: Benzodiazepine withdrawal symptoms and propranolol. Lancet 1(8219):520–522, 1981

27

The Hallucinogens and Cannabis

Robert N. Pechnick, Ph.D.
J. Thomas Ungerleider, M.D.
Mark S. Gold, M.D.
Michelle Tullis, Ph.D. candidate
Kimberly Frost-Pineda, M.P.H.

The Hallucinogens

Robert N. Pechnick, Ph.D.
J. Thomas Ungerleider, M.D.

Hallucinogens that are likely to be abused include the ergot hallucinogen lysergic acid diethylamide (LSD), which is the prototype of these drugs of abuse; other indolealkylamines, such as psilocybin ("magic mushrooms") and dimethyltryptamine (DMT); and the phenalkylamines, including mescaline, dimethoxymethylamphetamine (DOM; also known as "STP"), and the so-called stimulant hallucinogens methylenedioxyamphetamine (MDA) and methylenedioxymethamphetamine (MDMA; also known as "X" or "Ecstasy"). (The hallucinogen-like drugs marijuana and phencyclidine are covered in the second part of this chapter and in the second part of Chapter 28, respectively.) The hallucinogens, called psychotomimetics or psychedelics ("mind-manifesting"), are a group of drugs that produce thought, mood, and perceptual disorders. Depending on dosage, expectation (set), and environment (setting), they also can induce euphoria and a state similar to a transcendental experience.

The term *hallucinogen* means "producer of hallucinations." Many drugs can cause auditory and/or visual hallucinations. These hallucinations may be present as part of a delirium, accompanied by disturbances in judgment, orientation, intellect, memory, and emotion (e.g., an organic brain syndrome). Such delirium also may result from drug withdrawal (e.g., sedative-hypnotic withdrawal or delirium tremens in alcohol withdrawal). In the context of substance abuse, however, the collective term hallucinogens generally refers to a group of compounds that alter consciousness without delirium, sedation, excessive stimulation, or impairment of intellect or memory. The label hallucinogen actually is inaccurate, because true LSD-induced hallucinations are rare. What are commonly seen are illusory phenomena. An *illusion* is a perceptual distortion of an actual stimulus in the environment: to "see" someone's face melting is an illusion; to "see" a melting face when no one is present is a hallucination. Consequently, some investigators have called these drugs "illusionogenic." Those who use the term *psychedelic* (a term coined in 1957 by Osmond), or "mind-manifesting," for hallucinogens have been criticized as being "prodrug," much as those who use the term *hallucinogen* have been accused of being "antidrug" (Osmond 1957). The term *psychotomimetic*, meaning a producer of psychosis, also has been widely used.

No abstinence syndrome occurs—and thus, no detoxification is required—after the repeated use of hallucinogens, and there are few specific pharmacological interventions available for the treatment of acute toxic effects. Therefore, in this chapter part we focus on the general acute and chronic effects of these drugs and on the psychosocial interventions necessary to treat the adverse reactions. Again, LSD will be discussed as the prototypical hallucinogen.

Psychological Effects

When hallucinogens are taken orally, the psychic phenomena noted vary considerably, depending on the amount consumed and the set and the setting of both the subject and the observer. The overall psychological effects of the hallucinogens are quite similar; however, the rate of onset, duration of action, and absolute intensity of the effects can differ. Both Hofmann (1961) and Hollister (1978) described the effects of LSD in great detail. The absorption of LSD from the gastrointestinal tract and other mucous membranes occurs rapidly, with drug diffusion to all tissues, including the brain and across the placenta to the fetus. The onset of psychological and behavioral effects occurs approximately 30–60 minutes after oral administration and peaks at from 2 to 4 hours postadministration, with a gradual return to the predrug state in 8–12 hours. DMT produces similar effects but is inactive after oral administration and must be injected, sniffed, or smoked. It has a very rapid onset and a short duration of action (60–120 minutes). Thus, DMT previously was known as the "businessman's LSD" (i.e., one could have a psychedelic experience over the lunch hour and be back at work in the afternoon). In contrast, the effects of DOM have been reported to last for over 24 hours. The various hallucinogens also differ widely in potency and slope of the dose-response curve. Thus, some of the apparent qualitative differences between hallucinogens may be due, in part, to the amount of drug ingested relative to its specific dose-response characteristics. LSD is one of the most potent hallucinogens known, with behavioral effects occurring in some persons after doses as low as 20 µg. Typical street doses range from 70 to 300 µg.

Perceptual alterations are notable with the hallucinogens. The initial subjective effect may be a colorful display of geometric patterns appearing before one's closed eyes. Distorted human, animal, or other forms may be projected onto the visual fields. With the eyes open, the color of perceived objects becomes ever more intense. Afterimages are remarkably prolonged; fixed objects may undulate and flow. Such illusions are common and may be given personal or idiosyncratic meaning. Auditory hallucinations are seldom described, but hyperacusis is commonly reported. Greater sensitivity to touch is regularly noticed, and sometimes taste and smell are altered. Synesthesia is frequently described, with an overflow from one sense modality into another; colors are "heard" and sounds are "seen." Subjective time is frequently affected; users often feel that time is standing still. Hypersuggestibility and distractibility are notable, perhaps because the critical functions of the ego become diminished or are absent.

The emotional responses to the hallucinogens can vary markedly. Initial apprehension or mild anxiety is common, but the most frequent response is one of euphoria. Elation and a "blissful calm" have also been described. Less frequently, tension and anxiety culminating in panic have occurred. Mood is labile, shifting easily from happiness to depression and back. Prolonged laughter or tears may seem inappropriate emotional responses to seemingly innocuous situations. Complete withdrawal (catatonic states) and severe paranoid reactions have been encountered. An alternating intensification and fading out of the experience is present, with the subject going deeply in and out of the "intoxicated" state.

Performance on tests involving attention, concentration, and motivation is impaired. Thought processes are significantly altered under the influence of hallucinogenic drugs. A loosening of associations is regularly noted. Thoughts are nonlogical and fantasy laden and flood consciousness; on the other hand, a complete absence of thought occurs on occasion. Intelligence test scores drop, but this may be due to a lack of motivation to perform or a preoccupation with the unusual experiences. Orientation typically is not impaired, but judgments are not reliable. Paranoid grandiosity—and, less frequently, persecutory ideation—is common.

Changes in ego functioning may be imperceptible at the lower dosage ranges; however, the ego can be completely disrupted when a large amount of the hallucinogen has been ingested. At first one observes the ego's usual defense mechanisms operating to cope with these perceptions. Eventually, the ego may become overwhelmed to the point that depersonalization occurs. Current external events may not be differentiated from remote memories. The body image is frequently distorted, and parts of the body may seem to become larger or smaller, or to disappear completely.

Chronic personality changes, with a shift in attitudes and evidences of magical thinking, also can occur after the use of hallucinogens. An atypical schizophrenic-like state may persist, but whether the use of hallucinogens causes or only unmasks a predisposition to this condition is unclear. There is always the associated risk that self-destructive behavior may occur during both the acute and the chronic reaction—for example, thinking one can fly and jumping out of a window. In addition, the hallucinogenic drugs interact in a variety of nonspecific ways with the personality, which may particularly impair the developing adolescent (D. H. Miller 1973). Today, many persons who use LSD chronically eventually come to use a variety of drugs (polydrug or multiple-drug use), particularly the sedative-hypnotics and stimulants. This situation is a marked departure from the pattern of LSD use seen in the 1960s, when the LSD user's entire lifestyle was organized around the use of hallucinogens and involvement in the "psychedelic" subculture, adopting the motto "Turn on, tune in, and drop out."

Differential Diagnosis

The diagnosis of hallucinogen exposure is normally made from the patient's or an accompanying person's report. The diagnosis can be made clinically when a person is actively hallucinating, is delusional, and is describing illusions, changes in body size or shape, slowing of time, and a waxing and waning of these and related symptoms. Ordinarily, the person is able to report having taken a substance prior to the acute onset of the symptoms. The presence of dilated pupils, tachycardia, and quickened deep tendon reflexes increases the possibility that a hallucinogen has been consumed.

The routine clinical drug screen does not include testing for the hallucinogens in body fluids. However, these substances can be detected in the research laboratory in blood, and for longer periods in urine, by thin-layer chromatography, gas chromatography, fluorometry, or gas chromatography–mass spectrometry (Basalt 1982). A radioimmunoassay for LSD is also available. Shifts in body metabolism from hallucinogen ingestion are insufficient to induce specific abnormalities in blood chemistries, blood counts, or urine analyses.

The differential diagnosis of the psychotomimetic state includes consumption of deliriant drugs such as the atropine-like agents, phencyclidine (PCP), or tetrahydrocannabinol (THC) in marijuana. Many drugs can produce a toxic psychosis, but this state can readily be differentiated from the psychotomimetic picture. In the former condition, confusion is present and some aspects of orientation are impaired. With hallucinogens, the perceptual changes occur with a clear sensorium, with intact orientation and retention of recent and remote memory. In addition, the hallucinogens produce electroencephalographic arousal, whereas drugs that cause delirium result in slowing on the electroencephalogram (EEG) (Fink and Itil 1968). The THC-induced psychosis frequently occurs with drowsiness rather than with the hyperalertness characteristic of the LSD state. PCP psychosis is accompanied by marked neurological signs (e.g., vertical nystagmus, ataxia) and more pronounced autonomic effects than are seen with the psychotomimetics. Persons with amphetamine psychoses often fail to differentiate their perceptual distortions from reality, whereas persons who use LSD are usually aware of the difference.

The differential diagnosis also must distinguish between an acute schizophrenic reaction and a hallucinogen-induced (or other drug-induced) psychosis. The differentiation is not always easily made. It should be recalled that initial research interest in LSD arose because of the possibility that it might provide an artificially induced model of schizophrenia. Although the notion that LSD induces a "model psychosis" that resembles schizophrenia has several serious shortcomings, the use of the potent hallucinogens may have a variety of effects on the person who is predisposed to schizophrenia: 1) it may cause the psychosis to become manifest at an earlier age, 2) it may produce a psychosis that would have remained dormant if drugs had not been used, or 3) it may cause relapse in a person who had previously suffered a psychotic disorder (Bowers 1987).

It has also become more difficult to distinguish between LSD psychosis and paranoid schizophrenia, particularly because patients who in fact are paranoid often now complain of being poisoned with LSD, much as they once felt they were being talked about on radio or on television programs. Hallucinations in schizophrenic psychosis are usually auditory, in contrast to the hallucinations from psychotomimetics, which are predominantly visual. A history of mental illness; a psychiatric examination that reveals the absence of an intact, observing ego; auditory (rather than visual) hallucinations; and the lack of development of drug tolerance—all suggest schizophrenia. An organic brain syndrome in general makes the diagnosis of LSD psychosis less likely, especially if obtunded consciousness is also present. The brief reactive schizophrenic psychosis is also of sudden onset but usually follows psychosocial stressors and is associated with emotional turmoil.

Intervention

Intervention for Acute Adverse Reactions

A person's experience of the effects of the drug may be either pleasant or unpleasant; a perceptual distortion or illusion may be associated with intense anxiety in one person but be a pleasant interlude for another. Social factors, media presentations, and public fear have all shaped perceptions of the drug's effects. Persons who place a premium on self-control, advance planning, and impulse restriction may do particularly poorly on LSD. Prediction of who will have an adverse reaction is unreliable (Ungerleider et al. 1968). The occurrence of multiple previous good LSD experiences renders no immunity from an adverse reaction. Traumatic and stressful external events can precipitate an adverse reaction (e.g., being arrested and read one's rights in the middle of a pleasant experience may precipitate an anxiety reaction). Thus, acute adverse behavioral reactions generally are not related to dose but are a function of personal predisposition, set (attitude or expectation of what one will experience), and setting. Adverse reactions have occurred after doses of LSD as low as 40 µg, and no effects have been reported from a few persons using as much as 2,000 µg, although in general the hallucinogenic effects are proportional to dosage levels.

Acute dysphoric reactions, commonly known as "bummers" or "bad trips," are caused by loss of control, the inability to cope with ego dissolution, and/or marked environmental dissonance. The result is anxiety and, in some instances, panic. In terms of adverse physiological effects, LSD has a very high "therapeutic" index. The lethal dose in humans has not been determined, and the fatalities that have been reported usually are secondary to perceptual distortions with resultant accidental death. Overdose with the psychotomimetic drugs is rare. Instances are known of persons surviving 10,000 µg of LSD, 100 times the average dose. On the other hand, a few deaths have been reported from large amounts of the methoxylated amphetamine analogs (MDA and MDMA). Hemiplegia has been reported in some persons after taking LSD, possibly a result of the production of vasospasm (Sobel et al. 1971).

These acute anxiety/panic reactions usually end before medical intervention is sought. Symptoms of these acute reactions are best managed by using the hypersuggestibility of the hallucinogenic state to calm and reassure the person that he or she will be protected and that the condition will soon subside. Thus, the use years ago of a "guide," "sitter," or "babysitter" prevented marked anxiety from developing. Most LSD is metabolized and excreted within 24 hours, and most panic reactions are usually over within this time frame. Paranoid ideation, depression, "hallucinations," and occasionally a confusional state (organic brain syndrome) are the other commonly reported acute adverse reactions (Ungerleider 1968). Some of the adverse reactions that occur after ingesting hallucinogens can be due to other contaminants in the product, such as strychnine, PCP, or amphetamine.

Persons who use MDMA have reported nausea, jaw clenching and teeth grinding, increased muscle tension, and blurred vision, as well as panic attacks. A type of "hangover" the day after taking this drug has been described; it is manifested by insomnia, fatigue, drowsiness, sore jaw muscles, loss of balance, and headache.

Because the duration of the anxiety and paranoid reactions from hallucinogens varies, from an hour to as long as a few days, the patient may require unobtrusive protection for an extended period of time. Reassurance and support (i.e., the "talk down") are given in a quiet, pleasant environment, usually in a homelike setting. Because closing the eyes intensifies the state, the patient should sit up or walk about. Reminding the patient that a drug has produced the extraordinary ideas and feelings and that they will soon disappear may be helpful. The time sense distortion that makes minutes seem like hours should also be explained.

If drugs are needed for continuing panicky feelings, a benzodiazepine such as lorazepam can be given. The oral route can be used for administering such medication in mildly agitated patients; however, it can be difficult to convince severely agitated and/or paranoid patients to swallow a pill, in which case parenteral administration might be necessary. Severely agitated patients who fail to respond to a benzodiazepine may be given an antipsychotic. Caution must be used in administering antipsychotics, as they can lower the seizure threshold and elicit seizures, especially if the hallucinogen has been cut with an agent that has convulsant activity, such as strychnine. Phenothiazines, such as chlorpromazine, given orally or intramuscularly can end an LSD trip and have been found effective in treating LSD-induced psychosis (Cohen 1978; Dewhurst and Hatrick 1972; D. H. Miller 1973; Neff 1971). Because anticholinergic crises can develop when chlorpromazine is combined with other drugs with anticholinergic activity (PCP and DOM), haloperidol is a safer drug to use when the true nature of the drug ingested is unknown. Moreover, paradoxical reactions have been reported, with an increase in anxiety, after the administration of phenothiazines (Schwarz 1968). It has been suggested that a combination of intramuscular haloperidol and lorazepam is particularly effective in treating acute adverse reactions (P. L. Miller et al. 1992). Theoretically, selective serotonin type 2A receptor (5-HT_{2A}) antagonists should block the acute effects of hallucinogens, and antipsychotics with significant 5-HT_{2A} antagonist activity (clozapine, olanzapine, and risperidone) might also be effective (Aghajanian 1994). However, there is some indication that risperidone might exacerbate flashbacks (Abraham and Mamen 1996; Morehead 1997).

Acute paranoid states are adverse responses resulting from the hypervigilant state, overreading of external cues, and the unusual thoughts that occur in the course of the hallucinogenic experience. Although likely to be grandiose or megalomaniacal, these responses sometimes are instead manifested by suspiciousness and persecutory thoughts.

There is no generally accepted evidence of brain cell damage, chromosomal abnormalities, or teratogenic effects after the use of the indole-type hallucinogens and mescaline (Strassman 1984). However, controversy currently surrounds the possible neurotoxic effects of MDA and MDMA. The controversy centers on the suitability of extrapolating results from studies utilizing laboratory animals to human MDMA use, on how neurotoxicity is defined, and on the degree to which the neurochemical changes caused by exposure to MDMA diminish or disappear over time.

Drug interactions involving the hallucinogens do not appear to be an important source of adverse reactions. There are reports that the effects of LSD are reduced after the chronic administration of monoamine oxidase inhibitors or selective serotonin reuptake inhibitor (SSRI) antidepressants such as fluoxetine, whereas the effects of LSD are increased after the chronic administration of lithium or tricyclic antidepressants (Bonson and Murphy 1996; Bonson et al. 1996; Resnick et al. 1964; Strassman 1992).

Intervention for Chronic Adverse Reactions

The effects of the chronic use of LSD on personality and behavior must be differentiated from the clinical picture seen with personality disorders, particularly in those persons who use a variety of drugs in polydrug abuse–type patterns. Personality changes that result from LSD use may occur after a single experience, which is not the case with changes induced by other classes of drugs (with the possible exception of PCP) (Fisher 1968). In some persons with well-integrated personalities and with no previous psychiatric history, chronic personality changes also have resulted from repeated LSD use. The suggestibility that may come from many experiences with LSD may be reinforced by the social values of a particular subculture in which the drug is used. For instance, if one of these subcultures embraces withdrawal from society and a noncompetitive approach toward life, the person who "withdraws" after the LSD experience(s) may be suffering from a "side effect" that represents more of a change in social values than a physiological drug effect. Use of hallucinogens can lead to a diminution of a variety of acceptable social behaviors.

Schizophreniform reactions lasting from weeks to years have followed the psychotomimetic experience. The manifestations of psychosis may emerge closely following a dysphoric experience or may develop shortly after a positive one. These reactions are likely to be precipitated in characterologically predisposed persons who have decompensated because of the upsurge of repressed material that overwhelms their ego defenses. The management of these prolonged psychotic reactions does not differ from those of schizophrenia. Antipsychotics are used, particularly in a residential setting, when behavioral dysfunction makes it necessary. Efforts at self-medication are often made by patients with schizophreniform reactions, and serious polydrug abuse patterns have been seen (Wesson and Smith 1978). The prognosis of these psychotic states is usually favorable; however, a few of these states remain recalcitrant to treatment.

Chronic Anxiety and Depressive States

It is evident that to some persons (perhaps to all people under adverse circumstances) the LSD type of experience can be an unsettling one. In general, the psyche is capable of reconstituting itself surprisingly well within a reasonable period of time. A few persons continue to experience anxiety and depressive states for unusually long periods of time, however, and they may attribute these feelings to whatever psychotomimetic they took. It is difficult to know how much of the state that sometimes occurs is due to a disruption of psychological homeostasis and how much is because a fragile personality was exposed to the drug. At any rate, the anxiety and depression may persist despite psychiatric therapy and antianxiety and/or antidepressant medication.

Nonpharmacological antianxiety techniques such as relaxation exercises and behavior therapy may be helpful to reduce anxiety. One should not accede to the magical thinking of the patient that possibly another psychedelic session (or doubling the dose) might reshuffle the psychological fragments back into their premorbid pattern.

Flashbacks

A well-publicized adverse reaction unique to the hallucinogens is the flashback. Flashbacks have been renamed "hallucinogen persisting perception disorder" and assigned specific diagnostic criteria (American Psychiatric Association 1994). In the past, the use of variable definitions of what constitutes a flashback was a major problem (Frankel 1994), and it is hoped that the establishment of specific diagnostic criteria will facilitate the study and understanding of this problem.

Flashbacks are the apparently spontaneous recrudescence of the same effects that were experienced during the psychotomimetic state. These effects are usually brief visual, temporal, or emotional recurrences—complete with perceptive (time) and reality distortion—that may first appear days or months after the last drug exposure. They do not appear to be dose related—they can develop after a single exposure to the drug (Levi and Miller 1990). Because flashbacks appear suddenly, unexpectedly, and inappropriately, the emotional response to them may be one of dread. Even a previously pleasant drug experience may be accompanied by anxiety when the person realizes that there is no way to control its recurrence. Fear of insanity may arise, because no external cause for the strange, often recurrent phenomena is apparent. However, some individuals seem to enjoy the experience. Only a small proportion of users of LSD and other hallucinogens experience flashbacks (Shick and Smith 1970). Flashbacks may or may not be precipitated by stressors, fatigue, or use of another psychedelic such as psilocybin or marijuana. The administration of SSRI antidepressants has been reported to initiate or exacerbate flashbacks in some individuals with a history of LSD use (Markel et al. 1994).

The exact mechanism underlying flashbacks remains obscure. It is possible that these recurrences represent a response learned during a state of hyperarousal (Cohen 1981). LSD users have been shown to have long-term changes in visual function (Abraham 1982; Abraham and Aldridge 1993; Abraham and Wolf 1988). For example, a visual disturbance consisting of prolonged afterimages (palinopsia) has been found in individuals several years after the last reported use of LSD (Kawasaki and Purvin 1996). Such changes in visual function might underlie flashbacks. LSD users who experience flashbacks appear to have a higher lifetime incidence of affective disorder than do non-LSD-abusing substance abusers (Abraham and Aldridge 1994).

In time, flashbacks usually decrease in intensity, frequency, and duration. If no flashbacks have occurred during the 1–2 years since the last ingestion of the hallucinogen, it is unlikely that any more will occur. The most important aspect of treatment consists of reassurance that the condition will pass, that the brain is not damaged, and that the hallucinogen is not retained in the brain. Flashbacks can usually be handled with psychotherapy. If the patient is agitated because of repeated flashbacks, an anxiolytic drug is indicated. There is some evidence that clonidine might be useful in the treatment of flashbacks (Lerner et al. 1998); however, several reports have warned that risperidone may exacerbate flashbacks (Abraham and Mamen 1996; Morehead 1997).

Conclusions

Treatment of chronic hallucinogen abuse usually involves long-term psychotherapy to determine—*after* cessation of use—what needs are being fulfilled by the long-term use of the drug for the particular person. Support in the form of 12-Step-program meetings and family involvement also is crucial for reinforcement of the decision to remain abstinent. The patient's physical and mental status should be improved with the appropriate hygienic measures, and all substances with hallucinogenic activity, including marijuana, must be avoided.

References

Abraham HD: A chronic impairment of colour vision in users of LSD. Br J Psychiatry 140:518–520, 1982

Abraham HD, Aldridge AM: Adverse consequences of lysergic acid diethylamide. Addiction 88:1327–1334, 1993

Abraham HD, Aldridge AM: LSD: a point well taken. Addiction 89:763, 1994

Abraham HD, Mamen A: LSD-like panic from risperidone in post-LSD visual disorder. J Clin Psychopharmacol 16:238–241, 1996

Abraham HD, Wolf E: Visual function in past users of LSD: psychophysical findings. J Abnorm Psychol 97:443–447, 1988

Aghajanian GK: Serotonin and the action of LSD in the brain. Psychiatric Annals 24:137–141, 1994

American Psychiatric Association: Diagnostic and Statistical Manual of Mental Disorders, 4th Edition. American Psychiatric Association, Washington, DC, 1994

Basalt RC: Disposition of Toxic Drugs and Chemicals in Man. Davis, CA, Biomedical Publications, 1982

Bonson KR, Murphy DL: Alterations in responses to LSD in humans associated with chronic administration of tricyclic antidepressants, monoamine oxidase inhibitors or lithium. Behav Brain Res 73:229–233, 1996

Bonson KR, Buckholtz JW, Murphy DL: Chronic administration of serotonergic antidepressants attenuates the subjective effects of LSD in humans. Neuropsychopharmacology 14:425–437, 1996

Bowers MB Jr: The role of drugs in the production of schizophreniform psychoses and related disorders, in Psychopharmacology: The Third Generation of Progress. Edited by Meltzer HY. New York, Raven, 1987, pp 819–823

Cohen S: Psychotomimetics (hallucinogens) and cannabis, in Principles of Psychopharmacology. Edited by Clark WG, del Gudice J. New York, Academic Press, 1978, pp 357–371

Cohen S: The Substance Abuse Problems. New York, Haworth, 1981

Dewhurst K, Hatrick JA: Differential diagnosis and treatment of lysergic acid diethylamide-induced psychosis. Practitioner 209:327–332, 1972

Fink M, Itil TM: Neurophysiology of phantastica: EEG and behavioral relations in man, in Psychopharmacology: a Review of Progress, 1957–1967 (PHS Publ No 1836). Edited by Efrom DH (Editor-in-Chief), Cole JO, Levine J, et al. Washington, DC, American College of Neuropsychopharmacology/National Institute of Mental Health, U.S. Department of Health, Education and Welfare, 1968, pp 1231–1239

Fisher DD: The chronic side effects from LSD, in The Problems and Prospects of LSD. Edited by Ungerleider JT. Springfield, IL, Charles C Thomas, 1968, pp 69–79

Frankel FH: The concept of flashbacks in historical perspective. Int J Clin Exp Hypn 42:321–335, 1994

Hofmann A: Psychotomimetics: chemical, pharmacological and clinical aspects. Indian Medical Journal 55:84–85, 1961

Hollister LE (Chair): Clinical evaluation of naltrexone treatment of opiate-dependent individuals: report of the National Research Council Committee on Clinical Evaluation of Narcotic Antagonists. Arch Gen Psychiatry 35:335–340, 1978

Kawasaki A, Purvin V: Persistent palinopsia following ingestion of lysergic acid diethylamide (LSD). Arch Ophthalmol 114:47–50, 1996

Lerner AG, Finkel B, Oyffe I, et al: Clonidine treatment for hallucinogen persisting perception disorder (letter). Am J Psychiatry 155:1460, 1998

Levi L, Miller NR: Visual illusions associated with previous drug abuse. J Clin Neuroophthalmol 10:103–110, 1990

Markel H, Lee A, Holmes RD, et al: LSD flashback syndrome exacerbated by selective serotonin reuptake inhibitor antidepressants in adolescents. J Pediatr 125:817–819, 1994

Miller DH: The drug dependent adolescent, in Adolescent Psychiatry, Vol 2. Edited by Feinstein SC, Giovachini PL. New York, Basic Books, 1973, pp 70–97

Miller PL, Gay GR, Ferris KC, et al: Treatment of acute, adverse reactions: "I've tripped and I can't get down." J Psychoactive Drugs 24:277–279, 1992

Morehead DB: Exacerbation of hallucinogen-persisting perception disorder with risperidone. J Clin Psychopharmacol 17:327–328, 1997

Neff L: Chemicals and their effects on the adolescent ego, in Adolescent Psychiatry, Vol 1. Edited by Feinstein SC, Giovacchini PL, Miller AA. New York, Basic Books, 1971, pp 108–120

Osmond H: A review of the clinical effects of psychotomimetic agents. Ann N Y Acad Sci 66:418–434, 1957

Resnick O, Krus DM, Raskin M: LSD-25 action in normal subjects treated with a monoamine oxidase inhibitor. Life Sci 3:1207–1214, 1964

Schwarz CJ: The complications of LSD: a review of the literature. J Nerv Ment Dis 146:174–186, 1968

Shick JFE, Smith DE: An analysis of the LSD flashback. Journal of Psychedelic Drugs 3:13–19, 1970

Sobel J, Espinas O, Friedman S: Carotid artery obstruction following LSD capsule ingestion. Arch Intern Med 127:290–291, 1971

Strassman RJ: Adverse reactions to psychedelic drugs: a review of the literature. J Nerv Ment Dis 172:577–595, 1984

Strassman RJ: Human hallucinogen interactions with drugs affecting serotonergic neurotransmission. Neuropsychopharmacology 7:241–243, 1992

Ungerleider JT: The acute side effects from LSD, in The Problems and Prospects of LSD. Edited by Ungerleider JT. Springfield, IL, Charles C Thomas, 1968, pp 61–68

Ungerleider JT, Fisher DD, Fuller M, et al: The "bad trip"—the etiology of the adverse LSD reaction. Am J Psychiatry 124:1483–1490, 1968

Wesson DR, Smith DE: Psychedelics in Treatment Aspects of Drug Dependence. West Palm Beach, FL, CRC Press, 1978

Cannabis Use, Abuse, and Dependence

Mark S. Gold, M.D.
Michelle Tullis, Ph.D. candidate
Kimberly Frost-Pineda, M.P.H.

Cannabis sativa is Latin for "planted hemp." Compounds extracted from cannabis sativa are called *cannabinoids*. Marijuana is the most commonly available and used cannabinoid. Cannabinoids are usually smoked. Today, marijuana is the second most commonly smoked drug and the most frequently used illicit drug in the United States. The reasons for the popularity of marijuana are complex. Marijuana use is hotly debated. For some, it is a drug used occasionally to get high. Some consider it to be a medicine, and for others it is an addiction. Without rewarding brain effects, it is not likely that anyone would smoke marijuana, considering its multiple undesirable effects, which include bronchitis, memory problems, hoarseness, and sexual dysfunction. Although many users report that they smoke marijuana for relief from a diverse range of symptoms, marijuana is generally smoked for its euphoric effects and positive reinforcement. The cannabinoid identified as primarily responsible for the centrally reinforcing effects, mood, and behavior changes of cannabis is delta-9-tetrahydrocannabinol (THC, or Δ9-THC). Laboratory animals will self-administer tetrahydrocannabinol (THC), like other drugs of abuse, to experience the effects it produces on the putative brain reward neuroanatomy (Childers and Breivogel 1998; Gardner and Lowinson 1991; Tanda et al. 1997). Marijuana is more commonly smoked for the state it produces than for any state it may reverse. In this context, the drive for marijuana intoxication is similar to the drive for cocaine or alcohol.

Epidemiology

In the early 1960s, only 2% of all Americans had ever tried an illicit drug. According to the Monitoring the Future study (Johnston 1998), if the current rate of "first time" marijuana use by young people continues, along with the anticipated aging of current drug users, the need for drug abuse treatment will increase 57% by the year 2020. An incredible 400% increase in marijuana smoking takes place between ages 12–13 and ages 14–15 years. Eighty percent of current illicit drug users in the United States smoke marijuana or hashish either alone or in combination with other drugs. Age at first marijuana use is the most important predictor of future treatment need. Research has shown that peak marijuana initiation rates occur between 14 and 16 years of age and that initiation is unlikely after age 21 years.

According to the 1999 National Household Survey on Drug Abuse, marijuana use for young people ages 12–17 has decreased since 1997 (9.4% in 1997, 8.3% in 1998, and 7.0% in 1999). Despite this decrease, marijuana use is still widespread. In 1999, nearly a quarter (22%) of all eighth-graders said they had tried marijuana, and almost half (49.7%) of all 12th graders said they had tried marijuana (Figure 27–1) (Johnston et al. 1999).

The 1999 National Household Survey on Drug Abuse reported an increasing trend of marijuana use among young adults ages 18–25 years (12.8% in 1997, 13.8% in 1998, and 16.4% in 1999). The continuum of use includes experimental, occasional, daily, and chronic use. Typical users smoke marijuana on the weekend to relax or socialize. These individuals often smoke in social settings. The chronic user is compulsive to the point of smoking his or her first marijuana joint on awakening and continuing to smoke throughout the day.

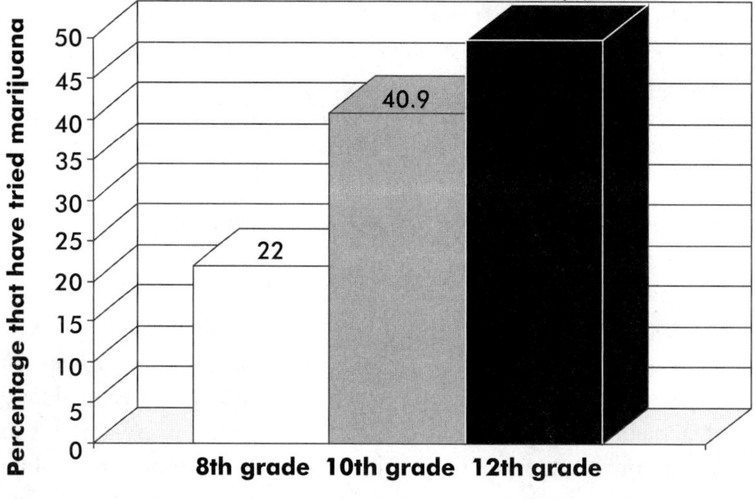

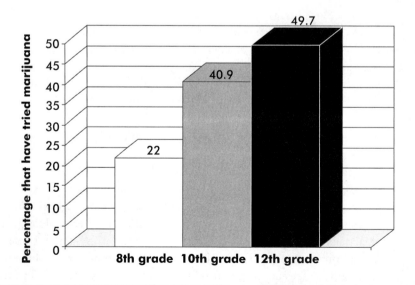

FIGURE 27–1. University of Michigan/National Institute on Drug Abuse (UM/NIDA) Monitoring the Future survey 1999: lifetime use of marijuana.
Source. Johnston et al. 1999.

TABLE 27–1. Monitoring the Future study: 1999 results for marijuana

Grade	Lifetime prevalence, %	Annual use, %	Use in past 30 days, %	Daily use, %
8	22.0	16.5	9.7	1.4
10	40.9	32.1	19.4	3.8
12	49.7	37.8	23.1	6.0

Source. Johnston et al. 1999.

Marijuana Content

The marijuana of today is not the same as that of the 1960s. There have been changes in marijuana importation, domestic production, hydroponics, and selective breeding. The THC content of marijuana is higher now than it was in the 1960s and may play a role in the increase in teen smoking. Increases in current or regular marijuana smoking in teens could also be attributable, at least in part, to cultural influences that minimize the danger and/or glamorize drug taking. In fact, 41% of teens and 53% of their parents state that American culture glamorizes the use of illegal drugs (National Center on Addiction and Substance Abuse 1996).

The Tobacco-Marijuana Connection

Cigarette smoking has typically preceded marijuana smoking. However, recent data from the University of Florida (Gold et al. 1999) showed that this trend may be reversing. Now it appears that some young people are initiating marijuana use first and then moving to tobacco. Others are initiating tobacco and marijuana use concurrently, years later than those who only smoke tobacco (Figure 27–2).

It appears that some teens are smoking marijuana first and then rapidly initiating tobacco smoking because of the discovery that nicotine not only sustains but also enhances the marijuana high. According to the 1999 National Household Survey on Drug Abuse, an estimated 66.8 million Americans (30%) smoked tobacco in the month before the interview. Among youth ages 12–17, 15.9% reported current cigarette use in 1999. Although this is not statistically different from 18.2% reported in 1998, but it is significantly lower than the 1997 rate of 19.9%.

Smoking tobacco potentiates the effects of marijuana and puts teens at high risk for other drug smoking. Our data (Gold et al. 1999) from a random sample of university students suggested that curiosity is the primary reason for initial marijuana use. Concurrent or alternating use with tobacco appears to make marijuana more inviting. Cigarettes may boost and sustain the marijuana high and may also reverse some of the more negative effects of marijuana, such as decreased arousal and attention. With the growing prevalence of marijuana use, the importance of alcohol as a gateway to marijuana appears to have declined. However, marijuana use as a precursor to both legal and illegal drug use appears to have increased (Golub and Johnson 1994).

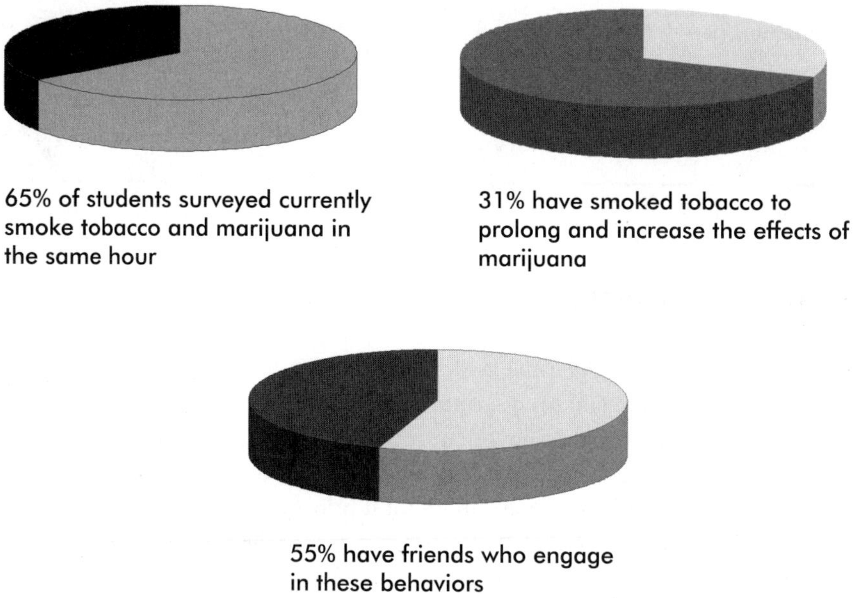
65% of students surveyed currently smoke tobacco and marijuana in the same hour
31% have smoked tobacco to prolong and increase the effects of marijuana
55% have friends who engage in these behaviors

FIGURE 27–2. Smoking behaviors among young people.
Source. Gold et al. 1999.

Clinical Psychopharmacology

Administration

Marijuana can be ingested orally, but the most common mode of administration is by smoking and inhalation. The principal psychoactive constituents Δ8-THC and Δ9-THC were isolated in the 1960s (Gaoni and Mechoulam 1964). In addition to these, marijuana smoke contains more than 400 other compounds. Δ9-THC is present in greater quantities in marijuana and more potent than Δ8-THC; therefore, most of the psychoactivity is attributed to Δ9-THC. The lack of a precise correlation between peak high and Δ9-THC has suggested the importance of THC metabolism in the high. Smoking delivers THC to the brain in seconds and is thus one of the quickest routes of administration. The intensity of central brain rewarding effects is usually correlated with the rapidity with which the drug reaches the brain. Marijuana is rapidly absorbed from the lungs, and THC and major metabolites can be traced throughout the brain and the rest of the body, including the hair and hails.

Intoxication

According to DSM-IV (American Psychiatric Association 1994), acute marijuana intoxication begins with a "high" feeling followed by the symptoms described in Table 27–2.

In addition to euphoria, users report an increase in appetite and a state of relaxation. Individual differences in intoxication are attributable to differences in THC concentration; previous use, including amount and frequency of use; the amount inhaled or ingested; and genetic and psychiatric factors. With smoking, intoxication develops within minutes; with oral ingestion, the time to intoxication is somewhat longer. The magnitude of the behavioral and physiological

TABLE 27–2. DSM-IV diagnostic criteria for cannabis intoxication

A. Recent use of cannabis.
B. Clinically significant maladaptive behavioral or psychological changes (e.g., impaired motor coordination, euphoria, anxiety, sensation of slowed time, impaired judgment, social withdrawal) that developed during, or shortly after, cannabis use.
C. Two (or more) of the following signs, developing within 2 hours of cannabis use:
  (1) conjunctival injection
  (2) increased appetite
  (3) dry mouth
  (4) tachycardia
D. The symptoms are not due to a general medical condition and are not better accounted for by another mental disorder.

Specify if:

With perceptual disturbances

changes depends on the dose, the method of administration, and the individual characteristics of the person using the substance, such as rate of absorption, tolerance, and sensitivity to the effects of the substance (American Psychiatric Association 1994).

Motor performance, ability to drive a car or an airplane, concentration, and alertness may be affected for hours to days. Because most cannabinoids, including Δ9-THC, are fat soluble, the effects of cannabis or hashish may occasionally persist or recur for 12–24 hours because of the slow release of psychoactive substances from fatty tissue or to enterohepatic circulation (Naditch 1974).

Adverse Psychiatric Reactions

Marijuana does not usually cause psychiatric disorders, but in an individual who is predisposed to a psychiatric illness, marijuana use may trigger panic attacks, paranoia, anxiety, and even psychosis (Novak 1980). These episodes are not necessarily indicative of a psychiatric diagnosis, because the symptoms typically subside after the user "comes down" from the high. However, patients with schizophrenia have relapsed to psychotic behavior after smoking marijuana. In their most extreme form, psychiatric manifestations of marijuana intoxication may result in emergency room or student health service presentations. Naive users (especially older individuals) and those exposed to high-potency marijuana tend to be the populations that most often seek treatment. Marijuana- and hashish-related emergency room visits have increased dramatically in the last few years. In 1999, total mentions of marijuana/hashish use in drug-abuse-related visits to hospital emergency departments exceeded mentions of heroin/morphine use for the first time (Office of Applied Studies, DAWN 2000). This changed the ranking of illicit drug mentions that had been the same since 1990. Panic, depersonalization, and psychosis are some of the reasons for emergency room visits. The user's previous marijuana use and mood and the dose and route of administration determine whether the smoker becomes euphoric or dysphoric.

Marijuana Use and Spontaneous Remission

Although marijuana use is usually time-limited, addiction appears to be at least as common as with alcohol. Who can stop and who cannot have been studied by Kandel and others. Kandel

(1975) concluded that the two most important predictors of stopping marijuana use were frequency of marijuana use and age. Frequent users were more persistent in their use and were more likely to become dependent. Cessation was more likely when marijuana was used for "social reasons," whereas using it to enhance positive feelings and reduce negative feelings was associated with persistent use. Cessation can be very difficult for depressed users.

Acknowledging the harmfulness of using marijuana has no impact on cessation. Postponing onset of marijuana use, reducing the extensiveness of use, increasing commitment to conventional social roles, and reducing delinquent participation are important interventions that appear likely to shorten marijuana use. Most people will stop using marijuana before age 30. Many of these smokers "grow out of" their marijuana use as a result of maturity, family, education, and employment. Frequent marijuana users may come to recognize that they are addicted and cannot quit without help. For depressed users, marijuana cessation increases negative feelings and affect, leading to relapse.

Medical Implications

Respiratory Effects

The effects of marijuana smoking on the respiratory system are similar to those of tobacco smoking. Chronic marijuana smoking (at least 4 days a week for 6–8 weeks) results in mild airway obstruction that may not be reversible, even with continued abstinence. Marijuana smoking can also cause lowered exercise tolerance, chronic cough, bronchitis, and decreased pulmonary function (Tashkin et al. 1976; Tilles et al. 1986). Lung function diminishes even more significantly with concurrent use of tobacco cigarettes. Both marijuana and tobacco increase the number of inflammatory cells in the lungs, but they differentially affect the activation of these inflammatory cells, possibly leading to differential effects on lung injury and physiological consequences, including altered alveolar epithelial permeability (Kelp et al. 1995). Cannabis smoke is highly irritating to the nasopharynx and bronchial lining and thus increases the risk for chronic cough and other signs and symptoms of nasopharyngeal pathology.

Immunological Effects

Animal studies have clearly established that marijuana and synthetic and endogenous cannabinoids change the natural function of immune cells (Klein et al. 1998). Cannabinoids are immunomodulators that alter immune system homeostasis. Cannabinoid receptors are found on white blood cells; however, it is not yet known whether marijuana use increases the risk of infection in healthy or immunosuppressed individuals.

Carcinogenic Effects

Epidemiological evidence strongly implicates cigarette smoking as a causative factor in pulmonary malignancy. Barsky et al. (1998) recently reported that marijuana appears to cause molecular damage to the lungs similar to that caused by cigarettes. Mainstream smoke from marijuana or tobacco is a highly concentrated aerosol of liquid particles that is formed by complex chemical reactions including hydrogenation, pyrolysis, oxidation, decarboxylation, dehydration, condensation, distillation, and sublimation. Smoking both marijuana and tobacco puts the smoker at greater risk for cancer than smoking either alone. Marijuana smoke contains even larger amounts of known carcinogens than tobacco, and heavy use may increase the risk of developing malignant disease. Risk of respiratory-system cancer (ranging from lips, mouth, pharynx, larynx, trachea, bronchi, to lungs) is significantly increased in smokers. Evidence links marijuana smoking with earlier onset and greater dysplastic changes in several types of head and neck malignancies (Barsky et al. 1998; Denissenko et al. 1996; Fligiel et al. 1997; Matthias et al. 1997). Recently, researchers found that THC may promote tumor growth by impairing the body's anti-tumor immunity system (Zhu et al. 2000). These researchers suggest that marijuana may even be a greater cancer risk than tobacco, because the tar portion of marijuana has greater concentrations of carcinogenic hydrocarbons that promote lung cancer.

Cardiovascular Effects

There is a causal relationship between cardiac and pulmonary vascular diseases and marijuana and tobacco smoking (Wu et al. 1988). In fact, some types of heart disease and pulmonary hypertension may be more common and/or more severe in marijuana smokers. Marijuana smoking almost immediately produces a significant increase in heart rate (Stillman et al. 1976), with inversion or flattening of the T wave on electrocardiogram (ECG), elevation of the ST segment, and increase in the amplitude of the P wave with occasional premature ventricular contractions. Fortunately, these changes in cardiac function can usually be reversed by abstinence.

Sexual Dysfunction and Related Issues

Initiation of marijuana smoking has been occurring at younger ages. Naturally, the toxic effects of marijuana are greater on developing than on developed organisms. Marijuana is reported to decrease plasma testosterone, sperm count, and sperm motility (Kolodny et al. 1974). Marijuana is antiandrogenic, and many of its components, including THC, bind to androgen receptors. Whether these antiandrogenic effects result in decreased libido or impaired fertility is not clear (Dupont and Voth 1995).

Women who smoke marijuana during pregnancy often have babies with low birth weights, and those with the highest consumption of marijuana have the lowest-birth-weight babies. One study found numerous abnormal responses, including increased startle reflex, tremors, poor self-quieting, and failure to habituate to light, in newborns whose mothers used marijuana during pregnancy (Jones and Chernoff 1984). In addition, THC has been shown to cross the placental barrier, and it accumulates in mother's milk (Fehr and Kalant 1983). Prenatal exposure to marijuana may also have long-term effects.

Marijuana and Pain

Recently, the brain has been found to have its own marijuana or THC receptors and chemicals like marijuana (Walker et al. 1999). Anandamide, a naturally occurring substance in the body that is similar to the active ingredient in marijuana, is an important part of the body's pain suppression system.

Dependence

Study findings (Warner et al. 1995) suggest that 9.2% of those who ever use marijuana will eventually meet DSM-IV criteria for dependence. Another study (Hall 1994) indicated that

20% of individuals who smoke several times meet these criteria. An increasing number of college students in the United States are presenting for treatment of their marijuana use, reporting loss of control of use, preoccupation with marijuana, inability to stop despite adverse consequences, narrowing of interests, and an uneasy feeling that they may be addicted. Marijuana acquisition and use become primary, and school, work, or recreational activities become secondary. Clinicians are evaluating and treating more marijuana-dependent patients than ever before. These patients typically establish a pattern of chronic use that gradually increases in both frequency and amount. According to researchers at the Center for Psychosocial Studies in New York, users often feel that marijuana improves their self-awareness and overall functioning. They also appear to use marijuana to avoid stress-inducing situations (National Institute on Drug Abuse 1997).

Marijuana-dependent patients report that they repeatedly fail at attempts to cut down, ration, or limit their use and that they are easily angered by questions relating to their marijuana use. They may feel guilty about their use and its consequences. Many marijuana-dependent individuals who seek treatment have experienced the loss of career, family, and friends. Some addicted persons report that they grow their own marijuana and smoke throughout the day, maintaining an intense personal relationship with their plants and paraphernalia. Like other addictions, marijuana addiction does not end after detoxification or after withdrawal; rather, the disorder can persist, and relapse is common. Individuals with cannabis dependence, like those with other addictions, are compulsive users.

The dependent cannabis smoker may experience any or all of the eight behavioral or psychological problems suggestive of dependence or addiction:

1. Repeated unsuccessful attempts at quitting, despite the desire to stop using
2. Tolerance (the same amount or the same potency has less effect)
3. A great deal of time spent getting, using, or recovering from the effects of marijuana, as well as use of the drug in greater quantities or more often than intended
4. Narrowing of interests to marijuana and marijuana-using friends
5. Reduction in important activities such as going to and performing at work or school
6. Reduction in caring for children or engaging in recreational activities due to marijuana
7. Emotional or psychological problems caused by marijuana use
8. Physical health problems caused by marijuana use

Withdrawal

Recent studies (Wickelgren 1997) suggest that marijuana influences the brain's stress and reward systems in the same way that opiates, nicotine, and cocaine do. Researchers at the Scripps Institute (Rodriguez de Fonseca et al. 1997) hastened THC withdrawal in rats with a cannabinoid antagonist that produced increases in corticotropin-releasing factor, anxiety, and stress. These results provide a neurochemical model for marijuana withdrawal that is consistent with the current understanding of drug withdrawal and the emotional symptoms commonly observed in marijuana users who abruptly discontinue use. The slow release of THC and active metabolites from lipid stores and other areas may explain the so-called carryover effects on driving and other reports of behavioral changes over time. Although acute withdrawal symptoms are rarely reported, thoughts and dreams about marijuana smoking, mental cloudiness, aggression, irritability, and other behavioral signs are commonly experienced for months after discontinuation of chronic marijuana smoking. It is logical to assume that brain cannabinoids decrease after prolonged marijuana smoking, as has been suggested in recent studies (Romero et al. 1997).

Overdose

THC is quite potent in comparison with most other psychoactive drugs. An intravenous dose of only 1–2 mg can produce profound mental and physiological effects. Despite their high psychoactivity and powerful pharmacological actions on multiple organ systems, cannabinoids have remarkably low lethal toxicity. In fact, lethal doses in humans are not known.

Although some advances have been made in identifying and testing an antagonist in animals, there has been little progress in determining which drugs activate the cannabinoid system indirectly by inhibiting the tissue uptake or metabolism of endogenous cannabinoids. Interestingly, new data suggest that nonsteroidal anti-inflammatory drugs inhibit anandamide hydrolysis; therefore, ibuprofen may cause special problems when used by marijuana smokers (Pertwee 1998).

Marijuana Abuse

According to the 1998 National Household Survey on Drug Abuse, 137,564 Americans were treated for marijuana abuse in 1994. Among participants who reported having used marijuana on 12 or more days in the previous year, 58% had one problem, 41% two, and 28% at least three problems that they attributed to their use. Among both past-year users and past-year users who had smoked on 12 days or more, the problems associated with use were greatest among the youngest age groups. Nearly 75% of children and teens (ages 12–17 years) who used marijuana on 12 or more days in the past year experienced significant problems related to their use, and 42% admitted three or more problems, including loss of control over use (National Household Survey on Drug Abuse 1998).

Neuropsychological Effects

College students who heavily smoke marijuana typically develop long-lasting and demonstrable neuropsychological deficits, including problems in executive functioning, attention, new-word learning, and verbal fluency that persist beyond intoxication (Pope and Yurgelun-Todd 1996). In our recent survey (Tullis et al. 1999), marijuana users had significantly lower grade point averages than nonusers. In addition to these studies, Lundavist (1995) studied approximately 400 cannabis users (duration of use ranging from 6 months to 25 years) over a 10-year period. Lundavist observed what he termed a cannabis-state-dependent set of cognitive processes that included weak analytic and synthetic skills, difficulty sorting and classifying information correctly, poor concentration, and problems differentiating time and space.

Behavioral Effects

Multiple brain systems are affected by marijuana use. Cerebral blood flow and cerebral metabolism are tightly coupled to brain function and used as indices of brain activity. In a recent study (Matthew et al. 1998), cerebral blood flow response to THC showed a marked increase in bilateral frontal regions, insula, and cingulate gyrus of the right hemisphere, peaking 30–60 minutes after intravenous infusion. Marijuana users also had decreased cerebral metabolism at baseline. Marijuana intoxication appears to impair time perception. A positron-emission tomography study (Matthew et al. 1998) showed an increase in cortical and cerebral blood flow following THC administration. Cerebral blood flow was decreased in those patients with a significantly altered time sense. Another recent study (Loeber and Yurgelun-Todd 1999) observed brain activity in long-term cannabis users and those with acute exposure. Images showed clear brain metabolism changes in chronic users, including decreased cerebral blood flow and brain activity. These findings suggest that chronic use may result in receptor-level changes, which influence neurotransmitter systems such as dopamine. Chronic use can cause changes in normal neurotransmitter levels. This alteration in dopamine leads to a reduction in brain activity, especially the frontal lobe and cerebellar cortex.

Additional studies may ultimately suggest that marijuana's most profound effects are in brain structures in which survival drives and emotions are centered and in the prefrontal regions, which sustain attention, shift focus, and promote adaptation to environmental change and new learning. The effects are often elusive and may be disguised by other addictive behaviors. In one study (Pope and Yurgelun-Todd 1996), heavy users exhibited significantly more impairment in attentional and executive functions than did light users. Researchers (Brooks et al. 1999) have shown that early adolescent marijuana use is associated with later problems, such as, limited acquisition of skills necessary for employment, increased risk of contracting HIV and increased risk of abusing other substances.

Treatment

Marijuana Treatment Research

Although little research has been done in the area of marijuana dependence treatment, contrary to popular belief, marijuana dependence does not always present in the context of polydrug abuse. Treatment for other drugs of abuse does not always recognize or effectively address marijuana abuse (Budney et al. 1997). Relapse prevention appears to play a key role in the success of treatment. The ritualistic and behavioral components inherent in marijuana use, like tobacco smoking, raise unique concerns for the treatment provider. Issues related to environmental cues, the frequency with which the drug is used, and the culture surrounding marijuana use should be incorporated into any treatment protocol.

Presentation for Treatment

In the college students we observed, treatment was sought only after deterioration of academic, social, and physical performance (Gold et al. 1999). Although changes are typically subtle, problems are usually first recognized by teachers, significant others, and friends. Students often fail to make an association between their marijuana use and their social, academic, and health problems. Early manifestations are behavioral:

- Non-drug-using friends feel estranged.
- Rigorous activities are dropped.
- Interests are narrowed.

- Marijuana acquisition and use become the major focus.
- Socialization is limited to contexts in which marijuana is acceptable.

Friends and loved ones may instigate a visit to a health care provider as a direct result of poor classroom attendance, poor grades, confrontations with the university judicial system, or concomitant psychiatric disorders.

We recently identified drug testing as a significant reason that college students are now seeking treatment for their marijuana use (Gold et al. 1999). Positive test results usually lead to a referral, but students also seek help in quitting before an interview or a test with a major national employer. Testing fears appear to be a new major concern, and according to our survey findings (Gold et al. 1999), many students seeking internships, employment, or admittance to higher education face the prospect of failing a pre-employment drug test. They worry that they may not be able to discontinue their marijuana use for even the 1 week or 1 month required to obtain a job. Fear of a positive drug screen can alter one's career path significantly, inhibiting application for employment or resulting in termination of employment in the event of a positive screen. Marijuana counseling should be facilitated with an open, nonjudgmental attitude and patience while the student undergoes the process of accepting the loss of his or her current lifestyle.

Diagnosis of Marijuana Dependence

Diagnosis of marijuana dependence is not specifically addressed in DSM-IV. Diagnosis of cannabis intoxication (see Table 27–2) does not immediately suggest dependence, just as acute alcohol intoxication does not prove dependence. However, marijuana dependence is more likely to be identified in smokers and those with recent marijuana use. To diagnose marijuana dependence, we have proposed using brief, office-based assessments similar to those commonly used to diagnose alcohol dependence. The following quick and reliable test (CAGE; Mayfield et al. 1974) can be administered easily in the physician's office:

1. Have you felt the need to Cut down on your marijuana use?
2. Are you easily Annoyed when questioned about your drug use?
3. Do you feel Guilty about your marijuana use?
4. Do you smoke first thing in the morning (Eye-opener)?

Pathological attachment despite adverse consequences and loss of control are hallmarks of marijuana dependence. However, when loss of control actually occurs is a question that most addicted persons cannot answer. Avoidance of activities that do not include marijuana is perhaps the best indicator and is manifested as changes in friends, sports, and school interests and initiation of amotivational behavior. Lack of clear thought processes, dreaming, and preoccupation with drug use provide the clinician with an opportunity for intervention and treatment. These early signs are not pathognomonic and mistakes can be made, but early intervention is crucial. Urine samples can confirm evidence of recent use.

Drug Testing

Urine tests generally identify cannabinoid metabolites. Because these substances are fat soluble, they persist in bodily fluids for extended periods and are excreted slowly. Routine urine tests for cannabinoids in individuals who casually use cannabis can be positive for

7–10 days; urine tests in individuals who heavily use cannabis may be positive for 2–4 weeks. With marijuana use on the rise, both government and private workplaces have implemented pre-employment drug testing. Urine is usually sent to laboratories for testing. Recently, self-contained urine-drug-testing kits have become available that seem to produce results consistent with gas chromatography/mass spectrometry at higher THC levels (Jenkins et al. 1995).

General Overview of Treatment Process

Treatment of marijuana dependence must be individualized for the highest probability of success. Addictions are chronic disorders like diabetes, not acute conditions such as a broken leg. Detoxification alone does not address the underlying disorder (O'Brien and McLellan 1996). Many chronic marijuana smokers successfully stop using for short periods, only to start again for no apparent reason. It is hard to imagine that physical dependence is driving this addictive behavior, but similar patterns are seen with other drugs, including alcohol, nicotine, cocaine, and heroin.

Before treatment begins, an accurate history and physical exam are essential, and all dependencies must be recognized. Twelve-Step programs based on the principles of Alcoholics Anonymous are at the core of most treatments.

The treatment of marijuana addiction has three general phases, all of which revolve around the addicted person's pathological attachment to the drug:

1. **The process of developing a willingness to enter treatment and a desire to stop using.** The first phase of treatment includes many important tasks, such as decreasing social tolerance for the use of marijuana as well as other drugs. The modern structured intervention is an organized approach to overcoming the most basic stages of denial to propel addicted people into treatment. In this phase, the clinician must approach the patient in an accepting and caring manner, even though confrontation may also be necessary to break through denial.
2. **The process of stopping use.** The second phase of treatment can take place on either an inpatient or an outpatient basis. Patients manifesting acute medical symptoms should be admitted and assessed for additional medical or psychiatric problems. Inpatient treatment is also essential for suicidal patients. Most marijuana-dependent patients, however, can receive outpatient treatment. During this phase, patients often grieve the loss of the drug and use defense mechanisms to resist treatment. Emotional support is paramount at this point.
3. **The process of remaining clean and sober.** It is during this third phase of treatment that relapse prevention and the 12-Step programs such as Alcoholics Anonymous and Narcotics Anonymous play their biggest role.

Marijuana Crisis Intervention

Many addicted persons will seek treatment in response to a crisis, be it physical, emotional, or drug-induced panic. The clinician should be able to respond to these individuals with crisis intervention skills. The clinician should be calm and reassuring on the basis of his or her experience with marijuana-related crisis. After assessment for suicidal ideation, a drug screen should be administered. Patients typically minimize their drug use, and the results will prove helpful even after the crisis is over. Many users admit to the least offensive drug, readily reporting recent alcohol, cigarette, and marijuana use but failing to mention the heroin they have been sniffing or the methylenedioxymethamphetamine (MDMA) they have been taking. After an initial assessment, admission to an inpatient treatment facility or detoxification unit may be needed if other drugs or significant medical or psychiatric problems are involved. If the patient is medically stable, the clinician should give immediate attention to the problem that precipitated the patient's seeking help. Using listening skills and allowing the patient to talk through the crisis will often defuse the situation. Reassurance that "This, too, shall pass" and use of cognitive and behavioral skills may be particularly effective.

Marijuana Inpatient Treatment

The least restrictive environment is generally recommended when patients are first attempting to stop using drugs. However, the patient's mental state, impulsivity, history, and safety must remain primary concerns. Outpatient treatment has the advantage of enabling addicted patients or drug abusers to incorporate and confront the everyday problems they will encounter without the use of drugs. Inpatient treatment, an intense program involving residential treatment or hospitalization, is appropriate when the patient has the following:

- Continuing drug use after outpatient treatment
- Medical and/or psychiatric complications
- A limited support system at home
- An intent to harm self or others
- A dual diagnosis requiring expertise in dealing with multiple issues

Group Therapy

Group therapy has become the most frequently used modality for all classes of drug abusers (Millman and Beeder 1994). This approach is extremely effective in helping those patients who are isolated from nonusers, who are in denial, or who have limited experience with detoxification and long-term abstinence. A viable peer group can be a part of the group process and can provide a major positive focus in the recovering person's life at a time when giving up marijuana is perceived as an overwhelming loss. Peers can provide a template for recovery through their own lives and experiences. Cathartic sharing coupled with confrontation allows users to recognize their typical defense mechanisms. Gestalt techniques are useful as well, enabling patients to "talk" to their drug-using friends, parents, or other people they may have difficulty with. A great deal of shame is often associated with drug use and consequent behavior. A group setting will offer support and validation of feelings.

Individual and Family Psychotherapy

Treatment with either relapse prevention or social support paradigms has been the outpatient approach used by many clinicians, because both are associated with substantial reductions in frequency of marijuana use and problems. However, treatment appears to be the most successful for those who smoke the least (Budney et al. 1997). In a study of 161 men and 51 women seeking treatment for marijuana use (Stephens et al. 1995), cognitive-behavioral relapse prevention treatment resulted in greater self-efficacy and a decrease in posttreatment marijuana use. Acknowledging the dangers of using marijuana had no effect on cessation. Overcoming denial is relevant to accepting the possibility that treatment has anything to offer. However, even though attitudes toward marijuana use affect tobacco smoking initiation, these attitudes do not appear relevant to successful cessation of tobacco use.

Individual and family psychotherapy may be particularly effective in helping patients accept the loss of time and goals that has resulted from their drug use, reconcile their ambitions with what may now be a reduced set of possibilities, and plan for the future. Individual work can help with the anger that addicted persons often direct at themselves and with the developmental and cognitive issues that, for example, a sober 20-year-old will need to face after spending adolescence and college under the influence. Individual sessions should address the following:

- Issues too painful to share in group therapy
- Goal setting
- Behavioral contracts, if needed
- Identification of problems specific to patient
- Issues related to dual diagnosis, if relevant
- Discussion of feelings about group process

Family psychotherapy can be a useful adjunct to individual and group counseling, especially if the patient has issues specific to the family. Often, the patient is the only one who receives treatment, and family members are left to deal with their pain on their own. A therapeutic environment is essential for all participants when addressing family issues, such as trust and anger, because these feelings have been anesthetized for so long in the marijuana user. A skilled clinician will be able to uncover the problems and facilitate growth among all participants.

Contingency Management

Contingency management treatment is a behavioral model that utilizes "contracts" between the treatment provider and the patient. This paradigm involves the use of positive reinforcement contingent on the continued cessation of marijuana use. The positive reinforcement may be anything that is considered a motivating stimulus in the patients' environment, such as money or reduced parole time in the case of patients who are on parole. The reinforcement is withdrawn if the contract is violated (Higgins et al. 1994).

Prevention and Intervention

While some researchers question the respective causes and effects to explain the current escalation in marijuana smoking, others have attempted to summarize what is known and to describe marijuana use and risk factors in a way that might be more protective (Bachman et al. 1998). Recent studies support the conclusion that youths do pay attention to credible information about the dangers of drug use and that the reduction in demand that occurred during the 1980s was a result of this approach (Bachman et al. 1997).

Prevention of smoking is the first priority. If that fails, delaying onset of marijuana use, reducing the extensiveness of use, increasing commitment to conventional social roles, and reducing delinquent participation are interventions that may shorten marijuana use.

Conclusions

Marijuana is an important drug of abuse associated with numerous physical and psychological consequences. Like most plants, cannabis sativa—marijuana—is a variable and complex mixture of biologically active compounds. Characterizing the clinical pharmacology of the constituents in cannabis is complicated, particularly when the plant is smoked or eaten in its natural form. It may be the "parent" drug of a number of effective medications, as the opium poppy is to morphine or opiates. Marijuana is usually smoked and thus serves as a potential "gateway" to other smokable drugs, from tobacco to opium. Regardless of whether progression to other drug use occurs, however, the subtlety of marijuana symptoms and user denial can create substantial problems. Predicting or measuring the loss of drive, memory, and motivation, as well as the altered quality of human relationships, is difficult. Pathological attachment to marijuana forms the basis of the marijuana dependence diagnosis. To the casual observer, marijuana is perceived as one more choice in the smorgasbord of recreational experience. For family members and concerned others, however, marijuana is the focus of considerable anxiety, and they experience it as a defrauder of family life, relationships, motivation, potential, time, and quality of life.

References

American Psychiatric Association: Diagnostic and Statistical Manual of Mental Disorders, 4th Edition. Washington, DC, American Psychiatric Association, 1994

Bachman JG, Wadsworth KN, O'Malley PM, et al: Smoking, Drinking, and Drug Use in Young Adulthood: The Impacts of New Freedoms and New Responsibilities. Mahwah, NJ, Lawrence Erlbaum, 1997

Bachman JG, Johnston LD, O'Malley PM: Explaining recent increases in students' marijuana use: impacts of perceived risks and disapproval, 1976 through 1996. Am J Public Health 88:887–892, 1998

Barsky SH, Roth MD, Kleerup EC, et al: Histopathologic and molecular alterations in bronchial epithelium in habitual smokers of marijuana, cocaine, and/or tobacco. J Natl Cancer Inst 90:1198–1205, 1998

Budney AJ, Kande DB, Cherek DR, et al: Marijuana use and dependence. Drug Alcohol Depend 45:1–11, 1997

Brook JS, Balka EB, Whiteman M: The risks for late adolescence of early adolescent marijuana use. Am J Public Health 89:1549–1554, 1999

Childers SR, Breivogel CS: Cannabis and endogenous cannabinoid systems. Drug Alcohol Depend 51:173–187, 1998

Denissenko MF, Pao A, Tang M, et al: Preferential formation of benzo(a)pyrene adducts at lung cancer mutational hotspots in P53. Science 274:430–432, 1996

Dupont RL, Voth EA: Legalization, harm reduction and drug policy. Ann Intern Med 123:461–465, 1995

Fehr KO, Kalant H (eds): Addiction Research Foundations. World Health Organization Meeting on Adverse Health and Behavioral Consequences of Cannabis Use. Toronto, Ontario, Addiction Research Foundation, May 1983

Fligiel SE, Roth MD, Kleerup EC, et al: Tracheobronchial histopathology in habitual smokers of cocaine, marijuana, and/or tobacco. Chest 112:319–326, 1997

Fride E: Anandamides: tolerance and cross-tolerance to delta-9-THC. Brain Res 697:83–90, 1995

Gaoni Y, Mechoulam R: Isolation, structure, and partial synthesis of an active constituent of hashish. Journal of American Chemistry Society 86:1646–1647, 1964

Gardner EL, Lowinson JH: Marijuana's interaction with the brain reward systems: update 1991. Pharmacol Biochem Behav 40:571–580, 1991

Gold MS, Tullis LM, Miller MD: Tobacco and marijuana smoking: a connection? (abstract). Biol Psychiatry 45:447, 1999

Golub A, Johnson BD: The shifting importance of alcohol and marijuana as gateway substances among serious drug users. J Stud Alcohol 55:607–614, 1994

Hall W: Health and Psychological Consequences of Cannabis Use (Monogr Series 25). Canbinn, Australia, Australian Government Publishing Service, 1994

Higgins ST, Budney AJ, Bickel WK: Applying behavioral concepts and principles to the treatment of cocaine dependence. Drug Alcohol Depend 34:87–97, 1994

Jenkins AJ, Darwin WD, Huestis MA, et al: Validity testing of the accupinch THC test. J Anal Toxicol 19:5–12, 1995

Johnston L: Monitoring the Future Study, University of Michigan. Ann Arbor, MI, National Institute on Drug Abuse, 1998

Johnston LD, O'Malley PM, Bachman JG: Drug trends in 1999 are mixed. University of Michigan News and Information Services: Ann Arbor, MI, December 1999 [On-line]. Available at: www.monitoringthefuture.org

Jones KL, Chernoff GF: Effects of chemical and environmental agents, in Maternal Fetal Medicine. Edited by Creasy RK, Resnik R. Philadelphia, PA, WB Saunders, 1984, pp 189–200

Kandel D: Stages in adolescent involvement in drug use. Science 190:912–914, 1975

Kelp E, Webber M, Taskin DP: Acute and chronic effects of marijuana smoking on pulmonary alveolar permeability. Life Sci 56:2193–2199, 1995

Klein TW, Friedman H, Specter S: Marijuana, immunity and infection. J Neuroimmunol 83:102–115, 1998

Kolodny RC, Masters WH, Kolodner RM, et al: Depression of plasma testosterone levels after chronic intensive marijuana use. N Engl J Med 290:872–874, 1974

Loeber RT, Yurgelun-Todd DA: Human neuroimaging of acute and chronic marijuana use: Implications for frontocerebellar dysfunction. Human Psychopharmacology Clinical & Experimental 14:291–304, 1999

Lundavist T: Specific thought patterns in chronic cannabis smokers observed during treatment. Life Sci 56:2141–2144, 1995

Matthew RJ, Wilson WH, Turkington TG, et al: Cerebellar activity and disturbed time sense after THC. Brain Res 797:183–189, 1998

Matthias P, Tashkin DP, Marques-Magallanes JA, et al: Effects of varying marijuana potency on deposition of tar and delta-9-THC in the lung during smoking. Pharmacol Biochem Behav 58:1145–1150, 1997

Mayfield DG, McLeon G, Hall P: The CAGE Questionnaire: validation of a new alcoholism screening instrument. Am J Psychiatry 131:1121–1123, 1974

Millman RB, Beeder AB: Cannabis, in The American Psychiatric Press Textbook of Substance Abuse Treatment. Edited by Galanter M, Kleber HD. Washington, DC, American Psychiatric Press, 1994, pp 91–109

Naditch MP: Acute adverse reactions to psychoactive drugs, drug usage and psychopathology. J Abnorm Psychol 83:394–403, 1974

National Center on Addiction and Substance Abuse at Columbia University (CASA): Quarterly Update, 1996. Available at: http://www.casacolumbia.org

National Household Survey on Drug Abuse: CDC's TIPS. August 1998. Available at: http://www.cdc.gov

National Household Survey on Drug Abuse: 1999 Report. Available at: http://www.DrugAbuseStatistics.samhsa.gov/

National Institute on Drug Abuse: NIDA Capsule Series (C-88-06 [Revised September 1997]). Rockville, MD, National Institute on Drug Abuse, 1997

Novak W: High Culture: Marijuana in the Lives of Americans. New York, Alfred A Knopf, 1980

O'Brien CP, McLellan AT: Myths about the treatment of addiction. Lancet 347:237–240, 1996

Office of Applied Studies, SAMHSA, Drug Abuse Warning Network, 1999 (03/2000 update) for DAWN ED

Pertwee RG: Pharmacological, physiological and clinical implications of the discovery of cannabinoid receptors. Biochem Soc Trans 26:267–272, 1998

Pope HG, Yurgelun-Todd D: The residual cognitive effects of heavy marijuana use in college students. JAMA 275:521–527, 1996

Rodriguez de Fonseca F, Carrera MRA, Navarro M, et al: Activation of corticotropin-releasing factor in the limbic system during cannabinoid withdrawal. Science 276:2050–2054, 1997

Romero J, Garcia-Palormero E, Castro JG, et al: Effects of chronic exposure to delta-9-THC on cannabinoid receptor binding and mRNA levels in several rat brain regions. Brain Res Mol Brain Res 46:100–108, 1997

Stephens RS, Wertz JS, Roffman RA: Self-efficacy and marijuana cessation: a construct validity analysis. J Consult Clin Psychol 63:1022–1031, 1995

Stillman R, Galanter M, Lemberger L, et al: Tetrahydrocannabinol (THC): metabolism and subjective effects. Life Sci 19:569–576, 1976

Tanda G, Pontieri FE, DiChiara G: Cannabinoid and heroin activation of mesolimbic dopamine transmission by a common mu1 opioid receptor mechanism. Science 276:2048–2050, 1997

Tashkin DP, Shapiro BJ, Lee EY, et al: Subacute effects of heavy marijuana smoking on pulmonary function in healthy young males. N Engl J Med 294:125–129, 1976

Tilles DS, Goldenheim PD, Johnson DC, et al: Marijuana smoking as cause of reduction in single-breath carbon monoxide diffusing capacity. Am J Med 80:601–606, 1986

Tullis LM, Miller MD, Gold MS: Effects of marijuana on the GPA of college students (abstract). Biol Psychiatry 45:448, 1999

Walker JM, Huang SM, Strangman NM, et al: Pain modulation by release of the edogenous cannabinoid anandamide. Proc Natl Acad Sci U S A 96:12198–12203, 1999

Warner LA, Kessler RC, Hughes M, et al: Prevalence and correlates of drug use and dependence in the United States: results from the National Comorbidity Survey. Arch Gen Psychiatry 52:219–229, 1995

Wickelgren I: Marijuana: harder than we thought? Science 276:1967–1968, 1997

Wu TC, Tashkin DP, Djahed B, et al: Pulmonary hazards of smoking marijuana as compared with tobacco. N Engl J Med 318:347–351, 1988

Zhu LX, Sharma S, Stolina M, et al: Delta-9-tetrahydrocannabinol inhibits antitumor immunity by a CB2 receptor-mediated, cytokine-dependent pathway. J Immunol 165:373–380, 2000

28

Stimulants and Related Drugs

Thomas R. Kosten, M.D.

Amrita K. Singha, Ph.D.

Michael F. Weaver, M.D.

Sidney H. Schnoll, M.D., Ph.D.

David M. McDowell, M.D.

Lori Pbert, Ph.D.

Sarah Reiff-Hekking, Ph.D.

Judith K. Ockene, Ph.D.

Stimulants

Thomas R. Kosten, M.D.
Amrita K. Singha, Ph.D.

Cocaine and amphetamine are psychoactive agents that increase central nervous system activity and produce powerful reinforcing effects (e.g., euphoria, elevated mood, a "high") that contribute to their high abuse liability. Since the peak of the cocaine epidemic in the mid-1980s, addiction to this stimulant has been a major public health concern. Recently, localized epidemics of amphetamine abuse have been developing, particularly in the western United States. The dangers associated with stimulant use are enormous and include increased risk of human immunodeficiency virus (HIV) infection, detrimental effects on the unborn and newborn, and increased crime and violence, as well as medical, financial, and psychological problems. Because of these consequences, the task of identifying, characterizing, and developing treatments is more important than ever.

Progress has been made in identifying and developing pharmacological and behavioral treatments for stimulant addiction. In this chapter subpart, we review the clinical characteristics resulting from stimulant use as a foundation for a discussion of the pharmacological and behavioral treatments. We conclude by providing specific treatment guidelines for managing stimulant-abusing individuals.

Support for this work was provided by National Institute on Drug Abuse grants P50-DA04060 and P50-DA09250 and the Veterans Administration Mental Illness Research, Education, and Clinical Center (MIRECC) to Dr. Kosten.
This chapter subpart is a revised version of our chapter "Stimulants," which appeared in Galanter MA, Kleber HD (eds): *The American Psychiatric Press Textbook of Substance Abuse Treatment,* 2nd Edition. Washington, DC, American Psychiatric Press, 1999, pp. 183–193.

Clinical Aspects of Stimulant Use

The rewarding effects of cocaine and amphetamine are influenced by the route of administration, with some routes (e.g., intravenous administration) producing a more immediate onset of euphoria. The preferred method of self-administering cocaine has been snorting and, more recently, smoking. Amphetamines come in a variety of forms (pill, liquid, or powder), but they are usually taken orally or intravenously. The effects from snorted cocaine generally occur within 15–20 minutes, whereas the effects from intravenously injected cocaine can be felt within minutes. Crack cocaine, a smokable form of cocaine obtained by processing cocaine hydrochloride with baking soda and water to produce a free base, produces euphoria within seconds. A smokable version of amphetamine ("ice" amphetamine), similar to cocaine, is also available that, because of its long duration of action, can produce euphoria lasting 12–24 hours.

Stimulant use can range from low dose to high dose and from infrequent to chronic or binge patterns. Depending on the dosage, pattern, and duration of use, stimulants can produce several drug-induced states that differ in their clinical characteristics. Moderate to high doses of stimulants can produce stimulant intoxication that may or may not be pleasant. The intoxicated person may show signs of hyperawareness, hypersexuality, hypervigilance, and psychomotor agitation. Often, the symptoms of stimulant-induced intoxication resemble mania. The intoxicated person should be monitored by medical staff until the symptoms of intoxication diminish. If the intoxication does not dissipate within 24 hours, mania may be present and treatment for manic disorder may be required (Gawin et al. 1994).

With increased dosage and duration of administration, stimulants can also produce a state of mental confusion and excitement known as *stimulant delirium*. Delirium involves disorientation and confusion, as well as anxiety and fearfulness. Extreme medical caution is needed when treating delirium, because such symptoms may indicate stimulant overdose. For instance, crack cocaine–addicted persons who overdose need careful monitoring for seizures, cardiac arrhythmias, stroke, and pulmonary complications. Overdose management has been reviewed in detail (see Gay 1982), but more recently a syndrome of hyperthermia and agitation has been described that resembles neuroleptic malignant syndrome (Kosten and Kleber 1988; Mittleman and Wetli 1984). Standard pharmacological management of overdose includes the use of antipsychotics; however, high doses of benzodiazepines may be safer alternatives for controlling the delirium and agitation, because in some cases of overdose, antipsychotics will worsen the hyperthermia and lead to fatality. Acute use of benzodiazepines can also help minimize the need for physical restraints.

During high-dose stimulant use, often seen during binge episodes, individuals can experience stimulant-induced psychosis characterized by delusions, paranoid thinking, and stereotyped compulsive behavior. When delusions are present, close clinical monitoring of the patient is essential, and short-term treatment with antipsychotics may be necessary to ameliorate the psychosis. Psychosis is more commonly induced by amphetamine than by cocaine, perhaps as a result of the difficulty in maintaining high chronic levels of cocaine in the body (King and Ellinwood 1997). Also, stimulant-induced psychosis in humans is related to the dose and duration of administration of amphetamine (Bell 1970) and cocaine (Satel et al. 1991) rather than to psychiatric predisposition.

Stimulant withdrawal, which occurs following cessation of cocaine or amphetamine use, can produce a wide range of dysphoric symptoms. Following binge use, individuals may initially experience a "crash" period characterized by symptoms of depression, anxiety, agitation, and intense drug craving (Gawin and Ellinwood 1988; Gawin and Kleber 1986). The crash period is followed by an intermediate withdrawal phase in which fatigue, a loss of physical and mental energy, and decreased interest in the surrounding environment are present (Gawin and Ellinwood 1988). During the late withdrawal phase, brief periods of intense drug craving can occur such that objects and people in the addicted person's life can become a conditioned trigger for craving and relapse. These withdrawal symptoms may be a target for pharmacological agents (see "Dopaminergic Agents," below).

Treatment of Stimulant Abuse

Although a great deal has been learned about the reward mechanisms underlying stimulant abuse, the development of effective treatment has lagged behind. There is virtually no controlled treatment literature for amphetamine abuse, partly due to the fact that amphetamine use was not as popular as cocaine use throughout the 1980s and early 1990s. However, epidemics of amphetamine abuse are on the rise, especially in the western United States. The pharmacological and behavioral treatment approaches used for cocaine abuse appear to be applicable to the treatment of amphetamine use.

Pharmacotherapy

Although no U.S. Food and Drug Administration (FDA)–approved agent is available for treating cocaine dependence, two major classes of medications have been investigated: 1) dopaminergic agonists and 2) antidepressants. Studies have been relatively brief for both types of agents and have focused on abstinence initiation rather than relapse prevention. In addition to dopaminergic agents and antidepressants, other compounds have been examined as potential treatment medication for cocaine dependence.

Dopaminergic Agents

Based on the theory that chronic cocaine use reduces the efficiency of central dopamine neurotransmission, a number of dopaminergic compounds, including amantadine, bromocriptine, mazindol, and methylphenidate, have been examined as treatment medications for cocaine abuse. It is thought that these dopaminergic agents might correct the dopamine dysregulation and alleviate the withdrawal symptoms that often follow cessation of stimulant use.

A number of studies have found amantadine to be effective in attenuating cocaine craving and use. For example, in cocaine-abusing methadone-maintained patients, Handelsman et al. (1988) reported decreases in urine cocaine metabolite levels and self-reported cocaine use following amantadine treatment, and Alterman et al. (1992) found that patients treated with amantadine had significantly greater rates of cocaine abstinence than those given placebo. Also, in a double-blind comparison of amantadine and bromocriptine for the treatment of acute cocaine withdrawal, Tennant and Sagherian (1987) found amantadine to be superior to bromocriptine. However, a placebo-controlled study comparing amantadine and placebo observed no differences between the treatment groups (Weddington et al. 1991). Amantadine was also compared with desipramine and placebo in a study of methadone-maintained patients (Kosten et al. 1992b). No differences were found between the three groups in treatment retention, cocaine craving, and cocaine-free urine samples, but attainment of 2 weeks of cocaine abstinence was significantly greater in the amantadine treatment group relative to the desipramine and placebo groups (Kosten et al. 1992b). Although these studies suggest that amantadine may be effective in the reduction of cocaine withdrawal symptoms and the initial attainment of cocaine abstinence, a more recent study found amantadine no more efficacious than placebo (Kampman et al. 1996).

The D_2 dopamine agonist bromocriptine has also been examined in the treatment of cocaine dependence. In a double-blind, placebo-controlled study with cocaine-dependent individuals, Giannini et al. (1987) found that bromocriptine significantly reduced cocaine craving compared with placebo. Tennant and Sagherian (1987) noted that bromocriptine blocked the euphorigenic effects of cocaine in several addicted individuals. Despite these positive results, bromocriptine has been reported to produce side effects such as headache, nausea, hypotension, and psychosis (Dackis et al. 1987; Turner et al. 1984), which makes this agent a poor treatment choice.

Mazindol, a catecholamine reuptake inhibitor, was initially associated with reduced cocaine use (Berger et al. 1989; Seibyl et al. 1992), but more recent studies failed to show significant therapeutic effects. For example, in a 1-week crossover study, no improvement in cocaine use or craving was found with mazindol (Kosten et al. 1993), and in double-blind studies, no differences were observed between mazindol and placebo treatment groups on self-report ratings, rates of relapse, or cocaine use (Margolin et al. 1995a; Stine et al. 1995).

The stimulant methylphenidate has also been examined as a treatment for cocaine dependence because of its low abuse liability relative to cocaine or amphetamine, its rapid onset of action relative to antidepressants, and its long duration of action relative to cocaine (Kosten and McCance-Katz 1995). Methylphenidate has been reported to have beneficial effects in cocaine-dependent individuals with attention-deficit/hyperactivity disorder (ADHD) (Khantzian et al. 1984). However, some researchers have found that methylphenidate produces a mild sense of stimulation that evokes an increased desire for cocaine in persons without ADHD (Gawin et al. 1985). Furthermore, a double-blind, placebo-controlled study found no difference between methylphenidate and placebo treatment groups in cocaine use (Grabowski et al. 1997).

Overall, these studies indicate that the rewarding effects and withdrawal symptoms induced by cocaine may be attenuated by fast-acting dopaminergic agents. However, more controlled studies are needed to better characterize the therapeutic efficacy of these agents and to assess additional compounds, including dopamine antagonists (e.g., flupenthixol).

Antidepressants

The second class of medications used to treat cocaine dependence—the antidepressants—is thought to downregulate synaptic catecholamine receptors, an action opposite to the presynaptic upregulation caused by chronic stimulant use (Gawin and Ellinwood 1988). Although antidepressants have a relatively benign side-effect profile, good patient compliance rates, and lack of abuse liability, they have a delayed onset of action ranging from 10 to 20 days (Kosten and McCance-Katz 1995). Therefore, the physician may consider beginning antidepressant treatment during early withdrawal and continuing for weeks or longer as clinically indicated.

Desipramine is the tricyclic antidepressant that has been studied most extensively as a treatment for cocaine dependence. Early studies using desipramine for cocaine treatment showed positive results (Gawin et al. 1989; Tennant and Rawson 1983), but placebo-controlled trials have not yielded impressive findings. A meta-analysis by Levin and Lehman (1991) of placebo-controlled studies showed that although desipramine did not improve retention in treatment, it did produce greater cocaine abstinence relative to placebo. Treatment with desipramine has been reported to produce "early tricyclic jitteriness syndrome" and cocaine craving, as well as relapse to cocaine use in some patients (Weiss 1988). Thus, desipramine should be used with caution in pharmacotherapy for stimulant dependence.

Another tricyclic antidepressant that has also been employed for cocaine pharmacotherapy is imipramine. In cocaine-using subjects, treatment with imipramine led to abstinence from cocaine in 80% of the subjects, but because participants were also treated with tyrosine and tryptophan, the precise contribution of imipramine's effects remains unclear (Rosecan 1983). A double-blind, placebo-controlled study with cocaine users found significant decreases in cocaine craving and high in the imipramine group relative to the placebo group; however, urine specimens for cocaine did not differ between the groups (Nunes et al. 1991). Moreover, secondary analyses of studies with imipramine and desipramine have suggested that depressed cocaine-abusing patients are more likely than nondepressed cocaine abusers to show significant reductions in cocaine abuse (Nunes et al. 1991; Ziedonis and Kosten 1991). Hence, imipramine's therapeutic efficacy in stimulant dependence needs further assessment, particularly in depressed cocaine-addicted subjects.

Several other antidepressants that exert their effects predominantly through serotonergic mechanisms have also been employed for cocaine pharmacotherapy. These include fluoxetine, sertraline, and trazodone hydrochloride. Although some researchers have reported that treatment with fluoxetine reduces cocaine craving and use in cocaine-abusing heroin-addicted patients (Batki et al. 1993; Pollack and Rosenbaum 1991), other investigators have not found fluoxetine to be an effective treatment agent for cocaine abuse (e.g., Covi et al. 1993; Grabowski et al. 1992; Oliveto et al. 1995). Only open studies of trazodone and sertraline have shown them to be effective in attenuating cocaine use and withdrawal symptoms (Kosten et al. 1992a; Small and Purcell 1985).

Bupropion, a "second generation" antidepressant, has also been examined for a possible role in cocaine pharmacotherapy. In an open pilot study, treatment with bupropion reduced cocaine use (Margolin et al. 1991) and attenuated several cocaine-induced positive subjective ratings during laboratory cocaine administration (Singha et al. 1997). However, a multisite placebo-controlled study failed to show that bupropion was more efficacious than placebo in reducing cocaine's effects (Margolin et al. 1995b).

Other Pharmacotherapeutic Agents and Approaches

In addition to the dopaminergic agents and antidepressants, a number of miscellaneous agents, including carbamazepine, disulfiram, and buprenorphine, have been examined for use in cocaine pharmacotherapy. Although carbamazepine has shown efficacy in reducing cocaine use (Halikas et al. 1991, 1992), other studies have failed to replicate this finding (Cornish et al. 1995; Kranzler et al. 1995; Montoya et al. 1995). Disulfiram, which is used in the treatment of alcoholism, has been effective in treating patients with comorbid cocaine and alcohol dependence (Carroll et al. 1993, 1998; McCance et al. 1995). For buprenorphine, studies have reported more negative than positive findings with regard to its effectiveness in treating cocaine-abusing opiate addicts (Fudala et al. 1991; Johnson et al. 1992; Kosten et al. 1989; Oliveto et al. 1994), although a recent study reported buprenorphine's efficacy in combination with desipramine for reducing cocaine abuse in patients with dual opioid and cocaine dependence (Oliveto et al. 1999). Clearly, more studies are needed to fully evaluate the usefulness of these agents in managing stimulant dependence.

Recent advances in the molecular biology of dopamine neuronal systems have led to innovative approaches to investigating cocaine's biochemical and behavioral effects. Giros and colleagues (1996) showed that rats, because they lack the dopamine transporter (DAT)–encoding gene, do not respond to cocaine either biochemically or behaviorally. Moreover, a study by Carrera et al. (1995) suggested that animals injected with a protein-conjugated analog of cocaine that triggers the immune system to produce cocaine antibodies had reduced cocaine concentrations in striatal tissue and lower psychomotor responses to stimulants compared with nonimmunized animals. Finally, Fox and colleagues (1996) demonstrated that a cocaine vaccine reduced cocaine self-administration in rats and decreased cocaine levels in the brains of immunized mice. These findings are exciting and suggest that vaccinations against cocaine's effects are possible. Future studies are needed to assess how these molecular approaches may be used to treat stimulant addiction in humans.

Behavioral Therapy

In addition to pharmacotherapy, a behavioral approach to relapse prevention has been used in the management of cocaine and amphetamine abuse (Anker and Crowley 1982; Boudin 1972; Higgins et al. 1991, 1993, 1994). The goal of this approach was to decrease behavior maintained by drug reinforcers and to increase behavior maintained by nondrug reinforcers by presenting rewards contingent on documented drug abstinence (positive contingencies) and withdrawing privileges contingent on documented drug use (negative contingencies).

Using the negative-contingency contract procedure, Anker and Crowley (1982) reported that more than 80% of the participants remained cocaine-free for the duration of their contracts, which averaged 3 months. However, more than one-half of these patients relapsed at the completion of their contracts. The investigators also found that more than 90% of the individuals who received psychotherapy instead dropped out of therapy or resumed cocaine use within 2–4 weeks of discontinuing therapy.

A series of studies have demonstrated that positive contingency management procedures in combination with a community reinforcement approach facilitate initial abstinence in cocaine-dependent persons. In the first study (Higgins et al. 1991), which lasted 12 weeks, the contingency management procedure consisted of vouchers with a monetary value that were presented to patients upon evidence of drug abstinence (i.e., cocaine-free urine). The vouchers increased in value for every consecutive drug-free urine test and were exchangeable for retail items and activities that the patient and therapist agreed upon. The community reinforcement approach consisted of reciprocal relationship counseling with a significant other, including engaging in activities that were purchased with vouchers for drug-free urine tests. Other components of the counseling included instruction in recognizing antecedents and consequences of drug use and changing the patient's behavior to increase the probability of drug abstinence (e.g., providing assistance with employment/career goals, developing new non-drug-related recreational activities). Treatment retention was significantly higher in the behavioral treatment group than in the standard drug counseling group: 85% of clients receiving the behavioral treatment achieved at least 3 weeks of abstinence, whereas only 33% of clients receiving standard drug abuse counseling did so.

In the second study in the series (Higgins et al. 1993), a 24-week trial, the contingency management procedure was modified to include vouchers exchangeable for goods and services during weeks 1–12 and lottery tickets during weeks 13–24. It was expected that a more intensive reward system (i.e., vouchers) would facilitate initial drug abstinence and that a less intensive reward system (i.e., lottery tickets) would continue to maintain sustained drug abstinence. As in the previous study, treatment retention was significantly higher in the behavioral treatment group than in the standard drug counseling group. Similarly, 68% and 42% of the clients in the behavioral treatment group achieved at least 8 and 16 weeks, respectively, of continuous cocaine abstinence, as opposed to 11% and 5% in the standard drug abuse counseling group. Moreover, cocaine abstinence did not precipitously decline when lottery tickets were substituted at week 13.

In the third study (Higgins et al. 1994), also a 24-week trial, cocaine-dependent individuals were randomized to receive either behavioral treatment without incentives or behavioral treatment with incentives (i.e., vouchers exchangeable for goods and services) during weeks 1–12. During weeks 13–24, clients in both groups received, in addition to behavioral treatment, a $1 lottery ticket for every drug-free urine test. The group that received the incentives showed significantly greater treatment retention and a longer duration of continuous abstinence than the group not receiving the incentives.

The voucher system was examined in a 12-week clinical trial among methadone-maintained cocaine abusers (Silverman et al. 1996). Relative to control subjects, the contingency group achieved a significantly longer duration of sustained cocaine abstinence. Overall, these findings suggest that incentives contingent on drug abstinence can be a powerful intervention tool for facilitating cocaine abstinence in cocaine abusers in methadone maintenance treatment.

Psychiatric Comorbidity

The rates of comorbid psychiatric disorders in stimulant abusers are significantly higher than community rates of depression, ADHD, and antisocial personality disorders (Gawin and Kleber 1984; Rounsaville et al. 1991; Weiss et al. 1986; Ziedonis and Kosten 1991). Because psychiatric disorders may increase the risk for drug use (e.g., individuals may self-medicate to alleviate psychiatric symptomatology), treatment needs to address both the stimulant addiction and the comorbid disorder. Certain pharmacotherapies may be particularly useful for stimulant-abusing patients with comorbid psychopathology. For example, treatment with antidepressants has reduced depressive symptoms, cocaine use, and craving in depressed cocaine-addicted patients (Nunes et al. 1990, 1991; Ziedonis and Kosten 1991). Also, methylphenidate and lithium have been reported to be effective in treating cocaine-addicted persons with ADHD (Khantzian et al. 1984) and with cyclothymia (Gawin 1986; Nunes et al. 1990), respectively. Unfortunately, psychiatric comorbidity has not yet shown a specific prognostic significance for behavioral therapies.

Summary of Treatment Considerations for Stimulant Abuse

Treatment of stimulant abuse requires a comprehensive assessment of the patient's psychological, medical, forensic, and drug use history. Moreover, because information obtained from chemically dependent persons may be incomplete or unreliable, it is important that patients receive a thorough physical, including blood and supervised urine samples for analysis. The clinician needs to be aware that polydrug abuse is common. Patients may ingest large amounts of one or more drugs at potentially lethal doses; it is therefore important that the physician be aware of the dangers of possible drug combinations, such as cocaine and alcohol or heroin (Goldsmith 1996).

Pharmacological intervention may be necessary during stimulant-induced drug states. For example, antipsychotics may be useful in controlling stimulant-induced psychosis or delirium, and anticraving agents with a rapid onset of action may be helpful during the early withdrawal period. During the late withdrawal phase, when depression may develop, antidepressants may be an appropriate treatment choice. Treatment medications can be administered on an inpatient or outpatient basis. However, if medications are used for outpatient treatment, it is critical to warn the patient of any potential adverse interactions between cocaine and the prescribed treatment medication. For example, high blood pressure could result from the release of epinephrine by cocaine combined with the reuptake blockade by the tricyclic (Fischman et al. 1976), although later in the course of treatment, tricyclics decrease the sensitivity of the postsynaptic adrenergic receptors (Charney et al. 1981).

The powerful rewarding effects of stimulants make them addictive and dangerous, creating a range of psychological, social, economic, and medical problems. To date, no effective treatment is available for stimulant dependence, although progress has been made in the development of pharmacological and behavioral techniques for cocaine and amphetamine addiction. Dopaminergic agents and antidepressants have shown some promise for reducing drug craving and preventing relapse. Behavioral techniques aimed at maintaining drug abstinence and preventing relapse have also shown favorable results. Although both pharmacological and behavioral interventions may be useful in treating addiction, Kosten (1989) suggested that individuals with significant medical risks, psychiatric comorbidity, and neuroadaptation from heavy stimulant use are particularly likely to benefit from pharmacological treatment. Further research is needed to address this issue and to identify other effective ways to treat, manage, and prevent stimulant use.

References

Alterman AI, Droba M, Antelo RE, et al: Amantadine may facilitate detoxification of cocaine addicts. Drug Alcohol Depend 31:19–29, 1992

Anker AL, Crowley TJ: Use of contingency contracts in specialty clinics for cocaine abuse, in Problems of Drug Dependence, 1981: Proceedings of the 43rd Annual Scientific Meeting, the Committee on Problems of Drug Dependence. NIDA Research Monograph 41 (NTIS Publ No 82-190760). Edited by Harris LS. Rockville, MD, National Institute on Drug Abuse, 1982, pp 452–459

Batki SL, Manfredi LB, Jacob P, et al: Fluoxetine for cocaine dependence in methadone maintenance: quantitative plasma and urine cocaine/benzoylecognine concentration. J Clin Psychopharmacol 13:243–250, 1993

Bell DS: The experimental reproduction of amphetamine psychosis. Arch Gen Psychiatry 127:1170–1175, 1970

Berger P, Gawin F, Kosten TR: Treatment of cocaine abuse with mazindol (letter). Lancet 1(8632):283, 1989

Boudin HM: Contingency contracting as a therapeutic tool in the deceleration of amphetamine use. Behav Res Ther 3:604–608, 1972

Carrera MR, Ashley JA, Parsons LH, et al: Suppression of psychoactive effects of cocaine by active immunization. Nature 378:727–730, 1995

Carroll K, Ziedonis D, O'Malley S, et al: Pharmacological interventions for alcohol- and cocaine-abusing individuals. Am J Addict 2:77–79, 1993

Carroll KM, Nich C, Ball SA, et al: Treatment of cocaine and alcohol dependence with psychotherapy and disulfiram. Addiction 93:713–727, 1998

Charney DS, Menkes DB, Heninger GR: Receptor sensitivity and the mechanism of action of antidepressant treatment. Arch Gen Psychiatry 38:1160–1180, 1981

Cornish JW, Maany I, Fudala PJ, et al: Carbamazepine treatment for cocaine dependence. Drug Alcohol Depend 38:221–227, 1995

Covi L, Hess JM, Kreiter NA, et al: Three models for the analysis of a fluoxetine controlled treatment in cocaine abuse, in Problems of Drug Dependence, 1993: Proceedings of the 55th Annual Scientific Meeting, The College on Problems of Drug Dependence. NIDA Research Monograph 141 (NIH Publ No 94-3749). Edited by Harris LS. Washington, DC, U.S. Government Printing Office, 1994, p 138

Dackis CA, Gold MS, Sweeny DR, et al: Single-dose bromocriptine reverses cocaine craving. Psychiatry Res 20:261–264, 1987

Fischman MW, Schuster CR, Resnekov I, et al: Cardiovascular and subject effects of intravenous cocaine administration in humans. Arch Gen Psychiatry 10:535–546, 1976

Fox BS, Kantak KM, Edwards MA, et al: Efficacy of a therapeutic cocaine vaccine in rodent models. Nat Med 2:1129–1132, 1996

Fudala PJ, Johnson RE, Jaffe JH: Outpatient comparison of buprenorphine and methadone maintenance, II: effects on cocaine usage, retention time in study, and missed clinic visits, in Problems of Drug Dependence, 1990: Proceedings of the 52nd Annual Scientific Meeting, The College on Problems of Drug Dependence. NIDA Research Monograph 105 (NIH Publ No 91-1663). Edited by Harris LS. Washington, DC, U.S. Government Printing Office, 1991, pp 576–588

Gawin FH: New uses of antidepressants in cocaine abuse. Psychosomatics 27 (suppl):24–29, 1986

Gawin FH, Ellinwood EH: Cocaine and other stimulants: actions, abuse, and treatments. N Engl J Med 318:1173–1182, 1988

Gawin FH, Kleber HD: Cocaine abuse treatments: an open pilot trial with lithium and desipramine. Arch Gen Psychiatry 41:903–910, 1984

Gawin FH, Kleber HD: Abstinence symptomatology and psychiatric diagnosis in chronic cocaine abusers. Arch Gen Psychiatry 43:107–113, 1986

Gawin FH, Riordan CA, Kleber HD: Methylphenidate treatment of cocaine abusers without attention deficit disorder: a negative study. Am J Drug Alcohol Abuse 11:193–197, 1985

Gawin FH, Kleber HD, Byck R, et al: Desipramine facilitation of initial cocaine abstinence. Arch Gen Psychiatry 46:117–121, 1989

Gawin FH, Khalsa ME, Ellinwood EH: Stimulants, in The American Psychiatric Press Textbook of Substance Abuse Treatment. Edited by Galanter M, Kleber HD. Washington, DC, American Psychiatric Press, 1994, pp 111–139

Gay GR: Clinical management of acute and chronic cocaine poisoning. Ann Emerg Med 11:562–572, 1982

Giannini AJ, Baumgartel P, Dimarzio LR: Bromocriptine therapy in cocaine withdrawal. J Clin Pharmacol 27:267–270, 1987

Giros B, Jaber M, Jones SR, et al: Hyperlocomotion and indifference to cocaine and amphetamine in mice lacking the dopamine transporter. Nature 379:606–612, 1996

Goldsmith RJ: The elements of contemporary treatment, in The Principles and Practice of Addictions in Psychiatry. Edited by Miller NS. Philadelphia, PA, WB Saunders, 1996, pp 392–399

Grabowski J, Elk R, Kirby K, et al: Fluoxetine and behavioral factors in treatment of cocaine dependence, in Problems of Drug Dependence, 1991: Proceedings of the 53rd Annual Scientific Meeting, the Committee on Problems of Drug Dependence. NIDA Research Monograph 119 (NIH Publ No [ADM] 92-1888). Edited by Harris LS. Washington, DC, U.S. Government Printing Office, 1992, p 362

Grabowski J, Roache J, Schmitz J, et al: Replacement medication for cocaine dependence: Methylphenidate. J Clin Psychopharmacol 17:485–488, 1997

Halikas J, Kuhn K, Carlson G, et al: The effect of carbamazepine on cocaine use. Am J Addict 1:129–139, 1992

Halikas JA, Crosby RD, Carlson GA, et al: Cocaine reduction in unmotivated crack users using carbamazepine versus placebo in a short-term, double-blind crossover design. Clin Pharmacol Ther 50: 81–95, 1991

Handelsman L, Chordia PL, Escovar IM, et al: Amantadine for treatment of cocaine dependence in methadone-maintained patients (letter). Am J Psychiatry 145:533, 1988

Higgins ST, Delaney DD, Budney AJ, et al: A behavioral approach to achieving initial cocaine abstinence. Am J Psychiatry 148:1218–1224, 1991

Higgins ST, Budney AJ, Bickel WK, et al: Achieving cocaine abstinence with a behavioral approach. Am J Psychiatry 150:763–769, 1993

Higgins ST, Budney AJ, Bickel WK, et al: Incentives improve outcome in outpatient behavioral treatment of cocaine dependence. Arch Gen Psychiatry 51:568–576, 1994

Johnson RE, Jaffe JH, Fudala PJ: A controlled trial of buprenorphine treatment for opioid dependence. JAMA 267:2750–2755, 1992

Kampman K, Volpicelli JR, Alterman A, et al: Amantadine in the early treatment of cocaine dependence: a double-blind, placebo-controlled trial. Drug Alcohol Depend 41:25–33, 1996

Khantzian EJ, Gawin F, Kleber HD, et al: Methylphenidate (Ritalin) treatment of cocaine dependence: a preliminary report. J Subst Abuse Treat 1:107–112, 1984

King GR, Ellinwood EH: Amphetamines and other stimulants, in Substance Abuse: A Comprehensive Textbook, 3rd Edition. Edited by Lowinson JH, Ruiz P, Millman RB, et al. Baltimore, MD, Williams & Wilkins, 1997, pp 207–223

Kosten TR: Pharmacotherapeutic interventions for cocaine abuse: matching patients to treatment. J Nerv Ment Dis 177:379–389, 1989

Kosten TR, Kleber TR: Rapid death during cocaine abuse: variant of the neuroleptic malignant syndrome? Am J Drug Alcohol Abuse 14:335–346, 1988

Kosten TR, McCance-Katz E: New pharmacotherapies, in American Psychiatric Press Review of Psychiatry, Vol 14. Edited by Oldham JM, Riba MB. Washington, DC, American Psychiatric Press, 1995, pp 105–126

Kosten TR, Kleber TR, Morgan CM: Treatment of cocaine abuse using buprenorphine. Biol Psychiatry 26:637–639, 1989

Kosten TR, Kosten TA, Gawin FH, et al: An open trial of sertraline for cocaine abuse. Am J Addictions 1:349–353, 1992a

Kosten TR, Morgan CM, Falcioni J, et al: Pharmacotherapy for cocaine-abusing methadone-maintained patients using amantadine or desipramine. Arch Gen Psychiatry 49:894–899, 1992b

Kosten TR, Steinberg M, Diakogiannis IA: Cross-over trial of mazindol for cocaine dependence. Am J Addict 2:161–164, 1993

Kranzler HR, Bauer LO, Hersh D, et al: Carbamazepine treatment of cocaine dependence: a placebo-controlled trial. Drug Alcohol Depend 38:203–211, 1995

Levin FR, Lehman AF: Meta-analysis of desipramine an adjunct in the treatment of cocaine addiction. J Clin Pharmacol 11:374–378, 1991

Margolin A, Kosten TR, Petrakis I, et al: Bupropion reduces cocaine abuse in methadone-maintained patients (letter). Arch Gen Psychiatry 48:87, 1991

Margolin A, Avants SK, Kosten TR: Mazindol for relapse prevention to cocaine abuse in methadone-maintained patients. Am J Drug Alcohol Abuse 21:469–481, 1995a

Margolin A, Kosten TR, Avants SK, et al: A multicenter trial of bupropion for cocaine dependence in methadone-maintained patients. Drug Alcohol Depend 49:125–131, 1995b

McCance EF, Price LH, Kosten TR, et al: Cocaethylene: pharmacology, physiology and behavioral effects in humans. J Pharmacol Exp Ther 274:215–223, 1995

Mittleman R, Wetli CV: Death caused by recreational cocaine use. JAMA 252:1889–1892, 1984

Montoya ID, Levin FR, Fudala PJ, et al: Double-blind comparison of carbamazepine and placebo for treatment of cocaine dependence. Drug Alcohol Depend 38:213–219, 1995

Nunes EV, McGrath PJ, Wager S, et al: Lithium treatment for cocaine abusers with bipolar disorders. Am J Psychiatry 147:655–657, 1990

Nunes EV, Quitkin FM, Brady R, et al: Imipramine treatment of methadone maintenance patients with affective disorder and illicit drug use. Am J Psychiatry 148:667–669, 1991

Oliveto AH, Kosten TR, Schottenfeld RS, et al: A comparison of cocaine use in buprenorphine and methadone-maintained cocaine users. Am J Addict 3:43–48, 1994

Oliveto AH, Kosten TR, Schottenfeld RS, et al: Desipramine, amantadine, or fluoxetine in buprenorphine-maintained cocaine users. J Subst Abuse Treat 12:423–428, 1995

Oliveto AH, Feingold A, Schottenfeld RS, et al: Desipramine in opioid-dependent cocaine abusers maintained on buprenorphine vs methadone. Arch Gen Psychiatry 56:812–820, 1999

Pollack MH, Rosenbaum JF: Fluoxetine treatment of cocaine abuse in heroin addicts. J Clin Psychiatry 52:31–33, 1991

Rosecan J: The treatment of cocaine abuse with imipramine, L-tyrosine, and L-tryptophan. Paper presented at the 7th World Congress of Psychiatry, Vienna, Austria, July 14–19, 1983

Rounsaville BJ, Anton SF, Carroll KM, et al: Psychiatric diagnosis of treatment seeking cocaine abusers. Arch Gen Psychiatry 18:43–51, 1991

Satel SL, Southwick SM, Gawin FH, et al: Clinical features of cocaine-induced paranoia. Am J Psychiatry 148:495–498, 1991

Seibyl JP, Brenner L, Krystal JH, et al: Mazindol and cocaine addiction in schizophrenia (letter). Biol Psychiatry 31:1179–1181, 1992

Silverman K, Higgins ST, Brooner RK, et al: Sustained cocaine abstinence in methadone maintenance patients through voucher-based reinforcement therapy. Arch Gen Psychiatry 53:409–415, 1996

Singha A, Oliveto A, McCance E, et al: Effects of cocaine prior to and during bupropion maintenance in cocaine abusers. Paper presented at the 59th Annual Scientific Meeting of the College on Problems of Drug Dependence, Nashville, TN, June 14–19, 1997

Small GW, Purcell JJ: Trazodone and cocaine abuse (letter). Arch Gen Psychiatry 42:524, 1985

Stine SM, Krystal JH, Kosten TR, et al: Mazindol treatment for cocaine dependence. Drug Alcohol Depend 39:245–252, 1995

Tennant FS, Rawson RA: Cocaine and amphetamine dependence treated with desipramine, in Problems of Drug Dependence, 1982: Proceedings of the 44th Annual Scientific Meeting, the Committee on Problems of Drug Dependence. NIDA Research Monograph 43 (DHHS Publ No [ADM] 83-1264). Edited by Harris LS. Rockville, MD, Department of Health and Human Services, 1983, pp 351–355

Tennant FS, Sagherian AA: Double-blind comparison of amantadine and bromocriptine for ambulatory withdrawal from cocaine dependence. Arch Intern Med 147:109–112, 1987

Turner TH, Cookson JC, Wass JAH, et al: Psychotic reactions during treatment of pituitary tumors with dopamine agonists. BMJ 289:1101–1103, 1984

Weddington WW Jr, Brown BS, Haertzen CA, et al: Comparison of amantadine and desipramine combined with psychotherapy for treatment of cocaine dependence. Am J Drug Alcohol Abuse 17:137–152, 1991

Weiss RD: Relapse to cocaine after initiating desipramine treatment. JAMA 260:2545–2546, 1988

Weiss RD, Mirin SM, Michael JL, et al: Psychopathology in chronic cocaine abusers. Am J Drug Alcohol Abuse 12:17–29, 1986

Ziedonis DM, Kosten TR: Pharmacotherapy improves treatment outcome in depressed cocaine addicts. J Psychoactive Drugs 23:417–425, 1991

Phencyclidine and Ketamine Abuse and Dependence

Michael F. Weaver, M.D.
Sidney H. Schnoll, M.D., Ph.D.

Phencyclidine (1-[1-phenylcyclohexyl]piperidine monohydrochloride), commonly referred to as PCP, was synthesized in the late 1950s. It is an arylcyclohexylamine that was the first of a new class of general anesthetics known as cataleptoid anesthetics or dissociative anesthetics. Phencyclidine can be manufactured easily in unsophisticated laboratories from simple materials. Ketamine, an arylcycloalkylamine related to phencyclidine, is less potent and shorter acting and is still used as a dissociative anesthetic in humans (Chen et al. 1959), in addition to its illicit use as a drug of abuse. This section focuses on ketamine intoxication, abuse, and dependence. For more information on the recreational use of ketamine, the reader is referred to McDowell's discussion of club drugs in the final subsection of this chapter.

Phencyclidine

Phencyclidine was originally described as a drug of abuse in the mid-1960s, but rapidly disappeared as a popular drug because of the unexpected reactions that often occurred following its use. In the late 1960s and early 1970s, phencyclidine emerged as a frequent contaminant of other drugs sold on the illicit market, most often in samples of hallucinogens and tetrahydrocannabinol (THC). Virtually all "THC extract" that used to be sold illicitly was actually phencyclidine, because phencyclidine is relatively easy to manufacture

This work was supported in part by National Institutes of Health grant AA00222-01A2 chemically compared with THC (Weaver et al. 1999). In the past few years, phencyclidine has once again become a sought-after drug of abuse. Patterns of phencyclidine abuse vary with time and location; it is primarily seen in large cities and its popularity tends to wax and wane. Phencyclidine is used mainly by adolescents and young adults. First use is usually between the ages of 13 and 15 years. Recent data suggest that although phencyclidine abuse is not widespread in the United States, it has become concentrated among post-high-school-age minority males in a limited number of cities (Thombs 1989). In some urban settings in the United States, phencyclidine abuse has been rivaled only by crack cocaine in popularity (Johnson and Jones 1990). Persons who use phencyclidine are usually polysubstance abusers, with more than 90% reporting use of other substances, mainly marijuana and alcohol (National Institute on Drug Abuse 1979). Chronic phencyclidine use does occur outside the young-adult age group and is not rare among psychiatric patients (Gorelick et al. 1987).

Phencyclidine can be taken by several routes: oral, intravenous, smoking, or insufflation ("snorting"). Whereas absorption with oral administration usually takes more than 1 hour, the effect with smoking is almost immediate. Smoking is becoming the most popular route, and inhalation produces a pharmacological profile similar to that of intravenous administration (Meng et al. 1996). This crystalline, water-soluble, lipophilic substance penetrates easily into fat cells and accumulates in adipose tissue as well as the brain (Misra et al. 1979). Phencyclidine's half-life is around 24 hours, depending on route of administration (Hurlbut 1991). It is one of the longest-acting drugs of abuse; a clinical episode of intoxication may take up to 6 weeks to completely resolve (Schuckit 1984). Metabolism takes place primarily in the liver by oxidation, hydroxylation, and conjugation with glucuronic acid (Wong and Biemann 1976). Only a small amount of the active drug is excreted directly in the urine.

Phencyclidine and analogs such as ketamine have multiple effects on the central nervous system (CNS). They selectively reduce the excitatory actions of glutamate on CNS neurons mediated by the *N*-methyl-D-aspartate (NMDA) receptor complex (Anis et al. 1983). These receptors are involved in synaptic transmission, long-term potentiation, seizure induction, ischemic brain damage, and perhaps neuronal plasticity. But phencyclidine's behavioral effects are not due simply to interaction with the NMDA-operated ion channel (Johnson and Jones 1990). Phencyclidine affects σ and μ opioid receptors (Giannini et al. 1984), blocks dopamine uptake (Bowyer et al. 1984), and inhibits serotonin uptake (Smith et al. 1977). Further elucidation of phencyclidine's action on these binding sites may play an important role in our understanding of its effects and potential benefits.

Clinically, the CNS effects result in a rise in blood pressure, heart rate, and respiratory rate. These catecholamine-mediated actions may be related to the panic reactions sometimes seen in persons who use phencyclidine. The effect of phencyclidine on reflexes probably leads to muscle rigidity, and its cholinergic effects lead to sweating, flushing, drooling, and pupillary constriction. Its serotonergic effects cause dizziness, incoordination, slurred speech, and nystagmus. Phencyclidine has been shown to bind to specific receptors in the liver, kidney, lung, heart, and brain (Weinstein et al. 1981).

Phencyclidine produces brief dissociative psychotic reactions similar to schizophrenic psychoses. These reactions are characterized by changes in body image, thought disorder, depersonalization, and autism. When taking higher doses, subjects have great difficulty differentiating between themselves and their surroundings. Other persons using phencyclidine will experience hostility, paranoia, violence, and preoccupation with death. Differences in the response to phencyclidine may be dose-related or based on the individual response of the user (National Institute on Drug Abuse 1979). The phencyclidine experience is regarded as pleasant only half the time and as negative or aversive the rest of the time, but many chronic users report that the unpredictability of the effects is one of its attractive features (Carroll 1985).

On the street, phencyclidine has been known by many names, such as "Angel Dust," "PCP," "Peace Pill," and "horse tranquilizer." The abundance of street names is probably related to the initial lack of popularity of the oral route. It has been suggested that a new drug with a bizarre name that is smoked or snorted can be assumed to be phencyclidine until proved otherwise.

Phencyclidine Intoxication

Clinical Characteristics and Diagnosis

Diagnosis of arylcyclohexylamine intoxication is based on behavioral changes that occur following ingestion of phencyclidine: belligerence, assaultiveness, impulsiveness, unpredictability, psychomotor agitation, and impaired judgment. Low-dose intoxication (5–10 mg) results in agitation, excitement, catalepsy, and mutism (Burns and Lerner 1976). With severe phencyclidine intoxication, patients are unresponsive and comatose, but their eyes remain open (Pearlson 1981). Although not discrete from one another, three stages for phencyclidine intoxication (Rappolt et al. 1980) have been described, depending on the dose taken: the stage of behavioral toxicity, the stuporous stage, and the comatose stage (Table 28–1). The patient may fluctuate between the stuporous stage and the behavioral toxicity stage over a 1- to 2-hour period. The comatose stage may last from 1 to 4 days, depending on the dose taken and the rate of excretion.

The differential diagnosis for phencyclidine intoxication should include head trauma, schizophrenia or acute psychosis, organic brain syndrome, mania, cerebrovascular accident, coma of metabolic origin, or other drug overdose. The presence of ataxia and nystagmus and the absence of dilated pupils are useful in ruling out the CNS stimulants and lysergic acid diethylamide (LSD) when evaluating the acutely agitated and confused patient. Phencyclidine is the only drug of abuse that causes a characteristic vertical nystagmus, although it can cause horizontal or rotary nystagmus as well. The presence of hyperreflexia and hypertension differentiates phencyclidine intoxication from sedative-hypnotic intoxication (National Institute on Drug Abuse 1979), although these signs may be present in acute withdrawal from sedative-hypnotic medications or alcohol. Naloxone may be given to rule out opioid intoxication.

Toxicology screening of blood and urine samples is important, although reliance on blood levels is hazardous because the active substance may be repeatedly released from fat stores. Phencyclidine testing should be done on body fluids of arrestees who exhibit impulsive, bizarre behavior or who have committed unexplained assaultive acts. Urine with a high pH may cause a false-negative result due to interference with the phencyclidine assay. Phencyclidine can also be detected in hair samples from chronic users (Slawson et al. 1996).

Management of Phencyclidine Intoxication

Because of poor judgment, the patient usually will require protective supervision in a nonstimulating environment that should include protection from self-injury. When possible, a careful history should be taken, including drugs taken, duration of use, time of last dose,

TABLE 28–1. Stages of phencyclidine intoxication

	Stage		
Findings	**1: Behavioral toxicity**	**2: Stupor**	**3: Coma**
Dose	2–5 mg	5–20 mg	>25 mg
Blood level	20–30 ng/mL	90–300 ng/mL	>300 ng/mL
Duration	1–2 hours	1–2 hours	1–4 days
Cognitive	Poor concentration, agitation	Catatonic (but eyes remain open), seizures	Coma, possible status epilepticus
Gaze	Blank stare	Fixed stare or roving eyes	Disconjugate
Pupil response	Variable, often miotic	Reactive	Dilated
Nystagmus	Horizontal, then vertical	Horizontal, vertical, rotary	Horizontal, vertical, rotary
Temperature	98–101°F	101–103°F	103–108°F (malignant hyperthermia)
Blood pressure and heart rate	Mild elevation	25% above normal	Twice normal
Respiration	Mild elevation	25% above normal	Periodic respirations, apnea
Deep tendon reflexes	Clonus	Crossed limb reflexes	Absent
Gag reflex	Increased	Repetitive swallowing, retching	Absent
Corneal reflex	Normal	Absent	Absent
Response to pain	Reduced pinprick sensation	Response only to deep pain	No response to deep pain
Musculature	Rigidity, spasm, ataxia, dysarthria, repetitive movements, grimacing, bruxism	Rigidity, twitching, myoclonus, spasticity	Myoclonus, opisthotonos
Nausea, diaphoresis, drooling	Mild	Moderate	Severe
Electroencephalogram (EEG)	Normal	Delta waves	Theta waves

adverse reactions to drugs, and psychiatric history. Obtaining history from companions or family members may be useful. Belongings should be carefully searched for the presence of drugs or paraphernalia that should be analyzed to assist in making the diagnosis.

Restraints should be avoided; Lahmeyer and Stock (1983) reported that the use of restraints may cause rhabdomyolysis that can lead to acute renal failure. If required, the preferred method of physical restraint for combative patients is total body immobilization by rolling the patient in a sheet (Aronow et al. 1980). Although the "talking down" technique has been used to treat acute hallucinogen reactions, this approach should be avoided in phencyclidine-intoxicated patients because it may intensify agitation.

Most patients with mild to moderate symptoms of acute phencyclidine intoxication will improve rapidly. Intoxicated patients should be observed until their mental status has remained normal for several hours (Baldridge and Bessen 1990). If symptoms continue to diminish and there is no cognitive impairment after 12 hours, the patient may be discharged from the emergency department (Woolf et al. 1980).

There is no specific antagonist for phencyclidine. If phencyclidine is taken orally, a gastric lavage can be done. Residual drug should be removed from the stomach and sent for analysis. An alternative to gastric lavage is the administration of activated charcoal to adsorb the phencyclidine that is secreted back into the acid environment of the stomach. Dialysis is ineffective in removing phencyclidine from the body (Rappolt et al. 1980).

The concentration of phencyclidine in body fluids and tissues is profoundly influenced by pH. Some phencyclidine is retained in fatty tissues and in the brain, where it escapes hepatic metabolism. Acidification of urine increases the excretion rate of phencyclidine roughly 100-fold because the drug is a weak base. Urine acidification is controversial, and the risks and benefits to the individual patient must be weighed before acidification is begun. If acidification is done prior to toxicological screens of urine and blood for the presence of other drugs, excretion and analysis for other drugs (e.g., barbiturates or salicylates) may be adversely affected. Urine acidification is contraindicated in the presence of myoglobinuria, renal insufficiency, severe liver disease, or concomitant abuse of barbiturates or salicylates (Woolf et al. 1980).

One approach to urine acidification is to administer Vitamin C (ascorbic acid) with intravenous fluids. Another approach is to use ammonium chloride. Urine pH needs to be checked two to four times each day. When the pH is 5.5, diuresis should be forced by using furosemide. After the patient regains consciousness, urine acidification should continue for a week by giving cranberry juice along with ammonium chloride (500 mg po qid) or ascorbic acid (1 g po tid). Ammonium chloride should be used with caution, because ammonia breakdown products may burden a damaged liver (Rappolt et al. 1980).

In a patient who is hypertensive secondary to phencyclidine, antihypertensive medications should be administered to reduce the patient's blood pressure. If the patient is severely agitated and poses a potential threat to self or others, haloperidol has been demonstrated to be effective in controlling the agitation. Lorazepam can also be used. Barbiturates may be more efficacious in treating the psychotomimetic effects of phencyclidine-like drugs (Olney et al. 1991).

Complications of Phencyclidine Intoxication

Phencyclidine overdose may initially go undetected as a result of the late onset of action of the orally ingested form. This should be suspected in those whose level of confusion seems to increase rather than decrease with time.

The association of seizures with phencyclidine use has been well documented (Alldredge et al. 1989). No medication is necessary to treat a single seizure; for repeated seizures, diazepam or lorazepam should be administered as needed. With intravenous administration, the duration of action of diazepam is shorter than that of lorazepam. Opisthotonos and acute dystonia usually clear as blood levels of phencyclidine decrease. If the problem persists, diazepam or lorazepam administered intravenously to relax the musculature is often effective.

Hypertension is treated with an intravenous drip of hydralazine (Apresoline) or phentolamine (2–5 mg over 5–10 minutes). For hyperthermia, hypothermic blankets or ice may be used. A urine sample should be obtained from the patient to evaluate for myoglobinuria, and serum should be obtained to test for elevated creatine phosphokinase levels to diagnose rhabdomyolysis, which may induce acute renal failure. Acidification of the urine is contraindicated in the presence of rhabdomyolysis or renal failure (either acute or chronic). Ischemic and hemorrhagic stroke have also been reported in association with phencyclidine (Gorelick 1990; Sloan et al. 1991).

Infants exposed to phencyclidine in utero may have intrauterine growth retardation and may require prolonged hospitalization. They are less likely to be born prematurely than are cocaine-exposed infants (Tabor et al. 1990).

Phencyclidine Delirium

Clinical Characteristics and Diagnosis

Acute delirium is the most common phencyclidine psychiatric syndrome that brings users to medical attention. The acute episode usually lasts 3–8 hours, but duration and severity are dose related. Phencyclidine delirium is characterized by clouded consciousness that waxes and wanes; this fluctuation may be attributable to periodic gastric secretion with enteric reabsorption of the drug (Hurlbut 1991). The clinical picture consists of insomnia, restlessness, hyperactivity, purposeless or bizarre behavior, agitation, and aggression. Initially, alterations of body image occur, with a loss of body boundaries and a sense of unreality. Feelings of estrangement and loneliness follow. The patient's mental state may fluctuate to include paranoia, mania, rapid thought and speech, grandiosity, and emotional lability. Some subjects become catatonic, with dreamlike experiences. Distortion of body image and depersonalization are universal reactions.

Three phases of phencyclidine psychosis have been described, each lasting about 5 days: 1) agitated phase, 2) mixed phase, and 3) resolution phase. Factors reported to influence the duration of each phase include individual susceptibility, degree of exposure to the drug, dosage of antipsychotic, and urine acidification. The psychosis may persist in some persons from 24 hours to several months or even years after the cessation of active phencyclidine use.

A phencyclidine psychosis in the presence of a clear sensorium is rare. It is important to examine the patient for the presence of horizontal or vertical nystagmus, ataxia, or slurred speech. These signs indicate phencyclidine intoxication rather than phencyclidine psychosis.

Management of Phencyclidine Delirium

The goals of treatment should include prevention of injury, facilitation of the excretion of phencyclidine in urine, and the amelioration of psychosis. The patient should be hospitalized in a closed psychiatric unit and assigned to a quiet room. All efforts should be made to avoid physical restraints. Because of the intense physical exertion often associated with the agitation seen in phencyclidine delirium, the patient should be given adequate hydration.

Urine acidification should be initiated and continue for at least 3 days after all evidence of psychosis has disappeared, and most patients will require a 3- to 10-day course of acidification. The use of antacids, which act as alkalinizing agents, should be avoided while attempts are being made to enhance excretion of phencyclidine by acidifying the urine.

Both benzodiazepines and haloperidol have been described as being useful in the treatment of phencyclidine delirium. Rosen et al. (1984) recommended that electroconvulsive therapy (ECT) be tried in psychotic patients who have used phencyclidine if they fail to respond to antipsychotic medications after 1 week of inpatient treatment. Further evidence of ECT's usefulness in phencyclidine-associated psychosis was reported by Grover et al. (1986). Following the resolution of the acute confusional psychotic state, a referral to long-term therapy is important.

There has been increasing interest in using phencyclidine as a model to study schizophrenia. Unlike the psychosis associated with amphetamines, phencyclidine-induced psychosis incorporates elements of both the positive (hallucinations, paranoia) and the negative (emotional withdrawal, motor retardation) symptoms of schizophrenia (Javitt and Zukin 1991). Other researchers have investigated positron-emission tomography of phencyclidine-using patients as a possible drug model for schizophrenia (Wu et al. 1991).

Phencyclidine Organic Mental Disorder

Clinical Characteristics and Diagnosis

Phencyclidine organic mental disorder is a mental impairment believed to result from chronic phencyclidine use. It is characterized by memory deficits and a state of confusion or decreased intellectual functioning with associated assaultiveness. Visual disturbances and speech difficulty, such as blocking (inability to retrieve the proper words), also occur. A differential diagnosis should rule out other possible causes of organicity. The course of the disorder may be quite variable. The reasons for this variability are not clear but may be related to residual drug being released from adipose tissues of the chronic user. The confusional state may last 4–6 weeks. The condition may improve with time if phencyclidine exposure does not recur and if residual phencyclidine is excreted by acidifying the patient's urine.

Management of Phencyclidine Organic Mental Disorder

The basic management plan involves protecting the patient from injury and helping the patient deal with disorientation by using a simple, structured, and supportive approach. Sensory input and stimuli must be kept to a minimum. A nonthreatening environment and nonjudgmental staff are of paramount importance. Excessive stimulation can result in agitation and violent behavior.

Phencyclidine Abuse and Dependence

Clinical Characteristics and Diagnosis

Diagnostic criteria for phencyclidine or similarly acting arylcyclohexylamine abuse include the following:

1. *Pattern of pathological use:* intoxication throughout the day; episodes of delirium or mixed organic mental disorder
2. *Impairment in social or occupational functioning due to substance use:* for example, fights, loss of friends, absence from work, loss of job, or legal difficulties (other than due to a single arrest for possession, purchase, or sale of the substance)
3. *Duration of disturbance of at least 1 month*

These criteria should be supported by the presence of phencyclidine or other arylcyclohexylamines in the blood or urine.

Regular users may spend a significant proportion of their time using the substance and experiencing its effects, sometimes using two to three times per day. Adverse consequences are common, and use frequently continues despite numerous psychological or medical problems. One of the worst problems occurs when individuals engage in dangerous behaviors due to lack of insight and judgment while intoxicated. Often, their behavior is aggressive, and they engage in frequent fights. Therefore, even in the absence of tolerance or withdrawal, there may be sufficient clinical findings to meet the criteria for dependence. Dependent individuals repeatedly fail to fulfill major obligations at school, work, or home. They also may engage in hazardous activities such as operating heavy machinery or a vehicle while intoxicated. This may result in legal difficulties. In addition, significant disruption of the individual's life may occur because of episodes of intoxication or the chaotic lifestyle that is associated with phencyclidine use. Although individuals who meet abuse but not dependence criteria use the drug less frequently, aggressive behavior is common in them as well.

Craving has been described by heavy chronic phencyclidine users. Physical dependence on phencyclidine can develop but probably requires long-term, regular exposure to relatively high levels (Gorelick et al. 1987). Tolerance to the disruptive effects of phencyclidine on operant behavior has been reported. A phencyclidine withdrawal syndrome in humans has not been clearly characterized. Phencyclidine withdrawal has been observed in animals within 4–8 hours after the drug is discontinued. In humans, because of a longer half-life, the withdrawal may not be seen for several days, if at all. Tennant et al. (1981) identified symptoms of depression, drug craving, increased appetite, laziness, and increased need for sleep occurring 1 week to 1 month after termination of drug use. Increased neuromuscular activity and bruxism are common. Diarrhea and abdominal pain have also been described (Balster and Woolverton 1981). Smith and Wesson (1978) reported that a significant number of persons who use phencyclidine experience profound depression from chronic use.

Management of Phencyclidine Abuse and Dependence

Treatment of phencyclidine abuse is often difficult because of patients' strong psychological dependence on the drug (Gorelick et al. 1987). Therapists should be cognizant of the fact that phencyclidine users display a wide range of behaviors, including flattened affect, depression, belligerence, and anxiety. Difficulties of treating phencyclidine abusers include impaired attention span and concentration, emotional lability, impulsiveness, poor group interaction, and low tolerance for confrontation (Bolter 1980). Phencyclidine-abusing individuals tend to be young and immature and have little tolerance for the usual confrontation techniques employed in therapeutic communities (De Angelis and Goldstein 1978). Chronic phencyclidine-abusing individuals exhibit characteristics similar to those of children with learning disabilities. They generally show overt impulsiveness, poor interpersonal relationships, and social maladjustment. These characteristics may be reversible if phencyclidine use stops and appropriate treatment is provided.

Because of the cognitive impairments associated with phencyclidine abuse, the treatment environment should provide a supportive structure. All staff members must be aware of the treatment plan to prevent the patient from playing one staff member against another (splitting). Phencyclidine-abusing patients may not initially join extensively in group therapy, individual therapy, or school or recreation programs. They may be belligerent toward treatment, especially on program entry. However, mixing phencyclidine abusers with other substance abusers appears to make clinical sense, since a majority of phencyclidine abusers and users also abuse other drugs (Gorelick and Wilkins 1989).

The following are important considerations when structuring a program responsive to phencyclidine-abusing patients: 1) there should be minimal confrontation or hostility-provoking behavior by staff; 2) patients should be provided with a nonthreatening, supportive environment in which they can begin to feel comfortable; and 3) minimal patient involvement in specific therapeutic intervention should be anticipated initially. Bolter (1980) suggested that the following management strategies may be effective at the beginning of treatment: 1) establish clear ground rules that are enforced; 2) keep decision making to a minimum; 3) accept some absentmindedness initially—directions may have to be repeated; 4) develop a short list of tasks with a regular routine; 5) avoid stressful situations; and 6) set realistic consequences for both positive and negative behavior and be consistent in the application of these consequences.

Caracci et al. (1983) recommended hospitalization for treatment of phencyclidine-induced depression with suicidal potential, because of poor compliance with regular clinic attendance and the high suicide risk.

During the course of outpatient therapy, educational and nutritional awareness will enhance the level of self-care of the patient. Vocational counseling and training may prove to be beneficial in enhancing self-esteem. Outpatient follow-up treatment is aimed at keeping the patient away from resuming drug use.

Using self-help groups has become an established and essential part of any successful treatment of phencyclidine and other drug dependence. Narcotics Anonymous (NA) groups have begun to gain increasing acceptance of phencyclidine users, and many patients have been able to use NA as part of a recovery program.

De Angelis and Goldstein (1978) found that persons who chronically abuse phencyclidine stay in treatment longer than persons who only occasionally use the drug. Individual, family, couples, and group therapies have been used with some success. Many persons who abuse phencyclidine have a sense of loss of contact with their bodies. Body awareness therapy, yoga, and progressive relaxation techniques help patients focus and help them improve attention span and concentration. Exercise can be helpful in restoring a healthy body image, so patients should be encouraged to seek out athletic activities.

Treatment of phencyclidine dependence and abuse, like all other chemical dependence problems, requires long-term treatment. Persistence and patience on the part of staff are necessary to achieve a satisfactory outcome.

Ketamine

Ketamine (2-[2-chlorophenyl]-2-[methylamino]-cyclohexanone) is a derivative of phencyclidine that was first synthesized in 1965. It also is a dissociative anesthetic that provides safe and effective sedation, analgesia, and amnesia (Harari and Netzer 1994). Ketamine has been used in ambulatory settings for distressing procedures such as dental work or bone marrow biopsies, and it is also used for burn ward procedures or genital examinations of children in cases of suspected sexual abuse. During ketamine anesthesia, respiration is maintained along with protective airway reflexes (gag and cough) so that endotracheal intubation is unnecessary (Green and Johnson 1990). Similar to phencyclidine, ketamine causes temporary increases in blood pressure and intracerebral pressure, as well as transient diplopia and nystagmus (Harari and Netzer 1994). Unlike phencyclidine, ketamine has an established place within the practice of medicine (White et al. 1982). However, it too has been taken for nonmedical recreational use and has potential for severe consequences of abuse.

Like phencyclidine, ketamine acts at the NMDA receptor complex to cause anesthesia as well as a range of behavioral effects. The exact mechanism responsible for ketamine's varied effects has not yet been determined. Research into the role of the NMDA receptor in anesthesia, analgesia, and behavior is ongoing.

Abuse of ketamine is still relatively uncommon. Recreational use has been concentrated among adolescents, often males, and is primarily a "party drug" at underground social events known as "raves," where it may be sold as MDMA (methylenedioxymethamphetamine, or "Ecstasy"). This deception is similar to how phencyclidine was often sold as THC or LSD. Use of ketamine has been concentrated primarily in large cities. Users have often abused or experimented with other drugs, especially hallucinogens (LSD, psilocybin, mescaline, peyote) or phencyclidine. Ketamine is known by several street names, including "ket," "Special K," "Cat Valium," or "Kit-Kat." Because ketamine abuse is still uncommon, there are currently no statistics available about prevalence of ketamine use and abuse in the United States.

There are a variety of routes by which ketamine can be taken: orally, intranasally as a spray or by insufflation ("snorting"), smoking, and injection (either intramuscularly or intravenously). The most common method of use is snorting (Delgarno and Shewan 1996). Once taken, the episode of subjective psychedelic experiences ("trip") lasts about an hour, regardless of route or dose (as long as the dose is at least one-eighth of a gram). The initial onset of effects ("rush") begins 1 to 10 minutes after snorting; however, it begins instantaneously if the drug is injected intravenously. The usual amount of ketamine snorted is comparable to a typical "line" of amphetamine or cocaine, consisting of one-sixteenth to one-fourth of a gram of active drug (Delgarno and Shewan 1996).

Ketamine Intoxication

Clinical Characteristics and Diagnosis

Diagnosis of ketamine intoxication is based on behavioral changes. Confirmation of intoxication is by toxicological analysis of blood or urine samples for the presence of ketamine and/or other drugs. Other causes of behavioral changes should be ruled out, such as intoxication with another drug, an acute psychotic break due to schizophrenia, or traumatic brain injury. These problems are often associated with the population that commonly uses ketamine.

Short-term effects of ketamine include profound changes in consciousness, dramatic feelings of dissociation (spiritual separation from the body), and altered perception that sometimes involves visual hallucinations (Hansen et al. 1988). The experience is described as being very intense, especially for first-time users. The aftereffects of a trip include a general feeling of well-being and relaxation, mild depression, a feeling of being mildly drained or "hung over," and nausea. Some users have reported very lucid dreams between episodes of ketamine use (Delgarno and Shewan 1996).

Multiple complications may occur as a direct result of ketamine use. Snorting may result in nosebleeds, eating or drinking shortly before use results in nausea and vomiting, or the rapid onset of the experience—especially in first-time users—may result in disorientation. Ketamine trips may be accompanied by a panic attack or extreme dissociation. Ketamine can induce a state of virtual helplessness and pronounced lack of coordination (known as "being in a 'K-hole'"), which can be problematic if the user is in a public setting (Jansen 1993). There is also potential for overdose, which is especially dangerous if ketamine is used in combination with depressants such as alcohol (Delgarno and Shewan 1996). Long-term adverse effects include psychological problems (Hurt and Ritchie 1994) such as dysphoria, apathy, or agitation; impairment of short-term memory function (Jansen 1990); and flashbacks (Soyka et al. 1993).

Management of Ketamine Intoxication

Ketamine intoxication should be managed in similar fashion to phencyclidine intoxication. A thorough history and physical examination, along with toxicology screening for the presence of ketamine, are important to establish the diagnosis. Patients with mild to moderate intoxication should improve rapidly with minimal supportive care; most do not even come into contact with the health care system. If the drug was taken orally, a gastric lavage should be performed to recover any pill fragments, then activated charcoal can be given to inactivate and absorb any residual drug in the intestines. Additional supportive care may be required for severe intoxication or overdose. This may require sedation with a benzodiazepine for anxiety, agitation, or harmful behavior. Haloperidol may be given for psychotic features of intoxication. Other complications are treated with additional supportive care, just as with phencyclidine intoxication.

Ketamine Abuse and Dependence

Clinical Characteristics and Diagnosis

Users report that they mainly use ketamine for relaxation, self-exploration, and pleasure (Delgarno and Shewan 1996)—the reasons usually cited for experimentation with phencyclidine or hallucinogens. Tolerance develops rapidly to the desired effects of ketamine, resulting in decreased length of the subjective experience, which necessitates an increase in dosage to maintain the maximal effect of the drug (Hurt and Ritchie 1994). Addicts may quadruple the amount used in order to achieve the full psychedelic experience sought. Despite the rapid development of tolerance to psychedelic effects, withdrawal symptoms do not appear to occur in humans (Delgarno and Shewan 1996), even after a period of daily use. Ketamine has the potential for compulsive, repeated intravenous use (Jansen 1990), and cases of ketamine dependence have been documented (Delgarno and Shewan 1996; Hurt and Ritchie 1994). Most ketamine users appear to be recreational users without developing dependence. One explanation is that the sheer intensity of the ketamine experience precludes frequent use (Delgarno and Shewan 1996). Another reason that dependence is not seen more often is that the scarcity of the drug renders addiction difficult (Delgarno and Shewan 1996). Ketamine is available on the street primarily through diversion from legitimate sources, such as hospitals or veterinary clinics.

Management of Ketamine Abuse and Dependence

Treatment of ketamine abuse and dependence is often difficult due to the young age of most users and polysubstance abuse. Ketamine dependence is uncommon, so there is very little literature available about appropriate long-term treatment strategies. Ketamine abuse and dependence are treated very much like phencyclidine abuse and dependence as described previously, since the population of users of these drugs is very similar. Successful treatment involves a supportive environment in a structured program.

References

Alldredge BK, Lowenstein DH, Simon RP: Seizures associated with recreational drug abuse. Neurology 39:1037–1039, 1989

Anis NA, Berry SC, Burton N, et al: The dissociative anesthetics ketamine and phencyclidine selectively reduce excitation of central mammalian neurons by N-methyl-D-aspartate. Br J Pharmacol 79:565–575, 1983

Aronow R, Miceli JN, Done AK: A therapeutic approach to the acutely overdosed PCP patient. Journal of Psychedelic Drugs 12:259–267, 1980

Baldridge EB, Bessen HA: Phencyclidine. Emerg Med Clin North Am 8:541–550, 1990

Balster RH, Woolverton WH: Tolerance and dependence to phencyclidine, in Phencyclidine (PCP): Historical and Current Perspectives. Edited by Domino EF. Ann Arbor, MI, NPP Books, 1981, pp 293–306

Bolter A: Issues for inpatient treatment of chronic PCP abuse. Journal of Psychedelic Drugs 12:287–288, 1980

Bowyer JF, Spuhler KP, Weiner N: Effects of phencyclidine, amphetamine and related compounds on dopamine release from and uptake into striatal synaptosomes. J Pharmacol Exp Ther 229:671–680, 1984

Burns RS, Lerner SE: Perspectives: acute phencyclidine intoxication. Clin Toxicol 9:477–501, 1976

Caracci G, Migoni P, Mukherjee S: Phencyclidine abuse and depression. Psychosomatics 24:932–933, 1983

Carroll ME: PCP, the dangerous angel, in The Encyclopedia of Psychoactive Drugs. Edited by Snyder SH. New York, Chelsea House, 1985

Chen G, Ensor CR, Russell D, Bohner B: The pharmacology of 1-(1-phenylcyclohexyl) piperidine HCl. J Pharmacol Exp Ther 127:241–250, 1959

De Angelis GG, Goldstein E: Treatment of adolescent phencyclidine (PCP) abusers. Am J Drug Alcohol Abuse 5:399–414, 1978

Delgarno PJ, Shewan D: Illicit use of ketamine in Scotland. J Psychoactive Drugs 28:191–199, 1996

Giannini AJ, Loiselle RH, Giannini MC, et al: Phencyclidine and the dissociatives. Psychiatr Med 3:197–217, 1984

Gorelick DA, Wilkins JN: Inpatient treatment of PCP abusers and users. Am J Drug Alcohol Abuse 15:1–12, 1989

Gorelick DA, Wilkins JN, Wong C: Diagnosis and treatment of chronic phencyclidine (PCP) abuse, in Phencyclidine: An Update. NIDA Research Monograph 64 (DHHS Publ No [ADM] 87-1443). Edited by Clouet DH. Rockville, MD, National Institute on Drug Abuse, 1987, pp 218–228

Gorelick PB: Stroke from alcohol and drug abuse: a current social peril. Postgrad Med 88:171–174, 177–178, 1990

Green SM, Johnson SE: Ketamine sedation for pediatric procedures, part 2: review and implications. Ann Emerg Med 19:1033–1046, 1990

Grover D, Yeragani VK, Keshanan MS: Improvement of phencyclidine-associated psychosis with ECT. J Clin Psychiatry 47:477–478, 1986

Hansen G, Jensen SB, Chandresh L, et al: The psychotropic effect of ketamine. J Psychoactive Drugs 20:419–425, 1988

Harari MD, Netzer D: Genital examination under ketamine sedation in cases of suspected sexual abuse. Arch Dis Child 70:197–199, 1994

Hurlbut KM: Drug-induced psychoses. Emerg Med Clin North Am 9:31–52, 1991

Hurt PH, Ritchie EC: A case of ketamine dependence (letter). Am J Psychiatry 151:779, 1994

Jansen KLR: Ketamine—can chronic use impair memory? International Journal of the Addictions 25:133–139, 1990

Jansen KLR: Non-medical use of ketamine (letter). BMJ 306:601–602, 1993

Javitt DC, Zukin SR: Recent advances in the phencyclidine model of schizophrenia. Am J Psychiatry 148:1301–1308, 1991

Johnson KM, Jones SM: Neuropharmacology of phencyclidine: basic mechanisms and therapeutic potential. Annu Rev Pharmacol Toxicol 30:707–750, 1990

Lahmeyer HW, Stock PG: Phencyclidine intoxication, physical restraints, and acute renal failure: case report. J Clin Psychiatry 44:184–185, 1983

Meng Y, Lichtman AH, Bridgen DT, Martin BR: Pharmacological potency and biodisposition of phencyclidine via inhalation exposure in mice. Drug Alcohol Depend 43:13–22, 1996

Misra AL, Pontani RB, Bartolomeo J: Persistence of phencyclidine (PCP) and metabolites in brain and adipose tissue and implications for long-lasting behavioral effects. Res Commun Chem Pathol Pharmacol 24:431–445, 1979

National Institute on Drug Abuse: Diagnosis and Treatment of Phencyclidine (PCP) Toxicity. Rockville, MD, National Institute on Drug Abuse, 1979

Olney JW, Labruyere J, Wang G, et al: NMDA antagonist neurotoxicity: mechanism and prevention. Science 254:1515–1518, 1991

Pearlson GD: Psychiatric and medical syndromes associated with phencyclidine (PCP) abuse. Johns Hopkins Med J 148:25–33, 1981

Rappolt RT Sr, Gay GR, Farris RD: Phencyclidine (PCP) intoxication: diagnosis in stages and algorithms of treatment. Clin Toxicol 16:509–529, 1980

Rosen AM, Mukherjee S, Shinbach K: The efficacy of ECT in phencyclidine-induced psychosis. J Clin Psychiatry 45:220–222, 1984

Schnoll SH: Street PCP scene: issues on synthesis and contamination. Journal of Psychedelic Drugs 12:229–233, 1980

Schuckit MA: Drug and Alcohol Abuse: A Clinical Guide to Diagnosis and Treatment, 2nd Edition. New York, Plenum, 1984, pp 152–160

Slawson MH, Wilkins DG, Foltz RL, et al: Quantitative determination of phencyclidine in pigmented and nonpigmented hair by ion-trap mass spectrometry. J Anal Toxicol 20:350–354, 1996

Sloan MA, Kittner SJ, Rigamonti D, et al: Occurrence of stroke associated with use/abuse of drugs. Neurology 41:1358–1364, 1991

Smith DE, Wesson DR: Barbiturate and other sedative hypnotics, in Treatment Aspects of Drug Dependence. New York, CRC Press, 1978, pp 117–130

Smith RC, Meltzer HY, Arora RC, Davis JM: Effect of phencyclidine on 3H-catecholamine and 3H-serotonin uptake in synaptosomal preparations from rat brain. Biochem Pharmacol 26:1435–1439, 1977

Soyka M, Krupinski G, Volki G: Phenomenology of ketamine-induced psychosis. Sucht 5:327–331, 1993

Tabor BL, Smith-Wallace T, Yonekura ML: Perinatal outcome associated with PCP versus cocaine use. Am J Drug Alcohol Abuse 16:337–348, 1990

Tennant FS, Rawson RA, McCann M: Withdrawal from chronic phencyclidine (PCP) dependence with desipramine. Am J Psychiatry 138:845–847, 1981

Thombs DL: A review of PCP abuse trends and perceptions. Public Health Reports, University of Maryland 104:325–328, 1989

Weaver MF, Jarvis MAE, Schnoll SH: Role of the primary care physician in problems of substance abuse. Arch Intern Med 159:913–924, 1999

Weinstein H, Maayuni S, Glick S, et al: Integrated studies on the biochemical, behavioral and molecular pharmacology of phencyclidine: a progress report, in Phencyclidine (PCP): Historical and Current Perspectives. Edited by Domino EF. Ann Arbor, MI, NPP Books, 1981, pp 131–175

White PF, Way WL, Trevor AJ: Ketamine, its pharmacology and therapeutic uses. Anaesthesia 56:119–136, 1982

Wong LK, Biemann K: Metabolites of phencyclidine. Clin Toxicol 9:583–591, 1976

Woolf DS, Vourakis C, Bennett G: Guidelines for management of acute phencyclidine intoxication. Critical Care Update 7:16–24, 1980

Wu JC, Buchsbaum MS, Bunney WE: Positron emission tomography study of phencyclidine users as a possible drug model of schizophrenia. Yakubutsu Seishin Kodo 11:47–48, 1991

Club Drugs

David M. McDowell, M.D.

Methylenedioxymethamphetamine (MDMA), ketamine, and gamma-hydroxybutyrate (GHB) are unique compounds, differing in terms of their pharmacological properties and their phenomenological effects. The common thread linking these disparate drugs is the people who take them. These substances are used throughout the world most frequently by a sophisticated adolescent or "20-something" constituency, and within a subculture of the gay community. The drugs are used and abused widely at urban social gatherings in both commercial and informal settings. They are most commonly used in nightclubs and all-night dance parties known as raves and at gay circuit parties. Attended primarily by affluent gay men, circuit parties are large social gatherings held in many different countries, usually on weekends and holidays. Both raves and circuit parties have become increasingly popular in recent years. Hence, these drugs, which we discuss extensively in this subchapter, and several other drugs, which we describe more briefly, are widely known as club drugs.

Raves have remained a locus where people use drugs. At raves, groups of young people (typically in their teens) dance to rapid, electronically synthesized music that has no lyrics (called techno). These events traditionally take place in unregulated and unlicensed locations such as stadiums, abandoned warehouses, and other clandestine locations. Since the early 1990s, the venues have become increasingly mainstream. At some of these events, as many as 70% of rave participants are using MDMA, ketamine, GHB, or other drugs such as marijuana and lysergic acid diethylamide (LSD) (McDowell and Kleber 1994). A recent study done at a circuit party revealed that more than 80% of the attendees had taken illicit drugs that day; the average number used was three substances (S. Lee and D. McDowell, "The Pattern and Incidence of Drug Use at a 'Circuit Party'" [manuscript submitted for publication], 1999).

This chapter subpart is a revised version of my chapter "MDMA, Ketamine, GHB, and the 'Club Drug' Scene," which appeared in Galanter MA, Kleber HD (eds): *The American Psychiatric Press Textbook of Substance Abuse Treatment,* 2nd Edition. Washington, DC, American Psychiatric Press, 1999, pp. 295–305.

Methylenedioxymethamphetamine

MDMA, better known as "Ecstasy," has also been known as "Adam," "XTC," and "X." A synthetic amphetamine analog with stimulant properties, the drug is easily distinguishable from chemically related substances in terms of its subjective effects (Hermle et al. 1993; Shulgin 1986). Recreational use of MDMA has been illegal since it was made a Schedule I drug on July 1, 1985. Despite its illegal status, the use of MDMA has skyrocketed in the past several years (Cohen 1998). MDMA damages brain serotonin (5-HT) neurons in laboratory animals (McCann and Ricaurte 1993). Although it is not known definitively whether MDMA is neurotoxic to humans, the weight of current scientific evidence indicates that this is probably the case (Gold and Miller 1997; Sprague et al. 1998). MDMA's appeal rests primarily on its psychological effect, a dramatic and consistent ability to induce in the user a profound feeling of attachment and connection. The compound's street name is perhaps a misnomer; the Los Angeles drug dealer who coined the term Ecstasy wanted to call the drug "Empathy" but asked, "Who would know what that means?" (Eisner 1986).

MDMA was patented in 1914 by Merck in Darmstadt, Germany (Shulgin 1990). The drug was not, as is sometimes thought, intended as an appetite suppressant but was originally developed as an experimental compound. MDMA was first used by humans probably in the late 1960s. It was discovered as a recreational drug by free-thinking pop aficionados ("New Age seekers"), people who liked its properties of inducing feelings of well-being and connection (Watson and Beck 1986). Given MDMA's capacity to induce feelings of warmth and openness, a number of practitioners and researchers interested in insight-oriented psychotherapy believed that it would be an ideal agent to enhance the therapeutic process. Before sale and use of the compound became illegal in 1985, it was used extensively for this purpose (Beck 1990). In the early 1980s, MDMA became increasingly popular. In 1989, production reached at least 30,000 tablets per month. The drug's capacity to induce feelings of connection as well as a psychomotor agitation that could be pleasurably relieved by dancing made it the ideal "party drug."

Despite widespread use during the early 1980s, the drug did not attract much attention from the media or from law enforcement officials. Until 1985, MDMA was not scheduled or regulated and was completely legal. A distribution network in Texas began an aggressive marketing campaign, and for a time, the drug was available over the counter at bars, at convenience stores, and even through a toll-free number. This widespread distribution attracted the attention of then–Texas Senator Lloyd Bensen. He petitioned the U.S. Food and Drug Administration (FDA), and the compound was placed on Schedule I on an emergency basis as of July 1, 1985. A series of three hearings was scheduled to determine MDMA's permanent status. The compound's possible neurotoxicity, combined with concern about illicit drug use in general, resulted in MDMA's permanent placement on Schedule I. Its clinical use is prohibited, and because of the intense regulation of Schedule I compounds, research with MDMA is very difficult to arrange. It remains on Schedule I today, and although some individuals believe that the drug should be more widely available for research, its status will not likely change in the foreseeable future (Cohen 1998).

Synthesis of MDMA is relatively simple and thus is often performed in illicit laboratories or even in domestic locations such as garages. In addition, the compound is often cut with other substances so that the purity varies substantially. In England, impure MDMA is known as "Snide-E." It currently sells in urban areas for $25–$35 for a 125-mg tablet, which produces the sought-after effect in most intermittent users (Green et al. 1995).

MDMA is usually ingested orally. Other methods of administration are much less popular. The usual single dose is 100–150 mg. The onset of effect begins about 20–40 minutes after ingestion and is experienced as a sudden, amphetamine-like "rush." Nausea, usually mild but sometimes severe enough to cause vomiting, often accompanies this initial feeling. The plateau stage of drug effects lasts 3–4 hours. The principal desired effect, according to most users, is a profound feeling of relatedness. Most users experience this feeling as a powerful connection to those around them, but this may include the larger world. In general, people taking the drug appear to be less aggressive and less impulsive. Users also experience a drastically altered perception of time and a decreased inclination to perform mental and physical tasks (Leister et al. 1992). Although the desire for sex can increase, the ability to achieve arousal and orgasm is greatly diminished (Buffum and Moser 1986). MDMA has thus been termed a sensual rather than a sexual drug. In addition, people taking the drug experience mild psychomotor restlessness, bruxism, trismus, anorexia, diaphoresis, hot flashes, tremor, and piloerection (Peroutka et al. 1988).

Common aftereffects can be pronounced, sometimes lasting 24 hours or more. The most dramatic *hangover effect* is a sometimes-severe anhedonia. The hangover effects of MDMA have many similarities with amphetamine withdrawal. MDMA users can experience lethargy, anorexia, decreased motivation, sleepiness, depressed mood, and fatigue, occasionally lasting for days. In a few instances, more severe effects have been reported, including altered mental status, convulsions, hypo- or hyperthermia, severe changes in blood pressure, tachycardia, coagulopathy, acute renal failure, hepatotoxicity, and death (Demirkiran et al. 1996).

There are numerous case reports of a single dose of MDMA precipitating severe psychiatric illness. MDMA probably induces a range of depressive symptoms and anxiety in some individuals, and for that reason, people with affective illness should be specifically cautioned about the dangers of using MDMA (McCann et al. 1994). Many of these reports represent single cases, and there may be other explanations for these occurrences. Still, the growing number of such adverse events is cause for concern.

MDMA's primary mechanism of action is as an indirect serotonergic agonist (Ames and Wirshing 1993). However, MDMA is considered a "messy drug" because it affects serotonin- and dopamine-containing neurons and a host of other neurotransmitter systems (Rattray 1991). MDMA is taken up by the serotonin cell through an active channel where it induces the release of serotonin stores. The drug also blocks reuptake of serotonin, contributing to its length of action. Although it inhibits the synthesis of new serotonin, this is an aftereffect and does not contribute to the intoxication phase. It may, however, contribute to sustained feelings of depression reported by some users and to a diminished magnitude of subjective effects when the next dose is taken within a few days of the first dose.

People who use MDMA on a regular basis tend not to increase their use as time goes on (Peroutka 1990). Because the drug depletes serotonin stores and inhibits synthesis of new serotonin, subsequent doses produce a diminished high and worsening of the drug's undesirable effects such as psychomotor restlessness and teeth gnashing. Many users who are at first enamored with the drug subsequently lose interest, usually citing the substantial side effects. An adage about Ecstasy reported on college campuses captures this phenomenon: "Freshmen love it, sophomores like it, juniors are ambivalent, and seniors are afraid of it" (Eisner 1993, p. 6). Those who continue to use the drug over longer periods of time usually tend to take the drug only periodically. MDMA's effects can be characterized as short term (lasting less than 24 hours) and long term (lasting more than 24 hours) (McKenna and Peroutka 1990).

In laboratory animals, ingestion of MDMA causes a decrease in the serum and spinal fluid levels of 5-hydroxyindoleacetic acid (5-HIAA) in a dose-dependent fashion (Shulgin 1990) and damages brain serotonin neurons (McCann and Ricaurte 1993). The dosage necessary to cause permanent damage to most rodent species is many times greater than that normally ingested by humans (Shulgin 1990). In nonhuman primates, the neurotoxic dosage approximates the recreational dosage taken by humans (McCann and Ricaurte I993). Like its close structural relative methylenedioxyamphetamine (MDA or "Eve"), MDMA has been found to damage serotonin neurons in all animal species tested to date (McCann et al. 1996). The closer a given mammal is phylogenetically to humans, the less MDMA is required to induce this permanent damage. Unequivocal data demonstrating that similar changes occur in the human brain do not exist, but the indirect clinical evidence is disconcerting (Green et al. 1995). For example, clear deficits and major neurotoxicity appear to be related to total cumulative dose in animals (Gold and Miller 1997). In addition, MDMA produces a 30%–35% drop in serotonin metabolism in humans (McCann et al. 1994). Even one dose of MDMA may cause lasting damage to the serotonin system. Furthermore, such damage might become apparent only with time or under conditions of stress. Users with no initial complications may nonetheless manifest problems over time (McCann et al. 1996). There have been reports of individuals with lasting neuropsychiatric disturbances after MDMA use (Creighton et al. 1991; McCann and Ricaurte 1991; Schifano 1991). Recently, there have been compelling reports of MDMA's negative effects on a variety of neurological measures (Burgess et al. 2000; Ricaurte et al. 2000; Schifano 2000). Until the full effect of widespread MDMA use is known, the risks must be taken seriously. The drug's potential neurotoxicity is the most significant concern about its use.

The treatment of MDMA abuse may be divided into the treatment of acute reactions to the drug and the treatment of chronic abuse. As discussed earlier, dehydration, coupled with the direct effects of MDMA, may be life threatening. The clinical characteristics of acute MDMA reactions resemble a combination of the serotonin syndrome and neuroleptic malignant syndrome (NMS). Caution should be used in adding antipsychotics for behavioral restraint, because these may exacerbate the syndrome. If the syndrome is treated aggressively and effectively, the patient usually recovers in a matter of days, although it may take longer; recovery is obviously impeded if more significant organ failure has occurred.

MDMA intoxication is associated with a number of psychiatric symptoms, particularly anxiety, panic, and depression. These symptoms are usually short-term sequelae and subside in a matter of days. Support and reassurance are often all that is needed to help the individual through this difficult time. If the symptoms are severe, brief pharmacotherapy, probably with benzodiazepines, is recommended.

Although physiological dependence on MDMA does not occur, some individuals use the drug compulsively and can be said to be dependent on it. For them, the standard approaches used in substance abuse treatment are recommended. These patients can be difficult to work with for many reasons. They are usually adolescents, and the many complications involved with this population must be considered (McDowell and Spitz 1999). Furthermore, they are more likely to be involved with the subculture that surrounds the drug, so that the very identity of the adolescent will need to be addressed in treatment. Healthy recreational alternatives need to be identified. Another complicating factor is that MDMA is often viewed as relatively benign in comparison with other drugs (Beck and Rosenbaum 1994). As a result and in contrast to the case for drugs that have more negative reputations, there is little urgency among the general public to eradicate MDMA.

Ketamine

Ketamine, also known as "Special K," "Super K," "Vitamin K," or just plain "K," has enjoyed a resurgence in popularity in recent years. Ketamine is a dissociative anesthetic. As its name implies, the drug causes a dose-dependent dissociative episode with feelings of fragmentation, detachment, and what one user described as "psychic/physical/spiritual scatter." It induces a lack of responsive awareness not only to pain but to the general environment, without a corresponding depression of autonomic reflexes and vital centers in the diencephalon. Someone who has recently used ketamine may exhibit catatonia, a flat face, an open mouth, fixed staring with dilated pupils ("sightless staring"), and rigid posturing. At higher dosages, the user enters a catatonic state colloquially known as a "K-hole" and characterized by social withdrawal, autistic behavior, an inability to maintain a cognitive set, impoverished and idiosyncratic thought patterns, and bizarre responses. Motor impairment is a marked feature of this state, and people in a K-hole are found on the edge of the dance floor, staring blankly into space, appearing nondistressed but seemingly incapable of communication.

Because of its high therapeutic index, only severe overdose presents substantial risk of significant morbidity and mortality and, as such, should be treated in the intensive care unit. Perhaps the most dangerous effects of ketamine are behavioral. Individuals may become withdrawn, paranoid, and very uncoordinated. In such cases, the physician must treat the overdose symptomatically, usually with calm reassurance and an environment as free from stimuli as possible.

Ketamine is an addictive drug. It is reinforcing in the classical sense. Numerous reports exist of individuals who became dependent on the drug and use it daily (Galloway et al. 1997). Such dependence should be treated in whatever traditional manner seems most appropriate. The clinician should evaluate the patient for any underlying psychiatric condition, and if such a condition is not found, then individual treatment should focus on the drug use issues. Readers wishing to learn more about the basic science of ketamine are referred to the excellent subchapter by Weaver and Schnoll.

Gamma-Hydroxybutyrate

GHB is sold as "liquid Ecstasy" and, in Great Britain, as "GBH" (for "grievous bodily harm"). It is found naturally in many mammalian cells. In the brain, the highest amounts are found in the hypothalamus and basal ganglia (Gallimberti et al. 1989). It may function as a neurotransmitter (Galloway et al. 1997). GHB is closely linked to gamma-aminobutyric acid (GABA) and is both a precursor and a metabolite of GABA. GHB, however, does not act directly on GABA receptor sites (Chin et al. 1992).

In the 1970s, GHB was used with little fanfare as a sleep aid. It has some demonstrated therapeutic efficacy, particularly in the treatment of narcolepsy (Lammers et al. 1993; Scrima et al. 1990). In addition, bodybuilders sometimes use it, hoping it will promote muscle growth because it increases episodic secretion of growth hormone. In 1990, after reports indicated that GHB may have contributed to the hospitalization of several California youths, it was banned by the FDA. Because it has not been scheduled by the Drug Enforcement Agency as a drug, *possession* of it is legal. Manufacturing GHB for sale to laboratories for research purposes or for sale to the public is prohibited by law.

In some European countries, GHB is available by prescription. Most of the GHB sold in the United States is of the bootleg variety, manufactured by nonprofessional "kitchen chemists." In fact, it is quite easy to manufacture, and several Internet sites are devoted to explaining the process. The unregulated nature of these operations arouses concern about the quality and safety of the GHB available for purchase. GHB has an extremely small therapeutic index, and as little as double the euphorigenic dose may cause serious central nervous system (CNS) depression. In recent years, it has been associated with several incidents of respiratory depression and coma. By the late 1990s, several deaths had been linked to GHB (Li et al. 1998).

GHB was first synthesized in 1960 by Dr. H. Laborit, a French researcher interested in exploring the effects of GABA in the brain. Laborit was attempting to manufacture a GABA-like agent that would cross the blood-brain barrier (Vickers 1969). During the 1980s, GHB was widely available in health food stores. It came to the attention of authorities in the late 1980s as a drug of abuse, and the FDA banned it in 1990 after reports of several poisonings with the drug (Chin et al. 1992). Since then, it has become more widely known as a drug of abuse associated with nightclubs and raves.

GHB is ingested orally, is absorbed rapidly, and reaches peak plasma concentrations in 20–60 minutes (Vickers 1969). The typical recreational dosage is 0.75–1.5 g; higher dosages result in increased effects. The high lasts for no more than 3 hours and reportedly has few lasting effects. Users of the drug report that GHB induces a pleasant state of relaxation and tranquility. Frequently reported effects are placidity, mild euphoria, and a tendency to verbalize. GHB, like MDMA, has been described as a sensual drug. Its effects have been likened to alcohol, another GABA-like drug (McCabe et al. 1971). Users report a feeling of mild numbing and pleasant disinhibition. This disinhibition may account for the reports that GHB enhances the experience of sex. The dose-response curve for GHB is exceedingly steep. The recommended or intoxicating dosage can result in severe adverse effects. The LD_{50} (i.e., lethal dose) is estimated at perhaps only five times the intoxicating dose (Vickers 1969). Furthermore, the drug has synergistic effects with alcohol and probably with other drugs. Therefore, small increases in the amount ingested may lead to significant intensification of the effects and to the onset of CNS depression. Overdose is a real danger. Users consuming alcohol, which impairs judgment and with which synergy is likely, are at even greater risk.

The most commonly experienced side effects of GHB are drowsiness, dizziness, nausea, and vomiting. Less common side effects include weakness, loss of peripheral vision, confusion, agitation, hallucinations, and bradycardia. The drug is a sedative and can produce ataxia and loss of coordination. As doses increase, patients may experience loss of bladder control, temporary amnesia, and sleepwalking. GHB induces a number of physiological and hormonal changes. The consequences of these physiological changes are unclear, as are the overall health consequences for individuals who use GHB.

Clinicians should remember to ask about GHB use, especially in younger people, for whom it has become a drug of choice. Because GHB is not detectable by routine drug screening, this history is that much more important. In cases of acute GHB intoxication, physicians should provide physiological support and maintain a high index of suspicion for intoxication with other drugs. A recent review (Li et al. 1998) suggested the following six features for the management of GHB ingestion with a spontaneously breathing patient:

1. Maintain oxygen supplementation and intravenous access.
2. Maintain comprehensive physiological and cardiac monitoring.

3. Attempt to keep the patient stimulated.
4. Use atropine for persistent symptomatic bradycardia.
5. Admit the patient if he or she is still intoxicated after 6 hours.
6. Discharge the patient if he or she is clinically well in 6 hours.

Often the most dangerous effects of GHB use have occurred with the use of other drugs. For example, concurrent use of sedatives or alcohol may increase the risk of vomiting, aspiration, or cardiopulmonary depression. For this reason, clinicians treating individuals who abuse or are dependent on GHB should be aware of its interactions with other drugs. Most patients who overdose on GHB recover completely if they receive proper medical attention. Some individuals have developed physiological dependence on GHB. The symptoms of withdrawal include anxiety, tremor, insomnia, and "feelings of doom," which may persist for several weeks after stopping the drug (Galloway et al. 1997). This complex of symptomatology suggests that benzodiazepines may be useful in treating GHB withdrawal. Currently, however, no well-controlled studies have examined the use of these or any other agents in the management of GHB withdrawal symptoms.

Conclusions

MDMA, ketamine, and GHB are by no means the only drugs found at clubs, raves, or circuit parties. They are, however, the most emblematic. Attendees also use more traditional drugs such as LSD and other hallucinogens. Marijuana is perennially popular, and alcohol use is also common. Some drug users have begun to experiment with flunitrazepam, a short-acting benzodiazepine better known by its street names, "Rohypnol," "Roofies," or "Ro." Because of the ability of this drug to interfere with short-term memory, it has become known in the media as the "date-rape drug." Slipped into the drink of an unsuspecting individual, it may indeed make the person feel very disinhibited and unable to remember much of what happened after ingestion. Furthermore, each week seems to bring a report of some "new" drug of abuse. Often this is just an older, well-known drug, packaged differently or with a new name. These drugs are used at clubs, often in combination, and often by very young people. This circumstance is cause for concern, for several reasons. The younger a person is when he or she begins to use drugs, and the more often he or she uses them, the more likely he or she is to develop serious problems with these or other substances. In the future we are likely to see more and more use of such drugs and the problems that come with their use.

References

Ames D, Wirshing W: Ecstasy, the serotonin syndrome, and neuroleptic malignant syndrome—a possible link? JAMA 269:869–870, 1993

Beck J: The public health implications of MDMA use, in Ecstasy: the Clinical, Pharmacological and Neurotoxicological Effects of the Drug MDMA. Edited by Peroutka S. Boston, MA, Kluwer Academic, 1990, pp 77–103

Beck J, Rosenbaum M: Pursuit of Ecstasy: The MDMA Experience. SUNY Series in New Social Studies on Alcohol and Drugs. New York, State University of New York Press, 1994

Buffum J, Moser C: MDMA and human sexual function. J Psychoactive Drugs 18:355–359, 1986

Burgess C, O'Donohoe A, Gill M: Agony and ecstasy: a review of MDMA effects and toxicity. Eur Psychiatry 15:287–294, 2000

Chin MY, Kreutzer RA, Dyer JE: Acute poisoning from gamma-hydroxybutyrate in California. West J Med 156:380–384, 1992

Cohen RS: The Love Drug: Marching to the Beat of Ecstasy. Binghamton, NY, Haworth, 1998

Creighton FJ, Black DL, Hyde CE: 'Ecstasy' psychosis and flashbacks. Br J Psychiatry 159:713–715, 1991

Demirkiran M, Jankovic J, Dean JM: Ecstasy intoxication: an overlap between serotonin syndrome and neuroleptic malignant syndrome. Clin Neuropharmacol 19:157–164, 1996

Eisner B: Ecstasy: The MDMA Story. Boston, MA, Little, Brown, 1986

Eisner B: Ecstasy: The MDMA Story, 2nd Expanded Edition. Berkeley, CA, Ronin Publishing, 1993

Gallimberti L, Gentile N, Cibin M, et al: Gamma-hydroxybutyric acid for treatment of alcohol withdrawal syndrome. Lancet 2(8666):787–789, 1989

Galloway GP, Frederick SL, Staggers FE, et al: Gamma-hydroxybutyrate: an emerging drug of abuse that causes physical dependence. Addiction 92:89–96, 1997

Gold M, Miller N: Intoxication and withdrawal from marijuana, LSD, and MDMA, in Manual of Therapeutics for Addictions. Edited by Miller N, Gold M, Smith D. New York, Wiley, 1997, pp 71–89

Green AR, Cross AJ, Goodwin GM: Review of the pharmacology and clinical pharmacology of 3,4-methylenedioxymethamphetamine (MDMA or "Ecstasy"). Psychopharmacology (Berl) 119:247–260, 1995

Hermle L, Spitzer M, Borchardt K, et al: Psychological effects of MDE in normal subjects. Neuropsychopharmacology 8:171–176, 1993

Lammers GJ, Arends J, Deckerck AC, et al: Gamma-hydroxybutyrate and narcolepsy: a double blind placebo controlled study. Sleep 16:216–220, 1993

Leister M, Grob C, Bravo G, et al: Phenomenology and sequelae of 3,4-methylenedioxymethamphetamine use. J Nerv Ment Dis 180:345–354, 1992

Li J, Stokes S, Woeckener A: A tale of novel intoxication. a review of the effects of γ-hydroxybutyric acid with recommendations for management. Ann Emerg Med 31:729–736, 1998

McCabe E, Layne E, Sayler D, et al: Synergy of ethanol and a natural soporific: gamma hydroxybutyrate. Science 71:404–406, 1971

McCann U, Ricaurte G: Lasting neuropsychiatric sequelae of methylenedioxymethamphetamine ("Ecstasy") in recreational users. J Clin Psychopharmacol 11:302–305, 1991

McCann U, Ricaurte G: Reinforcing subjective effects of 3,4-methylenedioxymethamphetamine ("Ecstasy") may be separable from its neurotoxic actions: clinical evidence. J Clin Psychopharmacol 13:214–217, 1993

McCann UD, Ridenour A, Shaham Y, et al: Serotonin neurotoxicity after (+/–)3,4-methylenedioxymethamphetamine (MDMA; "Ecstasy"): a controlled study in humans. Neuropsychopharmacology 10:129–138, 1994

McCann U, Slate S, Ricaurte G: Adverse reactions with 3,4-methylenedioxymethamphetamine (MDMA; "Ecstasy"). Drug Saf 15:107–115, 1996

McDowell D, Kleber H: MDMA, its history and pharmacology. Psychiatric Annals 24:127–130, 1994

McDowell D, Spitz H: Substance Abuse: From Principles to Practice. New York, Brunner/Mazel, 1999

McKenna D, Peroutka S: The neurochemistry and neurotoxicity of 3,4-methylenedioxymethamphetamine, "Ecstasy." J Neurochem 54:14–22, 1990

Peroutka S (ed): Ecstasy: The Clinical, Pharmacological and Neurotoxicological Effects of the Drug MDMA. Boston, MA, Kluwer Academic, 1990

Peroutka SJ, Newman H, Harris H: Subjective effects of 3,4-methylenedioxymethamphetamine in recreational abusers. Neuropsychopharmacology 1:273–277, 1988

Rattray M: Ecstasy: towards an understanding of the biochemical basis of the actions of MDMA. Essays Biochem 26:77–87, 1991

Ricaurte GA, Yuan J, McCann UD: (+/-)3,4-Methylenedioxymethamphetamine ('Ecstasy')-induced serotonin neurotoxicity: studies in animals. Neuropsychobiology 42:5–10, 2000

Schifano F: Chronic atypical psychosis associated with MDMA ("Ecstasy") abuse (letter). Lancet 338:1335, 1991

Schifano F: Potential human neurotoxicity of MDMA ('Ecstasy'): subjective self-reports, evidence from an Italian drug addiction centre and clinical case studies. Neuropsychobiology 42:25–33, 2000

Scrima L, Hartman P, Johnson F, et al: The effects of gamma-hydroxybutyrate on the sleep of narcolepsy patients: a double-blind study. Sleep 13:479–490, 1990

Shulgin A: The background and chemistry of MDMA. J Psychoactive Drugs 18:291–304, 1986

Shulgin A: History of MDMA, in Ecstasy: the Clinical, Pharmacological and Neurotoxicological Effects of the Drug MDMA. Edited by Peroutka S. Boston, MA, Kluwer Academic, 1990, pp 1–20

Sprague JE, Everman SL, Nichols DE: An integrated hypothesis for the serotonergic axonal loss induced by 3,4-methylenedioxymethamphetamine. Neurotoxicology 19:427–441, 1998

Vickers MD: Gamma-hydroxybutyric acid. Int Anaesthesiol Clin 71:75–89, 1969

Watson L, Beck J: New Age seekers: MDMA use as an adjunct to spiritual pursuit. J Psychoactive Drugs 23:261–270, 1986

Nicotine Withdrawal and Dependence

Lori Pbert, Ph.D.
Sarah Reiff-Hekking, Ph.D.
Judith K. Ockene, Ph.D.

Cigarette smoking is the leading preventable cause of illness and death in the United States, causing more than 430,000 deaths in the United States each year (Centers for Disease Control and Prevention 1999b). Forty-eight million adult Americans smoke cigarettes (Centers for Disease Control and Prevention 1999). Individuals with a current or past history of significant psychiatric problems, including depression, schizophrenia, and alcoholism, are much more likely to be smokers than are people in the general population and are less likely to stop smoking (Glassman 1993; Hughes 1995a; Ziedonis et al. 1994). Despite the enormous health consequences associated with smoking, health care professionals, including mental health professionals, often do not assess or treat nicotine dependence as part of routine care, even though there is significant evidence that brief smoking-cessation treatments can be effective (Fiore et al. 2000). Mental health professionals in particular have many opportunities to address both the physiological and the psychological aspects of nicotine dependence during the course of consultations on medical services, within inpatient psychiatric settings, and during psychotherapy.

Although nicotine, the psychoactive substance in tobacco, is not dangerous as an intoxicant, it is a highly addicting substance that may control significant aspects of a person's behavior. Nicotine shares a number of common factors with the other recognized euphoriants (e.g, cocaine, opiates, alcohol). It produces centrally mediated effects on mood and feeling states, is a reinforcer for animals, leads to drug-seeking behavior with deprivation, and shows similar patterns of persistence in the face of evidence that it is highly damaging to health (Benowitz 1983; Fagerstrom 1991; Henningfield 1984). As with other addicting substances, individual variability in the intensity of the dependence is wide, and although a large number of smokers successfully quit on their own, many others can benefit from a variety of interventions now available.

In this chapter subpart we examine current treatment strategies available to the mental health professional and present evidence-based treatment guidelines derived from the Agency for Healthcare Research and Quality's (AHRQ's) "Treating Tobacco Use and Dependence" guideline (Fiore et al. 2000) and the American Psychiatric Association's "Practice Guideline for the Treatment of Patients With Nicotine Dependence" (Hughes et al. 1996). Also discussed is nicotine dependence in combination with special clinical problems: alcoholism and other serious psychiatric disorders, in particular depression.

Diagnostic Criteria

Nicotine dependence is classified as a substance use disorder in DSM-IV (American Psychiatric Association 1994); the DSM-IV diagnostic criteria for nicotine withdrawal are presented in Table 28–2. Smokers who experience more intense withdrawal symptoms during their cessation attempts have a more difficult time stopping smoking (West et al. 1989). Symptoms begin within a few hours of abstinence or significant reduction of tobacco use, increase over 3–4 days, and then gradually decrease over 1–3 weeks (Gritz et al. 1992; Hughes and Hatsukami 1992). Change in appetite and problems with concentration appear to persist longer than do feelings of restlessness and irritability. Persons who take in more nicotine typically have stronger withdrawal symptoms, but considerable variability occurs (Hughes et al. 1990).

TABLE 28–2. DSM-IV diagnostic criteria for nicotine withdrawal

A. Daily use of nicotine for at least several weeks.

B. Abrupt cessation of nicotine use, or reduction in the amount of nicotine used, followed within 24 hours by four (or more) of the following signs:
 (1) dysphoric or depressed mood
 (2) insomnia
 (3) irritability, frustration, or anger
 (4) anxiety
 (5) difficulty concentrating
 (6) restlessness
 (7) decreased heart rate
 (8) increased appetite or weight gain

C. The symptoms in criterion B cause clinically significant distress or impairment in social, occupational, or other important areas of functioning.

D. The symptoms are not due to a general medical condition and are not better accounted for by another mental disorder.

Factors Supporting Smoking Behavior

Knowledge of the factors that affect smoking can help the clinician in deciding which strategies are most appropriate to recommend for a particular smoker. These factors are grouped into three categories: physiological, psychological, and social.

Physiological Factors

Nicotine exerts a number of neurochemical effects on the brain that are believed to contribute to the maintenance of cigarette smoking. It produces noradrenergic effects in the locus coeruleus, which are thought to involve the neurotransmitter norepinephrine and to mediate symptoms of withdrawal such as craving and irritability. Nicotine also exerts dopaminergic effects in the nucleus accumbens, which involve the release of dopamine and result in pleasurable feelings (Leshner 1996; Nisell et al. 1995). The smoker therefore takes in nicotine in order to avoid withdrawal symptoms and to obtain the pleasurable, immediate peripheral and central effects of nicotine (O. Pomerleau and Pomerleau 1984). Investigators have long noted that a smoker's primary use of cigarettes is to regulate emotional states (Tomkins 1966). Early laboratory studies conclude that smoking significantly reduces fluctuations or changes in mood or affect during stress (C. Pomerleau and Pomerleau 1987; Schachter 1978). However, more recent evidence suggests that smokers experience higher stress levels than nonsmokers and recent quitters and that the perceived reduction in tension and stress may be a function of the physiological dependence on nicotine (Parrott 1999). Although desire to end the symptoms of withdrawal largely interferes with initial efforts to quit smoking, the active benefits of nicotine—for example, improved concentration and the anorexic, stimulant, and perceived anxiolytic effects—clearly maintain the desirability of smoking and contribute to relapse for many persons.

Psychological Factors

The pleasurable physiological effects of nicotine become paired with the many activities and emotions associated with smoking (e.g., talking on the phone, driving, being in the work setting, feeling stressed or bored). These situations and emotions become "triggers" for the urge to smoke, and for many people smoking becomes a habitual behavior with little conscious forethought. Evaluating the functional uses of smoking for the person, such as a way to take a break from work or family chores or to handle daily stressors, can help identify areas in which the person will need to develop strategies other than smoking to help him or her function without cigarettes. In addition to identifying triggers, it is important to help the patient increase his or her self-efficacy, or confidence in handling such situations and emotions without cigarettes. Considerable evidence shows that high self-efficacy predicts success in stopping smoking, whether the person is dealing with specific problem situations or with withdrawal symptoms (Ward et al. 1997).

Social Factors

The social and cultural environments of smokers affect their ability to stop smoking. Individuals who experience more social support for cessation and have fewer smokers in their environment are more successful at stopping smoking (Gulliver et al. 1995; Ockene et al. 1982). As the percentage of smokers decreases among more highly educated groups, the "hard core" smoker may continue to smoke despite social pressures against doing so (Kristeller 1994) or may be a member of a social group in which there are social pressures to continue to smoke. The individual who is a member of the latter group and is one of the first in his or her group to stop smoking may have stronger personal reasons to quit than the other group members. Helping such individuals to address the social pressures to continue to smoke or including spouses or significant others in treatment may be particularly useful.

Assessment and Intervention

Assessment and intervention with the smoker are closely integrated, as gathering information about the person's smoking history and current smoking patterns increases self-awareness in a way that facilitates behavior change. To guide the clinician, the AHRQ has developed a clinical practice guideline titled "Treating Tobacco Use and Dependence" (Fiore et al. 2000). This guideline provides an assessment and intervention model for the treatment of nicotine dependence, as well as evidence-based treatment strategies that incorporate the National Cancer Institute's 5A's strategy: Ask, Advise, Assess, Assist, and Arrange follow-up. In the model proposed by AHRQ (Figure 28–1), it is recommended that smoking status be routinely assessed and documented at every clinical contact (Ask). All current smokers should be provided clear, strong, and personalized advice to stop smoking (Advise) and assessed for their willingness to quit at each contact (Assess). For those smokers who are willing to quit, further assessment should occur, taking into account the physiological, psychological, and social factors maintaining their smoking behavior, and brief intervention with follow-up should be provided (Assist and Arrange). When appropriate, referral should be made for more intensive treatment. Smokers who are not willing to quit should receive a brief motivational intervention to facilitate motivation and future quitting efforts. Additionally, individuals who have recently quit should be offered interventions to prevent relapse.

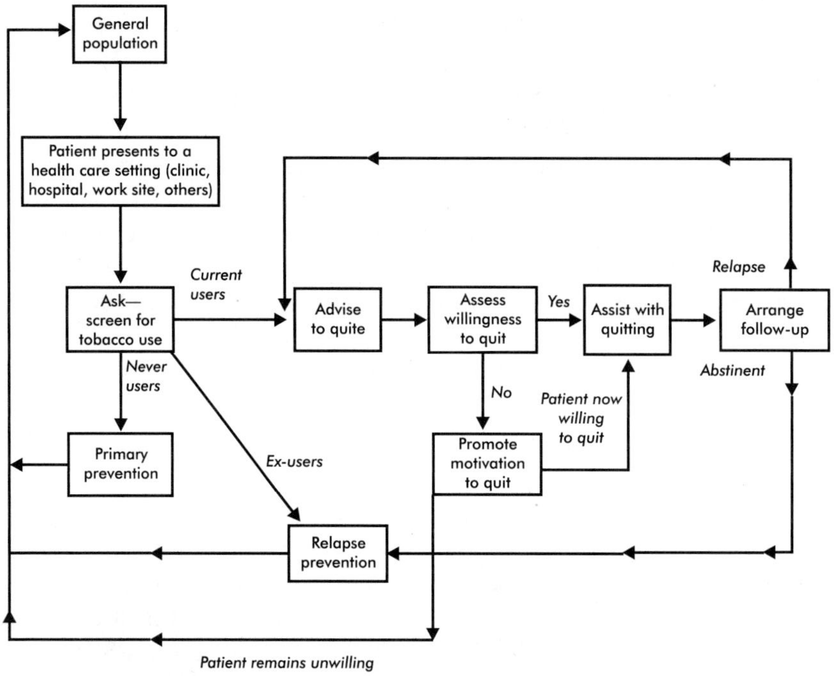

FIGURE 28–1. Model for nicotine dependence assessment and treatment.
Source. Reprinted from Fiore MC, Bailey WC, Cohen SJ, et al.: "Treating Tobacco Use and Dependence." Clinical Practice Guideline. Rockville, MD, U.S. Department of Public Health and Human Services, Public Health Service, Agency for Healthcare Research and Quality, June 2000. Used with permission.

Assessment of Motivation and Readiness to Quit

Once a smoker has been identified through the screening process and provided personalized advice to quit, the clinician will want to assess the person's motivation and readiness to quit. Nicotine dependence is a chronic, relapsing disorder, often requiring 5–7 attempts before maintained abstinence is achieved (U.S. Department of Health and Human Services 1990). Stopping smoking is therefore a long-term process of change that takes place in stages over time. Individuals typically proceed through the following stages of change: 1) precontemplation, 2) contemplation, 3) preparation, 4) action, and 5) maintenance (DiClemente et al. 1991). Different stages of change require different interventions on the part of the clinician.

Approximately 40% of smokers are not thinking about stopping smoking and are said to be in the *precontemplation* stage of change (Velicer et al. 1995). These smokers may be unaware of the risks of smoking, unwilling to consider making a change, or discouraged regarding their ability to quit. Many psychiatric patients fall into this stage of change (R. G. Hall et al. 1995; Ziedonis et al. 1994). For precontemplators, the clinician's goal is to introduce doubts into their intention to continue smoking by stimulating ambivalence, such as by increasing patients' perceptions of the risks and problems associated with their current behavior and the potential benefits of quitting. Exploring what individuals perceive as the positive aspects of smoking can help overcome the natural defensiveness and resistance that often accompany this stage of change. An effective approach with precontemplators is to develop discrepancy—a disconnect—between their reasons for smoking and their reasons for quitting, encouraging them to consider their contradictory beliefs and feelings in a sensitive, nonjudgmental manner.

Another 40% of smokers are ambivalent about stopping smoking. These smokers are in the *contemplation* stage of change (Velicer et al. 1995). They report thinking about quitting and seek information about smoking and stopping but are not ready to commit to quitting and express uncertainty regarding their desire or ability to stop. The clinician's goal with the contemplator is to help him or her to resolve ambivalence by tipping the balance in favor of quitting. Strategies that help with this process include 1) eliciting the smoker's thoughts regarding the potential negative consequences of smoking and benefits of quitting (e.g., personal and family health risks, financial cost, concern regarding role model for children); 2) determining barriers to quitting; 3) reviewing past quit attempts to identify problems that led to relapse and successful coping skills used in the past that can be applied to a future quit attempt; and 4) developing the smoker's confidence in his or her ability to stop smoking. Often, after exploring these issues, the individual may be ready to make a serious quit attempt or at least commit to an intermediate goal, such as reducing the number of cigarettes smoked.

The final 20% of current smokers are ready to stop smoking in the next month and are in the *preparation* stage of change (Velicer et al. 1995). Many of these individuals have made a serious quit attempt in the past year or have taken steps toward stopping, such as telling others of their intent to quit, cutting down on the number of cigarettes smoked, or imagining themselves as nonsmokers. The clinician's goal with the smoker in the preparation stage is to help the individual determine the best course of action to take and develop the strategies and skills needed to make a successful quit attempt. Individuals in the *action* and *maintenance* stages of change are no longer smoking. They are at particular risk for relapse during the action stage, and the best approach is to work on relapse prevention (refer to later section titled "Preventing Relapse and Maintaining Change").

Assisting the Smoker Who Is Ready to Quit

For the smoker who is ready to make a quit attempt, the clinician's role is to provide assistance in developing a quit plan and arranging follow-up to support the individual through the quitting process. In developing an individual treatment plan, the physiological, psychological, and social aspects of the patient's dependence need to be considered. The treatment plan should include the evidence-based strategies identified by the AHRQ clinical practice guideline (Fiore et al. 2000) and summarized in Table 28–3.

TABLE 28–3. Strategies for assisting smokers who are ready to quit

1. Set a *quit date*—preferably within the next 2 weeks.
2. Help patient *prepare for quitting:*
   a. *Inform* family, friends, and co-workers of intent to quit and request support.
   b. *Remove* cigarettes from environment.
   c. *Review* past quit attempts to identify high-risk situations and coping strategies.
   d. Prepare to *address anticipated challenges* to the planned quit attempt, including nicotine withdrawal symptoms.
3. Recommend use of *nicotine replacement therapy or non-nicotine pill, bupropion*, to all smokers unless contraindicated.
4. Give key *advice* regarding successful quitting:
   a. *Abstinence*—Total abstinence is essential.
   b. *Alcohol*—Consider limiting or abstaining from alcohol during the quitting process, as drinking alcohol is highly associated with relapse.
   c. *Other smokers in the household*—Consider quitting with significant others and/or developing specific plans to stay quit in a household where others smoke.
5. Provide *self-help materials.*
6. Schedule *follow-up contact*, either in person or by telephone—preferably during the first week after the quit date:

If abstinent at follow-up:
   a. Congratulate on success.
   b. Address problems encountered and challenges anticipated.
   c. Monitor pharmacological aids used.

If smoking occurred:
   a. Review circumstances leading to smoking.
   b. Elicit recommitment to total abstinence.
   c. Address problems encountered and challenges anticipated.
   d. Review appropriateness of pharmacological aids.
   e. Consider referral to a more intensive, specialized treatment program.

Source. Adapted from Fiore MC, Bailey WC, Cohen SJ, et al.: "Treating Tobacco Use and Dependence." Clinical Practice Guideline. Rockville, MD, U.S. Department of Public Health and Human Services, Public Health Service, Agency for Healthcare Research and Quality, June 2000. Used with permission.

Addressing Physiological Dependence

The AHRQ and American Psychiatric Association clinical practice guidelines provide strong evidence that nicotine replacement therapy and bupropion are effective treatments for nicotine dependence and should be offered to all smokers who are interested in quitting, unless contraindicated (Fiore et al. 2000; Hughes et al. 1996). A formal evaluation of physiological dependence is not necessary in order to recommend pharmacotherapy, but it can provide information on the individual's level of physiological dependence. The Fagerstrom Test for Nicotine Dependence (FTND; Heatherton et al. 1991) (Figure 28–2) is an excellent tool for assessing level of dependence and has demonstrated good reliability and validity (Heatherton et al. 1991). If the smoker reports having had significant withdrawal symptoms during prior quit attempts, has a pattern of relapsing within a few hours or days, and scores high on the FTND, nicotine dependence probably plays an important role in maintaining his or her smoking behavior. For all smokers, and especially highly dependent persons, nicotine fading, nicotine replacement therapy, or non-nicotine medication (bupropion) should be recommended. The clinician's role is to outline the benefits and drawbacks of nicotine fading and the medications available, to screen for contraindications, and to instruct the smoker in the appropriate use of the method or product selected.

Questions	Responses	Points
1. How soon after you wake up do you smoke your first cigarette?	Within 5 minutes	3
	6–30 minutes	2
	31–60 minutes	1
	After 60 minutes	0
2. Do you find it difficult to refrain from smoking in places where it is forbidden, e.g., in church, at the library, at the cinema?	Yes	1
	No	0
3. Which cigarette would you hate most to give up?	The first one in the morning	1
	All others	0
4. How many cigarettes/day do you smoke?	10 or less	0
	11–20	1
	21–30	2
	31 or more	3
5. Do you smoke more frequently during the first hours after waking than during the rest of the day?	Yes	1
	No	0
6. Do you smoke if you are so ill that you are in bed most of the day?	Yes	1
	No	0

FIGURE 28–2. Fagerstrom Test for Nicotine Dependence.
Source. Reprinted from Heatherton T, Kozlowski L, Frecker R, Fagerstrom K: "The Fagerstrom Test for Nicotine Dependence: A Revision of the Fagerstrom Tolerance Questionnaire." *British Journal of Addiction* 86:1119–1127, 1991. Used with permission.

Nicotine Fading: Brand Switching and Gradual Reduction

Nicotine fading (Foxx and Brown 1979) has two components: brand switching to a lower-nicotine-level cigarette and gradual reduction of number of cigarettes smoked. Brand switching to brands with lower nicotine levels one or more times over several weeks, in combination with reducing the number of cigarettes smoked by about one-half per week, can reduce withdrawal symptoms in the person who smokes heavily. However, the evidence does not support the efficacy of brand switching alone (Fiore et al. 2000; Law and

Tang 1995). In fact, a recent study (Massachusetts Department of Public Health 1998) has found that if smokers employ compensation techniques such as vent blocking, puffing more frequently, or inhaling more deeply when smoking lower-nicotine cigarettes, their nicotine yield will be considerably higher than that suggested by Federal Trade Commission ratings. Smokers should be cautioned about this possibility and advised to keep such compensation behaviors to a minimum during the nicotine fading process. On the other hand, contrary to the myth that a smoker needs to quit "cold turkey," there does not appear to be a significant difference in cessation rates between quitting "cold turkey" and gradually reducing the number of cigarettes smoked (Fiore et al. 2000; Hughes 1995b); therefore, patient preference should determine the approach selected. If nicotine fading is used, it should be combined with behavioral management strategies so that "lower need" cigarettes are eliminated first and awareness of the function of each cigarette is increased; this approach also increases the individual's confidence in his or her ability to eventually stop smoking.

Pharmacotherapy

To date, five pharmacological aids have been approved by the FDA for use in the treatment of nicotine dependence. These pharmacotherapies fall into two general categories: nicotine replacement therapies and a non-nicotine pill (bupropion) (refer to Hughes et al. 1999 and the American Psychiatric Association practice guideline [Hughes et al. 1996] for detailed descriptions of each of the products available, and to the clinician and patient product information sheets for product contraindications). It is important to emphasize to smokers that pharmacotherapies are not "magic bullets." Rather, they are used to help minimize or dampen withdrawal symptoms while smokers work to break the conditioned connections between smoking and the activities and emotions of their daily lives and to develop coping skills to replace the many functions of smoking. Table 28–4 provides a summary of the five pharmacological aids currently available.

The purpose of the four nicotine replacement therapies is to prevent or minimize the symptoms of withdrawal or cravings by replacing some of the nicotine that would otherwise be obtained from smoking. This allows the individual to focus on the behavioral and emotional aspects of stopping smoking. Nicotine replacement is then gradually reduced so as to minimize withdrawal symptoms experienced. All four forms of nicotine replacement therapy have been found to be equally efficacious, approximately doubling the quit rates seen with placebo. In most studies, nicotine replacement with concomitant supportive or behavior therapy has produced substantially higher quit rates than has either behavior therapy or nicotine replacement alone (Hughes 1991, 1995b); thus, use of such combinations should be encouraged but not required (Hughes et al. 1999).

Nicotine gum, approved in 1984, became available over the counter in the United States in 1995. Nicotine in the gum is absorbed in the buccal mucosa. The 2-mg gum is recommended for individuals who smoke fewer than 25 cigarettes per day, while the 4-mg gum is recommended for individuals who smoke at least 25 cigarettes per day. Scheduled dosing of 1–2 pieces per hour has been found to be more efficacious than as-needed use (Kilen et al. 1990). Proper chewing technique ("chew and park") is important to maximize the nicotine replacement obtained and to reduce potential side effects. The gum is chewed slowly for about 1 minute, then parked between the cheek and gum for a minute or two, then slowly chewed and parked for 30 minutes. Recommended length of treatment varies from 1 to 6 months.

TABLE 28–4. Comparison of current pharmacotherapies for nicotine dependence treatment

Product	Over-the-counter nicotine patches		Over-the-counter nicotine gum	Prescription nicotine inhaler	Prescription nicotine spray	Prescription bupropion hydrochloride SR tablet
Brand name	Nicotrol CQ	Nicoderm	Nicorette	Nicotrol inhaler	Nicotrol NS	Zyban
Product strengths	15 mg	21 mg, 14 mg, or 7 mg	2 mg, 4 mg	10 mg/cartridge	10 mg/ml	150 mg
Initial dosing	1 patch/16 hours	1 patch/24 or 16 hours	1 piece every 1 to 2 hours	6–16 cartridges/day	1–2 doses/hour (1 dose = 2 sprays or 1 per nostril)	150 mg/day (days 1–3); 300 mg/day (after day 3)
Maximum dosing	Same as above	Same as above	24 pieces/day	16 cartridges/day	5 doses/hour or 40 doses/day	300 mg/day
Time to peak plasma level	5–10 hours	5–10 hours	20–30 minutes	15 minutes	5–7 minutes	3 hours
Manufacturer's recommended treatment duration	6 weeks	10 weeks	12 weeks	12 weeks	12 weeks	7–12 weeks
Adverse reactions	50% experience mild skin reactions (rotate and use steroid cream); vivid dreams, sleep disturbances while on the patch 24 hours (remove at bedtime)		Mouth soreness, hiccups, dyspepsia, and jaw ache (usually mild and transient; correct technique)	40% experience mouth and throat irritation (resolved through regular use); dyspepsia	Local transient irritation in the nose and throat, watery eyes, sneezing and cough	Dry mouth; insomnia (avoid bedtime dose); shakiness and skin rash

TABLE 28–4. Comparison of current pharmacotherapies for nicotine dependence treatment *(continued)*

Product	Over-the-counter nicotine patches		Over-the-counter nicotine gum	Prescription nicotine inhaler	Prescription nicotine spray	Prescription bupropion hydrochloride SR tablet
Unique product contraindications	Severe eczema or other skin diseases that may be exacerbated by the patch; allergy to adhesive tape		Severe temporomandibular joint disease or other jaw problems; presence of dentures or other dental appliances	Allergy to menthol	Asthma, rhinitis, nasal polyps, or sinusitis	Seizure disorder; current use of bupropion (Wellbutrin); current or prior diagnosis of bulimia or anorexia nervosa; concurrent or recent use of monoamine oxidase inhibitors; bupropion allergy
Consumer information	1-800-699-5765	1-800-834-5895	1-800-419-4766	1-800-699-5765	1-800-699-5765	1-800-U-CAN-QUIT

The nicotine transdermal patch provides a more continuous delivery of nicotine than the gum. A patch is applied daily to the upper torso in the morning. Depending on the patch formulation used, it is removed either at bedtime (16-hour patch) or on waking (24-hour patch). Starting doses are 21 mg for the 24-hour patch and 15 mg for the 16-hour patch, with the dose gradually reduced over time. Six to 8 weeks of treatment is reasonable for most smokers, and tapering has not been found to be necessary (Fiore et al. 1994, 1996).

The nicotine inhaler addresses not only physical dependence but also the behavioral and sensory aspects of smoking. It delivers nicotine to the mouth and throat only, not to the lungs, through nicotine vapor inhaled from a plastic cartridge containing a nicotine plug. The recommended dosage is 6–16 cartridges/day for the first 6–12 weeks, followed by gradual reduction of the dose over the next 6–12 weeks. One dose is equivalent to frequent, continuous puffing for 20 minutes.

Nicotine nasal spray delivers nicotine to the bloodstream more rapidly than any other nicotine replacement therapy (although less rapidly than cigarettes), with peak blood levels occurring within 10 minutes of use (Gourlay and Benowitz 1997). Concern was initially raised that the nasal spray might have a significant dependency potential due to the rapid delivery of nicotine (Sutherland et al. 1992), but more recent studies have not found significant abuse liability (Hughes 1998; Schuh et al. 1997). The starting dosage is 1–2 doses/hour (1 dose = 2 sprays), with treatment for up to 8 weeks followed by stopping or tapering the dose for 4–6 weeks.

Bupropion SR (sustained-release bupropion) is an atypical antidepressant believed to work on the neurochemistry of addiction by enhancing dopamine levels and affecting the action of norepinephrine in the brain, both neurotransmitters believed to be involved in nicotine dependence (Ascher et al. 1995). As with nicotine replacement therapies, bupropion has been found to consistently double quit rates compared with placebo. Dosing begins 1 week prior to cessation to achieve steady-state blood levels, with 150 mg/day for the first 3 days, followed by a dose increase to the recommended dosage of 300 mg/day. An interval of at least 8 hours between doses is recommended to reduce the possibility of seizures. The recommended duration of treatment is 7–12 weeks. If the smoker has not made significant progress toward abstinence by the seventh week of therapy, he or she is unlikely to quit during this attempt, and treatment should be discontinued.

Addressing Psychological Dependence: Cognitive and Behavioral Interventions

Cognitive and behavioral interventions for smoking have been developed from cognitive and behavioral techniques used to treat a wide range of behavioral and addictive disorders (Bandura 1969; Goldfried and Davison 1976). Compared with no treatment, these interventions have been found to typically double the quit rates (Fiore et al. 1996; Law and Tang 1995; Schwartz 1992). The cognitive-behavioral approach encompasses assessment and intervention. First, past quit attempts are reviewed to identify reasons for attempting to quit, methods used (e.g., "cold turkey," tapering, pharmacological aids), problems experienced (including withdrawal symptoms), strategies that helped, and factors leading to relapse. The key is to assist the patient in reframing past efforts to stop smoking as learning experiences and to apply what was learned to the current quit attempt. Second, current smoking patterns are assessed. In what situations and in response to what feelings or emotions does the patient most feel like smoking? These are "high need" cigarettes. Asking the smoker to rate the level of need for each cigarette on a scale of 1 (low need) to 5 (high need) is often helpful. Behavioral self-monitoring, in which the patient records the time, place, situation, mood, thoughts, and need level associated with each cigarette smoked, can be very informative for both the patient and the clinician at this stage to identify specific areas requiring further attention.

Once anticipated problems and triggers are identified through review of past quit attempts and assessment of current smoking patterns, the patient can be helped to develop specific cognitive-behavioral coping strategies to address these problems and triggers, such as: 1) anticipate and avoid high-risk situations and cues that bring on an urge to smoke whenever possible; 2) remove oneself from the trigger situation; 3) substitute other behaviors incompatible with smoking cigarettes when urges arise (e.g., taking a walk, going to a smoke-free environment, deep breathing or other relaxation exercise); 4) use assertiveness, refusal skills, and other skills to manage the triggers; and 5) use cognitive restructuring to reshape positive beliefs about smoking or to counteract irrational thinking, replacing maladaptive thoughts with more constructive thoughts.

Addressing Social Influences

Three aspects of social influence are especially important: 1) the number of smokers among the patient's friends, family, and co-workers; 2) the quality of support for cessation that can be expected by the smoker; and 3) the extent to which the smoker is able to be assertive in resisting social pressures to smoke. Exploring the smoker's concerns about being tempted or even directly sabotaged by other smokers is important. Actively engaging the social support of friends, family, and/or co-workers may be easiest for the hospitalized smoker, as such a person is often recognized to have a heightened need to stop smoking. This is a time when a spouse also may try to quit or at least avoid smoking in the person's presence. A smoker may also have little confidence in his or her ability to turn down cigarettes if offered them or to be the first to quit in his or her social group.

Addressing Concerns About Weight Gain

Although the average weight gain for sustained quitters of 5–6 kilograms (Froom et al. 1998) does not present a medical risk equal to smoking a pack of cigarettes a day, weight gain is an issue that is important to many people and that represents a common reason for starting, continuing, and returning to smoking. Several factors have been implicated in weight gain, including an increase in metabolism from nicotine intake (Hofstetter et al. 1986; Perkins 1992), that may result in weight gain during the quitting process even without increased caloric intake (Fiore et al. 2000) and a heightened preference for sweets while smoking (Grunberg 1982). These biological factors, in combination with the use of food as a behavioral substitute, make it important to address weight gain explicitly in most treatment programs (Klesges et al. 1989; Wack and Rodin 1989). However, no published empirically tested treatment has successfully addressed the problem of weight gain while quitting. Dieting while attempting to quit increases the rate of relapse (Ockene et al. 2000). The AHRQ guideline (Fiore et al. 2000) suggests confronting issues of weight gain with patients before they quit and preparing them for the high probability of gaining weight. Additionally, it is important to remind the patient that quitting smoking is the current priority and that support is available if the patient would like to work on weight loss after successful cessation. A focus on weight loss should be delayed until the patient is no longer experiencing withdrawal symptoms and feels secure in his or her ability to remain smoke free. Encouraging patients to engage in sensible lifestyle changes such as increasing physical activity, eating plenty of fruits and vegetables, and avoiding alcohol is also suggested. There is evidence that increasing physical activity can help minimize weight gain and support maintenance (Bock et al. 1999; Froom et al. 1998).

Preventing Relapse and Maintaining Change

A major difficulty in smoking cessation, as with other substance abuse behaviors, is maintenance of the changed behavior. As many as 70% of those who stop smoking relapse within a year, with the strongest predictor of relapse being a slip within a relatively brief period of time (average 18–60 days) after cessation (Ockene et al. 2000). Up to 65% of persons who quit smoking on their own relapse within the first week of cessation (Hughes and Hatsukami 1992). Relapse prevention, a treatment technique originally developed by Marlatt and Gordon (1980) to help prevent relapse to alcohol abuse, has been adapted for use in the treatment of nicotine dependence (Lichtenstein and Brown 1985). However, the success of this approach with smokers is questionable; a recent review by Ockene et al. (2000) found studies showing both positive and negative results. Additionally, a recent meta-analysis (Irvin et al. 1999) concluded that relapse prevention treatment had effects that were strong and reliable for alcohol and polysubstance abuse but were much weaker for smoking. On the basis of a review of the literature, Ockene et al. (2000) made the following recommendations regarding maintenance of smoking cessation: 1) encourage smokers to use more intensive treatment programs, because they are the most effective; 2) although self-help interventions are widely used, they are limited in effectiveness when used alone and should be combined with more intensive interventions; 3) integration of telephone counseling into comprehensive treatments increases access to cessation and maintenance assistance; 4) pharmacotherapy doubles cessation outcomes and should be encouraged; 5) brief clinician-delivered interventions based on the clinical practice guidelines should be delivered routinely, as they increase long-term maintenance; and 6) dieting should be avoided during the quit attempt because it may undermine success in stopping smoking and maintaining abstinence.

Summary of Treatment Recommendations

To stop smoking, a smoker must perceive this change as beneficial and be confident that he or she can stop smoking. From a behavioral perspective, the smoker must learn new skills or enhance old skills that can be used in place of cigarettes to deal with problems as they arise. The person also needs to be able to attribute changes in smoking behavior to personal abilities and skills rather than to willpower or to the external aspects of treatment (Bandura 1977a, 1977b). From a pharmacological perspective, all smokers, and particularly those who demonstrate a high level of physiological dependence on nicotine, would benefit from nicotine replacement therapy or bupropion to allow them to work on the behavioral aspects of quitting while receiving some relief from the physiological withdrawal symptoms. Finally, the patient may benefit from intervention following a lapse to prevent relapse. For a more complete review of cognitive-behavioral interventions for smoking, the reader is directed to the American Psychiatric Association practice guideline (Hughes et al. 1996), the AHRQ clinical practice guideline (Fiore et al. 2000), and the review by Ockene et al. (2000).

Additional Treatment Issues

Smoking and Alcohol

Tobacco use and alcohol abuse are moderately to strongly related (Istvan and Matarazzo 1984; Kozlowski et al. 1993). Among identified alcoholic persons, the incidence of smoking has been 80%–90% in all studies; alcoholic persons also are more likely to smoke heavily (Bien and Burge 1990; Bobo 1989). Consequently, most patients seen in alcohol treatment programs will be smokers, many of them at a level that is acutely health endangering, a circumstance that underscores the need to treat nicotine dependence in this patient population.

Although some individuals in alcohol abuse treatment may be interested in a smoking cessation component to their treatment (Bobo 1989), many believe that attaining sobriety would be more difficult if they were simultaneously trying to stop smoking and become abstinent from alcohol (Bobo and Gilchrist 1983). Data obtained from individuals in substance abuse treatment suggested that it is difficult to quit smoking while undergoing substance abuse treatment but that working on smoking cessation does not increase relapse to alcohol use (Hughes et al. 1996; Kalman 1998). In fact, in some instances smoking cessation has been found to be associated with a *decreased* relapse to alcohol use (Kalman 1998; L. Sobell et al. 1992). Although it does not appear that smoking increases the rate of relapse to alcohol use, there is evidence that nicotine may interact with alcohol to increase tolerance to the more immediate effects of alcohol (e.g., feelings of intoxication) and enhance the reinforcing value of alcohol, thus setting the stage for high-risk drinking (Kalman 1998).

There is support for the notion that smoking may be used as a coping strategy to avoid alcohol use in response to urges to use alcohol during early sobriety (Kalman 1998). Kalman (1998) reviewed this literature and concluded that many alcoholic smokers in alcohol abuse treatment expect that they will smoke to help them remain abstinent from alcohol. Additionally, he noted that alcoholic individuals with greater nicotine dependence 1) more often report that they cope with drinking urges by smoking, 2) are more likely to have stronger urges to smoke when abstaining from alcohol; and 3) are more likely to be concerned about maintaining sobriety while quitting smoking. Kalman summarized this limited literature by stating that smoking cessation will be difficult for alcoholic smokers during the early phases of sobriety. The American Psychiatric Association practice guideline (Hughes et al. 1996) recommended that the timing of smoking cessation in relationship to alcohol abuse treatment should be determined by the patient.

Smoking and Psychiatric Disorders

Increasing attention is being paid to the role of smoking in psychiatric disorders in regard both to the role of the central nervous system effects of nicotine and to the apparent special value of smoking to psychiatric patients (Glassman 1993). Several studies showed a much higher prevalence of smoking in psychiatric populations (i.e., 50%–90%) (Breslau 1995; Hughes and Hatsukami 1986; Mathew et al. 1981; O'Farrell et al. 1983; Pohl et al. 1992), particularly in those with depression (Covey et al. 1998) and schizophrenia (Glassman 1993). The evidence is less clear regarding an increased prevalence in anxiety disorder populations (Glassman 1993; Parrott 1999). Some psychiatric patients may be actively self-medicating through their use of cigarettes (G. H. Hall 1980). There is evidence that smoking interacts with psychoactive medication. As noted by the American Psychiatric Association practice guideline (Hughes et al. 1996), abstinence from smoking increases blood levels of clomipramine, clozapine, desipramine, desmethyldiazepam, doxepin, fluphenazine, haloperidol, imipramine, oxazepam, nortriptyline, and propranolol. The guideline also notes that quitting smoking does not increase blood levels of amitriptyline, chlordiazepoxide, ethanol, lorazepam, midazolam, and triazolam, and that with alprazolam, chlorpromazine, and diazepam the effect of smoking abstinence on blood levels is unclear. In persons with schizophrenia, quitting smoking also may temporarily worsen drug-related movement disorders, and continued smoking may increase the required dosage of antipsychotics (Goff et al. 1992; Hughes et al. 1996; Menza et al. 1991; Newhouse and Hughes 1991).

Patients who are depressed or who have a history of depression are more likely to smoke, are less likely to quit (Anda et al. 1990; Covey et al. 1990; Glassman 1993), are at increased risk of experiencing dysphoric mood states and relapse of major depressive disorder after cessation (Covey et al. 1998), and may experience more extreme symptoms of withdrawal (Glassman 1993). Although the detrimental effect of depression on smoking cessation has been found in both men and women, it may be particularly important in the treatment of women because of the increased incidence of depression and dysphoric mood states in women (Borrelli et al. 1996). The period of time required for major depressive symptoms to return after stopping smoking varies by individual and may be as short as a few weeks or as long as a few months after quitting. Therefore, as noted in the American Psychiatric Association guideline (Hughes et al. 1996), individuals who have a history of depression or who report having experienced depression in association with previous quit attempts should be advised to consider psychotherapy or pharmacological treatment of depression if they begin to experience dysphoria. Additionally, because of the interaction between nicotine and antidepressant medication, smokers being treated pharmacologically for depression should undergo a reevaluation of psychotropic medication after cutting down or quitting, because decreasing nicotine intake may increase the level of antidepressant in the bloodstream (Hughes 1993).

A high rate of smoking and difficulty with cessation are also observed in patients with schizophrenia (Ziedonis et al. 1994). Nicotine may reduce drug-induced side effects experienced by these patients, and nicotine withdrawal symptoms can mimic drug-induced side effects (e.g., increased restlessness) as well. Because many individuals with schizophrenia are not interested in quitting smoking, motivational treatment approaches aimed at identifying personalized reasons for quitting and moving the individual from precontemplation through more advanced stages of change are warranted (Hughes et al. 1996).

Evidence is less strong for an association between smoking and anxiety disorders than for one between smoking and depression or schizophrenia (Breslau 1995; Glassman 1993). However, although smoking is often reported to be relaxing and calming, smokers report higher levels of stress than do nonsmokers and former smokers. It is likely that smoking adds to anxiety and stress by inducing mild withdrawal symptoms between cigarettes, thus generating feelings of tension, stress, and anxiety. The individual then smokes in response to the anxiety and stress created by a physiological need for nicotine. Once several weeks have passed after smoking cessation, stressed and anxious moods often stabilize at reduced levels compared with precessation. This reduction in stress does not occur for the individual who simply reduces his or her cigarette consumption; therefore, smokers should be made aware that smoking likely leads to increased feelings of stress and anxiety (Parrott 1999).

Although research is beginning to document the effects of smoking in psychiatric populations, little empirical evidence is available regarding the treatment of nicotine dependence in such patients (see Hughes et al. 1996 for a discussion of intervention issues). In the psychiatric patient for whom smoking cessation is critical for medical reasons, a comprehensive intervention plan—one that includes the treatment components outlined earlier in this chapter—is indicated. In particular, behavior therapy focused on the development of coping and social skills is important. Adjustment of medication may be needed as well, either in an attempt to decrease continued dependence on self-medication with nicotine or in response to possible interaction effects. As more inpatient services limit access to smoking or become smoke-free, use of the nicotine patch, particularly for persons who smoke heavily, is recommended. Additionally, a clear staff policy regarding smoking that does not undermine the smoke-free policy of the treatment unit is imperative. Providing assistance with smoking cessation within the context of a broader therapeutic alliance, monitoring for changes in psychiatric symptoms, and using motivational strategies with individuals in the precontemplation stage are also particularly important.

Modes of Intervention Delivery

Smoking interventions can be delivered through a variety of modalities, as reflected in the "Best Practices for Comprehensive Tobacco Control Programs" guideline published by the Centers for Disease Control and Prevention (CDC) in 1999. The CDC recommends that clinicians identify smokers, advise them to quit, and provide them with brief counseling within the course of routine care, as well as make available to them a full range of cessation aids and services, including pharmacological aids, behavioral counseling (group and individual), and follow-up visits (Centers for Disease Control and Prevention 1999a). And although one role for the mental health professional may be to refer smokers to more intensive treatment programs, it is important to keep in mind that only a small minority even of motivated smokers will attend such programs. In addition, a number of investigations and reviews (e.g., Fiore et al. 1996, 2000; Ockene et al. 1991, 1992) have demonstrated the value of brief counseling, particularly when accompanied by the use of pharmacological aids, such as nicotine replacement therapy or bupropion, and when some type of follow-up occurs, either in person or by telephone. Clinicians conducting brief counseling can supplement their intervention with a wide range of self-help materials and audiotapes now available. Of additional value to the clinician is the use of behavioral contracts, which can serve as an aid in establishing realistic goals and the steps by which to accomplish them. For example, the contract can specify a tapering schedule, a quit date, reasons for stopping, steps to follow in response to situational factors that could interfere with efforts to stop smoking, and a plan for follow-up. A stepped-care approach—in which, for example, less dependent smokers or smokers who are ready for action receive brief counseling and more dependent smokers or those who need more intensive help are referred to a smoking treatment specialist or a treatment group—can be used. For more intensive individual or group treatment, weekly contact for approximately 4 weeks and then biweekly contact for another 4 weeks provide both a reasonable frequency and the tapering of contact necessary for the patient to internalize control. For smokers with greater dependence or with other psychiatric problems, a longer and more intensive intervention may be necessary.

Conclusions

Cigarette smoking is the leading preventable cause of morbidity and mortality in the United States (Centers for Disease Control and Prevention 1996b), and nicotine dependence is classified as a substance use disorder in DSM-IV (American Psychiatric Association 1994). Health and mental health professionals have many opportunities within the context of routine care to work with patients who smoke to address nicotine dependence. There are now evidence-based treatment guidelines on which to base interventions, including treatment guidelines from the AHRQ (Fiore et al. 2000) and the American Psychiatric Association (Hughes et al. 1996). These guidelines help the clinician in assessing the unique needs of each smoker and assisting the smoker by addressing physiological, psychological and social dependence through pharmacotherapy and cognitive-behavioral intervention. From a behavioral perspective, the clinician can assist the smoker in developing or enhancing skills to manage stress and emotional and psychiatric problems without the use of cigarettes. From a pharmacological perspective, the clinician can recommend and supervise the use of nicotine replacement therapy or bupropion to provide some relief from the physiological withdrawal symptoms associated with quitting smoking. Compared with the general population, individuals with either a current or past history of significant psychiatric problems, including depression, schizophrenia, and alcoholism, are much more likely to be smokers and are less likely to stop smoking (Glassman 1993; Hughes 1995a; Ziedonis et al. 1994). Guidelines are available for working with smokers who also suffer from psychiatric and substance abuse problems. Because they have regular contact with individuals who are highly likely to be smokers and who have the most difficulty stopping smoking, mental health professionals are in an excellent position to treat nicotine dependence. They should utilize all opportunities to assist their patients.

References

American Psychiatric Association: Diagnostic and Statistical Manual of Mental Disorders, 4th Edition. Washington, DC, American Psychiatric Association, 1994

Anda RF, Williamson DF, Escobedo LG, et al: Depression and the dynamics of smoking: a national perspective. JAMA 264:1541–1545, 1990

Ascher JA, Cole JO, Colin J, et al: Bupropion: a review of its mechanisms of antidepressant activity. J Clin Psychiatry 56:395–401, 1995

Bandura A: Principles of Behavior Modification. New York, Holt, Rinehart, & Winston, 1969

Bandura A: Self-efficacy: toward a unifying theory of behavioral change. Psychol Rev 84:191–215, 1977a

Bandura A: Social Learning Theory. Englewood Cliffs, NJ, Prentice-Hall, 1977b

Benowitz N: The use of biologic fluid samples in assessing tobacco smoke consumption, in Measurement in the Analysis and Treatment of Smoking Behavior. NIDA Research Monograph 48 (DHHS Publ No [ADM] 83-1285). Edited by Grabowski J, Bell CS. Rockville, MD, National Institute on Drug Abuse, 1983, pp 6–26

Bien T, Burge R: Smoking and drinking: a review of the literature. Int J Addict 25:1429–1454, 1990

Bobo JK: Nicotine dependence and alcoholism epidemiology and treatment. Journal of Psychoactive Drugs 21:323–329, 1989

Bobo JK, Gilchrist LD: Urging the alcoholic client to quit smoking cigarettes. Addict Behav 8:297–305, 1983

Bock BC, Marcus BH, King TK, et al: Exercise effects on withdrawal and mood among women attempting smoking cessation. Addict Behav 24:399–410, 1999

Borrelli B, Bock B, King T, et al: The impact of depression on smoking cessation in women. Am J Prev Med 12:378–387, 1996

Breslau N: Psychiatric comorbidity of smoking and nicotine dependence. Behav Genet 25:95–101, 1995

Centers for Disease Control and Prevention: Best Practices for Comprehensive Tobacco Control Program—August 1999. Atlanta, GA, U.S. Department of Health and Human Services, Centers for Disease Control and Prevention, National Center for Chronic Disease Prevention and Health Promotion, Office on Smoking and Health, August 1999a

Centers for Disease Control and Prevention: Cigarette smoking among adults—United States, 1997. MMWR Morb Mortal Wkly Rep 48:993–996, 1999b

Covey LS, Glassman AH, Stetner F: Depression and depressive symptoms in smoking cessation. Compr Psychiatry 31:350–354, 1990

Covey LS, Glassman AH, Stetner F: Cigarette smoking and major depression, in Smoking and Illicit Drug Use. Edited by Gold MS, Stimmel B. Binghamton, NY, Haworth Medical Press, 1998, pp 35–46

DiClemente C, Prochaska J, Fairhurst S, et al: The process of smoking cessation: an analysis of precontemplation, contemplation, and preparation stages of change. J Consult Clin Psychol 59:295–304, 1991

Fagerstrom K: Towards better diagnoses and more individual treatment of tobacco dependence. Br J Addict 86:543–547, 1991

Fiore MC, Smith SS, Jorenby DE, et al: The effectiveness of the nicotine patch for smoking cessation: a meta-analysis. JAMA 271:1940–1946, 1994

Fiore M, Bailey W, Cohen S, et al: Smoking Cessation: Clinical Practice Guideline No 18. Report No AHCPR 96-0692. Rockville, MD, U.S. Department of Public Health and Human Services, Public Health Service, Agency for Health Care Policy and Research, April 1996

Fiore M, Bailey W, Cohen S, et al: Treating Tobacco Use and Dependence: Clinical Practice Guideline. Rockville, MD, U.S. Department of Public Health and Human Services, Public Health Service, Agency for Healthcare Research and Quality, June 2000

Foxx R, Brown R: Nicotine fading and self-monitoring for cigarette abstinence or controlled smoking. J Appl Behav Anal 12:111–125, 1979

Froom P, Melamed S, Benbasal J: Smoking cessation and weight gain. J Fam Pract 46:460–464, 1998

Glassman AH. Cigarette smoking: implications for psychiatric illness. Am J Psychiatry 150:546–553, 1993

Goff DC, Henderson DC, Amico E: Cigarette smoking in schizophrenia: relationship to psychopathology and medication side effects. Am J Psychiatry 149:1189–1194, 1992

Goldfried MR, Davison GC: Clinical Behavior Therapy. New York, Holt, Rinehart, & Winston, 1976

Gourlay SG, Benowitz NL: Arteriovenous differences in plasma concentration of nicotine and catecholamines and related cardiovascular effects after smoking, nicotine nasal spray, and intravenous nicotine. Clin Pharmacol Ther 62:453–463, 1997

Gritz ER, Berman B, Bastani R: A randomized trial of a self-help smoking cessation intervention in a nonvolunteer female population: testing the limits of the public health model. Health Psychol 11:280–289, 1992

Grunberg N: The effects of nicotine and cigarette smoking on food consumption and taste preferences. Addict Behav 7:317–331, 1982

Gulliver SB, Hughes JR, Solomon LJ, et al: An investigation of self-efficacy, partner support, and daily stresses as predictors of relapse to smoking in self quitters. Addiction 90:767–772, 1995

Hall GH: Pharmacology of tobacco smoking in relation to schizophrenia, in Biochemistry of Schizophrenia and Addiction: In Search of a Common Factor. Edited by Hemmings G. Baltimore, MD, University Park Press, 1980, pp 199–207

Hall RG, Duhamel M, McClanahan R, et al: Level of functioning, severity of illness, and smoking status among chronic psychiatric patients. J Nerv Ment Dis 183:468–471, 1995

Heatherton T, Kozlowski L, Frecker R, Fagerstrom K: The Fagerstrom Test for Nicotine Dependence: a revision of the Fagerstrom Tolerance Questionnaire. Br J Addict 86:1119–1127, 1991

Henningfield JE: Pharmacologic basis and treatment of cigarette smoking. J Clin Psychiatry 45 (12, sec 2):24–34, 1984

Hofstetter A, Schutz Y, Jequier E: Increased 24-hours energy expenditure in cigarette smokers. N Engl J Med 314:79–82, 1986

Hughes JR: Combined psychological and nicotine gum treatment for smoking: a critical review. J Subst Abuse 3:337–350, 1991

Hughes JR: Possible effects of smoke-free inpatient units on psychiatric diagnosis and treatment. J Clin Psychiatry 54:109–114, 1993

Hughes JR: Clinical implications of the association between smoking and alcoholism, in Alcohol and Tobacco: From Basic Science to Policy. NIAAA Res Monogr 30. Edited by Fertig J, Fuller R. Washington, DC, U.S. Government Printing Office, 1995a, pp 171–181

Hughes JR: Treatment of nicotine dependence: is more better? JAMA 274:1390–1391, 1995b

Hughes JR: Dependence on and abuse of nicotine replacement: an update, in Nicotine Safety and Toxicity. Edited by Benowitz NL. New York, Oxford University Press, 1998, pp 147–160

Hughes JR, Hatsukami D: Signs and symptoms of tobacco withdrawal. Arch Gen Psychiatry 43:289–294, 1986

Hughes JR, Hatsukami D: The nicotine withdrawal syndrome: a brief review and update. International Journal of Smoking Cessation 1:21–26, 1992

Hughes JR, Higgins ST, Hatsukami D: Effects of abstinence from tobacco: a critical review, in Research Advances in Alcohol and Drug Problems, Vol 10. Edited by Kozlowski LT, Annis HM, Cappell HD, et al. New York, Plenum, 1990, pp 317–398

Hughes JR, Fiester S, Goldstein MG, et al: Practice guideline for the treatment of patients with nicotine dependence. American Psychiatric Association. Am J Psychiatry 153 (10 suppl):1–31, 1996

Hughes JR, Goldstein MG, Hurt RD, et al: Recent advances in the pharmacotherapy of smoking. JAMA 281:72–76, 1999

Irvin JE, Bowers CA, Dunn ME, et al: Efficacy of relapse prevention: a meta-analytic review. J Consult Clin Psychol 67:563–570, 1999

Istvan J, Matarazzo J: Tobacco, alcohol and caffeine use: a review of their interrelationships. Psychol Bull 95:301–326, 1984

Kalman D: Smoking cessation treatment for substance misusers in early recovery: a review of the literature and recommendations for practice. Subst Use Misuse 33:2021–2047, 1998

Kilen JD, Fortmann SP, Newman B, et al: Evaluation of a treatment approach combining nicotine gum with self-guided behavioral treatments for smoking relapse prevention. J Consult Clin Psychol 58:85–92, 1990

Klesges R, Meyers A, Klesges L: Smoking, body weight and their effects on smoking behavior: a comprehensive review of the literature. Psychol Bull 106:204–230, 1989

Kozlowski LT, Henningfield JE, Keenan RM, et al: Patterns of alcohol, cigarette, and caffeine and other drug use in two drug abusing populations. J Subst Abuse Treat 10:171–179, 1993

Kristeller J: The hard-core smoker: finding a definition to guide intervention. Health Values 18:25–32, 1994

Law M, Tang JL: An analysis of the effectiveness of interventions intended to help people stop smoking. Arch Intern Med 155:1933–1941, 1995

Leshner AI: Understanding drug addiction: implications for treatment. Hosp Pract (Off Ed) 31(10): 47–54, 57–59, 1996

Lichtenstein E, Brown A: Current trends in the modification of cigarette dependence, in International Handbook of Behavior Modification and Therapy, 2nd Edition, Vol 2. Edited by Bellack AS, Hersen M, Kazdin AE. New York, Plenum, 1985, pp 575–612

Marlatt GA, Gordon JR: Determinants of relapse: implications for the maintenance of behavior change, in Behavioral Medicine: Changing Health Lifestyles. Edited by Davidson PO, Davidson SM. New York, Brunner/Mazel, 1980, pp 410–452

Marlatt GA, Gordon JR (eds): Relapse Prevention: Maintenance Strategies in the Treatment of Addictive Behaviors. New York, Guilford, 1985

Massachusetts Department of Public Health: 1997 Cigarette Nicotine Disclosure Report as Required by Massachusetts General Laws. Chapter 307B, CMR 660.000, January 16, 1998

Mathew RJ, Weinman ML, Mirabi M: Physical symptoms of depression. Br J Psychiatry 139:293–296, 1981

Menza MA, Grossman N, Van Horn M, et al: Smoking and movement disorders in psychiatric patients. Biol Psychiatry 30:109–115, 1991

Newhouse P, Hughes J: The role of nicotine and nicotinic mechanisms in neuropsychiatric disease. Br J Addict 86:521–525, 1991

Nisell M, Nomikos GG, Svensson TH: Nicotine dependence, midbrain dopamine systems and psychiatric disorders. Pharmacol Toxicol 76:157–162, 1995

Ockene J, Ockene I: Helping patients to reduce their risk for coronary heart disease: an overview, in Prevention of Coronary Heart Disease. Edited by Ockene I, Ockene J. Boston, MA, Little, Brown, 1992, pp 173–200

Ockene J, Benfari R, Hurwitz I: Relationship of psychosocial factors to smoking behavior change in an intervention program. Prev Med 11:13–28, 1982

Ockene J, Kristeller J, Goldberg R, et al: Increasing the efficacy of physician-delivered smoking interventions: a randomized trial. J Gen Intern Med 6:1–8, 1991

Ockene J, Kristeller J, Goldberg R, et al: Smoking cessation and severity of disease: the Coronary Artery Smoking Intervention Study. Health Psychol 11:119–126, 1992

Ockene JK, Emmons KM, Mermelstein RJ, et al: Relapse and maintenance issues for smoking cessation. Health Psychol 19 (1 suppl):17–31, 2000

O'Farrell TJ, Connors G, Upper D: Addictive behaviors among hospitalized psychiatric patients. Addict Behav 8:329–333, 1983

Parrott AC: Does cigarette smoking cause stress? Am Psychol 54:817–820, 1999

Perkins K: Metabolic effects of cigarette smoking. J Appl Physiol 72:401–409, 1992

Perry PJ, Miller DD, Arndt SV, et al: Haloperidol dosing requirements: the contribution of smoking and non-linear pharmacokinetics. J Clin Psychopharmacol 13:46–51, 1993

Pohl R, Yeragani VK, Balon R, et al: Smoking in patients with panic disorder. Psychiatry Res 43:253–262, 1992

Pomerleau C, Pomerleau O: The effects of a psychosocial stressor on cigarette smoking and subsequent behavioral and physiological responses. Psychophysiology 24:278–285, 1987

Pomerleau O, Pomerleau C: Neuroregulators and the reinforcement of smoking: towards a biobehavioral explanation. Neurosci Biobehav Rev 8:503–513, 1984

Schachter S: Pharmacological and psychological determinants of smoking. Ann Intern Med 88:104–114, 1978

Schuh KJ, Schuh LM, Henningfield JE, et al: Nicotine nasal spray and vapor inhaler: abuse liability assessment. Psychopharmacology (Berl) 130:352–361, 1997

Schwartz JL: Methods of smoking cessation. Med Clin North Am 76:451–476, 1992

Sobell L, Sobell M, Toneatto T: Recovery from alcohol problems without treatment, in Self-Control and Addictive Behaviors. Edited by Heather N, Miller WR, Greeley J. New York, Maxwell MacMillan, 1992, pp 198–242

Sutherland G, Stapleton JA, Russell MAH: Randomized controlled trial of nasal nicotine spray in smoking cessation. Lancet 340:324–329, 1992

Tomkins S: Psychological model for smoking behavior. Am J Public Health 56:17–20, 1966

Transdermal Nicotine Study Group: Transdermal nicotine for smoking cessation. JAMA 266:3133–3138, 1992

U.S. Department of Health and Human Services: The Health Benefits of Smoking Cessation. U.S. Department of Health and Human Services, Public Health Service, Centers for Disease Control, Center for Chronic Disease Prevention and Health Promotion, Office on Smoking and Health. DHHS Publ No (CDC) 90-8416, 1990, pp 580–616

Velicer WF, Fava JL, Prochaska JO, et al: Distribution of smokers by stage in three representative samples. Prev Med 24:401–411, 1995

Wack J, Rodin L: Smoking and its effects on body weight and the systems of caloric regulation. Am J Clin Nutr 35:366–380, 1989

Ward KD, Klesges RC, Halpern MT: Predictors of smoking cessation and state-of-the-art smoking interventions. Journal of Social Issues 53:129–145, 1997

West RJ, Hajek P, Belcher M: Severity of withdrawal symptoms as a predictor of outcome of an attempt to quit smoking. Psychol Med 19:981–985, 1989

Ziedonis DM, Kosten TR, Glazer WM, et al: Nicotine dependence and schizophrenia. Hospital and Community Psychiatry 45:204–206, 1994

29

Pharmacological Treatments for Narcotic and Opioid Addictions

Herbert D. Kleber, M.D.
Edward C. Senay, M.D.
Charles P. O'Brien, M.D., Ph.D.

Detoxification

Herbert D. Kleber, M.D.

The availability and purity of heroin are higher than they have been in decades, and the cost per pure milligram is lower. This increased purity has made it easier for individuals to begin heroin use by snorting or smoking, deluding themselves that if they are not injecting, they risk neither harm nor addiction. Physicians who may have been seeing relatively few heroin-addicted patients will once again need to pay attention to this problem and the various treatment methods. Although drug detoxification is often the route into treatment, many who begin this process do not complete it, and many who complete it do not go on to more definitive treatment. Some enter only to lower their level of dependence and to have an easier time supporting their habit, but others, especially younger addicted persons who have not yet frequently relapsed, fully believe that detoxification is all that is necessary.

Choice of Setting

Detoxification can take place in an inpatient, a partial hospitalization, or an outpatient setting. Outpatient detoxification, the least expensive of the three, enables patients to carry on their lives and encourages them to cope with the home environment and/or the work settings where they will be after they have become drug-free. Disadvantages to outpatient detoxification include a much lower completion rate, more temptations to use, more difficulty in dealing with other medical conditions, and a slower detoxification to avoid undue stress. Unfortunately, choice of program is usually made on the basis of insurance coverage and program availability rather than of what might be best for the patient's needs.

Factors Influencing Symptom Severity

The nature and severity of withdrawal symptoms are influenced by the following four factors:

1. *The specific drug used.* The general rule is, the longer the duration of the drug, the less intense but longer lasting the withdrawal symptoms. Rapidly metabolized drugs such as heroin are generally associated with more severe withdrawal phenomena, whereas drugs that bind tightly to the receptor, such as buprenorphine, or that are slowly excreted from the body, such as methadone, have a slower onset with a less intense but also more protracted withdrawal syndrome.
2. *The total daily amount used.* In general, the larger the daily amount, the more severe the withdrawal.
3. *The duration and regularity of use.* Clinically significant withdrawal usually requires daily use of an adequate amount for at least 3 weeks; duration much beyond 3 months does not appear to lead to greater withdrawal severity. The more intermittent the use, the less likelihood of severe withdrawal.
4. *Psychological factors.* In general, the greater the expectation that medication will be available to alleviate the symptoms, the more severe the withdrawal experience. General physical health and ability to handle stress can also influence withdrawal severity.

Symptoms and Signs of Opioid Withdrawal

Withdrawal phenomena tend to be the reverse of the acute agonistic effects of the opioid (Table 29–1). (For example, acute opioid use causes constipation and pupillary constriction, whereas withdrawal is associated with diarrhea and pupillary dilatation.)

TABLE 29–1. Symptoms and signs of opioid withdrawal

Early to moderate	Moderate to advanced
Anorexia	Abdominal cramps
Anxiety	Broken sleep
Craving	Hot or cold flashes
Dysphoria	Increased blood pressure
Fatigue	Increased pulse
Headache	Low-grade fever
Increased respiratory rate	Muscle and bone pain
Irritability	Muscle spasm (hence the term *kicking the habit*)
Lacrimation	Mydriasis (with dilated, fixed pupils at the peak)
Mydriasis (mild)	Nausea and vomiting
Perspiration	
Piloerection (gooseflesh)	
Restlessness	
Rhinorrhea	
Yawning	

Heroin withdrawal tends to begin with anxiety and craving about 8–10 hours after the last dose. This initial response progresses to dysphoria, yawning, lacrimation, rhinorrhea, perspiration, restlessness, and broken sleep. Later, waves of gooseflesh, hot and cold flashes, aching of bones and muscles, nausea, vomiting, diarrhea, abdominal cramps, weight loss, and low-grade fever occur. The skin may be exquisitely sensitive to the touch. Heroin withdrawal typically peaks between 36 and 72 hours after the last dose, and acute symptoms have substantially subsided by 5 days. Methadone withdrawal peaks between days 4 and 6, and symptoms do not substantially subside until 10–12 days after the last dose (Kleber 1996) (Table 29–2). During withdrawal from meperidine, craving is intense and symptoms occur earlier than in heroin withdrawal, but the autonomic signs, such as pupillary dilatation, are not particularly prominent. There is usually little nausea, vomiting, or diarrhea, but at peak intensity the muscle twitching, restlessness, and nervousness have been described as worse than those experienced during morphine withdrawal (Jaffe and Martin 1975).

TABLE 29–2. Usual frequency of use (as measured by duration between doses) in established habits of selected opioids and first appearance of withdrawal symptoms

Drug	Duration between doses (hours)	Appearance of nonpurposive withdrawal symptoms (hours)	Peak of severity of withdrawal symptoms (hours)
Meperidine	2–3	4–6	8–12
Hydromorphone hydrochloride (Dilaudid)	4–5	4–5	Approximately the same as morphine
Heroin	4	8–12[a]	36–72
Morphine	4–5	8–12	
Codeine	4	Approximately the same as morphine	
Methadone	8–12	36–72[b]	96–144

[a]The majority of the symptoms associated with heroin withdrawal are gone after 5–10 days.
[b]The majority of the symptoms associated with methadone withdrawal are gone after 14–21 days.

In withdrawal from any opioid, there may be a protracted abstinence syndrome with subtle disturbances of mood and sleep that can persist for weeks or months (Martin and Jasinski 1969). The fatigue, dysphoria, irritability, and insomnia increase the likelihood of relapse. Protracted abstinence may involve both conditioned and physiological factors (Satel et al. 1993).

Evaluation and Diagnosis

The initial evaluation determines whether detoxification is needed. Once the person is in treatment, a more complete assessment of psychosocial and physical status is necessary to devise an individual treatment plan. (For a review of the evaluation and diagnosis of opioid addiction, see Kleber 1999.)

The Interview

Drug History

For each substance currently used, the following information should be obtained:

- Length of time and frequency of use
- Date or time of last use
- Route
- Amount
- Cost
- Purpose of use (e.g., to get high, to relieve depression)

The clinician should obtain the name of each drug the patient has previously used, the patient's age when he or she started using the drug, the length of time the drug was used, and any adverse effects experienced. Any previous treatment should also be noted, including where treatment took place, what type of treatment was involved, and the outcome.

Other Medical History

Special attention should be given to the possible medical complications of drug abuse, especially illnesses that may complicate withdrawal or that have been ignored because of the patient's chaotic lifestyle. When gathering the above information, especially the drug history, a nonjudgmental attitude is more likely to elicit the necessary data. Disdainful behavior is likely to create difficulties, produce false information, and even drive away the patient.

Social Functioning

Material should be elicited on the following:

- Living arrangements
- Marital status
- Sexual orientation and functioning
- Employment and/or educational status
- Family members' (parents', siblings', spouse's, other key members') occupations, education, psychological state, and history of drug or alcohol problems (if any)
- Friends (in particular, whether there are non-drug-using friends in addition to drug-using ones)
- Recreational and leisure time activities
- Current and past legal status

The Addiction Severity Index (ASI; McLellan et al. 1980) is a useful instrument for gathering these data.

Psychological Status

In addition to factors that could complicate withdrawal, such as severe depression or suicidality, the psychiatrist can look for conditions for which special treatments exist (e.g., mania [lithium]). It is helpful, though difficult, to assess whether psychiatric conditions predate or postdate the drug abuse. Opioids may have an ameliorating effect on psychosis, and withdrawal can lead to exacerbation or sudden appearance of psychotic symptoms.

Laboratory Tests

The following laboratory tests are useful in the evaluation of opioid abuse and its management:

- Urine screen for drugs, including narcotics, barbiturates, amphetamine, cocaine, benzodiazepines, tricyclic antidepressants, phencyclidine (PCP), and marijuana
- Complete blood count and differential (leukocytosis is common and white blood cell counts above 14,000 are not unusual)
- Urinalysis
- Blood chemistry profile (e.g., SMA 20 with serum amylase and magnesium)
- VDRL (Venereal Disease Research Laboratory) test
- Human immunodeficiency virus (HIV) test (**Note:** Patient permission is necessary in many states.)
- Hepatitis antigen and antibody test
- Chest X ray
- Electrocardiogram (in patients over age 40)
- Pregnancy test (chest X ray should be deferred until results are obtained)
- Tuberculin skin test plus antigen testing (because HIV-positive individuals may have a false-negative purified protein derivative [PPD] test result)
- Any other test suggested by the history or physical

Technique of Withdrawal

The usual method of withdrawal is substitution and then withdrawal of methadone. The advantages of methadone for this purpose include its effectiveness in oral form and its extended duration of action. (Longer-acting opioids produce milder though longer-lasting withdrawal syndromes, can be given less often, and are associated with a smoother withdrawal.) Although methadone is used for withdrawal from narcotics such as heroin, morphine, hydromorphone hydrochloride (Dilaudid), and meperidine, it is often avoided for propoxyphene, pentazocine, codeine, or oxycodone withdrawals, which can be handled by gradually decreasing the dose of the agent itself or by use of clonidine.

U.S. Food and Drug Administration (FDA) guidelines for narcotic detoxification describe two types of detoxification: short-term and long-term. Short-term narcotic detoxification cannot exceed 30 days, and long-term detoxification should not exceed 180 days. Short-term detoxification is primarily for individuals addicted to opioids other than methadone. Long-term detoxification is used either for persons already on methadone and wishing to come off or, in some programs, for persons who are to be taken directly from heroin to long-term detoxification on methadone over a 6-month period. Prolonged detoxification may obviate long-term methadone maintenance, avoids some of the withdrawal symptoms experienced with more rapid detoxification, and provides a setting for psychosocial rehabilitation. However, the effectiveness of the long-term approach compared with short-term detoxification or methadone maintenance has not yet been demonstrated.

Initiation of Detoxification Using Methadone

When the patient has been taking narcotics for medical purposes, the narcotic dose can be converted into methadone equivalents, as shown in Table 29–3. When a patient presents with illicit drug use, the picture is very different. The amount of narcotics in illegal "bags" can vary from dealer to dealer, from city to city, and even from day to day. Under these circumstances, the physician must guess at the initial dose. The quality of street heroin has increased in the past few years—street heroin in some cities contains from 5% to more than 45%–50% heroin—but could just as easily decline again. In general, the initial dose of methadone needs to be high enough to adequately suppress withdrawal symptoms yet low enough to not threaten the patient's health or life in the event that the patient's habit is not as severe as anticipated. Because 40 mg of methadone has proven to be a fatal dose in some persons when given without adequate verification of prior habit, it is important that the *initial* dose be substantially below that level. A dose of 10–20 mg is large enough to control the illicit habit of many, if not most, users and yet small enough not to be particularly dangerous. The patient should be kept under observation so that the effect of the dose can be judged. The dose should suppress withdrawal symptoms within 30–60 minutes; if not, an additional 5–10 mg of methadone can be given. If withdrawal symptoms are not present, the patient should be observed for drowsiness or depressed respiration. When an initial dose of 10–20 mg is given, a similar amount may be given 12 hours later as needed. Although usually not practical in outpatient detoxification, this approach is not uncommon in inpatient or residential settings. Unless there is documented evidence of use in excess of 40 mg of methadone equivalent a day, the initial dose should not exceed 30 mg and the total initial 24-hour dosage should not exceed 40 mg.

TABLE 29–3. Drug relationships between opioids and methadone for detoxification

Methadone: 1 mg is equivalent to	
Codeine	30 mg
Dromoran	1 mg
Heroin	1–2 mg
Hydromorphone hydrochloride (Dilaudid)	0.5 mg
Laudanum (opium tincture)	3 mL
Leritine	8 mg
Levorphanol (Levo-Dromoran)	0.5 mg
Meperidine (Demerol)	20 mg
Morphine	3–4 mg
Paregoric	7–8 mL

There is some disagreement about whether to start the withdrawal regimen in the absence of withdrawal signs and symptoms. It is often difficult to know with certainty that a patient is currently physically addicted. The interview, physical examination, and laboratory tests do not usually prove a diagnosis of current narcotic dependence of sufficient severity to require withdrawal treatment, unless the clinician has observed the actual signs and symptoms of opioid withdrawal.

If definitive evidence of physical dependence is needed, the clinician can either wait until the patient develops withdrawal signs and symptoms or conduct a naloxone provocation test. One method is to inject 0.2 mg of naloxone subcutaneously and follow that dose with 0.4 mg in 30–60 minutes if the results from the first dose are inconclusive. Some physicians recommend an initial dose of 0.6–0.8 mg to speed up the process and to rule out false negatives. Because of the possibility of fetal injury or induced abortion, the naloxone test should not be done if the patient is pregnant.

The availability of trained medical personnel will often determine whether a methadone treatment program will prefer to wait for withdrawal signs to develop, use a naloxone challenge test, or use the combined evidence of the history, physical, and urine screen as interpreted by experienced personnel. The combined-evidence approach is most commonly used, but in doubtful situations the clinician should wait for withdrawal signs or use the naloxone test. When serious physical or emotional problems are present, it is not uncommon to temporarily maintain the person on methadone and to not begin withdrawal until some stability has been achieved with the acute problems.

Length of Withdrawal

The total dose necessary to stabilize a patient for the first 24 hours should be repeated on day 2, either in one dose for outpatients or in divided doses for inpatients, with corrections if the dose either is too sedating or fails to adequately suppress the abstinence syndrome. Although objective signs of opioid withdrawal rather than subjective complaints alone should determine the need for a higher dose, certain signs, such as pupillary dilatation, may be modified by the dosage of methadone and yet the patient may still be undermedicated. After the patient is stabilized, the dose is gradually withdrawn, either by decreasing by 5 mg per day or by decreasing by 5 mg per day until a dosage of 10 mg/day is reached and then decreasing by 2–3 mg per day. In general, inpatient withdrawal occurs over 5–10 days, whereas outpatient withdrawal may be extended over a longer period to decrease the chance of premature termination by the patient. Although insomnia, fatigue, and anxiety can linger for weeks or months, acute withdrawal is considered to be complete if there are no objective signs of acute opioid withdrawal 48 hours after the last dose of methadone. A mild rebound in withdrawal symptoms may occur after the final methadone dose; this generally recedes in a few weeks.

Withdrawal From Methadone Maintenance

For withdrawal from methadone maintenance, the technique used often depends on why the patient is being withdrawn. Patients in good standing trying to become drug-free should in general be withdrawn slowly over a 3- to 6-month period. The most difficult period is when the dosage gets below 25 mg/day, because at that level, methadone may not last the full 24 hours and some withdrawal symptoms may occur before the next dose. Split doses may help but are not always possible. Five to 10 mg per week can be withdrawn from the established methadone dose until the patient reaches 25 mg; at that point, withdrawal of no more than 5 mg per week is often recommended. Being discharged in bad standing from the program, leaving the geographic locale, or going to prison usually requires a more rapid detoxification process over a 10- to 30-day period. If the patient is on an inpatient or residential basis, use of divided doses is helpful, especially when the total dose is below 25 mg.

Supportive Measures and Medications

Even with gradual withdrawal, certain mild symptoms may persist. With the exception of α-adrenergic agonists such as clonidine, non-narcotic medications are generally ineffective in relieving the specific symptoms of opioid abstinence. If insomnia and other withdrawal symptoms are unusually severe, especially in older patients, relief can be provided by increasing the next dose of methadone and then instituting a slower withdrawal schedule.

Not only is insomnia itself difficult to tolerate, but it also weakens the patient's ability to deal with other withdrawal problems. Drugs that have been advocated for treatment of insomnia include flurazepam, oxazepam, zolpidem, diphenhydramine, chloral hydrate, and antidepressants such as trazodone. Because many narcotic-addicted persons also abuse benzodiazepine-type drugs, choice of such agents needs to be carefully made.

Nonpharmaceutical supports can also play a useful role. A warm, kind, and reassuring attitude in the treatment staff is most helpful. Involvement of patients in their own detoxification schedule has been found to be of positive value, and patients usually do not unfairly take advantage of this situation.

Other measures advocated include warm baths, exercise, and various diets. Unless specific nutritional deficiencies are present, there is no evidence that any one dietary regimen is more useful than any other. Because addicted persons are often malnourished, general vitamin and mineral supplements should be given.

Other Detoxification Agents and Methods

Withdrawal From Opioids Using Clonidine Hydrochloride

The antihypertensive α_2-agonist drug clonidine (Catapres) has been used to facilitate either withdrawal from heroin or methadone maintenance in both inpatient and outpatient settings (Charney et al. 1986; Gold et al. 1978; Kleber et al. 1985). Clonidine at dosages of 0.6–2.0 mg/day reduces many of the autonomic components of the opioid withdrawal syndrome, although craving, lethargy, insomnia, restlessness, and muscle aches are not well suppressed (Charney et al. 1981; Jasinski et al. 1985). Clonidine presumably acts by binding to α_2 autoreceptors in the brain (e.g., locus coeruleus) and spinal cord. The locus coeruleus is hyperactive during opioid withdrawal.

Patients maintained on 20 mg/day or less of methadone are about as successful with abrupt substitution of clonidine as with reduction of methadone 1 mg/day (Kleber et al. 1985). Persons addicted to heroin can also be successfully withdrawn using clonidine; in a recent study (O'Connor et al. 1997), 65% of such patients completed withdrawal and entered the next phase of treatment. The use of clonidine for controlling withdrawal has not yet been given official FDA approval, but clonidine has been so widely used, both in the United States and abroad, that it has become accepted as an alternative to gradual methadone reduction. Use of clonidine avoids the postwithdrawal rebound in symptoms commonly seen after methadone reduction.

Technique

A procedure for clonidine-aided detoxification is given in Table 29–4. On the first day, the opioid is withdrawn completely and clonidine is given in divided doses totaling 0.15–0.3 mg. Clonidine should be used with caution in patients with hypotension or patients receiving antihypertensive medications. Contraindications to clonidine include use of tricyclic antidepressants within the past 3 weeks, pregnancy, history of psychosis, or history of cardiac arrhythmias. Because clonidine can cause sedation, patients should be cautioned about driving and operating equipment.

TABLE 29–4. Clonidine-aided detoxification

Schedule for heroin, morphine, oxycodone, meperidine, and other short-acting opioids (outpatient/inpatient)		
Day 1	0.1–0.2 mg orally every 4–6 hours up to 1 mg	
Days 2–4	0.2–0.4 mg orally every 4–6 hours up to 1.2 mg	
Day 5 to completion	Reduce dosage by 0.2 mg/day, given in two or three divided doses. The nighttime dose should be reduced last. Or reduce total dosage by one-half each day, not to exceed 0.4 mg/day reduction.	
Schedule for methadone-maintained patients (20–30 mg/day methadone)		
Day 1	0.3 mg	
Day 2	0.4–0.6 mg	Total daily dosage, given in divided doses every 4–6 hours
Day 3	0.5–0.8 mg	
Day 4	0.5–1.2 mg	
Days 5–10	Maintain on above dosage	
Day 11 to completion	Reduce by 0.2 mg/day, given in two or three divided doses. The nighttime dose should be reduced last. If the patient complains of side effects, the dosage can be reduced by one-half each day, not to exceed 0.4 mg/day reduction.	

When clonidine is used on an outpatient basis, it is usually advisable not to give more than a 2-day supply at a time. Blood pressure should be checked when the patient is seen. If dizziness occurs, the patient should reduce the dose or lie down.

Lower clonidine doses are used on day 1 because narcotic withdrawal is less severe at that point and the patient usually needs time to adjust to the sedative effects. It is useful to give 0.1 mg clonidine as the initial dose and to observe the patient's reaction and blood pressure at least over the next hour. The total daily dose should be divided into three parts given at 4- to 6-hour intervals.

During the patient's withdrawal from methadone, clonidine doses are gradually increased over several days. In treating withdrawal from short-acting opioids, however, dosages of clonidine are increased (i.e., titrated to symptoms) as rapidly as is consistent with a concern for side effects. Clonidine-aided withdrawal from heroin usually takes 4–6 days, and from methadone, 10–14 days. Antiwithdrawal effects usually begin within 30 minutes and peak at 2–3 hours.

Insomnia is not usually a problem until day 3 or 4 of withdrawal from methadone or day 2 or 3 of withdrawal from short-acting opioids. Benzodiazepines may be used with caution both for the muscle aches and for the insomnia. In some settings, clonidine is administered via transdermal patches (Spencer and Gregory 1989). The clonidine patch is a 0.2-mm square applied as a self-adhesive bandage. It comes in three sizes that deliver an amount of clonidine equal to daily dosing with 0.1, 0.2, or 0.3 mg of oral clonidine. Oral clonidine is given during the first 2 days because the steady-state levels of transdermal clonidine are not reached for 24–48 hours after application of the patch. The patches are used for 7 days for heroin withdrawal and for 10 days or more for methadone withdrawal. Although clonidine can be an effective agent for opioid withdrawal, its usefulness is limited by its hypotensive effects. Lofexidine, another adrenergic agonist, has shown evidence in controlled studies of being approximately as efficacious as clonidine but causing less hypotensive and sedative effects (Carnwath and Hardman 1998; Kahn et al. 1997). Bearn et al. (1996) found that at a maximum dosage of 2 mg/day, lofexidine was approximately equivalent to methadone detoxification in regard to overall symptom relief.

Clonidine-Naltrexone Ultrarapid Withdrawal

Although clonidine can be an effective alternative to methadone for opioid withdrawal, it does not substantially shorten withdrawal. Combining clonidine and naltrexone can provide a safe, effective, and more rapid withdrawal for patients detoxifying from either heroin or methadone. The method makes use of the known ability of naltrexone to produce immediate withdrawal from an opioid as it displaces the opioid from the endogenous receptor. When clonidine is used as pretreatment and as needed after the naltrexone, symptoms are substantially relieved. For symptoms that are not adequately controlled, other medications, such as oxazepam for muscle spasm and antiemetics for nausea and vomiting, are employed. The method was described in detail by Vining et al. (1988), and O'Connor et al. (1995) provided an update in a paper aimed at primary practitioners. The clonidine-naltrexone rapid detoxification method is detailed in Table 29–5. Although a large majority of the patients were able to successfully complete detoxification, by 1 month later, however, there was no difference in treatment retention between the clonidine alone and the clonidine-naltrexone groups (O'Connor et al. (1995). The limitations of this method are 1) the need to monitor patients for 8 hours on day 1 because of the potential severity of naltrexone-induced withdrawal and 2) the need for careful blood pressure monitoring during the detoxification procedure. A recent review of 12 clonidine-naltrexone rapid detoxification studies found only 3 reporting outcome data after the acute detoxification (O'Connor and Kosten 1998).

Ultrarapid Opioid Detoxification Under Anesthesia/Sedation

The rate-limiting factor of the clonidine-naltrexone method is the ability to find medications that adequately relieve the symptoms of the precipitated withdrawal in the awake patient. The procedure was later shortened and advanced by carrying it out under a general anesthetic (an ironic throwback to the hibernation therapy of 1941, in which a patient was kept asleep for 1–3 days) (Loimer et al. 1989). Over the next 10 years, the technique was modified and improved (see Brewer 1997 for a review). The current method commonly uses naltrexone, the anesthetic propofol, the antiemetic ondansetron, the antidiarrheal octreotide, and clonidine and benzodiazepines for other withdrawal symptoms. Heavy sedation with midazolam is sometimes employed instead of anesthesia. Intubation is ordinarily used with anesthesia but not with heavy sedation. Occasionally, nalmefene is used instead of naltrexone. Some clinicians perform the procedure on an inpatient basis, others on an outpatient basis; some encourage naltrexone maintenance and/or therapy after detoxifica-

TABLE 29–5. Clonidine-naltrexone rapid detoxification

Day 0	Use of heroin or methadone as usual
Day 1	
9:00 A.M.	Clonidine, 0.2–0.4 mg orally Oxazepam, 30–60 mg orally
11:00 A.M.	Naltrexone, 12.5 mg orally Clonidine, 0.1–0.2 mg every 4–6 hours up to 1.2 mg Oxazepam, 30–60 mg every 4–6 hours as needed
Patient remains in clinic until 5:00 P.M.	
Day 2	
9:00 A.M.	Clonidine, 0.1–0.2 mg orally (then every 4–6 hours as needed up to 1.2 mg) Oxazepam, 30–60 mg (then every 4–6 hours as needed)
10:00 A.M.	Naltrexone, 25 mg orally
Patient may leave 2 hours after naltrexone administration.	
Day 3	
9:00 A.M.	Clonidine, 0.1–0.2 mg (then every 4–6 hours as needed, tapering total dosage by 0.2–0.4 mg/day) Oxazepam, 15–30 mg (then every 4–6 hours as needed)
10:00 A.M.	Naltrexone, 50 mg orally
Patient may leave 1 hour after naltrexone administration.	
After day 3[a]	Clonidine: continue 0.1–0.2 mg every 4–6 hours as needed over next 2–3 days Oxazepam: continue 15–30 mg every 4–6 hours as needed over next 2–3 days Naltrexone: 50 mg/day orally

[a]Administer adjuvant medications as needed. For muscle cramps: nonsteroidal anti-inflammatory drugs (NSAIDs; e.g., ibuprofen 600 mg orally every 6 hours or ketorolac 30 mg intramuscularly every 6 hours while on site); for nausea/vomiting: antiemetics (e.g., prochlorperazine 5 mg intramuscularly or 10 mg orally every 4–6 hours while on site or ondansetron 8 mg orally every 8 hours); for anxiety, insomnia, or muscle cramps: benzodiazepines (e.g., oxazepam 30–60 mg as needed, not to exceed 120 mg/day after day 1).

tion, and others simply refer the patient to Narcotics Anonymous. What tends to be common is the high price, usually ranging from $2,500 or more for the outpatient to $7,500 or more for the inpatient anesthesia method. Claims of high rates of abstinence months after detoxification have been made, but no objective verification has occurred. Until adequate controlled studies are carried out, the place for this technique in the spectrum of opioid detoxification procedures is unclear (Kleber 1998).

Buprenorphine

Buprenorphine, a partial μ opiate receptor agonist, is being used in a variety of approaches for treatment of narcotic addiction, including as a maintenance agent, as a transition from a full agonist such as methadone or heroin to a full antagonist such as naltrexone, and as a detoxification agent from an agonist such as methadone or heroin. The first step in detoxification is to transfer the patient from either heroin or methadone maintenance to buprenorphine. Detoxification can then be accomplished by gradual buprenorphine tapering, abrupt discontinuation, or discontinuation of buprenorphine and precipitation of withdrawal using naltrexone. In these methods, the patient is usually first stabilized on buprenorphine for a period that may be as brief as 3 days at relatively low dosages of 2 or 3 mg/day sublingually or for a longer-term maintenance period of 6 months or more at dosages of up to 16 mg/day. The sublingual form of buprenorphine is being considered by the FDA as a detoxification agent. If buprenorphine is stopped abruptly, the withdrawal syndrome is mild, although in some patients it may be protracted. In a recent study, patients were given buprenorphine 3 mg/day sublingually for 3 days followed by 25 mg of naltrexone plus clonidine on day 4 and 50 mg plus clonidine on day 5 (O'Connor et al. 1997). The buprenorphine group had milder withdrawal symptoms and were more likely to complete detoxification (81%) compared with those in the clonidine group (65%). The success of the buprenorphine group was equal to that of the clonidine-naltrexone comparison group (also 81%), but no difference in naltrexone retention was found at 8 days.

Acupuncture

Although acupuncture has been used for thousands of years in Chinese medicine to relieve pain, its use in the treatment of narcotic withdrawal dates only to the early 1970s (Wen and Cheung 1973). Programs that employ these methods tend to be enthusiastic about the results, but published reviews are generally more critical (Alling et al. 1990; Lipton et al. 1994; National Council Against Health Fraud 1991; Ter Riet et al. 1990; Ulett 1992). Thus, although acupuncture may be useful for some patients, clarification is needed regarding its duration and frequency and the nature of the psychosocial adjuncts. Washburn et al. (1993) suggested that light users of opioids stay in treatment longer than heavy users.

Special Problems Associated With Detoxification

Seizures

Opioid withdrawal or intoxication usually does not lead to seizures, but meperidine or propoxyphene intoxication may occasionally do so. A seizure, therefore, usually signifies undiagnosed sedative withdrawal (e.g., alcohol, barbiturate, benzodiazepine) or another medical condition (e.g., head injury, epilepsy); seizures may also be faked.

Mixed Addictions

Sedative dependence can lead to serious hazards, including seizures, toxic psychosis, hyperthermia, and even death. If sedative dependence is present, it is often useful to maintain the patient on methadone, withdraw the sedative gradually, and then withdraw the methadone. Withdrawal from stimulant-type drugs is less of a physical hazard than withdrawal from sedatives but can be associated with severe depression and even suicide.

Vomiting

Although vomiting can be a symptom of withdrawal, it can also occur without regard to the degree of physical abstinence and in spite of all kinds of supporting measures, including reintoxication with opioids. Vomiting can usually be handled by intramuscular injections of trimethobenzamide or perphenazine.

Other Medical Conditions

High fevers are not common in opioid withdrawal, although low-grade temperature elevation can occur. Acute febrile illnesses may temporarily increase the severity of withdrawal symptoms, necessitating higher doses of methadone. When serious medical problems are present, withdrawal should be very gradual to minimize stress. With certain illnesses (e.g., acute myocardial infarction, renal colic), the patient should be maintained on methadone until stable enough to permit withdrawal. The patient should also be evaluated carefully to determine whether longer-term maintenance is indicated. When withdrawal does take place, methadone three or four times a day instead of once or twice can minimize discomfort and stress.

Pregnancy

When pregnancy is complicated by heroin addiction, the patient and her physician are faced with the choice of which of several undesirable alternatives is the *least* undesirable. The best scenario would be for the patient to abstain totally from drugs, licit or illicit, during the pregnancy. Unfortunately, this is often unlikely to occur. On an outpatient drug-free regimen, many patients cycle in and out of heroin use, subjecting the fetus to periods of intoxication and withdrawal and a risk of spontaneous abortion, stillbirth, prematurity, and anomalies. The drug effects are compounded by the patient's lifestyle, poor prenatal care, inadequate diet, and drug adulterants. Residential placement to ensure a drug-free status is usually resisted or else hard to find. Narcotic antagonists have not yet been approved for maintenance during pregnancy. Methadone maintenance at the lowest dose possible remains the least undesirable option available for most such patients. The infant will be born addicted and may need to be withdrawn from the drug but should otherwise not have problems if there has been adequate obstetrical care during the pregnancy.

If withdrawal from methadone maintenance is necessary, it should be slow, with a reduction of no more than 5 mg every 1–2 weeks, and should take place during the middle trimester. During the first trimester, withdrawal may be especially deleterious to fetal development; during the third trimester, withdrawal may trigger premature labor. In deciding on the methadone dose, especially during the third trimester, the clinician must keep in mind that the woman's metabolism of methadone may be increased during that time, so higher doses may be needed to avoid withdrawal.

Conclusions

For most patients, detoxification from narcotics is only the first step in the long process of remaining abstinent from illicit drugs. Success is a function, therefore, of the number of patients retained and the likelihood that they will go on to longer-term treatment. Whatever method is chosen, appropriate psychosocial interventions and education must be provided to prepare the patient for this next step. The ideal detoxification method would be relatively short, inexpensive, and painless; would be able to be done on an outpatient basis; and would leave the patient with a desire to seek longer-term help. We are closing in on methods to address the pharmacological ramifications of opioid withdrawal and thus need to focus as well on what psychosocial interventions in combination with the pharmacological approaches will most likely keep the patient in treatment for both detoxification and the next stage. Compared with the methods of the 1940s, current methods are more rapid and cause less discomfort; however, they do not necessarily produce longer periods of abstinence.

References

Alling FA, Johnson BD, Elmoghazy E: Cranial electrostimulation (CES) use in the detoxification of opiate-dependent patients. J Subst Abuse Treat 7:173–180, 1990

Bearn J, Gossop M, Strang J: Randomised double-blind comparison of lofexidine and methadone in the in-patient treatment of opiate withdrawal. Drug Alcohol Depend 43:87–91, 1996

Brewer C: Ultra-rapid antagonist precipitated opiate detoxification under general anesthesia or sedation. Addiction Biology 2:291–301, 1997

Carnwath T, Hardman J: Randomised double-blind comparison of lofexidine and clonidine in the outpatient treatment of opiate withdrawal. Drug Alcohol Depend 50:251–254, 1998

Charney DS, Sternberg DE, Kleber HD, et al: The clinical use of clonidine in abrupt withdrawal from methadone: effects on blood pressure and specific signs and symptoms. Arch Gen Psychiatry 38:1273–1277, 1981

Charney DS, Heninger GR, Kleber HD: The combined use of clonidine and naltrexone as a rapid, safe, and effective treatment of abrupt withdrawal from methadone. Am J Psychiatry 143:831–837, 1986

Gold MS, Redmond DE Jr, Kleber HD: Clonidine blocks acute opiate withdrawal symptoms. Lancet 2(8090):599–602, 1978

Jaffe JH, Martin WR: Narcotic analgesics and antagonists, in The Pharmacological Basis of Therapeutics, 5th Edition. Edited by Goodman LS, Gilman A. New York, Macmillan, 1975, pp 245–324

Jasinski DR, Johnson RE, Kocher TR: Clonidine in morphine withdrawal: differential effects on signs and symptoms. Arch Gen Psychiatry 42:1063–1066, 1985

Kahn A, Mumford JP, Rogers GA, et al: Double-blind study of lofexidine and clonidine in the detoxification of opiate addicts in hospital. Drug Alcohol Depend 44:57–61, 1997

Kleber HD: Outpatient detoxification from opiates. Primary Psychiatry 1:42–52, 1996

Kleber HD: Ultrarapid opiate detoxification. Addiction 93:1629–1633, 1998

Kleber HD: Opioids: detoxification, in The American Psychiatric Press Textbook of Substance Abuse Treatment, 2nd Edition. Edited by Galanter M, Kleber HD. Washington, DC, 1999, pp 251–269

Kleber HD, Riordan CE, Rounsaville B, et al: Clonidine in outpatient detoxification from methadone maintenance. Arch Gen Psychiatry 42:391–394, 1985

Lipton DS, Brewington V, Smith M: Acupuncture for crack-cocaine detoxification: experimental evaluation of efficacy. J Subst Abuse Treat 11:203–215, 1994

Loimer N, Schmid RW, Presslich O, et al: Continuous naloxone administration suppresses opiate withdrawal symptoms in human opiate addicts during detoxification treatment. J Psychiatr Res 23:81–86, 1989

Martin WR, Jasinski DR: Physiological parameters of morphine in man: tolerance, early abstinence, protracted abstinence. J Psychiatr Res 7:9–16, 1969

McLellan AT, Luborsky L, Woody GE, et al: An improved diagnostic evaluation instrument for substance abuse patients: the Addiction Severity Index. J Nerv Ment Dis 168:26–33, 1980

National Council Against Health Fraud: Acupuncture: The position paper of the National Council Against Health Fraud. American Journal of Acupuncture 19:273–279, 1991

O'Connor PG, Kosten TR: Rapid and ultrarapid opioid detoxification techniques. JAMA 279:229–234, 1998

O'Connor PG, Waugh ME, Carroll KM, et al: Primary care-based ambulatory opioid detoxification: the results of a clinical trial. J Gen Intern Med 10:255–260, 1995

O'Connor PG, Carroll KM, Shi JM, et al: Three methods of opioid detoxification in a primary care setting. A randomized trial. Ann Intern Med 127:526–530, 1997

Satel SL, Kosten TR, Schuckit MA, et al: Should protracted withdrawal from drugs be included in DSM-IV? Am J Psychiatry 150:695–704, 1993

Spencer L, Gregory M: Clonidine transdermal patches for use in outpatient opiate withdrawal. J Subst Abuse Treat 6:113–117, 1989

Ter Riet GT, Kleijnen J, Knipschild P: A meta-analysis of studies into the effect of acupuncture on addiction. Br J Gen Pract 40:379–382, 1990

Ulett GA: Beyond Yin and Yang: How Acupuncture Really Works. St. Louis, MO, Warren H Breen, 1992

Vining E, Kosten TR, Kleber HD: Clinical utility of rapid clonidine-naltrexone detoxification for opioid abuse. British Journal of Addiction 83:567–575, 1988

Washburn AM, Fullilove RE, Fullilove MT, et al: Acupuncture heroin detoxification: a single-blind clinical trial. J Subst Abuse Treat 10:345–351, 1993

Wen HL, Cheung SYC: Treatment of drug addiction by acupuncture and electrical stimulation. American Journal of Acupuncture 1:71–75, 1973

Opioids: Methadone Maintenance

Edward C. Senay, M.D.

Properly prescribed methadone substantially reduces and frequently eliminates use of nonprescribed opioids in heroin-dependent populations (Dole and Nyswander 1965; Newman and Whitehill 1979). Because many addicted persons must commit crimes to get money for illegal opioids, an indirect effect of legal methadone is to reduce or to eliminate associated crime (Ball et al. 1988a). Methadone has no direct effect on low self-esteem, psychopathology, or the social problems that frequently accompany opioid dependence. A comprehensive program of services, in which methadone is prescribed as one of the services, may have desirable effects on some or all of these factors by changing the balance of forces on and in the addicted person. (For example, the addicted person with antisocial personality disorder has to steal less because of the methadone, thus avoiding arrests.)

The foregoing statements are supported by close to three decades of clinical experience and the largest scientific database ever gathered on any biopsychosocial problem (Senay 1989). The proper question to ask with respect to the clinical use of methadone is whether or not it is achieving the goal of reducing use of nonprescribed opioids. The quality of the program in which the methadone is used, the community in which the program is embedded, funding levels, regulatory interventions, and the availability of economic and educational opportunity—all must be examined if other effects are in question.

When properly prescribed, methadone is not intoxicating or sedating, is effective orally, suppresses narcotic withdrawal and "craving" for 24–36 hours, and does not have effects that interfere with ordinary activities such as reading a newspaper or with activities such as driving a car or operating an industrial machine in which safety is an issue. The methadone maintenance patient who is intoxicated from the methadone, by definition, is getting improperly prescribed, poorly monitored doses of methadone.

Results from methadone maintenance programs reveal that one-third of patients do well, one-third vacillate between good and bad performance, and one-third show no change from a lifestyle centered on drugs and crime. The clinician needs to appreciate the subtlety that before methadone there was no way to effect the positive outcome of the one-third of patients who do well or the successful periods of treatment for the one-third who vacillate. Methadone, for most opioid-dependent persons, is not a cure, but substantial benefits result from its proper use. For example, a growing body of evidence indicates that methadone maintenance programs have prevented many opiate-injecting persons from getting human immunodeficiency virus (HIV) (Barthwell et al. 1989; Novick et al. 1990), and there is substantial evidence that needle use and needle sharing are lessened when addicted persons enter methadone programs (Ball et al. 1988b).

Many addicted persons develop careers marked by periods of abstinence interspersed with periods of addiction. These persons use the treatment system to abort the episodes of addiction. Early in their career, addicted persons use all the treatment modalities—that is, drug free, therapeutic communities, methadone maintenance, and detoxification. As their career lengthens, addicted persons tend to use methadone maintenance preferentially over the other modalities. The clinical reality is that addicted persons often leave treatment before completing their recovery. But they will use the system for future episodes of addiction, and the net effect on their career is an amelioration that is significant for the addicted person and for the community.

Federal and State Eligibility Criteria for Methadone Maintenance

Methadone can be used for analgesia by any licensed physician. It cannot be used for the treatment of opioid dependence unless it is used by a physician working in a treatment facility licensed by a state. States can have criteria more stringent than those established by the U.S. Food and Drug Administration (FDA), but they cannot have less stringent criteria. States differ in eligibility criteria and in a variety of regulations on matters such as take-home methadone. By federal mandate, each state must have a single state agency that licenses and coordinates drug treatment and prevention programs. If there are questions about eligibility criteria, the designated state agency should be consulted. The FDA's eligibility criteria for methadone maintenance (21 CFR 291, 1994), defined as the use of methadone for the treatment of narcotic dependence for more than 90 days, are as follows:

a. **Current Physiologic Dependence on Opioids.** A one-year history of physiologic dependence on opioids must be present together with current physiologic dependence as demonstrated by positive urines for opioids, needle tracks and signs and symptoms of opioid withdrawal. The regulations do not specify any particular subset of the foregoing criteria for current physiologic dependence; it is a medical judgment that physiologic dependence exists. The regulations require that the judgment must be based on some of the criteria. An addict, for example, may never have used needles and can still have acquired a substantial degree of physiologic dependence by "snorting" i.e. insufflating opioids. The physiologic dependence on opioids must have existed episodically or continuously for a one year period. If the addict has a history of only six to seven months of dependence during a given year then the physician should consult with the single state agency before beginning a treatment regimen of methadone maintenance.
b. **Persons From Penal Institutions.** A person who has been in a penal institution is eligible for methadone maintenance after a period of incarceration without current physiologic dependence on opioids if eligibility criteria were met before entering the penal institution.

c. **Pregnant Patients.** Pregnant patients can be placed on MM [methadone maintenance] if currently physiologically dependent on opioids. There is no stipulation that the dependence must have existed for one year in the case of the pregnant addict, simply that physiologic dependence is current. A physician can place a pregnant addict, opioid dependent in the past, on MM without current physiologic dependence if return to opioid dependence is a threat.
d. **Previously Treated Patients.** For a two year period following an episode of MM patients may be readmitted without evidence of current physiologic dependence if the physician documents that return to opioid dependence is imminent.
e. **Persons Under 18 Years of Age.** Persons under 18 must have two documented attempts at drug detoxification or drug free treatment with a 1-week period between treatment episodes and they must show evidence of current physiologic dependence on opioids to be eligible for MM. A parent, legal guardian or responsible adult designated by state authority must also complete and sign an official FDA consent form (obtainable from the single state agency) to complete the eligibility criteria.

These criteria may vary in that a state can elect to be more stringent; for example, states can require 2 years of physiological dependence before methadone maintenance is legal, or they may make the rules for take-home methadone more stringent. FDA regulations permit programs to dispense one or two take-home doses of methadone after a 3- to 6-month period of good performance in treatment. Some states require longer periods of good performance, and some may not permit take-home doses at all.

If a patient has current physiological dependence on opioids but does not meet the FDA criteria just cited, then methadone can be used for detoxification for up to a 90-day period. This use is defined by FDA regulations as *methadone detoxification*.

Safety of Methadone

Close to three decades of clinical research have established that medically prescribed methadone is safe and that its routine use is remarkably free from serious problems. Common side effects are sedation, if the dose is too high; constipation, which can be treated by increasing fluid intake and using stool softeners; occasional transient ankle edema in females; excessive sweating; and changes in libido. All these effects tend to improve with the passage of time, but they may require dose reduction if they are very disturbing to the patient. There are four recorded cases of severe edema in methadone maintenance patients in the literature (O'Conor et al. 1991).

Daily administration of opioids increases the possibility of synergism with other psychoactive drugs. Patients who develop alcohol problems while on methadone may be required to take breathalyzer tests before methadone is administered. If levels are 0.05 mg% or above, methadone is not administered until levels are below 0.05 mg% or perhaps until the next visit. Persons who use multiple drugs while on methadone are, of course, at risk of lethal overdose because of synergism.

Studies of the biotransformation of methadone indicate wide interindividual variability in blood levels following identical dosing regimens. This research suggests that persons who respond poorly to treatment may not absorb methadone from the gastrointestinal tract normally (Kelley et al. 1978). Liver and renal disease may account for some of the individual variation. Any stress—for example, heavy alcohol or cocaine consumption, severe weather changes, or marital discord—can speed the biotransformation of methadone, which can lead, in a previously stable dosing regimen, to associated complaints of withdrawal toward the end of the 24-hour cycle.

A number of investigators, as reviewed by Gritz et al. (1975), have found that methadone does not interfere with reaction time; methadone maintenance patients did not appear to have memory deficits as tested by Gritz et al., but chronic administration of methadone was found to differentiate performance of patients from that of control subjects on tests of recall in that in the former, subtle recall deficits appeared on the more difficult tests. Clinically these effects are not detectable. In a study of driving records, Maddox et al. (1977) found no evidence that would argue for restricting driving privileges of persons while on methadone maintenance. Methadone maintenance clinics in our large cities have patients from most, if not all, occupations necessary to the daily life of large urban centers.

Rifampin, barbiturates, and tricyclic antidepressants may induce liver enzymes that speed the biotransformation of methadone. Patients taking these medications may need increases in the dose of methadone to maintain stability. Methadone can be used concurrently, with close monitoring, with therapeutic doses of antidepressants, antipsychotics, anticonvulsants, anxiolytics, sedative-hypnotics, lithium, or disulfiram (Ling et al. 1983). Methadone and clonidine should not be used concurrently because of the danger of synergism of their sedative effects.

Dosage

Initial Dose

If an opiate-addicted person gives a history of using low-potency heroin in the 3-week period preceding the examination and of using just once or twice a day—and if, in addition, he or she has minimal signs of opioid withdrawal—then an initial dose of 5 or 10 mg of methadone would be indicated. If 1) use in the preceding 3 weeks has been more frequent than once a day, *and* 2a) the potency of the heroin is estimated to be moderate to strong, *and* 2b) the patient has dilated pupils, rhinorrhea and tearing, then the initial dose should be in the 10-mg to 20-mg range. If the clinician is prescribing for someone using high doses of fentanyl or if there is obvious severe opioid withdrawal, as there may be in cases in some communities in which high-potency heroin is being used, then an initial dose of 20–40 mg should be employed.

If an addicted person is not going to be observed for a 1- to 2-hour period after an initial dose, then it is best to err on the low side, because there is evidence that at least some addicted persons entering treatment are not physically dependent despite the fact that they meet all the criteria for physical dependence, including positive results on urine analysis for morphine and positive signs of opioid withdrawal (Kanof et al. 1991; Senay and Schick 1978). A dose of 30–40 mg in these patients may induce a significant degree of sedation, and if there is use of heroin, alcohol, and/or other drugs, as there may be following the initial dose when the addicted person leaves the clinic, the possibility of an overdose exists. It is good practice to observe the patient for a 1- to 2-hour period after the first dose to see what the effects of the dose are on the signs of opioid withdrawal. Adjustments can then be made on the basis of clinical observation combined with the patient's report. All of the foregoing comments pertain to outpatient settings. Empirically, initial and maintenance doses in hospitalized patients can be lower than is necessary in outpatient settings.

Maintenance Dose

The maintenance dose of methadone must be individualized. The clinician and/or the staff should observe the effects of a given dose with the following endpoints in mind: 1) suppression of narcotic withdrawal, 2) no induction of euphoria or sedation, and 3) reduction or elimination of narcotic use as measured by self-reports and other reports and from the results of random, monitored (visually or by temperature) urine screens. Urine screens are particularly useful in the early phase of maintenance and with relapsing patients, and they are critical in evaluating the success of programs.

Federal regulations prohibit methadone dosages above 120 mg/day without special permission from the FDA and/or state regulatory authorities. Most methadone clinics have patients who are successful at both ends of the dose spectrum defined by federal regulation. Thus, there will be some patients who do well on 10–50 mg/day, whereas others will require doses at the other end of the spectrum. There is no rationale for forcing patients at the lower end of the dosage spectrum to higher doses, because this will have the consequence of prolonging the duration and increasing the severity of withdrawal if they want to detoxify. If one examines large numbers of addicted persons from a national perspective, it appears that better results are achieved at dosages in excess of 60 mg/day (Hargreaves 1983). A recent study (Strain et al. 1999) confirmed this earlier finding.

When administered chronically, methadone accumulates in pools in body tissues and there is a steady blood concentration. A given daily dose does not cause a sharp increase in blood levels. This accounts for the drug's inability to produce sedation or intoxication and for the fact that methadone is not an effective analgesic in methadone maintenance patients. The pool level may not decrease much following omission of a daily dose, which accounts for the fact that omission of a daily dose may not cause withdrawal. Optimal blood levels in a methadone maintenance patient are between 150 and 600 ng/mL (Dole 1988).

The clinician will encounter a spectrum whose ends are defined by two different populations of addicted persons. The first group of patients will try to manipulate endlessly for higher and higher doses. The second group will resist higher doses because of fears that methadone habits are "worse than heroin habits," "methadone gets in your bones," and the like. Most addicted persons will range between these two poles. With the former group it is good procedure to observe the patient for signs of withdrawal, such as dilated pupils, moist skin, runny nose, and tearing, 24 hours after the last dose of methadone. The signs of withdrawal should bear some relationship to the severity of complaints (other than "craving"). The clinician can then decide whether or not to increase the dose. If an increase in dose appears to be indicated, then it may be made in increments of 5 or 10 mg, depending on clinical judgment of what effects are desired. In a patient with severe complaints of withdrawal but no signs of withdrawal, one might prescribe a 5-mg increment; in a patient with severe complaints of withdrawal and positive signs, a 10-mg increment may be appropriate. Any change should be discussed with the patient, and the clinician should make it clear to the patient that as the dose goes up, the difficulty in withdrawing also goes up with respect to both the length of time that will be necessary for the patient to accomplish detoxification and the severity of withdrawal that will likely be experienced.

Positive urine sample results for opiates should prompt serious consideration of raising the methadone dose, because cessation of illegal opiate use is the first priority. Drug hunger or craving bears no constant relationship to narcotic withdrawal, and although the observation may indicate few or no signs of withdrawal, an increase in dosage is justified to attempt to stop the patient's illicit opiate use. Increments of 5 mg every few days should be employed until use of illegal opioids has diminished or disappeared or until legal ceilings have been reached. If the patient is willing, the clinician may request an exemption from the guidelines of the state agency to bring the methadone dosage higher than normally permitted, because it may be that the patient is a rapid metabolizer of methadone.

Clinical experience indicates that 6–24 months is a cutoff point for many addicted persons in that it appears to take that long for them to accomplish changes in lifestyle. For others, who may constitute one-third or more of a given clinic population, opioid use will continue. If the continuation is at a much reduced level and, particularly, if it means a relative or complete cessation of needle use or needle sharing, then this is a legitimate clinical outcome and the maintenance program should be continued. The administration of a daily dose of methadone, at almost any level, probably lessens the urgency of pressure to use narcotics and thus gives the addicted person a little more time for making judgments than would otherwise be the case. The addicted person may be better able to decline to use or to share needles and thus has a lower likelihood of contracting HIV.

What to do about the patient who is not doing well involves a number of considerations, including clinic policy, a clinical cost-benefit analysis, and pressure on the clinic for services. The challenge for the clinician is to find the factors responsible for the continued drug use. An addicted person whose family and extended family are involved in drug dealing may find family and neighborhood pressures too strong to overcome. For such a patient, a move to a new neighborhood may be the prescription. In others a divorce, change of jobs, or entrance to a controlled environment such as a therapeutic community may be considered. Most addicted persons in methadone maintenance programs will have to change friends if they want to get out of the drug culture.

For patients whose treatment was not successful, some clinics, at the end of a 6- to 12-month period, decrease the dose of methadone by 1–3 mg for each positive urine sample result so that the patient detoxifies himself or herself out of the program by continued drug use. In the age of HIV, such policies need to be reconsidered, because returning someone to needle use and possibly needle sharing creates risk of contracting HIV.

The scientific evidence, as reviewed by Cooper (1992), indicates that the clinician should explore dosage increases in treatment-refractory patients rather than dosage decreases. Program policies that limit the duration of methadone maintenance (to, e.g., 2 years) are difficult to justify in this age of HIV. Attempts to force patients who do not want to undergo withdrawal from successful methadone maintenance usually cause much suffering and, in the occasional case, may lead to the patient's incarceration and/or death. Patients who are being successfully maintained on methadone should be allowed indefinite maintenance, even lifelong if they so desire.

No rationale exists for blind withdrawal of methadone from a legally competent adult without his or her consent. In a blind detoxification, the patient's dosage is gradually reduced without the patient's being aware of when and how much the dose is being changed. Blind detoxification is probably the best regimen for most addicted persons who want to prepare to become drug-free. In these cases, however, the patient has agreed to the contract. Blind withdrawal without the patient's consent may result in much suffering with little or no clinical gain. The legally competent adult patient has a right to know his or her dose.

Structure of Methadone Programs

Methadone programs commonly have "cardinal" rules that prohibit drug dealing or selling of goods of any kind, threats of violence, carrying of weapons, display of gang colors, and so forth. The ability of the clinic administration to enforce these rules will determine the clinical context in which methadone is dispensed. Program results will not be as good as they can be if the clinic atmosphere is controlled by an uncaring administration or, alternatively, by clients who are not able to change from street life and who make the clinic an extension of the drug/street culture rather than a center governed by the culture of hope and recovery. In general, the program will have better results when the staff is stable; has either training or life experience, or both, that provides for sensitivity on racial, ethnic, and gender issues; and that has a board of directors that takes an active interest in the life of the clinic. Many clinics have formerly addicted persons as counselors, and studies indicate that these persons are effective in changing drug behavior but often have no formal training and are therefore not effective in other areas (e.g., mental health) important to the recovery process (of which methadone is just one component).

A number of behavior modification techniques have been demonstrated to have clinical usefulness, although the clinic system as a whole has not had the resources to put this new technology on line (S. H. Hall et al. 1991; O'Brien et al. 1991; Stitzer and Kirby 1991). The difficulties in applying this technology are discussed by Nolimal and Crowley (1990). A recently developed performance-based program (Kidorf et al. 1999) reported impressive results and retention rates.

Methadone and Pregnancy

The pregnant opioid-dependent patient presents a dilemma because clinical experience indicates that attempts to detoxify the patient carry substantial risk of death for her fetus. The human adult rarely dies or has convulsions from opioid withdrawal, but the human fetus/neonate undergoing opioid withdrawal is liable to have convulsions and to die. In the United States, several clinical centers have independently arrived at a policy of maintaining a pregnant opioid-dependent woman throughout her pregnancy and delivery on doses of methadone as *low* as possible. This regimen avoids fetal death from withdrawal and also avoids the death of neonates from withdrawal if high doses of methadone are used for maintenance throughout the pregnancy. Additional principles of management of the drug-dependent woman are given by Finnegan (1991).

Methadone and Medical/Surgical/Obstetric Problems

Experience has taught clinicians that opioid withdrawal is a major stress and that it is not wise to sum stresses on an individual. For this reason, the heroin-addicted person with a concurrent medical problem should be maintained on methadone during any acute medical stress. In the event that a given medical/surgical/obstetric patient is on methadone maintenance, the dose used for maintenance should be continued throughout the hospitalization. If the opioid-addicted person is a so-called street addict, then, in most cases, smooth control can be achieved with methadone 10–30 mg/day. Control of withdrawal is usually possible with once-a-day administration, but if problems arise at the end of the 24-hour withdrawal period, the clinician can split the total dose into two or three parts administered daily.

If anesthesia is necessary, the fact of the patient's current dependence on opioids should be communicated to the anesthesiologist. Pentazocine or other mixed agonist-antagonists, such as buprenorphine, are contraindicated for analgesia because they may have antagonist actions and cause or worsen withdrawal. Empirically, the opiate-addicted person will need regular analgesics in normal doses with normal frequencies, in addition to the daily dose of methadone, for the duration of the medical/surgical/obstetric treatment. When hospital treatment is complete, a decision can be made about detoxification. If an addicted person wants to be detoxified, referral to a drug abuse program should be the option of choice. Many patients will not want to be detoxified and will want to return to heroin use in their customary surroundings. There may be no other option, as drug abuse treatment programs in many areas of the country have long waiting lists and the option of withdrawal on medical-surgical wards is problematic. Methadone maintenance patients should be referred back to their programs of origin.

Psychiatric Aspects of Methadone Treatment

A number of studies indicate that opioid-dependent populations have rates of depressive symptoms perhaps three times higher than those found in community-based samples (Ginzburg et al. 1984). The daily administration of methadone does not appear to improve or to worsen the depression. Anxiety disorders and antisocial personality disorder also appear to be more frequent in opioid-dependent populations than in the general population. Methadone has no effect on antisocial personality disorder, but if an antisocial personality disorder patient is depressed, the depression may be treated and general functioning is improved. Some feel that methadone may have therapeutic effects on patients with schizophrenia or bipolar disorder. In my experience, if methadone does have such effects, they are quite variable from patient to patient and are not dramatic in any one patient (for a review of psychopathology and addiction, see Meyer 1986).

McLellan et al. (1993), in their study of randomly assigned groups who received methadone alone or methadone with two levels of enhanced services, found that the addition of counseling and professional services significantly improved treatment efficacy. Previous studies by McLellan (1986) found that psychiatric severity predicts treatment outcome, with patients with high psychiatric severity who had not responded to standard substance abuse treatment regimens and patients with low psychiatric severity doing well in all standard regimens, and patients with midrange psychiatric severity having differential responses to standard treatments.

New Drugs for Legal Substitution Treatment

Levomethadyl acetate (LAAM) is a long-acting congener of methadone that is being explored for use in legal substitution treatment. In a LAAM regimen, the opiate-addicted person needs only three-times-a-week administration, usually on Monday, Wednesday, and Friday, with the Friday dose being some 10% to 15% higher than the Monday or Wednesday dose. Take-home LAAM needs exploration, because intravenous LAAM has an onset of action that can be hours from the time of injection, in contrast to the onset of oral LAAM, which is similar to that of methadone. Addicted persons may not appreciate this difference and may keep injecting the drug, resulting in an overdose. Results with LAAM are equal to those with methadone, although a different subset of addicted patients seems to be helped by LAAM. Buprenorphine, a partial opioid mixed agonist-antagonist, is being explored in legal substitution and withdrawal treatment for opioid dependence.

References

Ball JC, Corty E, Bond H, et al: The reduction of intravenous heroin use, non-opiate abuse and crime during methadone maintenance treatment: further findings, in Problems of Drug Dependence, 1987: Proceedings of the 49th Annual Scientific Meeting, the Committee on Problems of Drug Dependence. NIDA Research Monograph 81 (DHHS Publ No [ADM] 88-1564). Edited by Harris L. Rockville, MD, National Institute on Drug Abuse, 1988a, pp 224–229

Ball JC, Lange WR, Myers E, et al: Reducing the risk of AIDS through methadone maintenance treatment. J Health Soc Behav 29:214–226, 1988b

Barthwell A, Senay E, Marks R, et al: Patients successfully maintained with methadone escaped human immunodeficiency virus infection (letter). Arch Gen Psychiatry 46:957–958, 1989

Cooper JR: Ineffective use of psychoactive drugs. JAMA 267:281–282, 1992

Dole VP: Implications of methadone maintenance for theories of narcotic addiction. JAMA 260:3025–3029, 1988

Dole VP, Nyswander ME: A medical treatment of diacetylmorphine (heroin) addiction. JAMA 193:646–650, 1965

Finnegan LP: Perinatal substance abuse: comments and perspectives. Semin Perinatol 15:331–339, 1991

Ginzburg HM, Allison M, Hubbard RL: Depressive symptoms in drug abuse treatment clients: correlates, treatment and changes, in Problems of Drug Dependence, 1983: Proceedings of the 45th Annual Scientific Meeting, the Committee on Problems of Drug Dependence. NIDA Research Monograph 49 (DHHS Publ No [ADM] 84-1316). Edited by Harris LS. Rockville, MD, National Institute on Drug Abuse, 1984, pp 313–319

Gritz ER, Shiffman SM, Jarvik ME, et al: Physiological and psychological effects of methadone in man. Arch Gen Psychiatry 32:237–242, 1975

Hall SH, Wasserman DA, Havassy B: Relapse prevention, in Improving Drug Abuse Treatment. NIDA Research Monograph 106 (DHHS Publ No [ADM] 91-1754). Edited by Pickens RW, Leukefeld CG, Schuster CR. Rockville, MD, National Institute on Drug Abuse, 1991, pp 279–292

Hargreaves WA: Methadone dose and duration for maintenance treatment, in Research on the Treatment of Narcotic Addiction: State of the Art. NIDA Treatment Research Monograph 70 (DHHS Publ No [ADM] 83-1281). Edited by Cooper J, Altman F, Brown BS, et al. Washington, DC, U.S. Government Printing Office, 1983, pp 19–79

Kanof PD, Aronson MJ, Ness R, et al: Levels of opioid physical dependence in heroin addicts. Drug Alcohol Depend 27:253–262, 1991

Kelley D, Welch R, McNeely N, et al: Methadone maintenance; an assessment of potential fluctuations in behavior between doses. International Journal of Addictions 13:1061–1068, 1978

Kidorf M, King V, Brooner R: Integrating psychosocial services with methadone treatment, in Methadone Treatment for Opioid Dependence. Edited by Strain EC, Stitzer ML. Baltimore, MD, Johns Hopkins University Press, 1999, pp 166–195

Ling W, Weiss DG, Charuvastra VC, et al: Use of disulfiram for alcoholics in methadone maintenance programs: a Veterans Administration cooperative study. Arch Gen Psychiatry 40:851–854, 1983

Maddox JF, Williams TR, Ziegler DA, et al: Driving records before and during methadone maintenance. Am J Drug Alcohol Abuse 4:91–100, 1977

McLellan AT: "Psychiatric severity" as a predictor of outcome from substance abuse treatments, in Psychopathology and Addictive Disorders. Edited by Meyer RE. New York, Guilford, 1986, pp 97–135

McLellan AT, Arndt IO, Metzger DS, et al: The effects of psychosocial services in substance abuse treatment. JAMA 269:1953–1959, 1993

Meyer RE (ed): Psychopathology and Addictive Disorders. New York, Guilford, 1986

Newman RG, Whitehill WB: Double-blind comparison of methadone and placebo maintenance treatments of narcotic addicts in Hong Kong. Lancet 2(8141):485–488, 1979

Nolimal D, Crowley TJ: Difficulties in a clinical application of methadone-dose contingency contracting. J Subst Abuse Treat 7:219–224, 1990

Novick DM, Joseph H, Croxson TS, et al: Absence of antibody to human immunodeficiency virus in long-term, socially rehabilitated methadone maintenance patients. Arch Intern Med 150:97–99, 1990

O'Brien CP, Childress AR, McLellan AT: Conditioning factors may help to understand and prevent relapse in patients who are recovering from drug dependence, in Improving Drug Abuse Treatment. NIDA Research Monograph 106 (DHHS Publ No [ADM] 91-1754). Edited by Pickens RW, Leukefeld CG, Schuster CR. Rockville, MD, National Institute on Drug Abuse, 1991, pp 293–312

O'Conor LM, Woody G, Yeh H-S, et al: Methadone and edema. J Subst Abuse Treat 8:153–155, 1991

Senay EC: Methadone maintenance, in Treatments of Psychiatric Disorders: A Task Force Report of the American Psychiatric Association, Vol 2. Washington, DC, American Psychiatric Association, 1989, pp 1342–1359

Senay EC, Schick JF: Pupillography responses to methadone challenge: aid to diagnosis of opioid dependence. Drug Alcohol Depend 3:133–138, 1978

Stitzer ML, Kirby KC: Reducing illicit drug use among methadone patients, in Improving Drug Abuse Treatment. NIDA Research Monograph 106 (DHHS Publ No [ADM] 91-1754). Edited by Pickens RW, Leukefeld CG, Schuster CR. Rockville, MD, National Institute on Drug Abuse, 1991, pp 178–203

Strain EC, Bigelow GE, Leibson IA, et al: Moderate- vs high-dose methadone in the treatment of opioid dependence. JAMA 281:1000–1005, 1999

Antagonist Treatment: Use of Naltrexone and Related Medications

Charles P. O'Brien, M.D., Ph.D.

Basic research in an effort to find better and nonaddicting analgesics has had the by-product of increasing our knowledge of the endogenous opioid system. These discoveries have already been translated into improvements in treatment of addiction using opiate antagonists and partial agonists. Our understanding of the biology of opiate effects, including opiate dependence, is well developed and probably more complete than our understanding of the biology of any other class of drugs of abuse (for a review, see O'Brien 1992). Of course, much remains to be learned about the chronic changes produced in opiate receptors and the cascade of subsequent intracellular changes produced after drug-receptor interactions. The changes during the development of tolerance and dependence are only beginning to be addressed (Nestler et al. 1993), but there is already considerable knowledge about the interaction between these receptors and both opiates (i.e., derivatives of the opium plant) and opioids (i.e., synthetic substances acting at opiate receptors).

This increased understanding has led to the classification of drugs into three basic categories, according to their interaction with opiate receptors:

1. agonists (e.g., heroin, methadone), which activate specific opiate receptors
2. antagonists (e.g., naloxone, naltrexone), which occupy opiate receptors but do not activate them
3. partial agonists (e.g., buprenorphine), which occupy opiate receptors but activate them only in a limited way and also may block the occupation of receptors by other substances, thus producing both agonist and antagonist effects

Of all the medications used in the treatment of opiate dependence, methadone, a long-acting agonist at the μ subtype of opiate receptor, has clearly had the greatest impact (see previous chapter subpart by Senay on methadone maintenance). Naltrexone, which became available for general use in 1985, is an antagonist, and its use therefore constitutes a distinctly different treatment from treatment with methadone. Naltrexone specifically blocks opiate receptors; while the drug is present, it prevents readdiction to heroin and other opiates and opioid drugs. Because it is so different from other available agents used in treatment of addictions, naltrexone is commonly misunderstood. Clinicians tend to confuse it with disulfiram (Antabuse) for the treatment of alcoholism or with methadone for agonist maintenance of opioid-addicted persons. As an antagonist, naltrexone has a mechanism of action that is specific, and to use this tool effectively, this mechanism should be clearly understood.

Despite naltrexone's pharmacological distinctiveness, the basic requirements for good treatment of addiction still apply. The administration of naltrexone should be included in a comprehensive treatment program with attention to the nonpharmacological variables that play a critical role in the overall addiction syndrome. The prescription of naltrexone alone will not be adequate. This medication should be part of an overall treatment program that includes individual or group psychotherapy, family therapy, contingency contracting, and possibly behavioral extinction of drug-conditioned responses.

Experience has shown that naltrexone will not appeal to the majority of opioid-dependent persons. Not more than 10%–15% of heroin addicts show any interest in a drug that prevents them from getting high (Greenstein et al. 1984). The vast majority prefer methadone treatment, but for those highly motivated patients who prefer to be opioid-free, naltrexone is an excellent alternative. Certain patients—such as health care professionals, middle-class addicted persons, and formerly addicted persons given an early parole from prison (Cornish et al. 1997)—may find naltrexone to be the treatment of choice.

Naltrexone is a very specific drug with a very high affinity for opiate receptors. It does not block the effects of nonopiate drugs such as cocaine or marijuana, although there is evidence that it diminishes the "high" produced by alcohol. This latter effect is thought to be mediated via the endogenous opiate system, which is activated by alcohol.

Of course, many patients use multiple drugs, and a common combination is heroin with cocaine. There is clinical evidence that taking the two drugs together—the "speedball" effect—enhances the euphoria. Heroin is also used by cocaine addicts to counteract some of the negative effects of cocaine. Those patients dependent on both opioids and cocaine may be treated with naltrexone, but they will need additional therapy to deal with their cocaine dependence.

Opioid Receptor Interactions

The opiates (e.g., heroin and morphine) as well as the synthetic opioids (e.g., methadone and meperidine) act through specific opioid receptors; these drugs are referred to as *agonists* (Reisine and Pasternak 1995). Antagonists such as naloxone or naltrexone also bind to these receptors but do not activate the receptor to initiate the chain of cellular events that produce so-called opiate effects. Naloxone and naltrexone are relatively pure antagonists in that they produce little or no agonist activity at usual doses. Partial agonists/antagonists such as nalorphine and buprenorphine, in contrast, produce significant agonist effects of their own. Not only do pure antagonists fail to produce opioid effects, but their presence at the receptor also prevents opioid agonists from binding to the receptor and producing pharmacological effects.

Because the antagonist competes for a binding site with the agonist, the degree of blockade depends on the relative concentrations of each and their relative affinities for the receptor site. Naltrexone has greatest affinity for the μ category of opiate receptors and thus can block virtually all of the effects of the usual doses of opiates such as heroin. In the presence of a full dose of naltrexone, there can be no opiate-induced euphoria, respiratory depression, pupillary constriction, or any other significant opiate effect (Martin et al. 1973; O'Brien et al. 1975).

There are four types of medical uses for opiate antagonists:

1. To reverse the effects of an opiate, particularly in the treatment of an opiate overdose. Naloxone is commonly used to counteract the effects of high-dose morphine anesthesia and to reverse opiate-induced respiratory depression in newborns. Naltrexone would also have this effect, but it is not used because of its long duration of action. If too much naloxone is given to an opiate-dependent person who has overdosed, the person will move from an overdose state to one of precipitated withdrawal.
2. To diagnose physical dependence on opioid drugs. An antagonist such as naloxone will displace the opiate from the receptors in a dependent person and produce an immediate withdrawal syndrome. For this purpose, the short duration of naloxone is again an advantage.
3. To prevent readdiction in a person who has been detoxified from opiate drugs. This is a major indication for naltrexone and will be discussed in detail in the section below.
4. To reduce the likelihood of relapse in alcoholic individuals who are also engaged in a behavioral treatment program. This is the newest indication for naltrexone and has led to greatly increased usage worldwide.

Naltrexone in Treatment of Opiate Addiction

Individuals who are currently dependent on opioids are exquisitely sensitive to opiate antagonists. This fact forms the basis of the naloxone test for opioid dependence mentioned above. The degree of sensitivity depends on the time since the last dose of opiate and the size of the opiate dose. Even a very small amount of naloxone or naltrexone can rapidly displace enough opioid from opiate receptors to precipitate a withdrawal syndrome. Thus, before starting naltrexone, it is important to be certain that an opioid-dependent person is fully detoxified. If the presence of physical dependence is in question, a small (0.4–0.8 mg) injection of naloxone can be given. In a dependent person, a withdrawal syndrome would immediately occur, although it would be short-lived (20–40 minutes).

There are several pharmacological options for detoxification. One approach is to gradually reduce doses of methadone for 5–10 days. At the other end of the spectrum, a rapid detoxification assisted by clonidine can have the opioid-dependent patient ready for naltrexone in as little as 48 hours (Kleber and Kosten 1984). The choice of psychopharmacological approach depends on the type of opioid agonist the patient was using (short-acting versus long-acting), the motivation of the patient, and the need for speed in returning the patient to work. The technique of very rapid opiate detoxification under general anesthesia has received a great deal of publicity in recent years, but there is no evidence that the increased risk is justified by a better long-term outcome (Kleber 1998).

Pharmacokinetic studies of naltrexone show a plasma half-life of the parent compound of 4–6 hours. An important active metabolite, 6-β-naltrexol, has a plasma half-life of 12 hours. With chronic administration, both peak and trough levels of 6-β-naltrexol increase. The pharmacological duration of naltrexone is actually longer than might be predicted by the plasma kinetics; this is supported by a positron-emission tomography (PET) study in human volunteers that showed substantial blockade of μ opiate receptor binding for more than 72 hours after a 50-mg dose (Lee et al. 1988). This observation was consistent with findings of an early study of duration of blockade of injected opiates. In that study, a double-blind investigation of former addicts maintained on naltrexone, a 150-mg dose of the drug was shown to be effective in attenuating the effects of opioids for 72 hours (O'Brien et al. 1975).

In the presence of naltrexone, heroin self-administration is no longer rewarding, and subjects are observed to stop taking available heroin (Mello et al. 1981). Although daily ingestion of naltrexone would provide the most secure protection against opioid effects, naltrexone administered as infrequently as two or three times per week will provide adequate protection against readdiction. The reduced frequency makes monitoring of the medication more practical over the long term. A depot formulation of naltrexone that gives effective blood levels for 30–60 days is currently undergoing clinical trials (Kranzler et al. 1998). This formulation will make adherence to the treatment regimen more consistent and presumably will improve the results of treatment of both heroin addiction and alcoholism. Tolerance to the antagonism of opioid effects does not appear to develop even after more than a year of regular naltrexone ingestion (Kleber et al. 1985).

Benefits of Opiate Antagonist Treatment

Naltrexone was approved by the U.S. Food and Drug Administration (FDA) on the basis of its clear pharmacological activity as an opiate antagonist. However, it has never been shown in large-scale double-blind trials to be more effective than placebo in the rehabilitation of opiate-addicted persons. In clinical trials with persons addicted to street heroin, the dropout rate is very high, just as it is in drug-free outpatient treatment of heroin addiction. Naltrexone clearly is not effective when simply prescribed as a medication in the absence of a structured rehabilitation program. Within a structured program, however, naltrexone appears to be effective, particularly with specific motivated populations. A randomized controlled trial (Cornish et al. 1997) among federal probationers showed that the impressions of naltrexone's efficacy can be confirmed by data collected in such motivated groups.

Naltrexone can permit addicted persons who have been recently detoxified to return to their usual environments secure in the knowledge that they cannot succumb to an impulsive wish to get "high." For many patients, this may be the first time in years that they have been able to exist outside of a hospital or prison in an opioid-free state. The subtle manifestations of the protracted opioid withdrawal syndrome are known to persist for months (Martin and Jasinski 1969). During this protracted withdrawal period, the patient's autonomic nervous system is unstable, and symptoms such as anxiety and sleep disturbances are common. Conditioned responses to environmental cues produced by previous drug use (O'Brien et al. 1986; Wikler 1965) also may contribute to relapse. Maintenance on naltrexone provides an ideal situation to extinguish these conditioned responses (O'Brien 1992; O'Brien et al. 1980) and to permit the protracted withdrawal syndrome to subside.

For a person recovering from opiate addiction who works in a field such as nursing, pharmacy, or medicine, there is an added benefit to naltrexone maintenance. When a health care professional returns to work after treatment for an opiate addiction, colleagues and supervisors tend to be suspicious of any unusual behavior. Knowing that the recovering individual is taking naltrexone helps to reduce this distrust Because these medical occupations often require continuing access to opioid drugs, there is a daily temptation for the formerly addicted professional to resume drug use. However, with a program of verified naltrexone ingestion as part of a comprehensive treatment program, the professional can return to work. Physicians who are recovering from addiction often cite this reduction of suspicion from colleagues as an important reason to continue naltrexone, in some cases for 5 years or more. Of course, the opiate-free period also permits the use of psychotherapy to deal with underlying or superimposed psychosocial problems.

A beneficial effect that may be produced by naltrexone is reduced craving for drugs. Reduced heroin craving (Sideroff et al. 1978) and, more recently, reduced alcohol craving (Anton et al. 1999; Volpicelli et al. 1992) have been reported, but the mechanism of this potential effect is completely unknown.

Like other treatments for addiction, naltrexone works best within a comprehensive program that deals with all aspects of the patient's problems (Resnick et al. 1979). Naltrexone is similar to methadone in this sense: both are medications that can reduce relapse to illicit drug use. There are significant differences between the two compounds, however. Methadone maintenance has been found to be an excellent treatment for the majority of persons who use street heroin and are seeking treatment, because it satisfies their drug craving. Methadone also enables them to stop committing crimes, because they no longer have an expensive drug habit to support. Persons who formerly used heroin can thus stabilize their lives, take care of their families, and find legal employment. Methadone does not block heroin's effects. However, there is cross-tolerance between heroin and methadone, and, thus, the patient maintained on an adequate dose of methadone will experience little reward from the usual dose of heroin. In addition to satisfying opioid craving, methadone may produce beneficial psychoactive effects.

In contrast to methadone, naltrexone cannot be given until all opioids have been metabolized and cleared from the body. Naltrexone does not produce opioid effects or any psychoactive benefits; patients are therefore without the feeling of opioids in their bodies. During the 24–72 hours of its effects, naltrexone will effectively block the actions of any opiate or opioid drug; thus, if the patient decides to resume heroin use, he or she cannot experience euphoria or calming from the use of heroin, as in the past.

Another important distinction between methadone and naltrexone is the absence of dependence with naltrexone. Naltrexone can be stopped abruptly at any time without concern about withdrawal symptoms. In a sense, this lack of dependence is a drawback to naltrexone in clinical practice, because the patient perceives no drug effect. Thus, there is no built-in reward, and there is no immediate penalty for stopping treatment. Some clinicians have actually experimented with small monetary payments contingent on patients' ingesting naltrexone in an effort to provide an external reward (Grabowski et al. 1979). Frequently, patients feel so good and overconfident about being opioid-free that they may prematurely assume that they no longer need naltrexone. They can stop naltrexone abruptly, but several days later they are again at risk for relapse to opioid use.

Naltrexone therapy is often confused with disulfiram (Antabuse) treatment for alcoholism. The medications are similar only in that both are taken to prevent relapse and both are nonaddicting. Disulfiram blocks the metabolism of alcohol but not its effects. If a person receiving disulfiram ingests alcohol, the normal degradation of alcohol is inhibited and acetaldehyde accumulates. Acetaldehyde produces flushing, nausea, and other noxious symptoms. These effects, of course, can be prevented by avoiding alcohol while taking disulfiram. In contrast, no such noxious effects result from the use of opioids in association with naltrexone treatment. The opioid effects are simply blocked or neutralized in a person receiving naltrexone treatment.

If a person not currently dependent on an opioid agonist receives an antagonist, there are usually no obvious effects. Theoretically, *something* should happen, because the antagonist blocks certain endogenous opioids (endorphins) that may serve to regulate mood, pain perception, and various neuroendocrine and cardiovascular functions. In fact, there have been reports of dysphoric reactions and endocrine changes in experimental subjects given naltrexone (Ellingboe et al. 1980; Mendelson et al. 1980). Spiegel et al. (1987) reported that naltrexone produced small decreases in appetite in human volunteers. Hollister et al. (1982) found adverse mood effects in nonaddicted volunteers who were given naltrexone. Crowley et al. (1985) noted similar effects in recently detoxified opioid-addicted persons. These dysphoric effects of naltrexone were reported after brief treatment (1 day to 3 weeks), and the number of subjects was very small. More recently, Kranzler et al. (2000) found significant side effects, including dysphoria and nausea, in a population of alcoholic patients receiving naltrexone at 50 mg/day.

In contrast, another study of healthy subjects reported no differences in mood effects between naltrexone and placebo (O'Brien et al. 1978). Moreover, most large-scale studies of recovering opiate-addicted or alcoholic persons have not found dysphoria or other mood changes to be a significant problem in the clinical use of naltrexone (Brahen et al. 1984; Greenstein et al. 1984; O'Malley et al. 1992; Tennant et al. 1984; Volpicelli et al. 1992, 1997; Washton et al. 1984). It may be that blocking endogenous opioids with naltrexone produces mood problems in some patients, and this may explain part of the early-dropout phenomenon. Those persons who continue on naltrexone for months or even years generally report no mood effects, although careful long-term studies of mood have not been conducted.

Nausea has been reported as a side effect in normal volunteers, alcoholic persons (Kranzler et al. 2000; Volpicelli et al. 1992), and post-opiate-dependent persons receiving naltrexone. Of course, if naltrexone is given too soon after the last dose of opiate, nausea could be produced as part of a precipitated withdrawal syndrome. Another side effect reported occasionally in male patients is an increase in spontaneous penile erections. This effect is presumed to be related to release of opiate-mediated inhibition of the hypothalamus permitting the release of luteinizing hormone (LH). Changes in sexual behavior have been difficult to assess in patients receiving naltrexone, because behavior on this agent is contrasted with the previous condition of suppression by opiates (i.e., while the person was using heroin).

Patients Suited for Antagonist Treatment

Health Care Professionals

Health care professionals have generally done well in naltrexone treatment programs. For example, Ling and Wesson (1984) reported the use of naltrexone in the management of 60 health care professionals for an average of 8 months. Forty-seven (78%) of the subjects were rated as much improved or moderately improved at follow-up. Washton et al. (1984) found that 74% of opioid-dependent physicians completed at least 6 months of treatment with naltrexone and were opioid-free and practicing medicine at 1-year follow-up. Roth et al. (1997) also reported excellent success among health care professionals treated with naltrexone and group therapy. The successful studies in the literature involved comprehensive treatment programs, with naltrexone providing a kind of structure around which psychotherapy was built.

The naltrexone treatment program should include a full medical evaluation, detoxification, psychiatric evaluation, family evaluation, and provision for ongoing therapy, as well as confirmed regular ingestion of naltrexone. Ongoing therapy usually involves marital therapy and individual therapy. Through use of this approach, a physician—whose drug use may have been discovered during a crisis—can be detoxified, started on naltrexone, and back at work practicing medicine in as little as 2 weeks. Of course, psychotherapy along with continued use of naltrexone may continue for several years, but disruption of the physician's family life and medical practice is minimized.

White-Collar Persons

Studies of psychotherapy outcome consistently show that patients coming into treatment with the greatest psychosocial assets tend to respond best to treatment. Thus, it is not surprising that patients with a history of recent employment and a good educational background do well on naltrexone in combination with psychotherapy. Some patients avoid methadone because of the required daily clinic visits, especially at the beginning of treatment. Naltrexone is not a controlled substance, and thus, greater flexibility is permitted. Although these patients may be strongly motivated to be drug-free, they are still susceptible to impulsive drug use. Using naltrexone as a kind of insurance is often very appealing to these persons.

Another practical reason that naltrexone has been successful in middle-class populations is that it can be prescribed by any licensed physician. Naltrexone use is not restricted to a special program for the treatment of addiction. So-called white-collar patients may object to attending such a clinic. It is recommended, however, that naltrexone be prescribed only by physicians who are familiar with the psychodynamics and behavior patterns of addicted individuals. Patients may appreciate the opportunity to be treated by an experienced practitioner in a private office rather than being restricted to a drug treatment clinic.

Tennant et al. (1984) described a group of suburban practitioners treating opioid dependence in a wide range of socioeconomic groups in southern California. They reported on 160 patients with an average history of opioid use of 10.5 years. The majority (63.8%) were employed; all patients in the study expressed a desire for abstinence-oriented treatment. Treatment was on an outpatient basis, and a naloxone challenge was given after completion of detoxification. After a graduated dose increase, naltrexone was given three times a week. Patients paid a fee or had the treatment covered by insurance. Each week, the patients received a urine screen for all drug classes and an alcohol breath test. Counseling sessions were held weekly.

The 160 opioid-addicted patients remained in treatment for a mean of 51 days (range: up to 635 days), but the majority were in short-term treatment. Only 27 (17%) remained longer than 90 days. During treatment, only 1%–3% of the tests for illicit drug or alcohol use were positive. Tennant et al. (1984) considered the program to be successful. However, they pointed out that despite long remissions on naltrexone, a patient can still relapse to opioid use after naltrexone is stopped. On the basis of follow-up results of naltrexone patients, Greenstein et al. (1983)

found that even a treatment period as short as 30 days was associated with a significant improvement in overall rehabilitative status at 6-month follow-up.

A study of patients in a higher socioeconomic group predictably found even better results. Washton et al. (1984) described naltrexone treatment of 114 businessmen who had been dependent for at least 2 years on heroin, methadone, or prescription opioids. The patients were mainly white males averaging 30 years of age with a mean income of $42,000 per year. A critical feature of this group was the presence of considerable external pressure to receive treatment, and almost half were in jeopardy of losing their jobs or of suffering legal consequences. The treatment program was oriented toward complete abstinence. It began with 4–10 weeks of inpatient treatment, during which detoxification and induction onto naltrexone were accomplished. Patients were also undergoing intensive individual psychotherapy and were involved in self-help groups. The importance of the posthospital phase was stressed, and all patients signed a contract for aftercare treatment.

Of the 114 patients who began the program, all completed naltrexone induction; 61% remained on the antagonist for at least 6 months with no missed visits or positive urine sample results. An additional 20% took naltrexone for less than 6 months but remained in the program with drug-free urine samples. Of the entire group, at 12- to 18-month follow-up, 64% were still opioid-free. Those who had stipulated pressure from their employers to get treatment did significantly better than the group without a clear-cut risk of loss of job.

Probationers in Work-Release Programs

It is well known that a large proportion of the inmates of prisons throughout the country are there because of drug-related crimes. Of course, relapse to drug use and consequent crime is common among these prisoners after they are released. One way to approach this recidivism and perhaps also to alleviate some of the overcrowding of our prison system is to use a work-release or halfway house program that enables prisoners to obtain an early release with the stipulation that they work in the community and live in a prison-supervised house. Naltrexone can be prescribed for those prisoners who were previously addicted to heroin. A pioneering model of such a program was established in Nassau County, Long Island, New York (Brahen et al. 1984), and the outcomes of 691 former inmates treated with naltrexone have been described. The treatment is provided within a work-release program in which the members live in a transitional house outside the prison and obtain employment in the community. Before the introduction of naltrexone into the program, the success of formerly opioid-addicted participants was limited because of their high relapse rate when they were placed in an environment where drugs were freely available.

In the Nassau County program, an inmate with a history of opioid addiction who wishes to volunteer for the program must first be stabilized on naltrexone. Random urine tests are also used to monitor the participants. Uncashed paychecks must be turned in as proof that attendance at work has been regular; a portion of the salary is applied to the cost of room and board. The participants are given supervision and counseling for problems that develop during this reentry period. Some participants try to use street heroin to get high despite the naltrexone, but because this fails, they eventually abandon these attempts. Participants are also offered continuance in treatment after their sentences have been served.

Since the introduction of naltrexone, the rehabilitation success rate of the formerly addicted participants in the program has been equal to that of inmates without a drug history.

Controlled studies of such programs have been difficult to implement. Cornish and colleagues (1997) conducted a random-assignment study among federal probationers convicted of drug-related crimes in Philadelphia, Pennsylvania. The probationers all received the same amount of parole counseling, but half were randomly selected to receive naltrexone as well. After 6 months outside of prison, the reincarceration rate for the group randomly selected for naltrexone was approximately half that for the control group (Figure 29–1).

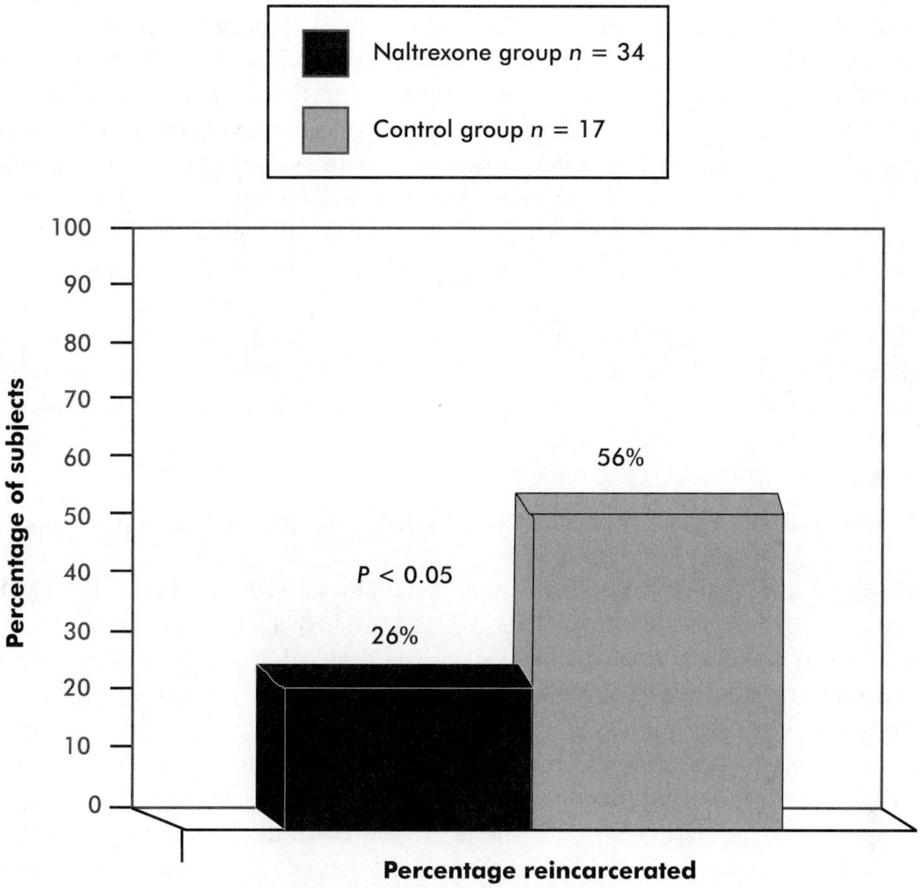

FIGURE 29–1. Subject reincarceration rates.

Patients in Heroin Addiction Programs

Although naltrexone can be used in the treatment of any opiate-dependent patient, it appeals most to those who are strongly motivated to become drug-free. Methadone, by contrast, requires much less motivation, because treatment involves only a relatively small and gradual shift from daily use of heroin to daily use of another opioid agonist, methadone. Naltrexone, however, requires a much bigger change: the person must genuinely wish to remain free of opiate effects. Unfortunately, most patients who assert strongly that they want to give up drugs are really ambivalent and have not thought through the consequences of their statements. Once they find themselves on a medication that makes it physically impossible for them to feel euphoric effects from heroin, they often change their minds.

The majority of persons addicted to street heroin are generally not interested in naltrexone treatment after learning how effectively it antagonizes opioids. Studies of the use of naltrexone in public drug treatment clinics have found that no more than 10%–15% of patients are willing to try naltrexone, and most of these persons drop out during the first month of naltrexone treatment (Greenstein et al. 1983; Hollister 1978; Judson and Goldstein 1984; O'Brien et al. 1975).

Among street heroin–using persons involved in crime to support their drug habit, it is difficult to predict who will respond well to treatment with naltrexone; however, the proportion of appropriate cases is almost certainly low. Publicly funded treatment programs may be discouraged by the cost of naltrexone (about $4 per tablet), although the main cost of the overall treatment is the counseling required to support patients after detoxification. Most naltrexone treatment programs have focused on patients who are employed or have good employment prospects, have a stable relationship with a spouse or family, and express willingness to enter into long-term psychotherapy or family therapy. Surprisingly, as mentioned earlier, even short-term (i.e., 30 days or more) treatment with naltrexone has been shown to be associated with improved outcome at 6-month follow-up (Greenstein et al. 1983). Of course, those willing to continue taking the antagonist for 6–12 months generally do well, but it is difficult to know to what degree the success is influenced by the patient's strong motivation, as evidenced by his or her remaining in treatment. It is probable that several factors interact to produce a good outcome, and that any single factor might not have been adequate in this regard.

Relapse Prevention Programs

When there is no "physical" dependence (as evidenced by a negative naloxone challenge), naltrexone can be started with an initial dose of 25 mg (one-half of a tablet). If no side effects occur within an hour, another 25 mg may be administered. The recommended dosage subsequently is 50 mg/day. After the first 1–2 weeks, it is usually possible to graduate to three doses per week (e.g., 100, 100, and 150 mg given on Monday, Wednesday, and Friday, respectively). It is critical that psychotherapy sessions be initiated early in treatment and that these involve family members and other significant figures in the patient's life. Ingestion of naltrexone must be monitored whenever possible rather than left to the patient's initiative. Confirmed dosing can occur in the clinic, but it is usually disruptive to the patient's rehabilitation to be required to come to the clinic or the physician's office for every dose. For this reason, it is important to involve significant figures in the patient's life to observe the ingestion of naltrexone and to report periodically to the therapist. In the case of physicians, for example, a colleague may have already confronted the patient with his or her drug problem and helped steer the patient into therapy. This colleague has sometimes been the chief of staff of the hospital where the patient works or the head of the patient's department. A family member or co-worker can also be enlisted after determining the existence of a constructive relationship.

Progress in treatment is determined by engagement in psychotherapy, performance on the job, and absence of drug abuse as confirmed by urine tests. The patient should be asked to agree to random urine tests, which are arranged by telephoning the patient and asking him or her to come in that day without prior notification. Patients who are doing well can eventually graduate to a schedule of only two doses of naltrexone per week, even though this will not provide full antagonist coverage over the entire interval between doses. However, the decreased frequency of visits reduces the patient's dependence on the therapist and diminishes interference with the patient's life. Although the degree of pharmacological blockade is reduced by the third or fourth day after the patient receives the drug, at this stage of therapy the patient is less likely to be testing limits by taking opiates. Moreover, the random urine testing should detect opiate use between naltrexone doses, which would then necessitate a return to more frequent dosing. A slip should not be treated as a failure of treatment; rather, it should be viewed as a symptom to be examined in therapy (i.e., grist for the therapeutic mill).

Patients of physicians in private practice are often given a prescription for naltrexone that can be filled at a pharmacy. Patients can eventually be trusted to take doses of naltrexone at home, but it is best that some doses be taken in the physician's office under direct observation. If a patient is pretending to take naltrexone and is using opiates, a dose in the office would precipitate a withdrawal reaction. Also, the treating physician should keep a supply of naltrexone tablets in his or her office to administer to patients. Patients who are physicians or pharmacists have been known to attempt to deactivate naltrexone tablets by treating them in a microwave oven. They could then appear to consume naltrexone in the presence of the treating physician or nurse but would be taking a relatively inert tablet.

Long-Term Effects of Opiate Antagonists on Opiate Receptors

Studies in rodents have shown that repeated doses of naloxone or naltrexone produce upregulation of μ opiate receptors (Yoburn et al. 1985) and transiently increased sensitivity to morphine. If this phenomenon were present in humans treated with naltrexone, formerly opiate-addicted persons would be at risk for overdose if they stopped naltrexone and returned to their usual dose of heroin. This question was addressed in an experiment by Cornish et al. (1993) with healthy volunteers. Administering a test dose of morphine, the authors determined the degree to which the normal respiratory response to a carbon dioxide stimulus was depressed. After 2 weeks of naltrexone at 50 mg/day, the subjects were retested for morphine sensitivity. No change in morphine's effects were found, indicating lack of detectable change in receptor sensitivity. Thus, the theoretical risk of overdose based on upregulation of opiate receptors does not seem to present a clinical problem for the use of naltrexone in preventing relapse to opiate dependence.

Effects of Opiate Antagonists on Blood Chemistry

Changes in laboratory test results have been examined in more than 2,000 patients involved in clinical trials with naltrexone (Hollister 1978; Pfohl et al. 1986). Despite the fact that addicted persons are generally unhealthy prior to naltrexone treatment, the studies in addiction treatment programs have not turned up significant laboratory abnormalities resulting from naltrexone treatment. Liver function tests are a matter of great concern because of the high frequency of hepatitis among addicted persons. As many as 70%–80% of addicted participants in methadone programs have some liver abnormalities, usually ascribed to past or present hepatitis.

Studies of nonaddicted groups at high doses of naltrexone have noted dose-related increments in transaminase levels that were all reversible when the drug was stopped. These subjects generally received 300 mg of naltrexone per day, or about six times the therapeutic dose for prevention of relapse to addiction (Pfohl et al. 1986). This finding highlights the need for caution in the treatment of addiction, although, in practice, transaminase elevations have not been observed at the lower dose levels used by persons recovering from addiction (Arndt et al. 1986).

Despite the evidence of its safety, naltrexone has a "Black Box Warning" on its package insert that has caused some physicians to be inappropriately concerned about the risk of prescribing it. Opioid-addicted persons with liver failure should not be treated with naltrexone, although those with minor abnormalities in liver function tests may receive naltrexone. Baseline laboratory tests should include a full battery of liver function studies, and monthly retesting should occur for the first 3 months. If no evidence of rising enzymes is observed, the tests can be repeated at 3- to 6-month intervals. Some clinicians have used the guideline that naltrexone should not be started if either the aspartate aminotransferase (AST; formerly called serum glutamic-oxaloacetic transaminase [SGOT]) level or the alanine aminotransferase (ALT; formerly called serum glutamic-pyruvic transaminase [SGPT]) level is greater than three times the normal level. Also, ongoing treatment should be stopped if the enzyme levels increase significantly, unless, of course, an alternative cause is found. Frequently, an alternative cause is excessive alcohol intake; when this is stopped, the enzyme levels usually return to normal.

Safety of Naltrexone in Women and Children

Another set of issues regarding the safety of any new drug concerns its use in pregnant women and in children. There have been no clinical trials of naltrexone specifically directed at these populations, and thus no definitive statements can be made. Studies of naltrexone in animals have generally not yielded data that could be interpreted as indicating potential risks for pregnant patients at clinical doses (Christian 1984), but there is always the possibility of a teratogenic effect specific to humans.

Drug Interactions

No systematic studies of nonopioid drug interactions with naltrexone have been reported, but with more than 20 years of clinical trials of naltrexone and 15 years of postmarketing experience, much anecdotal information is available. Naltrexone has been safely used in combination with disulfiram, lithium, selective serotonin reuptake inhibitors, and tricyclic antidepressants; if these agents are indicated, they apparently can be used in their normal way at their usual doses.

One adverse interaction that has been reported is that between thioridazine (Mellaril) and naltrexone. Maany et al. (1987) reported that sedation occurred when naltrexone was added to the regimens of two patients stabilized on thioridazine. No thioridazine plasma levels were available, but a likely explanation is that naltrexone impaired the degradation of thioridazine, resulting in increased plasma levels and increased sedation. If an antipsychotic is required in combination with naltrexone, a nonsedating agent would be preferable.

Treatment of Pain in Naltrexone-Maintained Patients

Patients are expected to remain on naltrexone for months or years to prevent relapse to opioid abuse. During this time. they may require surgery or treatment of trauma caused by an accident. The presence of naltrexone would not interfere with inhalation anesthesia, but the use of morphine would be affected. Also, opiates for immediate postoperative pain would be precluded or given in higher doses. For elective surgery, the naltrexone could be stopped several days before the operation. For emergency surgery, nonopioid anesthesia and postoperative pain medication could be used. If opiate medication is necessary, high doses of a short-acting opiate could be used to override the competitive antagonism produced by naltrexone. As naltrexone and its active metabolites are metabolized, the problem would be resolved. In practice, this issue is rarely a problem because nonopiate alternatives are available that can be used for these patients.

Looking to the Future

Depot Naltrexone

A major impediment to the more widespread use of naltrexone is the early-dropout rate. Patients express an apparently genuine desire for opiate-free treatment, but during the extremely vulnerable period within the first month after detoxification, they may miss an appointment, act on an impulse, and take a dose of heroin. There are no withdrawal symptoms from stopping naltrexone. Other patients simply become overly confident and feel that they do not need the protection of naltrexone. Even though the patient may later regret the sudden decision to stop naltrexone, the treatment process must start all over again with detoxification.

A delivery system for naltrexone that provides adequate antagonist protection for 30–60 days would protect the patient during the period when relapse is most likely. Currently, three versions of a slow-release depot preparation of naltrexone are undergoing clinical trials, and one study (Kranzler et al. 1998) in alcoholic patients has already been published.

Buprenorphine: Qualities of Both Methadone and Naltrexone

Buprenorphine is a partial μ opiate receptor agonist that is currently approved by the FDA as an injectable medication for pain. As an agonist, buprenorphine is 25–50 times more potent than morphine, but because it is a partial agonist, there is a limit to the opiate effects it can produce. Unlike agonists such as morphine and methadone, buprenorphine at higher doses does not produce progressively greater opiate effects and thus is less likely to cause an overdose. Buprenorphine is now extensively prescribed in France, largely by general practitioners. Current estimates are that as many as 50,000 patients in France receive buprenorphine with little of the strict supervision found in U.S. methadone programs. So far, the most important result of buprenorphine availability has been a dramatic reduction in the opiate overdose rate (Auriacombe et al. 1999).

In clinical trials in the United States, buprenorphine shows some of the features of both methadone and naltrexone. The agonist properties of buprenorphine cause it to be attractive as a maintenance treatment for a large proportion of opiate-addicted persons. Buprenorphine blocks opiate withdrawal and satisfies craving for opiates. If buprenorphine is discontinued abruptly, the withdrawal syndrome is very mild. Heroin, in contrast, has an intense but short-lived withdrawal syndrome, depending on the dose. The methadone withdrawal syndrome is significantly longer in duration. In addition to these opiate agonist effects, buprenorphine antagonizes the effects of other opiates in a manner comparable to naltrexone.

Buprenorphine has certain drawbacks as well. It is only one-fifteenth as potent by oral administration as by subcutaneous injection (Jasinski et al. 1989). By sublingual administration, the delivery system used in clinical trials for addiction, it is two-thirds as potent as subcutaneous injection. Buprenorphine has been found to block craving for approximately 24 hours, but this means that patients are required to come to the clinic daily and to hold the medication in the mouth without swallowing for at least 3–5 minutes. In busy treatment programs, such administration regimens can cause practical problems.

Based on its success in clinical trials to date (Bickel et al. 1988; R. E. Johnson et al. 1992), it appears that buprenorphine will likely receive FDA approval as an important new option for the treatment of opiate-dependent patients.

Opiate Antagonists in the Treatment of Alcoholism

An unexpected use for opiate antagonists was discovered in the late 1980s on the basis of animal models of alcohol consumption. Numerous studies in animals have shown that alcohol produces changes in the endogenous opioid system. Low doses of opiates have been reported to increase alcohol consumption in rodents (Hubbell et al. 1987; Reid and Hunter 1984), and opiate antagonists block or reduce preference for alcohol (DeWitte 1984; Hubbell et al. 1986; Samson and Doyle 1985; Volpicelli et al. 1986). The mechanism of these effects is not clear, but blocking opiate receptors consistently tends to decrease the ingestion of alcohol by laboratory animals previously choosing to drink this substance.

Although the effects of alcohol consumption on endogenous opioids appear to be quite complex and incompletely understood, experiments with naltrexone in human alcoholic patients showed important beneficial effects. Volpicelli et al. (1990, 1992), in a placebo-controlled study, found significant reductions in relapse to alcohol dependence in alcoholic outpatients treated with naltrexone after detoxification. All patients received intensive outpatient rehabilitation counseling in addition to naltrexone or placebo. Naltrexone-treated patients had about as many small slips to alcohol use as the patients randomly assigned to placebo. However, significantly fewer of the naltrexone patients continued to drink and to relapse to alcohol dependence during the 3-month trial. One interpretation of these results is that alcohol activates the endogenous opioid system, which forms part of the reinforcement of continued alcohol drinking. Because naltrexone blocks opiate receptors, the reinforcement via the opiate system would be attenuated and the probability of continued alcohol drinking would be reduced. O'Malley et al. (1991, 1992) reported results similar to those of Volpicelli et al. Other randomized clinical trials in alcoholic populations showed significant benefits for naltrexone (Anton et al. 1999; Kranzler et al. 1998; Volpicelli et al. 1997) and for nalmefene, another opiate antagonist (Mason et al. 1999). Of course, naltrexone alone is not necessarily effective, especially the oral form, for which adherence to the daily medication regimen may not be good. Naltrexone is considered to be adjunctive to a comprehensive treatment program that includes psychotherapy and attention to all facets of the alcohol dependence syndrome.

Conclusions

Naltrexone is a specific opiate antagonist that has a relatively long duration of action such that it can be used in the prevention of relapse to opiate dependence. It is safe and relatively nontoxic. Antagonist treatment is an important option that should be made available to well-motivated opiate-addicted persons who desire to become drug-free. As with all medications in the treatment of addiction, naltrexone must be used within a comprehensive treatment program that includes individual or family psychotherapy and urine testing for illicit drug use. Treatment should continue for at least 3 months following detoxification, and in many cases longer, because there is a significant risk of relapse continuing for several years.

Worldwide, more alcoholic persons than opiate-dependent persons are being treated with naltrexone. Controlled trials in alcoholic patients show that naltrexone may reduce the frequency of relapse among those engaged in an outpatient rehabilitation program.

An active program in medications development is currently being conducted by the National Institute on Drug Abuse and the National Institute on Alcohol Abuse and Alcoholism. Several agents currently under study will increase treatment options in the next several years. The partial agonist buprenorphine combines features of both methadone and naltrexone and will probably become available in 2001. A depot form of naltrexone that gives protection against relapse for 30–60 days is currently undergoing clinical trials (Kranzler et al. 1998).

References

Anton RF, Moak DH, Waid LR, et al: Naltrexone and cognitive behavioral therapy for the treatment of outpatient alcoholics. Am J Psychiatry 156:1758–1764, 1999

Arndt IO, Cacciola JS, McLellan AT, et al: A re-evaluation of naltrexone toxicity in recovering opiate addicts, in Problems of Drug Dependence, 1985: Proceedings of the 47th Annual Scientific Meeting, the Committee on Problems of Drug Dependence. NIDA Research Monograph 67 (NIH Publ No [ADM] 86-1448). Edited by Harris LS. Rockville, MD, National Institute on Drug Abuse, 1986, p 525

Auriacombe M, Franques P, Daulouède J, et al: The French experience: results from extensive delimited research studies and nation-wide sample surveys. Research and Clinical Forums 21:9–13, 1999

Bickel WK, Stitzer ML, Bigelow GE, et al: A clinical trial of buprenorphine: comparison with methadone in the detoxification of heroin addicts. Clin Pharmacol Ther 43:72–78, 1988

Brahen LS, Henderson RK, Copone T, et al: Naltrexone treatment in a jail work-release program. J Clin Psychiatry 45 (8 sec 2):49–52, 1984

Christian MA: Reproductive toxicity and teratology evaluation of naltrexone. J Clin Psychiatry 45 (8 sec 2):7–10, 1984

Cornish JW, Henson D, Levine S, et al: Morphine sensitivity in normal subjects after naltrexone treatment. Am J Addict 2:34–38, 1993

Cornish JW, Metzger D, Woody GE, et al: Naltrexone pharmacotherapy for opioid dependent federal probationers. J Subst Abuse Treat 14:529–534, 1997

Crowley TJ, Wagner JE, Zerbe G, et al: Naltrexone-induced dysphoria in former opioid addicts. Am J Psychiatry 142:1081–1084, 1985

DeWitte P: Naloxone reduces alcohol intake in a free-choice procedure even when both drinking bottles contain saccharin sodium or quinine substances. Neuropsychobiology 12:73–77, 1984

Ellingboe J, Mendelson JH, Kuehnle JC: Effects of heroin and naltrexone on plasma prolactin levels in man. Pharmacol Biochem Behav 12:163–165, 1980

Grabowski J, O'Brien CP, Greenstein RA: Effects of contingent payment on compliance with a naltrexone regimen. Am J Drug Alcohol Abuse 6:355–365, 1979

Greenstein RA, Evans BD, McLellan AT, et al: Predictors of favorable outcome following naltrexone treatment. Drug Alcohol Depend 12:173–180, 1983

Greenstein RA, Arndt I, McLellan AT, et al: Naltrexone: a clinical perspective. J Clin Psychiatry 45 (8 sec 2):25–28, 1984

Hollister LE: Clinical evaluation of naltrexone treatment of opiate-dependent individuals: report of the National Research Council Committee on Clinical Evaluation of Narcotic Antagonists. Arch Gen Psychiatry 35:335–340, 1978

Hollister LE, Johnson K, Boukhabza D, et al: Aversive effects of naltrexone in subjects not dependent on opiates. Drug Alcohol Depend 8:37–42, 1982

Hubbell CL, Czirr SA, Hunter GA, et al: Consumption of ethanol solution is potentiated by morphine and attenuated by naloxone persistently across repeated daily administrations. Alcohol 3:39–54, 1986

Hubbell CL, Czirr SA, Reid LD: Persistence and specificity of small doses of morphine on intake of alcoholic beverages. Alcohol 4:149–156, 1987

Jasinski DR, Fudala PJ, Johnson RE: Sublingual versus subcutaneous buprenorphine in opiate abusers. Clin Pharmacol Ther 45:513–519, 1989

Johnson RE, Jaffe JH, Fudala PJ: A controlled trial of buprenorphine treatment of opioid dependence. JAMA 267:2750–2755, 1992

Judson BA, Goldstein A: Naltrexone treatment of heroin addiction: one year follow-up. Drug Alcohol Depend 13:357–365, 1984

Kleber HD: Ultrarapid opiate detoxification (editorial). Addiction 93:1629–1633, 1998

Kleber HD, Kosten TR: Naltrexone induction: psychologic and pharmacologic strategies. J Clin Psychiatry 45 (8 sec 2):29–38, 1984

Kleber HD, Kosten TR, Gaspari J, et al: Nontolerance to the opioid antagonism of naltrexone. Biol Psychiatry 20:66–72, 1985

Kranzler HR, Modesto-Lowe V, Nuwayser ES: Sustained-release naltrexone for alcoholism treatment: a preliminary study. Alcohol Clin Exp Res 22:1074–1079, 1998

Kranzler HR, Modesto-Lowe V, Van Kirk J: Naltrexone vs nefazodone for treatment of alcohol dependence: a placebo-controlled trial. Neuropsychopharmacology 22:493–503, 2000

Lee MC, Wagner HN, Tanada S, et al: Duration of occupancy of opiate receptors by naltrexone. J Nucl Med 29:1207–1211, 1988

Ling W, Wesson DR: Naltrexone treatment for addicted health-care professionals: a collaborative private practice experience. J Clin Psychiatry 45 (8 sec 2):46–48, 1984

Maany I, O'Brien CP, Woody GE: Interaction between thioridazine and naltrexone (letter). Am J Psychiatry 144:966, 1987

Martin WR, Jasinski DR: Physiological parameters of morphine in man: tolerance, early abstinence, protracted abstinence. J Psychiatry Res 7:9–16, 1969

Martin W, Jasinski D, Mansky P: Naltrexone: an antagonist for the treatment of heroin dependence. Arch Gen Psychiatry 28:784–791, 1973

Mason BJ, Salvato FR, Williams LD, et al: A double-blind, placebo-controlled study of oral nalmefene for alcohol dependence. Arch Gen Psychiatry 56:719–724, 1999

Mello NK, Mendelson JH, Kuehnle JC, et al: Operant analysis of human heroin self-administration and the effects of naltrexone. J Pharmacol Exp Ther 216:45–54, 1981

Mendelson JH, Ellingboe J, Kuehnle JC, et al: Heroin and naltrexone effects on pituitary-gonadal hormones in man: interaction of steroid feedback effects, tolerance and supersensitivity. J Pharmacol Exp Ther 214:503–506, 1980

Nestler EJ, Hope BT, Widnell KL: Drug addiction: a model for the molecular basis of neural plasticity. Neuron 11:995–1006, 1993

O'Brien CP: Opioid addiction, in Handbook of Experimental Pharmacology. Edited by Herz A, Akil H, Simon EJ. Berlin, Springer-Verlag, 1992, pp 803–823

O'Brien CP, Greenstein RA, Mintz J, et al: Clinical experience with naltrexone. Am J Drug Alcohol Abuse 2:365–377, 1975

O'Brien CP, Greenstein RA, Ternes J: Clinical pharmacology of narcotic antagonists. Ann N Y Acad Sci 311:232–240, 1978

O'Brien CP, Greenstein RA, Ternes J, et al: Unreinforced self-injections: effects on rituals and outcome in heroin addicts, in Problems of Drug Dependence, 1979: Proceedings of the 41st Annual Scientific Meeting, the Committee on Problems of Drug Dependence. NIDA Research Monograph 27 (DHEW Publ No [ADM] 80-901). Edited by Harris LS. Washington, DC, U.S. Government Printing Office, 1980, pp 275–281

O'Brien CP, Ehrman R, Ternes J, et al: Classical conditioning in human opioid dependence, in Behavioral Analysis of Drug Dependence. Edited by Goldberg S, Stolerman I. San Diego, CA, Academic Press, 1986, pp 329–356

O'Malley SS, Jaffe AJ, Chang G, et al: Naltrexone in the treatment of alcohol dependence: preliminary findings, in Novel Pharmacological Interventions for Alcoholism. Edited by Naranjo CA, Seller EM. New York, Springer-Verlag, 1991, pp 148–157

O'Malley SS, Jaffe AJ, Chang G, et al: Naltrexone and coping skills therapy for alcohol dependence: a controlled study. Arch Gen Psychiatry 49:881–887, 1992

Pfohl D, Allen J, Atkinson R, et al: TREXAN (naltrexone hydrochloride): a review of hepatic toxicity at high dosage, in Problems of Drug Dependence, 1985: Proceedings of the 47th Annual Scientific Meeting, the Committee on Problems of Drug Dependence. NIDA Research Monograph 67 (NIH Publ No [ADM] 86-1448). Edited by Harris LS. Rockville, MD, National Institute on Drug Abuse, 1986, pp 66–72

Reid LD, Hunter GA: Morphine and naloxone modulate intake of ethanol. Alcohol 1:33–37, 1984

Reisine T, Pasternak G: Opioid analgesics and antagonists, in Goodman & Gilman's The Pharmacological Basis of Therapeutics, 9th Edition. Edited by Hardman JG, Limbird LE. New York, McGraw-Hill, 1995, pp 521–555

Resnick RB, Schuyten-Resnick E, Washton AM: Narcotic antagonists in the treatment of opioid dependence: review and commentary. Compr Psychiatry 20:116–125, 1979

Roth A, Hogan I, Farren C: Naltrexone plus group therapy for the treatment of opiate-abusing health-care professionals. J Subst Abuse Treat 14:19–22, 1997

Samson HH, Doyle TF: Oral ethanol self-administration in the rat: effect of naloxone. Pharmacol Biochem Behav 22:91–99, 1985

Sideroff SI, Charuvastra VC, Jarvik ME: Craving in heroin addicts maintained on the opiate antagonist naltrexone. Am J Drug Alcohol Abuse 5:415–423, 1978

Spiegel T, Stunkard AJ, Shrager E, et al: Effect of naltrexone on food intake, hunger, and satiety in obese men. Physiol Behav 40:135–141, 1987

Tennant F, Rawson R, Cohen A, et al: A clinical experience with naltrexone in suburban opioid addicts. J Clin Psychiatry 45 (8 sec 2):42–45, 1984

Volpicelli JR, Davis MA, Olgin GE: Naltrexone blocks the post-shock increase of ethanol consumption. Life Sci 38:841–847, 1986

Volpicelli JR, O'Brien CP, Alterman AI, et al: Naltrexone and the treatment of alcohol dependence: initial observations, in Opioids, Bulimia, and Alcohol Abuse and Alcoholism. Edited by Reid LB. Berlin, Springer-Verlag, 1990, pp 195–214

Volpicelli JR, Alterman AI, Hayashida M, et al: Naltrexone in the treatment of alcohol dependence. Arch Gen Psychiatry 49:876–880, 1992

Volpicelli JR, Rhines KC, Rhines JS, et al: Naltrexone and alcohol dependence. Arch Gen Psychiatry 54:737–742, 1997

Washton AM, Pottash AC, Gold MS: Naltrexone in addicted business executives and physicians. J Clin Psychiatry 40 (8 sec 2):39–41, 1984

Wikler A: Conditioning factors in opiate addiction and relapse, in Narcotics. Edited by Wilner DI, Kassenbaum GG. New York, McGraw-Hill, 1965, pp 85–100

Yoburn BC, Goodman RR, Cohen AH, et al: Increased analgesic potency of morphine and increased brain opioid binding sites in the rat following chronic naltrexone treatment. Life Sci 36:2325–2332, 1985

30

Individual Treatment

Richard J. Frances, M.D.
Avram H. Mack, M.D.
Lisa Borg, M.D.
John E. Franklin, M.D.
Sheldon Zimberg, M.D., M.S.
George E. Woody, M.D.
Delinda E. Mercer, Ph.D.
G. Alan Marlatt, Ph.D.
Kimberly Barrett, Ed.D.
Marc Galanter, M.D.

Psychodynamics and the Treatment of Substance-Related Disorders

Richard J. Frances, M.D.
Avram H. Mack, M.D.
Lisa Borg, M.D.
John E. Franklin, M.D.

Concepts derived from psychodynamic theory have had an important influence on addiction treatment. Although some addiction treatment experts argue against the psychodynamic treatment of alcoholic patients (Vaillant 1995), we feel that psychoanalytic concepts can shed light on the rehabilitation process and can add depth to individual and group treatment. In this chapter subpart we focus on the application, indications, contraindications, and utility of psychodynamic approaches to patients with substance use–related disorders.

Historical Background

Freud's work in exploring the unconscious continues to inform psychoanalytic theory and practice. Recent theorists have emphasized ego psychology, object relations theory, self psychology, and the importance of affective states, self-esteem, and self-care, and these addi-

This chapter subpart is a revised version of our chapter "Psychodynamics," which appeared in Galanter MA, Kleber HD (eds): *The American Psychiatric Press Textbook of Substance Abuse Treatment,* 2nd Edition. Washington, DC, American Psychiatric Press, 1999, pp. 309–322.

tions have widened the application of psychodynamic ideas to addiction treatment.

Freud, Abraham, and Radó each stressed trauma-related developmental issues involving orality, regression toward infantile fixations, defenses against homosexuality, sexual and social inferiority, emotional immaturity, depressive tendencies, and insecurity as psychopathologic pathways leading to substance abuse (Lorand 1948). Glover noted the important role of aggressive drives in substance abuse (Glover 1932/1956). The question of primary versus secondary effects of alcoholism was argued as early as 1911, when Bleuler (1911/1921) hypothesized that drinking was often the cause of neurotic disturbances. Ferenczi (1912/1916), on the other hand, viewed alcoholism as an "escape into narcosis" from underlying psychodynamic causes, thus originating what has come to be called the "self-medication hypothesis."

As the focus of psychoanalytic theory has moved from its classical attention to drives to the modern focus on developmental and structural deficits and affective experience, psychoanalytic approaches to the addictions have been redrawn as well. The roles of ego defense, defense deficit, and affective experience have been included in this understanding. Krystal (1982) noted the substance abuser's inability to deal with overwhelming affect and described the patients' inability to label affect (i.e., "alexithymia"). In discussing the causes of substance abuse, Wurmser (1984) emphasized narcissistic collapse as resulting from the punctured grandiose or idealized self. Substances may indeed be used to assuage feelings of emptiness, boredom, rage, shame, depression, and guilt that result from narcissistic wounds. O. F. Kernberg (1991) described addictive behavior as a reunion with a forgiving parent, an activation of "all good" selfobject images, and a gratification of instinctual needs.

An important advance in the psychodynamic approach to the addictions has been the self-medication hypothesis, developed by Wieder and Kaplan (1969), Milkman and Frosch (1973), and Khantzian (1997), which postulates that individuals choose a substance on the basis of specific sought-after effects. Khantzian (1997) suggested that opiates are used to self-medicate rage and aggression, whereas cocaine is used to counter feelings of depressive worthlessness or to augment grandiosity. Alcohol may ward off fears of closeness, dependency, and intimacy and may allow acceptance of loving or aggressive feelings (Khantzian et al. 1990). Addicted patients often participate in self-defeating and self-destructive behavior leading to relapse because of their inability to anticipate danger and to consider the consequences of their actions (Dodes and Khantzian 1998). A recent view is that the addicted individual has a sense of helplessness and powerlessness, often in the face of intolerable affects, and that substance abuse restores a sense of control to which the person feels entitled (Dodes and Khantzian 1998).

Finally, one should not forget that the neural pathways that conduct the effects of substances (including the mesolimbic system and the ventral tegmental area) have been discovered and that further knowledge of their relation to the psyche will offer a welcome opportunity to advance psychoanalytic understanding in the future (Leshner 1997).

Application of Psychodynamics to Substance Abuse Treatment

A deeper understanding of the addictive process and the psychology of addiction can enhance the design of treatment programs and the conceptualization of the rehabilitation process, group psychotherapy, and self-help groups. Recovering patients are in a continuous state of conflict, with the desire to use substances (craving) counterposed against the wish to stay sober. Awareness of reasons not to drink strengthens that side of the conflict versus the craving side, and enhancing insight regarding the sources of the internal struggle is useful. When self-medication is the cause of substance abuse, other means of regulating affect must be found and other underlying psychiatric problems must be addressed. Cognitive-behavioral techniques that take into account the more complex motivational factors may be specifically tailored to a person's conflicts and defenses and are compatible with increased self-awareness, self-care, self-esteem, and the working through of conflicts.

Psychodynamically oriented psychotherapy, usually involving one or two sessions per week and often used in conjunction with Alcoholics Anonymous (AA) groups or network therapy, should be distinguished from psychoanalysis. Psychodynamically oriented treatment focuses on current conflicts as they relate to the past, rather than on childhood experiences. Initially, the therapist may confront denial and other defenses around drinking while supporting the patient's denial of anger, showing sensitivity to the patient's characteristic defenses and to his or her ego weaknesses and strengths. The treatment relationship is openly discussed and the negative transference interpreted. Many addicted patients have narcissistic traits or personality disorders involving a sense of entitlement and an inability to allow gratification of dependency needs. These patients need to accept their vulnerability and their need for others and to deal with their fears of shame and humiliation.

Indications and Contraindications

Positive characteristics for insight-oriented psychotherapy include high IQ, interest, insight, psychological mindedness, a desire to understand or find meaning in behavior, a capacity for intimacy, the ability to identify with a therapist, time (i.e., availability and commitment to the necessary duration of treatment), an awareness of conflicts and patterns of self-destructive behavior, and a desire to change aspects of the self that are not acceptable.

Patients will often select insight-oriented psychotherapy out of an interest in their own motivations, a sense that this form of treatment is likely to help them, or a wish for privacy and confidentiality. Some patients choose this modality because of a distaste for spiritual programs, a fear of groups, or an unwillingness to take medications, and/or because other treatments have failed.

There are a few contraindications to the use of psychodynamically oriented psychotherapy in substance abuse treatment. These include active use of substances, neuropsychiatric impairment, psychosis, and antisocial personality disorder that is not comorbid with other Axis I disorders.

General and Technical Aspects

Although some authors recommend waiting up to 1 year before beginning psychodynamic-oriented psychotherapy (Bean-Bayog 1988), we believe that, in general, it need not be delayed, because the greatest opportunity to develop an alliance is often early, while the patient is in crisis. Focusing on motivational aspects of treatment and confronting denial of the need for help are essential elements in initiating treatment, and supportive elements, such as confrontation, clarification, support of defenses, and building on ego strengths, are very important as well. Encouraging the patient to view him- or herself as a "recovering" person can boost self-esteem and provide stability.

Interpretations may help the patient work through resistances to accepting help. They may also provide a meaningful explanation for destructive patterns that can inspire a wish for change. The timing of interpretations, however, is crucial. Although the psychotherapist needs to consider the effects of intoxication, withdrawal, and the chronic organic effects of alcohol, these are not absolute contraindications to psychodynamic-oriented interpretations. Regardless of the stage of recovery, interpretations sometimes are indicated from the outset of treatment. A patient who initially projects blame and responsibility for his or her actions onto substances may later be able to accept responsibility for those actions. Defenses may need to be supported at first, including denial of affect related to some of the losses. Confrontation should initially concentrate on denial surrounding addiction but ultimately must be expanded to focus on other areas of the patient's world. In certain cases involving repeated treatment failure, however, an initial intervention may require active, across-the-board confrontation and interpretation of inconsistencies and denial to help the patient accept a need for change. For patients who have alexithymia or constricted affect, interpretations are aimed at increasing the patient's awareness of feeling states and helping him or her to connect thoughts and feelings without the use of substances.

Psychodynamic therapy sessions are usually conducted once or twice per week without the use of a couch; can begin in an inpatient, organized outpatient, or office practice setting; and can be either time-limited and focused or long term. The dialogue with the patient is active, with the therapist evidencing an attitude of empathic concern, flexibility, and sharing. Issues of dependency may be partially worked through, and ongoing positive identification with a therapist, sponsor, recovering friends, and AA is a major positive outcome in treatment. Some other positive attributes of the therapist that facilitate substance use disorder treatment include informed optimism, a capacity to tolerate anxiety and depression, a knowledge of addictions, intellectual curiosity, wisdom, persistence and patience, a capacity to listen, and impeccable honesty and integrity (Frances and Franklin 1989). The therapist listens to themes relating to the patient's intrapsychic conflicts, developmental impairments, and defenses with special attention to how these themes may apply to substance abuse and relapse prevention. The effects of regression need to be monitored carefully. A detailed developmental history includes attention to achievement of milestones and ego development; evaluation of temperament in the patient and significant caregivers and of the patient's capacity to identify with and separate from important figures of identification (including parents, siblings, or admired peers); and exploration of affect regulation, especially in relation to the use of substances. The therapist uses additional traditional tools, such as free association and exploration of "slips" and dreams in the search for meaning in the unconscious derivatives of behavior. For example, an unconscious wish to drink expressed in a "drunk dream" may help the patient realize the importance of increasing efforts at relapse prevention. Psychotherapists are advised never to promise patients that they will ever be able to return to controlled drinking once the underlying causes of their alcoholism are dealt with, or that they will not need additional help at some future date through 12-Step programs or additional psychotherapy.

Structure and boundaries, including abstinence, are important in helping the patient to reestablish control and self-regulation and to verbally express feelings rather than acting them out. Conventional limit setting may be enough; however, the therapist may also need to actively mobilize a family to bring a suicidal alcoholic patient to an emergency room or to the doctor's office after the patient has experienced a relapse. Psychodynamic strategies such as clarification and interpretation are used in tandem with directive approaches such as assertiveness training, social skills training, self-efficacy groups, modeling, positive reinforcement, cognitive therapy, and suggestion.

The phases of intervention with the addicted patient include initial screening, evaluation and intervention, rehabilitation, and aftercare. The first focus of treatment is often on conflicts around acceptance of addiction as a problem (the equivalent to Step 1 of AA), the patient's reluctance to acknowledge dependency and his or her need for treatment (the equivalent of Step 2 of AA), and conflicts resulting from the complications of alcoholism, including loss of employment, relationships, and health. The early goal is to maintain abstinence and prevent relapse. Initially, the patient may be coerced into seeking consultation by an employer, probation officer, family member, or physician, and considerable effort may be needed for the therapist to develop trust and a working alliance with the patient. The therapist's integrity, adherence to confidentiality, and ability to be helpful contribute to establishing trust. Therapy is the process by which a need for abusable substances is transformed into a need for people, including the therapist.

Paradoxically, the same patients who abuse drugs often refuse medications, in part out of a fear of being dependent on the therapist to obtain these medications. Major themes include specific conflicts over assertiveness, handling of aggression, and issues of control and disinhibition. The disinhibiting role of addictions in allowing risk-taking behavior, including increased sexual activity, may be an issue. On the other hand, substance abuse may play a role in distancing the person from his or her sexual life or substituting for sexual activity. Patients need to be closely watched for potential relapses. Laboratory tests may be useful in monitoring a patient's compliance. Meeting with the family, as well as drawing on other sources of collateral information, is essential in obtaining a history. Family members can aid in supporting treatment goals and are especially needed to confront patients who frequently dissimulate.

An Ego Psychological Model of Rehabilitation

An assessment of ego function needs to include an inventory of the patient's strengths. One way to combine positive insight with support is to help patients recall periods in their lives in which they had beliefs and values and to give them hope for a return to a higher level of functioning. Even very damaged, impaired individuals have or have had dreams in their lives. The stigma of the illness can also be lessened by discussing positive role models who have struggled with the same illness.

An ego psychological model can be applied to the biopsychosocial effects of addiction and to rehabilitation. Intoxication, chronic use, and psychosocial consequences may lead to regression and impairment of defenses, object relatedness, judgment, reality testing, and superego. The defenses initially encountered are usually the most primitive. With time and treatment, higher-level defenses may develop. For example, denial of alcohol's harmful effects on the liver can be replaced with curiosity and intellectualization about how liver damage occurs.

The Patient-Therapist Relationship

Many of the problems related to working with addicted patients relate to the challenge of establishing a positive therapeutic relationship between the patient and the therapist. Frequently, errors in treatment occur because of negative feelings and attitudes that therapists have toward addicted patients. Typical mistakes include providing inadequate empathy or overly identifying with patients. A major source of countertransference is a clinician's uncritical acceptance of roles projected onto him or her from the patient's transference.

In many cases, an understanding of the patient's specific transference—especially one that evokes countertransference problems or that prevents compliance with treatment—may be essential for good management and a successful alliance with the patient. Typical transference problems can result from growing up in a household in which the parents were addicted, inconsistent, and either overly harsh or indulgent. Children of alcoholic parents frequently have problems with authority figures and will often trust siblings, peers, and fellow alcoholic individuals more readily than teachers, nurses, doctors, or police. A patient's description of a therapist as cold, neglectful, uninvolved, or detached may be transference response to a parent who fits that description and may lead the therapist to behave in this way.

It is helpful for therapists to be able to interpret patients' negative transference and to know how to manage and appropriately use their own countertransference. Alcoholic patients frequently will try to evoke in their therapist feelings of fear, anger, and despair and will reenact relationships with alcoholic parents, siblings, and spouses through the transference. They may project critical attitudes onto their therapist and withhold information because they believe that the therapist will respond like a harsh parent. A patient's regarding or treating the therapist as a parent, sibling, or friend may have specific transference roots. The greater the therapist's awareness of what is happening, the more such issues can be brought into the treatment in a constructive way.

A second major source of countertransference problems in the treatment of addicted patients is a weak knowledge base on the part of the therapist. The more knowledgeable the therapist is about addiction psychiatry and about the patient, the less likely the therapist is to project his or her own problems onto the patient. Attitudinal problems on the part of the therapist can be reduced by good training and the experience of having worked through issues related to stigma. The more the therapist is in command of a treatment armamentarium, the less intimidated he or she will be in the face of what can be a daunting illness. Ultimately, patients are the best teachers. By listening carefully, the therapist can gain knowledge about the addictive experience, drug-using practices, and street language.

A third source of countertransference involves the mostly unconscious transference reactions a therapist may have toward a patient. These may relate to the therapist's own attitudes about substance use; his or her present or past problems with addiction; or his or her experience with a parent, spouse, or child with a substance use problem. The therapist's own envy, fear, hopes, and needs can adversely affect his or her prescribing practices and lead to overinvolvement, avoidance, hopelessness, jealousy, and burnout. Clinicians who have chosen to work in the addiction field because of their wish to overcome personal problems related to addictions may have special difficulty dealing with patients' problems if they have not completely worked out their own. Frequent mistakes include excessive self-disclosure of personal problems and a tendency not to see the specifics of a patient's problems clearly because of a need to see everyone as similar to oneself. A recovering clinician might consider a patient's problem minor compared with his or her own. Alternatively, some clinicians see every problem as relating to addiction. Such mistakes result in misdiagnosis and overdiagnosis.

Additional protection is provided by working in a team in which team members can point out one another's blind spots and assist in improving one another's technique. Feedback from patients and their families can be another source of guidance for the clinician who listens carefully. A wise clinician admits his or her mistakes, learns from them, and tries to avoid making the same ones in the future.

Importance of Treatment Outcome Research

Unfortunately, at present addiction treatment is as much an art as it is a science, because adequate treatment outcome studies are not yet available to guide treatment choice. Standardized practice guidelines have been developed by the American Psychiatric Association (1995), and these, combined with the improved diagnostic standardization in DSM-IV (American Psychiatric Association 1994), offer the potential for good research. Nonetheless, some studies already have yielded important findings. Woody et al. (1986, 1990) found meaningful differences in efficacy favoring professional supportive-expressive psychotherapy plus counseling over counseling alone in methadone-maintained patients. The same researchers observed no differences in treatment outcome between cognitive-behavioral and supportive-expressive therapies in this population, and they showed that among methadone maintenance patients undergoing psychotherapy, comorbidity with major depression and antisocial personality disorder was of higher prognostic value than comorbidity with antisocial personality disorder alone. O'Malley et al. (1996) compared psychotherapy for alcoholic patients with and without naltrexone as adjunctive therapy and found favorable results for combined treatment. And Carroll et al. (1994) reported that short-term cognitive-behavioral psychotherapy produced improvement in cocaine-dependent patients but noted that there was a delay between cessation of treatment and emergence of these beneficial effects.

The relationship between the cost and outcome of intervention is of great interest today. Humphreys and Moos (1996) found reduced substance-related health care costs in an AA study of veterans. In fact, O'Brien (1997) reported that treatment of some addictive disorders is currently more cost effective than that of asthma or diabetes mellitus.

Validation of psychodynamic psychotherapy and 12-Step programs has not been accomplished by formal efficacy studies, even though each of these modalities has a constituency that has reported favorable results. Clearly, research is needed to determine which kinds of interventions, including psychodynamic therapy, are most useful for which patient characteristics and which diagnoses. There is a danger that because of the difficulty of studying what often appears to be clinically subjective material, premature closure could lead to an overly narrowly based, inferior treatment as being all that is funded and made available.

Conclusions

Psychodynamic theory can have an important role in enriching and informing substance abuse treatment. Its rigid application, however, can be counterproductive. Use of psychodynamic understanding widens the range of patients that can be treated. A rich, descriptive clinical experience in this area improves our understanding of addicted patients and lays the groundwork for further study.

References

American Psychiatric Association: Diagnostic and Statistical Manual of Mental Disorders, 4th Edition. Washington, DC, American Psychiatric Press, 1994

American Psychiatric Association: Practice guideline for the treatment of patients with substance use disorders: alcohol, cocaine, opioids. Am J Psychiatry 152 (11 suppl):1–59, 1995

Bean-Bayog M: Alcoholism as a cause of psychopathology. Hospital and Community Psychiatry 39:352–354, 1988

Bleuler E: Alkohol und Neurosen [Alcohol and neuroses]. Jahrbuch für psychoanalytische und psychopathologische Forschungen 3:848–852, 1911 [Abstract in Psychoanalytic Review 8:443–444, 1921]

Carroll KM, Rounsaville BJ, Nich C, et al: One-year follow-up of psychotherapy and pharmacotherapy for cocaine dependence. Delayed emergence of psychotherapy effects. Arch Gen Psychiatry 51:989–997, 1994

Dodes LM, Khantzian EJ: Individual psychodynamic psychotherapy, in Clinical Textbook of Addictive Disorders, 2nd Edition. Edited by Frances RJ, Miller SI. New York, Guilford, 1998, pp 479–495

Ferenczi S: On the part played by homosexuality in the pathogenesis of paranoia (1912), in First Contributions to Psycho-Analysis. Boston, MA, Richard G Badger, 1916, pp 154–184

Frances RJ, Franklin JE Jr: Concise Guide to Treatment of Alcoholism and Addictions. Washington, DC, American Psychiatric Press, 1989

Glover E: On the aetiology of drug addiction (1932), in Selected Papers of Psychoanalysis, Vol 1: On the Early Development of Mind. Edited by Glover E. New York, International Universities Press, 1956, pp 187–215

Humphreys K, Moos RH: Reduced substance abuse-related health costs among voluntary participants in Alcoholics Anonymous. Psychiatr Serv 47:709–713, 1996

Kernberg OF: Transference regression and psychoanalytic technique with infantile personalities. Int J Psychoanal 72:189–200, 1991

Khantzian EJ: A clinical perspective of the cause-consequence controversy in alcoholic and addictive suffering. J Am Acad Psychoanal 15:521–537, 1987

Khantzian EJ: The self medication hypothesis of substance abuse disorders: a reconsideration and recent applications. Harv Rev Psychiatry 4:231–244, 1997

Khantzian EJ, Halliday KS, McAuliffe WE: Alcoholism and the Vulnerable Self: Modified Dynamic Group Therapy for Substance Abusers. New York, Guilford, 1990

Krystal H: Alexithymia and the effectiveness of psychoanalytic treatment. International Journal of Psychoanalytic Psychotherapy 9:353–388, 1982

Leshner AI: Addiction is a brain disease, and it matters. Science. 278:45–47, 1997

Lorand J: Summary of psychoanalytic literature on problems of alcoholism. Yearbook of Psychoanalysis 1:359–378, 1948

Milkman H, Frosch WA: On the preferential use of heroin and amphetamine. J Nerv Ment Dis 156: 242–248, 1973

O'Brien CP: A range of research-based psychotherapies for addiction. Science 278:66–69, 1997

O'Malley SS, Jaffe AJ, Chang G, et al: Six month follow up of naltrexone and psychotherapy for alcohol dependence. Arch Gen Psychiatry 53:217–224, 1996

Vaillant GE: The Natural History of Alcoholism Revisited. Cambridge, MA, Harvard University Press, 1995

Wieder H, Kaplan EH: Drug use in adolescents. Psychoanal Study Child 24:399–431, 1969

Woody GE, McLellan AT, Luborsky L, et al: Psychotherapy for substance abuse. Psychiatr Clin North Am 9:547–562, 1986

Woody GE, Luborsky L, McLellan AT, et al: Corrections and revised analyses for psychotherapy in methadone maintenance patients (letter). Arch Gen Psychiatry 47:788–789, 1990

Wurmser L: The role of superego conflicts in substance abuse and their treatment. International Journal of Psychoanalytic Psychotherapy 10:227–258, 1984

Individual Management and Psychotherapy for Alcoholism

Sheldon Zimberg, M.D., M.S.

Most psychiatrists have considered psychotherapy for alcoholism to be ineffective because *psychoanalytic* psychotherapy has been largely a failure (Zimberg 1982). Also, the rationale for psychoanalysis has been the mistaken belief that alcoholism is *always* a symptom of underlying psychological disorders, and that by uncovering these disorders and providing insight into their role in abusive drinking, the therapist can help end the patient's drinking problem. This has not proven to be the case, because alcoholism has multiple causes, including biological (i.e., genetic), sociocultural, and psychological factors. The ineffectiveness of psychoanalysis and the psychoanalytic rationale has resulted in psychotherapists' avoidance of alcoholic patients and a bias against psychiatry by those in the addictive disorders field and by many members of Alcoholics Anonymous (AA).

Tiebout (1962) and Fox (1965) pioneered a modified form of psychodynamic psychotherapy for the treatment of alcoholism. Although they used a psychodynamic understanding of alcoholism in their approach to psychotherapy, they avoided uncovering underlying psychological conflicts early in treatment and gave priority to the elimination of alcohol use as the first and necessary step in the psychotherapeutic approach.

Individual therapy is underutilized in the treatment of alcoholism, but it can be the most effective approach with individuals who are resistant to treatment or who have coexisting psychiatric disorders. The transference can develop into a dependent relationship with the therapist that can be used to influence the patient's drinking and to encourage

---

This chapter subpart is a revised version of my chapter "Individual Psychotherapy: Alcohol," which appeared in Galanter MA, Kleber HD (eds): *The American Psychiatric Press Textbook of Substance Abuse Treatment,* 2nd Edition. Washington, DC, American Psychiatric Press, 1999, pp. 335–341.

changes in the self-perceptions and self-destructive behaviors that characterize many alcoholic individuals' lives. Individual therapy can be the preferred approach for those who feel uncomfortable in groups or who fear being pressured to disclose intimate details about themselves to others. Alcoholic individuals are a heterogeneous group, and no one treatment modality can be effective for all patients.

Psychodynamics of Alcoholism

The psychological conflict observed in alcoholic individuals consists of low self-esteem together with feelings of worthlessness and inadequacy. These feelings are denied and repressed and result in unconscious needs to be taken care of and to be accepted. Because these dependent needs cannot be met in reality, they lead to anxiety and compensatory needs for control, power, achievement, and elevated self-esteem. Denial of this conflict is present, and reactive grandiosity and excessive narcissism develop as defense mechanisms. Alcohol tranquilizes the anxiety, but more importantly, it creates pharmacologically induced feelings of power, omnipotence, and invulnerability in men (McClelland et al. 1972) and enhanced feelings of femininity in women (Wilsnack 1976). When alcoholic individuals wake up after a drinking episode, they experience guilt and despair because they have not achieved anything more than before they drank, and their problems remain. They have a primitive, punishing superego, and their feelings of worthlessness are intensified. The conflict continues in a vicious circle, often with a progressive downward spiral leading to psychological dependence and eventually addiction to alcohol.

An individual who has such a psychological conflict is likely to become alcoholic if he or she has a genetic predisposition to alcoholism and if he or she lives in a society in which alcohol use is sanctioned as a way to feel better or in which there is considerable ambivalence regarding alcohol use. In any particular individual, one or more of these etiological factors may predominate and lead to alcoholism.

AA is effective because the alcoholic individual's narcissism is sublimated by the rescuing of other alcoholic individuals; therefore, the grandiosity is fulfilled and becomes socially useful, and much of the alcoholic individual's dependent needs are met by the group's acceptance. AA members recognize that their support of other alcoholic individuals helps them maintain their own sobriety.

The central problem in the psychotherapy of alcoholism is breaking through the reactive grandiosity that produces the patient's massive denial of profound feelings of inferiority and dependence, which permits the pattern of self-destructive drinking to continue.

Differential Diagnosis and Treatment of Coexisting Psychiatric Disorders

A cardinal rule for treating alcoholism is the recognition that alcoholic patients do not constitute a homogeneous group. Specific subpopulations of alcoholic individuals require specific treatments. No one treatment approach, even AA, will be successful for all alcoholic patients.

One alcoholic subpopulation consists of problem drinkers with age-related developmental problems for whom alcohol abuse is part of an adjustment reaction. Such groups include adolescent problem drinkers and the alcoholic elderly. The manifestations of alcoholism are different in these two groups, relating to the adjustment problems in adolescents (Fischer 1985) or the stresses of aging in the alcoholic elderly (Zimberg 1990).

Another large subpopulation of alcoholic individuals consists of those with coexisting psychiatric disorders, called *dual-diagnosis patients*. The high prevalence of comorbid psychiatric disorders in alcoholic populations (Regier et al. 1990) and the difficulty of treating them has become apparent. Many alcoholic individuals also use other substances of abuse.

Successful treatment of alcoholism and identification of problems other than alcoholism require a complete psychiatric history, a mental status examination, and a developmental and family history as part of the initial evaluation.

Another cardinal rule in alcoholism therapy is that an actively drinking alcoholic patient with psychiatric signs and symptoms must be detoxified from alcohol and observed to be alcohol-free for 3–6 weeks before an effective diagnosis of a coexisting psychiatric disorder can be made. This step is essential, because excessive use of alcohol can produce a large variety of psychiatric symptoms. Identification and treatment of these psychiatric complications are required for effective treatment of the alcoholism.

Dual-Diagnosis Typology

A dual-diagnosis typology was developed, on the basis of a study of 130 outpatients in mental health and substance abuse clinics and 38 inpatients in a state psychiatric institution, to facilitate the differential diagnosis and treatment of disorders in this complicated population (Hien et al. 1997; Zimberg 1999). Individuals with a primary psychiatric disorder who used substances only when psychiatrically symptomatic were designated Type I patients. Type II patients were primary substance abusers with substance-induced psychiatric symptoms that resolved with abstinence. Type III patients were those with long histories of psychiatric and substance use disorders that were not related temporally or in a cause-and-effect manner. Type III alcoholic individuals are the true dual-diagnosis patients. Hien et al. (1997) used a series of questions about current and past relationships between psychiatric disorders and substance use. This approach was found to be reliable and valid in various clinical settings.

Therapists must be able to make an effective differential diagnosis and provide appropriate treatment for alcoholism that coexists with major psychiatric disorders. Individual therapy is the most effective way to identify coexisting psychiatric disorders and provide appropriate treatment. If the therapist is a psychiatrist, he or she can provide medication and individual therapy. If the therapist is not a psychiatrist, he or she must refer the patient to a psychiatrist who is knowledgeable about alcoholism for psychiatric medication.

Pharmacological Treatment of Alcoholism in Individual Therapy

Pharmacological interventions in the treatment of alcoholism include the use of benzodiazepines in detoxification and the use of psychiatric medications in treatment of coexisting psychiatric disorders. These medications are not designed to specifically treat the behavioral aspects of drinking or the excessive consumption of alcohol.

Disulfiram has been used since the 1950s to modify some of the behavioral aspects of drinking, particularly impulsive drinking. It was introduced into the United States by Ruth

Fox (1965), one of the early pioneers of the psychiatric treatment of alcoholism. Disulfiram inhibits the enzyme involved in ethyl alcohol metabolism in the liver at the stage of acetaldehyde production. Acetaldehyde is a toxic substance that in sufficient quantities can produce the unpleasant physical consequences of a disulfiram-alcohol interaction. This interaction results in nausea, tachycardia, facial flushing, and dizziness and is subjectively unpleasant. The interaction is not life threatening if the dose of disulfiram is limited to 250–500 mg/day and the patient receives a medical examination before use to rule out cardiac problems and significant liver abnormalities.

Disulfiram is useful as a deterrent to alcohol use early in treatment in patients whose drinking has been impulsive, without planning or conscious craving. It can be of particular use if administered under supervision in an employee assistance program or by a spouse or significant other. Disulfiram requires several days to take effect after therapy is initiated, and its clinical effects extend 4–7 days after the drug is stopped if the patient has been using it for 4–6 weeks. This prolonged duration of effect can encourage patients to deal with their intentions to drink through individual therapy, AA meetings, or discussions with a sponsor.

The drug naltrexone, a long-acting opiate antagonist, is a more recent addition to the alcoholism treatment armamentarium. Two controlled studies have shown that this drug can significantly reduce alcohol consumption and alcohol craving (O'Malley et al. 1992; Volpicelli et al. 1992) in alcoholic patients. These studies were done in different geographic locations and involved different treatment populations.

The use of naltrexone (at a dosage of 50 mg/day) has been a useful adjunct in the treatment of alcoholism in which craving is a significant clinical symptom. The only serious side effect is liver toxicity, but this side effect is rare at the standard dosage. Baseline liver function tests should be obtained before the drug is prescribed, and liver function should be monitored monthly for up to 6 months. The initial positive findings of the value of naltrexone in alcoholism treatment have been substantiated in a review article (Weinrieb and O'Brien 1997) and a clinical study (Jaffe et al. 1996). The mechanism of naltrexone's effects on alcohol consumption is not clear, although most experts believe that the drug inhibits the effect of β-endorphin on the dopamine reward system (Terenius 1996).

Currently, I prescribe naltrexone for patients who have relapsed repeatedly and in whom craving appears to be a major factor in the relapses.

Indications and Advantages of Individual Therapy

Individual therapy provides distinct advantages over the more commonly used modality of group therapy. Among these advantages is the ability to observe patients more closely to permit the differential diagnosis of coexisting psychiatric disorders. When such psychiatric disorders are present, the therapist must provide the necessary treatments, or the patient will not recover from either the alcoholism or the coexisting disorder.

Individual therapy can facilitate a dependent transference with the therapist. This dependent relationship can be useful in influencing the patient to change his or her drinking behavior and other maladaptive approaches to life and problems. The early stages of treatment require the provision of suggestions, guidance, advice, and role modeling to effect change in the patient, and a dependent relationship with the treater providing these interventions can facilitate their acceptance. In individual therapy, the therapist is able to learn more about the patient more quickly than is possible in group therapy, and this information enables the therapist to time specific interventions for periods when the patient is likely to be most receptive. Premature interventions can result in anger and avoidance and, in extreme situations, can cause the patient to leave therapy. Knowledge of the patient is also important in regard to identifying cues or triggers that could lead to relapse drinking. In contrast to the more general discussion of relapse prevention principles that occurs in groups, individual therapy can facilitate cognitive relapse prevention strategies specific to the patient.

Individual therapy can be more effective for individuals who fear groups and/or who are unwilling to disclose very sensitive life traumas. Individual therapy, however, cannot provide the peer support and identification with recovering alcoholic patients that occurs in group therapy in which the group is made up of patients at various levels of recovery. However, individual therapy in combination with AA participation can provide the peer support so helpful to recovery.

Techniques of Individual Therapy

Early Stage of Treatment

The basis of the early stage of treatment is *intervention* with regard to drinking. The therapeutic contract must establish that the goal of treatment is to achieve abstinence. Most patients in early-stage treatment will reluctantly agree to this goal because they believe they "cannot drink," although they will likely test it with slips or provocative drinking. This behavior must be confronted and used to help the patient see his or her inability to control the impulse to drink. The use of disulfiram should be introduced as a method for controlling the impulse to drink. If the patient refuses such medication or the use of naltrexone, and craving is a major problem at this stage, a contract should be established specifying that if the patient can remain alcohol free, there is no problem; however, if the patient has one more slip, medication will be mandatory if treatment is to continue.

Patients should be encouraged to attend AA meetings. They should be helped to find meetings at which they feel comfortable with other members, who should be their peers. The AA message and settings are similar from group to group, but the membership may vary greatly. Although some alcoholic individuals can recover without AA, the elements provided by this program—peer support, alcoholism education, opportunities to identify with others recovering from alcoholism, and guidance on how to live without alcohol in our drinking society—are extremely helpful to most recovering patients.

The family should be involved early and encouraged to attend AA. They should learn about their *enabling* behaviors, encourage the patient's sobriety with their support and interest, and avoid covering up for or excusing the patient's drinking.

Thus, structure should be provided to the alcoholic patient early in treatment in the form of *scaffolding*. The scaffolding erected around a building under renovation does not itself provide structural support for the building's foundation but rather enables workers to enter the building from different directions and make the renovations inside. The changes produced are from *outside in*. In psychoanalytic treatment, the changes occur through insight and are from *inside out*. The therapist, the family, AA, and pharmacological interventions provide the structural components of *scaffolding therapy*.

The therapist provides direction, guidance, and cognitive suggestions to help the alcoholic patient learn to cope with unpleasant feelings, conflicts, problems, and stress without resorting to alcohol. Cognitive-behavioral strategies are suggested to encourage the patient to avoid situations, interpersonal relationships, and places that have been triggers to drinking in the past. Because such triggers are unique to each individual, the therapist must learn about the unique drinking triggers in each patient. The more the therapist learns, the more effective this approach will be. This avoidance strategy is extremely useful early in therapy, although it can be modified later as the patient develops better coping skills and changes his or her attitude about the need for alcohol. Anxiety- and stress-reduction techniques other than cognitive-behavioral approaches can be used early in therapy and can include meditation, self-hypnosis, biofeedback, and other relaxation techniques.

The major goals of scaffolding therapy are to help patients accept their problem with alcohol and learn to cope with their life and its problems without using alcohol. In some patients, the absence of the anesthetic effects of alcohol will cause problems that were once neglected to become more apparent and more painful. Patients should be helped to recognize that only with sobriety can they successfully deal with their problems. In some patients, early sobriety can produce a feeling of euphoria and omnipotence (called the "pink cloud" in AA). Giving up alcohol successfully seems to suggest that they can do anything. Therapists should guide their patients through this reaction-formation defense by helping them recognize their limitations and the possibilities for feeling and functioning better without alcohol in the future if sobriety is maintained.

Defenses observed in patients and in the transference should not be interpreted at this stage of treatment; instead, if possible, they should be utilized and redirected in the recovery process. Sublimation of the feelings of omnipotence through involvement in AA and helping others by qualifying to speak at AA meetings is an example of such redirection. Wallace (1985) has provided an excellent discussion of managing the "preferred defense structure of the alcoholic."

The early stage of treatment, with its active intervention in relation to drinking and helping the alcoholic individual adapt to life and its problems without drinking, typically requires about 6 months to 1 year to produce stability. The overt conflict of whether to drink becomes internalized, and the alcoholic individual enters the next stage of treatment with the belief that "I won't drink."

Middle Stage of Treatment

In the middle stage of treatment, the therapeutic effort is focused on helping the individual gain more independence, and the scaffolding system can be partially dismantled. Disulfiram or naltrexone can be discontinued but might be used intermittently when the patient anticipates some severe stress. The patient should be able to use these drugs when his or her control over the impulse to drink feels threatened by intense craving or other external or internal drink signals.

Attendance at AA should continue, but its frequency might diminish from daily to two or three times a week. Patients should be encouraged to actively speak at AA meetings to reinforce their determination to stay sober. According to AA, "You can't keep it unless you give it away."

The therapeutic approach should remain supportive, but the emphasis should shift to opportunities to change behavioral patterns that contributed to the patient's drinking. Greater attention should be focused on dealing with feelings such as anger and the need for control. Some interpretation of behavior and feelings could be made, but uncovering approaches and interpretation of the dependent transference should be avoided.

By helping the patient develop an ability to empathize, the therapist can help the patient become less egocentric and reach a more mature recognition of his or her limitations and the inability of others to respond to all of the patient's needs. Although the patient will feel more anxiety, he or she is usually able to cope without drinking because of stable internalized control over the impulse to drink. Drinking dreams and fantasies are common during this stage. Interpretation of these dreams and fantasies should deal with issues of controlling the impulse to drink.

After 1½ years in the middle stage, the alcoholic individual has generally established good internalized control over the impulse to drink. This is the stage that has been achieved by most successful AA members. Although these individuals may not possess insight into the psychological sources of the dependency conflict or an understanding of the serious interpersonal problems or profound feelings of anger that exist, they usually have good sobriety.

Late Stage of Treatment

Patients with severe anxiety, episodes of depression, or serious characterological problems are candidates for treatment in the late stage of treatment, in which a belief that "I don't have to drink" is the goal. Although the late stage is not necessary for maintaining sobriety, the conflict resolution achieved by patients who complete this stage can allow better outcomes. At this stage, the focus of therapy is on uncovering and reconstruction and is less supportive, directive, and cognitive. The transition should be gradual, because as the therapist becomes more passive and analytical, transference issues will surface that should be interpreted. Dreams and fantasies should be used to a greater degree, and memories and feelings from childhood should be examined as they relate to past and present behavior and feelings. Thus, a more traditional psychoanalytic approach can be used. The duration of this phase of treatment is indefinite but usually lasts an additional 1–2 years.

Termination of Treatment

Drinking slips can occur during the middle and late stages of treatment but are usually of short duration and without serious consequences. If they occur during the middle stage, drinking cues and control issues are reviewed. If the slips occur during the late stage, the role of unconscious conflicts in the slips should be explored to foster insight into and greater control over the impulse to drink.

Successful termination can occur in the middle stage or in the late stage when the patient and the therapist mutually agree that the patient has good internalized control over the impulse to drink and has experienced significant improvement in functioning. Because alcoholism is a lifelong condition and patients are never "cured," the door to return to treatment should be left open. Patients involved in AA should be encouraged to maintain their involvement, and those not involved should be encouraged to consider trying again in order to benefit from observing role models of successful recovery.

Transference and Countertransference

In individual therapy the transference relationship is intensified. It is usually based on dependency needs but includes some mistrust and hostility stemming from previous rejections and is therefore ambivalent. The patient may test the therapeutic relationship by drinking early in therapy. If such episodes can be dealt with in an understanding rather than a judgmental or punitive way, the transference can be shifted to the dependent relationship necessary for successful therapy. In a dependent transference, the patient is more receptive to guidance and suggestion as part of the scaffolding therapy.

A supportive and nonjudgmental, nonpunitive therapeutic relationship will produce a "corrective emotional experience" as described by Alexander (1946) and will foster the maintenance of long-term sobriety. After a stable sobriety has been maintained for 1½ years, the transference relationship can be explored and interpreted as part of the uncovering approaches used in the late stage of treatment. The late stage should be entered by mutual agreement, and the transition should be a slow process over weeks rather than an abrupt transition from support to insight-oriented therapy.

Countertransference refers to the therapist's reaction to the patient as if the patient were an important person in the therapist's life and/or the therapist's reaction to the patient's behavior in relation to the therapist's own feelings, needs, and self-image. The patient's early and provocative drinking and later slips can cause the therapist to feel frustrated and angry because of his or her need for the gratification of successful treatment. This anger and frustration is very common in therapists and is the major reason that many therapists refuse to treat alcoholic patients.

The reality is that the therapist cannot force, control, or seduce patients into achieving abstinence but can only offer them tools to assist them in achieving abstinence for themselves. The therapist's omnipotent need for successful treatment cannot compete against the patient's unconscious psychological need for omnipotence and control, or the treatment will fail. Only the patient can decide to work toward abstinence, using the therapist's help and guidance. Therapists who work with alcoholic patients must recognize their own limitations; otherwise, burnout, avoidance of alcoholic patients, and other adverse psychological reactions will result.

Outcome Studies

Few controlled studies have compared outcomes of individual and group therapy of alcoholism. In a review of this subject, Solomon (1982) reported slightly better outcomes for group therapy. However, patient characteristics appeared more predictive of outcome than did treatment modality. Woody et al. (1983) found individual therapy to be efficacious in opioid-addicted patients.

Clinical reports and my experience have indicated the value of individual therapy (Hoffman and Miller 1993; Kaufman 1989; Khantzian 1982; O'Malley and Carroll 1996; Wurmser 1984; Zimberg 1989). Group therapy, however, is more widely practiced than individual therapy in alcoholism treatment, particularly in hospital- and institution-based programs, because group therapy, with its peer involvement, can be very effective, is generally more cost-efficient, and more closely resembles the group model of the 12-Step programs.

However, the great heterogeneity of the alcoholic population suggests that no one modality of treatment can be effective for all patients. The literature indicates that different types of alcoholism require differing treatment approaches (Meyer 1989; Schuckit 1989). A major effort to determine which subpopulations of alcoholic individuals might do best with which specific type of treatment was undertaken in Project MATCH (Matching Alcoholism Treatments to Client Heterogeneity) (Project MATCH Research Group 1997). This project involved 1,726 alcohol-dependent outpatients and aftercare patients who had completed inpatient or day hospital treatment. The subjects were randomly assigned to one of three manually guided individual treatments: Cognitive-Behavioral Coping Skills Therapy, Motivational Enhancement Therapy, or Twelve-Step Facilitation Therapy. Ten patient characteristics comprised the matching variables: severity of alcohol involvement, client conceptual level, meaning seeking, motivational readiness to change, psychiatric severity, social support for drinking versus abstinence, sociopathy, typology, gender, and cognitive impairment.

This study found little difference in treatment outcome by type of treatment. All of the treatments produced improvement, but no treatment was superior to any other for the matched samples of patients. The only variable that appeared to affect outcome was psychiatric severity, with those with low severity doing better with Twelve-Step Facilitation Therapy.

A weakness of this study was that it did not include as matching variables the more mundane clinical and demographic variables—such as age, age at onset of alcohol problem, socioeconomic status, marital status, employment history, and ethnicity—that earlier studies have suggested may possess prognostic significance in regard to treatment outcomes of alcoholic patients (Kissin et al. 1968; Zimberg 1974). Therefore, the definitive matching study has yet to be done.

Conclusions

Individual therapy, both alone and in combination with AA involvement, can be very effective for alcoholic populations with diverse characteristics and is particularly useful for those with coexisting psychiatric disorders.

References

Alexander F, French TM: Psychoanalysis Therapy: Principles and Application. New York, Ronald Press, 1946

Fischer J: Psychotherapy of adolescent alcohol abusers, in Practical Approaches to Alcoholism Psychotherapy, 2nd Edition. Edited by Zimberg S, Wallace J, Blume SB. New York, Plenum, 1985, pp 295–313

Fox R: Psychiatric aspects of alcoholism. Am J Psychother 19:408–416, 1965

Hien D, Zimberg S, Weisman S, et al: Dual diagnosis subtypes in urban substance abuse and mental health clinics. Psychiatr Serv 48:1058–1063, 1997

Hoffman NG, Miller NS: Perspectives of effective treatment for alcohol and drug disorders. Psychiatr Clin North Am 16:127–140, 1993

Jaffe AJ, Rounsaville B, Chang G, et al: Naltrexone, relapse prevention, and supportive therapy matching with alcoholics: an analysis of patient treatment matching. J Consult Clin Psychol 64:1044–1053, 1996

Kaufman E: The psychotherapy of dually diagnosed patients. J Subst Abuse Treat 6:9–18, 1989

Khantzian EJ: Some treatment implications of the ego and self disturbance in alcoholism, in Dynamic Approaches to the Understanding and Treatment of Alcoholism. Edited by Bean MH, Zinberg NE. New York, Free Press, 1982, pp 103–188

Kissin B, Rosenblatt SM, Machover S: Prognostic factors in alcoholism. Psychiatry Res Rep Am Psychiatr Assoc 24:22–43, 1968

McClelland DC, Davis WW, Kalin R, et al: The Drinking Man. New York, Free Press, 1972

Meyer R: Typologies, in Treatments of Psychiatric Disorders: a Task Force Report of the American Psychiatric Association, Vol 2. Washington, DC, American Psychiatric Association, 1989, pp 1065–1072

O'Malley SS, Carroll KM: Psychotherapeutic considerations in pharmacological trials. Alcohol Clin Exp Res 20 (suppl 7):17A–22A, 1996

O'Malley SS, Jaffe AJ, Chang G, et al: Naltrexone and coping skills therapy for alcohol dependence: a controlled study. Arch Gen Psychiatry 49:881–887, 1992

Project MATCH Research Group: Matching Alcoholism Treatments to Client Heterogeneity: Project MATCH posttreatment drinking outcomes. J Stud Alcohol 58:7–29, 1997

Regier DA, Farmer ME, Rae DS, et al: Comorbidity of mental disorders with alcohol and other drug abuse. JAMA 264:2511–2518, 1990

Schuckit MA: Goals of treatment, in Treatments of Psychiatric Disorders: a Task Force Report of the American Psychiatric Association, Vol 2. Washington, DC, American Psychiatric Association, 1989, pp 1072–1076

Solomon SD: Individual versus group therapy: current status in the treatment of alcoholism. Advances in Alcohol and Substance Abuse 2:69–86, 1982

Terenius L: Alcohol addiction (alcoholism) and the opioid system. Alcohol 13:31–34, 1996

Tiebout HM: Intervention in psychotherapy. Am J Psychoanal 22:1–6, 1962

Volpicelli JR, Alterman AL, Hayashida M, et al: Naltrexone and the treatment of alcohol dependence. Arch Gen Psychiatry 49:876–880, 1992

Wallace J: Working with the preferred defense structure of the recovering alcoholic, in Practical Approaches to Alcoholism Psychotherapy, 2nd Edition. Edited by Zimberg S, Wallace J, Blume SB. New York, Plenum, 1985, pp 23–36

Weinrieb RM, O'Brien CP: Naltrexone in the treatment of alcoholism. Annu Rev Med 48:477–487, 1997

Wilsnack SC: The impact of sex roles and women's alcohol use and abuse, in Alcoholism Problems in Women and Children. Edited by Greenblat N, Schuckit MA. New York, Grune & Stratton, 1976, pp 264–271

Woody GE, Luborsky L, McLellan AT, et al: Psychotherapy for opiate addicts: does it help? Arch Gen Psychiatry 40:639–645, 1983

Wurmser L: More respect for the neurotic process: comments on the problem of narcissism in severe psychopathology; especially the addictions. J Subst Abuse Treat 1:37–45, 1984

Zimberg S: Evaluation of alcoholism treatment in Harlem. Q J Stud Alcohol 35:550–557, 1974

Zimberg S: The Clinical Management of Alcoholism. New York, Brunner/Mazel, 1982

Zimberg S: Individual management and psychotherapy, in Treatments of Psychiatric Disorders: a Task Force Report of the American Psychiatric Association, Vol 2. Washington, DC, American Psychiatric Association, 1989, pp 1093–1103

Zimberg S: Management of alcoholism in the elderly. Addiction Nursing Network 1:4–6, 1990

Zimberg S: A dual diagnosis typology to improve diagnosis and treatment of dual disorder patients. J Psychoactive Drugs 31:47–51, 1999

Individual Psychotherapy for Substance Use Disorders

George E. Woody, M.D.
Delinda E. Mercer, Ph.D.

Psychosocial treatments for substance-related disorders are used in almost all treatment programs. Drug counseling in a group therapy setting is probably the most common of these psychosocial treatments; however, individual counseling or psychotherapy and family therapy are also available in many drug-free rehabilitation, methadone maintenance, and detoxification programs (National Drug and Alcoholism Treatment Unit Survey 1982). The types of psychotherapy vary, but cognitive-behavioral, supportive-expressive, and interpersonal are well represented. In this chapter subpart, we focus on these and other individual-treatment models.

Despite the widespread use of psychotherapeutic approaches to treat chemical dependence, it is only within the last two decades that these approaches have been scientifically evaluated. Most of the earlier research on addiction treatment focused on pharmacotherapies, even though some form of psychosocial intervention was at least a part of almost every treatment program and in some cases constituted the entire program (Onken and Blaine 1990). This relative absence of research on psychosocial treatments for substance use disorders was due, at least in part, to the difficulties associated with the conduct of research in this area (Onken and Blaine 1990), which include issues of compliance with study procedures and of recruitment and retention of patients. These methodological problems have been discussed in detail elsewhere (Borkovec 1990; Howard et al. 1990; Lambert 1990) and will not be reviewed here.

This chapter subpart is a revised version of our chapter "Individual Psychotherapy: Other Drugs," which appeared in Galanter MA, Kleber HD (eds): *The American Psychiatric Press Textbook of Substance Abuse Treatment,* 2nd Edition. Washington, DC, American Psychiatric Press, 1999, pp. 343–351.

Psychotherapy Versus Drug Counseling

Throughout this chapter subpart, the term *psychotherapy* is used to describe a psychological treatment that aims to change problematic thoughts, feelings, and behaviors by creating a new understanding of the thoughts and feelings that appear causally related to the presenting problem(s). Change is believed to occur within the context of a supportive relationship with a skilled therapist, who provides the patient an opportunity to explore the underpinnings of maladaptive behaviors, thoughts, and feelings and then to change undesirable patterns that contribute to the patient's distress. When used in the treatment of addiction, psychotherapy addresses addictive behaviors and the thoughts and feelings that appear to promote, maintain, or result from the addiction. Along with cessation of substance use, psychotherapy addresses issues related to other aspects of patients' lives, under the assumption that some of these contribute to the use.

In contrast to psychotherapy, *drug counseling* is generally defined as the regular management of addicted patients with a strong focus on motivating them to change their behavior to adopt a drug-free lifestyle. Counseling includes giving support; educating the patient about drug effects; providing structure; monitoring behavior; encouraging abstinence; providing concrete services such as referral for job counseling, medical services, or legal aid; and fostering participation in self-help groups. Counseling continuously and persistently focuses on the addictive behavior, often using language and concepts derived from the 12-Step program model of Alcoholics Anonymous. Addiction counseling attempts to end the dependence by identifying daily problems and behaviors that contribute to substance use, educating the patient about drug effects, enhancing motivation, and delivering concrete services aimed at overcoming these problems.

In some ways counseling is similar to psychotherapy, although there are important differences. Counseling, like psychotherapy, attempts to help the patient deal with addiction-related consequences that have often become a part of his or her life. Like psychotherapy, it provides an ongoing supportive relationship with a skilled clinician; however, its approach is concrete and specific, in contrast to the indirect intrapsychic focus of psychotherapy.

Rationale for Using Psychotherapy to Treat Addiction

Psychotherapy, in one form or another, is commonly used either alone or in conjunction with medication for treating psychiatric disorders. It is reasonable to suppose that psychotherapy would have a place in the treatment of addiction, because subjective distress seems to contribute to, and result from, chemical dependence. Clinical observations indicate that some substances of abuse can alleviate certain psychiatric symptoms, at least temporarily, and this effect is likely to contribute to their use. Such use to relieve emotional distress has resulted in a theory of addictive behavior known as the "self-medication hypothesis" (Khantzian 1985). An example is opiate use by an anxious person. Opiates can cause a temporary relaxed state in which a person does not care so much about his or her current problems. Thus, an anxious person with many worries and concerns may find that his or her distress is reduced by opiates and may therefore be predisposed to repeatedly administer the drug when anxious.

A corollary of the self-medication hypothesis is that drug users with underlying non-substance-induced psychiatric symptoms who are attempting to treat themselves by repeated ingestion of psychoactive substances can be helped by psychotherapy, either alone or in combination with an appropriately selected psychotropic medication. Thus, the presence of a non-substance-induced psychiatric disorder identifies a subgroup of patients who may benefit from additional psychiatric treatment. These patients are often referred to as "dual diagnosis" patients because they have both a substance use disorder and another psychiatric disorder.

Consistent with the idea that some addicted patients need treatment for both the addiction and one or more other psychiatric disorders is the fact that psychiatric disorders co-occurring with substance use disorders have been found to have prognostic significance. Generally, the more severe the psychiatric symptoms, the more difficult to treat the addiction. Depression may be the exception to this rule, because a moderate level of depression has sometimes been shown to be associated with better outcomes, although the findings have not always been consistent on this point (Carroll et al. 1995).

In the following discussion of individual psychotherapy, a practical approach is emphasized that draws on both clinical experience and research findings. General factors that are important for the clinician when providing psychotherapy for addicted patients are first described, then modalities of individual psychotherapy and their relative efficacies, and finally treatment implications.

General Factors in Addiction Treatment

Therapists treating addiction should be familiar with the pharmacological and medical effects of abused drugs, the subculture of addiction and addictive lifestyles, and 12-Step programs. Possession of this knowledge is likely to increase the therapist's credibility in the eyes of the patient as well as help the therapist to better understand the current and past experiences of the patient.

Knowledge of Abused Drugs

It is important that therapists who treat persons with substance use disorders become familiar with both the "normal" and the adverse effects of abused drugs, their routes of administration, the drug combinations commonly used, and the typical patterns of use. This information can be useful in several ways.

For example, patients sometimes come to treatment while under the influence of drugs. This probably occurs most often on initial visits, but it can happen at any time. The patient's mental state can vary considerably, depending on whether he or she is intoxicated, withdrawing, or in the more "normal" state between these two extremes. The therapist needs to know how the patient's mood may be altered by recent drug intoxication or withdrawal and whether mental symptoms are substance induced or represent an underlying disorder.

Although substance-induced mental disorders are usually temporary, they may need to be treated aggressively with medication or close supervision to ensure the patient's safety. Conversely, psychiatric disorders can be masked by drug intoxication and thus become evident only when the acute drug effects wear off. This latter situation may occur more often with opiates than with other psychoactive medications, because opiates have antianxiety and weak antipsychotic effects (American Psychiatric Association 1994).

In an outpatient setting, when a patient arrives for a scheduled therapy session intoxicated with alcohol or drugs, the therapist's immediate response should be guided by his or her own judgment of the clinical situation (including severity of symptoms and degree of impairment). Severe intoxication may require referral for emergency admission or supervised monitoring. In most cases, assuming that no emergency or need for intensive monitoring exists, it is best to reschedule the appointment and to strongly discourage the patient from coming to treatment intoxicated. The decision to reschedule often involves finding a time when the patient agrees to try to come in a sober condition, because little psychotherapy can be done with the patient under the influence of a drug. Inability of the patient to comply with this request is probably an indicator that the addiction is so severe that the patient needs hospitalization or treatment in some other controlled setting with more structure and support.

Many patients use drugs in combination and become addicted to multiple substances. Common drug combinations are cocaine and alcohol, amphetamines and sedatives, alcohol and marijuana, and heroin with cocaine, amphetamines, benzodiazepines, or alcohol. Persons dependent on cocaine and alcohol often report that they drink to reduce anxiety resulting from cocaine. Methadone maintenance patients who abuse benzodiazepines typically report that they take the benzodiazepines immediately before or after the methadone in an attempt to produce a "high." Persons with such complex patterns of use can be unusually difficult to treat, because they may be under the influence of opposing pharmacological effects in addition to having other psychiatric problems. For example, patients may be withdrawing from one drug and intoxicated with another while also experiencing symptoms of a psychiatric disorder such as major depression or posttraumatic stress disorder.

It is also helpful to know what drugs are currently available in a particular locale. For example, new drugs can quickly appear ("Rohypnol" [flunitrazepam], "Ecstasy" [methylenedioxymethamphetamine; MDMA]) or older drugs can reappear (inhalants, amphetamines). In other cases, the price or availability of a drug may change, with serious clinical implications. An example is the recent increase in purity and lower price of heroin, which increases the chances for lethal effects, especially in persons with low levels of tolerance. Any of these changes can influence patterns of drug use, negatively affect the chances for recovery, and increase the adverse medical consequences of the use.

Knowledge of Subculture of Addiction and Lifestyles of Addicted Persons

It is also helpful for psychotherapists to be familiar with the lifestyles of addicted persons and the subculture in which addiction prevails. Such knowledge can be acquired either through talking with paraprofessionals or psychotherapists who treat these populations or through firsthand experience working with these individuals.

Lifestyles of addicted persons are quite diverse. For example, some persons with alcohol dependence may be able to function well enough in society to retain employment and family relationships, although these relationships are damaged by the dependence. On the other hand, persons addicted to heroin often live in a subculture of their own, and much of their time is spent in drug-related activities such as obtaining the drug, preparing to "shoot up," "nodding out," becoming "normal," and then experiencing withdrawal until their next dose.

The lifestyles of many cocaine-addicted persons are often midway between those of alcoholic persons and heroin-addicted persons. Persons with cocaine dependence frequently enter treatment while continuing to function in society, as evidenced by maintaining family relationships and holding a job. However, severe cocaine addiction leads to rapid disintegration of connections with non-drug-using society and usually immerses the addict in the subculture that typically surrounds use of "crack" cocaine. This involvement progresses as the person becomes increasingly absorbed with cocaine use and results in lost ties with normal social contacts and problems on the job.

The risk of infection with human immunodeficiency virus (HIV) is another lifestyle issue with serious treatment implications. For injection drug users (primarily heroin and amphetamine but also some cocaine users), there is a high level of risk associated with sharing needles and drug paraphernalia and engaging in increased levels of unprotected sex. Although these risky behaviors have become less prevalent in association with HIV-risk-reduction efforts, they are still common to some extent, particularly among those who use "shooting galleries" or who are not in treatment. High-risk sexual behavior has been identified as a particularly common problem among cocaine addicts, who use the drug very often (due to its short half-life) and often trade sex for cocaine or for money to buy cocaine.

Knowledge of Self-Help Programs

The 12-Step programs are widely available, free of charge, and extremely helpful in addiction treatment. As a result, referral to and participation in these groups are a part of most successful addiction treatment programs. Outcome results from 12-Step programs have been difficult to obtain, although recent studies have shown that 12-Step participation is associated with improved outcomes. Furthermore, the fact that these programs can be easily combined with psychotherapy or counseling seems to have an additive affect in enhancing outcomes (Fiorentine and Hillhouse 2000). Twelve-step programs are used throughout treatment and, perhaps more importantly, have been found helpful in preventing relapse after completion of a structured program of psychotherapy or counseling (Fiorentine 1999). These programs are abstinence oriented and foster a network of healthy social support. In addition, their philosophy imparts ideas that many recovering persons find useful in dealing with everyday life and attempting to establish and maintain a sober lifestyle.

Therapists treating addiction should be familiar with the following key aspects of the 12-Step philosophy: 1) the belief that addiction is a disease rather than bad behavior, 2) the idea that addiction damages the whole person—physically, mentally and spiritually—and that recovery must address all of those domains, 3) the idea that healing or recovery comes from connecting to something larger than oneself, 4) the paradox of surrendering power so as to ultimately be empowered to attain sobriety, 5) the idea that interpersonal support is critical for recovery, and 6) the belief that recovery is a lifelong process and that there should be continued personal growth.

Treatment Models

Psychotherapy probably has the best chance of being effective when it is integrated into an ongoing program that focuses directly on reducing or eliminating drug use and treating psychiatric symptoms that may accompany the dependence. Washton (1989) described the components of such a structured, progressive treatment program: it is abstinence oriented, provides education about the effects of drugs, fosters family involvement, includes frequent urine testing, offers both group and individual therapy, supports 12-Step participation, and encourages good physical health. In such a program, drug-focused counseling and psychotherapy are provided by the same person.

Another treatment model involves assigning the patient both an addiction counselor and a psychotherapist. The counselor handles the patient's more concrete needs by, for example, talking about current problems, supporting and encouraging efforts to reduce drug use, monitoring progress, providing liaison or consultation with medical personnel, providing job referrals, obtaining legal advice, encouraging limit setting by enforcing program rules, and keeping accurate records. The psychotherapist addresses cognitive, attitudinal, or interpersonal issues that contribute to the addiction. This model requires coordination of services and good personal relations between the psychotherapist and the counseling staff. In this regard, it is very helpful if the therapist demonstrates commitment to the overall program through activities such as working within the facility, interacting with other treatment staff, being involved in making decisions regarding the patient's treatment plan, and being familiar with the overall program procedures and policies.

Therapist Qualities and the Therapeutic Alliance

Therapist qualities appear to have an important impact on treatment outcome (Luborsky et al. 1985, 1986). Kleinman et al. (1990) found that therapist assignment was the strongest predictor of treatment retention for patients dependent on cocaine. Unfortunately, little evidence is available to indicate what type of therapist is likely to work best with and be most helpful to substance-abusing patients. This difficulty stems, in part, from the fact that persons who abuse substances constitute a heterogeneous group. Nonetheless, some guidelines can be offered from the few available studies that have examined therapist qualities and outcome.

Three qualities have emerged as predictive of outcome: the therapist's personal adjustment, the therapist's skill, and the therapist's interest in helping patients (Luborsky et al. 1985). All of these qualities probably have an impact on the therapist-patient relationship. Several studies have shown that therapists who from the beginning of treatment establish a positive relationship that is perceived by the patient as one of "helping" have a better chance of success than do therapists who form less-positive bonds (Luborsky et al. 1985). Related to these qualities is the therapist's interest in helping the patient and comfort with certain kinds of problems. Some therapists have strong negative reactions to the manipulative, antisocial, impulsive, and demanding behavior that is often seen in drug-abusing patients. Therapists with such predominantly negative reactions will probably not do well with these patients.

Therapists may occasionally need to extend themselves a little more with addicted patients than with other types of psychiatric patients. The dependency needs of addicted patients often express themselves in the physician-patient relationship, and an occasional appropriate, concrete supportive response is probably useful, especially in the early phases of treatment. Such a response may involve greeting the patient warmly on his or her entering the office, actively seeking to reestablish contact when an appointment is missed, acknowledging improvements when they occur, or seeing the patient occasionally at unscheduled times if the need occurs and the time is available.

Psychotherapy Techniques in Substance Abuse

Most of the techniques of individual psychotherapy for patients with substance use disorders have been adapted from models developed for treating other types of nonpsychotic psychiatric disorders, especially depression. It appears that to be effective, addiction therapies must integrate some of the more concrete behavioral strategies typically considered to be part of addiction counseling. Of course, adding such direct approaches is less necessary if the psychotherapy is offered in combination with addiction counseling than if the therapy is a "standalone" treatment. It is also important to have a good appreciation of the power of the dependence, with its attendant loss of control and the biopsychosocial consequences that often result.

Luborsky and colleagues (1995) identified certain special emphases that are particularly important in treating addiction with psychotherapy, regardless of the particular treatment model:

1. Much time and energy on the therapist's part are required to introduce the patient to treatment and to engage him or her in it.
2. The treatment goals must be formulated early and kept in sight.
3. Much attention must be given by the therapist to developing a positive relationship and supporting the patient.
4. The therapist must maintain awareness of the patient's compliance with the overall drug treatment program, and especially of any illicit drug use. This information should come from the patient's self-report and from urinalysis and breath tests, and may also be provided by family, friends, and other treatment staff.
5. If the patient is receiving pharmacotherapy in addition to psychotherapy, the therapist should keep abreast of the patient's compliance with and reactions to the medication. If the patient is receiving methadone or LAAM, attention should be given to when the patient feels therapy is best conducted (i.e., before or after the daily dose). Methadone or LAAM usually is such a central part of the patient's life that establishing an agreed-upon time for therapy around the dosing schedule could determine whether the patient engages in or drops out of therapy.

Efficacy Studies of Substance Abuse Therapies

A number of individual psychotherapy and counseling approaches have been tested for efficacy in research supported by the National Institute on Drug Abuse. Key points from these studies are briefly described here.

Cognitive-behavioral therapy, cognitive therapy, and relapse prevention therapy (Carroll et al. 1991a; Marlatt and Gordon 1985) are related and are based on the theory that learning processes play a critical role in the development of both addiction and other maladaptive behavior patterns. These therapies involve strategies and techniques to enhance self-control and foster abstinence—for example, self-monitoring to recognize and change false beliefs and to detect drug cravings when they first appear, identification of high-risk situations, and development of strategies for avoiding or coping with affects or situations that stimulate drug craving ("triggers") without resorting to use. A number of studies have reported positive results with these approaches, which have been delivered in both group and individual settings (Maude-Griffin et al. 1998).

Individual supportive-expressive (SE) psychotherapy (Luborsky 1984) derives from psychoanalytic therapy and has been modified to address substance use disorders, specifically opioid and cocaine dependence (Luborsky et al. 1995; Mark and Faude 1995). It has two main components: supportive techniques to help patients feel comfortable in discussing their concerns, and expressive (or interpretative) techniques to help patients identify and work through problematic interpersonal issues. Special attention is paid to the role of drugs in relation to feelings and behaviors and to how problems may be solved without resorting to drug use. Positive results with SE therapy were demonstrated in two studies that used this modality in combination with methadone maintenance and drug counseling for treatment of heroin-addicted patients. In these studies, patients with moderate to high levels of psychiatric symptoms demonstrated benefits greater than those obtained from drug counseling alone; patients with low levels of symptoms showed equal improvement with drug counseling and counseling plus psychotherapy (Woody et al. 1984, 1995). However, in a more recent study (Crits-Christoph et al. 1999) in cocaine-addicted patients who were not heroin dependent or receiving methadone maintenance, SE therapy plus group drug counseling was associated with significant reductions in cocaine use but was not as effective as group and individual drug counseling. In this study, all therapies, including SE, were equally effective in reducing the severity of self-reported psychosocial problems. However, SE therapy did not do as well as the other therapies in reducing acquired immunodeficiency syndrome (AIDS) risk behavior, as measured by the Risk Assessment Battery (Navaline et al. 1994).

Interpersonal psychotherapy (IPT) is another supportive/dynamic treatment that has shown effectiveness in some studies. It focuses on resolving current interpersonal problems and has been adapted for use in treating both opioid and cocaine dependence (Rounsaville et al. 1983, 1985). In one study of methadone-maintained, opioid-addicted patients, those receiving IPT improved, but not to a greater extent than those receiving drug counseling alone (Rounsaville et al. 1983). In a more recent study of cocaine addicts, patients receiving IPT improved, but not to the same degree as those receiving cognitive-behavioral therapy (Carroll et al. 1991b).

Motivational enhancement therapy (MET), another individual treatment that has been shown to be useful in treating alcohol dependence (Miller 1996; Project MATCH Research Group 1997), attempts to facilitate reduction or cessation of substance use by helping patients resolve their ambivalence about engaging in treatment and stopping substance use. Patients are encouraged to talk about the positive and negative aspects of use, with the therapist always looking for ways to help the patient tip the balance of ambivalence in the direction of abstinence. MET is usually time-limited, often involving only one to four sessions. MET is also quite versatile—it can be used at the initial stages of treatment only, as a "standalone" therapy throughout the treatment process, or in combination with other interventions.

Contingency management (CM) has been studied mainly for opiate and cocaine dependence and has been shown to be effective in reducing use. Community reinforcement (CR) (Higgins et al. 1994; Silverman et al. 1996a) uses CM principles and has been a focus of special interest, especially for treatment of cocaine dependence. In CM, patients typically receive one to two individual counseling sessions per week. They submit two or three weekly urine samples to be tested for unprescribed substances and receive vouchers that can be exchanged for retail goods as incentives for drug-negative urine tests in a stepwise fashion, with higher-value vouchers given as the number and consistency of negative urine test results increases.

Studies have shown that CM and CR facilitate engagement in treatment and abstinence from cocaine, heroin, and marijuana (Silverman et al. 1996a, 1996b; Calsyn and Saxon 1999). One problem with applying CM or CR beyond specially funded research programs is that community providers are not reimbursed for funds spent as incentives to reward patients for abstinence or compliance. Because of this problem, the most common use of CM is in methadone maintenance programs in which take-home doses are contingent on progress in treatment, as demonstrated by having consistently drug-free urine test results, keeping regular appointments, and showing other signs of progress.

Matching Patients and Treatments

It may be that specific psychotherapy models work better for some patients than for others. There is some evidence for this conclusion in the studies of psychotherapy with methadone patients, as discussed earlier. However, Crits-Christoph et al. (1999), in their recent study of treatments for cocaine dependence, failed to find that patients with higher levels of psychiatric symptoms did better with cognitive-behavioral or supportive-expressive psychotherapy than with drug counseling, as did Project MATCH (Matching Alcoholism Treatments to Client Heterogeneity) (Project MATCH Research Group 1997). Reasons for these inconsistent results are unclear, although the differences may be related to the fact that methadone is a powerful pharmacotherapy that substantially reduces drug use, thus making it easier for psychotherapists to focus on a wider range of issues than was possible in the cocaine and alcohol treatment studies, which did not use an effective pharmacotherapy. In any case, the discrepant findings highlight the importance of further exploring the question of patient-treatment matching in various treatment settings.

Other studies have found evidence that a greater intensity of services, especially in the beginning of treatment, leads to better outcomes. For example, Kleinman et al. (1990) reported a 50%–60% abstinence rate among cocaine-dependent subjects who were treated with a 12-Step-oriented, drug-focused therapy in inpatient and intensive day treatment for 1 month, followed by twice-weekly group drug counseling. The relatively high abstinence rate found in these studies compared very favorably with the 19% abstinence rate that was associated with once-weekly outpatient individual or group drug counseling or family therapy for cocaine addiction (Kleinman et al. 1990). These findings, taken collectively, suggest that psychosocial treatments may need to be delivered at a fairly high level of intensity for most persons with substance dependence, at least during the initial phases of treatment.

A related finding emerged from a study by McLellan and colleagues (1993). This study examined three levels of treatment services for methadone-maintained heroin-addicted patients: 1) minimal services (10 minutes of counseling once a month), 2) standard services (one drug counseling session per week, with referral to other sites for treatment of associated psychiatric, family, and vocational problems), and 3) enhanced services (weekly drug counseling plus psychotherapy, family therapy, and vocational services available on site). About 30% of the patients receiving minimal services had drug-free urine tests and did well, indicating that minimal psychosocial services plus methadone can be highly effective for a minority of patients, mainly those with few medical and psychiatric problems. The other two-thirds did not stop drug use and, as a result, were administratively transferred to the standard services. Upon transfer, most of these patients improved substantially within 6 weeks, with patients receiving enhanced services doing somewhat better than those in the standard treatment condition. Thus, a stepwise progression of improvement was associated with receiving increasing levels of psychosocial services, including psychotherapy for about two-thirds of the patients, thereby indicating that the intensity of counseling and the availability of additional services are important matching factors for most methadone-maintained heroin-addicted patients. Other studies have also found that more treatment is generally associated with better outcome (Fiorentine and Anglin 1996). However, the best way to intensify the treatment may be to provide a mix of drug-focused treatment and treatment to address associated problems, such as family, vocational, and psychiatric treatments (McLellan et al. 1997).

Research findings in regard to individual psychotherapy and counseling with methadone patients are consistent with results reported by other studies suggesting that only some substance abuse patients can be successfully treated with a purely psychotherapeutic approach (Carroll et al. 1994). Much research has been directed toward possible pharmacological treatments for addiction, and it seems likely that in many situations, optimal treatment involves a combination of—on the one hand—psychotherapy, counseling, or both and—on the other—an appropriate pharmacological intervention. Although such combinations currently are used mainly in methadone or LAAM programs, they are also employed in detoxification programs, where combined pharmacotherapy and psychosocial treatment is usually necessary (Alterman 1990).

Treatment Implications

In summary, most studies of individual psychotherapy, and of CM and CR therapy for substance use disorders, have found that these treatments are associated with reductions in substance use and improvements in other important areas (Carroll et al. 1991b; Crits-Christoph et al. 1999; Woody et al. 1983, 1995). However, it also appears that certain conditions must be met in order to maximize patients' chances of becoming engaged in therapy and attaining positive outcomes.

Usually, the chemically dependent patient requires more structure and greater frequency of visits than traditional psychotherapy provides. Pharmacological treatments may be needed in addition to psychotherapy, and the psychotherapy must often be integrated with other psychosocial interventions. In fact, psychotherapy appears to be most effective when combined with other treatment services, either in the context of a structured addiction treatment program (McLellan et al. 1993) or in a model in which the individual psychotherapist coordinates a continuum of ancillary services as needed (Khantzian 1987).

Frequent, observed urine and breath testing is an important aspect of the structure. Each of these tests for the presence of drugs of abuse encourages honesty and helps to hold the patient accountable for his or her behavior. Prompt feedback on drug-positive and drug-negative urine samples assures the patient that the therapist is concerned and is monitoring the patient's progress in recovery. Appropriate confrontation and analysis of what led to the drug use are important in the case of continuing or relapse to drug use, whether discovered through urine or breath testing or by the patient's self-report. Positive feedback for "clean" urine test results is a powerful reinforcer of abstinence.

Many clinicians find that involvement of family members and significant others in the treatment process is also helpful. Family members are usually informed of the nature and consequences of addiction and of the treatment process, and their support may be enlisted through occasional family meetings. Most counselors and therapists pay special attention to any factors in the family that may undermine treatment, such as addiction in a family member or the development of family crises in response to the patient's improvement. If such factors exist, family therapy in addition to individual treatment may be necessary. One controlled study of structural family therapy used in combination with drug counseling for patients on methadone maintenance showed positive results (Stanton and Todd 1982).

Most of the different therapy models offer helpful strategies. It may be that future studies will show that certain patient characteristics are associated with more improvement with one particular psychotherapy than with another. Studies have demonstrated that both therapist and patient qualities, including presence of comorbid psychiatric symptoms and disorders, can influence treatment outcome (Luborsky et al. 1985, 1986; McLellan et al. 1988).

A very positive effect of psychotherapy, counseling, and other treatments for substance use disorders is the reduction in HIV risk behaviors, a recent finding that appears to cut across all treatment modalities. This reduction is extremely important, particularly for some groups of drug users and also in the more general sense of benefit to the public health (Metzger et al. 1998).

Suggested guidelines for clinicians treating chemically dependent patients with psychotherapy are as follows:

1. Be familiar with the pharmacology of abused drugs, the subculture of addiction, and the key principles of self-help programs. Also, understand the power of the dependence and the loss of control that accompanies the addiction.
2. Be open to working with substance abuse patients and accepting of their problems. Establish a positive, supportive relationship with the patient.
3. Regardless of therapeutic orientation, integrate into the therapy some concrete, direct behavioral interventions that focus on eliminating drug use.
4. Formulate clear goals early in treatment and keep abreast of the patient's success with abstinence and compliance with other aspects of the treatment. Let the patient know that you recognize and appreciate his or her progress in therapy.
5. Try to involve the patient in group treatment and/or a 12-Step program in addition to the individual treatment.
6. Consider involving family members and significant others in the treatment process if they are available and willing.
7. Understand that the person recovering from addiction usually requires treatment resources in addition to psychotherapy. Therapy is most effective when it is provided in the context of a structured treatment program or when the individual therapist takes responsibility for connecting the patient to other services as needed.

References

Alterman AI: Day hospital versus inpatient cocaine dependence rehabilitation: an interim report, in Problems of Drug Dependence, 1990: Proceedings of the 54th Annual Scientific Meeting, The College on Problems of Drug Dependence. NIDA Research Monograph 105 (DHHS Publ No [ADM] 90-1663). Edited by Harris L. Rockville, MD, U.S. Department of Health and Human Services, 1990, pp 363–364

American Psychiatric Association: Diagnostic and Statistical Manual of Mental Disorders, 4th Edition. Washington, DC, American Psychiatric Association, 1994

Borkovec TD: Control groups and comparison groups in psychotherapy outcome research, in Psychotherapy and Counseling in the Treatment of Drug Abuse. NIDA Research Monograph 104 (DHHS Publ No [ADM] 91-1722). Edited by Onken LS, Blaine JD. Rockville, MD, U.S. Department of Health and Human Services, 1990, pp 50–65

Calsyn DA, Saxon AJ: An innovative approach to reducing cannabis use in a subset of methadone maintenance clients. Drug Alcohol Depend 52:167–169, 1999

Carroll KM, Rounsaville BJ, Keller D: Relapse prevention strategies for the treatment of cocaine abuse. Am J Drug Alcohol Abuse 17:249–265, 1991a

Carroll KM, Rounsaville BJ, Treece FH: A comparative trial of psychotherapies for ambulatory cocaine abusers: relapse prevention and interpersonal psychotherapy. Am J Drug Alcohol Abuse 17:229–247, 1991b

Carroll KM, Rounsaville BJ, Gordon LT, et al: Psychotherapy and pharmacotherapy for ambulatory cocaine abusers. Arch Gen Psychiatry 51:177–187, 1994

Carroll KM, Niche C, Rounsaville BJ: Differential symptom reduction in depressed cocaine abusers treated with psychotherapy and pharmacotherapy. J Nerv Ment Dis 183:251–259, 1995

Crits-Christoph P, Siqueland L, Blaine J, et al: Psychosocial treatments for cocaine dependence: results of the NIDA Cocaine Collaborative Study. Arch Gen Psychiatry 57:493–502, 1999

Fiorentine R: After drug treatment: are 12-step programs effective in maintaining abstinence? Am J Drug Alcohol Abuse 25:93–116, 1999

Fiorentine R, Anglin MD: More is better: counseling participation and the effectiveness of outpatient drug treatment. J Subst Abuse Treat 13:341–348, 1996

Fiorentine R, Hillhouse MP: Drug treatment and 12-step program participation: the additive effects of integrated recovery activities. J Subst Abuse Treat 18:65–74, 2000

Higgins ST, Budney AJ, Bickel WK, et al: Incentives improve outcome in outpatient behavioral treatment of cocaine dependence. Arch Gen Psychiatry 51:568–576, 1994

Howard KI, Cox WM, Saunders SS: Attrition in substance abuse comparative treatment research: the illusion of randomization, in Psychotherapy and Counseling in the Treatment of Drug Abuse. NIDA Research Monograph 104 (DHHS Publ No [ADM] 91-1722). Edited by Onken LS, Blaine JD. Rockville, MD, U.S. Department of Health and Human Services, 1990, pp 66–79

Khantzian EJ: The self-medication hypothesis of addictive disorders: focus on heroin and cocaine dependence. Am J Psychiatry 142:1259–1264, 1985

Khantzian EJ: The primary care therapist and patient needs in substance abuse treatment. Am J Drug Alcohol Abuse 14:159–167, 1987

Kleinman PH, Woody GE, Todd TC, et al: Crack and cocaine abusers in outpatient psychotherapy, in Psychotherapy and Counseling in the Treatment of Drug Abuse. NIDA Research Monograph 104 (DHHS Publ No [ADM] 91-1722). Edited by Onken LS, Blaine JD. Rockville, MD, U.S. Department of Health and Human Services, 1990, pp 24–34

Lambert MJ: Conceptualizing and selecting measures of treatment outcome: implications for drug abuse outcome studies, in Psychotherapy and Counseling in the Treatment of Drug Abuse. NIDA Research Monograph 104 (DHHS Publ No [ADM] 91-1722). Edited by Onken LS, Blaine JD. Rockville, MD, U.S. Department of Health and Human Services, 1990, pp 80–90

Luborsky L: Principles of Psychoanalytic Psychotherapy: A Manual for Supportive-Expressive (SE) Treatment. New York, Basic Books, 1984

Luborsky L, McLellan AT, Woody GE, et al: Therapist success and its determinants. Arch Gen Psychiatry 42:602–611, 1985

Luborsky L, Crits-Christoph P, McLellan AT: Do therapists vary in their effectiveness? findings from four outcome studies. Am J Orthopsychiatry 66:501–512, 1986

Luborsky L, Woody GE, Hole A, et al: Supportive-expressive dynamic psychotherapy for opiate drug dependence, in Dynamic Therapies for Psychiatric Disorders. Edited by Barber J, Crits-Christoph P. New York, Basic Books, 1995, pp 131–160

Mark D, Faude J: Supportive-expressive therapy of cocaine abuse, in Dynamic Therapies for Psychiatric Disorders. Edited by Barber J, Crits-Christoph P. New York, Basic Books, 1995, pp 294–331

Marlatt GA, Gordon J (eds): Relapse Prevention: Maintenance Strategies in the Treatment of Addictive Behaviors. New York, Guilford, 1985

Maude-Griffin PM, Hohenstein JM, Humfleet GL, et al: Superior efficacy of cognitive-behavioral therapy for urban crack cocaine abusers: main and matching effects. J Consult Clin Psychol 66:832–837, 1998

McLellan AT, Woody GE, Luborsky L, et al: Is the counselor an "active ingredient" in methadone treatment? An examination of treatment success among four counselors. J Nerv Ment Dis 176:423–430, 1988

McLellan AT, Arndt IO, Metzger DS, et al: Are psychosocial services necessary in substance abuse treatment? JAMA 269:1953–1959, 1993

McLellan AT, Alterman A, Metzger DS, et al: Similarity of outcome predictors across opiate, cocaine, and alcohol treatments: role of treatment services. J Consult Clin Psychol 62:1141–1158, 1997

Metzger DS, Navaline H, Woody GE: Drug abuse treatment as AIDS prevention. Public Health Rep 113 (suppl 1):97–106, 1998

Miller WR: Motivational Interviewing: research, practice and puzzles. Addict Behav 61:835–842, 1996

National Drug and Alcoholism Treatment Unit Survey (DHHS Publ No ADM-89-1626). Rockville, MD, U.S. Department of Health and Human Services, 1982

Navaline HA, Snider EC, Petro CJ, et al: Preparations for AIDS vaccine trials. An automated version of the Risk Assessment Battery (RAB): enhancing the assessment of risk behaviors. AIDS Res Hum Retroviruses 10 (suppl 2):S281–S283, 1994

Onken LS, Blaine JD: Psychotherapy and counseling research in drug abuse treatment: questions, problems, and solutions, in Psychotherapy and Counseling in the Treatment of Drug Abuse. NIDA Research Monograph 104 (DHHS Publ No [ADM] 91-1722). Edited by Onken LS, Blaine JD. Rockville, MD, U.S. Department of Health and Human Services, 1990, pp 1–5

Project MATCH Research Group: Matching Alcoholism Treatments to Client Heterogeneity: Project MATCH posttreatment drinking outcomes. J Stud Alcohol 58:7–29, 1997

Rounsaville BJ, Glazer W, Wilber CH, et al: Short-term interpersonal psychotherapy in methadone maintained opiate addicts. Arch Gen Psychiatry 40:629–636, 1983

Rounsaville BJ, Gawin FH, Kleber HD: Interpersonal psychotherapy (IPT) adapted for ambulatory cocaine abusers. Am J Drug Alcohol Abuse 11:171–191, 1985

Silverman K, Higgins ST, Brooner RK, et al: Sustained cocaine abstinence in methadone maintenance patients through voucher-based reinforcement therapy. Arch Gen Psychiatry 53:409–415, 1996a

Silverman K, Wong C, Higgins S, et al: Increasing opiate abstinence through voucher-based reinforcement therapy. Drug Alcohol Depend 41:157–165, 1996b

Stanton MD, Todd TC: The Family Therapy of Drug Abuse and Addiction. New York, Guilford, 1982

Washton AM: Cocaine Addiction: Treatment, Recovery, Relapse Prevention. New York, WW Norton, 1989

Woody GE, Luborsky L, McLellan AT, et al: Psychotherapy for opiate addicts: does it help? Arch Gen Psychiatry 40:639–645, 1983

Woody GE, McLellan AT, Luborsky L, et al: Psychiatric severity as a predictor of benefits from psychotherapy: the Penn-VA Study. Am J Psychiatry 141:1172–1177, 1984

Woody GE, McLellan AT, Luborsky L, et al: Psychotherapy in community methadone programs: a validation study. Am J Psychiatry 152:1302–1308, 1995

Relapse Prevention

G. Alan Marlatt, Ph.D.
Kimberly Barrett, Ed.D.

What Is Relapse Prevention?

Relapse prevention (RP) is a cognitive-behavioral treatment (Kendall and Hollon 1979) that combines behavioral skills training procedures with cognitive intervention techniques to assist persons in maintaining desired behavioral changes. Based in part on the principles of health psychology (e.g., Stone et al. 1979) and social-cognitive theory (Bandura 1986), RP uses a psychoeducational self-management approach to substance abuse, designed to teach clients new coping responses (e.g., alternatives to addictive behavior) and to help them modify maladaptive beliefs and expectancies concerning substance use and change personal habits and lifestyles. Background research and theory leading to the development of this model can be found in earlier publications on the RP approach (Marlatt 1979, 1982; Marlatt and George 1984; Marlatt and Gordon 1985; Sandberg and Marlatt 1991). Much of the material presented in this chapter subpart is drawn from these sources.

Initially, the RP model was developed as a behavioral maintenance program for use in the treatment of addictive behaviors (Marlatt 1978; Marlatt and Gordon 1980). In the addictions, the typical treatment goal of RP is either to refrain totally from performing a target behavior (i.e., the abstinence model) or to reduce the harm or risk of ongoing habits (i.e., the harm reduction model) (Marlatt and Gordon 1985; Marlatt and Tapert 1992; Weingardt and Marlatt 1998). Although the material presented in this chapter subpart is primarily directed toward substance use disorders, the RP model may have additional applications that extend beyond drug addiction. Problems such as excessive drinking, smoking, overeating, gambling, and high-risk sexual behaviors may be considered collectively as *addictive behaviors* (Donovan and Marlatt 1988). Because many treatment programs for these kinds of problems have high recidivism rates, the RP model has been applied to an increasingly broad range of behaviors as well as to dual-diagnosis populations such as substance abusers with posttraumatic stress disorder (PTSD), schizophrenia, or other serious psychiatric conditions (Bellack and DiClemente 1999; Daley 1989; Herman et al. 1997; Laws 1989; Roget et al. 1998; Sharkansky et al. 1999; Ward and Hudson 1998; Wilson 1992).

Treatment Goals and Philosophy in Relapse Prevention

The cornerstone of the RP approach is coping skills training (Chaney et al. 1978; Monti et al. 1989). In this approach, clients are taught behavioral and cognitive skills such as skills for resisting social pressure, increased assertiveness, relaxation and stress management, interpersonal communication, and so forth (Shiffman and Wills 1985).

Relapse prevention procedures can be applied in prevention and treatment efforts designed to prevent relapse or to manage ongoing relapse problems. Maintenance strategies are designed both to anticipate and to prevent the occurrence of relapse following treatment (e.g., to prevent a recently detoxified drug-abusing person from returning to habitual drug use), as well as to help clients cope with relapse if it occurs. The RP model is also used to facilitate changes in personal habits and lifestyle to reduce the risk of physical disease or other harm associated with the addictive behavior. In this case, the aim of the RP program is much broader in scope: to teach the person how to reduce lifestyle health risks and prevent the formation of additional unhealthy habit patterns. The central motif of this approach is one of *moderation*, a balanced lifestyle midway between the opposing extremes of behavioral excess and restraint. Viewed from this more global perspective, RP can be considered a component of the developing public health model of "harm reduction"—that is, behavior change programs designed to reduce the risk of ongoing addictive behavior problems (Marlatt 1998).

Harm reduction provides a pragmatic and humanistic alternative to the moral/criminal/disease model of addiction (Barrett and Marlatt 1999; Marlatt and Tapert 1992; Roberts and Marlatt 1999). The therapeutic focus shifts away from the actual occurrence of drug/alcohol use to the consequences of addictive behaviors. The black/white dynamics of abstinence and relapse, which traditionally have meant treatment failure and possible rejection from treatment for the client, are replaced with a model that accepts clients where they are in the change process, reducing barriers and stigmas in treatment for clients who are still unable or unwilling to achieve abstinence (Marlatt 1996). Harm reduction approaches incorporate motivational enhancement methods for promoting change and help to engage the client in an active partnership with the therapist in developing treatment goals and strategies for change (Miller and Rollnick 1991). Change is process-oriented and gradual, and success is defined not as a final outcome but rather as movement in the direction of less risk and harmful consequences to the client.

A harm reduction model also addresses a broader range of problems than do other models of addiction, treating the client as a whole person and seeing addictive and other harmful behaviors as interacting with additional psychological, interpersonal, and social/environmental problems that the client may be experiencing. The client thus learns to understand the relationship between the functions of his or her substance abuse and other problems as they occur in multiple contexts. Involving the family and addressing the family dynamics of addiction serve to enhance client motivation and engagement in treatment, linking RP and harm reduction models to systematically based interventions (Barrett and Marlatt 1999).

Definition of Lapse and Relapse

Broadly considered, *relapse* is defined as any discrete violation of a self-imposed rule or set of rules governing the rate or pattern of a selected target behavior. Total abstinence, the most stringent rule one can adopt, is thus violated by a single instance of a target behavior (e.g., the first drink or use of a substance). Viewed from this absolute "black/white" perspective, a single lapse is equated with total relapse (Figure 30–1). Although violation of the abstinence rule is the primary form of relapse we have studied in our research in substance abuse, other forms of relapse would also be included within the above definition. Violating rules governing caloric intake imposed by a diet would also constitute a relapse, as would exceeding alcohol consumption limits imposed in a drinking moderation program. Within this general definition of relapse, we distinguish between the first violation of the rules (the initial *lapse*) and the subsequent secondary effects in which the behavior may increase in the direction of the original pretreatment baseline level (a full-blown *relapse*). This distinction between lapse and relapse is illustrated in Figure 30–2, showing the "gray area" of a lapse experience.

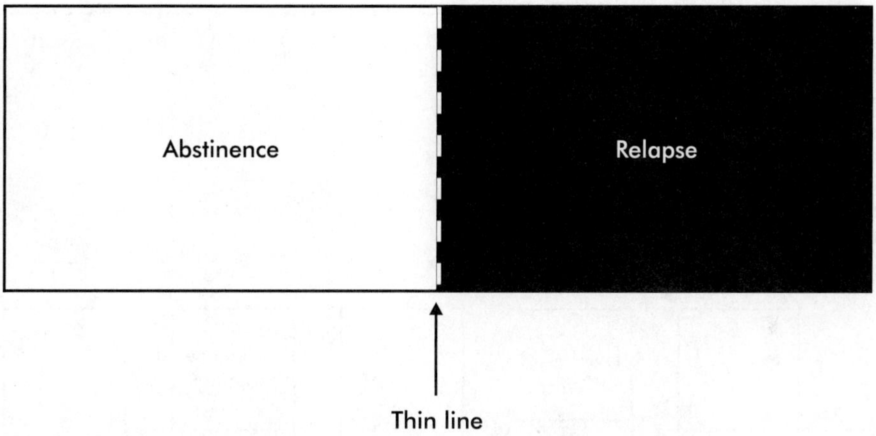

FIGURE 30–1. The "black/white" model of abstinence versus relapse.

Overview of High-Risk Situations for Relapse

In the following overview, we present only the highlights of the RP model. Further details on background research and theory leading to the assessment of high-risk situations can be found elsewhere (Cummings et al. 1980; Daley and Salloum 1999; Dimeff and Marlatt 1998; Donovan and Marlatt 1988; Maisto et al. 1999; Marlatt and Gordon 1985; Marlatt et al. 1999). A schematic representation of the relapse model is presented in Figure 30–3.

To begin, we assume that the person experiences a sense of perceived control while maintaining abstinence (or complying with other rules governing the target behavior). The target behavior is "under control" so long as it does not occur. For example, the longer the

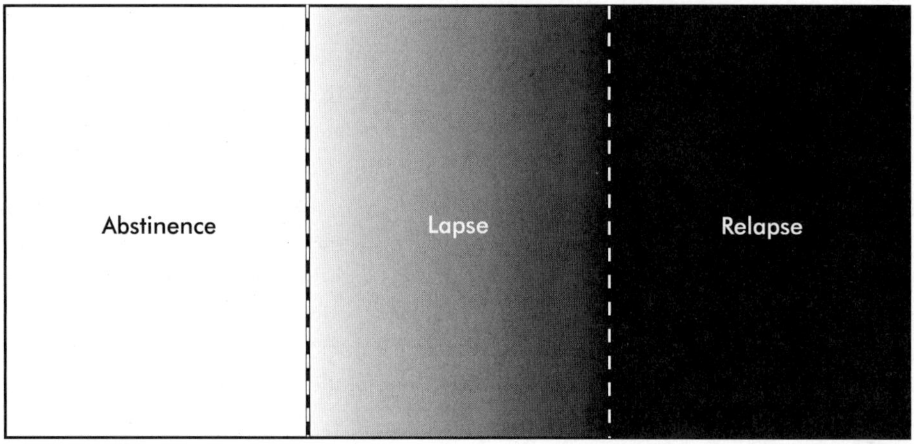

FIGURE 30–2. The "gray area" model of abstinence/lapse/relapse.

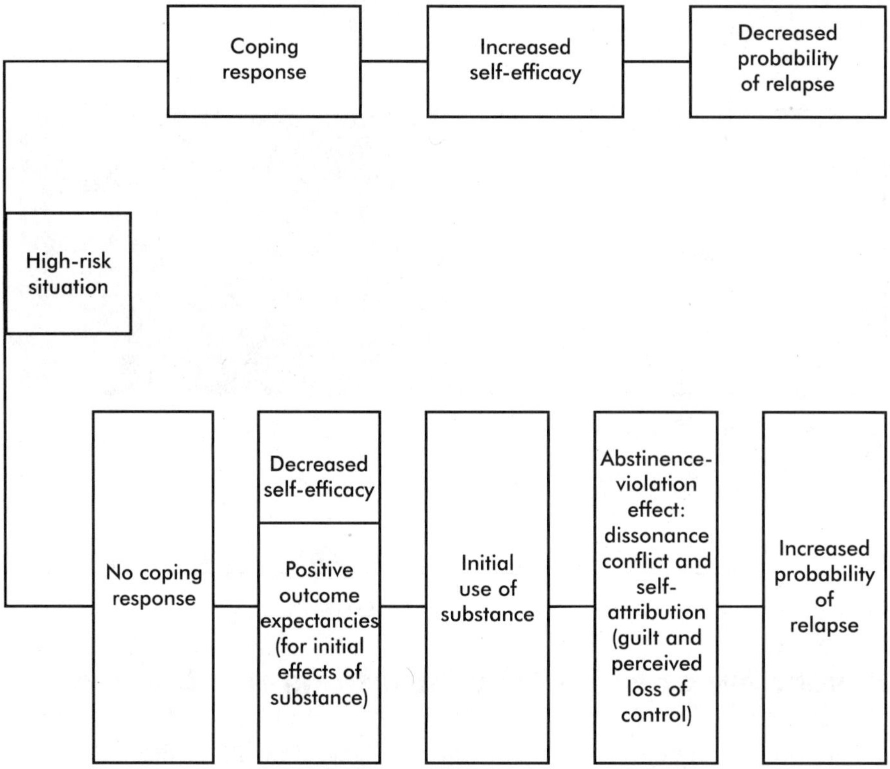

FIGURE 30–3. A cognitive-behavioral model of the relapse process.

period of successful abstinence, the greater the person's perception of self-control. This perceived control will continue until the person encounters a *high-risk situation*, defined broadly as any situation that poses a threat to the person's sense of control and increases the risk of potential relapse. In an analysis of 311 initial relapse episodes in clients with a variety of problem behaviors (i.e., problem drinking, smoking, heroin addiction, compulsive gambling, and overeating), three primary high-risk situations were associated with almost 75% of all the relapses reported (Cummings et al. 1980; Marlatt and Gordon 1985). The high-risk situations associated with the highest relapse rates are as follows:

1. *Negative emotional states* (35% of all relapses in the sample): situations in which the person is experiencing a negative (or unpleasant) emotional state, mood, or feeling such as frustration, anger, anxiety, depression, boredom, etc., prior to or simultaneously with the first lapse.
2. *Interpersonal conflict* (16% of all relapses): situations involving an ongoing or relatively recent conflict associated with any interpersonal relationship, such as marriage, friendship, family, or employer-employee relations. Arguments and interpersonal confrontations occur frequently in this category.
3. *Social pressure* (20% of all relapses): situations in which the person is responding to the influence of another person or group of people who exert pressure on the person to engage in the proscribed behavior. Social pressure may be either direct (e.g., direct interpersonal contact with verbal persuasion) or indirect (e.g., being in the presence of others who are engaging in the same target behavior, even though no direct pressure is involved).

In our analyses of relapse episodes, these same three high-risk situations are frequently found to be associated with relapse, which is indicative of a common risk factor for a variety of addictive behaviors (i.e., problem drinking, smoking, gambling, heroin use, or overeating). Other high-risk situations described by Marlatt and Gordon (1985) include negative physical states (withdrawal), testing personal control, and responsivity to substance cues (craving, urges) (see also el-Guebaly and Hodgins 1998; Grabowski et al. 1979). This pattern of findings lends support to our hypothesis that there are common triggers that frequently initiate the relapse process across a wide range of target behaviors.

If a person is able to execute an effective coping response in a high-risk situation (e.g., is assertive in counteracting social pressures), the probability of relapse decreases. A person who copes successfully with a high-risk situation is likely to experience a sense of mastery or perception of control. Successful mastery of one problematic situation is often associated with an expectation of being able to cope successfully with the next challenging event. The expectancy of being able to cope with successive high-risk situations as they develop is closely associated with Bandura's notion of "self-efficacy" (Bandura 1977), defined as the person's expectation concerning the capacity to cope with an impending situation or task.

What happens if a person is unable or unwilling to cope successfully with a high-risk situation? Perhaps the person has never acquired the coping skills involved or the appropriate response has been inhibited by fear or anxiety. Or perhaps he or she fails to recognize and respond to the risk involved before it is too late. For other persons, the anticipated rewards for indulgence may undermine motivation to resist temptation in the high-risk situation. Whatever the reason, if a coping response is not performed, the person is likely to experience a decrease in self-efficacy, frequently coupled with a sense of helplessness and a tendency to passively give in to the situation. "It's no use, I can't handle this" is a common reaction. As self-efficacy decreases in the precipitating high-risk situation, one's expectations for coping successfully with subsequent problem situations also drop. If the situation also involves the temptation to engage in the prohibited behavior (substance abuse) as a means of attempting to cope with the stress involved, the stage is set for a probable relapse. The probability of relapse is enhanced if the person holds positive expectancies about the effects of the substance involved. Positive outcome expectancies are a primary motivational determinant of alcohol and drug use (Marlatt and Rohsenow 1980).

The combination of being unable to cope effectively in a high-risk situation and positive outcome expectancies for the effects of the habitual coping behavior (substance use) greatly increases the probability that an initial *lapse* will occur. On the one hand, the person faces a high-risk situation with no coping response available; self-efficacy decreases as he or she feels less able to exert control. On the other hand, there is the lure of the old coping response—the drink or the drug. At this point, unless a last-minute coping response or a sudden change of circumstances occurs, the person may cross over the abstinence border. Whether the first lapse is followed by a total relapse depends in part on the person's attributions as to the "cause" of the lapse and the reactions associated with its occurrence.

The requirement of abstinence is an absolute dictum. Once someone has crossed over the line, there is no going back. From this black/white perspective (see Figure 30–1), a single drink or a single instance of using a drug is sufficient to violate the rule of abstinence: once the person has committed it, the deed cannot be undone. Unfortunately, many persons who attempt to stop a habit, such as using drugs or drinking, perceive quitting as occurring in this "once and for all" manner. To account for this reaction to the transgression of an absolute rule, we have postulated a mechanism called the *abstinence-violation effect*, or AVE (Curry et al. 1987; Marlatt and Gordon 1985). The AVE is postulated to occur under the following conditions. Before the first lapse, the person is personally committed to an extended or indefinite period of abstinence. The intensity of the AVE varies as a function of several factors, including the degree of prior commitment or effort expended to maintain abstinence, the duration of the abstinence period (the longer the period, the greater the effect), and the subjective value or importance of the prohibited behavior to the person. We hypothesize that the AVE is characterized by two key cognitive-affective elements: cognitive dissonance (i.e., conflict and guilt) and a personal attribution effect (i.e., blaming the self as the cause of the relapse). Persons who experience an intense AVE following a lapse often undergo a motivation crisis (demoralization reaction) that undermines their commitment to abstinence goals.

Covert Antecedents of Relapse

In the foregoing discussion of the immediate determinants and reactions to relapse, the high-risk situation is viewed as the precipitating or triggering situation associated with the initial lapse, or first "slip," following a period of abstinence or of controlled use. In many of the relapse episodes we have studied, the first lapse is precipitated in a high-risk situation that the person unexpectedly encounters. In most of these instances, the person is not expecting the high-risk situation to occur and/or is generally ill prepared to cope effectively with the circumstances as they arise. In other relapse episodes, however, the high-risk situation appears to be the last link in a chain of events leading up to the first lapse.

Why do some persons appear to "set up" their own relapse? From a cost-benefit perspective, a relapse can be seen as a rational choice (or a justified gamble). The benefit is swift in coming: a payoff of immediate gratification. The reward of instant gratification is seen to outweigh the cost of potential negative effects that may or may not occur sometime in the distant future. The person might think, "Why not take a chance, when this time the outcome might be different?" Cognitive distortions such as denial and rationalization make it much easier to set up one's own relapse episode; one may deny both the intent to relapse and the importance of long-range negative consequences. There are also a number of excuses one can use to rationalize the act of indulgence (e.g., "I was drunk and couldn't help myself").

Denial and rationalization are cognitive distortion mechanisms that go hand in hand in the covert planning of a relapse episode. These two defense mechanisms may combine to influence the person to make certain uninformed choices or decisions as part of a chain of events leading ultimately to relapse. We hypothesize that a person headed for a relapse often makes a number of minidecisions over time, each of which brings the person closer to the brink of succumbing to or creating a high-risk situation. The term *apparently irrelevant decisions* is used to describe these choices. An example is that of the abstinent drinker who buys a bottle of sherry to take home "just in case guests drop by."

One of the most tempting rationalizations is that the desire to yield to temptation is justified. Our research findings and clinical experience suggest that the degree of *lifestyle balance* has a significant impact on the person's desire for indulgence or immediate gratification (Marlatt and Gordon 1985). In this context, we are defining "balance" as the degree of equilibrium that exists in one's daily life between those activities perceived as external demands (or "shoulds") and those perceived as activities engaged in for pleasure or self-fulfillment (the "wants").

Assessment and Specific Intervention Strategies

In this section, we present highlights of RP assessment and intervention strategies. First, we discuss strategies designed to teach the client to recognize and cope with high-risk situations that may precipitate a lapse, and to modify cognitions and other reactions to prevent a single lapse from developing into a full-blown relapse. Explicitly focused on the high-risk situations for relapse, these procedures are referred to collectively as *specific RP intervention strategies*. Second, we go beyond the microanalysis of the initial lapse and present strategies designed to modify the client's lifestyle and to help the client identify and cope with covert determinants of relapse. We refer to these procedures as *global RP self-control strategies*.

Both specific and global RP strategies can be grouped in three main categories: skills training, cognitive reframing, and lifestyle intervention. *Skills training strategies* include both behavioral and cognitive responses to cope with high-risk situations. *Cognitive reframing* procedures are designed to provide clients with alternative cognitions concerning the nature of the habit-change process (e.g., to view it as a learning process), to introduce coping imagery to deal with urges and early warning signals, and to reframe reactions to the initial lapse (i.e., restructuring of the AVE). Finally, *lifestyle balancing strategies* (e.g., meditation, mindfulness, and exercise) are designed to strengthen the client's global coping capacity and to reduce the frequency and intensity of urges and cravings that are often the product of an unbalanced lifestyle.

The possibility of moderation as an alternative to abstinence is the single most controversial issue associated with treatment planning. Resistance to controlled drinking in the treatment of alcohol abuse and dependence has intensified in the traditional "disease model" or "chemical dependency" programs in the United States. Because a complete discussion of the controversy is beyond the scope of this chapter subpart, the reader is referred to other publications on the topic (e.g., Heather and Robertson 1987; Marlatt 1983). As a form of secondary prevention or harm reduction, controlled drinking may work best for those persons who are beginning to develop problems with their drinking, rather than as a remedial treatment program for persons who have developed a long-term dependence on alcohol (Baer et al. 1992; Kivlahan et al. 1990; Marlatt et al. 1998). Initial reduction of alcohol use rather than abstinence may also be used as a tool to motivate otherwise resistant clients to seek help (Miller and Rollnick 1991).

When abstinence has been identified as the goal of treatment, the overall aim of specific intervention procedures is to teach the client to anticipate and cope with the possibility of relapse: to recognize and cope with high-risk situations that may precipitate a slip, and to modify cognitions and other reactions to prevent a single lapse from developing into a full-blown relapse. A schematic overview of the specific RP intervention techniques is presented in Figure 30–4. The first step in the prevention of relapse is to teach the client to recognize high-risk situations that may precipitate or trigger a relapse. Here, the earlier one becomes aware of being involved in a chain of events that increases the probability of a slip or lapse, the sooner one can intervene by performing an appropriate coping skill. Clients are taught to recognize and respond to warning signals (i.e., discriminative stimuli) associated with entering a high-risk situation and to use these signals as reminders to engage in alternative or remedial action.

An essential aspect of teaching clients to better handle high-risk situations is to help them to identify and anticipate these situations. Earlier we discussed prototypical kinds of high-risk situations. However, ultimately the identification of high-risk situations is an individualized question requiring ideographic assessment procedures. *Self-monitoring procedures* (e.g., keeping a diary or daily tally) offer an effective method for assessing high-risk situations whenever it is possible to have clients keep a record of their addictive behavior for a baseline period prior to the onset of treatment.

Determining the adequacy of preexisting coping abilities is a critical assessment target. In a treatment outcome investigation aimed at teaching alcoholic persons to handle situational temptations, Chaney et al. (1978) devised the Situational Competency Test to measure coping ability. In this technique, the client is presented with a series of written or audiotaped descriptions of potential relapse situations. Each description ends with a prompt for the client to respond. Later, the client's responses to the scenes can be scored on a number of dimensions, including response duration and latency, degree of compliance, and specification of alternative behaviors. A similar technique involves the use of *self-efficacy ratings*, in which the client, and perhaps spouse, are presented with a list of potential relapse situations (Annis and Davis 1988). For each situation, the client uses a rating scale to estimate his or her subjective expectation of successful coping. Ratings across a wide range of situations enable the client to identify both problematic situations and skill deficits for which remedial training is needed. Results from these types of assessment tools can later dictate the focus of skills-training procedures.

Remedial skills training necessitated by identification of coping skill deficits is the cornerstone of the RP treatment program. When the person lacks coping skills, a variety of coping skills can be taught. The content of the skills training program is variable and will

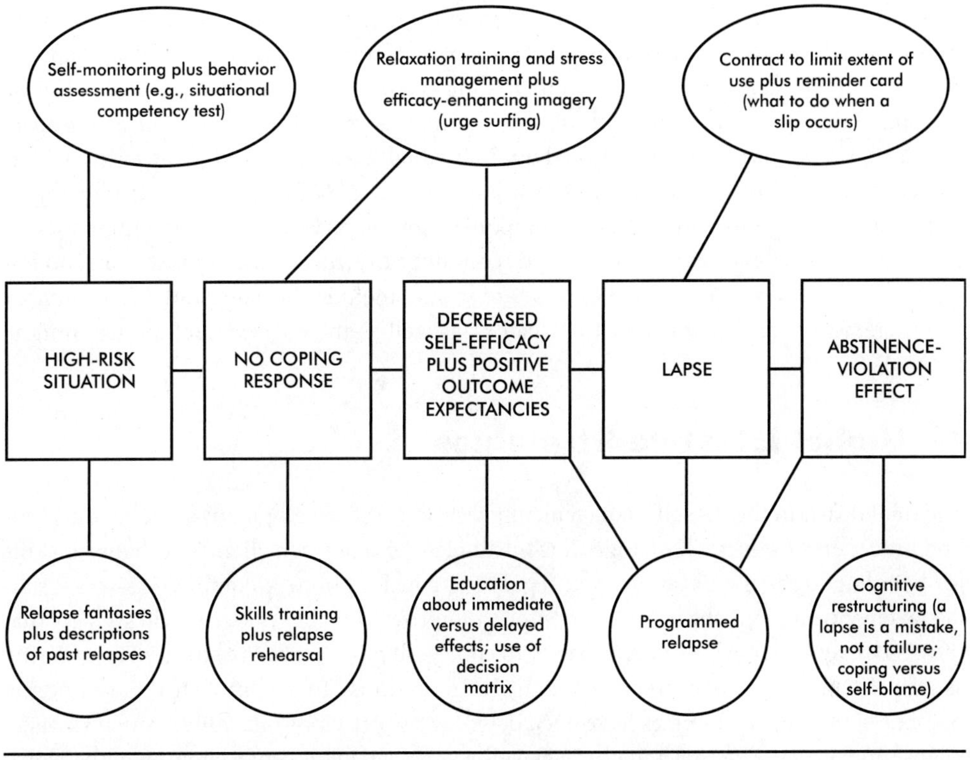

FIGURE 30–4. Relapse prevention: specific intervention strategies.

depend on the needs of the individual. Possible content areas include assertiveness, stress management, relaxation training, anger management, communication skills, marital therapy, and general social and/or dating skills.

Along with education about the long-range negative effects of excessive substance use on physical health and social well-being, a *decision matrix* allows clients to examine both the immediate and the delayed effects of substance use, which may help counter the tendency of clients to think only of the initial, pleasant short-term effects. In skills training, the actual teaching procedures are based on the work of McFall (1976) and other investigators. The range of methods includes behavior rehearsal, instruction, coaching, evaluative feedback, modeling, and role playing. In addition, cognitive self-instructional methods introduced by Meichenbaum (1977) have proved especially valuable. For troubleshooting and consolidating the newly acquired skills, regular homework assignments are an essential ingredient in skills training.

In some instances, it is impractical to rehearse the new coping skills in real-life situations. This problem can be surmounted through use of *relapse rehearsal methods*. In this procedure, the client is instructed to imagine being involved in actual high-risk situations and performing more adaptive coping behaviors and thoughts. The emphasis here is on active coping rather than on resisting temptation. The client is thus encouraged to visualize that he or she is successfully handling the difficult situation through effective coping instead of through exercising "willpower." To emphasize self-efficacy enhancement, the therapist can instruct the client to imagine that the rehearsed experience is accompanied by mounting feelings of competence and confidence.

That the client may fail to effectively employ these coping strategies and experience a slip must be anticipated. The client's reaction to the slip is a pivotal intervention point in the RP model because it determines the degree of escalation from a single, isolated lapse to a full-blown relapse. The first step in anticipating and dealing with this reaction is to devise an explicit therapeutic contract to limit the extent of use if a lapse occurs. The actual specifications of the contract can be worked out individually with the client. However, the fundamental method of intervention after a lapse is the use of cognitive restructuring to counteract the cognitive and affective components of the AVE. It may be helpful in this regard to have the client carry a wallet-sized reminder card with instructions to read and follow in the event of a slip. The text of this card should include the name and phone number of a therapist or treatment center to be called, as well as the cognitive reframing antidote to the AVE.

Global Lifestyle Strategies

The final thrust in the RP self-management program is the development of global intervention procedures for lifestyle change. It is insufficient to just teach clients mechanistic skills for handling high-risk situations and regulating consumption. A comprehensive RP self-management program should also attempt to improve the client's overall lifestyle so that the client may increase his or her capacity to cope with more pervasive stress factors serving as antecedents to the occurrence of high-risk situations. To accomplish this training, a number of treatment strategies have been devised to short-circuit the covert antecedents to relapse and promote mental and physical wellness. A schematic representation of the global self-control strategies employed in the RP approach is presented in Figure 30–5.

An effective way to induce clients to view lifestyle disequilibrium as a precursor of relapse is to have them self-monitor "wants" and "shoulds." By keeping a daily record of duties and obligations on the one hand and enjoyable pleasures on the other, the client becomes aware of the sources of imbalance. Next, the client is encouraged to seek a restoration of balance by engaging in healthy daily lifestyle habits, such as exercise, the practice of mindfulness (Astin 1997), or "positive addictions" (Glasser 1976). The advantage of this shift from negative (substance abuse) to positive addiction lies in the latter's capacity to contribute toward the person's long-term health and well-being while also providing an adaptive coping response for life stressors and relapse situations. As long-range health benefits accrue, the person begins to develop more self-confidence and self-efficacy.

Despite the efficacy of these techniques for counteracting feelings of deprivation that would otherwise predispose the person toward relapse, occasional urges and cravings may still surface from time to time. As indicated in Figure 30–5, various *urge control procedures* are recommended. Sometimes urges and cravings are directly triggered by external cues such as the sight of one's favorite beer mug in the kitchen cabinet. The frequency of these externally triggered urges can be substantially reduced by employing simple *stimulus control techniques* aimed at minimizing exposure to these cues. In some instances, avoidance strategies offer the most effective way of reducing the frequency of externally triggered urges.

In teaching clients to cope with urge and craving experiences, it is important to emphasize that the discomfort associated with these internal events is natural. Indeed, urges can be likened to waves in the sea: they rise, crest, and fall. Using this "urge surfing" metaphor, we encourage the client to wait out the urge, to look forward to the downside, and to maintain balance when the urge wave is peaking.

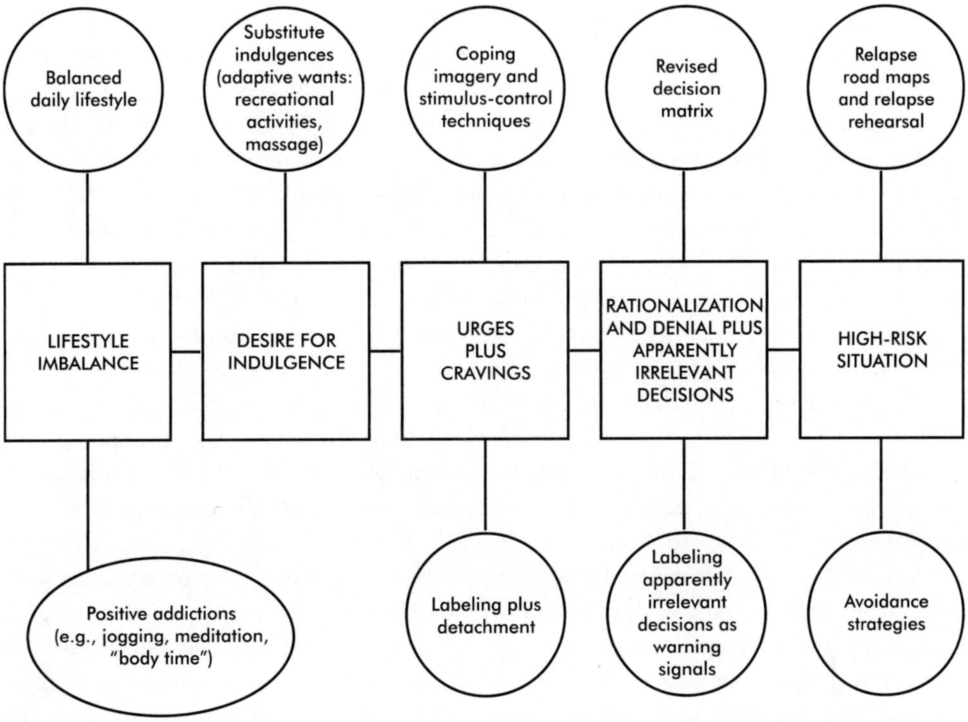

FIGURE 30–5. Relapse prevention: global self-control strategies.

Recall that urges and cravings may not always operate at a conscious level but may become masked by cognitive distortions and defense mechanisms. An important objective in these urge-control techniques is to enable the person to externalize urges and cravings and to view them with objective detachment. Training the client in the regular use of mindfulness meditation techniques (Kabat Zinn 1994; Nhât Hanh 1992) can help the client to observe the "rising" and "falling away" of desires while also staying focused and calm during stressful circumstances. Because mindfulness is a daily practice, the client will begin to experience improvement in his or her overall sense of well-being and connectedness to the environment. Another way to achieve this detachment is to encourage the client to deliberately label the urge as soon as it registers into consciousness. Urges should be viewed as natural occurrences in response to environmental and lifestyle forces rather than as signs of treatment failure and indicators of future relapse.

Relapse Prevention With Couples and Families

The use of RP techniques in combination with family therapy can help clinicians to assist their clients in understanding the functional relationship between their addictive behaviors and difficulties in close interpersonal relationships.

The importance of family involvement and social support in substance abuse treatment has been emphasized by a number of authors (Barrett and Rafton 1997; Catalano and Hawkins 1985; Jacob et al. 1983; Kaufman 1985; Kaufman and Kaufmann 1979; Moos et al. 1990; Steinglass 1999; Steinglass et al. 1987).

Several clinicians and researchers have recently extended the RP model to treatment with couples and families (Cawthra et al. 1991; Daley and Raskin 1991; McCrady 1989; O'Farrell 1991). Heath and Stanton (1998) describe family therapy as being integral to the most successful substance abuse treatment programs; they view family treatment as a critical component of RP. Alcohol Behavioral Couples Therapy (ABCT) is tailored to treat alcohol problems and is reported to produce both significant reductions in alcohol consumption and improvement in marital functioning (Epstein and McCrady 1998). O'Farrell et al. (1998) describe a study that used behavioral marital therapy plus RP in work with 59 couples in which the husband was alcoholic. Behavioral marital therapy with RP led to more days of abstinence and greater use of disulfiram (Antabuse) in the husbands, better adjustment in the wives, and more improvement in the marital relationship in comparison with behavioral marital therapy without RP.

Catalano et al. (1997) described a family intervention designed to reduce opiate-addicted parents' risk of relapse and their children's risk of substance use. Compared with controls receiving individual treatment, the parents who received the intervention had more frequent use of relapse coping skills, a stronger sense of self-efficacy, and lower levels of opiate use.

O'Farrell (1991) summarized promising results with couples who were treated with behavioral marital therapy in conjunction with RP. This combination of interventions with couples can be used to facilitate the initial motivation to change in the alcoholic person and to promote the use of problem-solving and communication skills to increase positive interactions between the partners. The program is designed to stabilize the marriage while the alcoholic spouse is trying to maintain sobriety and to teach both partners how to recognize and cope with triggers that could potentially lead to relapse. Available data show more days of abstinence and enhancement of the marital relationship in the recovery process when behavioral marital therapy and RP are combined.

Conclusions

In recent years, the application of RP in treatment research with a broad range of populations has brought growing empirical support to document the model's strength in facilitating behavior change and increasing the client's sense of efficacy and motivation for addressing a variety of problems.

Alcohol's role in precipitating relapse in sex offenders is emphasized in a number of studies (Fisher and Beech 1998; Monson et al. 1998; Ward and Hudson 1998), indicating that RP has an important role in reducing recidivism in sex offenders.

The success of RP in the treatment of cocaine-addicted populations has received growing empirical support (Carroll et al. 1999; McKay et al. 1997, 1998; Rawson et al. 1999; Schmitz et al. 1997; Weatherby et al. 1999). Treatment of high-risk behavior in HIV populations through the incorporation of RP strategies also shows promise (McCusker et al. 1997; Roffman et al. 1998).

References

Annis HM, Davis CS: Assessment of expectancies in alcohol dependent clients, in Assessment of Addictive Behaviors. Edited by Donovan DM, Marlatt GA. New York, Guilford, 1988, pp 84–111

Astin JA: Stress reduction through mindfulness meditation: effects on psychological symptomatology, sense of control, and spiritual experiences. Psychother Psychosom 66:97–106, 1997

Baer JS, Marlatt GA, Kivlahan DR, et al: An experimental test of three methods of alcohol risk reduction with young adults. J Consult Clin Psychol 60:974–979, 1992

Bandura A: Self-efficacy: toward a unifying theory of behavior change. Psychol Rev 84:191–215, 1977

Bandura A: Social Foundations of Thought and Action: A Social Cognitive Theory. Englewood Cliffs, NJ, Prentice-Hall, 1986

Barrett KS, Marlatt GA: Relapse prevention and harm reduction in the treatment of co-occurring addiction and mental health problems, in Comparative Treatments of Substance Abuse, New York, Springer, 1999, pp 176–192

Barrett KS, Rafton SA: The treatment of substance abuse in children and adolescents: a guide for educators and counselors, in Crisis Counseling in the Quality School Community: Applying William Glasser's Choice Theory. Edited by Palmatier LL. New York, Taylor & Francis, 1997, pp 175–204

Bellack AS, DiClemente CC: Treating substance abuse among patients with schizophrenia. Psychiatr Serv 50:75–80, 1999

Carroll KM, Nich C, Frankforter TL, et al: Do patients change in the ways we intend? Assessing acquisition of coping skills among cocaine-dependent patients. Psychological Assessment 11:77–85, 1999

Catalano RF, Hawkins JD: Project skills: preliminary results from a theoretically based aftercare experiment, in Progress in the Development of Cost-Effective Treatment of Drug Abusers. NIDA Research Monograph 58 (DHHS Publ No [ADM] 88-1401). Edited by Ashery RS. Rockville, MD, National Institute on Drug Abuse, 1985, pp 157–181

Catalano RF, Haggerty KP, Gainey RR, et al: Reducing parental risk factors for children's substance misuse: preliminary outcomes with opiate-addicted parents. Subst Use Misuse 32:699–721, 1997

Cawthra E, Borrego N, Emrick C: Involving family members in the prevention of relapse: an innovative approach. Alcoholism Treatment Quarterly 8:101–112, 1991

Chaney EF, O'Leary MR, Marlatt GA: Skill training with alcoholics. J Consult Clin Psychol 46:1092–1104, 1978

Cummings C, Gordon JR, Marlatt GA: Relapse: strategies of prevention and prediction, in The Addictive Behaviors. Edited by Miller WR. Oxford, UK, Pergamon, 1980, pp 291–321

Curry S, Marlatt GA, Gordon JR: Abstinence violation effect: validation of an attributional construct with smoking cessation. J Consult Clin Psychol 55:145–149, 1987

Daley DC (ed): Relapse: Conceptual, Research and Clinical Perspectives. New York, Haworth, 1989

Daley DC, Raskin M: Relapse prevention and treatment effectiveness studies, in Treating the Chemically Dependent and Their Families. Edited by Daley DC, Raskin M. Newbury Park, CA, Sage, 1991, pp 128–171

Daley DC, Salloum I: Relapse prevention, in Sourcebook on Substance Abuse: Etiology, Epidemiology, Assessment, and Treatment. Edited by Ott PJ, Tarter RE, Ammerman RT. Boston, MA, Allyn & Bacon, 1999, pp 255–263

Dimeff LA, Marlatt GA: Preventing relapse and maintaining change in addictive behaviors. Clinical Psychology: Science and Practice 5:513–525, 1998

Donovan DM, Marlatt GA (eds): Assessment of Addictive Behaviors: Behavioral, Cognitive, and Physiological Processes. New York, Guilford, 1988

el-Guebaly N, Hodgins D: Substance-related cravings and relapses: clinical implications. Can J Psychiatry 43:29–36, 1998

Epstein EE, McCrady BS: Behavioral couples treatment of alcohol and drug use disorders: current status and innovations. Clin Psychol Rev 18:689–711, 1998

Fisher D, Beech A: Reconstituting families after sexual abuse: the offender's perspective. Child Abuse Review 7:420–434, 1998

Glasser W: Positive Addiction. New York, Harper & Row, 1976

Grabowski J, O'Brien CP, Greenstein RA: Effects of contingent payment on compliance with a naltrexone regimen. Am J Drug Alcohol Abuse 6:355–365, 1979

Heath AW, Stanton MD: Family-based treatment: stages and outcomes, in Clinical Textbook of Addictive Disorders. Edited by Frances RJ, Miller SI. New York, Guilford, 1998, pp 496–520

Heather N, Robertson I (eds): Controlled Drinking, 2nd Edition. London, Methuen, 1987

Herman SE, BootsMiller B, Jordan L, et al: Immediate outcomes of substance use treatment within a state psychiatric hospital. J Ment Health Adm 24:126–138, 1997

Jacob T, Dunn NJ, Leonard K: Patterns of alcohol use and family stability. Alcohol Clin Exp Res 7:382–385, 1983

Kabat Zinn J: Wherever You Go, There You Are. New York, Saint Martin's, 1994

Kaufman E: Substance Abuse and Family Therapy. Orlando, FL, Grune & Stratton, 1985

Kaufman E, Kaufmann P: Family Therapy of Drug and Alcohol Abuse. New York, Gardner, 1979

Kendall PC, Hollon SD (eds): Cognitive-Behavioral Interventions: Theory, Research and Procedures. New York, Academic Press, 1979

Kivlahan DR, Marlatt GA, Fromme K, et al: Secondary prevention with college drinkers: evaluation of an alcohol skills training program. J Consult Clin Psychol 58:805–810, 1990

Laws R (ed): Relapse Prevention With Sex Offenders. New York, Guilford, 1989

Maisto SA, Carey KB, Bradizza CM: Social learning theory, in Psychological Theories of Drinking and Alcoholism. Edited by Leonard KE, Blane HT. New York, Guilford, 1999, pp 106–163

Marlatt GA: Craving for alcohol, loss of control and relapse: a cognitive-behavioral analysis, in Alcoholism: New Directions in Behavioral Research and Treatment. Edited by Nathan PE, Marlatt GA, Loberg T. New York, Plenum, 1978, pp 271–314

Marlatt GA: Alcohol use and problem drinking: a cognitive-behavioral analysis, in Cognitive-Behavioral Interventions: Theory, Research and Procedures. Edited by Kendall PC, Hollon SD. New York, Academic Press, 1979, pp 319–355

Marlatt GA: Relapse prevention: a self-control program for the treatment of addictive behaviors, in Adherence, Compliance and Generalization in Behavioral Medicine. Edited by Stuart RB. New York, Brunner/Mazel, 1982, pp 329–378

Marlatt GA: The controlled-drinking controversy: a commentary. Am Psychol 38:1097–1110, 1983

Marlatt GA: Harm reductions: come as you are. Addict Behav 21:779-788, 1996

Marlatt GA (ed): Harm Reduction. New York, Guilford, 1998

Marlatt GA, George WH: Relapse prevention: introduction and overview of the model. British Journal of Addiction 79:261–273, 1984

Marlatt GA, Gordon JR: Determinants of relapse: implications for the maintenance of behavior change, in Behavioral Medicine: Changing Health Lifestyles. Edited by Davidson PO, Davidson SM, New York, Brunner/Mazel, 1980, pp 410–452

Marlatt GA, Gordon JR (eds): Relapse Prevention: Maintenance Strategies in the Treatment of Addictive Behaviors. New York, Guilford, 1985

Marlatt GA, Rohsenow DR: Cognitive processes in alcohol use: expectancy and the balanced placebo design, in Advances in Substance Abuse, Vol 1. Edited by Mello NK. Greenwich, CT, JAI Press, 1980, pp 159–199

Marlatt GA, Tapert SF: Harm reduction: reducing the risk of addictive behavior, in Addictive Behaviors Across the Lifespan. Edited by Baer JS, Marlatt GA, McMahon B. Newbury Park, CA, Sage, 1992, pp 243–273

Marlatt GA, Baer JS, Kivlahan DR, et al: Screening and brief intervention for high-risk college student drinkers: results from a 2-year follow-up assessment. J Consult Clin Psychol, 66:604-615, 1998

Marlatt GA, Barrett K, Daley DC: Relapse prevention, in The American Psychiatric Press Textbook of Substance Abuse Treatment, 2nd Edition. Edited by Galanter M, Kleber HD. Washington, DC, American Psychiatric Press, 1999, pp 353–366

McCrady BS: Extending relapse prevention models to couples. Addict Behav 14:69–74, 1989

McCusker J, Bigelow C, Frost R, et al: The effects of planned duration of residential drug abuse treatment on recovery and HIV risk. Am J Public Health 87:1637–1644, 1997

McFall RM: Behavioral Training: A Skills-Acquisition Approach to Clinical Problems. Morristown, NJ, General Learning Press, 1976

McKay JR, Alterman AI, Cacciola JS, et al: Group counseling versus individualized relapse prevention aftercare following intensive outpatient treatment for cocaine dependence: initial results. J Consult Clin Psychol 65:778–788, 1997

McKay JR, McLellan AT, Alterman AI, et al: Predictors of participation in aftercare sessions and self-help groups following completion of intensive outpatient treatment for substance abuse. J Stud Alcohol 59:152–162, 1998

Meichenbaum D: Cognitive-Behavioral Modification. New York, Plenum, 1977

Miller WR, Rollnick S: Motivational Interviewing. New York, Guilford, 1991

Monson SM, Jones LM, Rivers PC, et al: Alcohol and sex offending: what do child sex offenders think about drinking? Journal of Addictions and Offender Counseling 19:15–27, 1998

Monti PM, Abrams DB, Kadden RM: Treating Alcohol Dependence. New York, Guilford, 1989

Moos RH, Finney JW, Cronkite RC: Alcoholism Treatment: Process and Outcome. New York, Oxford University Press, 1990

Nhât Hanh T: The Miracle of Mindfulness: A Manual of Meditation, Boston, MA, Beacon Press, 1992

O'Farrell TJ: Using couples therapy in the treatment of alcoholism. Family Dynamics of Addiction Quarterly 1:39–45, 1991

O'Farrell TJ, Choquette KA, Cutter HSG: Couples relapse prevention sessions after behavioral marital therapy for male alcoholics: outcomes during the three years after starting treatment. J Stud Alcohol 59:357–370, 1998

Rawson R, McCann M, Huber A, et al: Contingency management and relapse prevention as stimulant abuse treatment interventions, in Motivating Behavior Change Among Illicit-Drug Abusers: Research on Contingency Management Intervention. Washington, DC, American Psychological Association, 1999, pp 57–74

Roberts LJ, Marlatt GA: Harm reduction, in Sourcebook on Substance Abuse: Etiology, Epidemiology, Assessment, and Treatment. Boston, MA, Allyn & Bacon, 1999, pp 389–398

Roffman RA, Stephens RS, Curtin L, et al: Relapse prevention as an interventive model for HIV risk reduction in gay and bisexual men. AIDS Educ Prev 10:1–18, 1998

Roget NA, Fisher GL, Johnson ML: A protocol for reducing juvenile recidivism through relapse prevention. Journal of Addictions and Offender Counseling 19:33–43, 1998

Sandberg GG, Marlatt GA: Relapse prevention, in Clinical Manual of Chemical Dependence. Edited by Ciraulo DA, Shader RI. Washington, DC, American Psychiatric Press, 1991, pp 377–399

Schmitz JM, Oswald LM, Jacks SD, et al: Relapse prevention treatment for cocaine dependence: group vs individual format. Addict Behav 22:405–418, 1997

Sharkansky EJ, Brief DJ, Pierce JM, et al: Substance abuse patients with posttraumatic stress disorder (PTSD): identifying specific triggers of substance abuse and their associations with PTSD symptoms. Psychology of Addictive Behaviors 13:89–97, 1999

Shiffman S, Wills TA (eds): Coping and Substance Abuse. New York, Academic Press, 1985

Steinglass P: Family therapy: alcohol, in The American Psychiatric Press Textbook of Substance Abuse Treatment. Edited by Galanter M, Kleber HD. Washington, DC, American Psychiatric Press, 1999, pp 353–366

Steinglass P, Bennett LA, Wolin SJ, et al: The Alcoholic Family. New York, Basic Books, 1987

Stone GC, Cohen F, Adler NE: Health Psychology. San Francisco, CA, Jossey-Bass, 1979

Ward T, Hudson SM: A model of the relapse process in sexual offenders. Journal of Interpersonal Violence 13:700–725, 1998

Weatherby NL, McCoy HV, Metsch LR, et al: Crack cocaine use in rural migrant populations: living arrangements and social support. Subst Use Misuse 34:685–706, 1999

Weingardt KR, Marlatt GA: Sustaining change: helping those who are still using, in Treating Addictive Behaviors, 2nd Edition. Edited by Miller WR, Heather N. New York, Plenum, 1998, pp 337–351

Wilson PH (ed): Principles and Practice of Relapse Prevention. New York, Guilford, 1992

Network Therapy

Marc Galanter, M.D.

In this chapter subpart I describe a treatment modality designed to allow the practitioner to treat addictive disorders in the ambulatory setting. The approach, called *network therapy* (Galanter 1993, 1999), was developed specifically to bring addicted patients to a successful recovery, an outcome that traditional office therapy often fails to bring about. Network therapy can be defined as an approach to addiction rehabilitation in which specific family members and friends are enlisted to provide ongoing support and to promote attitude change. Network members are part of the therapist's working "team" and are not themselves the subjects of treatment.

The effectiveness of ambulatory therapy can be enhanced by a patients' drawing on his or her immediate network, which may consist of the spouse, some friends (perhaps a friend from work), and/or the family of origin. Components of the network are part of the natural support system that usually operates without professional involvement. However, when these components are brought to act in concert, the strength of their social influence can serve as a therapeutic device that can complement individual or group therapy and 12-Step programs such as Alcoholics Anonymous as well.

The Problem Confronting the Clinician

To frame a psychosocial therapy using network support, we must first define the target problem clearly and then consider the particulars of how the network exerts its influence. From a clinician's perspective, the problems of *relapse* and *loss of control*, embodied in the criteria for substance dependence in DSM-IV (American Psychiatric Association 1994), are central to the difficulty of treating addiction. Because addicted patients are typically under pressure to relapse to ingestion of alcohol or drugs, they are seen as poor candidates for stable attendance and tend to drop out. "Loss of control" has been used to describe addicted persons' inability to reliably limit consumption once an initial dose of the addictive substance is taken (Gallant 1987).

Withdrawal feelings—and thus craving—can be elicited by cues that were previously associated with the addicted individual's use of the drug. Hence, exposure to the smell of liquor in a bar can precipitate a "need" to drink in an alcoholic person, and seeing the "works" for injecting heroin or going by a "shooting gallery" can lead a heroin-addicted person to relapse (Ludwig et al. 1974). Very often, modulations in mood state constitute the conditioned stimuli for drug seeking, and the substance-abusing person can become vulnerable to relapse through reflexive responses to a specific affective state. Such seeking of drugs to regulate specific affects was described in the clinical context by Khantzian (1985) as *self-medication.* These responses, however, are not necessarily mentioned spontaneously by the patient in a conventional therapy, because the triggering stimulus may not be associated with a memorable event and the drug use may avert emergence of memorable distress.

More dramatic is the phenomenon of affect regression, which Wurmser (1977) observed among addicted patients studied in a psychoanalytic context. Wurmser pointed out that when addicted individuals suffer narcissistic injury, they are prone to a precipitous collapse of ego defenses and the consequent experience of intense and unmanageable affective flooding. In the face of such vulnerability, these persons handle stress poorly and may turn to drugs for relief. This vulnerability can be considered in light of the model of conditioned withdrawal, whereby drug seeking can become an immediate reflexive response to stress, undermining the stability and effectiveness of a patient's coping mechanisms.

This model helps to explain why relapse is such a frequent and unanticipated aspect of addiction treatment. Exposure to conditioned cues—ones that were repeatedly associated with drug use—can precipitate reflexive drug craving during the course of therapy, and such cue exposure can also initiate a sequence of conditioned behaviors that leads addicted individuals to relapse into drug use.

Use of Social Network Support

The use of social support as a means of addressing relapse is evident in the potential of family treatment for alcohol problems as reported by the Institute of Medicine, which concluded that "research data support superior outcomes for family-involved treatment, enough so that the modal approach should involve family members and carefully planned interventions" (Institute of Medicine 1990, p. 84). Indeed, the idea of the therapist's intervening with family and friends to start treatment was introduced by Johnson (1986) as one of the early ambulatory techniques in the addiction field (Gallant 1987; Gitlow and Peyser 1980). More broadly, the availability of greater social support to patients has been shown to be an important predictor of positive outcome in addiction treatment (McLellan et al. 1983).

Galanter (1993) first reported a positive outcome with this approach in a clinical trial conducted in a series of 60 patients treated with network therapy. This trial involved one network session a week for the first month, with subsequent sessions held less frequently, typically on a bimonthly basis after a year of ambulatory care. Individual therapy was carried out concomitantly on a once- or twice-weekly basis. On average, the networks had 2.3 members, the most frequent participants being mates, peers, parents, or siblings.

A cohabiting couple will provide an example of how natural affiliative ties can be used to develop a secure basis for rehabilitation. Couples therapy for addiction has been described in both ambulatory and inpatient settings, and a stable marital relationship is found to be associated with a diminished likelihood of dropout and a positive overall outcome

(Kaufman and Kaufman 1979; McCrady et al. 1986; Stanton and Thomas 1982).

Disulfiram therapy has yielded relatively little benefit overall in controlled trials when the drug is prescribed for patients to take on their own recognizance (Fuller and Williford 1980). This lack of benefit results from the fact that this agent is effective only when it is ingested as instructed, typically on a daily basis. Alcoholic patients who forget to take required doses will likely resume drinking in time. Indeed, such forgetting often reflects the initiation of a sequence of conditioned drug-seeking behaviors.

Although patient characteristics have not been shown to predict compliance with a disulfiram regimen (Schuckit 1985), changes in the format of patient management have been found to have a beneficial effect (Brubaker et al. 1987). For example, the involvement of a spouse in observing the patient's consumption of disulfiram yields a considerable improvement in outcome (Azrin et al. 1982; Keane et al. 1984). Patients alerted to taking disulfiram each morning by this external reminder are less likely to experience conditioned drug seeking when exposed to addictive cues and are more likely to comply with the dosing regimen in subsequent days.

The technique of spousal involvement in monitoring the patient's dosing regimen also helps in clearly defining the roles in therapy of both the alcoholic patient and his or her spouse by not requiring the spouse to monitor drinking behaviors she or he cannot control. The spouse does not actively remind the alcoholic patient to take each dose. She or he merely notifies the therapist if she or he does not observe the pill being ingested on a given day. Decisions on managing compliance are then allocated to the therapist, thereby avoiding entanglement of the couple in a dispute over the patient's attitude and the possibility of surreptitious drinking.

A variety of other behavioral devices that have been demonstrated to improve outcome can be incorporated into this couples format. For example, it has been found that setting the first appointment as soon as possible after an initial phone contact improves outcome by undercutting the possibility of an early loss of motivation (Stark et al. 1990). The spouse can also be engaged in history taking at the very outset of treatment to minimize the introduction of denial into the patient's presentation of his or her illness (Liepman et al. 1989).

How Network Therapy Is Conducted

Network Membership

Networks generally consist of a number of members when a simple network employing the spouse and disulfiram therapy cannot be used. Once the patient has come for an appointment, the patient and therapist actively collaborate to establish a network. The patient and therapist, aided by those parties who join the network initially, must search for the right balance of members. The therapist must carefully choose appropriate network members, however, just as the platoon leader prudently selects those who will go into combat with him. The network will be crucial in determining the balance of the therapy. This process of building a network is not without problems, and the therapist must think in a strategic fashion of the interactions that may take place among network members. The following vignette illustrates the nature of the network's task.

> A 25-year-old graduate student had been abusing drugs since high school, in part drawing on funds from his affluent family, who lived in a city remote from the patient. At two points in the process of establishing his support network, the reactions of his live-in girlfriend

> were particularly important. Both he and she agreed to bring in his 19-year-old sister, a freshman at a nearby college. He then mentioned a "friend" of his, a woman whom he apparently found attractive, even though there was no history of an overt romantic involvement. The expression on his girlfriend's face suggested that she was uncomfortable with this option. The therapist, in deference to the girlfriend's discomfort about the patient's "friend" being included, moved on to evaluating the patient's uncle as an alternative. Initially the patient was reluctant; it later turned out that he perceived the uncle as a potentially disapproving representative of the parental generation. The therapist and girlfriend encouraged him to accept the uncle as a network member nonetheless, so as to round out the range of relationships within the group. In matter of fact, the uncle was caring and supportive, particularly after he was helped to understand the nature of the addictive process.

The Network's Task

The therapist's relationship to the network is that of a task-oriented team leader rather than a family therapist oriented toward restructuring relationships. The network is established to implement a straightforward task, that of helping the therapist to secure the patient's abstinence. The network must be directed with the same clarity of purpose with which a task force is directed in any effective organization. Competing and alternative goals must be suppressed or at least prevented from interfering with the primary task.

Unlike family members involved in traditional family therapy, network members are not led to expect symptom relief or self-realization for themselves. This approach prevents the development of competing goals for the network's meetings. It also assures the members protection from having their own motives scrutinized and thereby supports their continuing involvement without the threat of an assault on their psychological defenses. Because network members have kindly volunteered to participate, their motives must not be impugned. Their constructive behavior should be commended. It is useful to acknowledge appreciation for the contribution they are making to the therapy. There is always a counterproductive tendency on the part of network members to minimize the value of their contribution. The network must therefore be structured as an effective working group with good morale.

Specific Techniques

Yalom (1974) described anxiety-reducing tactics that he used in therapy groups with alcoholic patients to avert disruptions and promote cohesiveness. These tactics include setting an agenda for the session and using didactic instruction. In the network format, a cognitive framework can be provided for each session by starting out with the patient's recounting events related to cue exposure or substance use since the last meeting. Network members are then expected to comment on this report to ensure that all are engaged in a mutual task with correct, shared information. Their reactions to the patient's report are addressed as well. This format is illustrated in the following vignette:

> An alcoholic patient began one of his early network sessions by reporting a minor lapse to drinking. His recounting was disrupted by an outburst of anger from his older sister, who said that she had "had it up to here" with his frequent unfulfilled promises of sobriety. The psychiatrist addressed this source of conflict by explaining in a didactic manner how behavioral cues affect vulnerability to relapse. This didactic approach was adopted to counter the assumption that relapse is easily controlled and to relieve consequent resentment. The therapist then led the members in planning concretely with the patient how he might avoid further drinking cues in the period preceding their next conjoint session.

Patients undergoing detoxification from long-standing use of depressant medication often experience considerable anxiety, even when a gradual dosage reduction schedule is undertaken (American Psychiatric Association 1990). The expectation of distress, coupled with conditioned withdrawal phenomena, may cause patients to balk at completing a detoxification regimen (Monti et al. 1988). In individual therapy alone, the psychiatrist would have little leverage at this point. When individual therapy is augmented with network therapy, however, the added support can be invaluable in securing compliance under these circumstances.

> A patient elected to undertake detoxification from chronic use of diazepam at approximately 60 mg daily. In network meetings with the patient, her husband, and her friend, the psychiatrist discussed the patient's need for added support toward the end of her detoxification. As the daily dose was brought to 2 mg three times a day, however, the patient became anxious, said that she had never intended to stop completely, and insisted on being maintained permanently on that low dose. Network members supportively but explicitly pointed out that this had not been the plan. The patient then relented to the original detoxification agreement, and her dosage was reduced to zero over 6 weeks.

Patients are strongly inclined to deny their drinking problems during relapse. The network may be the only resource available to the psychiatrist through which he or she can communicate with a relapsing patient and assist in reestablishing abstinence.

> A patient suffered a relapse to drinking after 6 months of abstinence. One of the network members consulted with the psychiatrist and then stayed with the patient in his home for a day to ensure that he would not drink. The network member then brought the patient to the psychiatrist's office, where the patient, the other network members, and the psychiatrist reestablished a plan for abstinence.

Use of Twelve-Step Programs With the Network

Use of AA is desirable whenever possible. For the alcoholic patient, certainly, participation in AA is strongly encouraged. Groups such as Narcotics Anonymous, Pills Anonymous, and Cocaine Anonymous are modeled after AA and play a similarly useful role for persons who abuse drugs. One approach is to tell the patient that he or she is expected to attend at least two AA meetings a week for at least 1 month so as to familiarize him- or herself with the program. If after a month the patient is quite reluctant to continue the 12-Step meetings but other aspects of the treatment are going well, his or her nonparticipation may have to be accepted. Some patients are more easily convinced to attend AA meetings, whereas others may be less compliant. The therapist should mobilize the support network as appropriate in order to continue to press for the patient's involvement with AA for a reasonable trial.

Like family and group therapy, network therapy brings several people together to address a psychological problem. Approaches vary among practitioners of group and family modalities, with some therapists focusing on the individual patient and others trying to shape the family or group overall. In the network, by contrast, the focus is always kept on the individual patient and his or her addictive problem. In network therapy, unlike in family therapy, the practitioner avoids focusing on the patient's family history in the network sessions themselves, because an involvement in family conflicts can be disruptive to the network's primary task of helping to maintain the patient's abstinence.

Principles of Network Therapy Management

Starting the Network

The following points define major aspects of the initial encounter with the patient in which the therapist explains why and how the network is to be established:

1. It is important to see the alcohol- or drug-abusing person promptly, because the window of opportunity for openness to treatment is generally brief.
2. If the person is married, engage the spouse at the outset of treatment, preferably at the time of the first phone call. Point out that addiction is a family problem. For most drugs, you can enlist the spouse or significant other in ensuring that the patient arrives at your office with at least a day's sobriety.
3. In the initial interview, frame the exchange so that a good case is built for the grave consequences of the patient's addiction, and do this before the patient can introduce his or her system of denial. By doing this, you are not placing the spouse or other network members in the awkward position of having to contradict a close relation. Then make it clear that the patient needs to be abstinent, starting immediately.
4. When seeing an alcoholic patient for the first time, start him or her on disulfiram as soon as possible, in the office if you can. Have the patient continue taking disulfiram under the observation of a network member.
5. At the first session, start arranging for a network to be assembled, generally involving a number of the patient's family or close friends.
6. From the very first meeting, consider what is needed to ensure the patient's sobriety until the next meeting and plan a course of action for accomplishing that with the network. Initially, this course will include their immediate presence and a plan for daily AA attendance.
7. Include people who are close to the patient, have a long-standing relationship with him or her, and are trusted. Avoid enlisting network members with substance problems, because they will let you down when you need their unbiased support.
8. Build a balanced group. Avoid a network composed solely of the parental generation, of younger people, or of persons of the opposite sex.
9. Maintain a tone that is directive; that is, give explicit instructions to support and ensure abstinence.

Priorities of Ongoing Therapy

After the network is to be established, norms of behavior for the patient and each network member should be reinforced:

1. *Maintaining abstinence.* The patient and the network members should report at the outset of each session any events related to the patient's exposure to alcohol and drugs. The patient and network members should be instructed on the nature of relapse and should plan with the therapist how to sustain abstinence. Cues to conditioned drug seeking should be examined.
2. *Supporting the network's integrity.* The patient is expected to make sure that network members keep their meeting appointments and stay involved. The therapist sets meeting times explicitly and summons the network for any emergency, such as a relapse;

the therapist also does whatever is necessary to secure stability of the membership if the patient is having trouble with this function.

3. *Securing future behavior.* The therapist should combine any and all modalities necessary to ensure the patient's stability. Stability is enhanced by maintenance of a stable, drug-free residence; avoidance of substance-abusing friends; and attendance at 12-Step meetings, as well as by the patient's taking medications such as disulfiram or opioid-blocking agents, undergoing observed urinalysis, and receiving ancillary psychiatric care.

Research on Network Therapy

Studies of network therapy have demonstrated its effectiveness in treatment and in training. Among the studies summarized here, each addressed the approach from a different perspective: a clinical trial of office-based management of substance-dependent patients, investigations of network therapy's effectiveness in the training of psychiatric residents and then counselors who treat cocaine-addicted patients; and an evaluation of acceptance of the network approach in an Internet technology-transfer course.

An Office-Based Clinical Trial

A chart review was conducted of a series of 60 substance-dependent patients treated by the author, with follow-up through the period of treatment and up to 1 year thereafter (Galanter 1993). Primary drugs of dependence were alcohol, cocaine, opiates, and marijuana. In all but eight of the patients, networks were fully established. Forty-six of the 60 patients demonstrated full improvement (abstinence for at least 6 months) or major improvement (a marked decline in drug use to nonproblem levels).

Treatment by Psychiatry Residents

After a study examining reliability and validity of the network model (Keller et al. 1997), third-year psychiatry residents were trained to apply the technique to a total of 24 cocaine-addicted subjects, employing a treatment manual and videotape illustrations (Galanter et al. 1997a). Results of treatment were analyzed relative to reported findings with ambulatory treatment in comparable settings. Although inexperienced in drug treatment, the residents achieved results similar to those reported in the literature for experienced professionals. These comparisons supported the feasibility of successful training of psychiatry residents naive to addiction treatment and the subsequent efficacy of treatment in their hands.

Treatment by Addiction Counselors

Counselors in a community-based addictions treatment clinic received training in the application of network therapy techniques (Keller et al. 1999). Outcomes of 10 cocaine-dependent patients treated with network therapy in addition to the clinic's usual package of modalities were compared with those of 20 cocaine-dependent patients treated as usual. Patients who received network therapy were found to have better outcomes, as judged by the results of random urine tests and social adaptation. These study findings supported the feasibility of transferring network technology into community-based settings with the potential for enhancing outcomes.

Use of the Internet

Psychiatrists and other professionals were offered training by a distance learning method using the Internet, a medium that offers the advantage of not being fixed in either time or location (Galanter et al. 1997b). The sequence of material presented on the Internet was divided into three didactic "Sessions" followed by a set of questions, with a hypertext link to download relevant references and a certificate of completion. Of the initial cohort of 154 psychiatrists who completed the course, 70% indicated via e-mail response that it was clinically useful. This course continues to be posted on the Internet at www.med.nyu.edu/substanceabuse/course.

Summary of Research

These four studies support the use of network therapy as an effective treatment for addictive disorders. Their results are encouraging, given the relative ease with which different types of clinicians were engaged and trained in the network approach, and through the Internet as well. Because the approach combines a number of well-established clinical techniques, each packaged in a format adapted to delivery in typical clinical settings, it is apparently suitable for use by general clinicians as well as addiction specialists.

References

American Psychiatric Association: Task Force on Benzodiazepine Dependence, Toxicity, and Abuse—A Task Force Report of the American Psychiatric Association. Washington, DC, American Psychiatric Association, 1990

American Psychiatric Association: Diagnostic and Statistical Manual of Mental Disorders, 4th Edition. Washington, DC, American Psychiatric Association, 1994

Azrin NH, Sisson RW, Meyers R: Alcoholism treatment by disulfiram and community reinforcement therapy. J Behav Ther Exp Psychiatry 13:105–112, 1982

Brubaker RG, Prue DM, Rychtarik RG: Determinants of disulfiram acceptance among alcohol patients: a test of the theory of reasoned action. Addict Behav 12:43–52, 1987

Fuller RK, Williford WO: Life-table analysis of abstinence in a study evaluating the efficacy of disulfiram. Alcohol Clin Exp Res 4:298–301, 1980

Galanter M: Network therapy for addiction: a model for office practice. Am J Psychiatry 150:28–36, 1993

Galanter M: Network Therapy Alcohol and Drug Abuse, Expanded Edition. New York, Guilford, 1999

Galanter M, Keller DS, Dermatis H: Network therapy for addiction: assessment of the clinical outcome of training. Am J Drug Alcohol Abuse 23:335–368, 1997a

Galanter M, Keller DS, Dermatis H: Using the Internet for clinical training: a course on network therapy. Psychiatr Serv 48:999–1000, 1008, 1997b

Gallant DM: Alcoholism: A Guide to Diagnosis, Intervention, and Treatment. New York, WW Norton, 1987

Gitlow SE, Peyser HS (eds): Alcoholism: A Practical Treatment Guide. New York, Grune & Stratton, 1980

Institute of Medicine: Broadening the Base of Treatment for Alcohol Problems. Washington, DC, National Academy Press, 1990

Johnson VE: Intervention: How To Help Someone Who Doesn't Want Help. Minneapolis, MN, Johnson Institute Books, 1986

Kaufman E, Kaufman PN: Family Therapy of Drug and Alcohol Abuse. New York, Gardner, 1979

Keane TM, Foy DW, Nunn B, et al: Spouse contracting to increase Antabuse compliance in alcoholic veterans. J Clin Psychol 40:340–344, 1984

Keller DS, Galanter M, Weinberg S: Validation of a scale for network therapy: a technique for systematic use of peer and family support in addiction treatment. Am J Drug Alcohol Abuse 23:115–127, 1997

Keller DS, Galanter M, Dermatis H: Technology transfer of network therapy to community-based addiction counselors. J Subst Abuse Treat 16:183–189, 1999

Khantzian EJ: The self-medication hypothesis of addictive disorders: focus on heroin and cocaine dependence. Am J Psychiatry 142:1259–1264, 1985

Liepman MR, Nierenberg TD, Begin AM: Evaluation of a program designed to help family and significant others to motivate resistant alcoholics to recover. Am J Drug Alcohol Abuse 15:209–222, 1989

Ludwig AM, Wikler A, Stark LM: The first drink. Arch Gen Psychiatry, 30:539–547, 1974

McCrady BS, Noel NE, Abrams DB, et al: Comparative effectiveness of three types of spouse involvement in outpatient behavioral alcoholism treatment. J Stud Alcohol 47:459–467, 1986

McLellan AT, Woody GE, Luborsky L, et al: Increased effectiveness of substance abuse treatment: a prospective study of patient-treatment "matching." J Nerv Ment Dis 171:597–605, 1983

Monti PM, Rohsenow DJ, Abrams DB, et al: Social learning approaches to alcohol relapse: selected illustrations and implications, in Learning Factors in Substance Abuse. NIDA Research Monograph 84 (DHHS Publ No [ADM] 88-1576). Edited by Ray BA. Rockville, MD, Department of Health and Human Services, 1988, pp 141–159

Schuckit MA: A one-year follow-up of men alcoholics given disulfiram. J Stud Alcohol 46:191–195, 1985

Stanton MD, Thomas TC (eds): The Family Therapy of Drug Abuse and Addiction. New York, Guilford, 1982

Stark MJ, Campbell BK, Brinkerhoff CV: "Hello, May We Help You?" A study of attrition prevention at the time of the first phone contact with substance-abusing clients. Am J Drug Alcohol Abuse 16:67–76, 1990

Wurmser L: Mrs. Pecksniff's horse? Psychodynamics of compulsive drug use, in Psychodynamics of Drug Dependence. NIDA Research Monograph 12 (DHEW Publ No [ADM] 77-470). Edited by Blaine JD, Julius DS. Washington, DC, U.S. Government Printing Office, 1977, pp 36–72

Yalom ID: Group therapy and alcoholism. Ann N Y Acad Sci 233:85–103, 1974

31

Group and Family Treatments

Edward J. Khantzian, M.D.
Sarah J. Golden, Ph.D.
William E. McAuliffe, Ph.D.
Peter Steinglass, M.D.
Edward Kaufman, M.D.

Group Therapy for Psychoactive Substance Use Disorders

Edward J. Khantzian, M.D.
Sarah J. Golden, Ph.D.
William E. McAuliffe, Ph.D.

Group treatment modalities are almost universally adopted as the preferred or predominant therapeutic modality for patients with psychoactive substance use disorders. This preference for use of group modalities appears to hold despite the presumption that different ideologies or conceptualizations of problems often dictate different approaches. The field of substance abuse treatment is characterized by strong and often polarized etiological views of substance dependency in which biological, psychological, and/or social factors are often invoked and pitted against one another. Nevertheless, regardless of orientation or conceptualization, treatment approaches predominantly place persons together in groups to consider the nature of their addictive vulnerability and what course of action can be taken in response to it.

A systematic review of outcome or efficacy studies is beyond the scope of this chapter subpart. In fact, little systematic study has been undertaken to evaluate the efficacy of group treatment or to compare its efficacy with that of other treatments. However, a number of more recent studies indicate that treatment efficacy and outcome are improved by better matching of patient characteristics, needs, and vulnerabilities to the different individual and group methods employed in substance abuse treatment (Carroll et al. 1998;

This chapter subpart is a revised version of our chapter "Group Therapy," which appeared in Galanter MA, Kleber HD (eds): The American Psychiatric Press Textbook of Substance Abuse Treatment, 2nd Edition. Washington, DC, American Psychiatric Press, 1999, pp. 367–378.

Cooney et al. 1991; Khantzian et al. 1990; Martin et al. 1996; McAuliffe and Albert 1992; Poldrugo and Forti 1988).

In this subchapter we review theoretical and clinical aspects of the various group treatments commonly employed and examine the commonalities as well as the differences in these group approaches. We stress the specific needs of substance-dependent persons, their special vulnerabilities, and the characteristic and characterological problems they present that are associated with their addiction. We also demonstrate how group therapy can help patients with psychoactive substance use disorders to effectively access, target, and modify the factors that govern their dependency on alcohol and drugs.

Groups and Addiction

Groups are effective in treatment because they embody an appreciation of the healing power of connection with others. Groups address the universal need to belong and at the same time counter the tendency to believe one is unique in one's plight and distress. Elements of information, support, understanding, and confrontation act as important, if not powerful, antidotes to and respite from the shame, isolation, and loneliness that is so central a determinant of addictive illness. Whether the aim of the group is education or therapy, persons can be extraordinarily helpful to each other in the group context (Herman 1992; Khantzian 1986, 1995; Tuttman 1990; Yalom 1983).

Overview and a Review

As we have indicated, each group approach reflects a particular view of addiction. Self-help groups, epitomized by Alcoholics Anonymous (AA), constitute one of the most widely recognized and successful group approaches. These groups are so widely used not only because they were some of the first to be established but also because they were more clear and effective in providing practical explanations and solutions. AA was and still is successful because it offers a corrective psychological, spiritual, and moral approach to the problem of addiction. Founded in 1935 by Bill Wilson and Dr. Bob in an attempt to help each other, AA derived from a model of Christian fellowship that fostered self-examination, acknowledgment of character defects, restitution, and "*working with others*" (Orford 1985; emphasis added). AA targets deficits, and attitudes about self and others embodied in character traits and styles, that make interdependence, experience, and expression of feelings and self-care difficult. Participation in AA counters and transforms these difficulties by effectively advocating acceptance of and surrender to a higher power and by challenging human self-centeredness (Khantzian 1994; Khantzian and Mack 1989).

The concept of an individual's submitting to a group's treatment ideology has perhaps found its fullest expression in therapeutic communities for the treatment of addiction. Synanon, established in the 1960s to address heroin addiction, aggressively used the group modality to change attitudes through confinement, structure, daily work assignments, and often demanding interpersonal confrontation (Cherkas 1965). This "total" group approach, in which every aspect of daily life is regimented, continues to thrive in such programs as Daytop Village and Phoenix House.

Other major group approaches in the treatment of addiction have developed from the cognitive-behavioral and psychoanalytic/psychodynamic clinical traditions. From these schools of thought have emerged both individual and group therapies for addiction. In the following discussion, we focus on the group models. One form of cognitive-behavioral group therapy, the psychoeducational group, uses the group format to inform and teach addicted persons about the behavioral, medical, and psychological consequences of addiction. Such groups are a staple of most rehabilitation programs (Nace 1987) and are often seen as the "first step" of a more comprehensive treatment program. By raising awareness of the consequences of addictive behavior through informational materials, didactic presentations, and group discussions, this method is intended both as education and as "persuasion," an attempt to show group members how addiction "complicate[s] their lives" (Drake et al. 1991). As agencies of persuasion, these groups encourage members to commit to further treatment.

Cognitive-behavioral theory holds that addiction is learned behavior that is reinforced by contingencies such as the pleasurable effects of drugs (McAuliffe and Ch'ien 1986). The addictive behavior is conditioned and then generalized to a range of stimuli in the environment that continue to perpetuate the addiction. The treatment for addiction thus involves learning to recognize and avoid these stimuli and, ultimately, to extinguish conditioned responses to these stimuli. Cognitive-behavioral therapy aims to develop alternative thoughts and behaviors in response to the conditions that have triggered "addictive" responses. Based on such an understanding, McAuliffe and associates (McAuliffe and Ch'ien 1986) developed a cognitive-behavioral group treatment for substance abuse (Recovery Training/Self Help [RTSH]) to prevent relapse. RTSH uses a curriculum, a didactic group format, and discussion groups to recognize social and environmental cues that lead to relapse. Based on these assumptions and a similar format, McAuliffe and Albert (1992) developed an outpatient cessation model for early recovery from cocaine dependence.

A number of group models have emerged from the psychoanalytic/psychodynamic tradition. Most relevant for the treatment of addiction have been those groups that have a psychodynamic, interpersonal focus and that address the addicted person's particular needs for safety and structure in the group setting (Brown and Yalom 1977; Khantzian et al. 1990, 1995; Matano and Yalom 1991; Vannicelli 1982; Yalom 1974).

In the psychoanalytic/psychodynamic tradition, addiction is understood as the person's "solution" to the problem of psychological vulnerability. Contemporary psychoanalytic theory has elaborated on these vulnerabilities as defects of self, both intrapsychic and characterological, that can lead to addiction in an attempt by the person to regulate and medicate the distress caused by the defect (Kohut 1977; Meissner 1986; Wurmser 1978). Khantzian (1974, 1978, 1985, 1995, 1997, 1999) has addressed the particular psychological and narcissistic vulnerabilities of the potential "addict"; Khantzian's "self-medication" hypothesis holds that addiction results when a person seeks to relieve the suffering and distress resulting from deficits in ego capacities involving affects, self-esteem, self-care, and relationships with others as these deficits play themselves out in everyday life. Heightening awareness of self and changing characteristic patterns of handling these vulnerabilities in everyday situations are addressed in the psychodynamic group treatment of addiction.

Perhaps the most important aspect of Khantzian's model is that it is "modified" dynamic group therapy (Khantzian et al. 1990, 1995). The therapy is modified in that the vulnerabilities and difficulties of the addicted person are recognized in the format of the treatment; the group model is one that establishes maximum safety for addicted persons in requiring and helping to maintain abstinence, in providing outreach and support, in using an active style of leadership, and in always addressing the potential for drug and psychological relapse. Structure and containment are emphasized rather than confrontation. This group model has been studied experimentally as part of the Harvard Cocaine Recovery Project (Khantzian et al. 1990).

Group Therapy as Treatment of Choice

Group psychotherapy was described by Alonso (1989) as "the definitive treatment for producing character change" (p. 1), because in a group setting, as Alonso explained, the "cost of character defenses is illuminated and presents a conflict which can render the same traits dystonic and thus available to interpretation and change" (p. 8). Similarly, group therapy was described by Matano and Yalom (1991) as "the treatment of choice for chemical dependency" (p. 269). Matano and Yalom attributed this choice to the "power of groups—the power to counter prevailing cultural pressures to drink, to provide effective support to those suffering from the alienation of addiction, to offer role modeling, and to harness the power of peer pressure, an important force against denial and resistance" (pp. 269–270).

Our own work with modified dynamic group therapy and the work of R. H. Klein and associates (1991) place a premium on helping group members recognize their characterological and personality problems. The group provides a "supportive holding environment" that fosters conditions for examining the character flaws that perpetuate the group members' suffering and addictive behavior.

Special Needs of the Addicted Person in Group Therapy

Whether persons are seen as vulnerable to addiction because they are narcissistically compromised through early experiences of deprivation and damage, with the persistent feelings of shame, loneliness, depression, defectiveness, and emptiness described by Kohut (1977) and Meissner (1986); whether they are understood to be narcissistically vulnerable and impaired *secondary* to the addiction (Vaillant 1983); or whether they are thought to have some "common shared factor" responsible for both the addiction and their character problems (Flores 1998)—the addicted person faces particular difficulties in the therapeutic process. A narcissistically vulnerable person may crave empathy and contact with others and yet fear and reject such contact (Liebenberg 1990). The characteristically "uneven and inconsistent" way in which cocaine-addicted persons relate suggests their dilemma upon entering therapy: "They may be alternately charming, seductive, and passively expectant, or they may act aloof, as if they do not need other people. Their supersensitivity may be evident in deferential attitudes and attempts to gain approval and acceptance, but they may rapidly shift and become ruthless and demanding in their dealings with others" (Khantzian et al. 1990, p. 40).

R. H. Klein and colleagues (1991) outlined the relevant issues involved in providing outpatient group psychotherapy for persons with character disorders with comorbid addiction: 1) these persons must be viewed as having a dual diagnosis; 2) the "recurrent dangers these individuals pose to themselves and/or to others" must be recognized; and 3) "their intense demands, during repeated crises," "their propensity for acting out anxiety and aggression, and [their] tendency to split clinicians and systems," and the difficult countertransference these patients can evoke must all be addressed (p. 99). Taking action, rather than bearing affect or anxiety or talking about things, is the preferred "expressive mode" in these patients, and the acting out may well involve relapsing to the addictive behavior (e.g., drinking, using drugs, gambling). Other characteristic acting-out behaviors may include splitting and violations of boundaries and of the group contract (e.g., attempting to conduct group business outside the group either with therapists or with other group members).

Matano and Yalom (1991) identified the tendency of alcohol-abusing persons to externalize, to "see themselves as being influenced or controlled primarily by external events," and, by way of compensation, to employ the defenses of "defiance, grandiosity, and counterdependency" (pp. 288–289). Because they do not experience themselves as being effective or in control, these persons rebel against control experienced as coming from outside. These defenses, or characteristic ways of coping, are taken into account in tailoring the group therapy to the needs of the addicted person.

Khantzian (1986, 1995, 1999) identified four areas of psychological vulnerability in the addicted person that may be viewed as disturbances or deficits in ego functioning and that potentiate characterological problems: 1) regulation of affects, 2) self-care (i.e., the capacity to protect oneself from undue risk or danger), 3) relationships with others, and 4) self-esteem. The difficulty in regulating affects manifests itself in an intensity of unmodulated feeling, often dysphoric, or in being unable to identify one's own emotions. Self-care deficits find their expression in poor attention to health, engagement in high-risk behaviors such as unsafe sex, and a general lack of concern for emotional and physical self-preservation. Relationships with others can be problematic in many ways—tumultuous, dependent, or lacking because of the individual's isolation and withdrawal. Finally, self-esteem is compromised or shaky, and this problem may manifest itself as idealization or devaluing of others, feelings of shame and inadequacy, or bravado and grandiosity.

In group treatment modified for the special needs of the addicted person, these four dimensions of everyday intrapsychic and social life become the organizing foci for understanding the addicted person's distress, behavioral difficulties, characteristic ways of handling problems, and possibilities for change. These foci provide a clarity and structure for handling complex issues with action-oriented, crisis-prone, and affectively constricted or volatile group members.

Features of Group Psychotherapy With Addicted Persons

Specific features of group therapy for the addicted person derive from a consideration of the person's special needs and have been discussed by several authors in the literature of addiction and group psychotherapy (Brown and Yalom 1977; Flores 1998; Golden et al. 1993; Khantzian et al. 1990, 1992; Matano and Yalom 1991; McAuliffe and Albert 1992; Vannicelli 1982, 1988; Yalom 1974). In addition, the emerging literature of group psychotherapy of the "difficult" patient—one whose character defenses and acting-out behavior challenge the traditional group therapy format—contributes to our understanding of what is needed in the group psychotherapy of addicted persons (Fenchel and Flapan 1985; R. H. Klein et al. 1991; Leszcz 1989; Liebenberg 1990; Rice and Rutan 1987; Roth et al. 1990; W. N. Stone and Gustafson 1982). Finally, the literature of dual diagnosis of major mental illness and substance use disorder offers guidance in modifying group therapy for this population (Addington and el-Guebaly 1998; Levy and Mann 1987; Minkoff and Drake 1991; Weiss et al. 1999).

Pregroup Preparation

Preparation for group therapy increases motivation, reduces premature dropouts, and eases fears and resistances. Khantzian and colleagues (1990) pointed out that the therapist can play a critical role at this point in establishing optimistic and realistic member expectations regarding the efficacy of the group. The therapist (in this case, for a psychodynamic group treating cocaine addiction) not only "acquaints the new members with the established ground rules, which include strict confidentiality, attendance and promptness, and abstinence from drugs and alcohol," but also discusses the benefits of group therapy, defines the focus of the group, acknowledges the difficulty of joining groups, "explains the work of therapy," and helps new members to identify their goals (Khantzian et al. 1990, pp. 46–48). Reaching out to the prospective group members, anticipating what will follow, and concretely outlining the expectations provide necessary structure to allay overwhelming anxiety in group members.

Structure and Safety

Structure and safety in a group for addicted persons are provided in a number of ways. The group contract initially serves as an organizing feature, and as the group progresses, the contract will be tested and perhaps hotly debated, which is part of the work of the group. Shared norms, explicitly stated and reiterated, also provide structure. Abstinence from the problematic addictive behavior, a commitment to talking about feelings and problems rather than acting on them in the group, and agreement about the goals of the treatment are important. Maintaining enhanced structure in a psychodynamically oriented group means explicitly endorsing certain group norms, adopting an active leadership style for the therapist, and, as in Khantzian's modified dynamic group therapy model, keeping the group's focus on specific character and interpersonal problems.

Treaters of addiction must place at a premium, and remain eternally vigilant around issues and themes of, sobriety, self-preservation, and self-care (Khantzian et al. 1992, 1995; Matano and Yalom 1991). Emphasis is placed on support and on alertness for early signs of psychological relapse such as the company patients keep and potentially risky environments. At the same time, group leaders act as facilitators, catalysts, and modulators to ensure optimal interaction and to discourage member overactivity or premature self-disclosure. In doing so, the group leader creates conditions for listening, empathy, participation, and patience for the invariable resistances that occur, as well as toleration of the anxiety and discomfort that group participation can repeatedly evoke.

Confrontation Versus Support

Matano and Yalom (1991) point to the dangers of an overly confrontational approach in the group. Although the necessity of increasing the addicted person's honesty with him- or herself and others is real, the group leader's attempt to "break down" denial can backfire, causing the patient to "leave the treatment program or to dissemble compliance while inwardly retreating" (p. 291). The key is to treat addicted patients like "other patients—that is, by relating to them in an empathic, supportive, and understanding manner" (p. 291). A central task of the group leader is thus to "manage" the anxiety that the group process, particularly confrontation, inevitably stimulates in the group members and to keep it at a tolerable level.

Leszcz (1989), discussing the group treatment of the characterologically difficult patient, views the group as first of all providing a holding environment, a place that is reliable, constant, and accepting, where group members can "relate in a nonrelated way, until they are able to ascertain that it is safe" (p. 326). The confrontation itself is spelled out as "a forceful, but supportive pressure on the patient to acknowledge something that is conscious or preconscious, but avoided because of the distress that it involves" (p. 327).

The group model of Khantzian and colleagues (1990, 1995) encourages an understanding of addictive behavior as an attempt to deal with feelings and experiences and as an adaptation that has outlived its usefulness. In their resistance to change, group members are guided "to appreciate how their ways of coping and the crises they precipitate are linked to the past; they need to acknowledge their painful feelings from the past and in the present, and to support each other in finding alternative ways to cope with their painful feeling states and problems in living" (p. 76). In other words, the group members, although they are held responsible for their choices and actions and are asked to look squarely at themselves, are not blamed and judged.

The group modality offers a particular advantage when it comes to confrontation: group members are more likely to respond to confrontation by their peers—that is, as Leszcz (1989) noted, "group members are less restricted in their range of responses and may be better able to use humor, cajole, or shock one another to force attention to a disavowed issue" (p. 327).

The Group Therapist

The therapist in the group therapy of addiction has an active, demanding role to play. Concerns for safety and structure require an alert presence and a readiness to manage and help to modulate anxiety, to address acting-out behavior, and to intervene if it is necessary to set limits and uphold the group contract, even as building cohesion and developing the work of the group proceed. This active mode of leadership is important because addicted persons with histories of neglect and trauma "do not respond well to the traditions of therapeutic passivity… [but] instead they need therapists who can actively and empathically help to engage them and each other around their vulnerabilities and the self-defeating defenses and behaviors they adopt to avoid their distress and suffering" (Khantzian et al. 1990, p. 162).

The therapist may become the focus of anger and dependency, the mediator of struggles, and the unintentional voice of the superego. Co-therapists are split into good and evil. Countertransference feelings may be difficult, especially when helplessness and fear are evoked, as they often are in these groups (R. H. Klein et al. 1991). Undergoing supervision, taking opportunities to share the work, using concurrent therapies or supports (when indicated) for the group members, working as part of a team or a program—all help to make group therapy for addiction possible and effective.

Conclusions

Current group approaches to the treatment of addictions have emerged from several traditions; self-help fellowships, the psychoeducational cognitive-behavioral modality, and the psychodynamic, interpersonal tradition. Although group approaches have evolved from these diverse theoretical and ideological viewpoints, there is a dearth of controlled studies of efficacy and outcome that could support a particular school of thought. Conceptually and pragmatically, practitioners working with addicted persons have come to similar conclusions regarding these patients' special needs in a group setting. If addicted persons are to receive the full benefit of treatment, their characterological and psychological vulnerabilities must be recognized and addressed. Traditional treatments are then modified, particularly if they do not already provide the high degree of structure and safety necessary for engaging and holding the addicted person. The group approach—in its powerful capacity to support and confront, to comfort and challenge, and to involve its members in encounters that vividly heighten awareness of interpersonal and characterological problems and provide a safe place for change—is now viewed as the treatment of choice for the addicted person. Special features of group therapy for the treatment of addiction are an emphasis on outreach and preparation for involvement in the group, a high degree of structure and active leadership, a concern for safety (particularly an awareness of the risk of relapse to the addictive behavior), a balance between confrontation and support, and a goal of moving beyond the initial cohesiveness of the group members' identification as "addicts" to helping them discover common bonds in living ordinary life.

References

Addington J, el-Guebaly N: Group treatment for substance abuse in schizophrenia. Can J Psychiatry 43:843–845, 1998

Alonso A: Character change in group therapy. Paper presented at Psychiatric Grand Rounds, The Cambridge Hospital, Cambridge, MA, September 1989

Brown S, Yalom ID: Interactional group therapy with alcoholics. J Stud Alcohol 38:426–456, 1977

Carroll KM, Nich C, Ball SA, et al: Treatment of cocaine and alcohol dependence with psychotherapy and disulfiram. Addiction 93:713–727, 1998

Cherkas MS: Synanon Foundation—a radical approach to the problem of addiction. Am J Psychiatry 121:1065–1068, 1965

Cooney NL, Kadden RM, Litt MD, et al: Matching alcoholics to coping skills or interactional therapies: two-year follow-up results. J Consult Clin Psychol 59:598–601, 1991

Drake RE, Antosca LM, Noordsy DL, et al: New Hampshire's specialized services for the dually diagnosed. New Dir Ment Health Serv 50:57–67, 1991

Fenchel GH, Flapan D: Resistance in group psychotherapy. Group 9(2):35–47, 1985

Flores PJ: Group Psychotherapy With Addicted Populations. New York, Haworth, 1998

Golden S, Halliday K, Khantzian EJ, et al: Dynamic group therapy for substance abuse patients: a reconceptualization, in Group Psychotherapy in Clinical Practice. Edited by Alonso A, Swiller HI. Washington, DC, American Psychiatric Press, 1993, pp 271–287

Herman JL: Trauma and Recovery. New York, Basic Books, 1992

Khantzian EJ: Opiate addiction: a critique of theory and some implications for treatment. Am J Psychother 28:59–70, 1974

Khantzian EJ: The ego, the self and opiate addiction: theoretical and treatment considerations. International Review of Psycho-Analysis 5:189–198, 1978

Khantzian EJ: The self-medication hypothesis of addictive disorders: focus on heroin and cocaine dependence. Am J Psychiatry 142:1259–1264, 1985

Khantzian EJ: A contemporary psychodynamic approach to drug abuse treatment. Am J Drug Alcohol Abuse 12:213–222, 1986

Khantzian EJ: How AA works and why it's important for clinicians to understand. J Subst Abuse Treat 11:157–165, 1994

Khantzian EJ: Self-regulation vulnerabilities in substance abusers: treatment implications, in The Psychology and Treatment of Addictive Behavior. Edited by Dowling S. New York, International Universities Press, 1995, pp 17–41

Khantzian EJ: The self-medication hypothesis of substance use disorders: a reconsideration and recent applications. Harv Rev Psychiatry 4:231–244, 1997

Khantzian EJ: Treating Addiction as a Human Process. Northvale, NJ, Jason Aronson, 1999

Khantzian EJ, Mack JE: Alcoholics Anonymous and contemporary psychodynamic theory, in Recent Developments in Alcoholism, Vol 7. Edited by Galanter M. New York, Plenum, 1989, pp 67–89

Khantzian EJ, Halliday KS, McAuliffe WE: Addiction and the Vulnerable Self: Modified Dynamic Group Therapy for Substance Abusers. New York, Guilford, 1990

Khantzian EJ, Halliday KS, Golden S, et al: Modified group therapy for substance abusers: a psychodynamic approach to relapse prevention. Am J Addict 1:67–76, 1992

Khantzian EJ, Golden SJ, McAuliffe WE: Group therapy for psychoactive substance use disorders, in Treatments of Psychiatric Disorders, 2nd Edition. Edited by Gabbard GO. Washington, DC, American Psychiatric Press, 1995, pp 832–839

Klein RH, Orleans JF, Soul CR: The Axis II group: treating severely characterologically disturbed patients. Int J Group Psychother 41:97–115, 1991

Kohut H: Preface, in Psychodynamics of Drug Dependence. NIDA Research Monograph 12 (DHEW Publ No [ADM] 77-470). Edited by Blaine JD, Julius DA. Washington, DC, U.S. Government Printing Office, 1977, pp vii–ix

Leszcz M: Group psychotherapy of the characterologically difficult patient. Int J Group Psychother 39:311–335, 1989

Levy MS, Mann DW: A change in orientation: therapeutic strategies for the treatment of alcoholism. Psychotherapy: Research and Practice 24:786–793, 1987

Liebenberg B: The unwanted and unwanting patient: problems in group psychotherapy of the narcissistic patient, in The Difficult Patient in Group. Edited by Roth B, Stone W, Kibel H. Madison, CT, International Universities Press, 1990, pp 311–322

Martin K, Grannandrea P, Rogers B, et al: Group intervention with pre-recovery patients. J Subst Abuse Treat 13:33–41, 1996

Matano RA, Yalom ID: Approaches to chemical dependency: chemical dependency and interactive group therapy—a synthesis. Int J Group Psychother 41:269–293, 1991

McAuliffe WE, Albert J: Clean Start. New York, Guilford, 1992

McAuliffe WE, Ch'ien JMN: Recovery training and self help: relapse-prevention program for treated opiate addicts. J Subst Abuse Treat 3:9–20, 1986

Meissner WW: Psychotherapy and the Paranoid Process. New York, Jason Aronson, 1986

Minkoff K, Drake RE (eds): Dual Diagnosis of Major Mental Illness and Substance Disorder (New Dir Ment Health Serv No 50). San Francisco, CA, Jossey-Bass, 1991

Nace EP: The Treatment of Alcoholism. New York, Brunner/Mazel, 1987

Orford J: Excessive Appetites: a Psychological View of Addictions. New York, Wiley, 1985

Poldrugo F, Forti B: Personality disorders and alcoholism treatment outcome. Drug Alcohol Depend 21:171–176, 1988

Rice CA, Rutan JS. Inpatient Group Psychotherapy. New York, Macmillan, 1987

Roth B, Stone W, Kibel H (eds): The Difficult Patient in Group. Madison, CT, International Universities Press, 1990

Stone WN, Gustafson JP: Technique in group psychotherapy of narcissistic and borderline patients. Int J Group Psychother 32:29–47, 1982

Tuttman S: Principles of psychoanalytical group therapy applied to the treatment of borderline and narcissistic disorders, in The Difficult Patient in Group. Edited by Roth B, Stone W, Kibel H. Madison, CT, International Universities Press, 1990, pp 7–29

Vaillant G: The Natural History of Alcoholism. Cambridge, MA, Harvard University Press, 1983

Vannicelli M: Group psychotherapy with alcoholics: special techniques. J Stud Alcohol 43:17–37, 1982

Vannicelli M: Group therapy aftercare for alcoholic patients. Int J Group Psychother 38:337–353, 1988

Weiss RD, Najavits LM, Greenfield SF: A relapse prevention group for patients with bipolar and substance use disorders. J Subst Abuse Treat 16:47–54, 1999

Wurmser L: The Hidden Dimension: Psychodynamics of Compulsive Drug Use. New York, Jason Aronson, 1978

Yalom ID: Group psychotherapy and alcoholism. Ann N Y Acad Sci 233:85–103, 1974

Yalom ID: Inpatient Group Psychotherapy. New York, Basic Books, 1983

Family Therapy for Alcoholism

Peter Steinglass, M.D.

During the past three decades, a growing clinical and research literature on family issues in alcoholism has pointed to the important role of family factors in the onset and clinical course of this condition (Jacob and Seilhammer 1987; Lawson and Lawson 1998; Steinglass and Robertson 1983). Considerable interest has been generated not only in investigating family aspects of alcoholism but also in applying family therapy techniques to its treatment. Thirty years ago, alcoholism clinicians by and large ignored families. The current picture is dramatically different. One is now hard pressed to find a credible alcohol addiction treatment program that does not at least give lip service to the importance of including family members in the treatment plan.

The increasing use of family-oriented treatment approaches to alcoholism has also been supported by the growing evidence of the efficacy of these approaches (Edwards and Steinglass 1995; O'Farrell 1992). These findings, both from case reports (Treadway 1989; Usher et al. 1982) and from treatment outcome research (Jacobson et al. 1989; Liepman et al. 1989a; McCrady et al. 1982, 1986; O'Farrell et al. 1985, 1992; Steinglass 1979; Zweben et al. 1988), have added a wealth of clinical data to more systematic research findings regarding alcoholism and the family. A meta-analysis conducted by Edwards and Steinglass (1995) of 21 outcome studies with designs adequate to be included in such an analysis yielded compelling evidence that 1) the involvement of a nonalcoholic spouse in a treatment program significantly improves participation rates of alcoholic family members in treatment and 2) such involvement also has a positive effect on the likelihood that these individuals will alter their drinking behavior after treatment.

But beyond the data from outcome studies, families with alcoholic members are themselves endorsing the concept of family therapy for alcoholism. Thus, pressure on the part of the nonpatient members of "alcoholic families" for increased services—the dramatic growth of the Adult Children of Alcoholics (ACOA) movement is perhaps the best example here—has brought home the need for alcoholism specialists to master family interviewing skills and to be able to provide therapeutic services to families as well as individuals.

As R. L. Collins (1990) noted, clinical wisdom has increasingly concluded that 1) response to treatment on the part of the alcoholic person is better when family members are included (this seems particularly true when spouses are incorporated in the treatment process); 2) isolation of the alcoholic person from his or her family, which is often a concomitant of chronic alcoholism, is reversed by using a family therapy approach; and 3) identification of parallel problems that frequently exist, such as sexual difficulties, parenting issues, and family violence, is often facilitated by inclusion of the family unit, thereby making the treatment more comprehensive.

Family Therapy Approaches to Alcoholism

General Issues

As will shortly be discussed, family-oriented clinicians have by now proposed a wide variety of models for incorporating family perspectives into both the assessment/diagnostic phase and the intervention phase of alcoholism treatment. However, whatever their theoretical orientation, all clinicians working with alcoholic patients from a family perspective must keep in mind four aspects of these conditions that invariably influence family life:

1. *The chronicity of the disorder.* Clinicians usually encounter alcoholism problems many years after these problems have reached pathological proportions. Relationships among the condition itself, the alcoholic family member, and the rest of the family have usually reached some steady state. The precipitating event leading to a request for treatment is often a crisis that has temporarily disrupted this steady state (e.g., a medical crisis, a drunk-driving arrest, a confrontation by an employer because of deterioration in work functioning). However, therapy, to be successful, must combat and overcome long-standing patterns of behavior that have become rigid over time. These patterns of behavior obviously include family interaction patterns.
2. *The use of a psychobiologically active drug.* Because the family's alcoholic member is chronically ingesting a psychobiologically active substance that both acts as a depressant and significantly impairs cognition and verbal communication, family behavior patterns have gradually been adopted to accommodate these defects. These patterns are often not immediately apparent and therefore represent a challenge to the family therapist during the initial phases of treatment.
3. *Sober-intoxicated cycling of interactional patterns.* Direct observations of interactional behavior of alcoholic families have indicated that these families manifest two quite distinct interactional styles: one when the alcoholic member is sober and another when the alcoholic member is intoxicated (Steinglass et al. 1977). It has been suggested, therefore, that a unique feature of the alcoholic family is its dual-state interactional style. It has further been suggested that family therapists must develop strategies for accessing information about the intoxicated interactional state in order to understand behaviors that have developed in these families. (One such strategy, developed by Liepman et al. [1989a], will be described in the next section.)
4. *Intergenerational transmission of alcoholism.* Alcoholism is a familial condition. Most likely, both genetic and psychosocial factors contribute to the intergenerational transmission of alcoholism. Family therapists must understand that their interventions are

appropriately directed not only at containing alcoholic behavior as it is currently being manifested but also at attending to the needs of children within the family, with the goal of disrupting possible intergenerational transmission of the condition (Wolin et al. 1980). Thus, family therapy might be considered unique among the various psychological therapies for alcoholism in that it explicitly addresses prevention of the disorder in at-risk children in addition to providing intervention for currently existing alcoholism problems (Bennett et al. 1987; Cermak 1986).

Overview of Treatment Models

Over the past three decades, family therapists have employed a number of conceptual models for designing treatment strategies for alcoholism. The best known of these is the *family systems* approach, a model in which principles of general systems theory are applied to families. In this approach, particular attention is paid to ways in which families, as behavioral systems, regulate their internal and external environments and how patterns of interactional behavior change over time. Both structural and strategic approaches to family therapy, as well as newer constructivist approaches, use family systems theory as their conceptual base.

A second approach that has been widely used is the *family behavioral* model, in which classical conditioning principles are extended to interpersonal behavior. Concepts of reciprocity, coercion, and reinforcement are applied to an analysis of the contingencies that help explain patterns of interactional behavior.

A third approach focuses particular attention on constructs of *social systems* and *social networks,* using a variety of family interventions to support a treatment plan targeted at the alcoholic individual as the primary patient. Here, the family's involvement is undertaken to obtain a more complete and accurate alcoholism history, to increase the likelihood of engaging the patient in treatment, to increase the patient's compliance with biological treatments (e.g., disulfiram), and to increase social supports for the patient during the postdetoxification period.

Although family therapy approaches to alcoholism have lagged behind family therapy for other psychiatric and medical conditions (e.g., schizophrenia, eating disorders, child behavioral disorders), by now virtually every one of the abovementioned conceptual approaches has been applied to treatment of alcoholism. For example, the family systems approach forms the underpinnings of the therapy approaches suggested by Steinglass et al. (1987), Treadway (1989), and Berenson (1979), among others. (A manualized version of a family systems treatment approach, developed by Shoham and colleagues [Rohrbaugh et al. 1996], has been researched in a controlled clinical trial of family systems versus behavioral treatment approaches for alcoholism [Beutler et al. 1997].)

Behavioral approaches, on the other hand, are the basis for the marital therapy approach advocated by McCrady and colleagues (1982, 1986) and O'Farrell and colleagues (O'Farrell 1993; O'Farrell and Cutter 1984; O'Farrell et al. 1985). (The study by Beutler et al. [1997] mentioned above also included a cognitive-behavioral couples treatment as one of its comparison treatments. A detailed manual describing this approach was prepared as part of the study [Wakefield et al. 1996] and is the clearest explication to date of behavioral principles applied to couples therapy for alcoholism.)

Family stress and coping concepts are perhaps best represented by the family functioning model proposed by Kaufman and Pattison (1981) and by the network therapy approach advocated by Galanter (1993). (Galanter has also prepared a manualized version of his network therapy model, so by now all of the major family-oriented approaches to alcoholism treatment have been specified in manual form.) In each of these areas—family systems, cognitive-behavioral, and family stress and coping—these different conceptual models have been used 1) to suggest strategies for assessment in which family data become important components of the diagnostic process and 2) to guide the treatment intervention approaches.

Family Systems Approaches to Assessment and Detoxification

Of the various family therapy approaches to the treatment of alcoholism outlined above, it is the family systems approach that is perhaps the most unique. I will therefore describe in somewhat greater detail how the first two phases of treatment—assessment and detoxification—are implemented in a family systems therapy approach.

Assessment Strategies

In the typical clinical situation, therapists are guided in their assessment approaches by the need to answer two fundamental questions: 1) What is wrong here? (i.e., the question of diagnosis) and 2) How should the clinical problem be treated? Treatment evaluation typically includes assessment of patient strengths and weaknesses, as well as a review of treatment options.

Family therapists obviously undertake the same assessment process, but rather than focus on each family member separately, they emphasize a family-level evaluation. Toward that goal, the assessment phase is typically carried out via conjoint interviews of the entire family and/or of important subunits (especially the marital dyad). In many regards, the material covered in these interviews parallels that covered in an individual assessment of an alcoholic patient. With family-level evaluation, however, the clinician has available the multiple perspectives of all family members, and the database therefore tends to be both richer and far more reliable than is the case with assessment of the alcoholic individual alone.

This ability to obtain multiple perspectives has proven especially valuable in assessing the impact of intoxicated behavior on such family regulatory behaviors as conjoint problem-solving styles, daily routines, and family rituals. A key aspect of the family systems model for treatment of alcoholism posits that differences in patterns of interactional behavior in the presence versus absence of active drinking must be understood *as a prerequisite* to undertaking detoxification. Otherwise, the complex ways in which alcohol-related behaviors have become incorporated into family life will not be understood, and, as a consequence, removal of alcohol may inadvertently destabilize rather than improve family life.

Consequently, interest has been generated in the development of assessment techniques for specifically addressing these differences. In some instances, an opportunity to assess behavior under "wet" (alcohol present) conditions is afforded by the alcoholic family member appearing for a treatment session in an intoxicated state. The therapist can use this opportunity to observe differences in interaction patterns regarding such variables as activity/passivity of various family members, interaction rates, range of affective expression, levels of direct conflict, verbal content (especially as regards raising of problem areas not previously mentioned), interactional distance, prevailing mood, and degree of interpersonal engagement. For example, an observation that a marital couple seems more emotionally engaged during such a session might lead to speculations that the couple is inadvertently using this engagement to carry out problem solving during periods of intoxication, a factor that might presumably then become a reinforcer of subsequent episodes of drinking.

At the same time, it is important to note that studies of such differences in patterns of interactional behavior under wet versus dry conditions, despite having established that such differences do exist, remain speculative as to the functional or adaptive consequences of this biphasic quality of family life (Jacob and Leonard 1988; Jacob et al. 1983; Liepman et al. 1989b; Steinglass et al. 1977). Also important to underscore here is that individual families differ in their response to the presence of an intoxicated member. (For example, one family might forcefully engage the intoxicated member, whereas another family might avoid or isolate the intoxicated member.) This interfamilial variability in response also suggests that the direction of changes in interactional patterns during wet conditions may vary considerably from family to family as well.

Further, it might also be the case that the concept that alcohol use might have adaptive consequences for family behavior would be true only for certain *subtypes* of alcoholic families (e.g., the "neurotic/enmeshed" or "disintegrated" families described by Kaufman [1985b] or the "stable wet" families described by Steinglass [1980]). However, for these families, at least, an assessment strategy that allows the therapist to carefully observe and delineate behavior sequences in families under wet conditions might be quite useful.

One such technique for more systematically carrying out such an enterprise has been suggested by Liepman et al. (1989c), a technique they have called "family behavior-loop mapping." In this technique, sequential behaviors are mapped to construct circular loops, with particular emphasis placed on determining which aspects of the sequence occur as the alcoholic family member moves from "dry" to "wet" to "dry" conditions in cyclical fashion.

An analysis of these loops is then useful not only in developing a better appreciation of the interface between drinking behavior and patterns of family interaction but also in identifying specific behavioral sequences that might be addressed in a behaviorally oriented or systemically oriented family therapy approach.

Family Detoxification

The family systems model of alcoholism treatment shares with virtually all other treatment approaches the assumption that meaningful psychotherapeutic work can only proceed after the alcoholic family member, the so-called identified patient, has stopped drinking. However, the approach to detoxification in the family systems model is fundamentally different from other treatment approaches in two ways: 1) the goal for this treatment phase is *family-level* detoxification (including, of course, abstinence on the part of the alcoholic identified patient), and 2) the central technique for accomplishing detoxification is the establishment of a contract *with the entire family* to achieve an alcohol-free environment at a family, as well as individual, level. (The most complete description of this approach to treatment can be found in Steinglass et al. [1987].)

The underlying rationale for family detoxification could be stated as follows. Whether or not the alcoholism started because of the behavior of one individual within the family, by the time the alcoholism reaches its chronic phase it has become a central organizer of important aspects of family life. For the marital couple being treated, it is likely that important aspects of their interaction patterns are now inexorably linked to patterns of alcohol consumption on the part of the identified patient. Daily routines may be paced to drinking patterns. Interaction rates, problem solving, and so forth all have been shaped by the types of behaviors the couple manifest when drinking is occurring. Each spouse has developed strong opinions and feelings about the reasons for and implications of alcoholic drinking, and these views have become fixed. Associated behaviors (e.g., physical violence, inconsistent marital and extramarital sexual behavior, impaired work performance) and their exigencies have required family attention and responses. These responses may also have placed heavy demands on family emotional and financial resources. In all these ways, alcoholism has invaded family life and dictated the shape and flavor of life within the family. The cessation of drinking by the identified patient will therefore have profound implications for all members of the family. Hence, the entire family has a stake in how the detoxification process unfolds. Further, because chronic alcoholism is now driving (i.e., organizing) much of family life, detoxification will at least initially be a *destabilizing* event for the family. For these reasons, it is important that the detoxification process be framed from a family as well as an identified patient perspective. Consequently, treatment has the twofold goal of 1) facilitating a cessation of drinking on the part of the alcoholic family member and 2) establishing an "alcohol-free" psychosocial environment for the family. It is this second part of the overall goal that differentiates the family systems approach from more traditional individual-oriented treatments. The term *psychosocial environment* as applied to the family refers to all settings in which the family interacts and behaves as a unit, including at home and in relationships with friends and relatives.

To accomplish the above aims, Steinglass et al. (1987) suggest a multiphase process that centers on the development of a written contract conjointly constructed by the family and the therapist—the *family detoxification contract.* The process begins with the therapist's explaining to the couple the rationale and need for detoxification as the first step in successful treatment, and then proceeds through a series of steps in which the couple identifies what has to be done to achieve an alcohol-free environment and assigns tasks to accomplish these goals.

As a first step, a contract is developed that is intended to ensure that no drinking occurs at home and that the household environment is made totally alcohol-free. Once this first step has been accomplished (a contract has been designed *and* successfully implemented), the family environment metaphor is expanded to include the environments of the extended family and the family's social and work networks. The contract first aims at detoxifying the family's daily routines and then moves on to ensure that the family's external boundaries are protected from any new alcohol invasion and, finally, that when the family moves into the outside world, it does so within a protective bubble that still keeps it alcohol-free (essentially taking an alcohol-free environment with them as they as a family unit venture out into the world).

Once the contract moves beyond the simple extrapolation of the family environment concept as analogous to the household and daily routines, the complexity of the interactions increases. The number of possible combinations and permutations exceeds the ability of the contract to anticipate all possible situations, so instead the contract focuses on a delimited number of "modal" exchanges between the family and the outside world that serve as examples of how the contract terms should be interpreted in such circumstances. Critical here is the ability of the therapist to identify with the couple two or three situations that in the past would have been "high risk" situations vis-à-vis drinking. Once these high-risk situations are identified, the couple then rehearses with the therapist an alternative way of handling the situation that will protect the alcohol-free family environment.

Finally, the therapist uses two additional techniques throughout the process of contracting that are designed to reinforce and solidify the terms of the contract itself. These techniques are 1) urging the family to make the terms of the contract "public" by sharing with friends or relatives that the contract has been established and is in effect and 2) using *rehearsing* techniques to *anticipate* any problems the couple might have with implementation of the details of the contract.

To summarize, the success of family-level detoxification depends on six integrated components: 1) the detoxification contract; 2) a core set of metaphors around which the detoxification contract is framed; 3) a multistage strategy for implementing the scope of detoxification; 4) "public disclosure" to reinforce the meaning and importance of the detoxification contract; 5) a prospective, anticipatory stance to identify potential challenges to abstinence; and 6) ample rehearsal of strategies to effectively meet these potential challenges to abstinence.

The family detoxification component is the most unique aspect of the systems treatment model. By asking the couple to work together on the framing of the contract and by establishing as the treatment goals the metaphor of an alcohol-free family environment, the therapist is automatically reframing the entire alcoholism issue in family rather than individual terms. Although not challenging that it is the identified patient who has actually been consuming the alcohol, the therapist is dramatically reinforcing the concept that the chronic alcohol abuse has in important ways taken over family life. Thus, at the same time this phase of treatment is aimed at the important goal of cessation of drinking as a necessary prerequisite for further treatment, the essential reframing work is also being carried out that will place the couple in a position to subsequently reevaluate how to reorganize family life to put in place the necessary relapse-prevention tools and structures.

Some Obstacles to Family Therapy Implementation in Alcoholism Treatment Settings

Despite the clear-cut advances in the development of clinical models incorporating family systems principles discussed previously, and despite the compelling evidence of the profound impact of chronic alcoholism on family life, it is still the case that family therapy is often relegated to a peripheral position in traditional alcoholism treatment programs. A number of factors can be pointed to as likely contributors to this situation.

The current politics of substance abuse treatment (i.e., an emphasis on viewing addictions treatment as a subspecialty with self-contained addictions treatment programs) has undermined the ability of experienced family therapists and experienced substance abuse clinicians to meet on a common ground. For example, it would be highly unusual for a family therapist to be included as a faculty member in a certified alcoholism counselor (CAC) training program. Typically, therefore, the "family" component offered in an alcoholism or drug abuse rehabilitation program is being administered by therapists with only elementary-level training in family interview skills and conjoint therapy techniques. Concern must also be expressed about the tendency to provide uniform, "prepackaged" treatment modules for families, as if all families with alcoholism and/or drug abuse problems have comparable issues and psychodynamics.

In addition, these family treatment modules are rarely informed by either advances in family systems treatment approaches or the growing body of research findings about alcoholism and the family. For example, family researchers have delineated major within-group differences in alcoholic families and have proposed interesting typologies of families based on drinking patterns (Dunn et al. 1987; Jacob and Leonard 1988; Steinglass 1981), family developmental issues (Steinglass et al. 1987), or family functional status (Kaufman and Pattison 1981). The clinical relevance and implications of these typologies have also been thoroughly described. Yet few treatment programs seem cognizant of these research-based clinical treatment models, preferring instead to impose standardized programs on families independent of the heterogeneity of this clinical population.

Further, the tendency in many treatment programs to compartmentalize individual and family-focused treatment components precludes the implementation of systems-oriented treatment techniques. For example, in many treatment programs, psychiatrists work exclusively with the identified patient, leaving to other professionals the tasks of evaluating and providing services for families. Psychiatrists, who often are poorly trained in family interviewing techniques, are therefore more comfortable treating the identified patient alone. Because of this separation of treatment responsibilities, the psychiatrist is likely to view the family as adjunctive to the treatment process and more likely to focus attention solely on the clinical parameters of the individual alcoholic patient. For families, however, the issues center on how to cope with the challenges of a chronic, episodic illness. Although they can usually be co-opted into supporting a treatment plan primarily designed to address the needs of the alcoholic family member, they often do so at the expense of their own needs and developmental priorities. In this sense, treatment success for the alcoholic family member can at the same time result in developmental distortions and arrest for the rest of the family.

References

Bennett LA, Wolin SJ, Reiss D, et al: Couples at risk for transmission of alcoholism: protective influences. Fam Process 26:111–129, 1987

Berenson D: The therapist's relationship with couples with an alcoholic member, in The Family Therapy of Drug and Alcohol Abuse. Edited by Kaufman E, Kaufmann P. New York, Gardner, 1979, pp 233–242

Beutler LE, Shoham V, Jacob T, et al: Family versus behavioral treatment of alcoholism, a final report on Grant No I-RO-11108486. Washington, DC, National Institute of Alcoholism and Alcohol Abuse, 1997

Cermak TL: Diagnosing and Treating Co-Dependence. Minneapolis, MN, Johnson Institute Books, 1986

Collins RL: Family treatment of alcohol abuse: behavioral and systems perspectives, in Alcohol and the Family: Research and Clinical Perspectives. Edited by Collins RL, Leonard KE, Searles JS. New York, Guilford, 1990, pp 285–308

Dunn NJ, Jacob T, Hummon N, et al: Marital stability in alcoholic-spouse relationships as a function of drinking pattern and location. J Abnorm Psychol 96:99–107, 1987

Edwards ME, Steinglass P: Family therapy treatment outcomes for alcoholism. J Marital Fam Ther 21:475–509, 1995

Galanter M: Network Therapy for Addiction: a New Approach. New York, Basic Books, 1993

Jacob T, Leonard KE: Alcoholic-spouse interaction as a function of alcoholism subtype and alcohol consumption interaction. J Abnorm Psychol 97:231–237, 1988

Jacob T, Seilhammer R: Alcoholism and family interaction, in Family Interaction and Psychopathology: Theories, Methods and Findings. Edited by Jacob T. New York, Plenum, 1987, pp 535–580

Jacob T, Dunn N, Leonard KE: Patterns of alcohol abuse and family stability. Alcohol Clin Exp Res 7:382–385, 1983

Jacobson NS, Holtzworth-Munroe A, Schmaling KB: Marital therapy and spouse involvement in the treatment of depression, agoraphobia, and alcoholism. J Consult Clin Psychol 57:5–10, 1989

Kaufman E, Pattison EM: Different methods of family therapy in the treatment of alcoholism. J Stud Alcohol 42:951–971, 1981

Lawson A, Lawson G: Alcoholism and the Family. Gaithersburg, MD, Aspen, 1998

Liepman MR, Nirenberg TD, Begin AM: Evaluation of a program designed to help families and significant others to motivate resistant alcoholics into recovery. Am J Drug Alcohol Abuse 15:209–221, 1989a

Liepman MR, Nirenberg TD, Doolittle RH, et al: Family functioning of male alcoholics and their female partners during periods of drinking and abstinence. Fam Process 28:239–249, 1989b

Liepman MR, Silvia LY, Nirenberg TD: The use of family behavior loop mapping for substance abuse. Family Relations 38:282–287, 1989c

McCrady BS, Moreau J, Paolino TJ Jr, et al: Joint hospitalization and couples therapy for alcoholism: a four-year follow-up. J Stud Alcohol 43:1244–1250, 1982

McCrady BS, Noel NE, Abrams DB, et al: Comparative effectiveness of three types of spouse involvement in outpatient behavioral alcoholism treatment. J Stud Alcohol 47:459–467, 1986

O'Farrell TJ: Families and alcohol problems: an overview of treatment research. Journal of Family Psychology 5:339–359, 1992

O'Farrell TJ (ed): Treating Alcohol Problems: Marital and Family Interventions. New York, Guilford, 1993

O'Farrell TJ, Cutter HSG: Behavioral marital therapy couples groups for male alcoholics and their wives. J Subst Abuse Treat 1:191–204, 1984

O'Farrell TJ, Cutter HSG, Floyd FJ: Evaluating behavioral marital therapy for male alcoholics: effects of marital adjustment and communication from before to after treatment. Behavior Therapy 16:147–167, 1985

O'Farrell TJ, Cutter HSG, Choquette KA, et al: Behavioral marital therapy for male alcoholics: marital adjustment during the two years after treatment. Behavior Therapy 16:147–167, 1992

Rohrbaugh MJ, Shoham V, Spungen C, et al: Family systems therapy in practice: a systemic couples therapy for problem drinking, in Comprehensive Textbook of Psychotherapy: Theory and Practice. Edited by Bongar B, Beutler LE. New York, Oxford University Press, 1996, pp 228–253

Steinglass P: An experimental treatment program for alcoholic couples. J Stud Alcohol 40:159–182, 1979

Steinglass P: The alcoholic family at home: patterns of interaction in dry, wet, and transitional stages of alcoholism. Arch Gen Psychiatry 38:578–584, 1981

Steinglass P, Robertson A: The alcoholic family, in The Biology of Alcoholism, Vol 6: The Pathogenesis of Alcoholism: Psychosocial Factors. Edited by Kissin B, Begleiter H. New York, Plenum, 1983, pp 243–307

Steinglass P, Davis DI, Berenson D: Observations of conjointly hospitalized "alcoholic couples" during sobriety and intoxication: implications for theory and therapy. Fam Process 16:1–16, 1977

Steinglass P, Bennett LA, Wolin SJ, et al: The Alcoholic Family. New York, Basic Books, 1987

Treadway D: Before It's Too Late: Working With Substance Abuse in the Family. New York, WW Norton, 1989

Usher ML, Jay J, Glass DR Jr: Family therapy as a treatment modality for alcoholism. J Stud Alcohol 43:927–938, 1982

Wakefield P, Williams RE, Yost E, et al: Couples Therapy for Alcoholism: Cognitive-Behavioral Treatment Manual. New York, Guilford, 1996

Wolin SJ, Bennett LA, Noonan DL, et al: Disrupted family rituals: a factor in the intergenerational transmission of alcoholism. J Stud Alcohol 41:199–214, 1980

Zweben A, Pearlman S, Li S: A comparison of brief advice and conjoint therapy in the treatment of alcohol abuse: the results of the Marital Systems Study. British Journal of Addiction 83:899–916, 1988

Family Therapy in Substance Abuse Treatment

Edward Kaufman, M.D.

Substance abuse has a profound effect on the family, and the family is a critical factor in the treatment of substance-abusing patients. In this chapter subpart I focus on the role of family therapy in substance abuse treatment. Family therapy cannot stand alone in the treatment of serious substance abuse. However, it is a valuable and often necessary adjunct to treatment, particularly when integrated into a comprehensive program. There are three basic phases of treatment involving the family: 1) developing a system for establishing and maintaining a drug-free state, 2) establishing a workable method of family therapy, and 3) dealing with family readjustment after the cessation of substance abuse.

Establishing and Maintaining a Drug-Free State

Family treatment of substance abuse begins with development of a system to achieve and maintain abstinence. This system, together with specific family therapeutic techniques and knowledge of family patterns commonly seen in families with a substance-abusing member, provides a workable, therapeutic approach to substance abuse.

Family treatment of substance abuse must begin with an assessment of the extent of the substance dependence as well as the difficulties it causes for the individual and the family. The quantification of substance abuse history can take place with the entire family present; persons who abuse substances often will be honest in this setting, and "confession" is a helpful way to begin communication. Moreover, other family members can often

The author wishes to acknowledge the assistance of Laura Lowe in the preparation of this manuscript.

provide more accurate information than the substance-abusing family member, known as the identified patient. However some identified patients will give an accurate history only when interviewed alone. In taking a drug abuse history, it is important to know the patient's current and past use of every type of abusable drug as well as alcohol, including details about quantity, quality, duration, expense, how intake was supported and prevented, physical effects, tolerance, withdrawal, and medical complications. At times, other substance-abusing persons within the family, both in the past and currently, are identified, and their own use and its consequences should be quantified without putting the family on the defensive. It is also essential to document the family's patterns of reactivity to drug use and abuse. Previous attempts at abstinence and treatment are reviewed to determine components of success and failure. The specific method necessary to achieve abstinence can only be decided on after the extent and nature of substance abuse are quantified.

Establishing a System for Achieving a Drug-Free State

It is critical first to establish a system for enabling the substance-abusing identified patient to become drug-free so that family therapy can take place effectively. The specific methods employed to achieve abstinence vary according to the extent of use, abuse, and dependence. Mild to moderate abuse in adolescents can often be controlled if both parents can agree on clear limits and expectations and on how to enforce them. Substance abuse in older persons may also stop if they are aware of the medical or psychological consequences to themselves or of the effects on their family.

If substance abuse is moderately severe or intermittent and unaccompanied by physical dependence (e.g., occasional use of hallucinogens or weekend cocaine abuse), the family is offered a variety of measures, such as regular attendance at Alcoholics Anonymous (AA), Narcotics Anonymous (NA), Cocaine Anonymous (CA), or Co-Anon for the identified patient and Al-Anon or Nar-Anon for family members (Kaufman 1985).

Some persons whose substance abuse is mild to moderate but who are resistant to self-help groups may find that another method (e.g., religion, exercise regimen, relaxation techniques, career change) helps them stay off drugs. If these methods fail, short-term hospitalization or treatment in a 20-hour or more weekly intensive outpatient program may be necessary to establish a substance-free state and to begin effective treatment, even with nondependent patients. In more severe cases of drug abuse and dependence, more aggressive methods are necessary to establish a substance-free state. However, if the substance abuse is so severe that the identified patient is unable to attend sessions without being under the influence of drugs, if social or vocational functioning is severely impaired, if there is drug-related violence, or if physical dependence is present, the first priority in treatment is to stop the substance abuse immediately. This involves persuading the family to pull together to achieve at least temporary abstinence. Often, abstinence is best achieved in a hospital setting. Thus, if the abuse pattern is severe, hospitalization will be established as a requirement very early in therapy.

Establishing a Method for Maintaining a Drug-Free State

The family is urged to adopt a system that will enable the identified patient to continue to stay free of abusable substances. This system is part of the therapeutic contract made early in treatment. A lifetime commitment to abstinence is not required. Rather, the "one day at a time" approach of AA is recommended; the patient is asked to establish a system for abstinence that is committed to for only one day at a time but that is renewed daily using the basic principles of AA (the 12 Steps). When the substance-abusing person has a history of past or present drug dependence, therapy is most successful when total abstinence is advocated.

Many persons must initially shop for a 12-Step group in which they feel personally comfortable. Every person recovering from substance abuse is strongly encouraged to attend small study groups that work on AA's 12 Steps, as well as larger meetings that often have speakers and are open for anyone to attend. In heroin-addicted persons, abstinence can also be achieved by drug-aided measures such as methadone maintenance or naltrexone blockade (see Chapter 29 in this volume). These medications work quite well in conjunction with family therapy, because work with the family enhances compliance, and the blocking effects that these medications exert on the primary drug of abuse help calm the family system so that family and individual therapy can take place.

Hospitalization also calms down an overreactive family system. Another advantage of hospitalization is that it provides an intensive 24-hour-a-day orientation to treatment. This total immersion in treatment for a 14- to 30-day period may provide the impetus for the drug-abusing person to get off and stay off drugs, particularly if effective, comprehensive aftercare is provided. Persons who have been dependent on illicit drugs for more than a few years generally do not do well in short-term programs, although these programs may buy time so that effective individual and family therapy can occur. For drug-dependent persons who repeatedly fail in outpatient and short-term hospital programs, insistence on long-term residential treatment is the only workable alternative. Most families, however, will not accept this until other methods have failed. Toward this end, the therapist must be willing to maintain long-term ties with the family, even through multiple treatment failures. On the other hand, it may be more helpful to terminate treatment if the identified patient continues to abuse chemicals, because continuing family treatment implies that change is occurring when it is not. One way to maintain therapist-family ties while not condoning substance abuse is to work with the family without the identified patient present (as will be described in the next section). In other cases, it is more effective to terminate treatment until all family members are willing and able to adopt a workable program for enforcing abstinence. Families who believe that therapy is being terminated in their best interest often return a few months or years later, ready and willing to commit to abstinence from drugs of abuse (Kaufman 1985).

Working With Families With Continued Drug Abuse

The family therapist is in a unique position in regard to continued substance abuse and other manifestations of the identified patient's resistance to treatment, including total nonparticipation. The family therapist still has a highly motivated patient—the family. One technique that can be used with an absent or highly resistant patient is the "intervention" (Johnson 1973), which was developed for use with alcoholic persons but can be readily adapted to work with persons who abuse other drugs, particularly those who are middle class, involved with their nuclear families, and currently employed.

In this technique, the family (excluding the identified patient) and significant network members (e.g., employer, fellow employees, friends, and neighbors) are coached to confront the identified patient with concern, but without hostility, about the destructiveness of his or her drug abuse and behavior. They agree in advance on what treatment is necessary and then insist on it. As many family members as possible should be included, because the breakthrough for acceptance of treatment may come from an apparently uninvolved family member such as a grandchild or a cousin. The involvement of the employer is crucial and, in some cases, may be sufficient in and of itself to motivate the drug-abusing person to seek treatment. The employer who clearly makes treatment a precondition of continued employment, who supports time off for treatment, and who guarantees a job on completion of the initial treatment course is a very valuable ally. The employer's model is also a very helpful one for the family members, who need to be able to say, "We love you, and because we love you, we will not continue to live with you if you continue to abuse drugs. If you accept the treatment being offered to you and continue to stay off drugs, we will renew our lifetime commitment to you" (Kaufman 1985).

If the substance-abusing person does not meet the above criteria for an intervention or if the intervention has failed, the therapist is left with the problems of dealing with a substance-abusing family. Berenson (1979) offers a workable three-step therapeutic strategy for dealing with the spouses or other family members of persons who continue to abuse substances or who are dependent on substances. The first step is to calm the family by explaining problems, suggesting solutions, and teaching coping mechanisms. The second step is to create an external supportive network for family members so that the emotional intensity is not all invested in the relationship with the identified patient or redirected to the therapist. Two types of support systems are available to spouses: a self-help group in the Al-Anon, Nar-Anon, or Co-Anon model; and a significant others (SO) group led by a trained therapist. The third step involves giving the spouse three choices: 1) keep doing exactly what you are doing, 2) detach or emotionally distance yourself from the drug-abusing spouse, or 3) physically separate or physically distance yourself.

As part of the initial contract with a family, it is suggested that the identified patient's partner remain in individual treatment, Al-Anon, Co-Anon, Nar-Anon, or a spouse group even if the identified patient drops out. Other family members are also encouraged to continue in family therapy and support groups. It should be reemphasized that whenever we maintain therapy with a family wherein serious drug abuse continues, we have the responsibility of not maintaining the illusion that a family is resolving problems when in fact they are really reinforcing them. On the other hand, even when the substance-abusing family member does not participate in treatment, the therapist may be quite helpful to the rest of the family.

Motivating the Entire Family to Participate

Although in the previous section I described how to deal with a family when the identified patient is resistant to treatment participation, it should be obvious that treatment works best when the entire family is available for therapy. Once the family therapist has knowledge of the substance-abusing family, a program for dealing with substance abuse, and a workable personal method of family therapy, it becomes remarkably easy to get the entire family to come in for treatment. The person who calls for an initial appointment is generally the one who is best able to mobilize the entire household to attend a therapy session. However, in some cases the therapist may have to contact one or more family members directly. If a reluctant family member claims to be no longer involved with the family, the therapist can truthfully point out to this person that he or she would be valuable because of his or her objectivity. If the family member says that his or her relationship with the family is too painful, then the therapist can emphasize the potential helpfulness of that person's joining the family therapy. The therapist may emphasize his or her own inability to help the family unless the member attends. Reluctant family members can also be asked to attend to protect their interests, to prevent a skewed view, to ensure that all views are expressed, and to preserve fairness, and can even be asked to attend a therapy session without any obligation to participate (Bauman 1981). Most family members will agree to a single evaluative visit. It then becomes imperative for the therapist to establish a contract with the family that all members feel will relieve their pain as well as that of the identified patient.

The concept of the family as a multigenerational system necessitates that the entire family be involved in treatment. The family members necessary to perform optimum treatment consist of the entire household and any relatives who maintain regular (i.e., approximately weekly) contact with the family. Use of a multigenerational approach involving grandparents, parents, spouse, and children at the beginning of family therapy as well as at certain key points throughout treatment is advised. However, the key unit with substance-abusing persons younger than about age 24 years is the identified patient and his or her siblings and parents. The critical unit with married substance-abusing persons older than 24 years is the identified patient and his or her spouse. However, the more dependent the identified patient is on the parents, the more critical is work with the parents.

Family therapy limited to any dyad is most difficult. The mother–addicted son dyad is almost impossible to treat; someone else, such as a lover, grandparent, aunt, or uncle, should be brought in if treatment is to succeed. If absolutely no one else is available from the natural family network, then surrogate family members in multiple family therapy groups can provide support and leverage to facilitate restructuring maneuvers (Kaufman and Kaufmann 1977).

Treatment for drug-addicted persons and their spouses has been less effective than treatment for alcoholic couples (Kaufman 1985). This finding led Stanton and Todd (1982) to suggest that family treatment of narcotic-addicted males begin with their parents and that work with the addicted person and spouse as a couple should not begin until the addicted person's parents can "release" him to the spouse. An essential aspect of treating couples with children is focusing on their functions as parents. Therapy involving children has the distinct advantage of helping the parents develop parenting skills.

Substance-abusing women with young children are often best treated in programs that can house the children jointly, provide child care, and attend directly to parenting and child care issues.

An Integrated Approach to a Workable System of Family Treatment

Family Diagnosis

Accurate diagnosis is as important a cornerstone of family therapy as it is of individual therapy. In family diagnosis, we look at family interactional and communication patterns and relationships. In assessing a family, it is helpful to construct a map of their basic alliances and roles (Minuchin 1974). We also examine the family rules, boundaries, and adaptability. We look for coalitions, particularly transgenerational ones; shifting alliances; splits; cutoffs; and triangulation. We observe communication patterns, confirmation and disconfirmation, unclear messages, and conflict resolution. We note the family's stage in the family life cycle. We also note mind reading (i.e., predicting reactions and reacting to them before they happen, or "knowing" what someone thinks or wants), double binds, and fighting styles. It is helpful to obtain an abbreviated three-generation genogram that focuses on the identified patient, his or her parents and progeny, and the spouse's parents.

The genogram (Bowen 1971) has become a basic tool in many family therapy approaches. A genogram is a pictorial chart of the persons involved in a three-generational relationship system. In stepfamilies, the initial genogram must include the noncustodial parent(s) and the geographical location and family situation of all children from prior marriages, because this information may be extremely significant.

Overview of Family Treatment Techniques

Each of the systems of family therapy currently in use is briefly summarized below, with an emphasis on the application of these techniques to substance abuse. The family therapy systems are classified into four schools: structural-strategic, psychodynamic, Bowen's systems, and behavioral. Any of these types of family therapy can be applied to treatment of substance abuse if these systems' common family patterns are kept in mind and if a method to control substance abuse is implemented.

Structural and Strategic Family Therapy

Structural and strategic family therapy approaches are combined because they were developed by many of the same practitioners and because shifts between the two are frequently made by the therapist, depending on the family's needs.

The thrust of structural family therapy is to restructure the family system by creating interactional change within the session. The therapist actively becomes a part of the family, yet retains sufficient autonomy to restructure the family (Stanton 1981).

In the strategic family therapy approach, symptoms are viewed as maladaptive attempts to deal with difficulties, which develop a homeostatic life of their own and continue to regulate family transactions. The strategic therapist works to substitute new behavior patterns for the destructive, repetitive cycles. The techniques used in strategic therapy (Stanton 1981) include the following:

1. Using tasks with the therapist responsible for planning a strategy to solve the family's problems.
2. Putting the problem in solvable form.
3. Placing considerable emphasis on change outside the sessions.
4. Learning to take the path of least resistance so that the family's existing behaviors are used positively.
5. Using paradox, including restraining change and exaggerating family roles.
6. Allowing change to occur in stages. (The family hierarchy may be shifted to a different, abnormal one before being reorganized into a new functional hierarchy.)
7. Using metaphorical directives in which the family members do not know they have received a directive.

Psychodynamic Family Therapy

The psychodynamic approach to family therapy has rarely been applied to treatment of substance-abusing persons, because they usually require a more active, limit-setting emphasis on the here and now than is typically associated with psychodynamic techniques.

However, if certain basic limitations are kept in mind, psychodynamic principles can be extremely helpful in the family therapy of these patients.

The symptoms of the identified patient are viewed in the context of his or her own remote past as well as that of every family member. The goal is to change the entire family system so that dysfunction does not occur in other family members once the symptoms of the identified patient have been alleviated.

Two cornerstones support the implementation of psychodynamic techniques: the therapist's self-knowledge and a detailed family history. Every family member will internalize a therapist's good qualities, such as warmth, trust, trustworthiness, assertion, empathy, and understanding. Likewise, they may incorporate less-desirable qualities such as aggression, despair, and emotional distancing. It is absolutely essential that a therapist thoroughly understand his or her own emotional reactions as well as those of the family.

Important elements of psychodynamic family therapy include interpreting countertransference, overcoming resistance, working through, and interpreting projective identification.

A specific psychodynamic technique that is often helpful with substance-abusing persons is the family-of-origin technique, as developed by Framo (1981). In this technique, the therapist works with the family of the substance-abusing adult to help them understand how past difficulties are being replayed in the present and to begin to shift these transferential problems.

Bowen's Systems Family Therapy

In Bowen's (1971) approach, the cognitive is emphasized and the use of affect is minimized. Systems theory focuses on *triangulation*, which implies that whenever there is emotional distance or conflict between two persons, tensions will be displaced onto a third party, issue, or substance. Drugs are frequently the subject of triangulation.

Behavioral Family Therapy

Behavioral family therapy is commonly used with substance-abusing adolescents. Its popularity may be attributed to the fact that it can be elaborated in clear, easily learned steps.

Noel and McCrady (1984) developed seven steps in the therapy of alcoholic couples that can readily be applied to married drug-abusing adults and their families:

1. *Functional analysis*. Families are taught to understand the interactions that maintain drug abuse.
2. *Stimulus control*. Drug use is viewed "as a habit triggered by certain antecedents and maintained by certain consequences" (Noel and McCrady 1984). The family is taught to avoid or change these triggers.
3. *Rearrangement of contingencies*. The family is taught techniques to provide reinforcement for efforts at helping the identified patient achieve a drug-free state by frequent reviewing of positive and negative consequences of drug use and by self-contracting for goals and specific rewards for achieving these goals.
4. *Cognitive restructuring*. The identified patient is taught to modify self-derogatory, retaliatory, or guilt-related thoughts. The identified patient questions the logic of these "irrational" thoughts and replaces them with more "rational" ideation.
5. *Alternatives to drug use*. The identified patient is taught techniques for refusing drugs through role-playing and covert reinforcement.

6. *Problem solving and assertion.* The identified patient and family are helped to decide whether a given situation calls for an assertive response and then, through role-playing, to develop effective assertive techniques.
7. *Maintenance planning.* The entire course of therapy is reviewed and the new armamentarium of skills emphasized. The identified patient is encouraged to practice these skills regularly as well as to reread handout materials that explain and reinforce these skills.

Families can also be taught through behavioral techniques to become aware of their nonverbal communication in order to make nonverbal messages concordant with verbal ones and to learn to express interpersonal warmth nonverbally as well as verbally (Stuart 1980).

Specific Structural Techniques

In this subsection, I cite those family therapy techniques that I have found most useful in my work with substance-abusing persons. Many of these approaches evolved from the structural family work of Minuchin (1974) and Haley (1976). Although these strategies are described individually, most "techniques," as implemented in clinical practice, are a fusion of several approaches.

Establishing the Contract

The contract is an agreement to work on mutually agreed-on, workable issues. The contract should always promise help with the identified patient's problem before it is expanded to other issues.

The primary contract is drafted with the family at the end of the first interview. In establishing a contract, the family chooses a system for achieving abstinence and agrees to pursue that system after it has been agreed on as part of the initial evaluation.

The family should be provided with the beginnings of a system of shifting overreactivity to substance abuse in the initial contract. They may be coached to disengage from the identified patient, using strength gained from support groups and the therapist. At times, this disengagement can be accomplished only with powerful restructuring or paradoxical interventions.

Joining

In joining, the therapist adjusts him- or herself in a number of different ways to affiliate with the family system. Joining with only one part of a family may severely stress or change the rest of the family. The therapist must make contact with *all* family members so that they will comply with the therapist even when they sense that he or she is being unfair (Kaufman 1985). The therapist should join by respecting and not challenging the initial defensiveness that is so common in these families.

Joining begins in the first moment of the session when the therapist makes the family comfortable through social amenities, chatting with each member. Three types of joining techniques are used: maintenance, tracking, and mimesis (Minuchin 1974).

Using Actualization

In actualization, the family members are directed to talk to each other rather than to the therapist and to enact transactional patterns rather than describe them. Many families try to look as good as possible when they enter therapy. Actualizations unleash sequences that are beyond the family's control and permit the therapist to see the family as it really is. Three progressively elaborated types of actualization are utilized (Minuchin and Fishman 1981). The first involves sequences that evolve spontaneously as families are permitted to be themselves during sessions. The second type, therapist-planned scenarios, permits further natural interactions that may make use of latent issues that are close to the surface and are beginning to erupt in sessions. In the third, and the most change-oriented, type of actualization, the family enacts in the therapy session a pattern that is outside the family's repetitive, maladaptive system and that demonstrates new ways of problem solving.

Marking Boundaries

Each individual and each subsystem are encouraged to preserve their appropriate boundaries. Each person should be spoken to, not about, and no one should talk, feel, think, answer, or act for anyone else. Each family member is encouraged to tell his or her own story and to listen to and acknowledge the communications of others. Nonverbal checking and blocking of communications should also be observed and, when appropriate, pointed out and halted. The most important boundary shift in family therapy involves weakening the ties between an overinvolved parent and child and strengthening the boundary that protects the parents as a unit and supports them against parents, in-laws, and the rest of the world external to the nuclear family. When boundaries are strengthened around a system, that system's functioning invariably improves.

Assigning Tasks

Tasks can be used to help gather information, intensify the relationship with the therapist, continue the therapy outside of sessions, and give family members the opportunity to behave differently (Haley 1976). Tasks that work in the framework of family goals, particularly those involving changing the symptoms of the identified patient, should be chosen. Tasks should involve everyone in the family and bring gains to each member. A task should be successfully completed in session before being assigned as homework. When assigned, tasks should be specific, clear, and concise.

Reframing

In reframing (Minuchin and Fishman 1981), the therapist takes information received from the family and transforms it into a format that will be most helpful to changing the family. Reframing is achieved by focusing material as it is received, selecting the elements that will facilitate change, and organizing the information in such a way as to give it new meaning. Perhaps the most common use of reframing involves viewing the symptoms of the identified patient in the context of the entire family system.

Using Paradoxical Techniques

Paradoxical techniques work best with chronically rigid, repetitive, circular, highly resistant family systems, particularly those that have had many prior therapeutic failures (Papp 1981). Paradox is not used when family motivation is high, resistance is low, and the family responds readily to direct interventions. Paradox is also not used in crisis situations such as cases of violence, suicide, incest, or child abuse; the therapist in these cases needs to provide structure and control. Paradox is often used to slow progress so that a family is chafing at the bit to move faster or to exaggerate a symptom to emphasize the family's need to extrude it. A person's behavior is not prescribed without relating it to its function in the family system. At times, psychodynamic interpretations can be made in a paradoxical way that gives greater impact in order to reach and change the family.

Balancing and Unbalancing

Balancing techniques, which tend to support a family, are conceptually similar to Minuchin and Fishman's (1981) complementarity. While supporting the family, these authors challenge the family's view of symptoms as part of a linear hierarchy, instead emphasizing the reciprocal involvement of symptom formation. In using balancing as a technique, the therapist emphasizes mutual responsibility and assigns tasks that involve change in all parties. Unbalancing involves changing or stressing the existing hierarchy in a family.

Creating Intensity

For creating intensity, verbal devices are used to ensure that the therapist's message is heard and incorporated by the family. One simple way to be heard is to repeat either the same phrase or different phrases that convey the same concept. Another way of creating intensity is through isomorphic transactions that use many different interventions to attack the same underlying dysfunctional pattern.

Family Readjustment After the Cessation of Substance Abuse

Once the substance abuse has stopped, the family may enter a "honeymoon" phase in which major conflicts are denied. The family may maintain a superficial harmony based on relief and suppression of negative feeling. On the other hand, when the drug-dependent person stops using drugs, other family problems may be uncovered, particularly in the parents' marriage or in other siblings. These problems, which were present all along but obscured by the identified patient's drug use, will be "resolved" by the identified patient's return to symptomatic behavior if the problems are not dealt with in family therapy. In the latter case, the family then reunites around the identified patient according to their old, familiar pathological style.

Too many treatment programs in the substance abuse field focus their efforts on 28-day intensive programs while minimizing family aftercare. Many of these programs include a 1-week intensive family educational and therapeutic experience, but with less focus on the family in aftercare than on the identified patient. These intensive short-term programs have great impact on the family system, but only temporarily. The pull of the family homeostatic system will draw the identified patient and/or other family members back to symptomatic behavior. The family must be worked with for months and often years after substance abuse first abates if a drug-free state is to continue. In addition, ongoing family therapy is also necessary for the emotional well-being of the identified patient and other family members.

In my experience, family therapy as described in this final subpart reduces the incidence of premature dropout from treatment, acts as a preventive measure for other family members, serves as an extended "healthy family," and creates structural family changes that prevent the return of drug abuse.

References

Bauman MH: Involving resistant family members in therapy, in Questions & Answers in the Practice of Family Therapy, Vol 1. Edited by Gurman A. New York, Brunner/Mazel, 1981, pp 16–19

Berenson D: The therapist's relationship with couples with an alcoholic member, in The Family Therapy of Drug and Alcohol Abuse. Edited by Kaufman E, Kaufmann P. New York, Gardner, 1979, pp 233–242

Bowen M: Family therapy and family group therapy, in Comprehensive Group Psychotherapy. Edited by Kaplan HI, Sadock BJ. Baltimore, MD, Williams & Wilkins, 1971, pp 384–421

Framo JL: The integration of marital therapy with sessions with family of origin, in Handbook of Family Therapy. Edited by Gurman AJ, Kniskern DP. New York, Brunner/Mazel, 1981, pp 133–158

Haley J: Problem-Solving Therapy (New Strategies for Effective Family Therapy). San Francisco, CA, Jossey-Bass, 1976

Johnson V: I'll Quit Tomorrow. New York, Harper & Row, 1973

Kaufman E: Family system variables in alcoholism. Alcohol Clin Exp Res 8:4–8, 1985

Kaufman E, Kaufmann P: Multiple family therapy: a new direction in the treatment of drug abusers. Am J Drug Alcohol Abuse 4:467–468, 1977

Minuchin S: Families & Family Therapy. Cambridge, MA, Harvard University Press, 1974

Minuchin S, Fishman HC: Family Therapy Techniques. Cambridge, MA, Harvard University Press, 1981

Noel NE, McCrady BS: Behavioral treatment of an alcohol abuser with the spouse present, in Power to Change: Family Case Studies in the Treatment of Alcoholism. Edited by Kaufman E. New York, Gardner, 1984, pp 23–77

Papp P: Paradoxical strategies and countertransference, in Questions and Answers in the Practice of Family Therapy, Vol 1. Edited by Gurman A. New York, Brunner/Mazel, 1981, pp 128–133

Stanton MD: An integrated structural/strategic approach to family therapy. J Marital Fam Ther 7:427–439, 1981

Stanton MD, Todd TC: The Family Therapy of Drug Abuse and Addiction. New York, Guilford, 1982

Stuart RB: Helping Couples Change. New York, Guilford, 1980

32

Special Programs and Populations

Chad D. Emrick, Ph.D.
Roger D. Weiss, M.D.
Jonathan I. Ritvo, M.D.
James H. Shore, M.D.
George De Leon, Ph.D.
Kathleen T. Brady, M.D., Ph.D.
Robert J. Malcolm, M.D.

Alcoholics Anonymous and Other Twelve-Step Groups

Chad D. Emrick, Ph.D.

Since its founding in 1935, Alcoholics Anonymous (AA) has grown into a worldwide organization with an estimated nearly 2 million members in almost 99,000 groups in over 140 countries (C. D. Emrick, personal communication, November 4, 1999). Its success as a social movement is indisputable, with the organization exercising considerable influence on the professional community and government agencies and programs, as well as on the general public. The shape of public policy and opinion has been substantially determined by the depiction in film, on television, and in the print media of AA's primacy and potency in helping "alcoholics" "recover" from "alcoholism." The primary purpose of this chapter subpart is to inform health care providers about pertinent findings from recent quantitative research on AA and to amplify these findings with observations from contemporary clinical writings concerning the organization. On the basis of these findings, suggestions are given to caregivers for making maximum use of AA and other 12-Step groups. In this chapter subpart, the term *12-Step group* is used to refer to any group

The author wishes to express his appreciation to Keith Humphreys, Dick Longabaugh, Barbara McCrady, Rudolf Moos, and Scott Tonigan for providing him with manuscripts that were difficult, if not impossible, to obtain elsewhere. Valuable assistance in conducting the literature review was also provided by Nancy Harris. The author is quite indebted to Nancy Moore, who not only brought her expert computer and editing skills to the preparation of the manuscript but also provided invaluable support and encouragement throughout the project. A special note of appreciation goes to Scott Tonigan, who was central to the acquisition of the research reports reviewed in this chapter and who also contributed substantially to the conceptualization of the project.

whose structure and function are guided by the Twelve Steps and Twelve Traditions of AA (see the Appendix to this subpart).

AA's Philosophy, Structure, and Therapeutic Processes

AA's philosophy, though rooted in the Judeo-Christian tradition, contains thought elements that are consonant with a variety of religious and philosophical traditions. Thus, people with a wide spectrum of beliefs can find a home in this organization. The organization itself is structured around the Twelve Steps and the Twelve Traditions. Therapeutic processes are played out in "working" the steps, having (for some members) one-to-one guidance and support from a senior member (identified as a "sponsor"), and participating in group meetings that possess therapeutic processes akin to those found in professionally led psychotherapy groups (Emrick et al. 1977).

The process of going through the Twelve Steps is adumbrated here for the reader who is unfamiliar with these steps. In Step One, members adopt the perspective that they cannot control their drinking behavior through conscious, deliberate effort. In Step Two, members incorporate the belief that only a Power greater than themselves can help them become free of alcohol dependence. In Step Three, members surrender to this Higher Power—and in so doing let go of their struggle with drinking behavior as well as with the thoughts, feelings, physical sensations, and behavioral predispositions that are associated with such behavior. In Step Four, members undertake a self-analysis of fear, guilt, and resentment that are often major contextual factors in drinking behavior. One's resentments are given especial attention, and members are guided through procedures for developing a less blaming, more self-responsible perspective with regard to resentments and associated actions. In Step Five, members share the product of their self-analysis with their Higher Power and another individual. In Steps Six and Seven, more letting go of an active struggle with one's inner life is prompted. Whatever behaviors are identified in Steps Four and Five as dysfunctional are viewed as beyond the scope of the individual to change directly. Rather, the individual lets go of a deliberate struggle, "turning over" these behaviors to a Higher Power to effect change. In Steps Eight and Nine, members extend the development of responsibility to their interpersonal relationships. Responsibility is taken for harm caused others (by omission and commission), and restitution to those one has harmed is undertaken, unless restitution efforts would bring harm either to the member or to someone else. Because self-awareness is inevitably limited, members are encouraged, once they have made amends for the harmful actions of which they are aware, to look the harmed individual square in the face and ask him or her to identify harmful acts that the member has forgotten. Responsibility is then extended to these behaviors. In Steps Ten and Eleven, activities are engaged in that serve to maintain the therapeutic gains achieved in taking the earlier steps. Finally, in Step Twelve, the healing gained through involvement in the program (referred to as a "spiritual awakening") is maintained by helping newcomers to the organization and by serving to sustain the organization itself. Increasing one's awareness of, acceptance of, and enactment of the paradoxes of life is at the core of spiritual awakening within the context of active AA involvement. A member's philosophical perspective on life becomes infused with such paradoxical truths as "In order to win, one has to lose" and "In order to give, one has to receive." It is from this place of awareness that experienced members help new members and contribute through service activities to the maintenance of the organization.

The Twelve Traditions of AA are intended to preserve AA as an organization that is completely dedicated to helping individuals live life free of alcohol. Central to AA is an essentially anarchistic organizational structure. There are no permanent leaders, and leaders are instructed to "serve but never govern." Each group maintains autonomy, owns no property, and receives income only from voluntary contributions. Members are to avoid identifying themselves to the public media as members of AA. AA does not "give endorsements, make alliances, or enter public controversies" (Alcoholics Anonymous World Services 1976, p. xix). AA is not to solicit new members through any promotional activity. By virtue of its organizational structure, AA has been able to avoid usurpation of power by any individual or faction of members. Such avoidance has been strongly contributive to AA's remarkable success as a social movement.

Demographics of Current AA Membership

Findings from the most recent triennial survey of AA members in North America reveal the demographics of the current membership (Alcoholics Anonymous World Services 1997). The average age of AA members is 44 years; 13% of members are age 30 years or younger, and 12% are age 61 years or older. Sixty-seven percent of members are men, and 40% of members age 30 years or younger are women. Married persons make up 39% of the membership, and 28% of members are single, 24% are divorced, 6% are widowed, and 3% are separated. Eighty-six percent of members are white, 5% are black, 4% are Hispanic, and 4% are Native American. Only 7% of the membership are unemployed. Twenty-nine percent hold professional/technical, managerial/administrative, or health professional positions.

When given the chance to identify three factors most responsible for joining AA, 51% of members reported that they had sought the support of AA on their own, whereas 48% were influenced to begin participation in AA by an AA member, 40% were influenced by a treatment facility, 16% by a counseling agency, and 8% by an individual health care provider. A total of 73% of members reported that their physicians knew they belonged to AA. Eighty-six percent of members reported that they belonged to a "home group" (a group identified as being primary for the member). Members reported attending an average of more than two AA meetings per week. Seventy-six percent of members had an AA sponsor, and 67% of members had obtained a sponsor within 90 days of attending an AA meeting. A total of 45% of members have been sober for more than 5 years, 28% have been sober for 1–5 years, and 27% have been sober for less than a year. The average duration of sobriety among active members is more than 6 years. Of the 60% of members who reported having received some type of treatment or counseling before attending an AA meeting, 77% said that the treatment or counseling played an important role in directing them to the organization. After beginning participation in AA, 62% of members received some type of treatment or counseling, with 85% of those members indicating that this treatment or counseling played an important part in their recovery.

Who Attends Twelve-Step-Group Meetings?

Multiple variables—both individual and social/interpersonal—have an effect on who attends 12-Step-group meetings and who does not. Findings concerning the relative severity of drinking problems of those who choose to go to AA meetings depend, at least in part, on the sample being studied. For example, in a meta-analysis of the AA literature, Tonigan et al. (1996) found that for outpatient samples, measures of drinking severity were modestly predictive of AA attendance, with greater severity predicting attendance. For inpatient samples, no relationship between drinking severity and AA meeting attendance was found.

As with data concerning severity of alcohol problems, the data are inconsistent with respect to the role the support system of the person with a drinking problem plays in seeking the resources of AA. Generally, however, research findings indicate that an individual with a drinking problem, particularly when that person is not being treated in a residential setting, is more likely to join and become involved in AA if family and friends provide weak or inconsistent support for overcoming the problem or if familial and friendship networks are impoverished. This observation appears valid inasmuch as AA is a social network that supports abstinence and encourages the development of helping relationships among its members.

Ethnicity also appears to affect the decision to become involved in AA, although no consistent pattern has been found. In one sample, among those involved in the criminal justice or welfare systems, whites were more likely than blacks or Hispanics to have attended AA meetings. However, in samples drawn from primary health care settings, blacks were more likely than whites or Hispanics to attend AA meetings (Caetano 1993). In another study (Kessler et al. 1997), blacks were less likely than whites to participate in self-help groups for substance abuse (mostly 12-Step groups). In an additional study, Hispanics were found to attend AA meetings less frequently than were whites (Arroyo et al. 1998).

Finally, it has been found that women with substance abuse disorders are more likely than men with these disorders to participate in self-help (mostly 12-Step) groups (Kessler et al. 1997).

The complex and inconsistent findings concerning the relationship between personal and contextual variables and the selection of AA as a resource provide the health care professional with few, if any, clear guidelines for determining who will be a good match for AA or a similar 12-Step group. For now, health care practitioners should keep in mind that *any given individual patient may or may not be a suitable candidate for AA or another 12-Step group*. Generally, the more severe the individual's drinking or other identified problem and the fewer the individual's interpersonal supports among family and friends (particularly in the case of an outpatient), the more likely the person is to join AA or another 12-Step group.

Frequency of Use of Twelve-Step Programs

Although AA and other 12-Step programs appear to be increasingly used, particularly by women, the level of participation in AA and other 12-Step groups by individuals with substance use disorders may still be modest. Hasin and Grant (1995) found that less than 6% of a sample of individuals who formerly drank alcohol who responded to the 1988 National Health Interview Survey (about half of whom met DSM-IV [American Psychiatric Association 1994] criteria for a diagnosis of alcohol use disorder) had attended AA meetings. In reporting data from another national survey, Hasin (1994) observed that less than 4% of the sample of individuals who currently or formerly drank alcohol (only a portion of whom were or had been dependent on alcohol) had attended AA meetings. These data highlight the opportunity that exists for increased use of AA and other 12-Step programs in the treatment of substance use disorders.

Although apparently relatively few individuals who have substance use disorders attend meetings of AA or other 12-Step groups, evidence indicates that most of those persons with substance use disorders who do seek treatment go to 12-Step-group meetings.

Attitudes of Health Care Practitioners Toward Twelve-Step Programs

Most physicians consider participation in AA an effective treatment for alcoholism, yet physicians often lack belief in the benefits of other forms of alcoholism treatment, despite scientific proof that other treatments can be beneficial. Such lack of belief may result in the underuse of effective professionally delivered treatments for individuals with substance use disorders.

Mental health treatment providers and substance abuse counselors vary in their endorsement of 12-Step groups, although many believe in the effectiveness of these programs. Depending on his or her theoretical orientation, the mental health treatment provider views 12-Step groups more or less as salient therapeutic resources. Similarly, substance abuse treatment providers vary in the degree to which they endorse the spiritual thinking found in the philosophy of AA, their level of endorsement varying according to variables such as their own involvement in 12-Step groups, their religious affiliation, and their educational background.

Effectiveness of AA

Ample research data document the effectiveness of AA (and, by extension, other 12-Step groups) in helping individuals maintain a lifestyle free of substance abuse. In effect, research evidence substantiates the intuitive knowledge that 12-Step-group members and their families and friends (as well as large numbers of health care providers) possess concerning the effectiveness of 12-Step programs.

Outcome Studies

The results of a meta-analysis of 107 studies on AA (Emrick et al. 1993) suggested that "professionally treated patients who attend AA during or after treatment are more likely to improve in drinking behavior than are patients who do not attend AA, although the chances of drinking improvement are not overall a great deal higher" (p. 57). Also, a positive relationship between AA affiliation and psychological health was observed.

Most salient among the recent original research findings on AA's effectiveness are the findings of investigators at the Center for Health Care Evaluation in Menlo Park, California. In one of their studies (Humphreys et al. 1997), 515 subjects from an original sample of 631 individuals with previously untreated drinking problems were followed up at 1 year. Of those in the sample who attended AA meetings but did not receive inpatient or outpatient professional treatment, significant improvement was found on all measures of drinking problems as well as on several other measures of functioning. A total of 395 subjects in this sample were followed up at 8 years, at which time it was found that the number of AA meetings attended during the first 3 years of follow-up was positively related to remission from alcohol problems 8 years after the beginning of the project. AA attendance in the first 3 years of the study also predicted, at 8-year follow-up, lower levels of depression as well as higher-quality relationships with friends and partners or spouses. Of particular note is that inpatient professional treatment services, which some in the sample received, failed to predict any measure of outcome at the 8-year follow-up. Although outpatient professional treatment was found to predict drinking outcome at 8-year follow-up, no other benefits of such treatment were observed. This comparison of AA and outpatient professional treatment leads to the obvious conclusion that, at least for this sample of persons with previously untreated drinking problems, AA's therapeutic benefits had a broader effect on alcoholic individuals' lives than did outpatient professional treatment. Humphreys et al. (1997) concluded that, compared with professionally delivered inpatient or outpatient treatment, "AA probably helped more people more substantially in this sample" (p. 237).

This same research group evaluated the effects of different types of aftercare treatment 1 year after inpatient treatment in a large sample of veterans (Finney et al. 1999; Moos et al. 1999; Ouimette et al. 1998, 1999). Followed up were 3,018 veterans who had been treated for substance abuse in an inpatient setting. The majority of patients, all of whom were male, were non-Caucasian. Eighty-three percent of the sample were dependent on alcohol, with about 52% of those with alcohol problems being dependent on other substances. They were evaluated with regard to their outcome status approximately 1 year after being discharged from the inpatient program. Participation in AA or Narcotics Anonymous (NA) in the 3 months prior to the 1-year follow-up was associated with a greater likelihood of being abstinent, free of substance use problems, free of significant distress and psychiatric symptoms, and employed. These findings held even when controlling for the influence of aftercare treatment, and they applied as much to dually diagnosed patients as to those with only substance use disorders (for the results pertaining to dually diagnosed patients, see Ouimette et al. 1999). Statistical analyses suggested that 12-Step involvement after inpatient treatment helped maintain the gains made during inpatient treatment (Finney et al. 1999). These results led the researchers to conclude that "overall, 12-Step attendance and involvement were more strongly related to positive outcomes than was outpatient treatment attendance" (Ouimette et al. 1998, p. 519).

Treatment Cost

Humphreys and Moos (1996) assessed the effectiveness of AA in another way. The per-person treatment costs for individuals with alcohol problems who sought help as outpatients from professional providers of alcoholism treatment were compared with the costs of treatment for individuals with drinking problems who initially chose to go to AA meetings. Costs were assessed for a 3-year period. Over the course of the study, some individuals within both groups required detoxification and inpatient or residential treatment. Furthermore, some persons who initially went to AA meetings also had outpatient treatment and vice versa. When all cost factors were calculated, those individuals who initially attended AA incurred per-person treatment costs that were 45% lower than the costs incurred by those individuals who initially sought outpatient treatment. AA appears to be considerably less costly in helping at least some individuals with alcohol problems.

Mechanisms of Effectiveness

Clinical writings assert that AA and, by extension, other 12-Step groups are effective because these groups (particularly AA) are readily and widely available, provide a philosophy for living, and present a structured community of individuals who are living life without alcohol. Twelve-step groups are normative organizations that help individuals experience, express, and manage feelings, in part through giving members the opportunity to express feelings in group meetings without fear of negative feedback from others. The groups also help members develop the capacity for self-regulation, increase their sense of self-efficacy, perceive the continuity of time, improve a sense of relationship to others, discover their purpose in life or meaning of life, find a way to connect with the unknown reality that exists outside themselves, engage in self-examination and self-expression, increase their ability to listen to others, and repair vulnerabilities in self-care.

Twelve-Step groups teach members healthy strategies for interpreting stressful events and experiences and for behaving in response to those events and experiences. For example, participants are taught to distinguish between controllable and uncontrollable events. Active cognitive coping strategies are provided for dealing with uncontrollable events (e.g., members are instructed to think, "This, too, shall pass," when they are faced with a situation they cannot change). For events which are controllable, use of active behavioral coping strategies is encouraged (e.g., members are taught to deal immediately and actively with interpersonal conflict). No matter the controllability of the event, members are urged to reduce their use of avoidant and destructive coping strategies, such as turning to alcohol or drugs.

In several research efforts (Humphreys et al. 1994; Morgenstern et al. 1996; Snow et al. 1994), data have been collected pertaining to the operational ingredients in AA's effectiveness. These data indicate that the more current and actively involved an individual is in AA, the more he or she uses a variety of therapeutic or adaptive processes, including behavioral change processes such as avoidance of high-risk situations and the use of active cognitive and behavioral coping strategies.

Health Care Providers and Twelve-Step Groups

Facilitating Affiliation and Involvement

Because AA and, by extension, other 12-Step groups can play a vital part in recovery from chemical dependency, health care practitioners need to prepare their patients for active participation in these groups. Empirical support for this suggestion comes from two recent major research efforts, both of which show that 12-Step–oriented treatment results in a higher percentage of patients involving themselves in 12-Step groups and that this involvement, in turn, produces higher abstinence rates (Humphreys et al. 1999; Project MATCH Research Group 1998).

To be successful in their efforts, professionals must have an accurate understanding of the nature of 12-Step groups. Practitioners need to understand, for example, that AA does *not* assert that "(1) there is only one form of alcoholism or alcohol problem; (2) moderate drinking is impossible for everyone with alcohol problems; (3) alcoholics should be labeled, confronted aggressively or coerced into treatment; (4) alcoholics are riddled with denial and other defense mechanisms; (5) alcoholism is purely a physical disorder; (6) alcoholism is hereditary; (7) there is only one way to recover; or (8) alcoholics are not responsible for their condition or actions" (Miller and Kurtz 1994, p. 165). Also, clinicians must educate their patients about the difference between religion and spirituality, because AA is often perceived to be a form of religion. AA is essentially a "spiritual program of living" (Miller and Kurtz 1994, p. 165) or "a way of life" (Gold 1994, p. 97). This is the case because "there is no dogma, theology, or creed to be learned" in AA (Chappel 1993, p. 181). Knowledgeable clinicians would do well to keep this understanding in mind as they assist their patients in preparing for AA participation.

Practitioners can also assist their patients in becoming beneficially involved in 12-Step groups by offering basic instruction about the meaning and purpose of each of the Twelve Steps and Twelve Traditions of AA. Further, professionals may facilitate involvement by having contact with their patients' sponsor, encouraging their patients to choose home groups and to attend 12-Step-group meetings frequently (particularly at the beginning of participation), and offering their patients guidance in becoming actively involved in the 12-Step community.

Learning How to Integrate Twelve-Step Programs and Professional Treatment

Health care professionals can further enhance the effective use of AA and other 12-Step programs by acquiring knowledge about how best to integrate these programs and professional treatment (see, e.g., Zweben 1995). Integration is advised because persons with substance use disorders who combine these two systems of care appear to have better outcomes (at least with respect to substance abuse) than do those who avail themselves of only one form of help.

A common theme in writings regarding integrating 12-Step programs and professional treatment is the need for professionals to learn the language and culture of such programs in order to understand in what ways the two systems differ and where the commonalities in concepts and processes exist. For example, both systems facilitate the development of cognitive and behavioral change processes; only the language used to foster this development differs. By possessing a working knowledge of the language and culture of both systems, health care providers can become more skilled in aiding their patients to use both forms of help simultaneously, alternately, or sequentially. As recent research data suggest, the most effective way to promote use of both types of care is to fashion a professional treatment approach that is consonant with that found in the 12-Step-group environment (Humphreys et al. 1999).

Tailoring Facilitation Efforts to Specific Groups

Professionals must tailor their facilitation efforts to the unique characteristics of the particular 12-Step groups in which their patients are to become involved. Given the fact that heterogeneity has been found to exist among different AA groups, a patient may find one particular group in his or her community to be compatible with individual needs and other groups to be inappropriate. Health care providers are encouraged to help patients understand the heterogeneity of groups and, therefore, the need to attend meetings of several groups before deciding which group (or groups) is most suitable.

Becoming Knowledgeable About Special-Population Considerations

A number of reports have identified points of consideration (as well as guidelines, in some cases) for facilitating AA involvement by individuals with special characteristics. These reports focused on the following special populations: veterans with posttraumatic stress disorder (Satel et al. 1993), lesbians (Hall 1994), adolescents (Kennedy and Minami 1993), persons with dual diagnoses (Kurtz et al. 1995), women (Sandoz 1995), persons with substance use disorders without a high degree of need to affiliate with others in a group (Smith 1993), and individuals within particular ethnic groups (Caetano 1993). The health care provider needs to become knowledgeable about, and sensitive to, these special-population issues to be maximally effective in facilitating 12-Step-group involvement among his or her patients.

Matching Patients to Twelve-Step Groups

An intuitively appealing—although practically difficult—approach to facilitating use and increasing effectiveness of 12-Step programs is to determine which patients are most appropriate for these programs. The Project MATCH (Matching Alcoholism Treatments to Client Heterogeneity) Research Group (1998) suggested three matching strategies that health care providers need to keep in mind when considering a referral to AA or another 12-Step group:

1. For drinkers who have a social system that is supportive of drinking, facilitating participation in AA (through Twelve-Step Facilitation Therapy) appears to result in better drinking outcome than does trying to motivate the individual to give up drinking (through Motivational Enhancement Therapy) or providing treatment based on cognitive-behavioral theory (i.e., Cognitive-Behavioral Coping Skills Therapy) (Longabaugh et al. 1998; Project MATCH Research Group 1998).
2. Alcohol-dependent individuals who have high levels of anger at the start of treatment may benefit more from a nonconfrontational approach to acquire motivation to change their drinking behavior (i.e., Motivational Enhancement Therapy) than from treatment that encourages them to attend AA (i.e., Twelve-Step Facilitation Therapy). Actively exhorting angry clients to attend AA may provoke an angry response, thereby lowering the chance of a good treatment outcome (Project MATCH Research Group 1998).
3. Those inpatients who have relatively high dependence on alcohol may benefit more from a 12-Step-group–oriented aftercare treatment than from treatment based on cognitive-behavioral theory (Project MATCH Research Group 1997).

An intriguing addendum to these matching strategies is found in a recent publication by Winzelberg and Humphreys (1999). In their study of 3,018 male substance-abusing inpatients, clients who were low in religious behaviors were less likely to be referred to a 12-Step mutual aid group. However, such individuals responded positively to 12-Step-group referrals if made and subsequently experienced better substance abuse outcomes. It appears, therefore, that health care providers should not be hesitant about encouraging their less religious clients to get involved in 12-Step groups. As Winzelberg and Humphreys (1999) noted, "A nonreligious patient may benefit from referral to AA or NA more than either the clinician or the patient expects" (p. 794).

Although not of the stature of a proposed matching strategy, another Project MATCH finding merits mention here. Problem drinkers treated in residential settings who scored high on a measure assessing the degree to which a person searches for meaning in life had better drinking outcomes, at least for a period of time, when they received aftercare treatment oriented toward AA participation rather than comparison aftercare treatments (Tonigan et al. 1997b). Because this finding is quite tentative, further research needs to be undertaken before the "meaning in life" variable can serve as a guide in making clinical decisions. Nonetheless, clinicians are encouraged to be sensitive to the interplay between a patient's search for meaning in life and the treatment that patient receives.

Matching AA Members to Professional Treatment

How are health care providers to approach their patients who have been involved previously in 12-Step groups and are now seeking the services of a professional? Does prior 12-Step-group involvement influence receptivity to certain types of treatment? Project MATCH data include relevant information concerning these questions.

Tonigan et al. (1997a) found that outpatients who had been involved in AA prior to professional treatment appeared to be more compatible with Twelve-Step Facilitation Therapy than with either Motivational Enhancement Therapy or Cognitive-Behavioral Coping Skills Therapy.

Matching strategies along these lines may be identified for 12-Step groups other than AA should researchers and clinicians undertake collaborative efforts to mine these groups for relevant data.

Twelve-Step Programs Are Not Always Helpful

The health care practitioner must keep in mind that any intervention having the power to help some people possesses the potential to harm others. Should a health care provider assume that 12-Step-group participation "can't hurt," he or she may fail to intervene appropriately if a patient claims to be worsening through his or her involvement in the 12-Step community. Quite often, such a complaint is an expression of resistance to a beneficial membership, in which case helping the patient overcome the resistance to active membership is appropriate. On the other hand, the organization may truly be having a negative effect on the patient, as evidenced by increased drug use; exacerbation of depressive symptoms such as helplessness, guilt, or inadequacy perceptions; or lack of improvement in family or social relationships.

If the health care practitioner determines that 12-Step-group involvement is having a negative effect on a patient, the practitioner needs to work with the patient to reverse such effects. One obvious course of action is to assist the patient in finding alternative treatments. Insisting that a patient continue attendance at 12-Step-group meetings when he or she is being harmed by such attendance is equivalent to instructing a patient to continue taking medication that not only is failing to improve his or her condition but also is causing harmful side effects. Good medical and other professional practice proscribe such behavior.

Alternatives to Twelve-Step Groups

Given that AA and other 12-Step groups are not always effective and may even be harmful to certain individuals, what community group alternatives are available to assist substance-abusing persons in dealing with their disorders? Rational Recovery (RR) is one alternative to 12-Step groups (see Galanter et al. 1993), as are Women for Sobriety (see Kaskutas 1996) and Secular Organizations for Sobriety/Save Our Selves (SOS) (see Connors and Dermen 1996).

Certainly, RR and other alternatives to AA are worthy of the health care provider's attention and are organizations to which the practitioner should consider making referrals, when appropriate.

Conclusions

In this chapter subpart, a wide spectrum of issues have been covered concerning AA and other 12-Step groups. Information has been presented regarding the philosophy, structure, and therapeutic processes of AA; the demographics of the current North American membership of AA; the degree to which AA and other 12-Step programs are being used; the beliefs and attitudes held by health care providers concerning AA and other 12-Step groups; the effectiveness of AA and the mechanisms of effect; ways to enhance the use of 12-Step programs; matching of patients to 12-Step groups; referral of patients involved in 12-Step groups to appropriate professional treatment; the limitations of 12-Step groups; and alternatives to 12-Step groups.

A virtual explosion of new findings concerning AA and other 12-Step groups has resulted from the research reviewed here. Health care providers, armed with greater knowledge than ever before about AA and other 12-Step groups, can now offer their patients even wiser counsel regarding such groups.

References

Alcoholics Anonymous World Services: Alcoholics Anonymous: The Story of How Many Thousands of Men and Women Have Recovered From Alcoholism, 3rd Edition. New York, Alcoholics Anonymous World Services, 1976

Alcoholics Anonymous World Services: Alcoholics Anonymous 1996 Membership Survey. New York, Alcoholics Anonymous World Services, 1997

American Psychiatric Association: Diagnostic and Statistical Manual of Mental Disorders, 4th Edition. Washington, DC, American Psychiatric Association, 1994

Arroyo JA, Westerberg VS, Tonigan JS: Comparison of treatment utilization and outcome for Hispanics and non-Hispanic Whites. J Stud Alcohol 59:286–291, 1998

Caetano R: Ethnic minority groups and Alcoholics Anonymous: a review, in Research on Alcoholics Anonymous: Opportunities and Alternatives. Edited by McCrady BS, Miller WR. New Brunswick, NJ, Rutgers Center of Alcohol Studies, 1993, pp 209–231

Chappel JN: Long-term recovery from alcoholism. Psychiatr Clin North Am 16:177–187, 1993

Connors GJ, Dermen KH: Characteristics of participants in Secular Organizations for Sobriety (SOS). Am J Drug Alcohol Abuse 22:281–295, 1996

Emrick CD, Lassen CL, Edwards MT: Nonprofessional peers as therapeutic agents, in Effective Psychotherapy: A Handbook of Research. Edited by Gurman AS, Razin AM. Oxford, UK, Pergamon, 1977, pp 120–161

Emrick CD, Tonigan JS, Montgomery H, et al: Alcoholics Anonymous: what is currently known? In Research on Alcoholics Anonymous: Opportunities and Alternatives. Edited by McCrady BS, Miller WR. New Brunswick, NJ, Rutgers Center of Alcohol Studies, 1993, pp 41–76

Finney JW, Moos RH, Humphreys K: A comparative evaluation of substance abuse treatment, II: linking proximal outcomes of 12-Step and cognitive-behavioral treatment to substance use outcomes. Alcohol Clin Exp Res 23:537–544, 1999

Galanter M, Egelko S, Edwards H: Rational Recovery: alternative to AA for addiction? Am J Drug Alcohol Abuse 19:499–510, 1993

Gold MS: Neurobiology of addiction and recovery: the brain, the drive for the drug, and the 12-Step fellowship. J Subst Abuse Treat 11:93–97, 1994

Hall JM: The experiences of lesbians in Alcoholics Anonymous. West J Nurs Res 16:556–576, 1994

Hasin DS: Treatment/self-help for alcohol-related problems: relationship to social pressure and alcohol dependence. J Stud Alcohol 55:660–666, 1994

Hasin DS, Grant BF: AA and other helpseeking for alcohol problems: former drinkers in the US general population. J Subst Abuse 7:281–292, 1995

Humphreys K, Moos RH: Reduced substance-abuse-related health care costs among voluntary participants in Alcoholics Anonymous. Psychiatr Serv 47:709–713, 1996

Humphreys K, Finney JW, Moos RH: Applying a stress and coping framework to research on mutual help organizations. Journal of Community Psychology 22:312–327, 1994

Humphreys K, Moos RH, Cohen C: Social and community resources and long-term recovery from treated and untreated alcoholism. J Stud Alcohol 58:231–238, 1997

Humphreys K, Huebsch PD, Finney JW, et al: A comparative evaluation of substance abuse treatment, V: substance abuse treatment can enhance the effectiveness of self-help groups. Alcohol Clin Exp Res 23:558–563, 1999

Kaskutas LA: Pathways to self-help among Women for Sobriety. Am J Drug Alcohol Abuse 22:259–280, 1996

Kennedy BP, Minami M: The Beech Hill Hospital/Outward Bound Adolescent Chemical Dependency Treatment Program. J Subst Abuse Treat 10:395–406, 1993

Kessler RC, Mickelson KD, Zhao S: Patterns and correlates of self-help group membership in the United States. Social Policy 27:27–46, 1997

Kurtz LF, Garvin CD, Hill EM, et al: Involvement in Alcoholics Anonymous by persons with dual disorders. Alcoholism Treatment Quarterly 12:1–18, 1995

Longabaugh R, McCrady B, Fink E, et al: Cost effectiveness of alcoholism treatment in partial vs inpatient settings. Six-month outcomes. J Stud Alcohol 44:1049–1071, 1983

Longabaugh R, Wirtz PW, Zweben A, et al: Network support for drinking, Alcoholics Anonymous and long-term matching effects. Addiction 93:1313–1333, 1998

Miller WR, Kurtz E: Models of alcoholism used in treatment: contrasting AA and other perspectives with which it is often confused. J Stud Alcohol 55:159–166, 1994

Moos RH, Finney JW, Ouimette PC, et al: A comparative evaluation of substance abuse treatment, I: treatment orientation, amount of care, and 1-year outcomes. Alcohol Clin Exp Res 23:529–536, 1999

Morgenstern J, Kahler CW, Frey RM, et al: Modeling therapeutic response to 12-Step treatment: optimal responders, nonresponders, and partial responders. J Subst Abuse 8:45–59, 1996

Ouimette PC, Moos RH, Finney JW: Influence of outpatient treatment and 12-Step group involvement on one-year substance abuse treatment outcomes. J Stud Alcohol 59:513–522, 1998

Ouimette PC, Gima K, Moos RH, et al: A comparative evaluation of substance abuse treatment, IV: the effect of comorbid psychiatric diagnoses on amount of treatment, continuing care, and 1-year outcomes. Alcohol Clin Exp Res 23:552–557, 1999

Project MATCH Research Group: Project MATCH secondary a priori hypotheses. Addiction 92:1671–1698, 1997

Project MATCH Research Group: Matching Alcoholism Treatments to Client Heterogeneity: Project MATCH three-year drinking outcomes. Alcohol Clin Exp Res 22:1300–1311, 1998

Sandoz CJ: Gender issues in recovery from alcoholism. Alcoholism Treatment Quarterly 12:61–69, 1995

Satel SL, Becker BR, Dan E: Reducing obstacles to affiliation with Alcoholics Anonymous among veterans with PTSD and alcoholism. Hospital and Community Psychiatry 44:1061–1065, 1993

Smith AR: The social construction of group dependency in Alcoholics Anonymous. Journal of Drug Issues 23:689–704, 1993

Snow MG, Prochaska JO, Rossi JS: Processes of change in Alcoholics Anonymous: maintenance factors in long-term sobriety. J Stud Alcohol 55:362–371, 1994

Tonigan JS, Toscova R, Miller WR: Meta-analysis of the literature on Alcoholics Anonymous: sample and study characteristics moderate findings. J Stud Alcohol 57:65–72, 1996

Tonigan JS, Miller WR, Connors GJ: Prior Alcoholics Anonymous Involvement and Treatment Outcome: Matching Findings and Causal Chain Analyses, Vol 8 (Project MATCH Monogr). Bethesda, MD, National Institute on Alcohol Abuse and Alcoholism, 1997a

Tonigan JS, Miller WR, Connors GJ: The Search For Meaning in Life as a Predictor of Treatment Outcome, Vol 8 (Project MATCH Monogr). Bethesda, MD, National Institute on Alcohol Abuse and Alcoholism, 1997b

Winzelberg A, Humphreys K: Should patients' religiosity influence clinicians' referral to 12-Step self-help groups? Evidence from a study of 3,018 male substance abuse patients. J Consult Clin Psychol 67:790–794, 1999

Zweben JE: Integrating psychotherapy and 12-Step approaches, in Psychotherapy and Substance Abuse: A Practitioner's Handbook. Edited by Washton AM. New York, Guilford, 1995, pp 124–140

Appendix

The Twelve Steps of Alcoholics Anonymous

1. We admitted we were powerless over alcohol—that our lives had become unmanageable.
2. Came to believe that a Power greater than ourselves could restore us to sanity.
3. Made a decision to turn our will and our lives over to the care of God *as we understood Him*.
4. Made a searching and fearless moral inventory of ourselves.
5. Admitted to God, to ourselves and to another human being the exact nature of our wrongs.
6. Were entirely ready to have God remove all these defects of character.
7. Humbly asked Him to remove our shortcomings.
8. Made a list of all persons we had harmed, and became willing to make amends to them all.
9. Made direct amends to such people wherever possible, except when to do so would injure them or others.
10. Continued to take personal inventory and when we were wrong promptly admitted it.
11. Sought through prayer and meditation to improve our conscious contact with God, *as we understood Him*, praying only for knowledge of His will for us and the power to carry that out.
12. Having had a spiritual awakening as the result of these steps, we tried to carry this message to alcoholics, and to practice these principles in all our affairs.

The Twelve Traditions of Alcoholics Anonymous

1. Our common welfare should come first; personal recovery depends upon AA unity.
2. For our group purpose, there is but one ultimate authority—a loving God as He may express Himself in our group conscience. Our leaders are but trusted servants; they do not govern.
3. The only requirement for AA membership is a desire to stop drinking.
4. Each group should be autonomous except in matters affecting other groups or AA as a whole.
5. Each group has but one primary purpose—to carry its message to the alcoholic who still suffers.
6. An AA group ought never endorse, finance, or lend the AA name to any related facility or outside enterprise, lest problems of money, property, and prestige divert us from our primary purpose.
7. Every AA group ought to be fully self-supporting, declining outside contributions.
8. Alcoholics Anonymous should remain forever nonprofessional, but our service centers may employ special workers.
9. AA, as such, ought never be organized; but we may create service boards or committees directly responsible to those they serve.
10. Alcoholics Anonymous has no opinion on outside issues; hence the AA name ought never be drawn into public controversy.
11. Our public relations policy is based on attraction rather than promotion; we need always maintain personal anonymity at the level of press, radio, and films.
12. Anonymity is the spiritual foundation of all our traditions, ever reminding us to place principles before personalities.

Inpatient Treatment

Roger D. Weiss, M.D.

The term *inpatient treatment* actually refers to a variety of forms of treatment that may take place in a number of different settings. Inpatient treatment may involve detoxification, rehabilitation, or a combination of the two; it may occur either in a medical or a general psychiatric setting or on a specialized chemical dependency unit. Although many clinicians in the field recommend that addicted patients be treated in a specialized setting, I am aware of no studies that have carefully compared the efficacy of substance use treatment on a specialized unit with that of treatment in a general psychiatric setting.

The recognition of the frequent comorbidity of addictive disorders and other psychiatric illness (Brooner et al. 1997; Kessler et al. 1997; Mirin et al. 1991) has fostered the establishment of numerous "dual diagnosis" inpatient units that treat patients with coexisting mental illness and substance use disorders. One potential problem with the grouping of such "dual diagnosis" patients is the fact that patients with coexisting mental illness and substance use disorders are quite heterogeneous (Weiss et al. 1992). Thus, although such patients are grouped together to create greater cohesion on an inpatient unit, this desired result may not, in fact, occur. Although treating dually diagnosed patients together may work well in some settings, it is important to recognize the potential limitations of this approach.

Treatment of dual diagnosis patients may occur on a unit in which the focus is primarily psychiatric, on a substance abuse unit with a psychiatric consultant, or on a unit that

This work was supported by grant DA00326 from the National Institute on Drug Abuse and a grant from the Dr. Ralph and Marian C. Falk Medical Research Trust.

attempts to integrate principles of psychiatric and chemical dependency treatment. Minkoff (1989), for example, argued for the latter approach; he posited that many concepts traditionally associated with chemical dependency treatment (e.g., acceptance of a chronic illness, the need to overcome denial and shame, the importance of asking for help) are equally useful in the treatment of patients with other primary psychiatric disorders.

Virtually all inpatient substance abuse programs in the United States advocate abstinence from all drugs of abuse, including alcohol, as a foundation of treatment. The most common form of inpatient treatment in this country is the "Minnesota Model" (Cook 1988a), so named because of its development in that state in the 1950s. After initially undergoing detoxification, patients in programs based on this model attend educational lectures derived from the disease concept of chemical dependency. The patients are typically taught about the harmful consequences of drugs and alcohol, the effects of substance abuse on the family, the use of relapse-prevention techniques, and the importance of making lifestyle changes. Many of the therapy groups in Minnesota Model programs are based on principles of Alcoholics Anonymous (AA) and Narcotics Anonymous. Thus, such programs frequently emphasize the importance of spirituality in the recovery process. Indeed, orienting patients to AA and establishing continued AA and group therapy involvement after discharge are major goals of such programs. Patients are often asked to recount their substance abuse histories in front of other patients and staff members, in a forum similar to AA meetings. This exercise is designed to help patients confront and accept the adverse effects of their substance use and to overcome minimization or denial of the severity of their problems. Minnesota Model programs rely strongly on group therapy and peer confrontation and heavily employ persons recovering from substance abuse as counselors. Systems interventions, including involvement of employers and family members, are also frequently utilized in these programs. Psychiatrists are involved to a variable extent in Minnesota Model programs; the degree of integration between the psychiatric staff and the counseling staff can range from cooperation and integration to mutual distrust.

The "comprehensive and dogmatic ideology" of Minnesota Model programs (Cook 1988b) has been described alternately as one of their most powerful therapeutic tools and as their biggest drawback. For example, some patients who object to the spiritual aspects of these programs or who find AA distasteful, for whatever reason, may be accused of being resistant to treatment, when, in fact, they are merely resistant to AA. Despite these criticisms, however, Minnesota Model programs remain extraordinarily popular in the United States.

A few hospitals in this country practice chemical aversion counterconditioning therapy (Institute of Medicine 1990), in which the pairing of an emetic drug with the patient's favored alcoholic beverage induces the patient to associate drinking with nausea and vomiting. Although uncontrolled research on this procedure has reported favorable outcomes (Neuberger et al. 1980), controlled investigations have been less encouraging (Richard 1983). At present, there is some disagreement regarding the overall efficacy of chemical aversion counterconditioning in the inpatient treatment of substance use disorders (Thurber 1985; G. T. Wilson 1987).

Rationale for Inpatient Treatment

Inpatient treatment offers several advantages over less intensive programs. First, a hospital setting provides a high level of medical supervision and safety for persons who require intensive physical and/or psychiatric monitoring. Thus, for patients with dangerous medical or psychiatric conditions, inpatient treatment in a hospital setting is indicated. The intensity of inpatient treatment may also be helpful to patients who have not responded to lesser measures, such as those who are too discouraged or unmotivated to regularly attend outpatient treatment. Moreover, inpatient treatment may benefit some persons by increasing their awareness of the triggers that place them at risk to return to substance abuse. For example, the intensity and degree of discomfort that some patients feel in a 24-hour-a-day treatment setting may precipitate drug urges. Patients' experiencing urges in a protected setting, where they cannot act on their urges, may help them to learn either to avoid such situations in the future or to cope with them effectively. Moreover, inpatient treatment can help to interrupt a cycle of drug use; for some persons the safety of an inpatient environment and the respite from a barrage of conditioned cues may help bolster their motivation to stop alcohol and drug use.

The protectiveness of an inpatient treatment unit also represents one of its potential disadvantages, however. Because one major determinant of craving is drug availability (Meyer and Mirin 1979), inpatients may not experience drug urges simply because they are living in a drug-free environment. Therefore, they may be unprepared to cope with the drug urges that they will encounter upon discharge to a setting in which drugs are again available. Many inpatient programs therefore gradually expose patients to such triggers by discharging them to "step-down" facilities such as partial hospital programs.

Other disadvantages of inpatient treatment, namely cost and disruption of work and/or family life, are obvious. Thus, inpatient treatment should generally be utilized only when less intensive treatment methods either have failed or are considered too risky to attempt.

Determination of Need for Patient Hospitalization

The implementation of cost-containment efforts, when combined with data challenging the effectiveness of inpatient treatment, has led to the creation of numerous lists of indications for inpatient treatment. Such criteria have been developed by insurers, managed care companies, hospitals, and professional groups. For example, one relatively recent attempt to define criteria for inpatient treatment (American Society of Addiction Medicine 1996) listed six areas that should be assessed in determining whether a patient requires hospital care or less intensive treatment. The areas recommended for assessment are 1) acute intoxication and/or withdrawal potential, 2) biomedical conditions and complications, 3) emotional and behavioral conditions or complications, 4) treatment acceptance/resistance, 5) relapse/continued use potential, and 6) recovery/living environment. Although one may argue with the specific criteria contained in this or any other publication, it is necessary to recognize the importance of a multidimensional assessment in determining the optimal treatment setting for a chemically dependent patient.

When this assessment has been completed, the clinician must ultimately consider two major issues in deciding whether or not to hospitalize a patient: 1) the danger of imminent harm to the patient or others, and 2) the likelihood that the patient would achieve treatment success in a less restrictive environment. These issues are frequently quite difficult to evaluate in substance-abusing persons. For example, although patients with homicidal threats or a recent suicide attempt are clearly candidates for hospitalization, danger to self or others may occur in substance-abusing persons in the absence of overt threats or acts. Patients who regularly drive while intoxicated, share needles with others, or commit violent crimes to support their drug habits may also represent a risk to themselves or society. Because one function of inpatient treatment is the protection of the chemically dependent patient and the people around him or her during a period of acute danger, deciding when to hospitalize persons whose behavior represents a chronic or recurrent danger is quite complicated.

Another area in which an inpatient setting may provide safety is during the process of detoxification. This is particularly true for patients being detoxified from alcohol and/or sedative-hypnotic drugs, because withdrawal from these agents may be accompanied by serious medical consequences, including seizures, delirium, and death. A number of studies have shown that outpatient alcohol detoxification can be accomplished safely and effectively in some circumstances (M. N. Collins et al. 1990; Hayashida et al. 1989). However, inpatient detoxification is still commonly employed because of the risk of potentially serious medical sequelae of withdrawal, in combination with the potential unreliability of this patient population. For example, some patients undergoing outpatient detoxification may concomitantly use alcohol and other drugs that lower seizure threshold (e.g., cocaine). Although detoxification from therapeutic doses of benzodiazepines is frequently performed on an outpatient basis, patients with mixed benzodiazepine and alcohol dependence or patients who have been abusing benzodiazepines are often detoxified as inpatients. Moreover, although opioid withdrawal is generally less medically dangerous than sedative-hypnotic or alcohol withdrawal, the discomfort that many opioid-dependent persons experience in attempting detoxification may diminish the effectiveness of outpatient treatment because of frequent relapses. Some patients who are unable to successfully detoxify from opioids as outpatients may thus be admitted to complete the withdrawal process. Complicated detoxification regimens such as those for patients who are dependent on two or more classes of drugs should generally be administered in a hospital because of the need for frequent adjustment of such regimens. Similarly, patients with significant organ (e.g., cardiac, cerebral, or hepatic) dysfunction should generally be detoxified in a hospital.

As can be seen in the latter examples of indications for hospitalization, there is frequently overlap between the use of the hospital for protection and its use to reap the benefits of maximally intensive treatment. Indeed, some persons are hospitalized because of their failure to benefit from less intensive treatment.

Studies comparing inpatients and outpatients typically show that the former have more severe substance use histories and a greater prevalence of medical, psychosocial, and vocational difficulties (Harrison et al. 1988; Skinner 1981). Of course, these data may reflect referral patterns and do not necessarily indicate which populations fare best in which settings. Indeed, a number of studies have now been conducted in which alcohol- or drug-dependent patients were randomly assigned to inpatient treatment or a less intensive alternative. Although these studies have generally shown little difference in outcome (Longabaugh 1988; W. R. Miller and Hester 1986), methodological flaws in some of these studies may have affected the results (Pettinati et al. 1993; Sell 1995). For example, a well-known study by Longabaugh et al. (1983) concluded that persons treated as inpatients or in a partial hospital setting had similar outcomes. However, both groups of patients in this study were initially treated as inpatients. Another frequently cited study, by Edwards et al. (1977), concluded that a session of outpatient "advice" was as effective as inpatient treatment.

However, later analysis of the data from this study showed that patients with more severe alcohol dependence responded better to inpatient treatment than to outpatient treatment (Nace 1990). More recent studies of randomized treatment have again shown some disagreement regarding the role of inpatient treatment. Walsh et al. (1991) found inpatient treatment to be more effective than assignment to AA meetings for alcohol-dependent persons referred for treatment by their employee assistance programs. In contrast, O'Brien et al. (1990) found that partial hospital treatment of cocaine-dependent persons was as effective as inpatient treatment. More recently, Budde et al. (1992) found that cocaine-dependent patients who were hospitalized had better 1-year outcomes on measures of cocaine use and psychopathology than did patients who entered outpatient treatment, despite the fact that the former group had experienced more severe problems before entering treatment. At this time, studies are needed to determine patient-treatment matching characteristics (McLellan et al. 1983) so that we can better identify which groups of patients are most likely to respond best to which specific types of treatment. Simple comparisons of inpatient versus outpatient treatment, as if it could be determined which one is categorically superior, have been called nonsensical (Weddington and McLellan 1994).

Outcome of Inpatient Treatment

General Findings

A number of follow-up studies from inpatient treatment programs have shown impressive success rates. For example, Gilmore et al. (1986) and Wallace et al. (1988) administered 6-month follow-up questionnaires to patients treated at several Minnesota Model treatment centers. These authors found that 57%–73% of those who completed the assessments were abstinent at 6 months. However, in both treatment samples, patients who were discharged prematurely or (in the latter study) were unmarried were excluded from the follow-up study. In a 4-year follow-up of inpatients treated at the Carrier Foundation, approximately half of the study sample had favorable outcomes (Pettinati et al. 1982). However, fluctuations in outcome status were common, and only one-quarter of patients were continuously abstinent for all 4 years. Finally, a Department of Veterans Affairs study of nearly 75,000 alcoholic men found that patients who completed extended formal inpatient alcoholism treatment had lower mortality rates in the 3 years following discharge than did patients who had shorter inpatient stays or patients who were hospitalized without receiving alcoholism treatment (Bunn et al. 1994). Unfortunately, all of these studies were uncontrolled and thus subject to bias. Although an increasing number of controlled trials have been conducted in recent years, these studies, as mentioned earlier, have not been immune to methodological flaws. Thus, continued research on this topic is needed.

Patient Characteristics

Although some authors have claimed that inpatient treatment of substance-abusing persons is often not superior to less intensive treatment, some subgroups of patients do appear to respond best to hospitalization. These include patients with greater severity of substance-related problems, less social stability, and greater psychiatric comorbidity (McKay et al. 1991). In general, most studies of inpatient treatment have found that the following groups have a better prognosis: patients who are older, those who are married, those who are abusing alcohol rather than other drugs, and those who have family members participating in their treatment (Harrison et al. 1991). Patients with histories of injection drug use or antisocial behavior tend to fare less well in treatment outcome studies (Harrison et al. 1991).

Program Characteristics

Relatively little research has been conducted on characteristics of inpatient treatment programs that affect outcome. Some authors have argued that patient characteristics are more important than programmatic variables in determining treatment outcome (Armor et al. 1976). However, Cronkite and Moos (1978) conducted a path analysis of treatment outcome for 429 alcoholic patients treated in five different programs and concluded that program-related characteristics influenced treatment outcome substantially.

A number of characteristics of inpatient substance abuse treatment have been examined to determine their impact on treatment outcome (Adelman and Weiss 1989), although many of the studies examining these characteristics either have been uncontrolled or, when controlled, have not included a carefully matched control group. In a study of the impact of the *referral process* on outcome, employed alcoholic persons who were forced by their employers to enter treatment fared better than employed persons who volunteered for treatment (K. S. Chopra et al. 1979). Moberg et al. (1982) also found that *involving a patient's employer* during hospitalization had a beneficial effect on treatment outcome.

There is evidence that the *milieu orientation* of a program may also affect treatment efficacy. Stinson et al. (1979) randomly assigned 466 patients to two alcoholism treatment programs, one of which emphasized intensive individualized treatment, with a high staff-to-patient ratio, and the other of which had a lower staff-to-patient ratio and emphasized peer group interaction. Patients who entered the latter program had better treatment outcome, suggesting the potential importance of peer support in alcoholism treatment programs.

Characteristics of staff members have been examined in several studies. For example, Valle (1981) found that the interpersonal skills of alcoholism counselors in an inpatient treatment facility had a significant effect on treatment outcome. Similar data from outpatient studies (McLellan et al. 1988) corroborated this finding. Smart and Gray (1978) showed that *degree of medical orientation* may also influence treatment outcome. In their study of 792 alcoholic patients in five different inpatient treatment programs, these authors attributed 30% of the variance in dropout rates to treatment variables. They found that patients in the more medically oriented facilities were most likely to complete treatment.

One of the major components of virtually all inpatient treatment programs is *an emphasis on group therapy and AA meetings*. Because of the near universality of these aspects of inpatient treatment, little research has been done on their relative contribution to treatment outcome. However, some specific types of groups have been examined, and positive results have been reported for groups teaching social skills (Eriksen et al. 1986) and coping skills (Vogel et al. 1997). Other specific interventions that have been reported as beneficial include the administration of thermal and electromyogram biofeedback (Denney et al. 1991) and the use of patient-authored treatment contracts (as opposed to staff-authored or mutually authored contracts) in treatment planning (Vannicelli 1979). Physical exercise has also been shown in one study to reduce anxiety and depression in patients hospitalized for substance use disorders, although the long-term effects of exercise on outcome are not clear (Palmer et al. 1988).

Although several studies have shown the positive impact of *aftercare attendance* on outcome, some researchers have questioned whether the aftercare program itself improves treatment outcome or whether the patients who are likely to have good outcomes are also those who attend aftercare more often. Two studies using cross-lagged analyses have supported the former hypothesis (Costello 1980; Vannicelli 1978). However, McLatchie and Lomp (1988) disputed this theory. They randomly assigned 155 patients who had completed a 4-week inpatient alcoholism treatment program to one of three aftercare groups: 1) mandated aftercare; 2) voluntary aftercare, in which patients could decide whether or not to attend; and 3) a condition in which patients were dissuaded from attending aftercare. No differences were found among groups with respect to relapse to drinking, lifestyle satisfaction, or level of anxiety. However, it should be noted that 66% of patients in the voluntary group did request aftercare.

Finally, the correlation between *length of stay* and inpatient treatment outcome has long been a controversial subject. Although some research, as mentioned previously, has found inpatient treatment to offer no more benefit than a session of outpatient advice (Edwards et al. 1977), and one study (Rae 1972) correlated longer hospital stays with poorer outcome, other studies (Finney et al. 1981; McLellan et al. 1982) reported a positive correlation between length of stay and treatment response. However, many of these findings are difficult to evaluate because of the lack of randomization or poor comparability of study groups. Gottheil et al. (1992) examined 131 alcoholic male veterans who were treated in an inpatient program with a recommended length of stay of 90 days. The authors found that patients with less severe impairment, as measured by the Addiction Severity Index (McLellan et al. 1980), fared best. Moreover, in these patients, a longer hospital stay resulted in better treatment outcome. Patients with the most severe problems, on the other hand, did not benefit from increased length of stay.

Conclusions

The role of inpatient treatment for patients with substance use disorders remains a complex and controversial issue, with public health, political, philosophical, and financial ramifications. It is clear, however, that attempting to formulate simplistic guidelines about the use of this treatment modality serves no one's best interest. Thus, the question of whether inpatient treatment is effective should continue to shift to a more difficult but critical question: For which patients is inpatient treatment effective, at what time(s), and for how long? To that end, current research in this area, such as that being performed by McLellan et al. (1992), is attempting to define the "active" and "inert" ingredients of inpatient (and outpatient) treatment in order to discern which aspects of inpatient (and outpatient) treatment are truly effective for particular subgroups of patients. As future research helps to clarify these issues, it is hoped that inpatient treatment can attain a more stable and well-defined place in the therapeutic approach to patients with substance use disorders.

References

Adelman SA, Weiss RD: What is therapeutic about inpatient alcoholism treatment? Hospital and Community Psychiatry 40:515–519, 1989

American Society of Addiction Medicine: Patient Placement Criteria for the Treatment of Substance-Related Disorders. Chevy Chase, MD, American Society of Addiction Medicine, 1996

Armor DJ, Polich JM, Stambul H: Alcoholism and Treatment. Santa Monica, CA, Rand Corporation, 1976

Brooner RK, King VL, Kidorf M, et al: Psychiatric and substance use comorbidity among treatment-seeking opioid abusers. Arch Gen Psychiatry 54:71–80, 1997

Budde D, Rounsaville B, Bryant K: Inpatient and outpatient cocaine abusers: clinical comparisons at intake and one-year follow-up. J Subst Abuse Treat 9:337–342, 1992

Bunn JY, Booth BM, Cook CAL, et al: The relationship between mortality and intensity of inpatient alcoholism treatment. Am J Public Health 84:211–214, 1994

Chopra KS, Preston DA, Gerson LW: The effect of constructive coercion on the rehabilitative process: a study of the employed alcoholics in an alcoholism treatment program. J Occup Med 21:749–752, 1979

Collins MN, Burns T, Van Den Berk PAH, et al: A structured programme for out-patient alcohol detoxification. Br J Psychiatry 156:871–874, 1990

Cook CCH: The Minnesota Model in the management of drug and alcohol dependence: miracle, method or myth? Part I: the philosophy and the programme. British Journal of Addiction 83:625–634, 1988a

Cook CCH: The Minnesota Model in the management of drug and alcohol dependence: miracle, method or myth? Part II: evidence and conclusions. British Journal of Addiction 83:735–748, 1988b

Costello RM: Alcoholism aftercare and outcome: cross-lagged panel and path analysis. British Journal of Addiction 75:49–53, 1980

Cronkite RC, Moos RH: Evaluating alcoholism treatment programs: an integrated approach. J Consult Clin Psychol 46:1105–1119, 1978

Denney MR, Baugh JL, Hardt HD: Sobriety outcome after alcoholism treatment with biofeedback participation: a pilot inpatient study. Int J Addict 26:335–341, 1991

Edwards G, Orford J, Egert S, et al: Alcoholism: a controlled trial of "treatment" and "advice." J Stud Alcohol 38:1004–1031, 1977

Eriksen L, Björnstad S, Götestam KG: Social skills training in groups for alcoholics: one-year treatment outcome for groups and individuals. Addict Behav 11:309–329, 1986

Finney JW, Moos RH, Chan DA: Length of stay and program component effects in the treatment of alcoholism: a comparison of two techniques for process analyses. J Consult Clin Psychol 49:120–131, 1981

Gilmore K, Jones D, Tamble L: Treatment Benchmarks. Center City, MN, Hazelden, 1986

Gottheil E, McLellan AT, Druley KA: Length of stay, patient severity and treatment outcome: sample data from the field of alcoholism. J Stud Alcohol 53:69–75, 1992

Harrison PA, Hoffman NG, Gibb L, et al: Determinants of chemical dependency treatment placement: clinical, economic, and logistic factors. Psychotherapy: Theory, Research and Practice 25:356–364, 1988

Harrison PA, Hoffman NG, Streed SG: Drug and alcohol addiction treatment outcome, in Comprehensive Handbook of Drug and Alcohol Addiction. Edited by Miller NS. New York, Marcel Dekker, 1991, pp 1163–1197

Hayashida M, Alterman AI, McLellan AT, et al: Comparative effectiveness and costs of inpatient and outpatient detoxification of patients with mild-to-moderate alcohol withdrawal syndrome. N Engl J Med 320:358–365, 1989

Institute of Medicine: Broadening the Base of Treatment for Alcohol Problems. Washington, DC, National Academy Press, 1990

Kessler RC, Crum RC, Warner LA, et al: Lifetime co-occurrence of DSM-III-R alcohol abuse and dependence with other psychiatric disorders in the National Comorbidity Survey. Arch Gen Psychiatry 54:313–321, 1997

Longabaugh R: Longitudinal outcome studies, in Alcoholism: Origins and Outcome. Edited by Rose RM, Barrett J. New York, Raven, 1988, pp 267–280

Longabaugh R, McGrady B, Fine E, et al: Cost effectiveness of alcoholism treatment in partial vs inpatient settings: six-month outcomes. J Stud Alcohol 44:1049–1071, 1983

McKay JR, Murphy RT, Longabaugh R: The effectiveness of alcoholism treatment: evidence from outcome studies, in Psychiatric Treatment: Advances in Outcome Research. Edited by Mirin SM, Gossett JT, Grob MC. Washington, DC, American Psychiatric Press, 1991, pp 143–158

McLatchie BH, Lomp KGE: An experimental investigation of the influence of aftercare on alcoholic relapse. British Journal of Addiction 83:1045–1054, 1988

McLellan AT, Luborsky L, Woody GE, et al: An improved diagnostic evaluation instrument for substance abuse patients: the Addiction Severity Index. J Nerv Ment Dis 168:26–33, 1980

McLellan AT, Luborsky L, O'Brien CP, et al: Is treatment for substance abuse effective? JAMA 247:1423–1428, 1982

McLellan AT, Luborsky L, Woody GE, et al: Predicting response to alcohol and drug abuse treatments: role of psychiatric severity. Arch Gen Psychiatry 40:620–625, 1983

McLellan AT, Woody GE, Luborsky L, et al: Is the counselor an "active ingredient" in substance abuse rehabilitation? An examination of treatment success among four counselors. J Nerv Ment Dis 176:423–430, 1988

McLellan AT, O'Brien CP, Metzger D, et al: Is substance abuse treatment effective—compared to what? in Addictive States. Edited by O'Brien CP, Jaffe J. New York, Raven, 1992, pp 231–252

Meyer RE, Mirin SM: The Heroin Stimulus: Implications for a Theory of Addiction. New York, Plenum, 1979

Miller WR, Hester RK: Inpatient alcoholism treatment: who benefits? Am Psychol 41:794–805, 1986

Minkoff K: An integrated treatment model for dual diagnosis of psychosis and addiction. Hospital and Community Psychiatry 40:1031–1036, 1989

Mirin SM, Weiss RD, Griffin ML, et al: Psychopathology in drug abusers and their families. Compr Psychiatry 32:36–51, 1991

Moberg DP, Krause WK, Klein PE: Post-treatment drinking behavior among inpatients from an industrial alcoholism program. Int J Addict 17:549–567, 1982

Nace EP: Inpatient treatment of alcoholism: a necessary part of the therapeutic armamentarium. The Psychiatric Hospital 21:9–12, 1990

Neuberger OW, Matarazzo JD, Schmitz RE, et al: One-year follow-up of total abstinence in chronic alcoholic patients following emetic counterconditioning. Alcoholism 4:306–312, 1980

O'Brien CP, Alterman A, Walter D, et al: Evaluation of treatment for cocaine dependence, in Problems of Drug Dependence, 1989: Proceedings of the 51st Annual Scientific Meeting, the Committee on Problems of Drug Dependence. NIDA Research Monograph 95 (DHHS Publ No [ADM] 90-1663). Edited by Harris LS. Rockville, MD, National Institute on Drug Abuse, 1990, pp 78–84

Palmer J, Vacc N, Epstein J: Adult inpatient alcoholics: physical exercise as a treatment intervention. J Stud Alcohol 49:418–421, 1988

Pettinati HM, Sugerman AA, DiDonato N, et al: The natural history of alcoholism over four years after treatment. J Stud Alcohol 43:201–215, 1982

Pettinati HM, Meyers K, Jensen JM, et al: Inpatient vs outpatient treatment for substance dependence revisited. Psychiatr Q 4:173-182, 1993

Rae JB: The influence of the wives on the treatment outcome of alcoholics: a follow-up study at two years. Br J Psychiatry 120:601–613, 1972

Richard GP: Behavioral treatment of excessive drinking. Unpublished doctoral dissertation, University of New South Wales, New South Wales, Australia, 1983

Sell J: Academic outcome studies: the research and its misapplication to managed care of alcoholism. Alcoholism Treatment Quarterly 13:17–31, 1995

Skinner HA: Comparison of clients assigned to in-patient and out-patient treatment for alcoholism and drug addiction. Br J Psychiatry 138:312–320, 1981

Smart RG, Gray G: Multiple predictors of dropout from alcoholism treatment. Arch Gen Psychiatry 35:363–367, 1978

Stinson DJ, Smith WG, Amidjaya I, et al: Systems of care and treatment outcomes for alcoholic patients. Arch Gen Psychiatry 36:535–539, 1979

Thurber S: Effect size estimates in chemical aversion treatments of alcoholism. J Clin Psychol 41:285–287, 1985

Valle SK: Interpersonal functioning of alcoholism counselors and treatment outcome. J Stud Alcohol 42:783–790, 1981

Vannicelli M: Impact of aftercare in the treatment of alcoholics: a cross-lagged panel analysis. J Stud Alcohol 39:1875–1886, 1978

Vannicelli M: Treatment contracts in an inpatient alcoholism treatment setting. J Stud Alcohol 40:457–471, 1979

Vogel PA, Eriksen L, Bjornelv S: Skills training and prediction of follow-up status for chronic alcohol dependent inpatients. Eur J Psychiatry 11:51–63, 1997

Wallace J, McNeill D, Gilfillan D, et al: Six-month treatment outcomes in socially stable alcoholics: abstinence rates. J Subst Abuse Treat 5:247–252, 1988

Walsh DC, Hingson RW, Merrigan DM, et al: a randomized trial of treatment options for alcohol-abusing workers. N Engl J Med 325:775–782, 1991

Weddington WW, McLellan AT: Substance abuse treatment (letter). Hospital and Community Psychiatry 45:80, 1994

Weiss RD, Mirin SM, Frances RJ: The myth of the typical dual diagnosis patient. Hospital and Community Psychiatry 43:107–108, 1992

Wilson GT: Chemical aversion conditioning as a treatment for alcoholism: a re-analysis. Behav Res Ther 25:503–516, 1987

Community-Based Treatment

Jonathan I. Ritvo, M.D.
James H. Shore, M.D.

In this chapter subpart we discuss community-based substance abuse treatment from two perspectives. The first perspective, the community's role in treatment, encompasses substance abuse identification and intervention ranging from noncoercive brief interventions in primary care settings to coercive interventions through social service agencies and criminal courts. The second perspective, specific non-hospital-based treatment services, encompasses outpatient treatment programs, outpatient detoxification, community residential facilities, and case management approaches.

Community Intervention

Brief Intervention in Primary Care Settings

Studies in the primary care setting have shown repeatedly that professional attention, discussion, education, and follow-up regarding alcohol consumption and its consequences reduce heavy drinking (Bien et al. 1993; Institute of Medicine 1990). The most recent confirmations of this effect come from an eight-site multinational study by the World Health Organization (WHO) Brief Intervention Study Group (1996) and from a study performed in primary care practices in southern Wisconsin (Fleming et al. 1997). In the latter study, at 1-year follow-up, the intervention group, which had received two 15-minute physician advice sessions and a telephone follow-up by nurse, showed significant ($P \leq 0.001$) reductions in comparison with control subjects in number of drinks, episodes of binge drinking, and frequency of excessive drinking in the previous month.

The screening/brief intervention strategy appears particularly valuable for reducing morbidity in individuals who drink heavily but are not yet symptomatic and therefore are not yet candidates for professional alcohol treatment. The mild to moderate alcohol problems targeted in these studies are more prevalent than dependence. Therefore, the repeatedly replicated findings of brief intervention studies in primary care have profound implications for public health and general medical practice. They indicate major cost-effective health benefits both from the use of screening instruments to identify individuals who drink heavily and from the investment of physician time to inform these patients about the benefits of reducing their drinking.

Brief Intervention in Colleges

The brief intervention approach is also appropriate for problem drinking among college students. A report of the Institute of Medicine (1990) recommended a harm-reduction approach designed to foster moderate and safe drinking practices through the use of personalized feedback "containing non-judgmental normative information." It was postulated that this approach would speed up the normal maturational process of increasing personal responsibility for drinking practices. Marlatt et al. (1998) described programs at the University of Washington for accomplishing this goal with college students who drink heavily. These programs do not involve diagnosis of alcoholism, labeling of problem drinking, or prescribing of abstinence. They present risks, benefits, choices, normative data, and personalized feedback as well as strategies and standards for moderate and safe drinking. Outcome analysis showed that first-year students identified as heavy drinkers who received a brief motivational intervention of this type demonstrated greater reductions in their drinking rates and drinking problems than did control subjects. Both the intervention and the control groups, as well as their peers who did not drink heavily, showed reduction in drinking over the study period, consistent with the postulated maturational effect.

Social Service Agency Intervention

Child Protective Services

MacMahon (1997) reviewed the cases of 53 San Mateo County, California, infants who were reported to child protective services because of urine screens positive for illicit substances in the newborn nursery. As a result of the hospital report, all mothers were court-ordered to participate in a drug rehabilitation program and to undergo urine monitoring. The 44% who complied with treatment had repeatedly drug-free urine tests. All mothers with repeatedly drug-free urine regained custody of their infants. Forty-six percent of infants were returned to their mothers within a week of birth, and 76% were living with a relative within the first month. Seventeen percent were eventually adopted, and another 17% entered long-term guardianships with relatives. Failure of family reunification was most strongly predicted by a history of failed drug treatment, previous involvement with child protective services, or previous removal of a child because of substance abuse and was highly correlated with noncompliance with current treatment and positive urine test results. For a few mothers, the threat of losing custody of their child in the final disposition hearing at 18 months was critical in motivating treatment. In this county with progressive services, the process of identifying maternal substance abuse in the newborn nursery, with intervention and follow-up by child protective services and the courts and referral to substance abuse treatment, appears to work as intended in the best interests of the child.

Byrd et al. (1999) described a less effective intervention system in Rochester, New York, in which child protective services accepted referral of only about half of the newborns whose urine tested positive for cocaine, and only 36% of mothers of cocaine-positive infants participated in drug treatment. The authors characterized maternal drug treatment services in the community as minimal. They presented no data on urine monitoring, treatment compliance, or the relationship of treatment to retaining custody.

Disability and Public Support

Substance abuse by recipients of public support has been an area of recent societal concern and legislative action. Shaner et al. (1995) documented increased cocaine use, psychiatric symptomatology, and hospitalization among cocaine-dependent schizophrenic individuals around the first of the month, when they received their support payments. In contrast, Frisman and Rosenheck (1997) found no increased drug and alcohol use among homeless mentally ill veterans who received disability payments. Other reports have linked the receipt of large lump-sum retroactive disability payments with negative treatment events, namely premature, abrupt termination of long-term residential substance abuse treatment (Satel et al. 1997) and missed visits and positive urine tests during methadone maintenance (Herbst et al. 1996).

Herbst et al. (1996) also found that use of a representative payee (an agency or individual appointed to receive and manage disability payments for the use and benefit of the disabled individual) protected against the negative effect on treatment of large lump-sum retroactive payments. Rosenheck et al. (1997) found that use of representative payees had a positive effect on homelessness but not on substance abuse in homeless mentally ill individuals. Neither report presented data on the practices of the payees or whether the payees were agencies or individuals.

Ries and Comtois (1997) described a successful community mental health center program that managed benefits for some of its chronically mentally ill, substance-abusing patients as part of their treatment. Case managers served as representative payees. The form and frequency of disbursement depended on the patient's functional stability, sobriety, and treatment participation. Compared with a control group of patients in the same program who were not on payee status, the payee-managed patients were more likely to be male and to have a diagnosis of schizophrenia, a history of high inpatient utilization, high psychiatric and substance abuse severity, and lower functional stability. However, during the time they were payee-managed, this group showed no difference from the control group in hospitalization, homelessness, or incarceration and attended outpatient services twice as frequently.

Until 1997, Social Security regulations required a representative payee whenever substance abuse contributed to a beneficiary's disability. The Contract With America Administration Act of 1996 disqualified beneficiaries for whom substance abuse contributed to disability. As an unintended consequence, this provision made it more difficult to appoint payees for beneficiaries with substance use disorders (Rosen and Rosenheck 1999). An additional obstacle is the Department of Veterans Affairs (VA) policy prohibiting its programs and clinicians from serving as representative payees (Satel 1995). Considering the role of money in access to substances and in relapses, greater coordination of policy and practice between entitlement/support programs and local treatment services regarding the representative payee mechanism could add considerable leverage to substance abuse treatment.

For the substance-abusing individual, disability benefits may be a mixed blessing. Before supporting an application for disability benefits, the clinician needs to consider potential negative aspects: disincentive to work, ineligibility for many rehabilitation programs, loss of the structuring of time and the rewards for sobriety provided by work, and availability of money for addictive substances. For the substance-abusing patient receiving disability payments, the clinician should weigh the benefits of including a representative-payee arrangement as part of the treatment plan.

Adult Protective Services

Adult protective services seldom use their guardianship capacity to address the substance abuse/payee problem. In addition, judges are reluctant to appoint conservators for financial incompetence attributable solely to substance use (Satel 1995). For example, in Denver, even when the substance-abusing individual has dementia, understaffed and underfunded adult protective services may choose not to become involved unless the patient is elderly (J. I. Ritvo, personal observations, 1989–1999). The nonelderly alcoholic patient with dementia who needs chronic custodial care but is long estranged from family and unwelcome in nursing homes, as well as unwanted by adult protective services, the public mental health system, or state hospitals, poses a difficult problem and often is left to receive care through emergency and acute hospital services.

Interventions Through the Criminal Justice System

The criminal justice system should be an ideal community setting for substance abuse identification and intervention. The National Center on Addiction and Substance Abuse at Columbia University (CASA) (1998) estimated that 1.2 million prisoners (70% of America's prison population) are alcohol and drug abusers and addicts, as are another 2 million probationers (Tauber 1998).

Drug Courts

Beginning in Miami in 1989, drug treatment courts have demonstrated that coerced treatment can be effective and have provided a model for cooperation between the criminal justice system and addiction treatment services. Between 1994 and 1998, the number of these courts expanded from 12 to almost 400 (Tauber 1998). The drug-court model depends on the collaboration of judges, prosecutors, public defenders, and community treatment programs to apply the leverage of the criminal justice system to the treatment of the drug-abusing offender.

Table 32–1 presents features of the drug-court model. The judge plays a key role by administering sanctions—often, brief jail stays—for positive urine screens or missed treatment appointments. Two drug-court judges have called this "smart punishment" (Hora et al. 1999). Satel (1998) pointed out that these sanctions conform to basic principles of behavioral therapy by "being swift and sure but not necessarily severe." The drug court's use of sanctions can also be conceptualized as shoring up the offender's weakened ego with firm, consistent limits that better promote emotional growth and mature accountability than do traditional court sanctions, which more closely follow the model of the offender's rigid, harsh, and unpredictable primitive superego. Reviewing the emerging research literature on drug courts, Belenko (1998) concluded that these courts engaged and retained felony offenders in treatment, saved money for the criminal justice system, and were associated with reduced recidivism and drug use both during and after the drug-court program.

Most drug-court programs target the least serious felonies (typically crack or cocaine possession). An exception is Brooklyn's Drug Treatment Alternative to Prison program, which offers the option of deferred prosecution and admission to long-term (15–24 months) residential treatment to defendants arrested for felony drug sales who have prior nonvio-

TABLE 32–1. Standard features of the drug-court model

1. Judicial supervision of structured community-based treatment
2. Timely identification of defendants in need of treatment and referral to treatment as soon as possible after arrest
3. Regular status hearings before the judicial officer to monitor treatment progress and program compliance
4. Increased defendant accountability through a series of graduated sanctions and rewards
5. Mandatory periodic drug testing
6. Dismissal of charges or reduction of sentence upon successful treatment completion
7. Provision of aftercare and support services following treatment to facilitate reentry into the community

Source. Belenko 1998; CASA 1998.

lent felony convictions and a drug abuse problem. Program completers have lower rearrest rates than do program noncompleters or control subjects (CASA 1998). Recently, some courts have reported successful engagement of a broader spectrum of the offender population through use of multitrack systems. In these courts, the more serious offenders begin with jail time and then enter the traditional drug-court model under the supervision of probation (Tauber 1998). Realizing the potential of probation and parole to offer surveillance, monitoring, and contingencies for treatment will require investment in substance abuse training for probation and parole officers and immediate access to comprehensive treatment services that can also address issues of poverty, employment, health, and drug-free housing (CASA 1998).

Drunk Driving

Alcohol use patterns among drunk drivers range from social drinking to incipient problem drinking to alcohol dependence. In the late 1960s and early 1970s, the Alcohol Safety Action Programs of the National Highway Traffic Safety Administration expanded the interventions for drunk driving from jail and license actions to education and rehabilitation. Evaluation revealed that social drinkers might benefit from alcohol-safety schools, that education and rehabilitation programs had a small effect on recidivism (compared with no intervention) and no effect on subsequent accidents, and that license sanctions were superior to rehabilitation alone in reducing accidents and convictions (Hagen 1985).

In the 1970s and 1980s, many states adopted statutes, called administrative per se laws, that permit swift license suspension for drivers who fail sobriety tests. Retrospective studies have shown decreases in recidivism and subsequent accidents involving offenders after initiation of these laws (McArthur and Kraus 1999). For drunk drivers, education and rehabilitation serve as adjuncts to, but not replacements for, community intervention in the form of license sanctions.

Non-Hospital-Based Treatment Services

The 1990s saw a major change in the substance abuse treatment paradigm. In the 1980s, the Minnesota Model of 28-day residential treatment followed by aftercare and participation in Alcoholics Anonymous was the treatment standard and was supported by generous insurance coverage of inpatient treatment. The pressure to provide less costly, less restrictive treatment increased interest in community-based treatment, as opposed to hospital-based treatment, and led to limiting inpatient and intensive residential (Minnesota Model) treatment to cases involving more severe complications or in which "life is in danger or other forms of treatment have failed" (Book et al. 1995). The standard of care now emerging involves individualized treatment determined through the matching of a patient's biopsychosocial needs to a continuum of levels of care and a spectrum of specific services (Gastfriend and McLellan 1997). In this section, we discuss the portion of the continuum of care levels based in the community.

We conceptualize three types of service components characterizing different levels of care: residential, addiction-focused, and comprehensive. Residential services provide room and board. Addiction-focused services encompass the general social support functions of the treatment milieu as well as specific treatments directed toward substance abuse disorders. Comprehensive services are usually provided by specialized professionals such as psychiatrists, other physicians, nurses, social workers, vocational rehabilitation counselors, and family therapists and address problems that are comorbid with or secondary to addiction—problems in areas such as physical and mental health, finances, housing, employment, and family relationships.

Day Hospital and Intensive Outpatient Treatments

Day or partial hospital programs evolved from inpatient programs through the subtraction of the overnight residential component. In the 1980s, comparisons of day and inpatient programs for alcoholic patients who were physically and psychiatrically stable demonstrated equivalent outcomes and a 50% cost savings for day programs (Longabaugh et al. 1983; McLachlan and Stein 1982). With cocaine-dependent patients, day programs have had more difficulty with retention in early treatment, and inpatient programs have had more difficulty with the transition to aftercare. The net result is equivalent outcomes at 6–7 months (Alterman et al. 1994; Schneider et al. 1996). The intense cue reactivity common in cocaine addiction and the lack of a deterrent such as disulfiram may explain why this finding appears specific to cocaine.

McKay et al. (1994) described and evaluated a 4-week (27 hours/week) day hospital rehabilitation program at the Philadelphia VA, with most of the features of Minnesota Model programs, for individuals who abused alcohol or cocaine. Continuity of care, with up to 5 months of twice-weekly aftercare, and an emphasis on 12-Step group participation were important features of the program. Alterman et al. (1994) compared the outcomes of 56 cocaine-dependent patients in this day program with the outcomes of 55 patients undergoing 28-day inpatient treatment at another Pennsylvania VA, located 35 miles away in Coatesville. After 28 days of inpatient treatment at Coatesville, patients returned to the twice-weekly aftercare program of the Philadelphia VA day program. Although the inpatient program had better treatment retention than the day hospital in the first 28 days, the difference between the groups largely disappeared when the inpatients returned to Philadelphia for aftercare. At 7 months, there was no difference in outcome. Obviously, the goal of facilitating the transition to ongoing self-help-group involvement is more practical for community-based programs than for residential programs at a distance from the patient's community.

The distinction between intensive outpatient and day or partial hospital programs is not always precise. McKay et al. (1997) used the term *intensive outpatient* to refer to the 27-hour-per-week Philadelphia VA day program (described in the previous paragraph as a day hospital). Guidelines published by the American Society of Addiction Medicine (1996) require 9 hours per week of structured programming for intensive outpatient programs and 20 hours per week for partial hospital programs, which are described as having more immediate access to medical and psychiatric services. McClellan et al. (1997) used a similar minimum criterion of 9 hours per week (three sessions per week) to define 10 intensive outpatient programs. They then compared these programs with 6 "traditional" outpatient programs that offered no more than two 2-hour sessions per week. All programs were non–hospital based and oriented toward abstinence. Patients in the intensive outpatient programs engaged in more severe substance use and had more social and health problems. They received more addiction-focused treatment but not more comprehensive services related to medical, employment, family, or social problems. At 6 months, patients in both kinds of programs showed notable improvement in substance use, personal health, and social functioning. These research findings should prompt referring clinicians to examine individual intensive outpatient programs before assuming that they are intensive in terms of providing comprehensive services. Day or partial hospital programs may better serve patients who have a substantial need for comprehensive services. Intensive outpatient programs, which often have evening schedules, may better serve patients for whom continued employment or attendance at school is indicated during treatment.

Community Residential Facilities

Community residential facilities (CRFs), often called halfway houses, typically receive patients, from inpatient treatment or detoxification services, who are not yet ready for independent living and who need the supervision and support of a living environment committed to sobriety. Moos et al. (1995) studied the 127 CRFs receiving the most VA referrals in 1991. Facilities generally had a 12-Step orientation and averaged 30 residents and a 42-day length of stay. Longer lengths of stay were associated with lower rates of readmission to inpatient facilities. Study patients were severely and chronically ill and were more ill than were patients in CRFs in 1987. For one VA hospital, CRF placement improved involvement in aftercare for patients returning from out-of-town inpatient treatment (Hitchcock et al. 1995). In general, halfway houses and CRFs ease the transition between inpatient and independent living for the substance-abusing individual with limited sober social support or limited sober housing resources.

Detoxification Services

Detoxification Centers

The Uniform Alcoholism and Intoxication Treatment Act promulgated by the National Conference of Commissioners on Uniform State Laws in 1971 sought to replace the criminal justice solution to public drunkenness with medical alternatives. Persons incapacitated by alcohol were to be taken home or to health care or treatment facilities instead of being arrested and held in "drunk tanks." By 1980, more than half of the states had implemented major provisions of the Act (Finn 1985). This legislation led to the development of detoxification centers as the medical alternative to the "drunk tank."

Detoxification centers developed along two major models, medical and nonmedical/

social, the latter relying on rest, comfort, and support, with minimal use of medication or medical examination and supervision (Whitfield et al. 1978). The social model initially predominated both because of its low cost and because of some hospitals' refusal to provide detoxification services (Finn 1985). Over time, the distinction between the two models blurred. As benzodiazepine therapy became the standard treatment for alcohol withdrawal, some nonmedical detoxification centers were "medicalized," adopting protocols by which nurses could administer benzodiazepines. Although the Uniform Alcoholism and Intoxication Treatment Act encouraged voluntary, community-based treatment through a continuum of services, Finn (1985) concluded that it did little to rehabilitate the "skid row alcoholic." It replaced one revolving door with another. The detoxification center is certainly more hospitable and humane than the "drunk tank"; however, decriminalization does nothing to address the conditions that perpetuate the problem, such as inadequate shelter, poverty, and vocational and social handicaps.

Outpatient Detoxification

Mild to moderate alcohol withdrawal can be managed on an outpatient basis with safety and efficacy, although the dropout rate is higher than for inpatient detoxification (Hayashida et al. 1989). Wiseman and colleagues (1997) reported that providing housing and starting psychosocial treatment during detoxification resulted in improved retention. In their study, 5% of patients undergoing outpatient detoxification required transfer to inpatient facilities. Outpatient cost can be as little as 10% of inpatient cost (Hayashida et al. 1989).

Case Management

The goals of case management are to ensure continuity of care and to integrate other functions of the treatment system (Institute of Medicine 1990). Case management can involve performing patient advocacy, shepherding patients through bureaucratic "red tape," improvising to fill gaps in services, conducting outreach to engage and retain patients in treatment, providing basic services such as transportation, and developing an individualized supportive, therapeutic relationship. A wide variety of persons can perform case management functions: psychiatrists, primary care physicians, social workers, case workers, probation officers, college counselors, substance abuse counselors and other therapists, Alcoholics Anonymous sponsors, trained laypersons, or even the patient him- or herself (Institute of Medicine 1990). Physician health programs, similar programs for dentists, nurses, and other health professionals, and employee assistance programs are community institutions that perform case management and continuity-of-care functions. Programs for health care professionals perform these functions by integrating community identification, patient advocacy, relations with licensing boards, assessment and referral for professional treatment, and ongoing monitoring.

Multiple factors contribute to whether patients will require case management to achieve optimal therapeutic results. On the patient's side, these factors include motivation or resistance, experience, knowledge, intelligence, and other internal and external resources or deficits. On the system's side, relevant variables include the complexity of the system, the accessibility of the relevant components, and how well the components are integrated with one another and match the patient's needs. Perhaps most important, many patients need individualized, caring long-term relationships that may not be present elsewhere in treatment. Given the variation in the types of case management and in the settings, populations, and systems in which they are applied, it is not surprising that the literature on the efficacy of case management for substance-abusing patients is inconsistent.

The most intensive case management approaches have been used in the treatment of substance abusers with severe and chronic mental illness (i.e., the dually diagnosed). The term *assertive community treatment* (ACT) describes outpatient programs that combine assertive outreach, medication management, integration of treatment, rehabilitation and support, a multidisciplinary team approach, low client-to-staff ratios (in the range of 12:1 or 8:1), extended or round-the-clock service hours, and a long-term commitment to clients (Drake et al. 1998). ACT and other intensive case management programs that also use stepwise motivational approaches to substance abuse and that integrate mental health and substance abuse counseling and services through the same staff have shown better treatment retention and better long-term outcomes than have short-term intensive dual diagnosis programs or programs that provide mental health and substance abuse treatment and services separately (Drake et al. 1998).

Case management approaches less intensive than ACT have been effective in engaging and helping substance-abusing individuals who are not seeking treatment. Rhodes and Gross (1997) found that noncoerced case management offered to arrestees who were using illicit drugs other than marijuana decreased drug use and recidivism and increased use of substance abuse treatment. It is noteworthy that this study attributed its case management effect more to personalized supportive relationships than to referral activity. A study of the "chronic public inebriates" who were the most frequent users of the King County (Seattle, Washington) Detoxification Center found that intensive outreach-oriented case management improved financial and residential stability and reduced use of alcohol and detoxification center admissions in this "revolving door" population (Cox et al. 1998). For homeless substance-abusing persons seeking treatment, case management approaches that are more office-based, more time-limited, and more directed toward arranging rather than directly providing services have not demonstrated a differential effect beyond the general short-term improvement that accompanies seeking treatment for substance abuse (Braucht et al. 1995; Stahler 1995; Stahler et al. 1995).

Summary

In this chapter subpart, we reviewed substance abuse identification and intervention in a variety of community settings and examined both the community-based portion of the continuum of levels of care and the case management approaches that serve to integrate the complex treatment system for the individual patient. We described instances, such as in drug courts and child protective services in some communities, in which the relationship between community institutions and treatment services has been fruitful. We highlighted promising community interventions, in primary care settings and colleges, that we hope will be disseminated, and we identified community institutions, such as the criminal justice system and public support programs, in which much of the potential for community-based substance abuse treatment remains to be realized.

References

Alterman AI, O'Brien CP, McLellan AT: Effectiveness and costs of inpatient versus day hospital rehabilitation. J Nerv Ment Dis 182:157–163, 1994

American Society of Addiction Medicine: Patient Placement Criteria for the Treatment of Substance-Related Disorders, 2nd Edition. Chevy Chase, MD, American Society of Addiction Medicine, 1996

Belenko S: Research on drug courts: a critical review. National Drug Court Institute Review 1:1–42, 1998

Bien TH, Miller WR, Tonigan JS: Brief interventions for alcohol problems: a review. Addiction 88:315–336, 1993

Book J, Harbin H, Marques C, et al: The ASAM and Green Spring alcohol and drug detoxification and rehabilitation criteria for utilization review. Am J Addict 4:187–192, 1995

Braucht GN, Reichardt CS, Geissler LJ, et al: Effective services for homeless substance abusers. J Addict Dis 14:87–109, 1995

Byrd RS, Neistadt AM, Howard CR, et al: Why screen newborns for cocaine: service patterns and social outcomes at age one year. Child Abuse Neglect 23:523–530, 1999

CASA (National Center on Addiction and Substance Abuse at Columbia University): Behind Bars: Substance Abuse and America's Prison Population. New York, National Center on Addiction and Substance Abuse at Columbia University, 1998

Cox GB, Walker RD, Freng SA, et al: Outcome of a controlled trial of the effectiveness of intensive case management for chronic public inebriates. J Stud Alcohol 59:523–532, 1998

Drake RE, Mercer-McFadden C, Mueser KT, et al: Review of integrated mental health and substance abuse treatment for patients with dual disorders. Schizophr Bull 24:589–608, 1998

Finn P: Decriminalization of public drunkenness: response of the health care system. J Stud Alcohol 46:7–23, 1985

Fleming MF, Barry KL, Manwell LB, et al: Brief physician advice for problem alcohol drinkers: a randomized controlled trial in community-based primary care practices. JAMA 277:1039–1045, 1997

Frisman LK, Rosenheck R: The relationship of public support payments to substance abuse among homeless veterans with mental illness. Psychiatr Serv 48:792–795, 1997

Gastfriend DR, McLellan AT: Treatment matching: theoretical basis and practical implications. Med Clin North Am 81:945–966, 1997

Hagen RE: Evaluation of the effectiveness of educational and rehabilitation efforts: opportunities for research. J Stud Alcohol 46 (suppl 10):179–183, 1985

Hayashida M, Alterman A, McLellan AT, et al: Comparative effectiveness and cost of inpatient and outpatient detoxification of patients with mild to moderate alcohol withdrawal syndrome. N Engl J Med 320:358–365, 1989

Herbst MD, Batki SL, Manfredi LB, et al: Treatment outcomes for methadone clients receiving lump-sum payments at initiation of disability benefits. Psychiatr Serv 47:119–120, 142, 1996

Hitchcock HC, Stainback RD, Roque GM: Effects of halfway house placement on retention of patients in substance abuse aftercare. Am J Drug Alcohol Abuse 21:379–390, 1995

Hora PF, Schma WG, Rosenthal JTA: Therapeutic jurisprudence and the drug treatment court movement: revolutionizing the criminal justice system's response to drug abuse and crime in America. Notre Dame Law Review 74:439–537, 1999

Institute of Medicine: Broadening the Base of Treatment for Alcohol Problems. Washington, DC, National Academy Press, 1990

MacMahon JR: Perinatal substance abuse: the impact of reporting infants to child protective services. Pediatrics 100:E1, 1997

Marlatt GA, Baer JS, Kivlahan DR, et al: Screening and brief intervention for high-risk college student drinkers: results from a 2-year follow-up assessment. J Consult Clin Psychol 66:604–615, 1998

McArthur DL, Kraus JF: The specific deterrence of administrative per se laws in reducing drunk driving recidivism. Am J Prev Med 16 (1 suppl):68–75, 1999

McKay JR, Alterman AI, McLellan AT, et al: Treatment goals, continuity of care and outcome in a day hospital substance abuse rehabilitation program. Am J Psychiatry 151:254–259, 1994

McKay JR, Cacciola JS, McLellan AT: An initial evaluation of the psychosocial dimensions of the American Society of Addiction Medicine criteria for inpatient versus intensive outpatient substance abuse rehabilitation. J Stud Alcohol 58:239–252, 1997

McLachlan JFC, Stein RL: Evaluation of a day clinic for alcoholics. J Stud Alcohol 43:261–272, 1982

McLellan AT, Hagan TA, Meyers K, et al: "Intensive" outpatient substance abuse treatment: comparison with "traditional" outpatient treatment. J Addict Dis 16:57–84, 1997

Moos RH, Pettit B, Gruber VA: Characteristics and outcomes of three models of community residential care for substance abuse patients. J Subst Abuse 7:99–116, 1995

Rhodes W, Gross M: Case management reduces drug use and criminality among drug-involved arrestees: an experimental study of an HIV prevention intervention (National Institute of Justice Res Rep). Washington, DC, U.S. Department of Justice, Office of Justice Programs, 1997. Available at: http://www.ncjrs.org/txtfiles/155281.txt

Ries RK, Comtois KA: Managing disability benefits as part of treatment for persons with severe mental illness and comorbid drug/alcohol disorders: a comparative study of payee and non-payee participants. Am J Addict 6:330–338, 1997

Rosen MI, Rosenheck R: Substance use and assignment of representative payees. Psychiatr Serv 50:95–98, 1999

Rosenheck R, Lam J, Randolph F: Impact of representative payees on substance use by homeless persons with serious mental illness. Psychiatr Serv 48:800–806, 1997

Satel SL: When disability benefits make patients sicker. N Engl J Med 333:794–796, 1995

Satel SL: Observational study of courtroom dynamics in selected drug courts. National Drug Court Institute Review 1:43–72, 1998

Satel S, Reuter P, Hartley D, et al: Influence of retroactive disability payments on recipients' compliance with substance abuse treatment. Psychiatr Serv 48:796–799, 1997

Schneider R, Mittelmeier C, Gadish D: Day versus inpatient treatment for cocaine dependence: an experimental comparison. J Ment Health Adm 23:234–245, 1996

Shaner A, Eckman TA, Roberts LJ, et al: Disability income, cocaine use and repeated hospitalization among schizophrenic cocaine abusers. N Engl J Med 333:777–783, 1995

Stahler GJ: Social interventions for homeless substance abusers: evaluating treatment outcomes (editorial). J Addict Dis 14:xv–xxvi, 1995

Stahler GJ, Shipley TF Jr, Bartelt D, et al: Evaluating alternative treatments for homeless substance-abusing men: outcomes and predictors of success. J Addict Dis 14:151–167, 1995

Tauber J: The future of drug courts: comprehensive drug court systems. National Drug Court Institute Review 1:86–97, 1998

Whitfield CL, Thompson G, Lamb A, et al: Detoxification of 1,024 alcoholic patients without psychoactive drugs. JAMA 239:1409–1410, 1978

WHO Brief Intervention Study Group: A cross-national trial of brief interventions with heavy drinkers. Am J Public Health 86:948–955, 1996

Wiseman EJ, Henderson KL, Briggs MJ: Outcomes of patients in a VA ambulatory detoxification program. Psychiatr Serv 48:200–203, 1997

Therapeutic Community Treatment

George De Leon, Ph.D.

Therapeutic communities (TCs) have been used in the treatment of substance-abusing persons for three decades. Originating as an alternative to conventional medical and psychiatric approaches, the TC has established itself as a major psychosocial treatment modality for thousands of chemically involved persons.

Today, the term *therapeutic community* is generic, describing a variety of short- and long-term residential programs as well as day treatment and ambulatory programs serving a wide spectrum of drug and alcohol abuse patients. It is the traditional long-term residential prototype, however, that has documented effectiveness in rehabilitating substance-abusing persons.

The Traditional Therapeutic Community

Traditional TCs are similar in planned duration of stay (15–24 months), structure, staffing pattern, perspective, and rehabilitative regimen, although they differ in size (e.g., 30–600 beds) and client demography. Staff is composed of TC-trained clinicians and other human services professionals. Primary clinical staff are usually former substance abusers themselves who were rehabilitated in TC programs. Other staff consist of professionals providing medical, mental health, vocational, educational, family counseling, fiscal, administrative, and legal services.

A version of this chapter subpart was published as "Therapeutic Communities" in *The American Psychiatric Press Textbook of Substance Abuse Treatment,* 2nd Edition. Edited by Galanter M, Kleber HD. Washington, D.C., American Psychiatric Press, 1999, pp. 447–462. This chapter subpart is a revision of longer discussions of therapeutic community treatment published previously (De Leon and Rosenthal 1989).

TCs accommodate a broad spectrum of drug-abusing individuals. Although they originally attracted narcotics-addicted persons, today a majority of their client populations are nonopioid substance–abusing persons who have differing lifestyles and are from various social, economic, and ethnic/cultural backgrounds and whose drug problems are of varying severity.

In the TC, drug abuse is viewed as a deviant behavior, reflecting impeded personality development or chronic deficits in social, educational, and economic skills. The antecedents of this use lie in socioeconomic disadvantage, poor family effectiveness, and psychological factors. Thus, the principal aim of the therapeutic community is a global change in lifestyle: abstinence from illicit substances, elimination of antisocial activity, development of employability, and development of prosocial attitudes and values. The rehabilitative approach requires multidimensional influence and training, which in most cases can only occur in a 24-hour residential setting.

The traditional TC can be distinguished from other major drug treatment modalities in three broad ways. First, in the TC a comprehensive offering of interventions and services is coordinated in a single treatment setting. Vocational counseling, work therapy, recreation, group and individual therapy, and educational, medical, family, legal, and social services all occur within the TC. Second, the primary "therapist" and teacher in the TC is the community itself, consisting of peers and staff who role-model successful personal change. Staff members also serve as rational authorities and guides in the recovery process. Thus, the community as a whole provides a crucial 24-hour context for continued learning in which individual changes in conduct, attitudes, and emotions are monitored and mutually reinforced in the daily regimen. Third, the TC approach to rehabilitation is based on an explicit perspective of the substance use disorder, the client, the recovery process, and healthy living. It is this perspective that shapes the TC's organizational structure, staffing, and treatment process.

View of the Disorder

Drug abuse is viewed as a disorder of the whole person, affecting some or all areas of functioning. Cognitive and behavioral problems are evident, as are mood disturbances. Thinking may be unrealistic or disorganized; values are confused, nonexistent, or antisocial. Frequently there are deficits in verbal expression, in reading and writing, and in marketable skills.

The problem is the person, not the drug. Addiction is a symptom, not the essence of the disorder. In the TC, chemical detoxification is a condition of entry into the TC, not a goal of treatment. Rehabilitation focuses on maintaining a drug-free existence.

View of the Person

Residents of the TC are distinguished along dimensions of psychological dysfunction and social deficits. Vocational and educational problems are marked; mainstream values are either missing or unpursued. Usually these clients emerge from a socially disadvantaged sector where drug abuse is more a social response than a psychological disturbance. Their TC experience is better termed *habilitation*, that is, the development of a socially productive, conventional lifestyle for the first time in their lives. Among clients from more advantaged backgrounds, drug abuse is more directly expressive of psychological disorder or existential malaise. For these persons, the word *rehabilitation* is more suitable, emphasizing a return to a lifestyle previously lived, known, and perhaps rejected.

Notwithstanding these social differences, substance-abusing residents of the TC share important similarities. Either as cause or as consequence of their drug abuse, all reveal features of personality disturbance and impeded social functioning. Thus, all residents in the TC follow the same regimen. Individual differences are recognized in specific treatment plans that modify the emphasis, not the course, of residents' experience.

View of Recovery

In the TC, recovery involves a change both in lifestyle and in personal identity. The primary psychological goal is to change the negative patterns of behavior, thinking, and feeling that predispose one to drug use; the main social goal is to develop the skills, attitudes, and values of a responsible drug-free lifestyle. Stable recovery, however, depends on a successful integration of these social and psychological goals. Behavioral change is unstable without insight, and insight is insufficient without felt experience.

Motivation

Recovery depends on pressures to change, whether they be externally applied or arise internally. Some clients are driven by stressful external pressures, whereas others are driven by more intrinsic factors. For all, however, remaining in treatment requires continued motivation to change. Thus, elements of the rehabilitation approach are designed to sustain motivation or to detect early signs of premature termination.

Self-Help and Mutual Self-Help

Strictly speaking, treatment is not *provided* but rather is *made available* to the person in the TC environment through its staff and peers and the daily regimen of work, groups, meetings, seminars, and recreation. However, the effectiveness of these elements depends on the resident, who must constantly and fully engage in the treatment regimen. Self-help recovery means that the resident makes the main *contribution* to the change process. Mutual self-help emphasizes the fact that the main messages of recovery and personal growth are mediated by peers through confrontation and sharing in groups, through their functioning as role models, and through their supportive, encouraging friendship in daily interactions.

Social Learning

A lifestyle change occurs in a social context. Thus, recovery depends not only on what has been learned but on how and where learning occurs. This assumption is the basis for the community itself collectively serving as "teacher." Learning is active, by doing and participating. A socially responsible role is acquired by acting the role. What is learned is identified with the persons involved in the learning process, with peers providing their support and with staff functioning as credible role models. Sustained recovery requires a perspective on self, society, and life that must be continually affirmed by a positive social network of others within and beyond residency in the TC.

Treatment as an Episode

Residency in the TC is a relatively brief period in a person's life, and its influence must compete with the influences of the years before and after treatment. For this reason, unhealthy "outside" influences are minimized until the person is better prepared to engage these on his or her own. Life in the TC is necessarily intense, its daily regimen demanding, and its therapeutic confrontations unmoderated.

View of Right Living

TCs adhere to certain precepts that constitute a view of healthy personal and social living. For example, TCs hold unambiguous *moral* positions regarding social and sexual conduct. Explicit right and wrong behaviors are identified, for which there exist appropriate rewards and sanctions. These include antisocial behaviors and attitudes, the negative values of the street or jails, and irresponsible or exploitative sexual conduct.

Guilts—in regard to self, to significant others, and to the larger community outside the TC—are central issues in the recovery process. Although referring to moral matters, guilts are special psychological experiences that, if not addressed, maintain the individual's disaffiliation from peers and block the self-acceptance that is necessary for authentic personal change.

Certain values are stressed as essential to social learning and personal growth. These values include truth and honesty (in word and deed), healthy work ethic, self-reliance, earned rewards and achievements, personal accountability, responsible concern ("brother's/ sister's keeper"), social manners, and community involvement.

Treatment helps the resident focus on the personal present ("here and now") versus the historical past ("there and then"). Past behavior and circumstances are explored only to illustrate the current patterns of dysfunctional behavior, negative attitudes, and outlook. Residents are encouraged and trained to assume personal responsibility for their present reality and destiny.

Profiles of Clients in Therapeutic Communities

The majority of persons entering TCs have histories of multiple drug use including marijuana, opiates, alcohol, and nonprescription medication, although in recent years most persons entering the TC for treatment report cocaine/crack or heroin as their primary drug of abuse. Persons newly admitted to TCs reveal a considerable degree of psychosocial dysfunction in addition to their substance abuse.

Social Profiles

Clients in traditional programs are usually male (70%–75%), but female admissions are increasing. Most community-based TCs are integrated across gender, race/ethnicity, and age (with most residents over 21), although the demographic proportions differ by geographic regions and in certain programs.

Most persons who are admitted to TCs are from broken homes, have poor work histories, and have engaged in criminal activities. Among adult admissions, less than one-third were employed full-time in the year before treatment, more than two-thirds have been arrested, and 30%–40% have had a history of prior drug treatment (De Leon 1984; Hubbard et al. 1984; D. D. Simpson and Sells 1982).

Psychological Profiles

Persons entering TCs for treatment differ in demography, socioeconomic background, and drug use patterns, but their psychological profiles obtained with standard instruments appear remarkably uniform (e.g., Biase et al. 1986; De Leon 1984; De Leon et al. 1973; Holland 1986). Typically, symptom measures on depression and anxiety are higher than the norm, socialization scores are poor, and IQ is in the dull-to-normal range. Self-esteem is markedly low, and scores on the Minnesota Multiphasic Personality Inventory (MMPI; Hathaway and McKinley 1943) deviate from the norm.

The psychological profiles of persons entering TCs for treatment mirror features of both psychiatric and criminal populations. For example, the character disorder elements and poor self-concept of delinquent and repeat offenders are present, along with the dysphoria and confused thinking of emotionally unstable or psychiatric populations.

Clinical Characteristics

The main clinical characteristics of addicted persons entering TCs for treatment reflect immaturity and/or antisocial dimensions. These characteristics include low tolerance for all forms of discomfort and for delay of gratification; problems with authority; inability to manage feelings (particularly hostility, guilt, and anxiety); poor impulse control (particularly control of sexual or aggressive impulses); poor judgment and reality testing concerning consequences of actions; unrealistic self-appraisal in terms of a discrepancy between personal resources and aspirations; prominence of lying, manipulation, and deception as coping behaviors; and personal and social irresponsibility (i.e., inconsistency or failures in completing expected obligations). Additionally, significant numbers of TC residents have marked deficits in education, communication skills, and marketable skills.

These clinical characteristics do not necessarily depict a uniform "addictive personality." However, many of these features are typical of conduct disorder in the younger substance-abusing person that later evolves into adult character disorder. Nevertheless, whether antecedent or consequent to serious drug involvement, these characteristics are commonly observed to be correlated with chemical dependency. More importantly, TCs require a positive change in these characteristics because such change is essential for stable recovery.

Psychiatric Diagnoses

In diagnostic studies of TC admissions in which the Diagnostic Interview Schedule (DIS; Robins et al. 1981) was utilized, over 70% of the admission sample were found to have a lifetime (i.e., before the last 30 days) non-drug-related psychiatric disorder in addition to substance abuse or dependence. One-third of the sample had a current (i.e., within the past 30 days) and past history of mental disorder in addition to their drug abuse. The most frequent non-drug-related diagnoses were phobias, generalized anxiety, psychosexual dysfunction, and antisocial personality. There were only a few cases of schizophrenia, but affective disorders occurred in more than one-third of those persons studied (De Leon 1993; Jainchill 1989, 1997; Jainchill et al. 1986).

That the psychological and psychiatric profiles reveal few psychotic features and relatively low variability in symptoms or personality characteristics reflects several factors: the TC exclusionary criteria for admission, the common characteristics among all substance-abusing persons, and some degree of self-selection among those who seek admission to residential treatment. Nevertheless, clients do differ, which is evident in their dropout and success rates, discussed later in this chapter subpart.

Contacts and Referrals

Clients voluntarily contact TCs through several sources—self-referral, social agencies, and treatment providers—and through active recruitment by the program. Outreach teams (usually, trained graduates of TCs and selected human services staff) recruit in hospitals, jails, courtrooms, social agencies, and the street, conducting brief orientations or face-to-face interviews to determine receptivity to the TC.

Among adolescents, 40%–50% have been criminal justice referrals to treatment compared with 25%–30% of adults (De Leon 1988a; National Institute on Drug Abuse 1980). For some programs, legal referrals constitute considerably higher percentages of all admissions (e.g., Pompi and Resnick 1987). Although the majority of admissions to TCs are voluntary, many of these persons come to treatment under various forms of perceived pressures from family/relationships, employment difficulties, or anticipated legal consequences (e.g., Condelli 1989; De Leon 1988b).

Detoxification

With few exceptions, admissions to residential treatment do not require medically supervised detoxification. Thus, traditional TCs do not usually provide this service on the premises. Most persons who primarily abuse opioids, cocaine, alcohol, barbiturates, or amphetamines have undergone medical or self-detoxification prior to seeking admission to the TC. A small proportion require detoxification during the admission evaluation, and they are offered the option of detoxification at a nearby hospital.

Criteria for Residential Treatment

Traditional TCs maintain an "open door" policy with respect to admission to residential treatment. This policy understandably results in a wide range of treatment candidates, not all of whom are equally motivated, ready, or suitable for the demands of the residential regimen. Relatively few are excluded, as the policy of the TC is to accept persons who elect residential treatment, regardless of the reasons influencing their choice. However, there is one major guideline for excluding clients: community risk. Community risk refers to the extent to which clients present a management burden to the staff or pose a threat to the security and health of the community or others.

Specific exclusionary criteria most often include histories of arson, suicide, and serious psychiatric disorder. Psychiatric exclusion is usually based on documented history of psychiatric hospitalizations or prima facie evidence of psychotic symptoms on interview (e.g., frank delusions, thought disorder, hallucinations, confused orientation, or signs of serious disorder of affect). An important differential diagnostic issue concerns drug-related mood or mental states. For example, disorientation, dysphoria, and thought or sensory disorders clearly associated with hallucinogens, phencyclidine (PCP), and sometimes cocaine may not exclude an otherwise suitable person from the TC. When diagnosis remains in question, most TCs will utilize a psychiatric consultation after admission. Appropriate referral, however, is based on the client's suitability or risk rather than on diagnosis alone.

Generally, persons on regular psychotropic regimens will be excluded because use of these agents usually correlates with chronic or severe psychiatric disorder. Medication for medical conditions is acceptable in TCs. Clients with disabilities or those who require prosthetics are also accepted for admission, providing they can meet the participatory demands of the program. Physical examinations and laboratory workups (blood and urine profiles) are obtained after admission to residency. Because of concern about communicable disease in a residential setting, some TCs require that the client undergo tests for conditions such as hepatitis and tuberculosis before entering the facility as a resident or at least in the first few weeks after admission.

Policy concerning testing for human immunodeficiency virus (HIV) status and management of acquired immunodeficiency syndrome (AIDS) emphasizes voluntary testing with counseling, special education seminars on health management and sexual practices, and special support groups for residents who are HIV-positive or who have a clinical diagnosis of AIDS.

Suitability for the Therapeutic Community

A number of persons seeking admission to the TC may not be ready for treatment in general or suitable for the demands of a long-term residential regimen. Assessment of these factors on admission provides a basis for treatment planning in the TC, or sometimes appropriate referral. Although motivation, readiness, and suitability per se are not criteria for admission to the TC, the importance of these factors often emerges after entry to treatment, and these factors, if not identified and addressed, are related to early dropout (De Leon and Jainchill 1986; De Leon et al. 1994).

The Therapeutic Community Approach

The TC utilizes the diverse elements and activities of the community to foster rehabilitative change.

Structure of the Therapeutic Community

The TC structure is composed of relatively few staff and stratified levels of resident peers—junior, intermediate, and senior—who constitute the community or family in the residence. This peer-to-community structure strengthens each resident's identification with a perceived and ordered network of others. More importantly, it arranges relationships of mutual responsibility to others at various levels in the program.

The daily operation of the community itself is the task of the residents working together under supervision of the staff. The broad range of resident job assignments illustrates the extent of the self-help process. These assignments include conducting all house services (e.g., cooking, cleaning, kitchen service, minor repair), serving as apprentices, running all departments, and conducting house meetings, certain seminars, and peer encounter groups.

The TC is managed by staff who monitor and evaluate client status, supervise resident groups, assign and supervise resident job functions, and oversee house operations. Clinically, staff conduct therapeutic groups (other than peer encounters), provide individual counseling, organize social and recreational projects, and confer with residents' significant others. They decide matters of resident status, discipline, promotion, transfers, discharges, furloughs, and treatment planning.

The new client enters a setting of upward mobility. Resident job functions are arranged in a hierarchy according to seniority, clinical progress, and productivity. Job assignments begin with the most menial tasks (e.g., mopping the floor) and lead vertically to levels of coordination and management. Indeed, clients come in as patients and can leave as staff. This social organization of the TC reflects the fundamental aspects of its rehabilitative approach: work as education and therapy, mutual self-help, peers as role models, and staff as rational authorities.

Work as Education and Therapy

Work and job changes have clinical relevance for residents in TCs, most of whom have not successfully negotiated the social and occupational world of the larger society. Vertical job movements carry the obvious rewards of status and privilege. However, lateral job changes are more frequent, providing exposure to all aspects of the community.

Job changes in the TC are singularly effective therapeutic tools, providing both measures of and incentives for behavioral and attitudinal changes. Lateral or downward job movements create situations that require demonstrations of personal growth. These movements are designed to teach new ways of coping with reversals and changes that appear to be unfair or arbitrary.

Mutual Self-Help

The essential dynamic in the TC is mutual self-help. In their jobs, groups, meetings, recreation, and personal and social time, residents are the ones who continually transmit to one another the main messages and expectations of the community.

Peers as Role Models

Peers as role models and staff as role models and rational authorities (see the subsection immediately below) are the primary mediators of the recovery process. All community members—roommates, older and younger residents, and junior, senior, and directorial staff—are expected to be role models. This participation as role models has two main attributes.

Resident role models "act as if." The resident behaves as the person he or she should be rather than as the person he or she has been. These attitudes and values include self-motivation, commitment to work and striving, positive regard for staff as authority, and an optimistic outlook toward the future. In the TC, "acting as if" is not just an exercise in conformity but an essential mechanism for more complete psychological change. Feelings, insights, and altered self-perceptions often follow rather than precede behavior change.

Role models display responsible concern. This concept is closely akin to the notion of "I am my brother's/sister's keeper." Showing responsible concern involves willingness to confront others whose behavior is not in keeping with the rules of the TC, the spirit of the community, or the knowledge consistent with growth and rehabilitation.

Staff as Rational Authorities

Staff foster the self-help learning process through their managerial and clinical functions and in their psychological relationship with the residents. TC clients often have had difficulties with authorities, who have not been trusted or perceived as guides and teachers. Thus, TC clients need a successful experience with an authority figure who is viewed as credible (i.e., recovered), supportive, corrective, and protective in order to gain control over themselves (personal autonomy). Implicit in their role as rational authorities, staff provide the reasons for their decisions and explain the meaning of consequences. They exercise their powers to teach and guide and to facilitate and correct, rather than to punish, control, or exploit.

The Therapeutic Community Process: Basic Program Elements

The recovery process may be defined as the interaction between treatment interventions and client change. Unlike other treatment approaches, however, the TC is a community milieu whose daily regimen consists of structured and unstructured activities and social intercourse occurring in formal and informal settings, all of which constitute the treatment interventions in the process.

The typical day in a TC is highly structured, beginning at 7 A.M. and ending at 11 P.M. During this time, residents participate in a variety of meetings, job functions (work therapy), encounter and other therapeutic groups, individual counseling, and recreation. The interplay of these activities contributes to the TC process and may be conceived of as involving three main elements: therapy-education, community enhancement, and community and clinical management.

Therapy-Education

Therapeutic-educative activities consist of various group processes and individual counseling. These activities provide an opportunity for residents to express feelings, resolve personal and social issues, and divert negative acting-out. The activities increase communication and interpersonal skills and can be used to examine and confront behavior and attitudes and to offer instruction in alternate modes of behavior.

Group processes. Four main forms of group activity are used in the TC: encounters, probes, marathons, and tutorials. All attempt to foster trust, personal disclosure, intimacy, and peer solidarity so as to facilitate therapeutic change. The focus of the encounter is behavioral. Its approach is confrontation, and its objective is to modify negative behavior and attitudes directly. Probes and marathons have as their primary objective significant emotional change and psychological insight. Tutorial groups stress learning of skills. In addition, other ad hoc groups are used when needed, and counseling is provided to balance the needs of the individual with those of the community.

Encounters. Encounters are the cornerstone of group process in the TC. The term *encounter* is generic, describing a variety of forms that utilize confrontational procedures as their main approach. The basic encounter is a peer-led group composed of 12–20 residents who meet at least three times weekly, usually for 2 hours in the evening. The basic objective of each encounter is to heighten individual awareness of specific attitudes or behavioral patterns that should be modified.

Probes. Probes are staff-led group sessions composed of 10–15 residents, conducted to obtain in-depth clinical information on clients early in their residency (2–6 months). These sessions usually last from 4 to 8 hours. Their main objectives are to increase staff understanding of the resident's background for the purposes of treatment planning and to increase openness, trust, and mutual identification. The probe emphasizes support, understanding, and empathy from the other group members. Probes go much beyond the here-and-now behavioral incident, which is the material of the encounter, to past events and experiences.

Marathons. Marathons are extended group sessions whose objective is to initiate resolution of life experiences that have impeded the resident's development. During their

18 months of residence, every client participates in several marathons. These groups are conducted by all staff, who are assisted by senior residents with marathon experience. Marathons are usually composed of large groups of selected residents and meet for 18–36 hours. Considerable experience, both personal and professional, is required to ensure safe and effective marathons.

The intimacy, safety, and bonding in the marathon setting facilitate emotional processing (working through) of a significant life event and encourage the person to continue to address the importance of certain life-altering issues of the past. These issues are identified in counseling, probes, or other groups and may include catastrophic events of violence, sexual abuse, abandonment, illness, deaths of significant others, and so forth. A wide variety of techniques are employed, including elements from psychodrama, primal therapy, and pure theater, to have an impact.

Tutorials. Tutorials are directed primarily toward training or teaching. Tutorial groups, usually staff-led, consist of 10–20 residents who address certain themes, including personal growth concepts (e.g., self-reliance, maturity, relationships), job skills training (e.g., managing the department or the reception desk), and clinical skills training (e.g., use of encounter tools).

Other groups. The four main groups described above are supplemented by a number of ad hoc groups that convene as needed. These groups vary in focus, format, and composition. For example, gender, ethnic, or age-specific theme groups may utilize encounter or tutorial formats. Dormitory, room, or departmental encounters may address issues of daily community living. Additionally, sensitivity training, psychodrama, and conventional gestalt and emotionality groups are employed to varying extents.

Individual counseling. One-to-one counseling balances the needs of the individual with those of the community. Peer exchange is ongoing and constitutes the most consistent form of informal counseling in TCs. Staff counseling sessions are both formal and informal and are usually conducted as needed. The staff's approach to counseling in the TC is not traditional, as is evident in the main features of their approach: transpersonal sharing, direct support, minimal interpretation, didactic instructions, and concerned confrontation.

Community Enhancement

Community enhancement activities, which facilitate assimilation into the community, include the four main facilitywide meetings: the morning meeting, seminars, the house meeting, and the general meeting. The morning meeting, seminars, and the house meeting are held each day, and the general meeting is convened when needed.

Morning meeting. The morning meeting convenes all residents of the facility and the staff on the premises after breakfast, usually for 30 minutes, to initiate the day's activities with a positive attitude, motivate residents, and strengthen unity. This meeting is particularly important in that most residents of TCs have never adapted to the routine of an ordinary day.

Seminars. Seminars are convened every afternoon, usually for 1 hour. The seminar serves the purpose of collecting all residents together at least once during the working day. A clinical aim of the seminar is to balance each resident's emotional and cognitive experience. Most seminars are conducted by residents, although sometimes staff and outside speakers lead the seminar. Of the various meetings and group processes in the TC, the seminar is unique in its emphasis on listening, speaking, and conceptual behavior.

House meeting. The house meeting is convened nightly after dinner, usually for 1 hour, and is coordinated by a senior resident. The main aim of this meeting is to transact community business, although social pressure is judiciously employed to facilitate individual change through public acknowledgment of positive or negative behaviors.

General meeting. General meetings are convened only when needed, usually to address negative behavior, attitudes, or incidents in the facility. Conducted by staff, general meetings reaffirm the motivation and purpose of the community.

Community and Clinical Management

The activities composing the community and clinical management element maintain the physical and psychological safety of the environment and ensure that resident life is orderly and productive. The main activities are privileges, disciplinary sanctions, and surveillance, including the house run and urine testing.

Privileges. In the TC, privileges are explicit rewards that reinforce the value of achievement. Privileges are accorded by overall clinical progress in the program. Displays of inappropriate behavior or negative attitude can result in loss of privileges; these privileges can be regained by demonstrated improvement. Privileges range from telephone calls and letter writing earlier in treatment to overnight furloughs later in treatment.

Although the privileges offered in the TC are quite ordinary, it is their social and psychological relevance to the client that enhances their importance. Moreover, because substance-abusing persons often cannot distinguish between privilege and entitlement, the privilege system in the TC teaches that productive participation or membership in a family or community is based on an earning process. Finally, the concrete feature of privilege as reward is particularly suitable for persons with histories of performance failure or noncompletion.

Disciplinary sanctions. TCs have their own specific rules and regulations that guide the behavior of residents and the management of facilities. The explicit purpose of implementing these rules is to ensure the safety and health of the community. However, the implicit aim is to train and teach residents through the use of discipline. In the TC, social and physical safety are prerequisites for psychological trust. For example, breaking one of the TC's cardinal rules—such as no violence or threat of violence—can bring immediate expulsion. Even threats as minor as the theft of a toothbrush or a book must be addressed.

Verbal reprimands, loss of privileges, or speaking bans may be selected for less severe infractions; job demotions, loss of residential time, and expulsion may be invoked for more serious infractions. Although often perceived as punitive, contracts have as their basic purpose to provide a learning experience by compelling residents to attend to their own conduct, to reflect on their own motivation, to feel some consequence of their behavior, and to consider alternative forms of acting under similar situations. The entire facility is made aware of all disciplinary actions. Thus, contracts deter violations and provide vicarious learning experiences for others.

Surveillance. The most comprehensive method for assessing the overall physical and psychological status of the residential community is the house run. Several times a day, staff and senior residents walk through the entire facility from top to bottom, examining its overall condition. This single procedure has clinical implications as well as management goals. House runs provide global "snapshot" impressions of the facility: its cleanliness, planned routines, safety procedures, morale, and psychological tone. They illuminate the psychological and social functioning of individual residents and of peer collections.

Most TCs utilize unannounced random or incident-related urine-testing procedures. The voluntary admission of drug use initiates a learning experience, which includes exploration of conditions precipitating the infraction. Denial of actual drug use, either before or after urine testing, can block the learning process and may lead to termination or dropping out.

When positive results from urine sample testing are detected, actions may involve loss of time, radical job demotions, loss of privileges for specific periods, or expulsion. Review of the "triggers" or reasons for drug use is also an essential part of the action taken.

The Therapeutic Community Process: Program Stages and Profiles

Individual change is a developmental process that can be understood as a passage through stages of incremental learning. There are three major program stages that characterize change in long-term residential TCs: induction-orientation, primary treatment, and reentry.

Stage I: Induction-Orientation (0–60 Days)

The main goals of this initial phase of residency are further assessment and orientation to the TC. The aim of orientation is to assimilate the individual into the community through full participation and involvement in all of its activities. Rapid assimilation is crucial at this point when the client is most ambivalent about the long tenure of residency.

Formal seminars and informal peer instruction focus on reducing anxiety and uncertainty through information and instruction concerning cardinal rules (e.g., no use of drugs, no violence or threat of physical violence); house regulations (e.g., maintaining manners; no leaving the facility; no stealing, borrowing, or lending) or expected conduct (e.g., appropriate speech and dress, punctuality, attendance); program essentials (e.g., structure organization; job functions; the privilege system and its process stages, as well as its philosophy and perspective); and therapeutic community tools (e.g., encounter and other groups).

Successful passage through the initial stage is reflected mainly in clients' retention in the program. The fact that clients remain 30–60 days indicates that they have adhered to the rules of the program enough to meet the orientation goals of this stage and have passed the period of highest vulnerability to early dropout.

Stage II: Primary Treatment (2–12 Months)

Primary treatment consists of three phases that roughly correlate with time in the program (2–4 months, 5–8 months, and 9–12 months). These phases are marked by plateaus of stable behavior that signal the need for further change. The daily therapeutic-educational regimen, meetings, groups, job functions, and peer and staff counseling remain the same throughout the year of primary treatment. However, client progress is reflected at the end of each phase in terms of three interrelated dimensions of change: community/status, development/maturity, and overall psychological adjustment.

Stage III: Reentry (13–24 Months)

Early reentry phase (13–18 months). The main goal of the early reentry phase, during which clients continue to live in the facility, is preparation for healthy separation from the community. Emphasis on rational authority decreases under the assumption that the client has acquired a sufficient degree of self-management. This degree of self-management is reflected in more individual decision making about privileges, social plans, and life design. Particular emphasis is placed on life skills seminars, which provide didactic training for life outside the community. Attendance is mandated for sessions on budgeting, job seeking, use of alcohol, sexuality, parenting, use of leisure time, and so on.

During this phase, development of individual plans is the collective task of the client, a key staff member, and peers. These plans are comprehensive blueprints for long-term psychological, educational, and vocational efforts that include goal attainment schedules, guidance on methods of improving interpersonal and family relationships, and counseling on issues of social and sexual behavior. Clients may be attending school or holding full-time jobs, either within or outside the TC. Still, they are expected to participate in house activities when possible and to carry some community responsibilities (e.g., facility coverage at night).

Later reentry phase (19–24 months). The goal of the later reentry phase is to complete a successful separation from residency. Clients are on "live out" status, are involved in full-time jobs or educational pursuits, and are maintaining their own households, usually with live-out peers. They may attend such aftercare programs as Alcoholics Anonymous or Narcotics Anonymous and/or take part in family or individual therapy. Contact is gradually reduced to weekly telephone calls and monthly visits with a primary counselor.

Graduation

Completion marks the end of active program involvement. Graduation itself, however, is an annual event conducted in the facility for completees usually 1 year beyond their residency. Thus, the TC experience is preparation rather than a cure. Residence in the program facilitates a process of change that must continue throughout life, and what is learned in treatment is the tools to guide the individual on a steady path of continued change. Completion or graduation, therefore, is not an end but a beginning.

Aftercare

Until recently, long-term TCs have not formally acknowledged aftercare as a definable period following program involvement. Many contemporary TCs now offer explicit aftercare components within their systems or through linkages with outside agencies.

Research and Evaluation

Effectiveness of the Therapeutic Community Approach

A substantial evaluation literature has documented the effectiveness of the TC approach in rehabilitating drug-abusing individuals (e.g., Condelli and Hubbard 1994; De Leon 1984,

1986; National Institute on Drug Abuse 1980; D. D. Simpson 1990; D. D. Simpson and Curry 1997; D. D. Simpson and Sells 1982; Tims and Ludford 1984; Tims et al. 1994).

A consistently positive relationship has been found between time spent in residential treatment and posttreatment outcome status (e.g., De Leon 1984; D. D. Simpson and Sells 1982; D. D. Simpson, Joe, and Brown 1997). For example, in one study, 2-year posttreatment success rates exceeded 75% among graduates and approximately 50% among dropouts who had remained at least a year in residential treatment (De Leon et al. 1982). A few studies that investigated psychological outcomes uniformly showed significant improvement in clients at follow-up (e.g., Biase et al. 1986; De Leon 1984; Holland 1983). The outcome studies reported were completed with an earlier generation of substance-abusing clients, primarily opioid-addicted individuals.

Retention in the Therapeutic Community Program

A high dropout rate is the rule for all drug treatment modalities. For TCs, retention is of particular importance because, as noted above, research on TCs has established a firm relationship between time spent in treatment and successful outcome. However, most persons admitted to TC programs leave residency, many before treatment influences are presumed to be effectively rendered. The key findings from reviews of the TC retention research (e.g., De Leon 1986, 1991; Lewis and Ross 1994) are briefly summarized in the following subsections.

Rates of Dropping Out

Rates of dropping out are highest (30%–40%) in the first 30 days of admission but decline sharply thereafter (De Leon and Schwartz 1984). This temporal pattern of dropping out is uniform across TC programs (and other modalities). In long-term (15- to 24-month) residential TCs, completion rates average 10%–20% of all admissions. One-year retention rates range from 15% to 40%.

Predictors of Dropping Out

There are no reliable client characteristics that predict dropping out of the TC program, with the exception of severe criminality and/or severe psychopathology, which are correlated with an earlier time of dropping out. However, some studies point to the importance of dynamic factors in predicting retention in treatment, such as perceived legal pressure, motivation, and readiness for treatment (e.g., Condelli and De Leon 1993; De Leon 1988b; De Leon et al. 1994; Hiller et al. 1998; Hubbard et al. 1988).

Although a legitimate concern, retention in treatment should not be confused with treatment effectiveness. TCs are effective for those who remain long enough for treatment to have an influence on them. Obviously, however, a critical issue for TCs is maximizing their holding power so that more clients will benefit. Recent developments have facilitated empirical studies into the hitherto underinvestigated area of treatment process. These include formulations of the essential elements of the TC approach and of the stages of recovery in the TC (De Leon 1995, 1996a). Preliminary findings based on these formulations illuminate some active ingredients in the treatment process (Melnick and De Leon 1999; Melnick et al. 2000).

Evolution of the Therapeutic Community: Modifications and Applications

The traditional TC model described in this chapter subpart is actually the prototype of a variety of TC-oriented programs. Today, the TC modality consists of a wide range of programs serving a diversity of clients who use a variety of drugs and present complex social/psychological problems in addition to their substance abuse.

Client differences, as well as clinical requirements and funding realities, have encouraged the development of modified residential TCs with shorter planned durations of stay (3, 6, and 12 months) as well as TC-oriented day treatment and outpatient ambulatory models. (A more complete description of the modifications and applications of the TC are provided elsewhere [G. De Leon 1997].) Correctional, medical, and psychiatric hospitals and community residence and shelter settings, overwhelmed with alcohol and illicit drug abuse problems, have implemented TC programs within their institutional boundaries.

Most community-based traditional TCs have expanded their social services or incorporated new interventions to address the needs of their diverse clients. These include family services; primary health care expanded particularly for HIV-positive and AIDS patients (e.g., Barton 1994; De Leon 1996b; McKusker and Sorensen 1994); aftercare services for special populations such as inmate substance abusers (e.g., Lockwood and Inciardi 1993); relapse prevention training (e.g., Lewis and Ross 1994) and 12-Step components (De Leon 1990–1991); and mental health services, including psychiatric medication (Carroll and McGinley 1998). In some cases, these additions enhance but do not alter the basic TC regimen. In other cases they significantly modify the TC model itself. For example, contemporary TCs typically include or offer family services, primary health care and mental health services, relapse prevention training, and 12-Step components.

The cross-fertilization of personnel and methods from the traditional TC, mental health services, and human services portends the evolution of a new TC: a general treatment model that is applicable to a broad range of populations for whom affiliation with a self-help community is the foundation for effecting the process of individual change.

References

Barton E: The adaptation of the therapeutic community to HIV/AIDS, in Proceedings of the Therapeutic Communities of America Planning Conference: Paradigms: Past, Present and Future, Chantilly, VA, December 6–9, 1992. Providence, RI, Manisses Communications Group, 1994, pp 66–70

Biase DV, Sullivan AP, Wheeler B: Daytop miniversity phase 2 college training in a therapeutic community: development of self-concept among drug free addict/abusers, in Therapeutic Communities for Addictions: Readings in Theory, Research and Practice. Edited by De Leon G, Ziegenfuss JT. Springfield, IL, Charles C Thomas, 1986, pp 121–130

Carroll JFX, McGinley JJ: Managing MICA clients in a modified therapeutic community with enhanced staffing. J Subst Abuse Treat 15:565–577, 1998

Condelli WS: External pressure and retention in a therapeutic community. International Journal of Therapeutic Communities 10:21–33,1989

Condelli WS, De Leon G: Fixed and dynamic predictors of retention in therapeutic communities for substance abusers. J Subst Abuse Treat 10:11–16, 1993

Condelli WS, Hubbard RL: Client outcomes from therapeutic communities. Therapeutic Community: Advances in Research and Application. NIDA Research Monograph 144 (NIH Publ No 94-3633).

Edited by Tims FM, De Leon G, Jainchill N. Rockville, MD, National Institute on Drug Abuse, 1994, pp 80–98

De Leon G: The Therapeutic Community: Study of Effectiveness. NIDA Treatment Research Monograph (Publ No [ADM] 84-1286). Rockville, MD, National Institute on Drug Abuse, 1984

De Leon G: Adolescent substance abusers in the therapeutic community: treatment outcomes, in Bridging Services: Drug Abuse, Human Services and the Therapeutic Community. San Francisco, CA, Abacus Printing, 1986, pp 195–201

De Leon G: Legal pressure in therapeutic communities, in Compulsory Treatment of Drug Abuse: Research and Clinical Practice. NIDA Research Monograph 86 (DHHS Publ No [ADM] 88-1578). Edited by Leukefeld CG, Tims FM. Rockville, MD, National Institute on Drug Abuse, 1988a, pp 160–177

De Leon G: The therapeutic community: enhancing retention in treatment. Final Report of NIDA Grant Project R01-DAO3860, 1988b

De Leon G: Aftercare in therapeutic communities. Int J Addict 25:1229–1241, 1990–1991

De Leon G: Retention in drug free therapeutic communities, in Improving Drug Abuse Treatment. NIDA Research Monograph 106 (DHHS Publ No [ADM] 91-1754). Edited by Pickens RW, Leukefeld CG, Schuster CR. Rockville, MD, National Institute on Drug Abuse, 1991, pp 218–244

De Leon G: Cocaine abusers in therapeutic community treatment, in Cocaine Treatment: Research and Clinical Perspectives. NIDA Research Monograph 135 (DHHS Publ No [ADM] 93-3639). Rockville, MD, National Institute on Drug Abuse, 1993, pp 163–189

De Leon G: Integrative recovery: a stage paradigm. Substance Abuse 17:51–63, 1996a

De Leon G: Therapeutic communities: AIDS/HIV risk and harm reduction. J Subst Abuse Treat 13:411–420, 1996b

De Leon G (ed): Community as Method: Therapeutic Communities for Special Populations and Special Settings. Westport, CT, Greenwood, 1997

De Leon G: The Therapeutic Community: Theory, Model, and Method. New York, Springer, 2000

De Leon G, Jainchill N: Circumstances, motivation, readiness and suitability (CMRS) as correlates of treatment tenure. J Psychoactive Drugs 8:203–208, 1986

De Leon G, Rosenthal MS: Treatment in residential therapeutic communities, in Treatments of Psychiatric Disorders: A Task Force Report of the American Psychiatric Association, Vol 2. Edited by Karasu TB. Washington, DC, American Psychiatric Press, 1989, pp 115–138

De Leon G, Schwartz S: The therapeutic community: What are the retention rates? Am J Drug Alcohol Abuse 10:267–284, 1984

De Leon G, Skodol A, Rosenthal MS: Phoenix House. Changes in psychopathological signs of resident drug addicts. Arch Gen Psychiatry 23:131–135, 1973

De Leon G, Jainchill N, Wexler H: Success and improvement rates 5 years after treatment in a therapeutic community. Int J Addict 17:703–747, 1982

De Leon G, Melnick G, Kressel D, et al: Circumstances, motivation, readiness and suitability (the CMRS Scales): predicting retention in therapeutic community treatment. Am J Drug Alcohol Abuse 20:495–515, 1994

Hathaway SR, McKinley JC: Minnesota Multiphasic Personality Inventory. Minneapolis, MN, University of Minnesota, 1943

Hiller ML, Knight K, Broome KM, et al: Legal pressure and treatment retention in a national sample of long-term residential programs. Criminal Justice and Behavior 25(4):463–481, 1998

Holland S: Evaluating community based treatment programs: a model for strengthening inferences about effectiveness. International Journal of Therapeutic Communities 4:285–306, 1983

Holland S: Measuring process in drug abuse treatment research, in Therapeutic Communities for Addictions: Readings in Theory, Research and Practice. Edited by De Leon G, Ziegenfuss JT. Springfield, IL, Charles C Thomas, 1986, pp 169–181

Hubbard RL, Rachal JV, Craddock SG, et al: Treatment outcome prospective study (TOPS): client characteristics and behaviors before, during, and after treatment, in Drug Abuse Treatment Evaluation: Strategies, Progress, and Prospects. NIDA Research Monograph 51 (DHHS Publ No [ADM] 84-1329), Special Issue on Research Analysis and Utilization System (RAUS). Edited by Tims FM, Ludford JP. Rockville, MD, National Institute on Drug Abuse, 1984, pp 42–68

Hubbard RL, Collins JJ, Rachal JV, et al: The criminal justice client in drug abuse treatment, in Compulsory Treatment of Drug Abuse: Research and Clinical Practice. NIDA Research Monograph 86 (DHHS Publ No ADM 88-1578). Edited by Leukefeld CG, Tims FM. Rockville, MD, National Institute on Drug Abuse, 1988, pp 57–79

Jainchill N: The relationship between psychiatric disorder, retention in treatment, and client progress among admissions to a residential drug-free modality. Doctoral dissertation, New York University, New York, NY, 1989

Jainchill N: Therapeutic communities for adolescents: the same and not the same, in Community as Method: Therapeutic Communities for Special Populations and Special Settings. Edited by De Leon G. Westport, CT, Greenwood Publishing Group. 1997, pp 161–177

Jainchill N, De Leon G, Pinkham L: Psychiatric diagnosis among substance abusers in therapeutic community treatment. J Psychoactive Drugs 18:209–312, 1986

Lewis BF, Ross R: Retention in therapeutic communities: challenges for the nineties, in Therapeutic Community: Advances in Research and Application. NIDA Research Monograph 144 (NIH Publ No 94-3633). Edited by Tims F, De Leon G, Jainchill N. Rockville, MD, National Institute on Drug Abuse, 1994, pp 99–116

Lockwood D, Inciardi JA: CREST Outreach Center: a work release iteration of the TC model, in Innovative Approaches in the Treatment of Drug Abuse: Program Models and Strategies. Edited by Inciardi J, Tims FM, Fletcher BW. Newport, CT, Greenwood, 1993, pp 61–69

McKusker J, Sorensen JL: HIV and therapeutic communities, in Therapeutic Community: Advances in Research and Application. NIDA Research Monograph 144 (NIH Publ No 94-3633). Edited by Tims FM, De Leon G, Jainchill N. Rockville, MD, National Institute on Drug Abuse, 1994, pp 232–258

Melnick G, De Leon G: Clarifying the nature of therapeutic community treatment: the Survey of Essential Elements Questionnaire (SEEQ). J Subst Abuse Treat 16:307–313, 1999

Melnick G, De Leon G, Hiller ML, et al: Therapeutic communities: diversity in treatment elements. Subst Use Misuse 35:1819–1847, 2000

National Institute on Drug Abuse: CODAP (Client Oriented Data Acquisition Process): 1979 Annual Data. NIDA Statistical Series (DHEW Publ No [ADM] 81-1-25). Rockville, MD, National Institute on Drug Abuse, 1980, p 395

Pompi KF, Resnick J: Retention in a therapeutic community for court referred adolescents and young adults. Am J Drug Alcohol Abuse 13:309–325, 1987

Robins LN, Helzer JE, Croughhan J, et al: National Institute of Mental Health Diagnostic Interview Schedule: its history, characteristics, and validity. Arch Gen Psychiatry 38:381–389, 1981

Simpson DD: 12-year follow-up: outcomes of opioid addicts treated in therapeutic communities, in Therapeutic Communities for Addictions. Edited by De Leon G, Ziegenfuss JT. Springfield, IL, Charles C Thomas, 1990, pp 109–120

Simpson DD, Curry SJ (eds): Special Issue: Drug Abuse Treatment Outcome Study. Psychology of Addictive Behaviors 11, 1997

Simpson DD, Sells SB: Effectiveness of treatment for drug abuse: an overview of the DARP research program. Advances in Alcohol and Substance Abuse 2:7–29, 1982

Simpson DD, Joe GW, Brown BS: Treatment retention and follow-up outcomes in the Drug Abuse Treatment Outcome Study (DATOS). Psychology of Addictive Behaviors 11:294–307, 1997

Tims FM, Ludford JP (eds): Drug Abuse Treatment Evaluation: Strategies, Progress, and Prospects. NIDA Research Monograph 51 (DHHS Publ No ADM 84-1329), Special Issue on Research Analysis and Utilization System (RAUS). Rockville, MD, National Institute on Drug Abuse, 1984

Tims FM, De Leon G, Jainchill N (eds): NIDA Research Monograph, Special Issue on Therapeutic Community Research. Rockville, MD, National Institute on Drug Abuse, 1994

Dual-Diagnosis Populations

Kathleen T. Brady, M.D., Ph.D.
Robert J. Malcolm, M.D.

The term *dual diagnosis* in the context of substance use disorders has generally been used to refer to the co-occurrence of a psychiatric disorder with a substance use disorder. This co-occurrence is probably more accurately captured by using the term *comorbid disorders,* because many individuals meet criteria for both a substance use disorder and a number of other psychiatric disorders. Data from the National Comorbidity Study (Kessler et al. 1994) indicated that psychiatric morbidity is highly concentrated; more than half of all lifetime psychiatric disorders occur in the 14% of the population who have a history of three or more comorbid psychiatric disorders. Two epidemiological surveys have examined the prevalence of psychiatric and substance use disorders in community samples: the National Institute of Mental Health Epidemiologic Catchment Area (ECA) study (Regier et al. 1990) conducted in the early 1980s and the National Comorbidity Study (NCS) conducted in 1991 (Kessler et al. 1994). Data from the ECA study estimated that 45% of individuals with an alcohol use disorder and 72% of individuals with a drug use disorder had at least one co-occurring psychiatric disorder (Regier et al. 1990). In the NCS, approximately 78% of alcohol-dependent men and 86% of alcohol-dependent women met lifetime criteria for another psychiatric disorder, including drug dependence (Kessler et al. 1994).

The relationship between substance use and psychiatric disorders is a complex one. This relationship can be characterized in a number of ways: 1) substance use and psychiatric disorders may co-occur by coincidence, 2) substance use may cause psychiatric conditions or increase the severity of psychiatric symptoms, 3) psychiatric disorders may cause or increase the severity of substance use disorders, 4) both disorders may be caused by a third condition, or 5) substance use and withdrawal may produce symptoms that mimic those of a psychiatric disorder (Meyer 1989). In any individual case, different facets of this complex relationship may be operating. This complexity can lead to difficulties in the accurate diagnosis and optimal management of individuals with comorbid conditions.

Of primary concern is the fact that comorbidity has been associated with poor outcome and poor treatment response (Keitner et al. 1991; Keller et al. 1986). For this reason, accurate diagnosis and aggressive treatment of comorbidity may also directly influence patterns of treatment service availability and reimbursement. Assessment of comorbidity is likely to be an important factor in providing the most cost-effective care. An understanding of comorbidity is essential to the development of effective treatment and prevention efforts.

General Diagnostic Considerations

One of the most difficult challenges in the area of comorbidity is diagnosis. It is clear that substance use and withdrawal can mimic nearly every psychiatric disorder. Substances of abuse have profound effects on neurotransmitter systems involved in the pathophysiology of most psychiatric disorders and, with chronic use, may unmask a vulnerability or lead to organic changes that manifest as psychiatric disorder. The best way to differentiate substance-induced, transient psychiatric symptoms from psychiatric disorders that warrant treatment is through observation of symptoms during a period of abstinence. Transient substance-related states will improve with time. The most controversial issue in this discussion is the amount of time in abstinence necessary for accurate diagnosis. It is likely that the minimum amount of time necessary for diagnosis will vary according to the comorbid condition being diagnosed. For alcohol-induced depression and anxiety, symptom resolution appears to occur 2–4 weeks after last use (Brown and Schuckit 1988; Thevos et al. 1991). Other psychiatric disorders are less well studied in this regard. It is likely, however, that one could make a diagnosis of schizophrenia, mania, an eating disorder, or other disorders that have symptoms clearly distinguishable from substance withdrawal with less than 2–4 weeks of abstinence.

There are many unanswered questions concerning accurate diagnosis of comorbid substance use and psychiatric disorder. A period of abstinence is optimal for diagnosis, but the necessary minimum time frame is not established. A family history of psychiatric illness, clear onset of psychiatric symptoms before onset of the substance use disorder, and sustained psychiatric symptoms during lengthy periods of abstinence in the past can all weigh in favor of making a psychiatric diagnosis in cases that are unclear.

General Treatment Considerations

The optimal treatment approach for individuals with substance use and psychiatric comorbidity is an area of active investigation. In general, treatment efforts addressing psychiatric and substance use disorders have developed in parallel. There is much work to be done in investigating the appropriate integration of treatment modalities from both fields to design treatments specifically tailored for patients with comorbidity. Psychosocial treatments are powerful interventions for both substance use and psychiatric disorders. There are common themes in the psychosocial treatments from both fields that can be built upon to optimize outcome.

Research in pharmacotherapies for both substance use and psychiatric disorders is progressing rapidly. This is also an area where integration of information from both the psychiatric and substance abuse fields has led to the testing of strategies targeting individuals with both disorders. Specific comorbid disorders will be discussed in detail below, but general principles in choosing a pharmacological agent include particular attention to potential toxic interactions of psychotherapeutic agents with drugs and alcohol should relapse occur, and assessment of the abuse potential of the agent being use. In Table 32–2, some of these potential interactions with common psychotropic agents are delineated.

TABLE 32–2. Interactions of psychotropic drugs and substances of abuse

Therapeutic agent	Potential risks/interactions in substance users
Antidepressants	
Tricyclic antidepressants	Chronic alcohol use may induce metabolism, decreasing drug levels
	Additive cardiotoxicity with cocaine
Monoamine oxidase inhibitors	Tyramine present in alcoholic beverages may induce pressor response (hypertensive crisis)
	Potentiation of sympathomimetic effects of stimulants
	Toxic interaction with meperidine (hypertensive crisis)
Selective serotonin reuptake inhibitors	Specific interactions not documented
	May decrease alcohol consumption
Mood stabilizers	
Lithium	Specific interactions not documented
Valproic acid	Potential for liver toxicity
Carbamazepine	Potential for liver toxicity
Antipsychotics	Possible increased risk for akathisia/dystonia
	Risk for hyperpyrexia in combination with stimulants
Benzodiazepines	Abuse potential
Stimulants	
Methylphenidate	Abuse potential
Amphetamine	Abuse potential
Pemoline	Potential for liver toxicity

In this chapter subpart, an overview of clinically relevant comorbidities of psychiatric and substance use disorders will be presented. For every category of psychiatric diagnosis discussed, prevalence rates, differential diagnosis, and information on pharmacotherapeutic and psychotherapeutic treatment options will be briefly reviewed when possible. Recommendations for clinical practice will be delineated.

Psychotic Disorders

Prevalence

Psychotic symptoms may co-occur with substance use disorders as a direct result of chemical intoxication and/or withdrawal or from a primary underlying psychotic disorder. A number of studies have demonstrated that as many as 50% of treatment-seeking schizophrenic patients have alcohol or illicit drug dependence and more than 70% are nicotine dependent (Dixon et al. 1991; Shaner et al. 1993; Ziedonis et al. 1994). Recent epidemiological surveys indicate that individuals with schizophrenia are at substantially greater risk (odds ratio 4.5) of having a substance use disorder relative to the general population (Kessler et al. 1994; Regier et al. 1990). The relationship between psychosis and substance use is complex. Individuals with schizophrenia may use substances to decrease the negative symptoms of schizophrenia (depression, apathy, anhedonia, passivity, social withdrawal, poverty of thought), to combat the overwhelming positive symptoms of schizophrenia (typically auditory hallucinations and paranoid delusions), or to attempt to ameliorate the adverse effects of antipsychotic medication (dysphoria, akathisia, sedation).

Diagnosis

Differential diagnosis frequently involves differentiating a substance-induced psychotic disorder (SIPD) from a primary psychotic disorder (PPD). Certain drugs of abuse (psychostimulants, hallucinogens, marijuana, and possibly industrial inhalants) can probably cause or increase the susceptibility to the development of a psychotic episode. Variables that might support a diagnosis of SIPD rather than PPD would be younger age at onset of psychosis, a family history of drug use, male gender, and better premorbid adjustment (Boutros and Bowers 1996). The most helpful factor in accurate diagnosis is careful history concerning symptoms during abstinent periods and observation during monitored abstinence.

A number of studies (Shaner et al. 1993) suggest that substance use often goes undetected among individuals with schizophrenia. Diagnosis of comorbid substance abuse can be improved by conducting routine toxicology screening and by involving family members in the diagnostic interview. Aggressive screening for substance use is important, because substance abuse has a negative impact on the course and prognosis of schizophrenia. Studies have demonstrated that substance use can exacerbate existing psychosis, resulting in repeated hospitalizations and an increased risk of suicide, violence, poverty, and homelessness (Brady et al. 1990; Breakey et al. 1974). Wilkins (1997) found the onset of psychosis to be an average of 4 years earlier when drug use preceded psychotic symptoms, thus supporting a diathesis-exposure model. Alcohol and marijuana may actually hasten the appearance and worsen the severity of tardive dyskinesia (Wilkins 1997).

Treatment

The optimal management of patients with comorbid schizophrenia and substance use involves both pharmacotherapy and psychotherapy. Although few empirical data are available on specific pharmacotherapeutic strategies, atypical antipsychotic agents such as clozapine and olanzapine may better target the negative symptoms of schizophrenia and may also result in fewer side effects compared with the more traditional antipsychotics, thus reducing patients' tendency to self-medicate with substances of abuse (Wilkins 1997). Several small case series in patients with schizophrenia and substance use disorders have reported positive responses to clozapine (Buckley et al. 1994; T. P. George et al. 1995). Management of dysphoric affect in substance abuse patients may be an important part of successful treatment. Siris and co-workers (1991) reported preliminary evidence that adjunctive antidepressant medication added to antipsychotic medication may be useful in some stable dysphoric, substance-abusing schizophrenia patients. A group of investigators studying adjunctive desipramine treatment in a small group of cocaine-abusing patients with schizophrenia found that the desipramine-treated group had better retention in treatment and fewer cocaine-positive urine drug screens than did the placebo-treated group (Ziedonis et al. 1992).

Disulfiram must be used with caution in this comorbid population because it may increase central levels of dopamine by blocking dopamine-β-hydroxylase and therefore exacerbate psychosis (Wilkins 1997). The use of naltrexone to decrease alcohol consumption in psychotic individuals is an intriguing idea that has not been explored in a systematic manner.

The psychotherapeutic management of the schizophrenic substance abuser is critical. Close monitoring via urinalysis and breathalyzer along with clear limit setting is important. Feedback should be given in an empathic and nonjudgmental manner. The confrontational group process approach often used for substance abusers has little value in the treatment of the schizophrenic substance abuser (Kosten and Ziedonis 1997) and may exacerbate psychosis. Ziedonis and Trudeau (1997) noted the problem of poor motivation to quit substances with many schizophrenic patients and suggest a dual diagnosis, treatment-matching strategy based on motivation levels, substance of abuse, and illness severity.

Treatment should involve psychoeducation, motivational enhancement, social skills training, psychopharmacology (with a strong focus on reducing side effects), vocational rehabilitation, and family involvement. In certain geographic areas, there are specialized Alcoholics Anonymous (AA)/Narcotics Anonymous (NA) groups for people with a dual diagnosis, known as MICA (mentally ill, chemically addicted) groups or "double trouble meetings," where people with schizophrenia may feel less threatened and more comfortable with discussing psychiatric symptoms and medication issues.

Affective Disorders

Prevalence

Symptoms of mood instability and depression are among the most common psychiatric symptoms seen in individuals with substance use disorders. In the ECA data set, 32% of individuals with an affective disorder also had a comorbid substance use disorder. Of the individuals with major depression, 16.5% had an alcohol use disorder and 18% had a drug use disorder; 56.1% of individuals with bipolar disorder had a substance use disorder (Regier et al. 1990). Using the NCS data set, an odds ratio was calculated to determine the relative risk of co-occurrence of affective disorders and substance use disorders. The odds ratio for co-occurrence of substance use with any affective disorder was 2.3, the odds ratio for major depression was 2.7, and the odds ratio for bipolar disorder was 9.2 (Kessler et al. 1994). In both of these studies, bipolar disorder was the Axis I diagnosis most likely to co-occur with a substance use disorder.

Studies in treatment-seeking samples have found variable estimates of the comorbidity of affective illness with substance use disorders. As discussed below, diagnostic issues at the interface of affective illness and substance use disorders are particularly complex. Estimates of the prevalence of depressive disorders in treatment-seeking alcoholics range from 15% to 67% (Hasin et al. 1988; Powell et al. 1982). In studies of cocaine-dependent individuals, estimates of affective comorbidity range from 33% to 53% (Nunes et al. 1991; Rounsaville et al. 1991; Weiss et al. 1988). Bipolar spectrum disorders appear to be more prevalent (20%–30%) in cocaine-dependent samples than in alcoholic samples. In opiate-dependent samples, rates of lifetime affective disorder (primarily depressive disorders) range from 16% to 75% (Brooner et al. 1997; Milby et al. 1996; Mirin et al. 1988; Rounsaville et al. 1982). In individuals seeking treatment for affective disorders, studies indicate that 30%–50% of individuals with depressive disorders and 50%–70% of individuals with bipolar disorder have a lifetime substance use disorder (Hasin et al. 1985; Miller and Fine 1993).

Diagnosis

Diagnosing an affective disorder in the presence of substance abuse can be particularly difficult. Stimulant, alcohol, marijuana, and hallucinogen intoxication can cause symptoms indistinguishable from mania or hypomania, and withdrawal states often produce symptoms of mood lability and depression. Addictive use of drugs is also associated with lifestyles and behaviors that lead to multiple losses and stressors, which in turn may result in depressed affect that is appropriate and transient.

As many as 98% of individuals presenting for substance abuse treatment have some symptom of depression (Jaffe and Ciraulo 1986). In one study, depressive symptoms were monitored over a 1-month period in 171 individuals presenting for alcohol treatment (Dorus et al. 1987). Whereas on admission 67% had high depression ratings on the Hamilton Rating Scale for Depression (Hamilton 1960), by discharge only 16% had ratings in the depressed range. Obviously, assessments conducted too early in the recovery process may lead to overdiagnosis and unnecessary treatment. On the other hand, promising new data indicate that, in some cases, appropriate treatment of depression can improve substance-related outcomes. For this reason, underdiagnosis also presents a risk. To obtain the best assessment, a careful history must be taken. Affective symptoms that predate the onset of substance use, a strong family history of affective disorder, and/or symptoms that have persisted during abstinent periods in the past are clinical features that should influence treatment decisions.

Mania is often easier to diagnose than depression in the substance abuser. During active drug use, urine drug screens can be useful for evaluating substance-induced mania. Withdrawal states generally do not mimic mania. Manic symptoms that persist for a number of days after the last substance use are not likely to be substance induced, given that substance-induced mania generally lasts only for the duration of the drug's pharmacological effect. Long-acting stimulants (methamphetamine), appetite suppressants, and hallucinogens may be an exception to this rule, as manic symptoms resulting from intoxication with these substances may last for several days.

Treatment

Studies of tricyclic antidepressants (TCAs) indicate that antidepressant treatment may be helpful in individuals with comorbid alcohol dependence and depression. In a 12-week placebo-controlled trial of imipramine treatment in actively drinking alcoholic outpatients with depression (McGrath et al. 1996), imipramine treatment was associated with an improvement in depression and a decrease in alcohol consumption. Mason and colleagues (1996) found that treatment of alcoholics with secondary depression (onset of depression after alcohol dependence) with desipramine led to a decrease in depression and an increase in length of abstinence.

Research investigating the use of selective serotonin reuptake inhibitors (SSRIs) in the treatment of alcoholism has also shown promise. The serotonin system has been implicated in control of alcohol intake (Amit et al. 1991). A number of selective serotonin agents have been shown to have a modest effect in decreasing alcohol consumption in problem drinkers and alcoholics (Gorelick 1989). A recent study investigating the use of fluoxetine in a group of alcoholics with major depression had positive results (Cornelius et al. 1997). Compared with those in the placebo group, individuals in the fluoxetine group had significantly greater improvement in both depressive symptoms and alcohol consumption. This study is particularly important because the clinical improvement was more robust than that seen with the TCA studies, and the SSRIs have less potential for toxicity and interaction with drugs of abuse than do the TCAs.

Several trials of TCAs have been performed with opioid-dependent patients. Doxepin has been shown in several case study series to relieve symptoms of depression, anxiety, and drug craving (Weiss and Mirin 1989) in methadone-maintained patients. It must be noted that methadone maintenance clinics have reported abuse of amitriptyline and other sedating TCAs. TCA plasma-level monitoring is important in methadone-maintained patients because patients receiving methadone and desipramine have been found to have an increase in plasma desipramine levels (Weiss and Mirin 1989).

The use of TCAs in cocaine-dependent patients has focused primarily on the treatment of cocaine dependence rather than the treatment of depression. Several studies using desipramine have shown improvement in anhedonia and cocaine craving and increased initial abstinence in nondepressed patients, and one small study showed improvement in depressed patients (Rao et al. 1995). Clinicians should be aware, however, that desipramine may have an activating effect in cocaine-dependent individuals, which can precipitate relapse. Also, TCAs may have additive cardiotoxicity in combination with cocaine should relapse occur (Weiss and Mirin 1989). Other antidepressants have shown preliminary efficacy in the treatment of cocaine dependence, but none have been explored specifically in depressed cocaine-dependent individuals.

There are very little published data on the treatment of bipolar disorder complicated by substance abuse. Agents that are generally used for the treatment of bipolar disorder include lithium and the anticonvulsant medications carbamazepine and valproate. Lithium has been used as the standard treatment for bipolar disorder for several decades; however, substance abuse may be a predictor of poor response to lithium (Bowden 1995; O'Connell et al. 1991). Bipolar patients with concomitant substance use disorders appear to have more mixed and/or rapid-cycling episodes and, therefore, may respond better to anticonvulsant medications (e.g., valproate) than to lithium therapy (Calabrese et al. 1992; Freeman et al. 1992). In an open-label pilot study, Brady et al. (1995a) found valproate to be safe and effective in bipolar patients with concurrent substance dependence. Weiss et al. (1998) reported better medication compliance with valproate than with lithium in a group of substance-abusing patients with bipolar disorder.

Psychotherapeutic interventions are useful in the treatment of both affective and substance use disorders and are a critical element in the treatment of patients with comorbidity. There is, however, little consensus concerning the most appropriate psychotherapeutic treatment. A wide range of psychotherapeutic interventions have been used in the treatment of affective disorders. These include psychodynamic, interpersonal, cognitive-behavioral (CB), and family therapies (American Psychiatric Association 1994b). Judgments concerning the effectiveness of these treatments are primarily based on clinical consensus rather than on controlled clinical trials; however, formal studies of several of these treatments are currently being conducted. For the treatment of substance use disorders, CB, motivation enhancement, and 12-Step therapies all have demonstrated efficacy (Project MATCH Research Group 1997).

The psychotherapeutic/psychosocial strategies used in the treatment of comorbid individuals should be specifically tailored and contain elements of effective treatment from both the substance abuse and affective disorders areas. Many of the principles of CB therapy are common to the treatment of affective disorder as well as substance use disorders. AA and NA are available in all communities, and active participation can be a major factor in an individual's recovery. Emphasis on developing therapies to specifically treat individuals with comorbid affective and substance use disorders by combining therapeutic techniques used to treat both disorders will be a fruitful area for further work.

Anxiety Disorders

Data from the NCS indicated that approximately 36% of individuals with anxiety disorders also have a substance use disorder (Kessler et al. 1994). In the ECA data set, the odds ratio for co-occurrence of any anxiety disorder with any substance use disorder was 1.7, but this number differed substantially among anxiety disorder diagnoses (Regier et al. 1990). Because the anxiety disorders are such a heterogeneous group and the issues concerning diagnoses, treatment, and prevalence differ substantially between disorders, each disorder will be discussed in a separate subsection.

Panic Disorder

In the ECA survey, 36% of individuals with panic disorder had lifetime substance use disorder (Regier et al. 1990). In the NCS, the odds ratio for co-occurring drug and alcohol dependence with panic disorder was 2.0 (Kessler et al. 1996). The estimated prevalence of panic disorder and agoraphobia in treatment-seeking samples of alcoholics is quite variable, with estimates ranging from 5% to 42% (Kushner et al. 1990). This variability is, in part, related to diagnostic difficulties. As mentioned earlier, anxiety symptoms in general, and panic attacks in particular, are commonly seen in withdrawal states. Alcohol, sedative-hypnotic, and opiate withdrawal are all marked by hyperexcitability of the noradrenergic systems, which also occurs with panic attacks.

While self-medication with alcohol/drugs of abuse to decrease anxiety associated with panic has been posited by some to explain the high comorbidity of panic and substance use disorders, some substances of abuse (cocaine/marijuana/other stimulants) may actually induce panic attacks during periods of acute intoxication, and for other substances (alcohol, sedative-hypnotics, opiates) panic attacks may occur as a part of withdrawal syndromes. Several reports have noted that both marijuana and cocaine can precipitate panic attacks in patients without previous panic disorder (Aronson and Craig 1986; Louie et al. 1989). Subjects suffering from both alcoholism and panic disorder are unable to distinguish among a number of symptoms common to both disorders (D. T. George et al. 1988). Eliciting a good history of panic symptoms in the absence of acute use and withdrawal will help differentiate symptoms of panic that are substance induced.

The most widely used classes of pharmacotherapeutic agents for the treatment of panic disorder are the TCAs, the SSRIs, the monoamine oxidase inhibitors (MAOIs), and the benzodiazepines (Lydiard et al. 1988). TCAs have been the mainstay of treatment in the non-substance-abusing panic patient, but controlled trials in substance-using patients have not been reported. Benzodiazepines are generally contraindicated in substance-using populations because of their abuse potential. This is a controversial issue, and some investigators report successful use of benzodiazepines in patients with substance use disorders without evidence of abuse (Adinoff 1992). Benzodiazepines may be considered as adjuncts during the early treatment phase when activation and latency of onset of the antidepressants are issues of concern. If one chooses to prescribe a benzodiazepine to a patient with comorbid substance use, limited amounts of medication should be given and there should be close monitoring for relapse. As a rule, it seems best to avoid benzodiazepine use in this population.

MAOIs are also difficult to use in patients with comorbid substance use disorders. Dietary restrictions are necessary because of the interaction with tyramine in the diet, which may result in a hypertensive crisis. Moreover, MAOIs in combination with stimulant drugs may precipitate a hypertensive crisis.

Clinical trials have demonstrated the efficacy of the SSRIs in the treatment of panic disorder in non-substance-using patients (Lydiard et al. 1988). In 1996 paroxetine (Paxil) was approved by the FDA for use in the treatment of panic disorder. As mentioned earlier, the SSRIs have been shown by some investigators to have modest effects in decreasing alcohol consumption. These drugs, therefore, are a logical choice for the patient with comorbid panic disorder and alcoholism, but controlled clinical trials have not been conducted. Because of difficulty in using benzodiazepines and MAOIs in the substance-abusing population, and the proven efficacy of both TCAs and SSRIs in treating panic disorder, these drugs should be considered the treatment of choice in patients with comorbid panic and substance use disorders.

Panic disorder is quite responsive to nonpharmacological treatment. CB techniques, such as exposure and systematic desensitization, have been shown to be particularly effective in the treatment of panic disorder (Barlow 1988; Barlow and Lehman 1996). Relaxation therapy and supportive therapy can also be helpful in some cases (Jansson and Ost 1982). It is particularly important to maximize these nonpharmacological treatments in patients with substance use disorders. The ability to self-regulate subjective states and the confidence that can result from successful mastery through therapy can be helpful to individuals in recovery. Many of the techniques used in anxiety disorders have overlap with therapies known to be successful in the treatment of substance use disorders. Therefore, combination therapy can be quite feasible. Finally, by learning therapeutic anxiety-reducing strategies patients may be able to acquire alternative coping strategies and break out of the mind-set of using external agents to combat intolerable subjective states.

Generalized Anxiety Disorder

For generalized anxiety disorder (GAD) and substance use disorders, diagnostic issues are particularly complex. The DSM-IV criteria for GAD require that symptoms occur for at least 6 months without being directly related to physiological effects of a substance or a general medical condition (American Psychiatric Association 1994a). Symptoms of GAD have substantial overlap with acute intoxication with stimulants and withdrawal from alcohol, sedative-hypnotics, and opiates, and often the 6-month period of abstinence may be difficult to ascertain. While many substance-using individuals report anxiety symptoms consistent with GAD, they may not meet diagnostic criteria for GAD because of difficulty in distinguishing symptoms of anxiety from substance-related symptoms. In the NCS data, the odds ratio for co-occurrence of GAD with alcohol dependence was 3.7 (Kessler et al. 1996).

The treatment of GAD complicated by a substance use disorder is challenging. Benzodiazepines are effective in the treatment of GAD; however, as previously discussed, their abuse potential limits utility in the substance-abusing population. Buspirone is a nonbenzodiazepine anxiolytic with no abuse potential that has been studied for the pharmacological treatment of GAD with comorbid alcohol dependence. In two double-blind, placebo-controlled trials, anxious alcoholics decreased alcohol consumption and improved symptoms of anxiety during treatment with buspirone (Kranzler et al. 1994; Tollefson et al. 1992). However, in a third study, buspirone was found to have no effect on alcohol consumption or anxiety symptoms (Malcolm et al. 1992). Although the data remain somewhat contradictory, because of the low abuse potential and reports of success in well-controlled studies, buspirone remains a good choice in individuals with comorbid GAD and substance use disorders. There are no systematic trials of TCAs or SSRIs in the treatment of GAD in individuals with substance use disorders, but these agents have been useful in non-substance-abusing populations (Lydiard et al. 1988).

As mentioned in the section concerning panic disorder, nonpharmacological treatments for anxiety disorder can be very useful. GAD can be effectively managed using relaxation, coping skills, and CB therapy techniques (Barlow 1988; Barlow and Lehman 1996; Jansson and Ost 1982). Pharmacotherapy and psychotherapy are likely to complement one another in maximizing patient outcomes. Nonpharmacological treatment strategies in conjunction with judicious pharmacotherapeutic management should be encouraged.

Social Phobia

Social phobia is defined as a marked and persistent fear of situations in which an individual is exposed to unfamiliar people or to the scrutiny of others. The studies examining the interface of alcohol abuse and dependence with social phobia found rates of comorbidity ranging from 8% to 56% (Kushner et al. 1990). Consistent with the self-medication hypothesis, socially phobic patients report the use of alcohol to reduce social anxiety, and in most studies the onset of social phobia occurs prior to the onset of alcohol abuse and/or dependence (Marshall 1994). Social phobia in drug dependence is not well studied, but in one study, Myrick and Brady (1996) found a lifetime prevalence of social phobia in a cocaine-dependent population to be 13.9%. In nearly all cases, the social phobia preceded the cocaine dependence.

As social phobia may interfere with an individual's ability to engage effectively in treatment, early recognition is paramount to an improved chance of recovery. Frequently, the diagnosis is missed unless specific symptomatology is thoroughly assessed. A lengthy period of abstinence may not be needed as the fear of interaction in a social situation is not a specific feature of substance use or withdrawal. However, the social fears that occur only during periods of intoxication with marijuana or stimulants should not be considered sufficient to meet diagnostic criteria for social phobia.

Many agents have been investigated in the treatment of uncomplicated social phobia, but there are no studies examining the psychopharmacological treatment of individuals with comorbid social phobia and substance use. Of these agents, the MAOIs, the reversible inhibitors of monoamine oxidase (RIMAs), the SSRIs, and the benzodiazepines have documented efficacy (Lydiard et al. 1988). Several other agents, such as bupropion, ondansetron, buspirone, and venlafaxine, may also have efficacy but have not been well studied. In choosing a medication for the treatment of comorbid social phobia and substance abuse, the SSRIs would probably be first choice as they are efficacious, require no dietary restrictions, and are without the potential toxic interactions of the MAOIs. As previously mentioned, SSRIs may have the additional benefit of producing modest decreases in alcohol consumption.

Psychotherapeutic treatment is important. It may be difficult for socially phobic patients to participate in group therapy or 12-Step programs. A treatment plan that emphasizes CB therapy may prove to be more effective. Although there are no published studies systematically examining these treatments in patients with comorbid social phobia and substance use, several types of nonpharmacological treatments such as systematic desensitization, imaginal flooding, graduated exposure, social skills training, and cognitive approaches have proven effective in non-substance-using individuals with social phobia (Heimberg et al. 1990).

Posttraumatic Stress Disorder

The prevalence of comorbid posttraumatic stress disorder (PTSD) and substance use disorders is high. In the NCS, approximately 30%–50% of men and 25%–30% of women with lifetime PTSD had a co-occurring substance use disorder (Kessler et al. 1995). In treatment-seeking samples of substance abusers, the lifetime prevalence is between 36% and 50%, and the current prevalence of PTSD is between 25% and 42% (Dansky et al. 1994; Grice et al. 1995; Triffleman et al. 1994).

It is likely that drug use (in particular, cocaine use) and repeated withdrawal (in particular alcohol, sedative-hypnotic, and opiate withdrawal) exacerbate symptoms of PTSD. Cocaine use is associated with paranoia, hypervigilance, sleep disturbance, and autonomic arousal, all of which are features of PTSD. Anxiety and autonomic nervous system hyperactivity are characteristic of alcohol, sedative-hypnotic, and opiate withdrawal. These withdrawal syndromes and symptoms of PTSD are believed to have origins in excessive firing of the locus coeruleus (Kosten and Krystal 1988). It is possible that common pathophysiological mechanisms are responsible for the symptom overlap and exacerbation in individuals with comorbid PTSD and substance dependence. While this symptom overlap may make diagnosis difficult, the presence of a traumatic event and intrusive symptoms related to this event are unique to PTSD and should be particularly emphasized in evaluation.

Pharmacotherapy is playing an increasingly important role in the treatment of PTSD. The most rational pharmacotherapeutic regimen depends on the symptom constellation exhibited by the individual. Although there are uncontrolled reports of positive therapeutic benefit with a number of agents, TCAs and MAOIs have been shown in double-blind, placebo-controlled trials to improve intrusive and depressive symptoms of PTSD (Davidson 1992). A recently published placebo-controlled study found fluoxetine (an SSRI) to be an effective treatment for PTSD (van der Kolk et al. 1994). As mentioned in the discussion of other disorders, this is of particular interest because these agents may also have a modest effect in reducing alcohol consumption, are well tolerated, and are relatively nontoxic in interaction with alcohol. Unfortunately, none of the trials mentioned above included individuals with substance use disorders. There is one report of an open trial of sertraline treatment in a small group of individuals with comorbid PTSD and alcohol dependence that resulted in decreased alcohol consumption and decreased symptoms of PTSD (Brady et al. 1995b).

The appropriate psychotherapeutic approach to comorbid PTSD and substance use disorders remains unclear. CB therapies have demonstrated efficacy in the treatment of PTSD, but a widely accepted treatment approach in substance abuse treatment settings has been to defer treatment of trauma-related issues until the substance use disorder is in remission. In this light, it is noteworthy that a number of case studies in the literature indicate that successful treatment of symptoms of PTSD can lead to reductions in alcohol and drug abuse (Fairbank and Keane 1982; Polles and Smith 1995). For some patients relief of PTSD symptoms may improve the chances of recovery from substance abuse. This area clearly warrants further investigation.

Obsessive-Compulsive Disorder

The coexistence of obsessive-compulsive disorder (OCD) and substance use disorders is understudied. Rasmussen and Tsuang (1986) reported that 12% of OCD probands in a clinical population they investigated had a lifetime history of alcoholism. Eisen and Rasmussen (1989) screened 50 patients with a diagnosis of alcohol dependence or abuse and found that 6% met DSM-III-R (American Psychiatric Association 1987) criteria for OCD, three times the lifetime prevalence of OCD in the general population.

There are no controlled trials or case reports of the treatment of comorbid OCD and substance use. Clomipramine and SSRIs are both efficacious in the treatment of OCD (Lydiard et al. 1988). However, toxic interactions with alcohol, stimulants, and central nervous system (CNS) depressants are also more likely to occur with clomipramine. Consequently, SSRIs are likely to be the first line of treatment in individuals with OCD and a substance use disorder because there are fewer side effects or risks for toxic interactions.

The use of psychotherapeutic techniques in combination with pharmacotherapy is important in the treatment of OCD (Cottraux et al. 1990). CB therapies including thought stopping, exposure, and response prevention have convincingly and reliably been shown to be extremely effective in the treatment of OCD (Fals-Stewart et al. 1993). Again, a synergistic effect of the pharmacotherapy and psychotherapy might be expected.

Attention-Deficit/Hyperactivity Disorder

The co-occurrence of attention-deficit/hyperactivity disorder (ADHD) and psychoactive substance use disorders has received much recent attention. In summarizing data from a number of studies of adults and adolescents with substance use disorders, a mean rate of 23% of subjects with ADHD was found (Wilens et al. 1994). Investigations of substance use disorders in adults with ADHD have estimated rates of alcohol use disorders between 17% and 45% and drug abuse or dependence between 9% and 50% (Wilens et al. 1994). Comorbid conduct disorder or antisocial personality disorder is a clear risk factor for the development of a substance use disorder.

In making the diagnosis of ADHD in adults, there must be evidence that the ADHD symptoms first appeared in childhood and have persisted over time. DSM-IV requires that symptoms first appear before age 7. Numerous rating scales, such as the Brown Attention Scale and the Wender Utah Rating Scale (Ward et al. 1993), are available to assist in making a diagnosis of ADHD. As with many comorbid conditions, diagnostic issues are problematic. Because attentional problems may be a common occurrence during withdrawal states and acute intoxication, assessment of symptoms must be made during abstinence. Because the symptoms must first occur in childhood, careful screening for childhood symptoms may be of help in differentiating withdrawal states from ADHD. The period of abstinence required for diagnostic accuracy has not been well explored.

Treatment of patients with comorbid ADHD and substance use disorders must focus on stabilizing the substance use disorder first. As above, it is impossible to evaluate the severity and types of symptoms during active drug use and withdrawal. Pharmacotherapy plays an important role. Stimulants are ordinarily the first-line drug of choice for uncomplicated ADHD in children and adults. However, because of the abuse potential of the stimulant drug, the risks of abuse in this patient population may outweigh potential benefits. However, several case studies indicate that appropriate treatment of the ADHD can abate the substance use (Cocores et al. 1987; Khantzian 1983). Prospective controlled trials of stimulant treatment within this subgroup of substance abusers are needed. It has been suggested that pemoline (Cylert), because of its longer half-life, may have less abuse potential than methylphenidate or dextroamphetamine. Recent evidence concerning hepatotoxicity with pemoline is, however, of concern. TCAs and bupropion may be helpful in treating ADHD as well as any coexisting depression. Antihypertensive medications like clonidine and propranolol have been helpful in decreasing impulsivity and aggression (Wilens et al. 1994).

Psychotherapy should address psychoeducation surrounding ADHD, substance use disorders, interpersonal difficulties, low self-esteem, impulsivity, and time management. Behavioral treatments to improve focus and attention can be helpful in the treatment of childhood ADHD but are understudied in the treatment of adult ADHD. As with other comorbid conditions, it is important to maximize nonpharmacological treatment approaches.

Impulse-Control Disorders

Impulse-control disorders and substance use disorders share common phenomenological, clinical, and neurobiological features. Both are marked by specific urges and irresistible impulses. In both disorders, these feelings are associated with tension or dysphoria, which is often immediately relieved by engaging in the desired behavior. There are also some common neurobiological abnormalities in both impulse-control disorders and substance use disorders. The serotonergic system is often implicated. Studies have correlated a central serotonin deficit (low cerebrospinal fluid [CSF] 5-hydroxyindoleacetic acid [5-HIAA] concentrations) with impulsivity among alcoholic, impulsive, violent offenders and fire setters (Linnoila et al. 1983; Virkkunen et al. 1989). As previously mentioned, abnormalities in the serotonergic system have also been found in substance use disorders, particularly alcoholism (Amit et al. 1991).

The comorbidity between impulse-control disorders and substance use disorders is high. A number of studies have found elevated rates of substance use disorders in individuals with impulse-control disorders. In four studies of impulsive, violent offenders, rates of lifetime substance use disorders range from 19% to 100% (Linnoila et al. 1983; Salomon et al. 1994; Virkkunen et al. 1989). In three studies of compulsive buyers, 37% had lifetime substance use disorders (Christenson et al. 1994; McElroy et al. 1994; Scholsser et al. 1994). In several studies of sex offenders with paraphilias, greater than 60% met lifetime criteria for a substance use disorder (Black et al. 1997; Galli et al. 1995; Kruesi et al. 1992). Pathological gambling is probably the best studied of the impulse-control disorders. Studies of pathological gamblers have revealed approximately 50% prevalence rate of alcohol and other substance abuse/dependence (Ramirez et al. 1983). Studies of individuals in substance abuse treatment centers have revealed 9%–14% incidence of comorbid pathological gambling (Lesieur and Rosenthal 1991). Studies show that pathological gamblers have significantly greater problems with impulsivity and inability to resist craving than do alcoholics or cocaine abusers who are not pathological gamblers (Castellani and Rugle 1995).

For the impulse-control disorders, the relationship between the disorders is likely to be complex, dictating the need for simultaneous treatment of both disorders. These disorders are likely to operate in a synergistic fashion. In the case of pathological gambling, gambling puts the chemically dependent individual in situations where alcohol and drugs are readily available. Drug and alcohol use are likely to disinhibit the gambler and, therefore, worsen the course of the gambling disorder.

Treatment for impulse-control disorders is underinvestigated. Because of the probable involvement of the serotonin system in the pathophysiology of both impulse-control and substance use disorders, pharmacotherapeutic treatment has focused on the use of SSRIs. There have been several controlled clinical trials indicating benefit with the use of the SSRIs in a variety of types of impulse-control disorders (Kafka 1994; Swedo et al. 1989). As previously mentioned, the SSRIs have been implicated in the control of drinking and have been shown to decrease alcohol consumption in some studies (Gorelick 1989); for this reason, they may be useful pharmacotherapeutic agents for individuals with these comorbidities. Psychotherapeutic approaches are also not well studied. Gamblers Anonymous was established in 1957, and like AA, it endorses the disease concept along with total abstinence as a spiritually based 12-Step program offering fellowship (Cusack et al. 1993). Individual and group psychotherapy should focus on delaying the decision-making process, teaching methods to regulate impulses, and slowing down the sequence of moving from impulse to action (Castellani and Rugle 1995).

Eating Disorders

There is a high comorbidity between eating disorders, particularly bulimia, and substance use disorders. Studies report that approximately 20%–25% of women with a lifetime diagnosis of bulimia also have a history of alcohol or drug abuse/dependence (Holderness et al. 1994). A family history of substance use disorder is also common in individuals with bulimia (Bulik 1987). Substance use disorders are less common in individuals with anorexia.

Phenomenological similarities in both disorders include craving, impulsivity, loss of control, and the secrecy and denial surrounding the behavior (Varner 1995). In both disorders, individuals often use the food or drug in response to specific urges and feel relief of tension or negative affect with use. A family history of substance abuse is common in individuals with bulimia.

In addition to the more typical substances of abuse, there is within the eating-disorder population the possibility of dependence on diuretics, emetics (syrup of ipecac being most common), laxatives, thyroid hormones, diet pills (or other amphetamine-like substances), and benzodiazepines (often used to self-medicate insomnia with eating disorders). Diuretics, emetics, and laxatives may result in electrolyte imbalances; dehydration; gastrointestinal, cardiac, and neuromuscular complications; and death (Bulik 1992).

Biological commonalities among these disorders have also been identified that can help guide pharmacological treatment efforts. The serotonin system is thought to be involved in regulating appetite as well as alcohol consumption. The notion of serotonergic mechanisms underlying all consummatory behaviors has been offered (Amit et al. 1991). The SSRIs have some efficacy in the treatment of bulimia. In the absence of any specific studies addressing pharmacological treatments in patients with comorbid substance use and eating disorders, SSRIs would be a reasonable first choice when a pharmacological agent is indicated.

For eating disorders, treatment must involve psychoeducation around the physical dangers of diuretics, emetics, laxatives, and diet pills, as well as their ineffectiveness as weight loss agents and their role in perpetuating the eating disorder (Bulik 1992). CB therapy should address emotion regulation, impulsivity, distress tolerance, all-or-none thinking patterns, interpersonal skills, problem solving, and low self-esteem. Family therapy may be helpful as well. Because CB therapy is also effective for substance use disorders, there are many commonalities between the treatment of these disorders. The development of CB therapies specifically tailored for individuals with both eating disorders and substance use disorders would be a fruitful area for research.

Personality Disorders

The personality disorders are among the most common comorbid disorders in substance abusers. Compared with substance-abusing individuals without personality pathology, those with personality disorders have been found to have an earlier onset of substance abuse, more severe complications of the substance abuse, and poorer treatment outcomes (Carroll et al. 1993; Yates et al. 1988). Of all the personality disorders, antisocial personality disorder (ASPD) is the best studied with regard to comorbidity with substance use.

In the ECA study (Regier et al. 1990), 14% of individuals with alcohol abuse or dependence and 18% of those with other substance dependence or abuse disorders met lifetime criteria for ASPD. In the NCS, 16.9% of men and 7.8% of women with alcohol dependence had ASPD (Kessler et al. 1994). Both the ECA study and the NCS focused on ASPD and did not include information regarding other personality disorders.

In a clinical population, 44% of a sample of 237 men and women meeting DSM-III-R criteria for recurrent opioid dependence also met criteria for ASPD (Brooner et al. 1993). In a study of 399 cocaine-dependent individuals seeking inpatient or outpatient treatment, Carroll et al. (1993) found that 7% of the sample had ASPD according to Research Diagnostic Criteria (RDC; Spitzer et al. 1978) and 53% of the sample met ASPD criteria according to DSM-III-R. The RDC's stringent requirements include the stipulations that childhood conduct disorder precede adult ASPD and that adult ASPD be independent of substance abuse. The DSM-III-R criteria are more inclusive. Substance-abusing individuals who met DSM-III-R criteria for ASPD had poorer treatment outcomes than those who did not. Nace and colleagues (1991) studied a sample of 100 consecutively hospitalized substance abusers and found that 57% had personality disorders. The majority of these patients had Cluster B diagnoses (antisocial, borderline, histrionic, and narcissistic). In an interesting study by Thevos and colleagues (1993), personality disorders in an alcoholic and a cocaine-dependent population were compared. The researchers found that the cocaine group was significantly more likely to meet criteria for an Axis II diagnosis than was the alcohol group (67% versus 40%).

The presence of personality disorder should be evaluated in every substance abuser because it can change treatment needs and alter prognosis. Substance abusers with ASPD have been shown to have a greater severity of substance dependence and more adverse medical sequelae of their substance use than other groups (Cadoret et al. 1984; Yates et al. 1988). Drug use usually occurs earlier in ASPD subjects than in non-ASPD subjects (Buydens-Branchey et al. 1989; Carroll et al. 1993). Individuals with ASPD and multiple substance abuse problems have higher rates of alcohol dependence than do non-ASPD individuals with substance abuse (Hesselbrock et al. 1985; Schuckit 1985). Substance abusers with ASPD have higher rates of human immunodeficiency virus (HIV)–related infection with intravenous drug use than do non-ASPD intravenous substance abusers (Brooner et al. 1993). Cocaine- and alcohol-dependent patients with the onset of ASPD in childhood or adolescence are more likely to engage in criminal and violent behaviors in adult life than non-ASPD individuals (Cacciola et al. 1994). Substance abuse and ASPD interact to produce a high cost to society in the form of medical care and criminal acts.

The co-occurrence of ASPD with substance abuse worsens treatment outcome. A pharmacological trial of cocaine-abusing ASPD individuals (Leal et al. 1994) found that retention was lower for the ASPD group and that those of the group who were still in treatment at the end of the study had a lower percentage of cocaine-free urine tests (7% versus 30%). Arndt and colleagues (1994), in a study of methadone-maintained cocaine-dependent men receiving placebo or desipramine, found that ASPD was a predictor of poor treatment response.

Treatment of the substance abuser with a personality disorder is challenging. Substance abusers with personality disorders are usually treated together with those without personality disorders, which can lead to problems for both groups. Walker (1992) came up with some excellent recommendations for borderline personality disorder (BPD) and ASPD patients with substance use disorders, but these have not been empirically tested for effectiveness. Linehan (1995) developed a specific behavior therapy program for BPD patients with substance abuse. This manual-driven behavior therapy addresses motivational deficits, behavioral and emotional self-regulation, and distress tolerance skills, as well as treatment of the substance abuse. This work requires replication in a larger population. Long-term treatment programs in therapeutic communities are frequently advocated for individuals with comorbid ASPD and substance abuse. However, relapse and dropout rates are often high (Ravndal and Vaglum 1991). Specific pharmacological treatment strategies have not been explored.

Conclusions

Evidence from multiple lines of investigation is converging to confirm that the substance use disorders and psychiatric disorders commonly co-occur. This co-occurrence presents challenges for diagnosis as well as optimal patient management. In terms of diagnosis, strategies designed to focus on features of the disorder or history most likely to be useful in making early diagnosis will be helpful. General principles emerging from the literature to guide treatment efforts include the combining of psychotherapeutic techniques from the psychiatric and substance use fields to design specifically tailored strategies for comorbid populations. Although much work remains to be done in exploring the most appropriate pharmacotherapeutic treatment for individuals with comorbid psychiatric and substance use disorders, the development of scientific techniques capable of elucidating the common neurobiological pathways in these disorders holds promise for the design of specifically targeted pharmacotherapeutic strategies. Recent studies have provided helpful information concerning diagnostic, pharmacotherapeutic, and psychotherapeutic strategies tailored for this population, but much work remains to be done in developing the optimal treatment for this prevalent group of disorders.

References

Adinoff B: Long-term therapy with benzodiazepines despite alcohol dependence disorder: seven case reports. Am J Addict 1:288–293, 1992

American Psychiatric Association: Diagnostic and Statistical Manual of Mental Disorders, 3rd Edition, Revised. Washington, DC, American Psychiatric Association, 1987

American Psychiatric Association: Diagnostic and Statistical Manual of Mental Disorders, 4th Edition. Washington, DC, American Psychiatric Association, 1994a

American Psychiatric Association: Practice guideline for the treatment of patients with bipolar disorder. Am J Psychiatry 151 (12 suppl):1–36, 1994b

Amit Z, Smith BR, Gill K: Serotonin uptake inhibitors: effects on motivated consummatory behaviors. J Clin Psychiatry 55:55–60, 1991

Arndt IO, McLellan AT, Dorozynsky L, et al: Desipramine treatment for cocaine dependence: role of antisocial personality disorder. J Nerv Ment Dis 182:151–156, 1994

Aronson TA, Craig TJ: Cocaine precipitation of panic disorder. Am J Psychiatry 143:643–645, 1986

Barlow DH: Anxiety and Its Disorders: The Nature and Treatment of Anxiety and Panic. New York, Guilford, 1988

Barlow DH, Lehman CL: Advances in the psychosocial treatment of anxiety disorders. Implications for national health care. Arch Gen Psychiatry 53:727–735, 1996

Black DW, Kehrberg LL, Flumerfelt DL, et al: Characteristics of 36 subjects reporting compulsive sexual behavior. Am J Psychiatry 154:243–249, 1997

Boutros NN, Bowers MB Jr: Chronic substance-induced psychotic disorders: state of the literature. J Neuropsychiatry Clin Neurosci 8:262–269, 1996

Bowden CL: Predictors of response to divalproex and lithium. J Clin Psychiatry 56:25–30, 1995

Brady KT, Anton R, Ballenger JC, et al: Cocaine abuse among schizophrenic patients. Am J Psychiatry 147:1164–1167, 1990

Brady KT, Sonne SC, Anton R, et al: Valproate in the treatment of acute bipolar affective episodes complicated by substance abuse: a pilot study. J Clin Psychiatry 56:118–121, 1995a

Brady KT, Sonne SC, Roberts JM: Sertraline treatment of comorbid posttraumatic stress disorder and alcohol dependence. J Clin Psychiatry 56:502–505, 1995b

Breakey WR, Goodell H, Lorenz PC, et al: Hallucinogenic drugs as precipitants of schizophrenia. Psychol Med 4:255–261, 1974

Brooner RK, Herbst JH, Schmidt CW: Antisocial personality disorder among drug abusers. Relations to other personality diagnoses and the five-factor model of personality. J Nerv Ment Dis 181:313–319, 1993

Brooner RK, King VL, Kidorf M, et al: Psychiatric and substance comorbidity among treatment-seeking opioid abusers. Arch Gen Psychiatry 54:71–80, 1997

Brown SA, Schuckit M: Changes in depression among abstinent alcoholics. J Stud Alcohol 49:412–417, 1988

Buckley P, Thompson P, Way L, et al: Substance abuse among patients with treatment-resistant schizophrenia: characteristics and implications for clozapine therapy [see comments]. Am J Psychiatry 151:385–389, 1994

Bulik CM: Drug and alcohol abuse by bulimic women and their families. Am J Psychiatry 144:1604–1606, 1987

Bulik CM: Abuse of drugs associated with eating disorders. J Subst Abuse 4:69–90, 1992

Buydens-Branchey L, Branchey MH, Noumair D, et al: Age of alcoholism onset, II: relationship to susceptibility to serotonin precursor availability. Arch Gen Psychiatry 46:231–236, 1989

Cacciola JS, Rutherford MJ, Alterman AI, et al: An examination of the diagnostic criteria for antisocial personality disorder in substance abusers. J Nerv Ment Dis 182:517–523, 1994

Cadoret R, Troughton E, Widmer R: Clinical differences between antisocial and primary alcoholics. Compr Psychiatry 25:1–8, 1984

Calabrese JR, Markovitz PJ, Kimmel SE, et al: Spectrum of efficacy of valproate in 78 rapid-cycling bipolar patients. J Clin Psychopharmacol 12:53S–56S, 1992

Carroll KM, Ball SA, Rounsaville BJ: A comparison of alternate systems for diagnosing antisocial personality disorder in cocaine abusers. J Nerv Ment Dis 181:436–443, 1993

Castellani B, Rugle L: A comparison of pathological gamblers to alcoholics and cocaine misusers on impulsivity, sensation seeking and craving. Int J Addict 30:275–289, 1995

Christenson GA, Faber RJ, de Zwaan M, et al: Compulsive buying: descriptive characteristics and psychiatric comorbidity [see comments]. J Clin Psychiatry 55:5–11, 1994

Cocores JA, Davies RK, Mueller PS, et al: Cocaine abuse and adult attention deficit disorder. J Clin Psychiatry 48:376–377, 1987

Cornelius JR, Salloum IM, Ehler JG, et al: Fluoxetine in depressed alcoholics: a double-blind, placebo-controlled trial [see comments]. Arch Gen Psychiatry 54:700–705, 1997

Cottraux J, Mollard E, Bouvard M, et al: A controlled study of fluvoxamine and exposure in obsessive-compulsive disorder. Int Clin Psychopharmacol 5:17–30, 1990

Cusack JR, Malaney KR, DePry DL: Insights about pathological gamblers. "Chasing losses" in spite of the consequences. Postgrad Med 93:169–176, 179, 1993

Dansky BS, Brady KT, Roberts JT: Post-traumatic stress disorder and substance abuse: empirical findings and clinical issues. Subst Abuse 15:247–257, 1994

Davidson J: Drug therapy of post-traumatic stress disorder [see comments]. Br J Psychiatry 160:309–314, 1992

Dixon L, Haas G, Weiden PJ, et al: Drug abuse in schizophrenic patients: clinical correlates and reasons for use. Am J Psychiatry 148:224–230, 1991

Dorus W, Kennedy J, Gibbons RD, et al: Symptoms and diagnosis of depression in alcoholics. Alcohol Clin Exp Res 11:150–154, 1987

Eisen JL, Rasmussen SA: Coexisting obsessive compulsive disorder and alcoholism. J Clin Psychiatry 50:96–98, 1989

Fairbank JA, Keane TM: Flooding for combat-related stress disorders: assessment of anxiety reduction across traumatic memories. Behavior Therapy 13:499–510, 1982

Fals-Stewart W, Marks AP, Schafer J: A comparison of behavioral group therapy and individual behavior therapy in treating obsessive-compulsive disorder [see comments]. J Nerv Ment Dis 181:189–193, 1993

Freeman TW, Clothier JL, Pazzaglia P, et al: A double-blind comparison of valproate and lithium in the treatment of acute mania. Am J Psychiatry 149:108–111, 1992

Galli VJ, Raute NJ, Kizer DL, et al: A study of the phenomenology, comorbidity, and preliminary treatment response of pedophiles and adolescent sex offenders (abstract). New Clinical Drug Evaluation Unit (NCDEU) 35th Annual Meeting, Orlando, FL, June 1995

George DT, Zerby A, Noble S, et al: Panic attacks and alcohol withdrawal: can subjects differentiate the symptoms? Biol Psychiatry 24:240–243, 1988

George TP, Sernyak MJ, Ziedonis DM, et al: Effects of clozapine on smoking in chronic schizophrenic outpatients. J Clin Psychiatry 56:344–346, 1995

Gorelick DA: Serotonin uptake blockers and the treatment of alcoholism. Recent Dev Alcohol 7:267–281, 1989

Grice DE, Dustan LR, Brady KT: Sexual and physical assault history and post-traumatic stress disorder in substance-dependent individuals. Am J Addict 4:297–305, 1995

Hamilton M: A rating scale for depression. J Neurol Neurosurg Psychiatry 23:56–62, 1960

Hasin D, Endicott J, Lewis C: Alcohol and drug abuse in patients with affective syndromes. Compr Psychiatry 26:283–295, 1985

Hasin DS, Grant BF, Endicott J: Lifetime psychiatric comorbidity in hospitalized alcoholics: subject and familial correlates. Int J Addict 23:827–850, 1988

Heimberg RG, Dodge CS, Hope DA, et al: Cognitive-behavioral group treatment of social phobia: comparison to a credible placebo control. Cognitive Therapy Research 14:1–23, 1990

Hesselbrock MN, Meyer RE, Keener JJ: Psychopathology in hospitalized alcoholics. Arch Gen Psychiatry 42:1050–1055, 1985

Holderness CC, Brooks-Gunn J, Warren MP: Co-morbidity of eating disorders and substance abuse review of the literature. Int J Eat Disord 16:1–34, 1994

Jaffe JH, Ciraulo KA: Alcoholism and depression, in Psychopathology and Addictive Disorders. Edited by Meyer RE. New York, Guilford, 1986, pp 293–320

Jansson L, Ost LG: Behavioral treatments for agoraphobia: an evaluative review. Clin Psychol Rev 2:311–336, 1982

Kafka MP: Sertraline pharmacotherapy for paraphilias and paraphilia-related disorders: an open trial. Ann Clin Psychiatry 6:189–195, 1994

Keitner GI, Ryan CE, Miller IW, et al: 12-month outcome of patients with major depression and comorbid psychiatric or medical illness (compound depression). Am J Psychiatry 148:345–350, 1991

Keller MB, Lavori PW, Coryell W, et al: Differential outcome of pure manic, mixed/cycling and pure depressive episodes in patients with bipolar illness. JAMA 255:3138–3142, 1986

Kessler RC, McGonagle KA, Zhao S, et al: Lifetime and 12-month prevalence of DSM-III-R psychiatric disorders in the United States. Results from the National Comorbidity Survey. Arch Gen Psychiatry 51:8–19, 1994

Kessler RC, Sonnega A, Bromet E, et al: Posttraumatic stress disorder in the National Comorbidity Survey. Arch Gen Psychiatry 52:1048–1060, 1995

Kessler RC, Nelson CB, McGonagle KA, et al: The epidemiology of co-occurring addictive and mental disorders: implications for prevention and service utilization. Am J Orthopsychiatry 66:17–31, 1996

Khantzian EJ: An extreme case of cocaine dependence and marked improvement with methylphenidate treatment. Am J Psychiatry 140:784–785, 1983

Kosten TR, Krystal J: Biological mechanisms in posttraumatic stress disorder: relevance for substance abuse, in Recent Developments in Alcoholism. Edited by Galanter M. New York, Plenum, 1988, pp 49–68

Kosten TR, Ziedonis DM: Substance abuse and schizophrenia: editors' introduction. Schizophr Bull 23:181–186, 1997

Kranzler HR, Burleson JA, Del Boca FK, et al: Buspirone treatment of anxious alcoholics: a placebo-controlled trial. Arch Gen Psychiatry 51:720–731, 1994

Kruesi MJ, Fine S, Valladares L, et al: Paraphilias: a double-blind crossover comparison of clomipramine versus desipramine. Arch Sex Behav 21:587–593, 1992

Kushner MG, Sher KJ, Beitman BD: The relation between alcohol problems and the anxiety disorders [see comments]. Am J Psychiatry 147:685–695, 1990

Leal J, Ziedonis D, Kosten T: Antisocial personality disorder as a prognostic factor for pharmacotherapy of cocaine dependence. Drug Alcohol Depend 35:31–35, 1994

Lesieur HR, Rosenthal RJ: Pathological gambling: a review of the literature. Journal of Gambling Studies 7:5–39, 1991

Linehan MM: Combining pharmacotherapy with psychotherapy for substance abusers with borderline personality disorder: strategies for enhancing compliance, in Integrating Behavioral Therapies With Medications in the Treatment of Drug Dependence. NIDA Research Monograph 150 (NIH Publ No 95-3899). Edited by Onken LS, Blaine JD, Boren JJ. Rockville, MD, National Institute on Drug Abuse, 1995, pp 129–142

Linnoila M, Virkkunen M, Scheinin M, et al: Low cerebrospinal fluid 5-hydroxyindoleacetic acid concentration differentiates impulsive from nonimpulsive violent behavior. Life Sci 33:2609–2614, 1983

Louie AK, Lannon RA, Ketter TA: Treatment of cocaine-induced panic disorder. Am J Psychiatry 146:40–44, 1989

Lydiard RB, Roy-Byrne PP, Ballenger JC: Recent advances in the psychopharmacological treatment of anxiety disorders. Hospital and Community Psychiatry 39:1157–1165, 1988

Malcolm R, Anton RF, Randall CL, et al: A placebo-controlled trial of buspirone in anxious inpatient alcoholics. Alcohol Clin Exp Res 16:1007–1013, 1992

Marshall JR: The diagnosis and treatment of social phobia and alcohol abuse. Bull Menninger Clin 58:A58–A66, 1994

Mason BJ, Kocsis JH, Ritvo EC, et al: A double-blind, placebo-controlled trial of desipramine for primary alcohol dependence stratified on the presence or absence of major depression [see comments]. JAMA 275:761–767, 1996

McElroy SL, Keck PE Jr, Pope HG Jr, et al: Compulsive buying: a report of 20 cases. J Clin Psychiatry 55:242–248, 1994

McGrath PJ, Nunes EV, Stewart JW, et al: Imipramine treatment of alcoholics with primary depression: a placebo-controlled clinical trial. Arch Gen Psychiatry 53:232–240, 1996

Meyer RE: Prospects for a rational pharmacotherapy of alcoholism. J Clin Psychiatry 50:403–412, 1989

Milby JB, Sims MK, Khuder S, et al: Psychiatric comorbidity: prevalence in methadone maintenance treatment. Am J Drug Alcohol Abuse 22:95–107, 1996

Miller NS, Fine J: Current epidemiology of comorbidity of psychiatric and addictive disorders. Psychiatr Clin North Am 16:1–10, 1993

Mirin SM, Weiss RD, Michael J, et al: Psychopathology in substance abusers: diagnosis and treatment. Am J Drug Alcohol Abuse 14:139–157, 1988

Myrick DH, Brady KT: Social phobia in cocaine-dependent individuals. Am J Addict 6:99–104, 1996

Nace EP, Davis CW, Gaspari JP: Axis II comorbidity in substance abusers [see comments]. Am J Psychiatry 148:118–120, 1991

Nunes EV, Quitkin FM, Brady R, et al: Imipramine treatment of methadone maintenance patients with affective disorder and illicit drug use. Am J Psychiatry 148:667–669, 1991

O'Connell RA, Mayo JA, Flatow L, et al: Outcome of bipolar disorder on long-term treatment with lithium. Br J Psychiatry 159:123–129, 1991

Polles AG, Smith PO: Treatment of coexisting substance dependence and posttraumatic stress disorder. Psychiatr Serv 46:729–730, 1995

Powell BJ, Penick EC, Othmer E, et al: Prevalence of additional psychiatric syndromes among male alcoholics. J Clin Psychiatry 43:404–407, 1982

Project MATCH Research Group: Matching Alcoholism Treatments to Client Heterogeneity: Project MATCH posttreatment drinking outcomes. J Stud Alcohol 58:7–29, 1997

Ramirez LF, McCormick RA, Russo AM, et al: Patterns of substance abuse in pathological gamblers undergoing treatment. Addict Behav 8:425–428, 1983

Rao S, Ziedonis D, Kosten T: The pharmacotherapy of cocaine dependence. Psychiatr Ann 25:363–368, 1995

Rasmussen SA, Tsuang MT: Clinical characteristics and family history in DSM-III obsessive-compulsive disorder. Am J Psychiatry 143:317–322, 1986

Ravndal E, Vaglum P: Psychopathology and substance abuse as predictors of program completion in a therapeutic community for drug abusers: a prospective study. Acta Psychiatr Scand 83:217–222, 1991

Regier DA, Farmer ME, Rae DS, et al: Comorbidity of mental disorders with alcohol and other drug abuse. Results from the Epidemiologic Catchment Area (ECA) Study [see comments]. JAMA 264:2511–2518, 1990

Rounsaville BJ, Weissman MM, Kleber H, et al: Heterogeneity of psychiatric diagnosis in treated opiate addicts. Arch Gen Psychiatry 39:161–168, 1982

Rounsaville BJ, Anton SF, Carroll K, et al: Psychiatric diagnoses of treatment-seeking cocaine abusers. Arch Gen Psychiatry 48:43–51, 1991

Salomon RM, Mazure CM, Delgado PL, et al: Serotonin function in aggression: the effect of acute plasma tryptophan depletion in aggressive patients. Biol Psychiatry 35:570–572, 1994

Schlosser S, Black DW, Repertinger S, et al: Compulsive buying: demography, phenomenology, and comorbidity in 46 subjects. Gen Hosp Psychiatry 16:205–212, 1994

Schuckit MA: The clinical implications of primary diagnostic groups among alcoholics. Arch Gen Psychiatry 42:1043–1049, 1985

Shaner A, Khalsa ME, Roberts L, et al: Unrecognized cocaine use among schizophrenic patients. Am J Psychiatry 150:758–762, 1993

Siris SG, Bermanzohn PC, Mason SE, et al: Antidepressant for substance-abusing schizophrenic patients: a minireview. Prog Neuropsychopharmacol Biol Psychiatry 15:1–13, 1991

Spitzer RL, Endicott J, Robins E: Research Diagnostic Criteria: rationale and reliability. Arch Gen Psychiatry 35:773–782, 1978

Swedo SE, Leonard HL, Rapoport JL, et al: A double-blind comparison of clomipramine and desipramine in the treatment of trichotillomania (hair pulling) [see comments]. N Engl J Med 321:497–501, 1989

Thevos AK, Johnston AL, Latham PK, et al: Symptoms of anxiety in inpatient alcoholics with and without DSM-III-R anxiety diagnoses. Alcohol Clin Exp Res 15:102–105, 1991

Thevos A, Brady KT, Grice DE, et al: A comparison of psychopathology in cocaine and alcohol dependence. Am J Addict 2:279–286, 1993

Tollefson GD, Montague-Clouse J, Tollefson SL: Treatment of comorbid generalized anxiety in a recently detoxified alcoholic population with a selective serotonergic drug (buspirone). J Clin Psychopharmacol 12:19–26, 1992

Triffleman EG, Marmar C, Delucchi KL: Childhood trauma and PTSD in substance abuse inpatients, in Problems of Drug Dependence, 1993: Proceedings of the 55th Annual Scientific Meeting of the College on Problems of Drug Dependence. Edited by Harris LS. Washington, DC, U.S. Government Printing Office, 1994

van der Kolk BA, Dreyfuss D, Michaels M, et al: Fluoxetine in posttraumatic stress disorder. J Clin Psychiatry 55:517–522, 1994

Varner LM: Dual diagnosis: patients with eating and substance-related disorders. J Am Diet Assoc 95:224–225, 1995

Virkkunen M, De Jong J, Bartko J, et al: Relationship of psychobiological variables to recidivism in violent offenders and impulsive fire setters: a follow-up study [published erratum appears in Arch Gen Psychiatry 46:913, 1989]. Arch Gen Psychiatry 46:600–603, 1989

Walker R: Substance abuse and B-cluster disorders, II: treatment recommendations. J Psychoactive Drugs 24:233–241, 1992

Ward MF, Wender PH, Reimherr FW: The Wender Utah Rating Scale: an aid in the retrospective diagnosis of childhood attention deficit hyperactivity disorder [published erratum appears in Am J Psychiatry 150:1280, 1993]. Am J Psychiatry 150:885–890, 1993

Weiss RD, Mirin SM: Tricyclic antidepressants in the treatment of alcoholism and drug abuse. J Clin Psychiatry 50 (suppl):4–11, 1989

Weiss RD, Mirin SM, Griffin ML, et al: Psychopathology in cocaine abusers: changing trends. J Nerv Ment Dis 176:719–725, 1988

Weiss RD, Greenfield SF, Najavits LM, et al: Medication compliance among patients with bipolar disorder and substance use disorder. J Clin Psychiatry 59:172–174, 1998

Wilens TE, Biederman J, Spencer TJ, et al: Comorbidity of attention-deficit hyperactivity and substance use disorders. Hospital and Community Psychiatry 45:421–435, 1994

Wilkins JN: Pharmacotherapy of schizophrenia patients with comorbid substance abuse. Schizophr Bull 23:215–228, 1997

Yates WR, Petty F, Brown K: Alcoholism in males with antisocial personality disorder. Int J Addict 23:999–1010, 1988

Ziedonis D, Richardson T, Lee E, et al: Adjunctive desipramine in the treatment of cocaine abusing schizophrenics. Psychopharmacol Bull 28:309–314, 1992

Ziedonis DM, Kosten TR, Glazer WM, et al: Nicotine dependence and schizophrenia. Hospital and Community Psychiatry 45:204–206, 1994

Ziedonis D, Trudeau K: Motivation to quit using substances among individuals with schizophrenia: implications for a motivation-based treatment model. Schizophr Bull 23:229–238, 1997

SECTION 5

Schizophrenia and Other Psychotic Disorders

Section Editors

Richard L. Munich, M.D.

Carol A. Tamminga, M.D.

Introduction

Schizophrenia presents as a heterogeneous and phasic illness, with defects and disabilities affecting perception, thinking, language, emotion, volition, and social behavior. The current consensus about its pathophysiology posits neuroanatomic and neurochemical abnormalities, which can be either genetically or environmentally induced. These neurobiological substrates can produce vulnerability in a particular person, which makes him or her sensitive to a variety of psychosocial and physical stressors. When a stressor coincides with the vulnerability, usually in late adolescence or early adult life, afflicted persons develop catastrophic changes in their neurochemical, cognitive, and interpersonal experiences. In the majority of cases, the condition usually steadily worsens. This complex and integrated view of the "schizophrenia process" has moved treatment from a monolithic dichotomy between somatic and psychosocial approaches to the broadly oriented but highly focused interventions detailed in the chapters in this section.

The section begins with a chapter by Gunvant Thaker and Carol Tamminga on treatment targets in schizophrenia and in schizophrenia spectrum disorders. Focusing on the symptom complexes that are the targets of drug and interpersonal treatment, the authors break down the manifestations of schizophrenia and its spectrum and discuss each complex individually with respect to its response to antipsychotic medications. The newer antipsychotic drugs have broader therapeutic action with fewer motor side effects; consequently, they are associated with better compliance. These therapeutic actions are then applied to positive and negative symptoms, conceptual disorganization, neuropsychological and neurophysiological deficits, regional cerebral blood flow and metabolic deficits, and the functional deficits of the nonpsychotic schizophrenic phenotype.

In Chapter 34, John Kane and Anil Malhotra summarize the clinical psychopharmacology of schizophrenia and related psychotic disorders. Treatment includes management of both the acute phase and the more chronic and maintenance phase. The appropriate regimens for treatment of both acute and chronic phases are currently undergoing reappraisal, with the recognition that optimal doses may be much lower than has been previously thought. The authors have included a section on managing the patient who does not respond or who has a partial response to antipsychotic drugs. Kane and Malhotra specifically focus on clozapine and the new generation of antipsychotic drugs and provide a discussion of tardive dyskinesia on maintenance strategies at the end of this section.

Modern treatment includes not only pharmacotherapy to alter the neurochemical aspects of vulnerability but also flexible individual and group psychotherapies, psychoeducation, and assertive case management to mitigate the impact of stress; rehabilitation to promote the development of resources; and social, cognitive, and vocational skills and learning strategies to enhance coping capacity (Andreasen 1994; Michels and Marzuk 1993; Mueser 1993). Thus, in Chapters 35 and 36, Wayne Fenton and Stephen Cole illustrate how individual, group, and family therapy approaches to schizophrenia spectrum disorders are tailored to the unique and phasic aspects of the disease process, the motivation of patients and their families, and the availability of resources. A key aspect of Fenton's chapter is the emphasis in all modalities on a flexible, patient-centered attitude on the part of the clinician—in individual psychotherapy, for example, moving from problem-solving strategies to supportive, reality-adaptive, expressive, insight-oriented, and interpretive strategies when appropriate. Finally, a substantial number of persons with schizophrenia and related disorders continue to live with their family of origin, and these families are welcomed into a full treatment partnership with patient and clinician.

Although rehabilitation in psychiatry is nearly 200 years old, the modern era of this field began in the 1970s with the work of William Anthony in Boston, J. K. Wing in England, and Robert Liberman in Los Angeles. Over the next two decades, these investigators and practitioners painstakingly helped define and develop the knowledge and technology required to integrate psychiatric rehabilitation into the contemporary treatment armamentarium. Charles Wallace, Robert Liberman, Alex Kopelowicz, and Daniel Yaeger, in Chapter 37, amply document the enlarging role for this modality, which is especially important because the ongoing worldwide shift from industrial to technological work skills will place an increasingly higher demand on cognitive skills; this in turn implies that persons afflicted with serious mental illness will require more rehabilitation services (Munich and Lang 1993).

More than 80% of treatments of persons with schizophrenia take place outside the traditional hospital setting. Appropriately, Richard Munich and William Sledge conclude the section on treatment of schizophrenia and related disorders in Chapter 38 by describing treatment systems and continua of care. As the authors point out, a system of care implies that the actual location of a patient's treatment depends on the phase of illness and on efforts to maximize contact with the patient's environment, to provide the least restrictive alternative, and to maintain continuity of treatment. The authors outline the role of hospitalization and its many alternatives, including case management, in giving shape to a continuum of care.

Schizophrenia is a tragic illness that tends to be persistent and to lead to both social and cognitive deterioration. Modern treatment methods and long-term outcome studies offer more hope for this illness than in the past, although much more remains to be done. Psychopharmacological intervention reduces delusions and hallucinations and can even reduce some negative symptoms. Nevertheless, many patients remain chronically ill. Clinicians using increasingly sophisticated and focused psychosocial interventions are making an effort to meet patients and their families where they are, to foster a new kind of alliance, and to offer treatments that will help reduce the residual psychosocial impairment that is so common in this illness.

References

Andreasen NC (ed): Schizophrenia: From Mind to Molecule. Washington, DC, American Psychiatric Press, 1994

Michels R, Marzuk PM: Progress in psychiatry. N Engl J Med 329:552–560, 1993

Mueser KT: Commentary on Liberman and Corrigan. Psychiatry 56:250–253, 1993

Munich RL, Lang E: The boundaries of psychiatric rehabilitation. Hospital and Community Psychiatry 44:661–665, 1993

33

Treatment Targets in Schizophrenia and Schizophrenia Spectrum Disorders

Gunvant K. Thaker, M.D.
Carol A. Tamminga, M.D.

Schizophrenia is presently conceptualized as a brain disease that presents with a combination of psychotic, affective, and cognitive symptoms (Carpenter and Buchanan 1994; Gottesman and Shields 1982; Kendler and Diehl 1993; Lenzenweger et al. 1991). Symptoms of schizophrenia are usually expressed over a lifelong course of episodic florid psychosis combined with residual disease phases (Bleuler 1978; Ciompi and Muller 1976). The boundary of schizophrenia is to a large extent defined by the presence or absence of overt psychosis, however many individuals with schizophrenia spectrum disorders experience no psychotic symptoms but have schizophrenia-like deficits in cognitive and other functions (Kendler et al. 1993; Kety et al. 1976; Siever and Gunderson 1983). The schizophrenia spectrum phenotype is characterized by mild psychotic-like symptoms, affective blunting, and cognitive symptoms. In earlier classification systems, persons with these symptoms were diagnosed with latent schizophrenia but now are included with those diagnosed with the schizophrenia spectrum disorders, as defined by schizotypal personality disorders or to a lesser extent paranoid and schizoid personality disorders.

Throughout the schizophrenia spectrum (diagnosis or phenotype), psychotic, affective, and cognitive symptoms can vary independently over the life course. All aspects of these clinical presentations represent targets for schizophrenia treatments. However, the symptom dimensions respond variably to available antipsychotic treatments, with psychosis most responsive and negative and cognitive symptoms most resistant to current therapies. Few individuals with schizophrenia lose all symptoms and recover completely, even with optimal treatment. Historically, individuals with schizophrenia spectrum personality disorders were not treated, but practices may be changing because data show that persons with schizophrenia may receive benefit from antipsychotic medications (Tsuang et al. 1999).

Neither the pathophysiological mechanism(s) nor the cause(s) of schizophrenia and its spectrum disorders are currently known. However, the clinical and biological characteristics of the disease have been vigorously explored for decades for clues leading to pathophysiology (Tamminga 1997). Phenomenological studies have carefully described the symptoms, lifetime course of the illness, neuropsychological performance, structure of the brain, and measures of brain function such as evoked potentials, eye movements, and in vivo brain imaging. Although the disease mechanism has not yet been discovered, considerable data characterizing persons with the illness or its phenotype have been collected and analyzed.

Despite the inadequate mechanistic understanding, treatments do exist for schizophrenia (Klein and Davis 1969; see Kane and Malhotra, Chapter 34, in this volume). These treatments are highly effective, especially in reducing certain types of symptoms, such as florid psychosis. The newer antipsychotic drugs, with broader therapeutic actions, provide better treatment than the conventional drugs (Tamminga 1998). Fewer motor side effects are associated with the newer drugs as well as consequent better compliance and ability to maintain adequate doses. Studies of the mechanism of action(s) of effective antipsychotic drugs (beyond dopamine receptor blockade) have not yet led to a full explication of actions, nor indirectly to disease pathophysiology. The discovery of proper treatment targets, derived directly from disease pathophysiology as it is discovered, is critical to provide not only symptomatic relief but full remission of symptoms and disability for persons with schizophrenia.

Phenomenology and Response to Treatment

Symptoms of schizophrenia in individuals have been noted in historical and creative writings over the millennia (Bleuler 1950, 1978; Schneider 1959; Thaker et al., in press). Although these manifestations have not inevitably been identified as illness in all historical eras, the descriptions of schizophrenia-like behaviors with their characteristic paranoia, thought disorder, or hallucinations are unmistakable nonetheless. Few treatments as we know them today were available before the mid-20th century. Early in that century, the schizophrenic psychoses were distinguished diagnostically from the primary affective psychoses. Thereafter, diagnosis in schizophrenia has been progressively refined. DSM-IV (American Psychiatric Association 1994) now clearly identifies the well-accepted diagnostic criteria for the illness.

It has become apparent that the characteristic symptoms of schizophrenia cluster together within subjects and across time (Table 33–1) (Lenzenweger et al. 1991). Cluster analyses of large cohorts of treated stable patients demonstrate that positive symptoms,

TABLE 33–1. Treatment targets in schizophrenia spectrum disorders

Symptom/ sign complex	Diagnostic group	Clinical significance	Treatment
Positive symptoms	Schizophrenia	Acute and distressing Can pose danger because of having lost touch with reality Can need aggressive and restrictive treatment	Partial to full response to typical as well as atypical antipsychotic medications Clozapine superior to traditional drugs in partial responders Atypical antipsychotic drugs can have superior effectiveness because of fewer motor side effects and consequently better compliance
	Spectrum	Can cause interpersonal problems	Some decrease in symptoms with low doses of antipsychotic medications Side effects discourage use of antipsychotic medications other than in select cases
Negative symptoms	Schizophrenia	Cause devastating disability because of lack of drive	Secondary negative symptoms respond better to atypical antipsychotic medications because of fewer motor side effects and better compliance than with typical antipsychotic drugs Deficit (primary and enduring negative) symptoms difficult to treat D-cycloserine and glycine show promise
	Spectrum	Social isolation common Occupational disability in a significant minority of subjects	No available treatments Effective drugs of primary negative symptoms may help
Conceptual disorganization	Schizophrenia	Can result in significant functional impairment	Antipsychotic medications reduce these symptoms to a variable extent, yet residual disorganization is common
	Spectrum	Core symptom marking the phenotype Can cause significant impairment in otherwise healthy subjects	Effects of available antipsychotic medications not adequately researched Anecdotal experience suggests that such treatment results in improved functioning to a marked extent generally not seen in schizophrenia

TABLE 33–1. Treatment targets in schizophrenia spectrum disorders *(continued)*

Cognitive deficits	Schizophrenia	Can significantly contribute to the functional impairment	Some improvement with antipsychotic and anticholinergic drug regimen is seen, although in some patients the treatment may cause or worsen the impairment Research in this area is sorely needed Newer classes of drugs show promise
	Spectrum	Core deficits marking the phenotype Can cause functional impairment	More research is needed
Neurophysiological deficits	Schizophrenia	Findings relatively stable over the course of illness Clinical significance unknown but the deficits likely to mark the enduring symptoms	Generally not affected by treatment of psychosis Can provide a model to test new classes of drugs for the enduring symptoms of schizophrenia
	Spectrum	Core sign marking the phenotype Clinical significance unknown	Can play a role in prevention strategies
Neuroimaging	Schizophrenia	A research tool to study pathophysiology and drug actions	Can provide a model to develop and test new classes of drugs
	Spectrum	As above	As above

negative symptoms, and cognitive dysfunctions run together as predominant symptom domains in persons with the illness (Carpenter and Buchanan 1994; Lenzenweger et al. 1991; Liddle 1990). Persons with schizophrenia may express predominantly at least one cluster, with or without prominent expression of symptoms from other clusters. At present, positive symptoms at least at illness onset are necessary for a diagnosis of schizophrenia. This requirement functions to exclude from the diagnosis and treatment all schizophrenia-like presentations (lacking only positive symptoms) and serves to create a more homogeneous disease class.

Positive Symptoms

Positive symptoms are easily recognized and include hallucinations, delusions, and paranoia. Hallucinations present over a severity continuum from episodic auditory, visual, tactile, or olfactory hallucinations (mild) to frequent hallucinatory experiences (moderate) to constant sensory preoccupation (severe). Illusions and perceptual distortions comprise the subthreshold symptoms experienced by individuals with the nonpsychotic phenotype. Delusions progress from limited paranoid formulations of events (mild) to broad formed delusions (moderate) to those delusions that can demand an action (severe). Ideas of reference and magical thinking are often experienced by individuals with schizotypal disorder. These positive symptoms in schizophrenia are typically characterized by "lack of insight," meaning a complete unawareness on the part of the affected person that the events are not real. This unawareness is perhaps more serious and disabling than the actual hallucination or delusion itself because the affected persons cannot distinguish between reality and their symptoms.

Positive symptoms are characteristically highly responsive to current antipsychotic drugs and show substantial improvement over time with treatment. Reduction in positive symptoms begins early after treatment is initiated, often directly after initial dosing, but may take 4–12 weeks to manifest full optimal response (Baldessarini et al. 1990; Beasley et al. 1996; Simpson et al. 1999). Clozapine shows superior efficacy on psychotic symptoms, often targeting those symptoms, which are otherwise unresponsive to conventional antipsychotic drugs in a significant group of patients (Kane et al. 1988; Rosenheck et al. 1997). The new antipsychotic agents in general have superior overall effectiveness in treating schizophrenia because of low rates of motor side effects and consequently better compliance and adequate dosing (Tamminga 1998).

Response of psychotic-like symptoms in schizophrenia spectrum persons to antipsychotic drug treatment has not been extensively studied because of the episodic and infrequent nature of the symptoms. The mild severity of their symptoms, the difficulties in distinguishing them from cultural norms, and the lack of interference in the individuals' function make these symptoms, in general, poor targets for clinical drug treatment or research trials. However, spectrum individuals have been identified whose work function is impaired by their symptoms. Here data from the few existing controlled studies suggest that symptoms decrease in severity with the antipsychotic drug therapy.

Negative Symptoms

Negative symptoms include lack of pleasure from social interactions and physical activity, resulting in isolation and withdrawal, restricted affect, and reduced drive and motivation. These "negative" manifestations of illness are associated with poor social and vocational adjustment in the community and, as such, powerfully restrict full rehabilitation and social reintegration of the affected persons. Adding a confusing element to the picture, negative symptoms can be caused by antipsychotic drugs themselves and hence are side effects of the traditional and to a lesser degree, if at all, the new antipsychotic treatments. Traditional antipsychotic treatments produce restricted facial expression, reduced emotional range, motor slowing associated with parkinsonism, and often sedation, thus causing secondary negative symptoms. Similarly, negative symptoms (e.g., social isolation as a result of paranoid thoughts) can occur as a result of psychosis. Determining the extent of primary negative symptoms, those that are independent of drug treatment, acute psychotic state, depression, or institutionalization, can be difficult. Evidence for the endurance of these negative symptoms over time, manifest across acute episodes and residual periods, is necessary for the diagnosis of primary and enduring negative symptoms, that is, deficit symptoms (Carpenter et al. 1988).

Specific treatments are not currently available for primary negative symptoms. Although conventional and new antipsychotic drugs diminish negative symptoms during acute episodes, this diminution may be secondary to the reduction of the acute psychosis. Some studies suggest that the newer antipsychotic drugs such as clozapine, risperidone, olanzapine, and the sulpiride derivative amisulpride might be superior to the conventional antipsychotic agents in treating negative symptoms (Danion et al. 1999; Ho et al. 1999; Pickar et al. 1992). However, it is likely that the overall superior effectiveness of the new antipsychotic drugs in treating psychotic symptoms, because of fewer motor side effects and better compliance, results in greater reductions in secondary negative symptoms compared with the conventional antipsychotic drugs. Verification of a treatment for primary negative symptoms will involve focusing on the primary negative symptoms over a treatment trial and documenting selective improvement. In such a longitudinal design, clozapine was found to be ineffective in treating the deficit symptoms (Buchanan et al. 1998). Recent trials using a similar study design have reported positive preliminary findings with glutamatergic agonists such as D-cycloserine or glycine (Goff et al. 1999; Heresco-Levy et al. 1999).

Primary negative symptoms are not limited to schizophrenia and are common in spectrum disorders; thus, an effective treatment of these symptoms is likely to benefit a broad range of people affected by the schizophrenia phenotype. Negative symptom treatments are likely to improve many of the functional disabilities experienced by a large number of individuals with schizophrenia and spectrum disorders (Green 1996).

Conceptual Disorganization

Conceptual disorganization in acute schizophrenia includes disorganized thought and behavior. Mild manifestations of this domain include concrete thinking and odd behavior (mild) and tangential speech (moderate); loose associations can be moderate or severe based on their pervasiveness. Word salad is the most severe presentation of thought disorder. Often these symptoms of conceptual disorganization are responsive to the typical and new antipsychotic drugs. But residual abnormalities are common even with optimal treatment and contribute significantly to the enduring disability associated with the illness. Conceptual disorganization as measured by communication deviancy is thought to be one of the core symptoms of schizophrenia associated with genetic vulnerability (Docherty et al. 1993). Mild conceptual disorganization is common in spectrum disorders, in which it is modestly associated with occupational dysfunction. Thus these symptoms make an attractive target for the development of drug treatments. Effective treatments for conceptual disorganization are likely to go a long way in alleviating the chronic disability associated with the schizophrenia diagnosis or phenotype. The extent to which the new antipsychotic drugs will improve this symptom domain remains to be clarified but appears promising.

Neuropsychological Deficits: Associated Symptoms and Response to Treatment

As a group, individuals with schizophrenia perform more poorly on most neuropsychological tests than do psychiatrically healthy individuals. This poor performance is likely partly the result of symptoms of schizophrenia (e.g., poor motivation or distraction resulting from psychotic symptoms). In addition, early onset of the illness and chronic institutionalization contribute to the generalized deficits in these patients (Chapman and Chapman 1973).

To identify the specific neurocognitive deficits associated with schizophrenia, it is important to examine the differential deficits associated with the illness (Chapman and Chapman 1973). A generalized neurocognitive deficit equally affects a person's performance in all tests; thus, measures that show selective excessive impairment in testing when applied in schizophrenia are more likely to be associated with the pathophysiology of schizophrenia. Within this context, abnormalities in abstraction, problem solving, and other "executive" functions have been particularly noted in individuals with schizophrenia (Goldberg et al. 1987). Similarly, persons with schizophrenia consistently perform poorly on tasks that require sustained attention or vigilance (Nuechterlein et al. 1992). Many studies document deficits in other types of memory, including explicit memory and verbal memory (Gold et al. 1994; Saykin et al. 1991). Working memory has received much attention in the schizophrenia literature. Working memory can be thought of as a mental notepad in which information is kept "on-line" for brief time periods as long as the information is relevant to the task being performed. Individuals with schizophrenia have difficulties maintaining working memory (Goldman-Rakic 1994). Because the ability to hold information on-line is critical for organizing future thoughts and actions in the context of the recent past, deficit in working memory can explain disorganization and functional deterioration observed in persons with the schizophrenia spectrum (Goldman-Rakic 1994).

A number of studies have shown that subjects with schizophrenia spectrum disorders and some of their unaffected first-degree relatives demonstrate many of the cognitive deficits observed in schizophrenia without any psychosis (Asarnow et al. 1991; Balogh and Merritt 1985; Braff 1981; Cornblatt et al. 1989; Green et al. 1997; Nuechterlein 1983; Park et al. 1995). These deficits include impairments in different dimensions of attention, language comprehension, verbal fluency, verbal memory, and spatial working memory. This pattern of findings has been documented by Cannon et al. (1994) and Faraone et al. (1995) in two comprehensive studies of relatives of patients with schizophrenia. Faraone et al. documented a somewhat lesser degree of global impairment than that seen by Cannon et al., and after adjusting for IQ, only measures of auditory attention, abstraction, and verbal memory differentiated relatives with schizophrenia from control subjects (Cannon et al. 1994; Faraone et al. 1995).

Current available drug treatments only marginally improve cognitive dysfunction in schizophrenia itself. Considerable study is currently under way to document the extent and target of cognitive improvement with the antipsychotic agents. Cognitive dysfunction is an important target for development of drug treatments because these symptoms are likely to be responsible for the enduring dysfunction found associated with schizophrenia (Green 1996). Many subjects with schizophrenia spectrum disorders and many first-degree relatives of schizophrenia probands show similar kinds of cognitive dysfunction. An effective drug treatment would be valuable in improving mental function in this broad group of individuals. Preliminary studies in which antipsychotic medications are administered to relatives of persons with schizophrenia have shown modest improvements in cognitive function over time (Tsuang et al. 1999). However, ethical and clinical issues need to be clarified before initiating extended research and clinical application of drug treatment in persons with schizophrenia spectrum disorders.

Neurophysiological Deficits: Associated Symptoms and Response to Treatment

In contrast to the neuropsychological studies, neurophysiological studies have identified abnormalities in information processing that can often be elicited in the absence of a behavioral response. Many studies have used signal averaging of electroencephalographic changes time-locked to sensory or cognitive events and evoked potential. Such event-related potentials have several time-bound segments that facilitate the examination of distinct aspects of information processing. One of the components is a reliable positive change in potential occurring around 300 msec after a task-relevant stimulus or an unexpected stimulus. This response is generally referred to as P300 evoked potential. It shows an increased latency and decreased amplitude in persons with schizophrenia. Although these electroencephalographic measures vary slightly with changes in symptoms, the P300 amplitude is small even in patients with schizophrenia in relative remission (Blackwood et al. 1991; Pfefferbaum et al. 1984). Other components of evoked potential are observed to be abnormal in schizophrenia. Mismatch negativity response occurring earlier than P300 is observed to have smaller amplitude in schizophrenia, suggesting an abnormality in the early response to stimulus novelty (Javitt et al. 1995).

Although several studies report significant correlations between abnormalities in information processing and clinical symptoms, it is unclear what, if any, role the information-processing deficits play in the development of clinical symptoms of schizophrenia. However, it is likely that information-processing abnormalities mark the more subtle but enduring features of the illness that tend to produce poor functional outcome rather than overt psychotic symptoms. As such, treatments for information-processing deficits might bring substantial improvements in schizophrenia outcome.

Neurophysiological paradigms that examine sensory gating provide a theoretical framework for understanding the development of the core symptoms of schizophrenia. Braff and others have proposed that schizophrenia is associated with an inability to gate sensory information, leading to sensory overload (Braff 1993; Freedman 1998). According to this hypothesis, positive symptoms develop as a result of misinterpretation or misidentification of unfiltered sensory information. Negative symptoms may occur as a result of the withdrawal from the sensory overload. Measures of sensory gating are obtained by examining a process called pre-pulse inhibition. In this test, a person's ability to inhibit a startle response to a strong sensory stimulus in the presence of a preceding weak pre-pulse stimulus is evaluated. In contrast to a comparison group of psychiatrically healthy individuals, persons with schizophrenia show poor pre-pulse inhibition.

Another test of sensory gating uses positive change in the evoked potentials 50 msec (P50) after each of the two auditory stimuli presented about 500 msec apart (Freedman 1998). Psychiatrically healthy subjects show a reduced evoked potential response to the second stimulus compared with that to the first stimulus. In contrast, the second P50 evoked potential response in schizophrenia is of similar amplitude as that to the first stimulus. This suggests that individuals with schizophrenia lack the normal ability to screen out redundant incoming sensory information. Interestingly, P50 gating is noted to be abnormal in a proportion of relatives of persons with schizophrenia, which suggests that the subtle neurophysiological deficit may be marking the genetic liability (Freedman et al. 1997).

Abnormality of smooth-pursuit eye movements is another neurophysiological deficit consistently observed in patients with schizophrenia as well as in a proportion of their first-degree relatives (Holzman et al. 1984; Thaker et al. 1996). Normally, humans are able to capture an image of a moving object onto the fovea, the most sensitive region of the retina, and approximately maintain the moving image on the fovea by generating smooth predictive eye movements that match the target velocity (Barnes and Asselman 1991). Recent data suggest that patients with schizophrenia and their first-degree relatives have difficulty maintaining an internal representation of the target velocity information and/or integrating this information into a predictive smooth-pursuit response (Thaker et al. 1998, 1999).

These neurophysiological deficits may provide an important framework for the development of new treatments for schizophrenia for several reasons:

- The abnormalities in these measures persist during psychotic symptom remission and are noted in a proportion of nonill relatives. This suggests that the dysfunctions can represent a fundamental abnormality associated with the schizophrenia phenotype and can occur in closer proximity to the genetic effects than positive psychotic symptoms.
- These deficits may mark functional impairments that are more enduring and perhaps more severe than the psychotic symptoms associated with the diagnosis of schizophrenia. Thus, treatments that target fundamental neurophysiological deficits can have a much larger impact on reversing the chronicity and disability associated with schizophrenia.
- In contrast to positive psychotic symptoms, many of the neurophysiological deficits can be modeled in animals, thus providing an opportunity to systematically develop and test novel treatments. Such attempts to develop novel treatments will obviously be helped by identification of schizophrenia genes.

Existing treatments of schizophrenia have generally been unsuccessful in treating neurophysiological and cognitive deficits in schizophrenia. In spite of some reports of effectiveness of the new antipsychotic agents in ameliorating some cognitive deficits, the bulk of the available data is not encouraging. Based on the possible role of nicotinic receptors in the P50 deficit, Freedman et al. (1997) tested effects of nicotine agonist on P50 and smooth-pursuit eye movement measures. Normalization of both neurophysiological deficits were noted in patients and their family members (Adler et al. 1992, 1993; Sherr et al. 1999).

Regional Cerebral Blood Flow/Metabolism Abnormalities: Associated Symptoms and Response to Treatment

We and others (Gur et al. 1995; Holcomb et al. 1996b; Liddle et al. 1992; Silbersweig et al. 1995; Wolkin et al. 1985) have been able to characterize abnormal regional cerebral metabolic patterns that accompany definable symptomatic states in schizophrenia. These patterns of cerebral dysfunction highlight those regions of schizophrenic brain in vivo that function abnormally by this quantifiable measure. Some studies have used correlational techniques between symptom measures states and regional cerebral blood flow (rCBF) to define brain regions most strongly associated with symptom states, for example, positive, negative, or cognitive symptoms (Liddle et al. 1992). Other studies have relied on a dichotomous subject technique, for example, doing functional brain imaging on psychotic versus nonpsychotic individuals or on individuals with primary negative versus nonnegative symptoms of schizophrenia (Holcomb et al. 1996a; Lahti et al. 1998). Both of these approaches have found reasonably coincident results, which suggest a localization of regional dysfunction with positive symptoms within limbic cortex and of negative symptoms within middle frontal and inferior parietal neocortex. This localization of dysfunction suggests either that these areas are merely used for the expressions of the symptoms or, possibly, that dysfunction in the area is generating the symptom. These kinds of functional data overall suggest that the central nervous system (CNS) abnormality in schizophrenia resides in distributed neural systems and that the different distributed systems involved determine the expressed symptoms. Specifically, studies from our laboratory show that an abnormal pattern of glucose metabolism involving the limbic cortex, especially the hippocampus and anterior cingulate region, is associated with positive symptoms in schizophrenia (Figure 33–1). Neuronal activation is reduced in these regions in schizophrenia at rest (Tamminga et al. 1992) and responds abnormally to task activation with mental activity (Holcomb et al. 1999). Furthermore, the degree of metabolic abnormality in the areas of the limbic cortex correlates with the magnitude of positive symptoms (Tamminga 1997). In contrast, primary negative symptoms are associated with middle frontal and inferior parietal cortex dysfunctions (Figure 33–2). Reductions in neuronal activity at rest and with task activation in these areas characterize the patterns of cerebral blood flow of schizophrenic persons with primary negative symptoms.

Schizophrenic persons with both positive and negative symptom profiles have both kinds of functional imaging abnormalities, whereas persons with positive-symptom-only schizophrenia tend to show only limbic cortex changes. Regional CBF markers for cognitive dysfunction are currently being sought but seem not as distinctly delineated. Whether these areas of cerebral abnormality represent the same or different regional tissue pathologies is unknown but being explored. It is tempting to turn to these specific cerebral areas to find the pathophysiology of these symptom domains in schizophrenia.

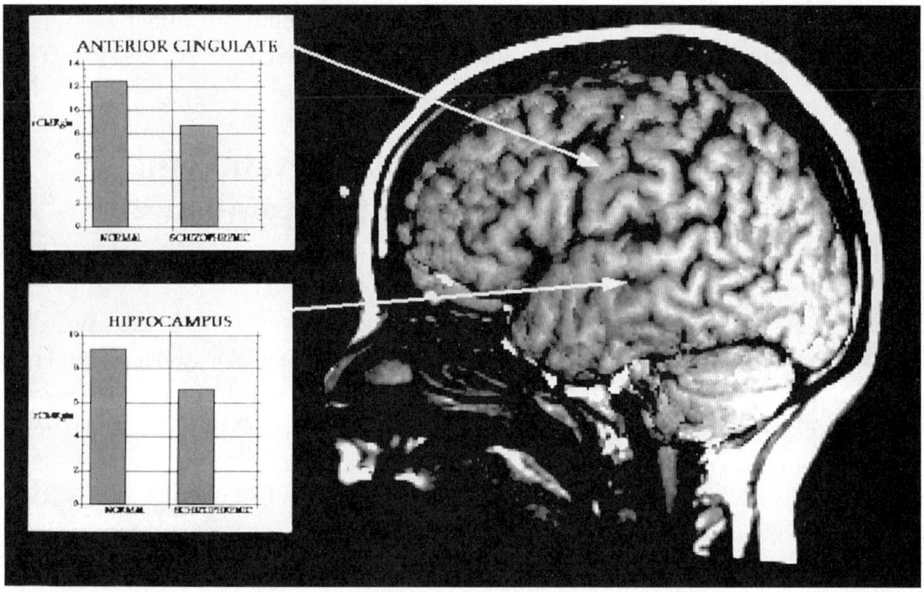

FIGURE 33–1. Magnetic resonance imaging view of the lateral brain surface. *Arrows* point to the regions where the anterior cingulate cortex (*top graph*) and the hippocampus (*bottom graph*) are located on the medial surface. The graphs show the levels of glucose utilization in the anterior cingulate cortex (*top*) and hippocampal cortex (*bottom*) in psychiatrically healthy (*N* = 12) and schizophrenic (*N* = 12) volunteers who are at rest and free of centrally active drugs. Metabolism in the volunteers with schizophrenia is reduced in both regions. Only these two regions showed significant differences between the two groups. rCMRglu = regional cerebral metabolic rate of glucose.

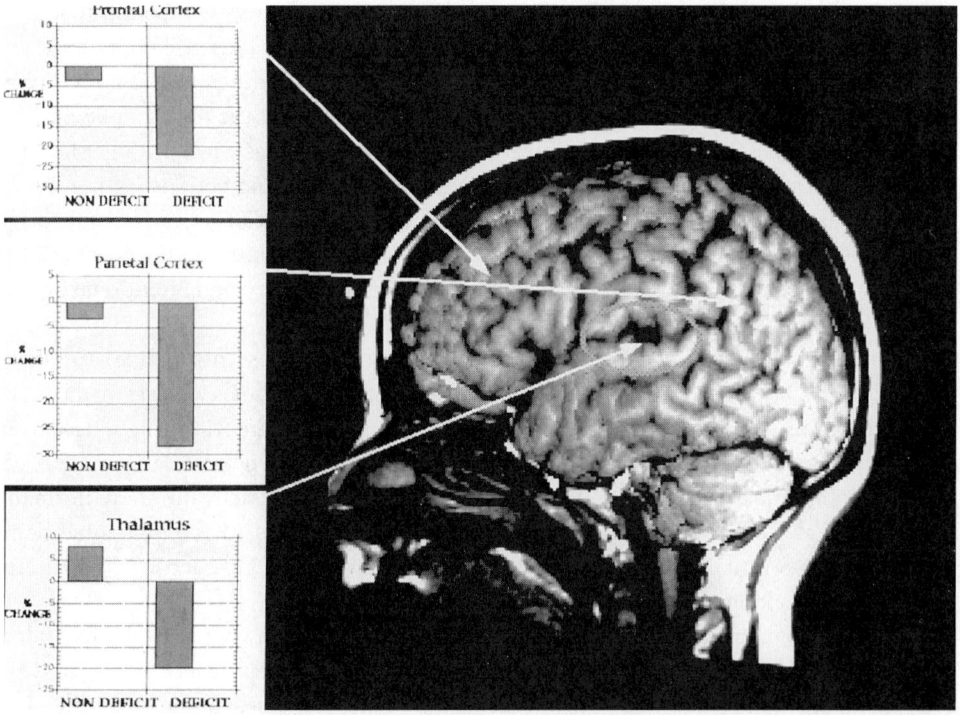

FIGURE 33–2. Magnetic resonance imaging view of the lateral brain surface. *Arrows* point to the frontal cortex (*top graph*), parietal cortex (*middle graph*), and the thalamus projection (*lower graph*). The graphs show the percentage change in glucose utilization in the schizophrenic volunteers with deficit ($N = 5$) and those with no deficit ($N = 7$) who were included in the experiment illustrated in Figure 33–1. Only the group of schizophrenic patients with deficit symptoms showed reduced glucose utilization in the frontal and parietal cortex and in the thalamus. Schizophrenic patients with no deficit showed glucose utilization in these regions similar to that of the psychiatrically healthy group.

Administration of antipsychotic drugs to persons with schizophrenia alters their patterns of induced cerebral metabolism in ways that are informative about the drugs' mechanism of action. Haloperidol is the best characterized of the conventional antipsychotics; it is predominantly a dopamine type 2 receptor antagonist at the doses used in schizophrenia. A dose of 10 mg haloperidol orally produces the following functional changes in cerebral metabolism/rCBF: 1) an increase in cerebral metabolism or rCBF in the caudate and putamen, 2) a similar functional increase in activation in the anterior thalamus, 3) a decrease in metabolism or rCBF in the anterior cingulate cortex, and 4) a decrease in metabolism or rCBF in the middle frontal cortex. This pattern of functional change in regional neural activity suggests that haloperidol may be having its primary action in the caudate putamen at the dopamine type 2 receptors and that this action is being transmitted through the already established basal ganglia–thalamocortical neural pathways through the thalamus to the anterior cingulate and the middle frontal cortex (Holcomb et al. 1996b). The regions affected by haloperidol are some of the same regions where schizophrenic symptoms themselves appear to be mediated, for example, the anterior cingulate and the middle frontal cortex. The temporal extent of haloperidol actions in these regions has a duration of 8–16 hours, consistent with the drug's half-life.

In preliminary study, olanzapine has demonstrated several contrasting functional actions consistent with its animal pharmacology (Bymaster et al. 1999) and clinical actions (Tollefson et al. 1997). Olanzapine appears to increase rather than decrease rCBF in the anterior cingulate cortex and the middle frontal cortex. These findings, albeit preliminary, suggest that this new antipsychotic, despite its standard action at the dopamine type 2 receptor, can have parallel additional clinical actions. Olanzapine has a much longer half-life than does haloperidol, and it produces metabolic in vivo imaging actions lasting 20–25 hours. The fact that olanzapine increases rather than decreases rCBF in the frontal cortex could underlie differences in therapeutic activity between olanzapine and the conventional antipsychotics such as haloperidol, especially on working memory and attentional abnormalities in schizophrenia.

Moreover, antipsychotic drugs alter and can in some cases "normalize" the task-induced rCBF CNS activation patterns. When schizophrenic individuals who are medication-free perform an auditory recognition task, they activate their anterior cingulate cortex poorly compared with psychiatrically healthy volunteers. But when those same individuals with schizophrenia are medicated, their anterior cingulate cortex activates more normally (Holcomb et al. 1999). This finding suggests the possibility that in vivo functional brain imaging might eventually substitute as a surrogate measure of drug response and be useful in new drug development for schizophrenia.

In vivo human brain imaging has provided psychiatric research with critical direct information about brain function in schizophrenia and its response to treatments. Patterns of rCBF in schizophrenia can be informative about the nature of the CNS defect in the illness and, furthermore, need to be developed as surrogate markers and/or targets of treatment. Already the patterns and changes in rCBF produced by antipsychotic medications are being characterized to provide surrogate markers of drug action. Subjects can be imaged either at rest or performing cognitive and/or motor tasks, depending on the questions asked, to characterize schizophrenia abnormalities and their response to treatment. These techniques have been applied in schizophrenia research in many different laboratories since 1974 (Buchsbaum et al. 1982; Holcomb et al. 1996a; Ingvar and Franzen 1974; Weinberger et al. 1986) and their results reviewed at regular intervals (Holcomb 1999; Holcomb et al. 1989).

Functional brain imaging studies performed at our institutions have used both fluorodeoxyglucose with positron emission tomography (PET) (to measure glucose utilization) and ^{15}O water with PET (to measure rCBF) to identify brain region of abnormal function in schizophrenia and to differentiate the abnormalities related to the illness from those rCBF changes induced by antipsychotic medication. Other brain imaging techniques, primarily receptor occupancy assessment, have been important, even critical, in development of drugs for CNS diseases. These imaging techniques, however, require knowledge of the proper receptor target, which is not always known in exploratory studies in schizophrenia. Functional brain imaging can identify both the region of altered rCBF activation patterns and additional performance abnormalities of the region in the illness. Additionally, effects of known therapeutic drugs can be assessed.

Schizophrenia Phenotype: Treatment of Functional Deficits

The functional significance of the neuropsychological and neurophysiological dysfunction observed in a proportion of relatives of patients with schizophrenia remains unclear. Meehl

(1962) named these subtle neurophysiological deficits associated with schizophrenia "schizotaxia" and argued that such physiological abnormalities would lead to cognitive slippage and result in subtle mental symptoms. Such mild symptoms could be coincident with those defined by DSM as schizophrenia spectrum personality disorders. Although some of the neurophysiological and cognitive deficits occur in relatives who do not meet the criteria for DSM-IV schizophrenia spectrum personality disorders, the smooth-pursuit abnormality is more prevalent in relatives who either meet the criteria or have subthreshold symptoms. Functional brain imaging is being applied in these studies to complement current techniques. The presence of unusual personality styles in themselves has little practical or clinical significance. Early studies have noted social isolation, poor occupational outcome, brief psychiatric hospitalizations, and suicide attempts in schizotypal patients (Stone 1993). However, these studies were conducted in patient samples, not nonpatient family groups. Here schizotypal patients had severe symptoms, many patients were recruited from inpatient settings, and the presence of DSM-III (American Psychiatric Association 1980) Axis I comorbidity was common.

More recently, investigators have noted that 25% of relatives who experience at least subthreshold schizophrenia spectrum personality disorder symptoms have poor occupational outcome (Thaker et al., in press). Treatment strategies based on the reversal of neurophysiological deficits may have a role in improving function in these psychotic and nonpsychotic affected subjects. Investigators have used low doses of traditional antipsychotic treatments and demonstrated a decrease in schizotypal symptoms in nonpsychotic subjects. The question remains whether such treatments will have any effect on the cognitive and functional deficits in this nonpsychotic group, particularly when antipsychotic drug treatments in schizophrenia have proven disappointing for reducing such deficits.

References

Adler LE, Hoffer LJ, Griffith J, et al: Normalization by nicotine of deficient auditory sensory gating in the relatives of schizophrenics. Biol Psychiatry 32:607–616, 1992

Adler LE, Hoffer LD, Wiser A, et al: Normalization of auditory physiology by cigarette smoking in schizophrenic patients. Am J Psychiatry 150:1856–1861, 1993

American Psychiatric Association: Diagnostic and Statistical Manual of Mental Disorders, 3rd Edition. Washington, DC, American Psychiatric Association, 1980

American Psychiatric Association: Diagnostic and Statistical Manual of Mental Disorders, 4th Edition. Washington, DC, American Psychiatric Association, 1994

Asarnow RF, Granholm E, Sherman T: Span of apprehension in schizophrenia, in Handbook of Schizophrenia: Neuropsychology, Psychophysiology, and Information Processing. Edited by Steinhauer SR, Gruzelier JH, Zubin J. Amsterdam, Elsevier, 1991, pp 335–370

Baldessarini RJ, Cohen BM, Teicher MH: Pharmacological treatment, in Schizophrenia: Treatment of Acute Psychotic Episodes. Edited by Levy ST, Ninan PT. Washington, DC, American Psychiatric Press, 1990, pp 61–118

Balogh DW, Merritt RD: Susceptibility to type A backward pattern masking among hypothetically psychosis-prone college students. J Abnorm Psychol 94:377–383, 1985

Barnes GR, Asselman PT: The mechanism of prediction in human smooth pursuit eye movements. J Physiol (Lond) 439:439–461, 1991

Beasley CM Jr, Sanger T, Satterlee W, et al: Olanzapine versus placebo: results of a double-blind, fixed-dose olanzapine trial. Psychopharmacology (Berl) 124:159–167, 1996

Blackwood DH, St. Clair DM, Muir WJ, et al: Auditory P300 and eye tracking dysfunction in schizophrenic pedigrees. Arch Gen Psychiatry 48:899–909, 1991

Bleuler M: Dementia Praecox or the Group of Schizophrenias. New York, International Universities Press, 1950

Bleuler M: The Schizophrenic Disorders: Long-Term Patient and Family Studies. New Haven, CT, Yale University Press, 1978

Braff DL: Impaired speed of information processing in nonmedicated schizotypal patients. Schizophr Bull 7:499–508, 1981

Braff DL: Information processing and attention dysfunctions in schizophrenia. Schizophr Bull 19:233–259, 1993

Buchanan RW, Breier A, Kirkpatrick B, et al: Positive and negative symptom response to clozapine in schizophrenic patients with and without the deficit syndrome. Am J Psychiatry 155:751–760, 1998

Buchsbaum MS, Ingvar DH, Kessler R, et al: Cerebral glucography with positron tomography. Arch Gen Psychiatry 39:251–259, 1982

Bymaster F, Perry KW, Nelson DL, et al: Olanzapine: a basic science update. Br J Psychiatry 174:36–40, 1999

Cannon TD, Mednick SA, Parnas J, et al: Developmental brain abnormalities in the offspring of schizophrenic mothers, II: structural brain characteristics of schizophrenia and schizotypal personality disorder. Arch Gen Psychiatry 51:955–962, 1994

Carpenter WT Jr, Buchanan RW: Schizophrenia. N Engl J Med 330:681–690, 1994

Carpenter WT Jr, Heinrichs DW, Wagman AM: Deficit and nondeficit forms of schizophrenia: the concept. Am J Psychiatry 145:578–583, 1988

Chapman LJ, Chapman JP: Problems in the measurement of cognitive deficit. Psychol Bull 79:380–385, 1973

Ciompi L, Muller C: Lifestyle and age of schizophrenics: a catamnestic long-term study into old age (in German). Monographien aus dem Gesamtgebiete der Psychiatrie Psychiatry Series 1:1–242, 1976

Cornblatt BA, Winters L, Erlenmeyer-Kimling L: Attentional markers of schizophrenia: evidence from the New York high risk study, in Schizophrenia: Scientific Progress. Edited by Schultz SC, Tamminga CA. New York, Oxford University Press, 1989, pp 83–92

Danion JM, Rein W, Fleurot O: Improvement of schizophrenic patients with primary negative symptoms treated with amisulpride. Amisulpride Study Group. Am J Psychiatry 156:610–616, 1999

Docherty NM, Hawkins KA, Hoffman RE, et al: Working memory, attention, and communication disturbances in schizophrenia DSM-III-R personality disorders in parents of schizophrenic patients. J Abnorm Psychol 48:60–62, 1993

Faraone SV, Seidman LJ, Kremen WS, et al: Neuropsychological functioning among the nonpsychotic relatives of schizophrenic patients: a diagnostic efficiency analysis. J Abnorm Psychol 104:286–304, 1995

Freedman R: Biological phenotypes in the genetics of schizophrenia. Biol Psychiatry 44:939–940, 1998

Freedman R, Coon H, Myles-Worsley M, et al: Linkage of a neurophysiological deficit in schizophrenia to a chromosome 15 locus. Proc Natl Acad Sci U S A 94:587–592, 1997

Goff DC, Henderson DC, Evins AE, et al: A placebo-controlled crossover trial of D-cycloserine added to clozapine in patients with schizophrenia. Biol Psychiatry 45:512–514, 1999

Gold JM, Hermann BP, Randolph C, et al: Schizophrenia and temporal lobe epilepsy: a neuropsychological analysis. Arch Gen Psychiatry 51:265–272, 1994

Goldberg SC, Schulz SC, Schulz PM, et al: Borderline and schizotypal personality disorders treated with low-dose thiothixene vs placebo. Arch Gen Psychiatry 43:680–686, 1986

Goldberg TE, Weinberger DR, Berman KF, et al: Further evidence for dementia of the prefrontal type in schizophrenia? A controlled study of teaching the Wisconsin Card Sorting Test. Arch Gen Psychiatry 44:1008–1014, 1987

Goldman-Rakic PS: Working memory dysfunction in schizophrenia. J Neuropsychiatry Clin Neurosci 6:348–357, 1994

Gottesman II, Shields J: Schizophrenia: The Epigenetic Puzzle. New York, Cambridge University Press, 1982

Green MF: What are the functional consequences of neurocognitive deficits in schizophrenia? Am J Psychiatry 153:321–330, 1996

Green MF, Nuechterlein KH, Breitmeyer B: Backward masking performance in unaffected siblings of schizophrenic patients: evidence for a vulnerability indicator. Arch Gen Psychiatry 54:465–472, 1997 (Published erratum appears in Arch Gen Psychiatry 54:846, 1997)

Gur RE, Mozley PD, Resnick SM, et al: Resting cerebral glucose metabolism in first-episode and previously treated patients with schizophrenia relates to clinical features. Arch Gen Psychiatry 52:657–667, 1995

Heresco-Levy U, Javitt DC, Ermilov M, et al: Efficacy of high-dose glycine in the treatment of enduring negative symptoms of schizophrenia (see comments). Arch Gen Psychiatry 56:29–36, 1999

Ho BC, Miller D, Nopoulos P, et al: A comparative effectiveness study of risperidone and olanzapine in the treatment of schizophrenia. J Clin Psychiatry 60:658–663, 1999

Holcomb HH: Images in neuroscience. Cognition. Perception, I. Am J Psychiatry 156:674, 1999

Holcomb HH, Links JM, Smith C, et al: Positron emission tomography: measuring the metabolic and neurochemical characteristics of the living human nervous system, in Brain Imaging Applications in Psychiatry. Edited by Andreasen NC. Washington, DC, American Psychiatric Press, 1989, pp 235–370

Holcomb HH, Cascella NG, Thaker GK, et al: Functional sites of neuroleptic drug action in the human brain: PET/FDG studies with and without haloperidol. Am J Psychiatry 153:41–49, 1996a

Holcomb HH, Gordon B, Loats HL, et al: Brain metabolism patterns are sensitive to attentional effort associated with a tone recognition task. Biol Psychiatry 39:1013–1022, 1996b

Holcomb HH, Lahti AC, Weiler M, et al: Neuroleptic treatment of schizophrenic patients: how do haloperidol and clozapine normalize brain blood flow patterns associated with a difficult tone recognition task? In Search for the Causes of Schizophrenia, Vol 4: Balance of the Century. Edited by Gattaz WF, Häfner H. Darmstadt, Germany, Steinkopff Verlag, 1999, pp 355–365

Holzman PS, Solomon CM, Levin S, et al: Pursuit eye movement dysfunctions in schizophrenia. Family evidence for specificity. Arch Gen Psychiatry 41:136–139, 1984

Ingvar DH, Franzen G: Abnormalities of cerebral blood flow distribution in patients with chronic schizophrenia. Acta Psychiatr Scand 50:425–462, 1974

Javitt DC, Doneshka P, Grochowski S, et al: Impaired mismatch negativity generation reflects widespread dysfunction of working memory in schizophrenia. Arch Gen Psychiatry 52:550–558, 1995

Kane J, Honigfeld G, Singer J, et al: Clozapine for the treatment-resistant schizophrenic: a double-blind comparison with chlorpromazine. Arch Gen Psychiatry 45:789–796, 1988

Kendler KS, Diehl SR: The genetics of schizophrenia: a current, genetic-epidemiologic perspective. Schizophr Bull 19:261–285, 1993

Kendler KS, McGuire M, Gruenberg AM, et al: The Roscommon Family Study, III: schizophrenia-related personality disorders in relatives. Arch Gen Psychiatry 50:781–788, 1993

Kety SS, Rosenthal D, Wender PH, et al: Mental illness in the biological and adoptive families of adopted individuals who have become schizophrenic. Behav Genet 6:219–225, 1976

Klein DF, Davis JM: Diagnosis and Drug Treatment of Psychiatric Disorders. Baltimore, MD, Williams & Wilkins, 1969

Lahti AC, Holcomb HH, Weiler MA, et al: Time course of rCBF changes after acute haloperidol in patients with schizophrenia (abstract). Schizophr Res 29:173, 1998

Lenzenweger MF, Dworkin RH, Wethington E: Examining the underlying structure of schizophrenic phenomenology: evidence for a three-process model. Schizophr Bull 17:515–524, 1991

Liddle PF: Syndromes of chronic schizophrenia. Br J Psychiatry 157:558–561, 1990

Liddle PF, Friston KJ, Frith CD, et al: Patterns of cerebral blood flow in schizophrenia. Br J Psychiatry 160:179–186, 1992

Meehl PE: Schizotaxia, schizotypy and schizophrenia. Am Psychol 17:827–838, 1962

Nuechterlein KH: Signal detection in vigilance tasks and behavioral attributes among offspring of schizophrenic mothers and among hyperactive children. J Abnorm Psychol 92:4–28, 1983

Nuechterlein KH, Dawson ME, Gitlin M, et al: Developmental processes in schizophrenic disorders: longitudinal studies of vulnerability and stress. Schizophr Bull 18:387–425, 1992

Park S, Holzman PS, Goldman-Rakic PS: Spatial working memory deficits in the relatives of schizophrenic patients. Arch Gen Psychiatry 52:821–828, 1995

Pfefferbaum A, Wenegrat BG, Ford JM, et al: Clinical application of the P3 component of event-related potentials, II: dementia, depression and schizophrenia. Electroencephalogr Clin Neurophysiol 59:104–124, 1984

Pickar D, Owen RR, Litman RE, et al: Clinical and biologic response to clozapine in patients with schizophrenia. Crossover comparison with fluphenazine. Arch Gen Psychiatry 49:345–353, 1992

Rosenheck R, Cramer J, Xu W, et al: A comparison of clozapine and haloperidol in hospitalized patients with refractory schizophrenia. Department of Veterans Affairs Cooperative Study Group on Clozapine in Refractory Schizophrenia. N Engl J Med 337:809–815, 1997

Saykin AJ, Gur RC, Gur RE, et al: Neuropsychological function in schizophrenia. Selective impairment in memory and learning. Arch Gen Psychiatry 48:618–624, 1991

Schneider K: Clinical Psychopathology. New York, Grune & Stratton, 1959

Sherr JD, Blaxton TA, Thaker GK: Nicotine nasal spray effects of specific components of smooth pursuit eye movements in schizophrenia (abstract). Society of Neuroscience Abstracts 658, 1999

Siever LJ, Gunderson JG: The search for a schizotypal personality: historical origins and current status. Compr Psychiatry 24:199–212, 1983

Silbersweig DA, Stern E, Frith C, et al: A functional neuroanatomy of hallucinations in schizophrenia. Nature 378:176–179, 1995

Simpson GM, Josiassen RC, Stanilla JK, et al: Double-blind study of clozapine dose response in chronic schizophrenia. Am J Psychiatry 156:1744–1750, 1999

Stone MH: Long-term outcome in personality disorders. Br J Psychiatry 162:299–313, 1993

Tamminga CA: Neuropsychiatric aspects of schizophrenia, in The American Psychiatric Press Textbook of Neuropsychiatry, 3rd Edition. Edited by Yudofsky SC, Hales RE. Washington, DC, American Psychiatric Press, 1997, pp 855–882

Tamminga CA: Principles of the pharmacotherapy of schizophrenia, in Neurobiology of Psychiatric Disorders. Edited by Bunney BS. New York, Oxford University Press, 1998, pp 272–285

Tamminga CA, Thaker GK, Buchanan R, et al: Limbic system abnormalities identified in schizophrenia using positron emission tomography with fluorodeoxyglucose and neocortical alterations with deficit syndrome. Arch Gen Psychiatry 49:522–530, 1992

Thaker GK, Cassady S, Adami H, et al: Eye movements in spectrum personality disorders: comparison of community subjects and relatives of schizophrenic patients. Am J Psychiatry 153:362–368, 1996

Thaker GK, Ross DE, Cassady SL, et al: Smooth pursuit eye movements to extraretinal motion signals: deficits in relatives of patients with schizophrenia. Arch Gen Psychiatry 55:830–836, 1998

Thaker GK, Ross DE, Buchanan RW, et al: Smooth pursuit eye movements to extraretinal motion signals: deficits in patients with schizophrenia. Psychiatry Res 88:209–219, 1999

Thaker GK, Adami HM, Gold JM: Functional deterioration in individuals with schizophrenia spectrum personality symptoms. J Personal Disord (in press)

Tollefson GD, Beasley CM Jr, Tran PV, et al: Olanzapine versus haloperidol in the treatment of schizophrenia and schizoaffective and schizophreniform disorders: results of an international collaborative trial. Am J Psychiatry 154:457–465, 1997

Tsuang MT, Stone WS, Seidman SV, et al: Treatment of nonpsychotic relatives of patients with schizophrenia: implications for research on prevention (abstract). Schizophr Res 36:299, 1999

Weinberger DR, Berman KF, Zec RF: Physiologic dysfunction of dorsolateral prefrontal cortex in schizophrenia, I: regional cerebral blood flow evidence. Arch Gen Psychiatry 43:114–124, 1986

Wolkin A, Jaeger J, Brodie JD, et al: Persistence of cerebral metabolic abnormalities in chronic schizophrenia as determined by positron emission tomography. Am J Psychiatry 142:564–571, 1985

34

Clinical Psychopharmacology of Schizophrenia and Psychotic Disorders

John M. Kane, M.D.
Anil K. Malhotra, M.D.

Pharmacological treatment is a critical component in the short- and long-term management of schizophrenia. Until the past decade, the mainstay of pharmacological treatment was the neuroleptic agents (or conventional agents), which provided antipsychotic efficacy with a variety of side effects ranging from the annoying to the potentially irreversible movement disorder tardive dyskinesia. The introduction of clozapine, a drug that provides superior antipsychotic efficacy in patients with treatment-resistant schizophrenia and has a markedly decreased propensity to induce neuromuscular side effects, has dramatically altered long-standing hypotheses of antipsychotic drug efficacy and led to the development of a new generation of antipsychotic medications. Overall, the new-generation antipsychotic drugs do provide clear advantages in terms of reducing adverse effects (particularly drug-induced parkinsonism, akathisia, and, it is hoped, tardive dyskinesia). Advantages in alleviating refractory symptoms, negative symptoms, depression, and suicidal behavior are found in some reports; however, further research is needed to establish the relative merits of specific drugs in regard to these various symptoms.

In this chapter, we review clinical management strategies in the acute treatment of schizophrenia, present data on the new generation of antipsychotic drugs, and discuss the current status of maintenance treatment in schizophrenia.

Acute Treatment

It is useful to consider different phases in treatment approaches to schizophrenia because to some extent the goals and challenges can differ. Acute treatment refers to that phase in which the patient has experienced a relapse or exacerbation of the illness, usually marked by an increase in positive symptoms such as delusions, hallucinations, or agitation. However, a marked increase in negative symptoms such as extreme withdrawal can also be involved. The concept of acute treatment would also apply to someone receiving medication for the first time or after a long period off medication. An episode or exacerbation can occur rapidly or gradually in a patient already receiving antipsychotics or a patient in a medication-free state. In addition, signs and symptoms can vary over time. Unfortunately, many symptoms of schizophrenia are subjective (e.g., hallucinations and delusions), and the ability or willingness of the patient to accurately describe these phenomena can vary over time.

Although many episodes of acute treatment occur in hospital settings, it is likely that with the availability of appropriate resources in the community many episodes could be treated on an outpatient basis. It is possible that with increasing emphasis on cost containment, hospitalization will be reserved for those persons who pose a danger to themselves or to others or who are lacking insight as to the need for treatment.

Once appropriate diagnostic, neuromedical, and psychosocial evaluations have taken place, the essential decisions in the acute treatment phase involve locus of care, choice of drug, drug dosage, and dosage escalation schedule, as well as the possible use of concomitant or adjunctive medication. It is important that the pharmacological treatment plan involve goals of treatment, assessment of efficacy and adverse effects, and alternative strategies if the treatment goals are not met. It is also important, as we will emphasize, to begin to plan for the appropriate maintenance strategy even before the acute treatment phase is over.

Drug Type

Several classes of antipsychotic drugs have been introduced over the past 40 years. The introduction of clozapine in 1990 made available for the first time a compound that had demonstrated some type of superiority over another compound in a large-scale controlled trial. Up until then, it was assumed that antipsychotic drugs were generally interchangeable in terms of efficacy, though they clearly differed in terms of adverse-effect profile. It is possible, however, that differences do exist among drugs, but the necessary methodology (including patient selection) has not been applied to this question. In general, available comparisons have involved group response data in random-assignment and parallel-group designs. These results do not necessarily rule out the possibility that a given person would respond differently to different drugs. Clinicians continue to assume or hope that there will be differences when they switch drugs in nonresponsive patients.

The most useful predictor of drug response is a detailed history of prior drug response. If a patient has responded well to a drug in the past, that would be a good justification for using that drug again with that patient. A history of adverse effects should also be considered when choosing a drug. Many clinicians still believe that highly sedating drugs should be used when patients are agitated or experiencing insomnia. No evidence suggests that high- or low-potency drugs differ in their efficacy in agitated patients and withdrawn and psychomotorically retarded patients.

When considering subsequent maintenance treatment, the clinician should give some thought to whether a long-acting injectable drug should be used. If the decision is made to use such a drug, it can be advantageous to introduce it before the patient is discharged from the hospital, even if only in a small test dose. (Clinical judgment should determine whether an oral test dose is necessary before initiating a depot drug.) Doing so can make the transition much easier. In our view, depot antipsychotic drugs are greatly underutilized. In the United States, haloperidol and fluphenazine are available in decanoate preparations that can be administered at intervals of 2–4 weeks. Many clinicians do not consider using these agents until patients have demonstrated noncompliance. However, because noncompliance is common and difficult to predict (Kane 1985), it would make sense to use these agents before noncompliance develops rather than just after a resulting relapse. (As yet, no long-acting, injectable, second-generation medications exist; therefore, the risks and benefits need to be weighed in a somewhat different context.)

Parenteral Antipsychotics

If patients are too disturbed to take oral medication, antipsychotics can be given intramuscularly. When given by this route, the drug is absorbed more rapidly, producing an effect more rapidly (i.e., within 30 minutes) than when given orally. This more rapid effect can be useful when a patient is severely agitated or violent. In addition, absorption is more rapid and bioavailability is greater with parenteral compared with oral medication. It is usually not necessary to continue intramuscular doses beyond the first several hours, and patients should be switched to oral medication as soon as that is feasible.

Most patients do not require more than one or two injections. At one time it was common to use repeated doses of intramuscularly administered medication to produce rapid tranquilization. However, this approach was associated with an unnecessary degree of adverse effects, and lower doses are just as effective. It is common to administer a relatively high-potency, short-acting benzodiazepine (e.g., lorazepam 1 mg) along with a low dose of a high-potency antipsychotic (e.g., haloperidol) to control acute and severe behavioral disturbances in patients with schizophrenia. It is not necessary to maintain benzodiazepine treatment beyond the very acute phase, because benzodiazepines are not effective antipsychotics by themselves and can produce dependency in some patients. In addition, patients should be observed for the unusual but potential paradoxical disinhibition that can occur with benzodiazepines.

Drug Dosage

Although antipsychotic drugs have been widely used for many years, debate continues about optimal doses (for both acute and maintenance treatment). This issue is important because antipsychotic drugs are associated with a variety of adverse effects that can be subjectively distressing, interfere with psychosocial and vocational adjustment, and contribute to some of the stigmata associated with this disease. In addition, adverse effects such as akathisia and akinesia can be mistaken for or exacerbate restlessness/agitation or negative symptoms, respectively.

In the early stages of antipsychotic drug development, it was evident that a dosage less than 400–600 mg/day of chlorpromazine was much less likely to prove superior to placebo than a dosage above that range (Klein and Davis 1969). Subsequently, considerable interest centered around examining the effects of the highest levels of tolerated doses to see if such doses could bring about either a more rapid or a greater degree of response. A number of studies were done comparing high-dose treatment (defined as greater than 2,000 mg chlorpromazine equivalents) with standard-dose treatment (Donlon et al. 1978; Ericksen et al. 1978; Neborsky et al. 1981; Quitkin et al. 1975; Rifkin et al. 1991). None of these studies found a significant superiority for high-dose treatment. Despite these findings we continue to see high-dose treatment employed in many clinical settings, particularly in patients who have had only poor or partial response to other psychopharmacological treatments.

Patients With No or Inadequate Response to Antipsychotic Drugs

One of the most frequent situations in which high doses of antipsychotic drugs are employed is when patients fail to respond adequately or continue to be violent and aggressive. It is certainly true that a substantial proportion of patients treated for 4–6 weeks with standard doses of antipsychotic drugs may not achieve adequate therapeutic response. In those trials conducted in the 1960s (Klein and Davis 1969), approximately 38% of patients derived little if any benefit from medication (including the slightly less than 10% considered unchanged or worse). In more recent trials the proportion of patients considered to have an inadequate response appears to be somewhat higher. Representative trials that attempted to exclude patients with refractory illness reported an average good response rate of 50% (Kinon et al. 1993; Levinson et al. 1990; Rifkin et al. 1991; Van Putten et al. 1990; Volavka et al. 1992).

We (Kane and Borenstein 1997) reviewed response rates in more than 700 haloperidol-treated patients participating in placebo-controlled, new drug development trials and found that the proportion of patients improving 30% or more on the Brief Psychiatric Rating Scale (BPRS; Overall and Gorham 1962) total score ranged from 12% to 45%. The patients participating in these trials were mostly male with an average age in the middle to late 30s, and most had six or more prior hospitalizations and were ill an average of 15 years.

When patients do not respond adequately, clinicians face the challenge of deciding whether and when to abandon the current treatment, to increase the dose, to add adjunctive medication, and/or to switch to another drug, as well as which drug to switch to. Despite the frequency of this situation, data by which to inform clinical practice are still inadequate. For years clinicians faced the dilemmas presented by conventional drugs and now those dilemmas are repeated with the new-generation antipsychotics. When drugs are initially developed, the pharmaceutical companies do not necessarily have an incentive to study a broad range of doses or to establish a maximum tolerated dose. As a result, clinicians sometimes tend to administer higher doses (assuming they are tolerated) in patients who are not adequately responding. This became such a widespread tendency with the conventional drugs that it was not uncommon for patients to be treated with extremely high doses of fluphenazine or haloperidol (or other mid- to high-potency drugs). Although some studies suggested that high-dose, or even "megadose," treatment might be beneficial in a proportion of patients with refractory disease, well-designed studies (Bjorndal et al. 1980; Prien and Cole 1968; Quitkin et al. 1975) have found little consistent advantage.

Remarkably few studies attempt to assess the value of switching from one antipsychotic drug to another. In addition, the merits of dosage escalation (or reduction) in patients whose disease responds only poorly or partially to the new-generation drugs need to be critically evaluated with well-designed studies.

We (Kinon et al. 1993) reported results from a study designed to compare the relative efficacy of treatment alternatives using conventional drugs in 156 patients who continued to exhibit clinically significant positive symptoms after a 4-week trial of fluphenazine 20 mg/day. At the end of 4 weeks of fluphenazine, 115 subjects had completed this portion of the trial and 68% had a score of moderate or greater on at least one psychotic item. Fifty-eight patients entered a second 4-week phase in which they were randomly assigned double-blind to continue taking fluphenazine 20 mg/day, have the dosage increased to 80 mg/day, or be switched to haloperidol 20 mg/day. Only 9% of subjects who completed this phase achieved the a priori response criteria and we did not observe a significant difference among the three alternatives.

It is possible, however, that further improvement would be observed with specific alternatives administered over a longer period of time than 4–8 weeks. Shalev et al. (1993) evaluated the proportion of patients with acutely exacerbated schizophrenia and who remained unimproved after consecutive administration of haloperidol, chlorpromazine, and perphenazine in randomly determined order. Two criteria were used concurrently to define therapeutic success: a decrease of 30% in a modified version of the BPRS and clinical improvement sufficient to permit discharge back into the community. Sixty patients completed the trial (58% were women, the mean age was 33, and the number of previous admissions averaged four). Each phase of the study averaged 28–33 days. Patients who did not improve during each 4-week period were switched to the next drug according to their predetermined schedule; however, if there was a "subthreshold" improvement, the drug was continued another week before determining ultimate response to that phase. The average daily dosages were 27–30 mg for haloperidol, 350–380 mg for chlorpromazine, and 36–47 mg for perphenazine.

The total improvement rate was 95% with only 3 of 60 patients remaining unimproved after the three phases of the study. Of the patients entering each phase of the trial, 67% improved after the first drug, 55% after the second, and 67% after the third. The differences in improvement rates among the phases were not statistically significant, nor were differences found between men and women. The differences in improvement rates among the three drugs over the entire trial were not statistically significant.

The disparity in results between these two trials might be at least in part a result of the differences in the criteria for good response. The Kinon et al. (1993) study required ratings of no more than "mild" on any psychotic item, whereas the Shalev et al. (1993) study required a 30% improvement on the total BPRS scale. In addition, the latter study used a 4-point version of the BPRS, so the rating scale data cannot easily be compared. It is also impossible to determine whether or not the improvement occurring in the second and third phases was in fact a result of the change in drug or the passage of additional time. In addressing this issue, the authors point out that it is difficult to maintain treatment of patients whose disease is responding poorly while the patients are taking the same drug for 12 weeks. It is notable that none of the drugs appeared superior in this context, despite some differences in receptor-binding profile.

Other treatment strategies for patients whose disease is not responding have included adjunctive treatments such as lithium, benzodiazepines, anticonvulsants, and electroconvulsive therapy. Although some patients may benefit from these strategies, the proportion of such patients is low (Christison et al. 1991). In treating patients whose disease responds poorly or partially to antipsychotic drugs, in order to assess the impact of a particular treatment trial it is critical that clinicians have a treatment plan that considers target symptoms, dosage, and duration. It is recommended that only one change in a given patient's pharmacological treatment be made at a time. It is also important to give patients an adequate amount of time to respond to an intervention. Some patients may require 4 weeks or more before they respond to a new drug regimen. Given that many alternative treatments used in patients with refractory disease do not have approved indications for schizophrenia, it is important that the rationale as well as potential benefits and risks be discussed with the patient and significant others and that these discussions be documented in the medical record.

Clozapine

Perhaps the best alternative for patients with refractory disease is clozapine. The introduction of clozapine into clinical practice in the United States in 1990 led to new perspectives on antipsychotic drug treatment, drug development, and outcome assessment. Clozapine was the first drug to demonstrate a qualitative difference in propensity to produce neuromuscular side effects (Casey 1989) and the first drug to show clear superiority over other antipsychotic drugs in the treatment of patients with refractory disease (Kane et al. 1988). As a result, an enormous amount of research has been conducted that aims to determine the neuropharmacological characteristics of clozapine that are responsible for these novel effects. Despite an extraordinary array of findings showing differences between clozapine and conventional drugs on neuroimaging, neurophysiological, and neurochemical measures, it is currently difficult to make definitive statements as to what characteristic(s) accounts for clozapine's clinical profile.

As a result of clozapine's adverse-effect profile (specifically, what initially appeared to be a 1%–2% risk of potentially fatal agranulocytosis, although incidence may now be as low as less than 0.5% in the first year of treatment), the use of this drug has generally been confined to patients with disease refractory to or intolerant of treatment. Therefore, any discussion of clozapine's clinical effects will largely focus on populations of patients with disease that is resistant to treatment.

Kane et al. (1988) reported on 267 patients who met strict criteria for having treatment-resistant schizophrenia. The patients' schizophrenia had to fail to respond to adequate trials of at least three antipsychotic drugs and a prospective, single-blind trial of haloperidol. Clozapine was associated with significantly greater improvement in both positive and negative symptoms. Using a priori criteria for improvement, Kane and colleagues found that 30% of clozapine-treated patients improved after 6 weeks in comparison with 4% of those receiving chlorpromazine. Since that report, a number of controlled trials have confirmed clozapine's superiority over conventional drugs in improving positive symptoms (Breier et al. 1994; J. M. Kane et al., submitted for publication; Pickar et al. 1992). However, clozapine's impact on primary negative symptoms or deficit state remains the subject of ongoing debate (Carpenter et al. 1995; Meltzer 1995). For example, in a 6-month double-blind comparison of clozapine and a modest dose of haloperidol (10 mg/day) in outpatients with poorly or partially responsive disease, we found that clozapine was superior in reducing positive symptoms but not negative symptoms (J. M. Kane et al., submitted for publication).

Two relatively long-term controlled trials have now been reported with clozapine. Essock et al. (1996) carried out an effectiveness trial of clozapine in which 227 state hospital inpatients with treatment-refractory disease were randomly assigned to nonblind, continued "usual care" or treatment with clozapine. No significant difference was found between clozapine and the usual care condition in the rate of discharge over the 24-month follow-up period, nor were there any significant differences on measures of psychopathology. However, clozapine-treated patients who were discharged were significantly less likely to be rehospitalized than the comparison group.

Rosenheck et al. (1997) conducted a 1-year randomized, double-blind comparative trial of clozapine and haloperidol in 423 patients at 15 Department of Veterans Affairs medical centers. Significantly more (57%) clozapine-treated patients continued on the assigned treatment for the whole year in comparison with only 28% in the haloperidol group. Also, significantly more haloperidol-treated patients discontinued treatment as a result of worsening of symptoms or lack of efficacy (51%) in comparison with the clozapine-treated patients (15%). Among patients taking clozapine, a 20% reduction in the total score on the Positive and Negative Syndrome Scale (PANSS; Kay et al. 1987) was seen in 24% of subjects after 6 weeks and 37% after 1 year. However, this was not significantly different from the 13% and 32%, respectively, who showed the same level of improvement while taking haloperidol.

The relapse data also deserve comment. In general, patients who relapse despite continued maintenance medications have not been considered as having refractory disease, but this is a subgroup of patients who are not responding optimally. Even with guaranteed medication delivery (i.e., depot drugs), approximately 15%–20% of patients will experience a relapse over a 1-year period (Kane 1996). Hardly any data exist to inform clinical strategies for the management of such patients. We (Pollack et al. 1998) observed, in a mirror-image analysis of hospitalization before and after taking clozapine in 81 patients, that the rate of hospitalization of those taking clozapine was significantly reduced. Clearly, given the mirror-image design, other factors may have contributed to this difference. A controlled trial with clozapine focusing on relapse prevention in patients who have relapsed on other drugs would be of considerable interest.

A series of reports suggests superiority for clozapine in a number of areas such as hostility and violence (Mallya et al. 1992), substance abuse (Albanese et al. 1994; Buckley et al. 1994), and suicidal behavior (Meltzer and Okayli 1995). These observations have been derived mainly from uncontrolled observations of patients with disease that is primarily chronic refractory or partially drug responsive, and these observations require confirmation.

New-Generation Antipsychotic Drugs

Risperidone

Risperidone was marketed in 1994 in the United States and has been widely used since then. Risperidone's efficacy was established in seven clinical studies of acutely psychotic patients (Borison et al. 1992; Ceskova and Svestka 1993; Chouinard et al. 1993; Claus et al. 1992; Heinrich et al. 1994; Marder and Meibach 1994; Muller-Spahn 1992). In the United States–Canadian multicenter trial, risperidone (6 or 16 mg/day) was superior to haloperidol (20 mg/day) in reducing total PANSS scores. At present, no evidence suggests that dosages higher than 6 mg/day offer any advantage. Moreover, higher doses are associated with a higher incidence of extrapyramidal side effects. In initial trials (Marder and Meibach 1994), risperidone appeared to be helpful for some patients with refractory disease. Flynn et al. (1998) described a series of cases of patients with treatment-resistant disease who were treated openly with either risperidone ($N = 29$, mean dose 7.75 mg) or clozapine ($N = 57$, mean dose 420 mg/day) over an average of 12 weeks. Using a response criterion of a 20% reduction in total PANSS score, 44% of the clozapine-treated and 28% of the risperidone-treated patients responded. Bondolfi et al. (1998) reported on 86 inpatients with treatment-refractory schizophrenia randomly assigned to an 8-week double-blind trial of risperidone or clozapine. The mean daily dosage for clozapine was 291 mg and for risperidone, 6.4 mg. The criterion for categorizing patients as improved was a 20% reduction in total PANSS score. At the end of the study, 67% of risperidone-treated patients and 65% of clozapine-treated patients met response criteria. Interpretation of these data is complicated by the use of a relatively low dose of clozapine and that the response rate is higher than usually reported in 8-week trials of clozapine in patients with treatment-refractory schizophrenia.

Additional data are necessary to clarify the relative value of risperidone in patients with treatment-refractory schizophrenia, and a number of relevant trials are currently under way.

Olanzapine

Olanzapine was marketed in the United States in 1996. Several large-scale trials have been conducted demonstrating olanzapine's efficacy in the treatment of schizophrenia. Most studies were controlled with placebo and/or haloperidol, but more recently studies are being reported comparing olanzapine to risperidone or clozapine. As is the case with all of the new antipsychotic drugs, in the initial studies done for drug regulatory purposes, the patient demographics were such that the efficacy results might have underestimated olanzapine's impact in younger patients and/or patients closer to the onset of the illness. In general, the studies demonstrate at least equivalent antipsychotic efficacy to haloperidol with some evidence of superiority on negative symptoms and depression (Beasley et al. 1996; Tollefson et al. 1997b, 1998). Although clear superiority was evident on propensity to induce neuromuscular side effects, olanzapine has a robust association with weight gain.

In addition, analysis of double-blind, continuation data from patients receiving olanzapine or haloperidol revealed a significantly lower incidence of treatment-emergent dyskinesia among olanzapine-treated patients (Tollefson et al. 1997a). The incidence observed with haloperidol was similar to that observed in incidence studies involving conventional antipsychotics (Kane 1995), which is helpful in supporting the validity of the findings.

In a recent study (Tran et al. 1997), olanzapine was compared with risperidone in schizophreniform, schizophrenia, and schizoaffective patients over a 28-week treatment period. The mean dosage of olanzapine was 16.9 mg/day and that of risperidone, 7.3 mg/day. Extrapyramidal side effects were more common in the risperidone group at week 8 and week 28. Olanzapine produced significantly greater improvement on the Scale for the Assessment of Negative Symptoms (SANS; Andreasen 1989) summary score, and significantly fewer patients taking olanzapine experienced a symptom exacerbation during one 28-week trial. The average dose of risperidone used in this study is somewhat greater than is generally recommended today for the treatment of psychosis, and this might have influenced the higher rate of adverse effects seen with risperidone. However, half of the patients taking risperidone were receiving dosages below 6 mg/day.

Studies are beginning to be reported examining olanzapine's potential for improving outcome in patients with treatment-refractory disease. In one open trial of olanzapine, 36% of patients achieved response criteria (Martin et al. 1997). In another, 48% of patients with treatment-refractory disease were reported to have responded to olanzapine (Baldacchino et al. 1998). Conley et al. (1998) have reported on an 8-week double-blind comparison of olanzapine and chlorpromazine in 84 subjects with treatment-refractory disease. No difference in efficacy was observed on measures of psychopathology. Seven percent of the olanzapine-treated patients responded according to a priori criteria, and no chlorpromazine-treated patients responded; however, this is a nonsignificant difference. The mean dosage of chlorpromazine was 1,173 mg/day. All olanzapine-treated patients received 25 mg/day. Overall, neither drug group experienced substantial change in the severity of psychosis from its baseline state. Breier and Hamilton (1999) reported on a subpopulation of patients meeting retrospectively applied criteria for treatment-refractory schizophrenia, selected from a large prospective, double-blind, 6-week study of olanzapine and haloperidol (Tollefson et al. 1997b). Olanzapine showed superiority over haloperidol on most of the major measures of psychopathology for those who completed the study. This study is limited by the retrospective nature of the determination of nonresponse, which relied on failure to respond to at least one 8-week trial of an antipsychotic during the previous 2 years and presence of a specified level of severity at baseline when subjects were still being treated with a prior antipsychotic. These criteria are not as clear or selective as those used in the study of Conley and colleagues (1998).

Quetiapine

The most recently marketed antipsychotic in the United States is quetiapine. This compound was also compared to placebo and conventional antipsychotics in a number of double-blind trials (Arvanitis et al. 1997; Peuskens and Link 1997). Superiority was demonstrated over placebo on measures of positive and negative symptoms. No significant superiority in efficacy was demonstrated in comparison with conventional drugs, but quetiapine was shown to produce low levels of extrapyramidal side effects and to be generally well tolerated. To date, no published data are available of patients with treatment-refractory disease. Concern about possible ophthalmological effects of quetiapine has led to recommendations of eye examinations at baseline and during follow-up.

In summary, as a class, the second-generation antipsychotics clearly have advantages over conventional drugs particularly in the area of adverse effects (with the exception of weight gain). Data with regard to positive and negative symptom efficacy are still inconsistent and limited by methodological considerations. When differences have been found between new compounds and standard agents (e.g., haloperidol), the effect sizes have generally been small to medium (Schooler 1998). Diminution of parkinsonian side effects can have important effects on appearance, subjective well-being, and functioning, so these gains are considerable. In addition, reducing the need for the adjunctive antiparkinsonism medications has potential benefits.

Other domains of outcome are now being explored as well. Increasing attention has been focused on cognitive dysfunction in schizophrenia, as it has been estimated that 75% of patients with schizophrenia exhibit some neuropsychological dysfunction (Gold and Harvey 1993). It has been shown that cognitive dysfunction can be more of an important determinant of poor social and vocational outcome than psychotic signs or symptoms can be (Green 1996). It also appears that some type of cognitive dysfunction precedes the overt onset of a schizophrenic illness (Erlenmeyer-Kimling et al. 1993). The new-generation antipsychotics appear to hold considerable promise in either improving or not worsening specific aspects of cognitive functioning. So far, there remain only a relatively small number of studies and few adequately controlled trials focusing on the impact of second-generation drugs on cognitive function.

Another critical area for assessing the ultimate impact of intervention strategies with the new antipsychotic drugs involves measures of functioning. Results from controlled trials (even with clozapine) are not as clear-cut as one would like, but this will become an increasingly important domain in comparing the impact of different treatment strategies.

Overall, still too few direct comparisons have been made of the new antipsychotic drugs against each other. Also no data provide biological predictors of response to enable clinicians to choose the ideal drug for a specific patient. It is hoped that pharmacogenomics may provide important guidance; however, we have not yet seen consistent results in this regard (Arranz et al. 1995; Malhotra et al. 1996).

Maintenance Treatment

Given the nature of schizophrenia and its long-term course, the role of maintenance treatment is absolutely critical. Because drug development relies heavily on acute effects in relatively short-term trials, far less research has been performed in the maintenance treatment arena. Although such trials are difficult to conduct, take a long time to complete, and can be expensive, it is producing and sustaining gains over the long term that will be critical in altering the course and improving functional outcome in this disease.

The importance of maintenance medication has been well established in numerous double-blind, placebo-controlled trials (Davis 1975; Gilbert et al. 1995; Kane and Lieberman 1987). Gilbert et al. (1995) reviewed 66 studies of antipsychotic withdrawal involving 4,365 patients. The mean cumulative relapse rate was 53% in patients withdrawn from treatment and 16% in those still receiving treatment over a mean follow-up of 9.7 months. If one focuses on patients who have been in remission for a year or more, available studies indicate that approximately 75% will relapse within 12–18 months after the discontinuation of antipsychotic medication (Davis et al. 1994; Kissling 1991). These data are particularly important for clinicians to appreciate because it is not uncommon for both patients and clinicians to develop a false sense of security regarding diminished need for medication when the patient has been in remission for a year or more. Current American Psychiatric Association (1997) guidelines recommend that individuals recovering from their first episode of illness should probably be treated for 1–2 years; however, 75% of patients will have relapses after therapy is discontinued. These guidelines should be revised as fears of long-term drug toxicity decline. Patients who have had two or more episodes should receive maintenance treatment for at least 5 years (American Psychiatric Association 1997), and many experts believe that these patients should be treated indefinitely (Davis et al. 1994). It has been difficult for us to identify subgroups of patients to whom these recommendations do not apply. It is also clear that 15%–20% of patients will relapse within a year despite guaranteed medication delivery (i.e., depot drugs). When rates of noncompliance are also taken into consideration, the frequency and consequences of relapse take on enormous public health significance (Weiden and Olfson 1995).

An important focus of research with conventional antipsychotic drugs has been to improve the overall benefit-to-risk ratio of long-term antipsychotic drug treatment by establishing optimal strategies. Studies comparing different fixed doses and comparing continuous with intermittent therapy have been conducted. Six studies involving different doses given for at least 1 year have been reported (Hogarty et al. 1988; Johnson et al. 1987; Kane et al. 1983, 1986b, 1993a; Marder et al. 1984, 1987; Schooler et al. 1997). All involved long-acting injectable medication given at intervals of 2–4 weeks. The results were similar in suggesting that low-dose maintenance treatment is feasible but that the risk of relapse during therapy is somewhat greater than if the maintenance dose is higher. Although lower doses were associated with fewer adverse effects in general, this relationship has not been clearly demonstrated with respect to tardive dyskinesia.

Intermittent treatment is a strategy intended to take advantage of the observation that many individuals do not experience a relapse until several months after the discontinuation of antipsychotic medication. This strategy includes the discontinuation of antipsychotic medication in stable outpatients who are in remission and the reinstitution of medication if and when prodromal signs of relapse occur. The aim of this "early intervention" is to prevent a full-blown psychotic relapse. The overall goal is to reduce the cumulative exposure to antipsychotic drugs and limit adverse effects. Five major studies have examined this strategy (Carpenter et al. 1991; Herz et al. 1991; Jolley et al. 1989, 1990; Pietzcker et al. 1993; Schooler et al. 1997). All of the patients in these trials were treated from 2 to 6 months before therapy was discontinued in those individuals who were assigned to the intermittent-treatment groups. The cumulative rates of relapse after 1 year in the groups that received continuous treatment were similar to those reported for the conventional doses of antipsychotic drugs in the trials involving low-dose therapy. The results with intermittent treatment, however, were relatively discouraging. The rates of relapse during the 1-year study follow-up interval were high, and in addition little benefit was found in terms of psychosocial adjustment, enhanced subjective well-being, or diminished incidence of tardive dyskinesia. In light of the overall twofold increase in the risk of relapse, this approach is difficult to justify. On the other hand, the intermittent approach may be useful in the treatment of those patients who adamantly refuse to take medication when in remission.

All of these studies involving alternative maintenance-treatment strategies have used depot antipsychotic drugs. The reason for this is that investigators attempting to make comparisons among different dosage levels or different strategies for administration need to be absolutely certain that the patient is taking the medication as prescribed. The only way that it has been possible to do this is by the administration of long-acting injectable medications; however, in clinical practice these drugs are used far less frequently (Glazer and Kane 1992). Now, with the introduction of a new generation of antipsychotic drugs that are associated with a lower risk of neuromuscular side effects, the clinician faces a dilemma in the treatment of patients who are potentially noncompliant. None of the new drugs are currently available in a long-acting injectable form. It is assumed that the reduction in adverse effects expected over long-term treatment with the new antipsychotic drugs will lead to a reduction in rates of noncompliance. However, this remains an as yet untested hypothesis, and it is also clear to clinicians and investigators that adverse effects of medication by no means explain all of the variance in the development of noncompliance. We continue, therefore, to be faced with the dilemma of increasing our certainty of preventing relapse but also increasing the potential risk of adverse effects such as tardive dyskinesia. It is hoped that new medication delivery methods will become available for the new-generation antipsychotic drugs in order to resolve this dilemma.

Another interesting aspect of long-acting injectable medication is the suggestion that, even after the discontinuation of such drugs, relapse rates are reduced because of the gradual withdrawal resulting from the pharmacokinetic properties of these agents. Viguera et al. (1997) reported that abrupt cessation of oral antipsychotic drugs was associated with a relapse rate of 50% within 30 weeks, with little additional risk thereafter up to 3.7 years. The risk was lower, however, after gradual discontinuation of oral treatment. A similar finding was reported by Gilbert et al. (1995) in their review of the literature on discontinuation of maintenance medication.

Depot medications, therefore, have the advantage of not only making it clear to family members and clinicians when medication has been discontinued (which may not necessarily be the case when an individual is receiving oral medication) but also providing some further protection against relapse for several weeks, thus allowing all interested parties to respond to this "crisis."

Tardive Dyskinesia

A significant adverse effect associated with maintenance treatment with conventional antipsychotic drugs, and to a lesser degree with the new generation of antipsychotic drugs, is tardive dyskinesia. Concern about tardive dyskinesia has played an important role in stimulating research on minimal effective dosage in addition to having an obvious impact on drug development goals. Research has helped to clarify the incidence of tardive dyskinesia, its course, and risk factors for its development. Prospective studies have suggested an incidence of 5% per year of antipsychotic exposure in young adults (Chakos et al. 1996; Kane et al. 1986a), with a substantially higher incidence in elderly persons (Saltz et al. 1991). The majority of cases are mild and not necessarily progressive even with continued antipsychotic exposure (Gardos et al. 1988). However, some patients develop a severe and disabling form of the condition. If medication can be discontinued, the prognosis is often favorable (Casey and Gerlach 1986), but discontinuation is often not feasible.

That clozapine, compared with other drugs, appears to be much less likely to cause tardive dyskinesia (Kane et al. 1993b) might suggest that the new antipsychotic drugs will also have a lower risk of tardive dyskinesia. Data available to date with risperidone (Jeste et al. 2000), olanzapine (Tollefson et al. 1997a), and quetiapine (Jeste et al. 1999) are encouraging in suggesting a significantly lower risk of tardive dyskinesia than the risk with conventional drugs. It is also important to keep in mind that some patients with schizophrenia may have abnormal, involuntary movements that are not the result of prolonged antipsychotic drug treatment.

Patients receiving chronic antipsychotic drug treatment should be evaluated on a regular basis (3- to 6-month intervals) for the possible development of abnormal, involuntary movements (Kane et al. 1992). Use of a rating scale such as the Abnormal Involuntary Movement Scale (AIMS; Guy 1976) can be helpful in providing a systematic screening tool and documentation of the examination. When evidence of tardive dyskinesia does develop, a differential diagnosis should ensue, because diagnoses should not be based on the results of a rating scale assessment. If no other cause is identified, the need for continued antipsychotic treatment should be carefully reviewed. When continued treatment is indicated and informed consent is obtained from the patient, an attempt should be made to use the lowest possible dose of the antipsychotic drug. If the condition is more than mild in severity, switching to clozapine should be considered (it remains to be seen whether other new-generation antipsychotic drugs would be an appropriate alternative as well). Considerable improvement and even remission of mild tardive dyskinesia can occur if the condition is detected early in its course and medication dosage is reduced.

Conclusions

Considerable progress is being made in our ability to use available agents in the most judicious manner and to develop new compounds that can improve our therapeutic options. More new antipsychotics are available and more potential antipsychotic drugs are under development now than at any time in the past several decades. It is expected that further advances in basic and clinical neuroscience will facilitate the development of more specific and efficacious treatments.

References

Albanese MJ, Khantzian EJ, Mercy FL, et al: Decreased substance use in chronically psychotic patients treated with clozapine. Am J Psychiatry 151:780–781, 1994

American Psychiatric Association: Practice guideline for the treatment of patients with schizophrenia. Am J Psychiatry 154 (4 suppl):1-63, 1997

Andreasen N: The Scale for the Assessment of Negative Symptoms (SANS): conceptual and theoretical foundations. Br J Psychiatry 155 (suppl 7):49–52, 1989

Arranz M, Collier D, Sodhi M, et al: Association between clozapine response and allelic variation in 5-HT 2A receptor gene. Lancet 345:281–282, 1995

Arvanitis LA, Miller DG, Seroquel Trial Thirteen Study Group: Multiple fixed doses of Seroquel (quetiapine) in patients with acute exacerbation of schizophrenia: a comparison with haloperidol and placebo. Biol Psychiatry 42:233–246, 1997

Baldacchino AM, Stubbs JH, Nevison-Andrews D: The use of olanzapine in non-compliant or treatment-resistant clozapine populations in hospital. Pharmaceutical Journal 260:207–209, 1998

Beasley CM, Tollefson G, Tran P, et al: Olanzapine versus placebo and haloperidol: acute phase results of the North American double-blind olanzapine trial. Neuropsychopharmacology 14:111–123, 1996

Bjorndal N, Bjerre M, Gerlach J, et al: High dosage haloperidol therapy in chronic schizophrenic patients: a double-blind study of clinical response, side effects, serum haloperidol, and serum prolactin. Psychopharmacology (Berl) 67:17–23, 1980

Bondolfi G, Dufour H, Patris M, et al: Risperidone versus clozapine in treatment-resistant chronic schizophrenia: a randomized double-blind study. Am J Psychiatry 155:499–504, 1998

Borison RL, Pathiraja AP, Diamond BI, et al: Risperidone: clinical safety and efficacy in schizophrenia. Psychopharmacol Bull 28:213–218,1992

Breier A, Hamilton SH: Comparative efficacy of olanzapine and haloperidol for patients with treatment-resistant schizophrenia. Biol Psychiatry 45:383–384, 1999

Breier A, Buchanan RW, Kirkpatrick B, et al: Effects of clozapine on positive and negative symptoms in outpatients with schizophrenia. Am J Psychiatry 151:20–26, 1994

Buckley P, Thompson P, Way L, et al: Substance abuse among patients with treatment-resistant schizophrenia: characteristics and implications for clozapine in therapy. Am J Psychiatry 151:385–389, 1994

Carpenter WT Jr, Hanlon TE, Heinrichs DW, et al: Continuous versus targeted medication in schizophrenic outpatients: outcome results. Am J Psychiatry 147:1138–1148, 1990 (Erratum published in Am J Psychiatry 148:819, 1991)

Carpenter WT Jr, Conley RR, Buchanan RW, et al: Patient response and resource management: another view of clozapine treatment of schizophrenia. Am J Psychiatry 152:827–832, 1995

Casey DE: Clozapine: neuroleptic-induced EPS and tardive dyskinesia. Psychopharmacology (Berl) 99:S47–S53, 1989

Casey DE, Gerlach J: Tardive dyskinesia: what is the long-term outcome, in Tardive Dyskinesia and Neuroleptics: From Dogma to Reason. Edited by Casey DE, Gardos G. Washington, DC, American Psychiatric Press, 1986, pp 75–97

Ceskova E, Svestka J: Double-blind comparison of risperidone and haloperidol in schizophrenia and schizoaffective psychoses. Pharmacopsychiatry 26:121–124, 1993

Chakos MH, Alvir JM, Woerner MG, et al: Incidence and correlates of tardive dyskinesia in first-episode schizophrenia. Arch Gen Psychiatry 53:313–319, 1996

Chouinard G, Jones B, Remington G, et al: A Canadian multicenter placebo-controlled study of fixed doses of risperidone and haloperidol in the treatment of chronic schizophrenic patients. J Clin Psychopharmacol 13:25–40, 1993 (Erratum published in J Clin Psychopharmacol 13:149, 1993)

Christison GW, Kirch DG, Wyatt RJ: When symptoms persist: choosing among alternative somatic treatments for schizophrenia. Schizophr Bull 17:217–245, 1991

Claus A, Bollen J, De Cuyper H, et al: Risperidone versus haloperidol in the treatment of chronic schizophrenic inpatients: a multicenter double-blind comparative study. Acta Psychiatr Scand 85:295–305, 1992

Conley RR, Tamminga CA, Bartko JJ, et al: Olanzapine compared with chlorpromazine in treatment-resistant schizophrenia. Am J Psychiatry 155:914–920, 1998

Davis JM: Overview: maintenance therapy in psychiatry, I: schizophrenia. Am J Psychiatry 132:1237–1245, 1975

Davis JM, Matalon L, Watanabe MD, et al: Depot antipsychotic drugs: place in therapy. Drugs 47:741–773, 1994 (Erratum published in Drugs 48:616, 1994)

Donlon PT, Meadow A, Tupin JP, et al: High vs standard dosage fluphenazine HCl in acute schizophrenia. J Clin Psychiatry 39:800–804, 1978

Ericksen SE, Hurt SW, Chang S, et al: Haloperidol dose, plasma levels, and clinical response: a double-blind study. Psychopharmacol Bull 14:15–16, 1978

Erlenmeyer-Kimling L, Cornblatt BA, Rock D, et al: The New York High-Risk Project: anhedonia, attentional deviants, and psychopathology. Schizophr Bull 19:141–153, 1993

Essock SM, Hargreaves WA, Covell NH, et al: Clozapine's effectiveness for patients in state hospitals: results from a randomized trial. Psychopharmacol Bull 32:683–697, 1996

Flynn SW, MacEwan GW, Altman S, et al: An open comparison of clozapine and risperidone. Pharmacopsychiatry 31:25–29, 1998

Gardos G, Cole JO, Haskell D, et al: The natural history of tardive dyskinesia. J Clin Psychopharmacol 8 (4, suppl):31S–37S, 1988

Gilbert PL, Harris NJ, McAdams LA, et al: Neuroleptic withdrawal in schizophrenic patients: a review of the literature. Arch Gen Psychiatry 52:173–188, 1995

Glazer WM, Kane JM: Depot neuroleptic therapy: an underutilized treatment option. J Clin Psychiatry 53:426–433, 1992

Gold JM, Harvey PD: Cognitive deficits in schizophrenia. Psychiatr Clin North Am 16:295–312, 1993

Green MF: What are the functional consequences of neurocognitive deficits in schizophrenia? Am J Psychiatry 153:321–330, 1996

Guy W: ECDEU Assessment Manual for Psychopharmacology (DHEW Publ No [ADM] 76-388). Rockville, MD, U.S. Department of Health, Education and Welfare, 1976

Heinrich K, Klieser E, Lehmann E, et al: Risperidone versus clozapine in the treatment of schizophrenic patients with acute symptoms: a double blind, randomized trial. Prog Neuropsychopharmacol Biol Psychiatry 18:129–137, 1994

Herz MI, Glazer WM, Mostert MA, et al: Intermittent vs maintenance medication in schizophrenia: two-year results. Arch Gen Psychiatry 48:333–339, 1991

Hogarty GE, McEvoy JP, Munetz M, et al: Dose of fluphenazine, familial expressed emotion, and outcome in schizophrenia results in a two-year controlled study: Arch Gen Psychiatry 45:797–805, 1988

Jeste DV, Glazer WM, Morgenstern H, et al: Rarity of persistent tardive dyskinesia with quetiapine treatment of psychotic disorders in the elderly patients. Paper presented at the annual meeting of the American College of Neuropsychopharmacology, Acapulco, Mexico, December 12–16, 1999

Jeste DV, Okamoto A, Napolitano J, et al: Low incidence of persistent tardive dyskinesia in elderly patients with dementia treated with risperidone. Am J Psychiatry 157:1150–1155, 2000

Johnson DA, Ludlow JM, Street K, et al: Double-blind comparison of half-dose and standard-dose flupenthixol decanoate in the maintenance treatment of stabilized out-patients with schizophrenia. Br J Psychiatry 151:634–638, 1987

Jolley AG, Hirsch SR, McRink A, et al: Trial of brief intermittent neuroleptic prophylaxis for selected schizophrenic outpatients: clinical outcome at one year. BMJ 298:985–990, 1989

Jolley AG, Hirsch SR, Morrison E, et al: Trial of brief intermittent neuroleptic prophylaxis for selected schizophrenic outpatients: clinical and social outcome at two years. BMJ 301:837–842, 1990

Kane JM: Compliance issues in outpatient treatment. J Clin Psychopharmacol 5:22S–27S, 1985

Kane JM: Tardive dyskinesia: epidemiological and clinical presentation, in Psychopharmacology: The Fourth Generation of Progress. Edited by Bloom FE, Kupfer DJ. New York, Raven, 1995, pp 1485–1495

Kane JM: Schizophrenia. N Engl J Med 334:34–41, 1996

Kane JM, Borenstein M: The use of placebo controls in psychiatric research, in Ethics in Neurobiological Research With Human Subjects: The Baltimore Conference on Ethics. Edited by Shamoo AE. Amsterdam, Gordon & Breach, pp 207–214, 1997

Kane JM, Lieberman JA: Maintenance pharmacotherapy in schizophrenia, in: Psychopharmacology: The Third Generation of Progress. Edited by Meltzer HY. New York, Raven, 1987, pp 1103–1109

Kane JM, Rifkin A, Woerner MG, et al: Low-dose neuroleptic treatment of outpatient schizophrenia, I: preliminary results for relapse rates. Arch Gen Psychiatry 40:893–896, 1983

Kane JM, Woerner M, Borenstein M, et al: Integrating incidence and prevalence of tardive dyskinesia. Psychopharmacol Bull 22:254–258, 1986a

Kane JM, Woerner MG, Sarantakos S: Depot neuroleptics: a comparative review of standard, intermediate, and low-dose regimens. J Clin Psychiatry 47 (suppl):30–33, 1986b

Kane JM, Honigfeld G, Singer J, et al: Clozapine for the treatment-resistant schizophrenic: a double-blind comparison with chlorpromazine. Arch Gen Psychiatry 45:789–796, 1988

Kane JM, Barnes TRE, Casey D, et al: Tardive Dyskinesia: An American Psychiatric Association Task Force Report. Washington, DC, American Psychiatric Association, 1992

Kane JM, Davis JM, Schooler NR, et al: A one-year comparison of four dosages of haloperidol decanoate. Schizophr Res 9:239–240, 1993a

Kane JM, Woerner MG, Pollack S, et al: Does clozapine cause tardive dyskinesia? J Clin Psychiatry 54:327–330, 1993b

Kay SR, Fiszbein A, Opler LA: The Positive and Negative Syndrome Scale (PANSS) for schizophrenia. Schizophr Bull 13:261–276, 1987

Kinon BJ, Kane JM, Johns C, et al: Treatment of neuroleptic resistant schizophrenic relapse. Psychopharmacol Bull 29:309–314, 1993

Kissling W (ed): Guidelines for Neuroleptic Relapse Prevention in Schizophrenia. Berlin, Germany, Springer-Verlag, 1991

Klein DF, Davis JM: Diagnosis and Drug Treatment of Psychiatric Disorders. Baltimore, MD, Williams & Wilkins, 1969

Levinson DF, Simpson GM, Singh H, et al: Fluphenazine dose, clinical response, and extrapyramidal symptoms during acute treatment. Arch Gen Psychiatry 47:761–768, 1990

Malhotra AK, Goldman D, Ozaki N, et al: Lack of association between polymorphisms in the 5-HT 2A receptor gene and the antipsychotic response to clozapine. Am J Psychiatry 153:1092–1094, 1996

Mallya AR, Roos PD, Roebuck-Colgan K: Restraint, seclusion and clozapine. J Clin Psychiatry 53:395–397, 1992

Marder SR, Meibach RC: Risperidone in the treatment of schizophrenia. Am J Psychiatry 151:825–835, 1994

Marder SR, Van Putten T, Mintz J, et al: Costs and benefits of two doses of fluphenazine. Arch Gen Psychiatry 41:1025–1029, 1984

Marder SR, Van Putten T, Mintz J, et al: Low- and conventional-dose maintenance therapy with fluphenazine decanoate: two-year outcome. Arch Gen Psychiatry 44:518–521, 1987

Martin J, Gomez J-C, Garcia-Bernardo E, et al: Olanzapine and treatment-refractory schizophrenia: results of an open-label study. J Clin Psychiatry 58:479–493, 1997

Meltzer HY: Clozapine: is another view valid? Am J Psychiatry 152:821–825, 1995

Meltzer HY, Okayli O: Reduction of suicidality during clozapine treatment of neuroleptic-resistant schizophrenia: impact on risk-benefit assessment. Am J Psychiatry 152:183–190, 1995

Muller-Spahn F: Risperidone in the treatment of chronic schizophrenic patients: an international double-blind parallel-group study versus haloperidol. Clin Neuropharmacol 15 (suppl 1):90A–91A, 1992

Neborsky R, Janowsky D, Munson E, et al: Rapid treatment of acute psychotic symptoms with high- and low-dose haloperidol: behavioral considerations. Arch Gen Psychiatry 38:195–199, 1981

Overall JE, Gorham DR: The Brief Psychiatric Rating Scale. Psychol Rep 10:799–812, 1962

Peuskens J, Link CG: A comparison of quetiapine and chlorpromazine in the treatment of schizophrenia. Acta Psychiatr Scand 96:265–273, 1997

Pickar D, Owen RR, Litman RE, et al: Clinical and biologic response to clozapine in patients with schizophrenia: crossover comparison with fluphenazine. Arch Gen Psychiatry 49:345–353, 1992

Pietzcker A, Gaebel W, Kopcke W, et al: Intermittent versus maintenance neuroleptic long-term treatment in schizophrenia: 2-year results of German multicenter study. J Psychiatr Res 27:321–339, 1993

Pollack S, Woerner MG, Howard A, et al: Clozapine reduces rehospitalization among schizophrenia patients. Psychopharmacol Bull 34:89–92, 1998

Prien RF, Cole JO: High dose of chlorpromazine in chronic schizophrenia. Arch Gen Psychiatry 18:482–495, 1968

Quitkin F, Rifkin A, Klein D: Very high dosage vs standard dosage fluphenazine in schizophrenia: a double-blind study of non-chronic treatment-refractory patients. Arch Gen Psychiatry 32:1276–1281, 1975

Rifkin A, Doddi S, Karajgi B, et al: Dosage of haloperidol for schizophrenia. Arch Gen Psychiatry 48: 166–170, 1991

Rosenheck R, Cramer J, Xu W, et al: A comparison of clozapine and haloperidol in hospitalized patients with refractory schizophrenia. N Engl J Med 337:809–815, 1997

Saltz BL, Woerner M, Kane JM, et al: Prospective study of tardive dyskinesia incidence in the elderly. JAMA 266:2402–2406, 1991

Schooler N: Comparing new anti-psychotic medications: what do the data say? Paper presented at the annual meeting of the Society of Biological Psychiatry, Toronto, May 1998

Schooler NR, Keith SJ, Severe JB, et al: Relapse and rehospitalization during maintenance treatment of schizophrenia. Arch Gen Psychiatry 54:453–463, 1997

Shalev A, Hermash H, Rothberg J, et al: Poor neuroleptic response in acutely exacerbated schizophrenic patients. Acta Psychiatr Scand 87:86–91, 1993

Tollefson GD, Beasley CM Jr, Tamura RN, et al: Blind, controlled, long-term study of the comparative incidence of treatment-emergent tardive dyskinesia with olanzapine or haloperidol. Am J Psychiatry 154:1248–1254, 1997a

Tollefson GD, Beasley CM Jr, Tran PV, et al: Olanzapine versus haloperidol and the treatment of schizophrenia and schizoaffective and schizophreniform disorders: results of an international collaborative trial. Am J Psychiatry 154:457–465, 1997b

Tollefson GD, Sanger TM, Lou Y, et al: Depressive signs and symptoms in schizophrenia: a trial of olanzapine and haloperidol. Arch Gen Psychiatry 55:250–258, 1998

Tran PV, Hamilton SH, Kuntz AJ, et al: Double-blind comparison of olanzapine versus risperidone in the treatment of schizophrenia and other psychotic disorders. J Clin Psychopharmacol 17:407–418, 1997

Van Putten T, Marder SR, Mintz J: A controlled dose comparison of haloperidol in newly admitted schizophrenic patients. Arch Gen Psychiatry 47:754–758, 1990

Viguera AC, Baldessarini RJ, Hegarty JD, et al: Clinical risk following abrupt and gradual withdrawal of maintenance neuroleptic treatment. Arch Gen Psychiatry 54:49–55, 1997

Volavka J, Cooper T, Czobor P, et al: Haloperidol blood levels and clinical effects. Arch Gen Psychiatry 49:354–361, 1992

Weiden PJ, Olfson M: Cost of relapse in schizophrenia. Schizophr Bull 21:419–429, 1995

35

Individual Psychotherapies in Schizophrenia

Wayne S. Fenton, M.D.

For most patients with schizophrenia, optimal treatment includes both pharmacological and psychosocial care. Individual, group, and family psychotherapy and psychoeducation are treatment modalities that, combined with appropriate antipsychotic medication, can enhance patient outcome, functioning, and well-being. As described in the American Psychiatric Association's "Practice Guideline for the Treatment of Patients With Schizophrenia" (American Psychiatric Association 1997), therapeutic efforts to treat schizophrenia must be comprehensive, multimodal, and empirically tailored to the individual patient's response and progress. Thus, specific psychosocial therapies are prescribed based on illness phase and severity, patient and family interest and motivation, and overall availability of treatment resources. The coordination of psychosocial treatments with medications, rehabilitation, and treatment settings is ideally done by a psychiatrist who can provide continuity of care over what for patients will be a prolonged course of illness. As is true in medicine generally, the individual physician-patient relationship provides the foundation for treatment of the person with schizophrenia.

Individual Psychotherapy

Historical Review

Psychodynamic and biological conceptions of schizophrenia have yielded two distinct therapeutic traditions of insight-oriented and supportive psychotherapy, each associated with specific assumptions about the nature of schizophrenia and appropriate therapeutic strategies.

Insight-oriented psychotherapy originated in the 1930s as a modification of psychoanalysis (McGlashan 1983b). The goals of insight-oriented psychotherapy include both the elimination of symptoms and the durable reshaping of repetitive maladaptive interpersonal patterns. Treatment is expected to include a thorough examination of the patient's life history and past relationships, a careful review of the realities of the patient's current relationships, and the development of a shared understanding of the historical roots and current operation of the patient's maladaptive behaviors. It is assumed that important past experiences shaping the patient's difficulties can be understood only by examining their repetition in the present. For this reason, examining transference in the doctor-patient relationship is a major focus in insight-oriented psychotherapy. A basic mistrust of and expectation of harm from others is most often described as the central psychological difficulty of patients with schizophrenia, leading to either isolation and withdrawal or a false and overly compliant effort to think and act as others wish (Fromm-Reichmann 1950).

The techniques of supportive therapy have been less extensively described than those of insight-oriented treatments (Winston et al. 1986; Zahniser et al. 1991). Supportive psychotherapy is based on the medical model in which the patient is seen as suffering from an organically based illness. The goals of treatment focus on the stabilization of acute disequilibrium, the reduction of symptoms, the strengthening of defenses, and the preservation of healthy aspects of the patient's functioning. Tracking and targeting symptoms for pharmacological treatment is a major clinical task of supportive psychotherapy. The overall technical approach is pragmatic, as the physician (based on his or her own medical and psychiatric expertise) helps the patient understand and adapt to reality.

Research Perspectives

In the United States, although some form of individual therapy, in combination with medication, is often provided to patients with schizophrenia, relatively few rigorous trials help define the most effective approaches. Reflecting ideological rivalries, early studies compared medications with psychotherapy alone. Five randomized clinical trials conducted during the 1960s and 1970s provided little or no evidence for the efficacy of individual psychotherapy as the sole treatment for schizophrenia (Fairweather et al. 1960; Grinspoon et al. 1972; Karon and O'Grady 1969; Karon and VandenBos 1970; May 1968; Rogers et al. 1967). In these studies, medication-treated patients fared better whether or not psychotherapy was offered to nonmedication comparison groups. Two later trials, however, suggested an additive therapeutic effect when a problem-oriented psychotherapy was provided along with appropriate pharmacotherapy (Hogarty and Goldberg 1973; Hogarty et al. 1974a, 1974b, 1979). In addition, high rates of noncompliance and relapse among medication-treated patients focused continued attention on psychological and psychosocial issues affecting treatment outcome (Kane 1983).

During the 1980s, investigators compared the combination of medication treatment and either intensive insight-oriented individual therapy (three times per week) or reality-adaptive supportive psychotherapy (once a week) among newly discharged patients with schizophrenia. Neither treatment emerged as superior, and more than two-thirds of patients dropped out of each treatment over the 2-year trial. As actually practiced, the different therapeutic techniques tended to converge; both included significant supportive elements, and for both, patient improvement was associated with the therapist's demonstration of a sound dynamic attunement to the patient's psychological concerns (Frank and Gunderson 1990; Glass et al. 1989; Gunderson et al. 1984; Stanton et al. 1984). These data suggested that the distinction between supportive and insight-oriented therapy was not salient for schizophrenia and underscored the need for new approaches more responsive to the patient's needs. A number of investigators and clinicians advocated the use of a pragmatic and broad-based psychotherapy that relies at various times on supportive, directive, educational, investigative, and insight-oriented strategies applied flexibly, depending on the individual patient's type of schizophrenia and phase of illness (Carpenter 1986; Coursey 1989; Dingman and McGlashan 1989; Greenfeld 1985; Katz 1989; Munich 1987).

Recent research has created a firmer empirical basis for individual psychotherapy (Fenton 2000b). Two major trends are discernible: Hogarty and colleagues (1995) tested personal therapy (PT), a broad strategic outline for individual therapy that matches techniques with individual patient progress; investigators from the United Kingdom developed a number of time-limited psychotherapeutic interventions that target specific problems encountered by patients with schizophrenia.

PT is a disorder-specific individual psychotherapy that can accommodate individual patient differences yet be operationalized for empirical testing (Hogarty et al. 1995). PT was designed for newly discharged patients with schizophrenia and includes three levels, each with explicitly defined goals and corresponding interventions. Patients spend as much time at each level as they require to meet advancement criteria, and they progress to more demanding treatment levels only after earlier goals are achieved. Beginning with therapeutic joining, the treatment focuses progressively on illness awareness, stress management, problem solving, and enhanced social and work skills. In a 3-year randomized clinical trial, fewer than 10% of patients dropped out of treatment, and about half of patients progressed through the most advanced level of PT. Although the functioning of patients receiving other treatments plateaued after 1 year, PT patients continued to show gains in social adjustment and role performance over 3 years with no evidence of a plateau. When applied before residential stability was achieved, however, PT was associated with an elevated risk of relapse (Hogarty et al. 1997a, 1997b).

PT provides an outline for a broad multiyear treatment effort. In contrast, time-limited and focal cognitive-behavioral interventions developed in the United Kingdom are designed as additions to usual care and to target specific problems. Compliance therapy, based on motivational interviewing, is an effective four- to six-session intervention for acutely ill inpatients that targets improved attitude toward medication and postdischarge compliance as treatment goals (Kemp et al. 1996, 1998). Targeted cognitive-behavioral therapy (CBT) is based on the observation that patients are able to discover, learn, and use coping strategies to reduce symptom severity or distress (Garety et al. 2000). Among acutely ill inpatients, intensive CBT with postdischarge booster sessions has reduced the duration of acute psychosis and level of residual symptoms (Drury et al. 1996a, 1996b). Outpatient CBT programs have demonstrated efficacy in reducing severity and distress associated with medication-resistant symptoms (Sensky et al. 2000; Tarrier et al. 1993a, 1993b) as well as days spent in the hospital (Tarrier et al. 1998). Outpatient CBT is most useful for patients who have some insight and who identify symptoms as dysphoric or distressing. For these patients, CBT added to routine care yields clinical gains and is cost-effective (Garety et al. 1997; Kuipers et al. 1997, 1998).

Current Clinical Practice: Flexible Psychotherapy

Although the techniques employed in empirically tested individual psychotherapies differ based on the treatment's specific goals, all effective individual psychotherapies share the following characteristics: 1) schizophrenia is understood as a biologically based disorder that can be partially managed by learned and practiced coping strategies; 2) a stress-vulnerability model is used to explain symptoms and illness course; 3) establishing a therapeutic alliance is a prerequisite for all other activities; 4) understanding the patient's subjective experience and strengthening natural coping mechanisms are emphasized; 5) treatment is modified flexibly based on individual patient needs and capacities; and 6) all interventions presuppose that patients are receiving ongoing supportive care and management, including attention to pharmacological treatment, human services needs, and rehabilitation.

Flexible psychotherapy is a disorder-specific treatment approach informed by current scientific conceptions of schizophrenia and consistent with available empirical treatment studies. This approach can be outlined in terms of a set of assumptions concerning the nature of schizophrenia, a hierarchy of clinical tasks and interventions that are likely to be required during different phases of illness, and a set of general technical strategies with which the therapist aims to guide treatment and strengthen collaboration. In this context, the term "psychotherapy" is expanded to include a wide range of activities occurring within a physician-patient relationship that provides continuity of care over a period of time.

Assumptions Underlying Flexible Psychotherapy

Vulnerability-Stress Model

Flexible psychotherapy is based on the vulnerability-stress model. In this model, clinical schizophrenia is viewed as occurring in individuals with varying degrees of biologically based vulnerability, and the emergence and progression of symptoms and disabilities are seen as the product of a dynamic interaction between these vulnerabilities and environmental stress or challenges (Meehl 1962, 1990; Zubin and Spring 1977).

Putative biomedical determinants of the vulnerability to schizophrenia include genetic predisposition; viral infections of the central nervous system; and intrauterine, parturitional, or postnatal neurological trauma (Andreasen 1999). At a psychophysiological level, vulnerability indicators observed can include deficits in information processing, inability to maintain a steady focus of attention, and deficient sensory inhibition and autonomic responsivity (Braff 1993). At a behavioral level, this may be manifest as impairments in social competence; a tendency toward cognitive slippage, disorganization, and perceptual distortions; and general coping deficits such as overvaluing threat, underappraising abilities, and using denial extensively (Meehl 1990). Although a variety of vulnerabilities have been hypothesized, none has been shown to be ubiquitous, so different etiological and vulnerability factors are likely operative in different patients.

Vulnerability to schizophrenia is likely a set of stable traits that shape development before illness onset and are present during both acute episodes and periods of remission. Vulnerability, however, is modified over time by environmental influences. Thus, for example, a stress sufficient to cause a relapse at one time may be less likely to do so at a later point when new coping strategies have been learned or better social supports are in place.

The stress side of the vulnerability-stress model assumes that a variety of environmental stressors can promote the emergence or recurrence of symptoms in vulnerable persons by precipitating subclinical states of dysfunction such as information-processing overload or deficient processing of social cues. This dysfunction can further exacerbate existing stressors, creating a negative feedback loop that ends in a full-blown psychotic decompensation (Nuechterlein et al. 1992). Learned coping strategies, effective environmental problem solving, supportive psychosocial interventions, and antipsychotic medications can act as protective factors capable of interrupting this process.

The specific stresses associated with illness onset or exacerbation are often highly individualized. They may be primarily biochemical (e.g., stimulant or hallucinogen abuse), developmental (e.g., leaving for college, joining the armed forces), social (e.g., breakup with a girlfriend, family or work tensions), or environmental (e.g., poverty, unemployment, eviction).

Heterogeneity of Schizophrenia

Both schizophrenia and the populations diagnosed with it are heterogeneous, and for this reason a single therapeutic approach applied rigidly to all patients is inadequate. The clinical diversity of schizophrenia in relation to vulnerabilities, risk factors, and course suggests that the disorder is likely heterogeneous in etiology (Carpenter et al. 1993; Tsuang et al. 1990). Clinical heterogeneity is partially mapped by schizophrenia subtypes. Paranoid schizophrenia, for example, is characterized by good premorbid functioning, a rapid onset at a later age, frequent delusions and hallucinations, and less intellectual impairment. The illness tends to be intermittent over the first several years and is associated with a good probability of recovery or good functional outcome. In contrast, the deficit form of schizophrenia is characterized by impaired premorbid functioning; an early and insidious onset; and an enduring and progressive loss of interest, motivation, and emotional reactivity that frequently results in lifelong disability (Fenton and McGlashan 1991a, 1991b, 1994). Although clinical subtypes linked to specific etiologies have not yet been isolated, available subtypes do appear to identify illnesses of greater or lesser severity or virulence.

In addition to the illness being heterogeneous, persons with schizophrenia themselves differ widely in adaptive capacities, intelligence, instrumental and verbal competence, and personality styles and traits. In general, the more adaptive skills (e.g., education, work experience, social relationships, independent living) acquired before illness onset, the greater the likelihood of maintaining or regaining functioning after the illness is established (Fenton and McGlashan 1987). For some patients, poor premorbid functioning may represent the product of the lifelong vulnerability to schizophrenia. For others, a severe form of schizophrenia may irreversibly erode good premorbid skills. Other patients with good premorbid abilities may fully maintain their skills and competence after or between episodes.

The manner in which individual differences in personality styles and traits are likely to influence the course of the illness has not yet been adequately investigated (Smith et al. 1993). Obsessive-compulsive symptoms, for example, are frequently associated with a poorer long-term course, whereas comorbid schizotypal or borderline features predict better long-term outcome (Fenton and McGlashan 1986; McGlashan 1983a, 1986). In addition, the presence of comorbid substance abuse has short- and long-term treatment implications (Drake et al. 1998; Turner and Tsuang 1990).

Phasic Illness Course

Schizophrenia symptoms and vulnerabilities are not static but in most cases develop, progress, and retreat through illness phases. Although systematic studies in this area are scarce, illness phases may include 1) prodromal periods during which an individual-specific constellation of symptoms that signals imminent clinical decompensation emerges; 2) acute or active phases associated with florid positive symptoms superimposed on preexisting deficits; 3) subacute or convalescent phases characterized by a lessening of positive symptoms, modest restoration of functioning, and, at times, postpsychotic depression; 4) moratoriums or adaptive plateaus characterized by the gradual restitution of identity and strengthening of confidence and skills; 5) change points representing shifts in functioning over a short time period that are self-motivated or initiated by others and carry the potential for either significant improvement or relapse; and 6) stable plateaus or end states characterized by enduring periods of stability that can range from complete remissions to residual states with varying degrees of fixed deficits and/or persistent positive symptoms (Strauss et al. 1985).

Clinical Tasks and Interventions

The clinical tasks, interventions, and goals required for the comprehensive treatment of schizophrenia are outlined in Table 35–1. All of the interventions aim to minimize the effect of vulnerabilities, strengthen adaptive capacities, and reduce the extent and effects of stress. The key question becomes the selection of interventions appropriate for a particular patient at a particular phase of illness. Although the therapeutic tasks can be ordered hierarchically in a way that roughly links goals and interventions to illness phase, in practice the psychotherapist should be prepared on short notice to shift gears based on changing circumstances and patient needs.

Although many of its tasks and interventions overlap with the areas of expertise of other service providers, this model assumes that an individual psychotherapist who is a psychiatrist is best suited to integrate the assessments and treatment interventions required at various times. This integration requires a thorough grounding in the psychopharmacology and the biological aspects of mental illness; the psychodynamics of schizophrenia; entitlement programs; and locally available medical, human services, and rehabilitative treatment resources. Although other professionals may be relied on to accomplish specific tasks, the physician-therapist should take an active interest in and consider himself or herself responsible for ensuring the results of these efforts. A narrow focus on psychopharmacological or psychological issues, for example, without attention to human services needs or a lack of environmental structure is inadequate.

Schizophrenia severity and subtype, the patient's premorbid functioning, and the patient's self-defined treatment goals are all relevant to the determination of appropriate treatment tasks. Establishing a supportive, ongoing treatment within a sheltered setting that minimizes stress and provides for basic human needs and asylum for an indefinite period is a humane and realistic goal for patients with severe hebephrenic and/or deficit forms of schizophrenia. For the majority of patients who reside in the community, some degree of psychoeducation and rehabilitation tasks should be achievable, with the aim of promoting

TABLE 35–1. Hierarchy of clinical tasks in the psychotherapy of schizophrenia

Clinical tasks	Psychiatric-medical stabilization	Psychosocial case management	Establishment of ongoing supportive treatment	Psychoeducation	Rehabilitation tasks	Insight-oriented tasks
Illness phase	Prodromal, onset, exacerbation, or relapse	Subacute and convalescence	Moratorium or adaptive plateau	Moratorium or change point	Stable plateaus	Selected patients with well-established stability
Clinical focus	1. Crisis intervention	1. Stresses and vulnerabilities	1. Treatment relationship and alliance	1. Understanding and acceptance of illness	1. Social, vocational, and self-care skills	1. Conflicts
	2. Medical and psychiatric diagnosis	2. Social supports	2. Mistrust, isolation, denial, suspiciousness	2. Human concerns associated with loss of functioning	2. Learning or relearning	2. Motivation
	3. Safety	3. Living arrangements	3. Damage to self-esteem	3. Self-management of illness	3. Establishment of realistic expectations	3. Interpersonal difficulties
	4. Acute symptom stabilization	4. Daily activities			4. Adaptation to deficits	4. Transference/ countertransference
		5. Economic resources			5. Recognition of fears and ambivalence	
Interventions	1. Psychiatric, medical, and neurological evaluation	1. Psychosocial evaluation	1. Continued medication	1. Support and teaching	1. Attention to details of self-care as well as social and work functioning	1. Discussion of feelings, fantasies, and conflicts
	2. Short-term psychopharmacological treatment	2. Evaluation of human services needs	2. Attention to side effects, complaints	2. Identification of individual-specific stresses	2. Modeling and encouraging the practice of new skills	2. Focus on meanings, past events, and life history

TABLE 35–1. Hierarchy of clinical tasks in the psychotherapy of schizophrenia *(continued)*

Clinical tasks	Psychiatric-medical stabilization	Psychosocial case management	Establishment of ongoing supportive treatment	Psychoeducation	Rehabilitation tasks	Insight-oriented tasks
Interventions *(continued)*	3. Supportive and directive communication	3. Linkage with social services, human services, and community treatment agencies	3. Direct assistance with situational problems	3. Identification of individual-specific prodromal and active symptoms	3. Direct intervention with family and/or employers	3. Examination of relationship with therapist (e.g., transference, countertransference
	4. Limit setting		4. Assertive outreach	4. Determination of lowest effective prophylactic medication dosage	4. Cognitive and/or social skills enhancement	4. Interpretation
			5. Reassurance, supporting defenses, positive regard		5. Support verbal rather than behavioral expression of fear or ambivalence	5. Possibly intermittent medication strategy
			6. Promotion of comfort with therapist and treatment		6. Maintenance medication	
Treatment goals	1. Rule out medical and neurological disorders	1. Assess and mobilize social support	1. Establish comfortable treatment routine	1. Collaborative self-monitoring and management of illness	1. Promote improvement in self-care as well as social and vocational skills	1. Construction of narrative life history
	2. Ensure patient safety	2. Ensure access to all appropriate entitlements	2. Promote trust in therapist and treatment	2. Self-recognition of prodromal symptoms	2. Encourage activities that enhance self-esteem through accomplishment and productivity	2. Working through of conflicts

TABLE 35–1. Hierarchy of clinical tasks in the psychotherapy of schizophrenia *(continued)*

Clinical tasks	Psychiatric-medical stabilization	Psychosocial case management	Establishment of ongoing supportive treatment	Psychoeducation	Rehabilitation tasks	Insight-oriented tasks
Treatment goals *(continued)*	3. Minimize impact of acute illness on life situation	3. Assess postepisode psychosocial service needs	3. Encourage sufficient acceptance of illness to allow cooperation with treatment	3. Coping strategies for managing stress	3. Help patient support highest level of functioning possible	3. Improved capacity for intimacy and productivity
	4. Effect rapid symptom reduction	4. Enlist cooperation of family or other caregivers	4. Support strengths	4. Avoidance of relapse	4. Encourage activities that improve quality of life	4. Integrating psychotic experience into expanded self-conception
			5. Monitor for relapse	5. Establishment of maintenance medication regimen		5. Help patient learn strategies to function despite deficits
Professional collaboration	1. Inpatient treatment team	1. Social work	1. Community support staff	1. Group therapist	1. Group therapist	1. Generally implies substantial progress in accomplishment and consolidation of earlier goals and tasks
	2. Residential alternatives to hospitalization	2. Health and human services intake personnel	2. Family	2. Self-help groups	2. Rehabilitation personnel, job coach	2. Separate psychopharmacologist, social worker, and/or family therapist sometimes useful

TABLE 35–1. Hierarchy of clinical tasks in the psychotherapy of schizophrenia *(continued)*

Clinical tasks	Psychiatric-medical stabilization	Psychosocial case management	Establishment of ongoing supportive treatment	Psychoeducation	Rehabilitation tasks	Insight-oriented tasks
Professional collaboration *(continued)*	3. Community crisis intervention team	3. Day treatment or community sup-port staff	3. Social service providers	3. Behavior therapist using educational models	3. Social, vocational, and self-care training providers	
	4. Internist			4. Family support groups	4. Family, employers, community support staff	
	5.Neurologist					

maximal functioning and quality of life while decreasing the frequency of relapses. A primary focus on the insight-oriented tasks is reserved for selected highly interested and motivated patients once clinical stability has been securely established.

Initiation of Psychotherapy

When scheduling an initial visit for a patient with schizophrenia, the therapist should set aside sufficient time (not uncommonly 2 hours) to conduct a thorough preliminary assessment. When the referral is initiated over the phone by someone other than the patient, it is useful to use this phone contact to gather enough clinical information to obtain a rough outline of the patient's history and current clinical status. Information about current and past suicidality and aggression, current symptom severity, and current medications should be sought with the aim of anticipating whether outpatient evaluation can proceed safely. If the patient initiates the appointment by phone, a brief preliminary phone conversation can be used to evaluate (albeit quite tentatively) the patient's condition before the first visit. If, based on these preliminary contacts, the need for hospitalization or short-term care in a nonhospital alternative setting appears possible, before the initial visit the physician should obtain specific knowledge concerning what short-term care resources the patient is eligible to access.

Patients with schizophrenia will often arrive for a first appointment accompanied by a family member, case manager, or other caregiver. After introduction to the patient and those arriving with him or her, the therapist may conduct the initial interview with the patient alone. Recognizing that the vulnerabilities associated with schizophrenia may make the initial meeting particularly anxiety-provoking for such patients, the therapist may need to make active efforts to attend to the patient's comfort by, for example, offering coffee, pointing out the specific place to sit, outlining what material will be discussed, and, if necessary, patterning the assessment interview with a specific set of questions. With the patient's permission, it will often be of value to then spend some time alone interviewing the accompanying family member or other caregiver. This interview can provide important additional information about the patient's situation and allow the person accompanying the patient to express specific concerns or worries in private.

By the end of the initial interview, a preliminary assessment across each of the major areas outlined in Table 35–1 should be accomplished. Areas that should be assessed include the following: 1) the need for further acute medical or psychiatric evaluation and stabilization; 2) the environmental supports available to the patient; 3) the patient's capacity to collaborate in treatment; 4) the patient's cognitive understanding of his or her illness and the the patient's ability to identify and self-manage symptoms; 5) the patient's strengths and weaknesses relating to social, vocational, and self-care skills and the patient's hopes and aspirations for the future; and 6) the role of damage to the patient's self-esteem from loss of functioning or stigma, interpersonal difficulties, and psychodynamic conflicts in the patient's current state.

A mutually agreed-upon plan for further assessment and/or treatment will ideally be the outcome of the initial visit. This plan should include the frequency and duration of visits, payment, medication regimen, and arrangements for the patient and/or other caregivers to reach the physician should an emergency arise between scheduled visits. Attention should be given to practical matters such as how the patient will get to the physician's office for follow-up visits and how and where prescriptions will be filled. If psychotherapy is recommended, it should not be assumed that the patient knows what this entails, so a general statement (e.g., "We will meet so that we can talk together, better understand your difficulties, and work with you on your medications to improve your situation") may be in order.

In addition to setting the stage for establishing a working relationship with the patient, the physician's management of the initial interviews should promote collaboration with the patient's family member(s), case manager, or other caregiver. Both the patient and the caregiver may be told that the patient's confidentiality will be respected, but that should the physician at any time believe a relapse is imminent or a dangerous situation is developing, the help of family and/or other caregivers will be solicited. Family members may be encouraged to contact the physician should they develop concerns, and the frequency of future family contacts might be outlined. The importance of the family's and/or caregiver's support to the outcome of treatment cannot be overestimated. This support will most likely be extended to a clinician who is felt to be empathic, responsive to family or caregiver concerns, and available. Many studies show that family psychoeducation is effective for reducing relapse in outpatients with schizophrenia, but these programs are not widely available in most mental health systems (Lehman and Steinwachs 1998). The physician-psychotherapist will need to assume responsibility for family education when professional or family-led psychoeducational programs are inaccessible.

Weekly psychotherapy visits for 45–50 minutes are most common in an outpatient setting, but the frequency of visits may be increased during periods of clinical instability or if insight-oriented psychotherapy is prescribed. Less frequent visits of shortened duration may be negotiated during periods of stability for patients who have learned to self-manage their illness or for those who find contact with a physician aversive, disorganizing, or irrelevant. The frequency and duration of psychotherapy are individualized. In most instances the tone of psychotherapy should be conversational. Free association is discouraged because many patients with schizophrenia already have difficulty screening marginal thoughts and fantasies from consciousness. Similarly, neutrality or excessive reticence on the part of the therapist is discouraged because it can easily be mistaken by the patient for indifference or dislike. A reasonable degree of self-disclosure on the therapist's part can help the patient assess the therapist as a person and can counter a patient's tendency toward excessive transference or distortion.

General Technical Strategies

The clinical focus of psychotherapy at any given time will be largely determined by the immediate problems facing the patient and by his or her progress in achieving the hierarchy of treatment goals outlined in Table 35–1. A set of general technical strategies that guide interventions in pursuit of these treatment goals have been articulated by Dingman and McGlashan (1989) as follows:

1. *Evaluation.* As described above, a thorough evaluation guides the treatment process during all illness phases. Initial medical and psychiatric evaluation include assessment of the role of identifiable physical conditions, accurate psychiatric diagnosis, assessment of dangerousness, determination of competence to consent to treatment, and evaluation of the responsiveness of symptoms to acute pharmacological treatment. If psychoeducational, rehabilitative, and investigative interventions will be used, an assessment of the patient's cognitive strengths and deficits will allow the therapist to design interventions that match the patient's cognitive capacities, interests, and personality style.

2. *Continuous reevaluation*. The phasic course of schizophrenia and the individual's changing adaptation to illness over time compel periodic reassessment of course, prognosis, phase of illness, and target problems. Providing concrete assistance with transportation may be helpful early to facilitate a stable ongoing treatment but later may promote unwarranted dependency and prolong disability. Longitudinal research has demonstrated the potential for improved functioning even among patients who have been ill for many years (Harding 1988), so illness chronicity should not be a rationalization for failure to conduct periodic reassessments of treatment needs and goals (McGlashan 1988).
3. *Timing*. Changes in the vulnerability of patients with schizophrenia over time require attention when particular therapeutic tasks are attempted. For many patients, to minimize stress and avoid relapse, relatively little beyond assessment, stabilization on medication, mobilization of social support, and establishment of supportive, ongoing treatment should be attempted during the first 6–12 months after an acute episode. When the patient is asymptomatic and shows signs of improved energy and concentration, vulnerability to relapse may be diminished and complex psychoeducational and rehabilitative elements may be introduced gradually.
4. *Titration*. Treatment interventions should be used with graded increases in intensity and complexity. In general, higher-level therapeutic tasks should be attempted only after completion and consolidation of earlier gains. Substantial rehabilitation efforts, for example, will rarely be possible until acute symptoms are stabilized and a supportive relationship is established. Treatment changes involving medication, housing, work, schooling, or psychosocial program participation, when indicated, should be pursued cautiously, modifying only one element at a time.
5. *Integration with psychopharmacology*. Each of the tasks of individual therapy outlined in Table 35–1 assumes the necessity of acute and prophylactic antipsychotic drugs for most patients. Decisions regarding pharmacological management will often be linked to the accomplishment of other psychotherapeutic tasks. Establishment of an ongoing treatment relationship and considerable psychoeducation, for example, should be accomplished before attempting maintenance medication reduction, initiation of a targeted (intermittent) medication strategy, or outpatient use of medications requiring frequent laboratory monitoring. Depot antipsychotics may be required for patients who are only tentatively able to maintain a supportive treatment relationship.

The Therapeutic Relationship

The quality of the physician's relationship with the patient will often be a major determinant of the success or failure of the overall treatment effort. Because of the patient's suspiciousness, withdrawal, and/or overwhelming ambivalence about human attachments, establishing a relationship with a patient with schizophrenia may be unusually difficult. The clinical literature in this area supports a number of general recommendations:

- A consistent, direct, and straightforward manner is advocated, whereas aloofness, rigidity, and an overly authoritarian posture are discouraged. A basic respect for the patient and curiosity in learning what the illness means to the patient should form the core of the physician's attitude. Such an attitude will often reveal that the patient's basic aspirations—to work and feel productive, to have family and friends, and to experience some measure of satisfaction—are similar to the physician's (Dingman and McGlashan 1989).

- Active and assertive efforts to build and maintain a relationship are often required and call for flexibility and resourcefulness on the therapist's part. The expectation that the patient can attend regularly scheduled psychotherapy sessions and collaborate with treatment will often be a goal, rather than a starting point, of treatment. Actively promoting the patient's comfort with the therapist by discussing neutral topics of shared interest; engaging in walks or playing games (e.g., cards, checkers); or providing concrete assistance with tasks such as banking, filling prescriptions, grocery shopping, or filling out forms may be useful early on in promoting a relationship. Similarly, actively structuring the content of therapy sessions by narrowing the focus and eliciting concrete details about the patient's current functioning and life situation may be of value. In outpatient settings, particularly early in the course of treatment, missed appointments should be anticipated and should be followed up with outreach efforts, including phone calls and/or home visits. A reminder phone call in advance of appointments may be required for some time.
- Persistence, patience, and the capacity to tolerate intense affects and ambiguous communication should characterize the therapist's approach. Excessive therapeutic zeal and unrealistic expectations for rapid and dramatic improvement will most often lead to disappointment. The therapist should communicate a willingness to "stick with" the patient through inevitable fluctuations associated with the illness's course. In this context, as in most psychotherapeutic work, recognizing and tolerating rather than acting on countertransference become important. It is not uncommon, for example, for a patient's initial indifference to engender a feeling of boredom or hopelessness in the therapist, for a patient's suspiciousness or accusations to generate feelings of defensiveness, or for a patient's noncompliance to provoke irritation or the impulse to abandon the patient. Steadfastness in these situations will often operate over time to consolidate a sense of working together toward common goals and provide a model for persisting in the face of adversity with which the patient may identify. At the same time, the therapist should be prepared, if needed, to set limits that unambiguously indicate that both his or her own and the patient's safety and self-interest will be protected.
- Many persons with schizophrenia are crisis-prone, and crises will not be confined to regular working hours. Ideally, the therapist—but when not possible, another treatment team member—should be available for crisis management. Because treatment at differing levels of care will often be required, to the extent possible the administrative context of the therapist's practice should allow continuity across inpatient or residential alternative, day treatment, and outpatient care settings. Fragmented systems that assign a different therapist based on treatment site disrupt the continuity of care. Thus, the therapist's versatility should include comfort both in using a range of interventions and in working in a variety of settings.

Suicide

Suicide is probably the single leading cause of premature death among persons with schizophrenia, with long-term rates of suicide estimated to be 10%–13% in this population (Caldwell and Gottesman 1990). Distressingly often, suicide in schizophrenia seems to occur "out of the blue" without prior warning or expressions of verbal intent (Breier and Astrachan 1984). Some data suggest that patients with the best prognosis for recovery (those with paranoid schizophrenia) can paradoxically also be at highest risk for suicide (Fenton and McGlashan 1997). These patients frequently declined from a higher level of premorbid functioning and had an intermittent illness that during periods of remission allowed them to retain the capacity to reflect on their life situation and illness. In the context of individual psychotherapy, these findings point to the importance of attunement to the human aspects of adapting to a severe and recurrent illness, including the potential for despair, damage to self-esteem, and hopelessness. An overall effort to assist the patient to acknowledge, bear, and put painful emotions and life experiences into perspective is frequently advocated, particularly for patients who recover from an episode with insight and recognition of what has happened (Rako and Mazer 1980). Specific recommendations for suicide prevention include recognizing actuarially defined high-risk patients (i.e., male; young; those with concurrent depression, recent loss or rejection, history of suicide attempts, limited external support), providing additional support during high-risk periods (e.g., immediately after hospital discharge), actively eliciting and searching for suicidal ideation, and utilizing specific targeted psychopharmacological and psychosocial interventions for comorbid depression and substance abuse (Fenton 2000a).

Medication Compliance

Medication noncompliance is common in illnesses for which long-term maintenance treatment is required, the medications cause uncomfortable side effects, and discontinuing medication makes the patient initially feel better (Diamond 1984). Rates of noncompliance in schizophrenia may be as high as 75% over several years of treatment (Corrigan et al. 1990). The assessment of noncompliance must be individualized and include attention to 1) patient-related factors (lack of insight, grandiosity, substance abuse comorbidity, disorganization, forgetfulness); 2) medication-related factors (dysphoric side effects, subtherapeutic or excessively high dosages, realistic concerns about side effects, overly complex regimens); 3) environment-related factors (inadequate support or supervision, practical problems such as lack of money or transportation, unappealing clinic settings); and 4) clinician-related factors (poor therapeutic alliance) (Fenton et al. 1997). The patient's health beliefs and the psychological meanings attached by the patient to medication are important considerations. The psychological meaning of medications is varied. For severely ill patients, global denial of illness or paranoid suspiciousness and fear of being poisoned or controlled may be operative. After the loss of control associated with acute psychosis, medications may be seized upon as one of the few potential ways to regain independence and control over aspects of one's life. A view of mental illness and the necessity of medication as a sign of weakness or moral inadequacy may be held by the patient and/or family and friends. For some patients, the removal of psychotic symptoms may be accompanied by intense shame, loneliness, and the need to face painful realities so that the return to a state of ego-syntonic psychosis is a serious temptation. For others, noncompliance can be related to the displacement of anger toward the therapist or family, can communicate that expectations are too high, or can express unconscious ambivalence or fear about increases in functioning, such as living independently or working. Psychodynamic factors such as these are often operative when patients discontinue medication immediately before taking a major step forward such as moving out of the hospital or beginning a job.

The psychotherapist should assume that most patients at some time will take more or less medication than prescribed and should work toward creation of a therapeutic relationship in which such experimentation can be openly discussed rather than hidden. Showing an active interest in medication by asking how much is being taken and attending to side effects is of value. During periods of clinical stability, allowing patients to self-regulate medication dosage within bounds can substantially enhance the therapeutic alliance (Diamond 1984). When denial is a major factor, enlisting the assistance of family and friends and arranging for the supervision of medication taking can be useful. When incorrect beliefs about mental illness are judged to be operative, psychoeducation with the patient, family, and friends is called for. When disorganization or cognitive deficits interfere with compliance, specific behavioral interventions can be of value (Corrigan et al. 1990; Falloon 1984). Dynamic exploration, attention to transference, and interpretation will be required when unconscious anger, fear, or ambivalence is judged to interfere with pharmacological treatment.

References

American Psychiatric Association: Practice guideline for the treatment of patients with schizophrenia. Am J Psychiatry 154 (4 suppl):1–63, 1997

Andreasen NC: A unitary model of schizophrenia: Bleuler's "fragmented phrene" as schizencephaly. Arch Gen Psychiatry 56:781–790, 1999

Braff DL: Information processing and attention dysfunctions in schizophrenia. Schizophr Bull 19:233–259, 1993

Breier A, Astrachan BM: Characterization of schizophrenic patients who commit suicide. Am J Psychiatry 141:206–209, 1984

Caldwell CB, Gottesman II: Schizophrenics kill themselves too: a review of risk factors for suicide. Schizophr Bull 16:571–589, 1990

Carpenter WT Jr: Thoughts on the treatment of schizophrenia. Schizophr Bull 12:527–539, 1986

Carpenter WT Jr, Buchanan RW, Kirkpatrick B, et al: Strong inference, theory testing, and the neuroanatomy of schizophrenia. Arch Gen Psychiatry 50:825–831, 1993

Corrigan PW, Liberman RP, Engel JD: From noncompliance to collaboration in the treatment of schizophrenia. Hospital and Community Psychiatry 41:1203–1211, 1990

Coursey RD: Psychotherapy with persons suffering from schizophrenia: the need for a new agenda. Schizophr Bull 15:349–353, 1989

Diamond RJ: Increasing medication compliance in young adult chronic psychiatric patients. New Dir Ment Health Serv 21:59–69, 1984

Dingman CW, McGlashan TH: Psychotherapy, in A Clinical Guide for the Treatment of Schizophrenia. Edited by Bellack AS. New York, Plenum, 1989, pp 263–282

Drake RE, Mercer-McFadden C, Mueser KT, et al: Review of integrated mental health and substance abuse treatment for patients with dual diagnosis. Schizophr Bull 24:589–608, 1998

Drury V, Birchwood M, Cochrane R, et al: Cognitive therapy and psychosis: a controlled trial, II: impact on recovery time. Br J Psychiatry 169:602–607, 1996a

Drury V, Birchwood M, Cochrane R, et al: Cognitive therapy and recovery from acute psychosis: a controlled trial, I: impact of psychotic symptoms. Br J Psychiatry 169:593–601, 1996b

Fairweather GW, Simon R, Gebhard ME, et al: Relative effectiveness of psychotherapeutic programs: a multi-criterial comparison of four programs for the three different patient groups. Psychological Monographs 74 (No 492):1–26, 1960

Falloon IRH: Developing and maintaining adherence to long-term drug-taking regimens. Schizophr Bull 10:412–417, 1984

Fenton WS: Depression, suicide and suicide prevention in schizophrenia. Suicide Life Threat Behav 30:34–49, 2000a

Fenton WS: Evolving perspectives on individual psychotherapy for schizophrenia. Schizophr Bull 26:47–72, 2000b

Fenton WS, McGlashan TH: The prognostic significance of obsessive-compulsive symptoms in schizophrenia. Am J Psychiatry 143:437–441, 1986

Fenton WS, McGlashan TH: Prognostic scale for chronic schizophrenia. Schizophr Bull 13:277–286, 1987

Fenton WS, McGlashan TH: Natural history of schizophrenia subtypes, I: longitudinal study of paranoid, hebephrenic, and undifferentiated schizophrenia. Arch Gen Psychiatry 48:969–977, 1991a

Fenton WS, McGlashan TH: Natural history of schizophrenia subtypes, II: positive and negative symptoms and long-term course. Arch Gen Psychiatry 48:978–986, 1991b

Fenton WS, McGlashan TH: Antecedents, symptom progression and long-term outcome of the deficit syndrome. Am J Psychiatry 151:351–356, 1994

Fenton WS, McGlashan TH: Symptoms, subtype and suicidality in patients with schizophrenia spectrum disorders. Am J Psychiatry 154:199–204, 1997

Fenton WS, Blyler CB, Heinssen RK: Determinants of medication compliance in schizophrenia. Schizophr Bull 23:637–651, 1997

Frank AF, Gunderson JG: The role of the therapeutic alliance in the treatment of schizophrenia. Arch Gen Psychiatry 47:228–236, 1990

Fromm-Reichmann F: Principles of Intensive Psychotherapy. Chicago, IL, University of Chicago Press, 1950

Garety PA, Fowler D, Kuipers E, et al: London–East Anglia randomized controlled trial of cognitive-behavioural therapy for psychosis, II: predictors of outcome. Br J Psychiatry 171:420–426, 1997

Garety PA, Fowler D, Kuipers E: Cognitive-behavioural therapy for medication-resistant symptoms. Schizophr Bull 26:73–86, 2000

Glass LL, Katz HM, Schnitzer RD, et al: Psychotherapy of schizophrenia: an empirical investigation of the relationship of process to outcome. Am J Psychiatry 146:603–608, 1989

Greenfeld D: The Psychotic Patient: Medication and Psychotherapy. New York, Free Press, 1985

Grinspoon L, Ewalt JR, Shader RI: Schizophrenia: Pharmacotherapy and Psychotherapy. Baltimore, MD, Williams & Wilkins, 1972

Gunderson JG, Frank AF, Katz HM, et al: Effects of psychotherapy in schizophrenia, II: comparative outcome of two forms of treatment. Schizophr Bull 10:564–598, 1984

Harding CM: Course types in schizophrenia: an analysis of European and American studies. Schizophr Bull 14:633–643, 1988

Hogarty GE, Goldberg SC: Drugs and sociotherapy in the aftercare of schizophrenic patients: one-year relapse rates. Arch Gen Psychiatry 28:54–64, 1973

Hogarty GE, Goldberg SC, Schooler NR, et al: Drug and sociotherapy in the aftercare of schizophrenic patients, II: two-year relapse rates. Arch Gen Psychiatry 31:603–608, 1974a

Hogarty GE, Goldberg SC, Schooler NR: Drug and sociotherapy in the aftercare of schizophrenic patients, III: adjustment of non-relapsed patients. Arch Gen Psychiatry 31:609–618, 1974b

Hogarty GE, Schooler NR, Urlich RF, et al: Fluphenazine and social therapy in the aftercare of schizophrenic patients: relapse analysis of a two-year controlled study of fluphenazine decanoate and fluphenazine hydrochloride. Arch Gen Psychiatry 36:1283–1294, 1979

Hogarty GE, Kornblith SJ, Greenwald D, et al: Personal therapy: a disorder-relevant psychotherapy for schizophrenia. Schizophr Bull 21:379–393, 1995

Hogarty GE, Greenwald D, Urlich RF, et al: Three year trials of personal therapy among schizophrenic patients living with or independent of family, II: effects on adjustment of patients. Am J Psychiatry 154:1514–1524, 1997a

Hogarty GE, Kornblith SJ, Greenwald D, et al: Three year trials of personal therapy among schizophrenic patients living with or independent of family, I: description of study and effects on relapse rates. Am J Psychiatry 154:1504–1513, 1997b

Kane JM: Problems of compliance in the outpatient treatment of schizophrenia. J Clin Psychiatry 44 (6 pt 2):3–6, 1983

Karon BP, O'Grady B: Intellectual test changes in schizophrenic patients in the first six months of treatment. Psychotherapy: Theory, Research and Practice 6:88–96, 1969

Karon BP, VandenBos GR: Experience, medication, and the effectiveness of psychotherapy with schizophrenics: a note on Drs. May and Tuma's conclusions. Br J Psychiatry 116:427–428, 1970

Katz HM: A new agenda for psychotherapy of schizophrenia: response to Coursey. Schizophr Bull 15:355–359, 1989

Kemp R, Haywood P, Applewhaite G, et al: Compliance therapy in psychotic patients: a randomized controlled trial. BMJ 312:345–349, 1996

Kemp R, Kirov G, Everitt P, et al: Randomised controlled trial of compliance therapy: 18 month follow-up. Br J Psychiatry 172:413–419, 1998

Kuipers E, Garety P, Fowler D, et al: London–East Anglia randomized controlled trial of cognitive-behavioural therapy for psychosis, I: effects on the treatment phase. Br J Psychiatry 171:319–327, 1997

Kuipers E, Fowler D, Garety P, et al: London–East Anglia randomized trial of cognitive-behavioural therapy for psychosis, III: evaluation and economic evaluation at 18 months. Br J Psychiatry 173:61–68, 1998

Lehman AF, Steinwachs DM: Patterns of usual care for schizophrenia: initial results from the Schizophrenia Patient Outcomes Research Team (PORT) Client Survey. Schizophr Bull 24:11–20, 1998

May PRA: Treatment of Schizophrenia: A Comparative Study of Five Treatment Methods. New York, Science House, 1968

McGlashan TH: The borderline syndrome, II: is it a variant of schizophrenia or affective disorder? Arch Gen Psychiatry 40:1319–1323, 1983a

McGlashan TH: Intensive individual psychotherapy of schizophrenia: a review of techniques. Arch Gen Psychiatry 40:909–920, 1983b

McGlashan TH: Schizotypal personality disorder: Chestnut Lodge follow-up study, VI: long-term follow-up perspectives. Arch Gen Psychiatry 43:329–334, 1986

McGlashan TH: A selective review of recent North American long-term followup studies of schizophrenia. Schizophr Bull 14:515–542, 1988

Meehl PE: Schizotaxia, schizotypy, schizophrenia. Am Psychol 17:827–838, 1962

Meehl PE: Toward an integrated theory of schizotaxia, schizotypy, and schizophrenia. J Personal Disord 4:1–9, 1990

Munich RL: Conceptual trends and issues in the psychotherapy of schizophrenia. Am J Psychother 61:23–37, 1987

Nuechterlein KH, Dawson ME, Gitlin M, et al: Developmental processes in schizophrenic disorders: longitudinal studies of vulnerability and stress. Schizophr Bull 18:387–425, 1992

Rako S, Mazer H: Semrad: The Heart of a Therapist. New York, Jason Aronson, 1980

Rogers CR, Gendlin EG, Kiesler DJ, et al (eds): The Therapeutic Relationship and Its Impact: Study of Psychotherapy With Schizophrenics. Madison, WI, University of Wisconsin Press, 1967

Sensky T, Turkington D, Kingdon D, et al: A randomized controlled trial of cognitive-behavioral therapy for persistent symptoms in schizophrenia resistant to medication. Arch Gen Psychiatry 57:165–172, 2000

Smith TE, Deutsch A, Schwartz F, et al: The role of personality in treatment of schizophrenic and schizoaffective disorder inpatients: a pilot study. Bull Menninger Clin 57:88–99, 1993

Stanton AH, Gunderson JG, Knapp PH, et al: Effects of psychotherapy in schizophrenia, I: design and implementation of a controlled study. Schizophr Bull 10:520–551, 1984

Strauss JS, Hafez H, Lieberman P, et al: The course of psychiatric disorder, III: longitudinal principles. Am J Psychiatry 142:289–296, 1985

Tarrier N, Beckett R, Harwood S, et al: A trial of two cognitive-behavioural methods of treating drug-resistant residual psychotic symptoms in schizophrenic patients, I: outcome. Br J Psychiatry 162:524–532, 1993a

Tarrier N, Sharpe L, Beckett R, et al: A trial of two cognitive-behavioural methods of treating drug-resistant residual psychotic symptoms in schizophrenic patients, II: treatment-specific changes in coping and problem-solving skills. Soc Psychiatry Psychiatr Epidemiol 28:5–10, 1993b

Tarrier N, Yusupoff L, Kinney C, et al: Randomised controlled trial of intensive cognitive behavior therapy for patients with chronic schizophrenia. BMJ 317:303–307, 1998

Tsuang MT, Lyons MJ, Faraone SV: Heterogeneity of schizophrenia: conceptual models and analytic strategies. Br J Psychiatry 156:17–266, 1990

Turner WM, Tsuang MT: Impact of substance abuse on the course and outcome of schizophrenia. Schizophr Bull 16:87–95, 1990

Winston A, Pinsker H, McCullough L: A review of supportive psychotherapy. Hospital and Community Psychiatry 37:1105–1114, 1986

Zahniser JH, Coursey RD, Hershberger K: Individual psychotherapy with schizophrenic outpatients in the public mental health system. Hospital and Community Psychiatry 42:906–913, 1991

Zubin J, Spring B: Vulnerability—a new view of schizophrenia. J Abnorm Psychol 86:103–126, 1977

36

Group and Family Psychotherapies in Schizophrenia

Stephen A. Cole, M.D., A.M.

Group Therapy

Persons with schizophrenia have deficits in attention focusing, information processing, and concept formation that can be remediated through cognitive, communication, and problem-solving training in group settings (Brenner et al. 1989; van den Bosch et al. 1992). Participation in interaction-oriented group therapy can assist isolated patients with schizophrenia to generate supportive social networks (Wallace 1984).

Group therapy was originally developed to enhance self-esteem and to alter attitudes and behavior through a corrective experience of supportive community feeling and positive "reflected appraisals" by group members (Adler 1967; Lewin 1947; Sullivan 1940). Group therapy requires a group of 6–12 persons and a leader or facilitator who helps the group members to use the group experience to achieve their goals (Powles 1964).

Group therapy in schizophrenia has been employed to

- *Provide insight* into unconscious processes, such as transference, resistance, and motivation (Selzer et al. 1992)
- *Test reality* by distinguishing between gross distortions and consensually validated perceptions or beliefs (Kanas 1985, 1986) and to control psychotic experiences through the

development of effective strategies of self-control (Breier and Strauss 1983; Falloon and Talbot 1981; Horowitz and Weisberg 1966)

- *Educate* about the illness, its treatment, and available community resources (Fenn and Dinaburg 1981; Kahn and Kahn 1992; Maxmen 1978, 1984)
- *Coordinate medication management* and the prompt response to the reemergence of symptoms of psychotic relapse (Herz et al. 1982; Olarte and Masnik 1981; Seaman 1981)
- *Prescribe activities* around the pursuit of a specific task or project (Anthony and Liberman 1986);
- *Improve skills* in communication, social relations, and problem solving via 1) a structured group process emphasizing disclosure, group discussion, feedback, and between-session task assignment (Kanas 1991; Malm 1982, 1990; O'Brien 1975; Steiner 1979), or 2) a cognitive-behavioral process focusing on the correction of distorted perceptions and ideas, the learning of ways to communicate without ambiguity, and the construction of effective behavioral strategies for solving problems (Benton and Schroeder 1990; Brady 1984; Curran et al. 1982; Liberman 1987; Liberman et al. 1980)
- *Render mutual aid* in self-help groups, where members share the experience of a common stigmatized condition and give each other encouragement and advice (Cole 1983)

Outcome Research

Outcome research has generated findings that can serve to guide the design of group treatment services for persons with schizophrenic disorders:

- *Persons with acute psychosis* are exquisitely sensitive to social overstimulation and thus should be treated with antipsychotic medication in low-stimulus environments (Ciompi 1983; Kanas et al. 1980; Keith and Matthews 1982; Leszcz et al. 1985; Pattison et al. 1967). Group therapy is inappropriate for this phase of illness.
- *Hospitalized persons in subacute and chronic phases of the disorder* cannot tolerate insight-oriented group therapy or stimulus-intensive milieu treatment (Bednar and Lawlis 1971; Fairweather et al. 1960; Kanas et al. 1980; Leszcz et al. 1985; Pattison et al. 1967; Paul and Lentz 1977; Schooler and Spohn 1982). However, supportive, interaction-oriented group therapy can facilitate early hospital discharge and increase community tenure for patients without prominent paranoid or deficit symptoms (Fairweather et al. 1960; Finch and Wallace 1977; Kanas 1991; Lukoff et al. 1986; Malm 1982, 1990; Otteson 1979). Persons with severe and persistent schizophrenia respond better to behaviorally oriented approaches, including token economies (Paul and Lentz 1977) and social skills training (Marder et al. 1996; Wallace and Liberman 1985).
- *High-functioning outpatients with schizophrenia* may benefit from interaction-oriented group therapy, which helps patients to understand the illness, use antipsychotic medication responsibly, apply reality testing to delusions and suspiciousness, and learn communication and problem-solving skills (Coons and Peacock 1970). This beneficial effect is maximized when all members of a group organized on an inpatient or partial hospitalization service are referred as an integral social unit to the same outpatient group (Kanas 1991; Malm 1990). Higher-functioning patients may respond adversely to social learning approaches that propose to train them in skills they already have acquired (Wallace 1984).

- *Ambulatory patients with severe and persistent disorders* are best approached with cognitive, communication, and problem-solving approaches that employ social learning principles to remediate specific deficits. Typically, group members learn assertiveness (Monti et al. 1980): how to initiate, continue, and end a conversation; how to cope more effectively with stressful situations (Liberman 1987); how to solve typical daily problems (Bellack et al. 1984; Coche and Flick 1975); how to set and attain goals (Barrowclough and Tarrier 1987); and how to neutralize encounters with relatives with high expressed emotion (EE) (Hogarty et al. 1991, 1992). The group process is employed to provide corrective feedback and social reinforcement for improvements in role-plays and rehearsals during the group session and for successful completion of homework task assignments (Douglas and Mueser 1990). These approaches should be restricted to patients with *good premorbid functioning and with intact memory without prominent negative symptoms* (Bellack et al. 1989; Benton and Schroeder 1990; McGlashan et al. 1990; Mueser et al. 1991).

Summary of Findings for Phase-Specific Interventions

The above findings point toward the following guidelines for group therapy of persons with schizophrenic disorders (see also Table 36–1):

- Insight-oriented approaches, except possibly for stable high-functioning outpatients, should not be used at all.
- Group therapy should not be used during acute psychosis.
- Once the acute episode has subsided and patients can engage in normal social conversation, interaction-oriented group therapy can be used for inpatients with good intermorbid functioning, whereas behaviorally oriented approaches should be used for patients with chronic schizophrenia who have good premorbid functioning without a preponderance of negative symptoms. For each modality, 9–12 daily or thrice-weekly sessions will be sufficient to initiate a group process that should be continued upon discharge.
- High-functioning outpatients can use interaction-oriented group approaches, whereas those with more severe and persistent disorders should be treated with cognitive remediation and behaviorally oriented skills training.

TABLE 36–1. Phase of schizophrenic illness and effectiveness of group therapy approach

Illness phase	Insight-oriented	Interaction-oriented	Social learning
Acute psychosis	–	0	0
Chronic hospitalized schizophrenia	–	±	+
Postacute hospitalized schizophrenia	0	+	+
Postacute, day hospitalization	0	±	+
Chronic, outpatient	0	±	+
High-functioning, outpatient	?	+	?
Negative-symptom, outpatient	0	–	?

Note. – = harmful; 0 = not helpful; ± = possibly helpful; + = definitely helpful; ? = data unclear.

Procedures and Techniques

Preparation

To counter the prevailing view that group therapy is second class, patients are told that they will gain a fuller understanding of their illness, learn survival skills, become more aware of themselves, and learn from group members who have coped with the same illness. Patients are provided a set of rules that stress the importance of attending regularly, being on time, remaining in the session until it ends, refraining from violence to persons or furniture, and keeping all information confidential.

Composition

Inpatient and outpatient groups should contain persons of similar levels of functioning; thus a group might have persons diagnosed with schizophrenia, schizoaffective disorder, and bipolar disorder who share either the capacity or incapacity for holding a job or living independently. Groups are matched for a balance of gender as well as ethnic and sociodemographic characteristics (O'Brien 1983). Other characteristics determining group composition include patients' level of attention, abstraction, affect tolerance, response to illness, developmental stage, and compliance with medication (Kahn and Kahn 1992).

Structure

Inpatient and partial-hospitalization groups contain 4–8 members; their meetings last 45–60 minutes and are conducted several times a week. Outpatient groups contain 5–10 members; their meetings last 60–90 minutes and are conducted weekly, twice monthly, or monthly. Inpatient group membership is open, as new members are admitted when their acute symptoms subside and old members are discharged. In the outpatient setting, membership may be kept open until the group reaches an optimal size and the inevitable early dropouts have departed and is then closed to facilitate cohesion. Time-limited groups of 12–16 weekly sessions can be organized for higher-functioning patients around specific themes, employing role-playing, homework assignments, and the sharing of coping strategies (Kahn and Kahn 1992; Kanas 1991).

Co-therapy

The inpatient and partial-hospitalization settings are conducive to co-therapy, which enables leaders to retain an objective and cool-headed approach to patients who are out of control and to provide one another with mutual encouragement and support. Co-therapy enables the leaders to demonstrate effective communication and to model correct behavior in role-play situations.

Training and Supervision

Typical group therapy training pairs a novice with an experienced co-therapist. It is crucial for group leaders to have access to supervision or consultation with colleagues when dealing with potentially psychotic patients (Cole 1987). Supervisors can help with co-therapy conflicts and coach trainees to remain hopeful in the face of patient passivity and slow rates of recovery. Access to a video camera or audiovisual studio with a one-way mirror can further enhance the process of training.

Leadership Techniques

- *Nonspecific techniques.* Exhibit an active sense of caring and unconditional positive regard, with a tolerant and nonjudgmental attitude (Slavson 1961; Steiner 1979; Wolman 1960).
- *Sense of expertise.* Convey a sound understanding of the schizophrenic disorders and an appreciation of the patient's experience of the illness (Maxmen 1984; Torrey 1983).
- *Low-key approach.* Avoid overstimulation through forced self-disclosure or applying social pressure (Drake 1986).
- *Psychoeducation.* Present a clear and understandable view of schizophrenic disorder, its prognosis, and its illness course, including steps patients can take to avoid relapse (Heinrichs 1984; K. G. Terkelsen, unpublished observations, September 1991).
- *Facilitation.* Encourage the discussion of current life situations, including events leading to hospitalization and difficulties with family, friends, co-workers, or other group members. As a group ethos develops, group members can share ways in which they have successfully coped with psychotic experiences, fostering cooperation with medical and psychosocial treatment.
- *Positive emphasis.* Stress the positive connotation of patient issues, emphasizing good intentions, accomplishments, and performances and encouraging group members to do likewise.
- *Personal responsibility.* In the interaction-oriented, high-functioning group, ask group members to speak clearly and directly, to make "I" statements, and to show interest in one another. Encourage group members to share experiences and to offer advice and moral support. Assist each member to develop and to be responsible for achieving a set of goals. Events occurring in the session can be used to illustrate member strengths and weaknesses. Group themes are highlighted, and group members are asked to summarize them. Leaders of interaction-oriented groups often combine psychodynamic and social learning techniques, such as modeling, role-playing, and communications training.
- *Effective communication.* Many patients are unable to ask effectively for what they want; others cannot find ways to neutralize emotional demands from significant others. Specific exercises teach members how to express positive and negative feelings, how to make requests, and how to listen responsively. Patients learn receiving, processing, and sending skills in problem-solving and role-playing exercises in which leaders serve as instructors, models, and coaches. Patients are trained to delineate problems, propose solutions, ask for group feedback, and ascertain the consequences of decided-upon strategies.
- *Medication monitoring.* Train patients to identify medication side effects and to anticipate target signs and symptoms preceding relapse (Herz 1984; Kane 1987; Schooler et al. 1997; Subotnik and Nuechterlein 1988).
- *Network formation.* An informal atmosphere is maintained, often with snacks being served and activities planned (e.g., going on a picnic, eating out in a restaurant, or visiting a local place of interest). Medication side effects or target symptoms may be discussed and prescriptions written at the end of the session. Group members may be encouraged to visit or telephone one another between sessions, as the group becomes an "invisible village," permitting otherwise isolated persons to build a supportive social network (Beels 1989).

A comparison of the techniques of supportive social learning and those of interaction-oriented group therapy based on typical group events is presented in Table 36–2.

TABLE 36–2. Comparison of supportive social learning with interaction-oriented group therapy

Event	Supportive social learning	Interaction-oriented group therapy
1. Leader opens the session.	Leader opens meeting, states group goals and methods, and asks for members' agendas of problems to be discussed.	Leader opens meeting and waits for members to make first remarks.
2. Leader closes the session.	Leader closes meeting after summarizing problems addressed and topics discussed.	Leader closes meeting after asking group members to summarize major group events and themes discussed.
3. Member brings up problem related to outside life.	Leader helps member to define skills amenable to improvement, elicits other members' suggestions, guides member through role-plays of possible solutions, and suggests "homework" task to continue practice of specific strategies.	Leader encourages other members to share similar experiences and to respond with opinions, suggestions, corrective feedback, and emotional support.
4. Member expresses intense feelings of anger, sadness, anxiety.	Leader helps member to identify specific situations or behavioral sequences that elicit these feelings and then asks group members to suggest alternative strategies. Typical interactional sequences are then role-played, first demonstrating problematic transactions and then possible alternatives.	Leader encourages other group members to share feelings and experiences evoked by the problem and helps speaker to identify underlying automatic thoughts and assumptions and to come up with possible solutions to original problem. These solutions are then role-played.
5. Member discusses conflict with other group member.	Leader helps member to view this as one example of a pattern of difficulty in social relations and uses this as opportunity to teach specific communication skills. Leader asks other group members to participate with patient in role-play that illustrates the problem and its solution.	Leader requests speaker and other group member to approach this conflict in a positive, constructive manner, asking each to present his or her point of view with an open and honest expression of feelings. Other group members are asked to give feedback and support.
6. Member expresses hostility toward leader or group member.	Leader restates purpose of group: to improve coping and problem-solving skills. Leader asks speaker to "reframe" remarks in a positive way and to view resentment as difficulty in making positive requests. Speaker engages in task to determine what he or she has trouble asking for, then in role-play to ask for it.	Leader elicits feedback from other group members and helps speaker to connect hostile feelings with underlying assumptions and group dynamics. Leader encourages speaker to "take the position of the other" to see positive aspect of negative viewpoint.

TABLE 36–2. Comparison of supportive social learning with interaction-oriented group therapy *(continued)*

Event	Supportive social learning	Interaction-oriented group therapy
7. Member expresses interest in socializing with other group members.	Leader decides to organize group outing and encourages member to telephone or meet with certain group members for specific purpose, such as practicing role-plays, coaching, or eliciting support.	Leader asks member to express reasons for wanting closer ties and to share these openly in direct conversation with affiliative objects. Leader discusses importance of positive group bonding to promote self-esteem and potential of "pairing" to lead to group fragmentation.
8. Member discusses delusions, suspiciousness, and/or hallucinations.	Leader points out that such experiences are indications that patient is experiencing a relapse and should seek psychiatric consultation immediately. Leader asks members to discuss their "target symptoms," which indicate when they are about to have a relapse. Leader stresses the importance of adherence to medication regimens, elicits discussion of side effects and other reasons for noncompliance, and refocuses topic to group task.	Leader remarks that these experiences indicate that the member may be experiencing a relapse and may require more medication and that he or she may be experiencing more stress than usual. The member is asked to discuss possible sources of current stress, and the group then suggests possible coping strategies. If the member's experiences are persistent and unresponsive to medication or stress, the group is asked to discuss ways in which they have coped with psychotic symptoms or made them "go away."
9. Member announces intention to discontinue medication.	Leader asks speaker to list reasons for stopping medication and then presents a cogent argument for continuing drug treatment, highlighting costs and benefits. Leader praises specific group members who remain compliant and encourages these group members to state their reasons for continuing medication.	Leader asks for reasons why speaker wants to stop and elicits group response. Leader helps speaker to weigh the advantages and possible disadvantages of proposed course of action. Leader suggests that speaker discuss this with prescribing physician.
10. New member joins group.	Leader introduces new member to group at beginning of the session, asks other members to introduce themselves, and then proceeds with day's agenda.	Leader introduces new member at beginning of group and asks old members to present thumbnail self-description. Near session's end, new member is asked to "go around," commenting on what has taken place, and old members are asked to respond.

TABLE 36–2. Comparison of supportive social learning with interaction-oriented group therapy *(continued)*

Event	Supportive social learning	Interaction-oriented group therapy
11. Group member leaves the room.	Leader continues with activity in progress, realizing that absent member needs to take "time-out" to reduce arousal level and will return when feeling calmer.	Leader asks group members to comment on member's departure and then has someone follow and bring back absent member. When departed member has returned, she or he is asked to discuss what prompted exit, and group members are asked to give feedback.
12. Group member is absent.	Leader notes absence and plans to telephone absent member to encourage attendance at next meeting. Other members are asked to place supportive phone calls.	Leader asks for others' ideas about why member has not come and for their feelings when people do not show up. Leader phones absent member. In next session, leader asks member to discuss his or her reasons for not attending and elicits response from other members.
13. Member states intention to drop out of group.	Leader stresses importance of continued membership: to learn communication and problem-solving skills and to benefit from social support during recovery from acute psychosis. Leader expresses hope that leave-taking will be temporary and assures member that he or she can return at any time. Leader elicits similar response from other group members.	Leader asks speaker to give specific reasons for wanting to leave group and asks for feedback from other group members, discussing issues of loyalty, commitment, identity, loss, etc.
14. Member recalls psychotic experience as a "bad dream."	Leader remarks that some patients cope with memories of psychosis by trying to forget them, whereas others see them as "experiences of significance" and try to learn from them. Members are asked to discuss the extent to which they have "sealed over" or "integrated" their experiences of psychosis.	Leader asks other group members to recall their psychotic experiences and how they have tried to forget them or integrate them into their ongoing experience of the world.

Family Treatment

Family EE, a measure of family criticism and overinvolvement, is associated with relapse in severely ill patients with poor premorbid functioning. Psychoeducational family management approaches can help to lower family EE and to reduce patient relapse. These methods teach patients and their family members to cope with the illness through a pragmatic understanding of the disease, of symptom and behavior management strategies, and of the local health care system. Group skills training can help patients to deal more effectively with relatives with high EE (Bellack et al. 1992; Hogarty et al. 1991, 1992). Combining group and family approaches within a program of supportive individual psychotherapy, antipsychotic medication, psychiatric rehabilitation, and assertive community outreach appears to hold the best hope for ameliorating the devastating effects of schizophrenia.

Family treatment suitable for work with patients with schizophrenia includes engagement of the family, psychoeducation, crisis management, linkage with inpatient and partial hospitalization staff, brief family therapy, multifamily therapy, and long-term outpatient treatment. Therapists frame the patient's problem as an acute episode of a biologically based illness triggered by acute or chronic stress and seek to engage the family in exploring ways in which they and the patient can reduce the level of stress and thereby lessen the chances of relapse. The work involves the modification of specific communication and problem-solving behaviors and helps the family to set realistic expectations for the patient's recovery. A survey of the family interactional correlates of schizophrenia will enable practitioners to anticipate typical transactional patterns and thereby tailor the model to specific situations. This approach to family treatment has been validated through controlled outcome studies (Falloon et al. 1985; Glick et al. 1990; Goldstein et al. 1978; Hogarty et al. 1986, 1991; Leff et al. 1982; MacCarthy et al. 1989; McFarlane et al. 1995b; Tarrier et al. 1988; Zastowny et al. 1992).

Family Burden

Since deinstitutionalization, families of psychiatric patients have endured considerable hardships coping with the psychotic and residual symptoms of schizophrenia (Creer and Wing 1975; Doll 1976; Fadden et al. 1987; Johnson 1990). These families have frequently become isolated from their communities and estranged from their patient-relatives (Beels et al. 1984; Kreisman and Joy 1975). In the past, mental health professionals have blamed families for either causing or triggering episodes of mental illness (Appleton 1974; Terkelsen 1983). However, since the establishment of the National Alliance for the Mentally Ill (NAMI) in 1979, families have begun to insist that professionals provide them with a more accurate understanding of severe and persistent mental disorders, their treatments, and available community resources (Cole 1987; Hatfield 1987; Holden and Lewine 1982; Lefley and Johnson 1990; Lefley and Wasow 1994; Reiser and Schorske 1994; Vine and Beels 1990). NAMI and the National Association for Research in Schizophrenia and Depression support research and governmental initiatives and have stimulated a widespread effort to develop new and effective treatment strategies that enlist families as partners in health care (Burland 1998).

In response both to families' needs and to the implications of the research on EE, model programs were developed to reduce family burden by educating the family and alerting its members to community resources and training them in effective coping strategies (Cole and Jacobs 1989; Kavanagh 1992; Strachan et al. 1986). Outcome research has shown that the psychosocial interventions employed succeeded not only in providing relief to families but also in reducing patient relapse (Falloon et al. 1985; Glick et al. 1990; Goldstein et al. 1978; Hogarty et al. 1986, 1991; Leff et al. 1982; MacCarthy et al. 1989; McFarlane et al. 1995b; Tarrier et al. 1988; Zastowny et al. 1992). These interventions have included social skills training for patients, health education for patients and families, family therapy and crisis intervention, and multiple-family and relatives' groups.

Family Interaction in Schizophrenia

Persons with persistent negative symptoms of schizophrenia show a lack of motivation, social withdrawal, and difficulties comprehending the contextual meanings of words. They can be confused by nonverbal cues and fail to communicate intended meanings to others. They might not respond predictably to positive reinforcement nor employ praise and attention to build supportive social ties, and they can have difficulty in performing social roles (Bellack et al. 1990; Wallace 1984). Many parents of persons with schizophrenic disorders have difficulties establishing a shared focus of attention and meaning (Wynne 1981). EE is strongly associated with increased posthospital relapse rates in male patients with chronic schizophrenia who are living in their parental homes (Brown et al. 1962, 1972; King and Dixon 1996; Kuipers and Bebbington 1988; Mintz et al. 1989; Vaughn and Leff 1976).

Hogarty (1985) and Falloon (1988) suggested that the criticism dimension of EE may represent a reactive, "state" phenomenon activated by the onset of disturbed patient behavior and diminishing as the patient appears to improve. It has been suggested that relatives who exhibit high EE in criticism interpret negative symptoms as willful behavior and doubt that schizophrenia is a legitimate illness (Barrowclough et al. 1987; Hooley 1985; Tarrier and Barrowclough 1986). Goldstein and Doane (1983) have suggested that emotional overinvolvement should be considered a "trait," a long-term adaptation to living with a chronically ill family member. Several writers have suggested that high EE can be viewed either as a normal family reaction to the burden posed by a poor prognosis patient "destined to relapse" (Lefley 1992; Parker et al. 1988; Stirling et al. 1991) or as a marker of enduring psychopathology (Goldstein et al. 1992).

The attitudinal and interactional correlates of EE are outlined in Table 36–3.

Family Work During Hospitalization

For many families, hospitalization is a last resort to be used only after outpatient management has failed. Patients in families with high EE are more likely to live at home and less likely to participate in outpatient treatment (Mintz et al. 1989). Brief hospitalization can be an opportunity to engage patients and families in programs of treatment and support. Psychoeducational family interventions define the patient's symptomatic behavior as a biologically based brain disorder and provide both the patient and family with cognitive, behavioral, and pharmacological strategies for coping more effectively (Cole and Jacobs 1989). Patients are viewed as experts in the subjective experience of schizophrenia (McGill et al. 1983); relatives are considered potential experts in its day-to-day management and are praised for doing their best to cope with the disorder (Steinglass 1987).

By the time the patient has come to the emergency room, the family is in a state of turmoil and confusion (Anderson 1977; Anderson and Reiss 1982; Bernheim and Lehman 1985; Biddle 1978; Cole and Jacobs 1989; Group for the Advancement of Psychiatry 1985;

TABLE 36–3. Attitudinal and interactional correlates of expressed emotion (EE)

Relatives' attitudes and behavior	
High-EE relatives	**Low-EE relatives**
See illness behavior as laziness	Accept psychosis as a disease process
Have unrealistic expectations	Understand the patient's limitations
Talk and interrupt more often	Listen to the patient
Express disagreement	Agree with the patient
Use peculiar language	Use clear language
Give intense and harsh criticism	Are emotionally neutral
Judge patient's behavior negatively	Are supportive and protective
Express personal rejections	Are accepting of the patient
Propose negative solutions to problems	Propose positive solutions to problems
Engage in negative escalations with patient	De-escalate potential conflicts
Show overconcern	May neglect patient
Patient's reactions	
High-EE family	**Low-EE family**
Expresses irritability	Appears calm
Denigrates self or criticizes others	Makes neutral statements
Becomes defensive or engages in ineffective counterattacks	Is able to react coolly in conflict situations without losing train of thought
Interactive pattern	
High-EE family	**Low-EE family**
Has parent that attacks and patient that counterattacks or makes excuses	Engages in problem-solving discussions

Source. Hahlweg et al. 1987; Kuipers et al. 1983; MacCarthy and Hemsley 1986; Miklowitz et al. 1983, 1984, 1986, 1989; Mueser et al. 1993; Strachan et al. 1986, 1989; Vaughn 1986.

Harbin 1979). Families in crisis are often receptive to help and change and may welcome assistance from an understanding, compassionate, and available therapist (Hill 1965; Parad and Caplan 1965; Rabkin 1972). If it is the patient's first psychotic break, the spouse and/or family members may blame themselves for the patient's condition and feel guilty for signing the patient into the hospital. They may not fully understand what has happened to the patient and may be afraid of losing their relative forever. Should the crisis be yet another of many breakdowns, the family may feel despairing and helpless over the patient's condition, isolated from society, and alienated from a health care system that has not succeeded in controlling the course of the illness. These families welcome the respite provided by hospitalization (Gould and Glick 1977; Greenley 1982; Withersty 1977).

The goals of engagement are to establish a working alliance, to educate the family about the patient's disorder, and to describe the policies of the inpatient unit. The first few meetings usually take place without the patient, to minimize disruptions and thereby allow a more open discussion of the patient's immediate past behavior. The therapist should carefully review past programs of outpatient management and endeavor to design a treatment plan that meets the current needs of both patient and family. The therapist collaborates with the family to identify problems, to recognize strengths and weaknesses, and to develop and implement problem-solving strategies (Epstein and Bishop 1981; Wynne et al. 1986, 1987).

The therapist should communicate an understanding of what it must be like to have a relative become psychotic. The family should be told that the patient has a chemical imbalance in the brain for which no one is to blame and then given a differential diagnosis. The therapist should show appreciation for the efforts that the patient's family and spouse have made to cope with severe and persistent mental illness. The patient should be told about the family meetings and their purpose and then be invited to join once the patient's therapist decides that the patient can participate in rational discourse. The family therapy team should be available on call to the family in event of an emergency.

Greenman et al. (1989) showed that program discharges against medical advice tend to occur more often when families cannot accept the notion that the patient is genuinely ill, cannot tolerate the separation imposed by hospitalization, or feel excessively guilty in the face of the patient's anger at being hospitalized. Educating family members and allowing them to unburden themselves can help to avoid premature patient release. Many families undergo a natural process of emotional separation when the patient is admitted and become reinvolved as discharge approaches (Stewart 1982). Drake and Sederer (1986) reported that loss of family support early in the course of inpatient treatment may lead to patient suicidal behavior. Thus the family therapist must also foster an ongoing supportive family involvement with the patient by beginning discussion of discharge planning at the point of admission.

Hospitalization and partial-hospitalization programs provide a controlled environment that facilitates a quick and accurate diagnostic assessment and the coordination of an individualized treatment plan for the acute episode and the aftercare period. The family therapist assumes the role of ombudsperson, presenting the family's point of view to the treatment team while keeping the family or the family's designated spokesperson abreast of the patient's response to treatment. The family should be informed of the hospital ward's rules, policies, and procedures either in a family meeting or during a "family night" in which several families meet with ward personnel (Scharfstein and Libbey 1982).

In coordinating communication between the family and staff, the family therapist can anticipate and prevent systemic conflicts when the treatment team temporarily assumes the function of primary caretaker. Individual-oriented clinicians can view themselves as protectors of the patient against a family perceived as intrusive and pathological (reviewed in Boyd 1979). These negative attitudes can be countered by including these staff members in family treatment sessions and by conducting in-service teaching of the principles of psychoeducational family treatment (Harbin 1982; Krajewski and Harbin 1982). Families might express disagreement with treatment, discharge, or aftercare plans to individual staff members or to higher-level administrators (Harbin 1978). Such conflicts can be avoided by working closely with the family and the treatment team and keeping each level of the system hierarchy informed of decisions made at other levels.

Families desperately hope that the patient will return to his or her premorbid functioning but fear an outcome of severe, persistent disability and dependency. The clinician should tell families and patients that recovery usually occurs several weeks to months after a first or second breakdown and in chronic disorders follows similar patterns after each acute episode. Strauss et al. (1985) proposed that the process of recovery involves periods of preparation with no observable progress alternating with bursts of obvious activity, "mountain climbing," when the patient may be overextended and vulnerable to social pressure. It is important for the therapist to present the patient's condition in a hopeful light and to advise the family not to push the patient to get well prematurely. The therapist should emphasize the patient's strengths and focus on what the patient and family can do to promote a gradual healing process.

Specific Family Treatment Approaches

Psychoeducational Workshop

The holding of periodic all-day, diagnosis-specific psychoeducational workshops for relatives or spouses will help to accomplish several objectives: 1) the workshop provides important scientific information in a more cost-effective format than working with individual families or spouses, 2) the workshop serves as an opportunity for relatives to share their experiences with professionals and other families, and 3) the workshop gives hesitant families the opportunity to follow the lead of more enthusiastic participants in searching for better ways to manage the patient's disorder. The morning session provides a description of the scientific basis of the disorder and its medical management; the afternoon session involves a discussion of the psychosocial aspects of symptom development and management, behavior control, recovery, and rehabilitation (Anderson et al. 1986b).

First-person accounts (published regularly in *Schizophrenia Bulletin* and as special articles in *Psychiatric Services*) of patients' and families' experiences in coping with the disorder are read aloud to the families in attendance at the workshop. Families are encouraged to set realistic expectations by comparing the patient's current level of functioning to her or his level of functioning 6 months ago, rather than to the functioning of an idealized, "normal" person. Families are asked to relate to the patient in a calm and logical manner, to set realistic goals and limits, and to give praise and attention for specific patient accomplishments. Families are encouraged to expand their social networks and are told of the benefits of joining support and advocacy groups for relatives of the mentally ill, such as local chapters of NAMI.

Brief Family Crisis Intervention

Family crisis treatment can begin during admission to the hospital or partial hospitalization program or upon discharge, once the patient's acute symptoms have subsided sufficiently to participate in family group sessions. Families of female patients who have schizophrenia with poor premorbid functioning respond well to brief family crisis intervention (Glick et al. 1985, 1990; Goldstein et al. 1978; Haas et al. 1990; Langsley and Kaplan 1968). The inpatient family intervention program of Clarkin et al. (1981) is staged for 6–10 problem-focused sessions during a patient's brief inpatient stay. The package includes psychoeducation; crisis management; and training in communicating, problem solving, and identifying early warning signs of relapse. The goals of treatment are that the family accept that the patient has a genuine biologically based illness triggered by stress, and that the family recognize, correct, and anticipate important stressful situations or interactive patterns contributing to the patient's breakdown and need for hospitalization. The patient's psychiatrist and primary therapist should attend these sessions to represent a biopsychosocial view of the patient's disorder and to facilitate the transmission of accurate information between the family and the treatment team.

At least one meeting, the "family consultation" (Wynne et al. 1986), should be devoted to making aftercare plans. A functional assessment of the patient will help to determine whether the patient would benefit from placement in assertive community treatment (ACT) (Allness and Knoedler 1998; Stein and Test 1980; Thompson et al. 1990) and/or psychosocial rehabilitation (Anthony and Liberman 1986; Linn 1989). Some patients may benefit from dosage-reduction medication strategies, which depend on the cooperation of the family to identify early warning signs of impending relapse (Carpenter et al. 1990; Herz et al. 1982; Kane et al. 1983; Schooler 1991; Schooler et al. 1997). Specific problems requiring continuing family care include persistent noncompliance or refusal to participate in rehabilitation programs as well as ongoing severe marital distress of the patient's parents or of the patient and spouse. As family consultant, the therapist should provide the family with sufficient information to make informed choices among potential family care options: 1) continuing in family treatment, 2) beginning multifamily treatment, 3) joining a peer-led family support group, 4) becoming involved in the local chapter of NAMI, or 5) opting out of further family involvement.

Outpatient Family Management

Several major demonstration projects with controlled research designs have measured the effectiveness of family treatment for patients with schizophrenia recently discharged from the hospital (Anderson et al. 1986a; Falloon et al. 1982, 1985; Goldstein 1981; Goldstein et al. 1978; Hogarty et al. 1986, 1991; Leff et al. 1982, 1985, 1989; MacCarthy et al. 1989; McFarlane et al. 1995a, 1995b; Tarrier et al. 1988). Each program controlled for medication and randomly assigned patients either to treatment as usual (usually individual supportive psychotherapy with medication management) or to family treatment. In all studies, the family intervention proved significantly more effective for reducing relapse and for training family members to become less critical of the patient (e.g., Doane et al. 1985; Falloon and Pederson 1985; Hogarty et al. 1986).

Hogarty and colleagues (1991) found no relapses in patients with families converting from high to low EE during the 2-year study, regardless of treatment condition. Moreover, family treatment achieved the most significant reduction in relapse because of its effectiveness in lowering EE and achieving medication compliance. Berkowitz et al. (1984) reported that family treatment helped relatives with high EE to become less pessimistic. Barrowclough and Tarrier (1987) suggested that parents become more optimistic as they perceive their patient-relatives setting and achieving behavioral goals. Tarrier and co-workers (1988) proposed that families with high EE require a program of treatment in which novel attitudes and strategies are observed, practiced, and embedded into their behavioral repertoire.

Findings of "second-generation" studies are as follows:

- Office-based family treatment is as effective as family therapy conducted in the family's home (Randolph et al. 1994; Zastowny et al. 1992).
- Both families with low EE and those with high EE benefit from behavioral family treatment (Randolph et al. 1994).
- Behavioral family treatment alone may not result in improved work skills or employment status and should be accompanied by a comprehensive program of psychiatric rehabilitation (Glynn et al. 1992).
- No advantage results when family treatment is offered to patients with schizophrenia

who are stable and living in the community (McCreadie et al. 1991). Family treatment is best begun shortly after hospital admission or discharge.

- Family treatment may offer no advantage when added to state-of-the-art programs of comprehensive community services (Linszen 1993, cited in Goldstein 1995).
- The inclusion of family treatment can diminish the benefits of individual, pragmatic "personal therapy" for relapse reduction and community adjustment (Hogarty et al. 1997a, 1997b).
- Short-term family approaches for schizophrenia are ineffective; at least 6 months of family treatment are required for efficacy (Baucom et al. 1998).

Techniques of Family Therapy

The techniques and strategies recommended here incorporate elements of behavioral, structural, problem-oriented, and strategic family therapies (Anderson et al. 1986a; Cole 1982; Epstein and Bishop 1981; Falloon 1981, 1984; Falloon et al. 1993; Haley 1987; Minuchin 1974; Mueser and Glynn 1995). Four major themes are emphasized in all psychoeducational approaches:

1. Families learn that they are not to blame for the patient's disorder.
2. Families learn to set realistic expectations for the patient, based on a clear understanding of the disorder.
3. Families learn how to respond to often exasperating patient behaviors with a cognitive, problem-solving approach.
4. Families learn to appreciate the importance of seeking the advice and support of other families with a severely mentally ill relative by attending a multifamily group or participating in community-based activities, such as those found within NAMI chapters (Burland 1998; Cole 1983; McFarlane 1983).

This treatment model recognizes the legitimacy of medical diagnosis and contrasts with approaches that hold families responsible for the patient's status as symptom bearer of a dysfunctional family system. This treatment model focuses on the modification of cognitive and behavioral patterns and seeks to reduce levels of stress and distress. Models of family therapy that explore the past can be upsetting to relatives; those that involve confrontation and escalation of stress can be overstimulating to patients.

Assessment

It is crucial to assess the family's strengths and areas of dysfunction (e.g., Epstein et al. 1978) and negotiate a set of problems to be addressed (e.g., Falloon et al. 1988; Mueser and Glynn 1995). The family should understand that for several months to a year after recovery from acute psychosis many patients with chronic schizophrenia might not tolerate stimulating programs of social interaction or rehabilitation (Hogarty et al. 1974, 1979).

Communication Training and Problem Solving

The therapy team should model clear, direct, and unambiguous communications (Falloon et al. 1988, 1993; Mueser and Glynn 1995) and help the patient and family to listen actively, to express feelings and opinions, and to make requests. The team should ask family members to use "I" statements and to recognize and clarify fuzzy verbal and nonverbal messages. The family is taught how to function as a team, recognizing problems, suggesting alternative solutions, trying them out, and thus progressively refining strategies.

Positive Connotation and Reinforcement

The family therapist should emphasizes the positive side of intentions and assume that family members are trying as hard as they can (Simon et al. 1985). Patients and family members are instructed to replace criticism of failure with immediate praise for the achievement of small steps toward stated goals.

Direct, Indirect, and Paradoxical Prescription

The family should be guided to invent new solutions to old problems. If a straightforward behavioral approach is ineffective, the therapist may directly suggest a solution, relate how another family solved a similar problem, or warn family members of the specific perils of changing their situation (Cole 1982; Cole and Jacobs 1989; Hoffman 1981; Watzlawick et al. 1974).

Neutralization of Negative, Hostile Affects

Escalating conflicts can be relieved by taking "time-outs," alternating who is in charge, acknowledging specific areas of expertise, and using some variant of Robert's Rules to set decorum in family negotiation sessions (Falloon et al. 1988).

Role Reallocation

Hospitalization involves at least a temporary disruption in the patient's execution of family role responsibilities and assumption of responsibilities by family members who might wish to rectify a situation in which they feel overburdened. Here, the therapist serves as coach or arbiter, helping the family to arrange for a more equitable distribution of labor (Tharp and Otis 1966).

Enactment and Rehearsal

Problem resolution often involves making simple changes in the patterns of family or dyadic interaction. The family enacts in the therapy session the most recent conflict as it actually occurred (Minuchin 1974). The therapist then suggests a small variation in the interactive behavioral sequence and has the family role-play this change in the office. The family is then sent home with an assignment to practice the change at home.

Strengthening of the Family Hierarchy

The family is shown how to establish a set of rules that define the limits of tolerable behavior, set expectations and deadlines, and provide clear rewards and penalties (Epstein et al. 1978). Parents are advised to suspend open hostilities in front of the children (Haley 1987).

Adjustment of the Degree of Affective Involvement

Underinvolvement. Low self-esteem sometimes accompanies relationships with family members who ignore one another's needs and feelings. Greater involvement may follow exercises that teach the principles of active, empathic listening (Falloon 1981; Falloon et al. 1988; Wallace et al. 1980).

Overinvolvement. Caretaker overinvolvement can be modified by 1) letting others share the caretaking, 2) having the caretaker spend more time with persons other than the sick member, and 3) encouraging the patient to assume more responsibility.

Identification of Early Warning Signs of Relapse

Medication side effects can interfere with patient functioning (Corrigan et al. 1990; Docherty and Fiester 1985). High-functioning, cooperative patients responsive to medication may maintain remission while reducing medication dosage. Family members can be trained to identify a specific set of target signs and symptoms preceding relapse that serve as indicators that the patient either restart medication or increase the dosage (Herz 1984; Kane 1987; Schooler et al. 1997; Subotnik and Nuechterlein 1988).

Multiple-Family Treatment

Multiple-family treatment (MFT) of schizophrenia has been used to 1) reduce social isolation, provide social support, and promote optimism (Atwood and Williams 1978; Leff 1994; McFarlane 1983, 1990; McFarlane and Dunne 1991); 2) provide information (Anderson et al. 1986b); and 3) reduce EE and family burden (Berkowitz et al. 1984; Kuipers et al. 1989). Two major studies comparing MFT with single-family therapy (SFT) have found no advantage for the more labor-intensive SFT approach. McFarlane et al. (1995b) found MFT more effective for reducing relapse of more severely ill patients compliant with medication. In a major five-center investigation of drug and family management, Schooler et al. (1997) found the more intensive assertive family management no more effective than monthly supportive psychoeducational family meetings. Birchwood et al. (1992) reported that family psychoeducation works best when delivered in a multifamily group setting.

In self-help–oriented MFT, professionals serve as sources of scientific information and as facilitators helping group members to share experiences and practical advice (Cole 1983, 1989; Cole et al. 1979; Gartner and Riessman 1982). A strong collective identity can then arise among family members sharing the common condition of having a close relative or friend with a schizophrenic disorder. Active participation by group members can reduce their social isolation and promote an active involvement in patient recovery through the development of a group consensus of how best to understand and cope with the disorder.

The professionally led multiple-relatives group intervention developed by investigators in England (Berkowitz 1984; Kuipers et al. 1989) and the multiple-family approaches developed in the United States (Atwood and Williams 1978; Beels 1975; Laqueur 1981; McFarlane 1983, 1990; Newmark 1991) provide an opportunity for families to continue to practice stress-reduction and problem-solving strategies introduced in the psychoeducational workshop within the secure and supportive atmosphere of the group. Patient-absent and patient-included multifamily group formats both have distinct advantages. The absence of patients in relatives-only groups permits relatives to freely unburden themselves and to ally with other group members who share their experiential knowledge of the frustrations of coping with severe and persistent mental disorder. Relatives-only groups promote stronger peer group identification and bonding than do groups that include patients. The presence of patients, however, can foster more tolerant attitudes toward patients, enabling relatives to view psychotic behavior more objectively, as relatives other than their own describe hallucinations and delusions.

Family members learn by "analogy and identification" (Laqueur 1981) and by modeling and spontaneous practice; they can then pass this understanding on to other patients and relatives (Gartner and Riessman 1982; McFarlane 1983, 1990). The group as a whole accumulates a repertoire of effective coping and management strategies that are passed on to succeeding generations of new members (Cole 1983; Cole et al. 1979; Markewich 1986; O'Shea and Phelps 1985; Walsh 1987). Professional group leaders in MFT provide scientific information and facilitate the sharing of experiences and practical advice. Many meetings are devoted to problem-solving discussions in which families enact typical stressful situations and suggest alternative ways to understand and solve their problems.

It is becoming clear that the positive effects of MFT cannot be realized in a time-limited format. Solomon et al. (1996, 1997, 1998) reported that a 10-session, structured, multiple-family education program resulted in improved medication compliance, but no change was reported in contact with community resources. Vaughan et al. (1992) found that 10 weekly sessions of a relatives' group offered no advantage over standard treatment for reducing patient relapse. In contrast, McFarlane et al.'s (1995a, 1995b) 2- and 4-year MFT projects resulted in lower relapse rates, improved patient functioning, and reduced family burden, compared with results found with SFT.

Single-Family Versus Multiple-Family Interventions

Mueser and Glynn (1995) have proposed that MFT be employed for families needing social support and SFT for families needing to learn problem-solving and coping skills. Males with schizophrenic or schizoaffective disorders who may be overstimulated by brief family crisis intervention should either be referred with their families to a multifamily support group (an MFT) or be seen in pragmatically oriented "personal therapy" while their relatives attend a family support group (Haas et al. 1990; Hogarty et al. 1997a, 1997b). Leff et al. (1989) reported that higher dropout rates from multiple-relatives groups diminish their advantage over individual family treatment for reducing EE. It is well known that dropout from medical care contributes to patient morbidity (Atwood and Beck 1985; Corrigan et al. 1990; Docherty and Fiester 1985; Haynes et al. 1979) and that dropout frequently occurs in psychiatric aftercare programs (Baekeland and Lundwall 1975; Katz et al. 1984). Families that initially appear hesitant to attend or that drop out after attending several MFT meetings may be engaged through individual family sessions at the office or in the family's home (MacCarthy et al. 1989).

Conclusions

The family intervention model is widely accepted for the treatment of patients with schizophrenic disorders. The strategies and techniques discussed derive from more than 30 years of family interaction studies and outcome research that have made us aware of the burdens families bear and of how managed change in family transactional patterns can help to reduce patient relapse. The psychoeducational approach begins when a family in crisis reaches out in fear and confusion and is greeted with understanding, compassion, and advocacy. The model recognizes the importance of treating the patient's acute symptoms with antipsychotic medication and emphasizes the importance of engaging the family as soon as possible. It places the family therapist in the role of both family advocate and mediator between the family and inpatient and partial hospitalization service systems.

The therapist encourages the family to attend a multifamily workshop providing information and social support. The family can then choose between single- and multiple-family approaches. For most of these families, it is crucial that family treatment and support be continued long after the patient leaves the hospital. Ongoing family treatment helps to improve family problem solving, to ensure access to community resources, to reduce isolation and instill hope, and to foster patient compliance with medication and rehabilitation. This program of family treatment will help to improve the patient's chances of remaining relapse-free and will thereby promote a more complete recovery from acute psychosis.

References

Adler KA: Adler's individual psychology, in Psychoanalytic Techniques: A Handbook for the Practicing Psychoanalyst. Edited by Wolman BB. New York, Basic Books, 1967, pp 299–337

Allness DJ, Knoedler WH: The PACT Model of Community-Based Treatment for Persons With Severe and Persistent Mental Illness: A Manual for PACT Start-Up. Arlington, VA, National Alliance for the Mentally Ill, 1998

Anderson CM: Family intervention with severely disturbed inpatients. Arch Gen Psychiatry 34:697–702, 1977

Anderson CM, Reiss DJ: Family treatment of patients with chronic schizophrenia: the inpatient phase, in The Psychiatric Hospital and the Family. Edited by Harbin HT. New York, SP Medical & Scientific Books, 1982, pp 79–101

Anderson CM, Griffin S, Rossi A, et al: A comparative study of the impact of education vs process groups for families of patients with affective disorders. Fam Process 25:185–206, 1986a

Anderson CM, Reiss DJ, Hogarty GE: Schizophrenia and the Family: A Practitioner's Guide to Psychoeducation and Management. New York, Guilford, 1986b

Anthony WA, Liberman RP: The practice of psychiatric rehabilitation: historical, conceptual, and research base. Schizophr Bull 12:542–559, 1986

Appleton WS: Mistreatment of patients' families by psychiatrists. Am J Psychiatry 131:655–657, 1974

Atwood N, Beck JC: Service and patient predictors of continuation in clinic-based treatment. Hospital and Community Psychiatry 36:865–869, 1985

Atwood N, Williams MED: Group support for the families of the mentally ill. Schizophr Bull 4:415–425, 1978

Baekeland F, Lundwall L: Dropping out of treatment: a critical review. Psychol Bull 82:738–783, 1975

Barrowclough C, Tarrier N: A behavioral family intervention with a schizophrenic patient: a case study. Behavioural Psychotherapy 15:252–271, 1987

Barrowclough C, Tarrier N, Watts S, et al: Assessing the functional value of relatives' knowledge about schizophrenia: a preliminary report. Br J Psychiatry 151:1–8, 1987

Baucom DH, Shoham V, Mueser KT, et al: Empirically supported couple and family interventions for marital distress and adult mental health problems. J Consult Clin Psychol 66:53–88, 1998

Bednar RL, Lawlis GF: Empirical research in group psychotherapy, in Handbook of Psychotherapy and Behavior Change. Edited by Bergin AE, Garfield S. New York, Wiley, 1971, pp 818–838

Beels CC: Family and social management of schizophrenia. Schizophr Bull 13:97–118, 1975

Beels CC: The invisible village. New Dir Ment Health Serv 42:27–40, 1989

Beels CC, Gutwirth L, Berkeley J, et al: Measurement of social support in schizophrenia. Schizophr Bull 10:339–411, 1984

Bellack AS, Turner SM, Hersen M, et al: An examination of the efficacy of social skills training for chronic schizophrenic patients. Hospital and Community Psychiatry 35:1023–1028, 1984

Bellack AS, Morrison RL, Mueser KT: Social problem solving in schizophrenia. Schizophr Bull 15:101–116, 1989

Bellack AS, Morrison RL, Wixted JT, et al: An analysis of social competence in schizophrenia. Br J Psychiatry 156:809–818, 1990

Bellack AS, Mueser KT, Wade J, et al: The ability of schizophrenics to perceive and cope with negative affect. Br J Psychiatry 160:473–480, 1992

Benton MK, Schroeder HE: Social skills training with schizophrenics: a meta-analytic evaluation. J Consult Clin Psychol 58:741–747, 1990

Berkowitz R: Therapeutic interventions with schizophrenic patients and their families: a description of a clinical research project. Journal of Family Therapy 6:211–233, 1984

Berkowitz R, Eberlein-Fries R, Kuipers L, et al: Educating relatives about schizophrenia. Schizophr Bull 10:418–429, 1984

Bernheim KF, Lehman AF: Working With Families of the Mentally Ill. New York, WW Norton, 1985

Biddle JR: Working with families within inpatient settings. Journal of Marriage and Family Counseling 4:43–51, 1978

Birchwood M, Smith J, Cochrane R: Specific and non-specific effects of educational intervention for families living with schizophrenia: a comparison of three methods. Br J Psychiatry 160:806–814, 1992

Boyd JH: The interaction of family therapy and psychodynamic individual therapy in an inpatient setting. Psychiatry 42:99–111, 1979

Brady JP: Social skills training for psychiatric patients. Am J Psychiatry 141:333–340, 491–498, 1984

Breier A, Strauss JS: Self-control in psychotic disorders. Arch Gen Psychiatry 40:1141–1145, 1983

Brenner HD, Boker W, Hodel B, et al: Cognitive treatment of basic pervasive dysfunction in schizophrenia, in Schizophrenia: Scientific Progress. Edited by Schulz SC, Tamminga CA. New York, Oxford University Press, 1989, pp 358–367

Brown GW, Monck EM, Carstairs GM, et al: Influence of family life on the course of schizophrenic illness. British Journal of Preventive and Social Medicine 16:55–68, 1962

Brown GW, Birley JLT, Wing JK: Influence of family life on the course of schizophrenic disorders: a replication. Br J Psychiatry 121:241–258, 1972

Burland J: Family-to-Family: a trauma-and-recovery model of family education, in Families Coping With Mental Illness: The Cultural Context. Edited by Lefley HP. San Francisco, CA, Jossey-Bass, 1998, pp 33–41

Carpenter WT Jr, Hanlon TE, Heinrichs DW, et al: Continuous versus targeted medication in schizophrenic outpatients: outcome results. Am J Psychiatry 147:1138–1148, 1990

Ciompi L: How to improve the treatment of schizophrenia: a multicausal concept and its theoretical components, in Psychosocial Intervention in Schizophrenia: An Interactional View. Edited by Stierlin H, Wynne L, Wirschung M. New York, Springer-Verlag, 1983, pp 53–66

Clarkin JF, Spencer JH, Peyser J, et al: Training Manual for Inpatient Family Intervention for Affective Disorders. New York, Payne Whitney Clinic, Cornell University Medical Center, 1981

Coche E, Flick A: Problem-solving training groups for hospitalized psychiatric patients. J Psychol 91:19–29, 1975

Cole SA: Problem-focused family therapy: principles and practical applications, in Psychopathology in Childhood. Edited by Lachenmeyer JR, Gibbs MS. New York, Gardner, 1982, pp 341–374

Cole SA: Self-help groups, in Comprehensive Group Psychotherapy, 2nd Edition. Edited by Kaplan HI, Sadock BJ. Baltimore, MD, Williams & Wilkins, 1983, pp 144–150

Cole SA (with Cole DS): Professionals who work with families of the chronic mentally ill: current status and suggestions for clinical training, in Families of the Mentally Ill: Coping and Adaptation. Edited by Hatfield A, Lefley H. New York, Guilford, 1987, pp 278–306

Cole SA: Group therapy in schizophrenia, in Treatments of Psychiatric Disorders: A Task Force Report of the American Psychiatric Association, Vol 2. Washington, DC, American Psychiatric Association, 1989, pp 1529–1542

Cole SA, Jacobs J: Family treatment of schizophrenia, in Treatments of Psychiatric Disorders: A Task Force Report of the American Psychiatric Association, Vol 2. Washington, DC, American Psychiatric Association, 1989, pp 1543–1567

Cole SA, O'Connor S, Bennett L: Self-help groups for clinic patients with chronic illness. Prim Care 6:325–340, 1979

Coons WH, Peacock EP: Interpersonal interaction and personality change in group psychotherapy. Canadian Psychiatric Association Journal 15:347–355, 1970

Corrigan PW, Liberman RP, Engel JD: From noncompliance to collaboration in the treatment of schizophrenia. Hospital and Community Psychiatry 41:1203–1211, 1990

Creer C, Wing JK: Living with a schizophrenic patient. Br J Hosp Med 7:73–82, 1975

Curran JP, Monti PM, Corriveau DP: Treatment of schizophrenia, in International Handbook of Behavior Modification and Therapy. Edited by Bellack AS, Hersen M, Kazdin AE. New York, Plenum, 1982, pp 433–466

Doane JA, Falloon IRH, Goldstein MJ, et al: Parental affective style and the treatment of schizophrenia: predicting course of illness and social functioning. Arch Gen Psychiatry 42:34–42, 1985

Docherty JP, Fiester SJ: The therapeutic alliance and compliance with psychopharmacology, in Psychiatry Update: American Psychiatric Association Annual Review, Vol 4. Edited by Hales RE, Frances AJ. Washington, DC, American Psychiatric Press, 1985, pp 607–632

Doll W: Family coping with the mentally ill: an unanticipated problem of deinstitutionalization. Hospital and Community Psychiatry 27:183–185, 1976

Douglas MS, Mueser KT: Teaching conflict resolution skills to the chronically mentally ill. Behav Modif 14:519–547, 1990

Drake RE: The adverse effects of intensive treatment of chronic schizophrenia. Compr Psychiatry 27:313–326, 1986

Drake RE, Sederer LI: Inpatient psychosocial treatment of chronic schizophrenia: negative effects and current guidelines. Hospital and Community Psychiatry 37:897–901, 1986

Epstein NB, Bishop DS: Problem-centered systems therapy of the family. J Marital Fam Ther 7:23–32, 1981

Epstein NB, Bishop DS, Levin S: The McMaster Model of Family Functioning. Journal of Marriage and Family Counseling 4:19–31, 1978

Fadden G, Bebbington P, Kuipers L: The burden of care: the impact of functional psychiatric illness on the patient's family. Br J Psychiatry 150:285–292, 1987

Fairweather GW, Simon R, Gebhard ME, et al: Relative effectiveness of psychotherapeutic programs: a multi-criterial comparison of four programs for the three different patient groups. Psychological Monographs 74:1–26, 1960

Falloon IRH: Communication and problem-solving skills training with relapsing schizophrenics and their families, in Family Therapy and Major Psychopathology. Edited by Lansky MR. New York, Grune & Stratton, 1981, pp 35–56

Falloon IRH: Developing and maintaining adherence to long-term drug-taking regimens. Schizophr Bull 10:412–417, 1984

Falloon IRH: Expressed emotion: current status (editorial). Psychol Med 18:269–274, 1988

Falloon IRH, Pederson J: Family management in the prevention of morbidity of schizophrenia: the adjustment of the family unit. Br J Psychiatry 147:156–163, 1985

Falloon IRH, Talbot RE: Persistent auditory hallucinations: coping mechanisms and implications for management. Psychol Med 11:329–339, 1981

Falloon IRH, Boyd JL, McGill CW, et al: Family management in the prevention of exacerbations of schizophrenia. N Engl J Med 306:1437–1440, 1982

Falloon IRH, Boyd JL, McGill CW, et al: Family management in the prevention of morbidity in schizophrenia. Arch Gen Psychiatry 42:887–896, 1985

Falloon IRH, Hole V, Mudray L, et al: Behavioral family therapy, in Affective Disorders and the Family. Edited by Clarkin JF, Haas GL, Glick ID. New York, Guilford, 1988, pp 117–133

Falloon IRH, Laporta M, Fadden G, et al: Managing Stress in Families. London, Routledge, 1993

Fenn HH, Dinaburg D: Didactic group psychotherapy with chronic schizophrenics. Int J Group Psychother 31:443–452, 1981

Finch BE, Wallace CJ: Successful interpersonal skills training with schizophrenic inpatients. J Consult Clin Psychol 45:885–890, 1977

Gartner AJ, Riessman F: Self-help and mental health. Hospital and Community Psychiatry 33:631–635, 1982

Glick ID, Clarkin JF, Spencer JH, et al: A controlled evaluation of inpatient family intervention, I: preliminary results of the six-month followup. Arch Gen Psychiatry 42:682–686, 1985

Glick ID, Spencer JH, Clarkin JF, et al: A randomized clinical trial of inpatient family intervention, IV: follow-up results with schizophrenia. Schizophr Res 3:187–200, 1990

Glynn SM, Randolph ET, Eth S, et al: Schizophrenic symptoms, work adjustment and behavioral family therapy. Rehabilitation Psychology 37:323–338, 1992

Goldstein MJ: Family therapy during the aftercare treatment of acute schizophrenia, in Family Therapy and Major Psychopathology. Edited by Lansky MR. New York, Grune & Stratton, 1981, pp 21–34

Goldstein MJ: Psychoeducation and relapse prevention. Int Clin Psychopharmacol 9 (suppl 5):59–69, 1995

Goldstein MJ, Doane JA: Family factors in the onset, course and treatment of schizophrenic spectrum disorders: an update on current research. J Nerv Ment Dis 170:692–700, 1983

Goldstein MJ, Rodnick EH, Evans JR, et al: Drug and family therapy in the aftercare of acute schizophrenics. Arch Gen Psychiatry 35:1169–1177, 1978

Goldstein MJ, Talovic SA, Nuechterlein KH, et al: Family interaction versus individual psychopathology: do they indicate the same processes in the families of schizophrenics? Br J Psychiatry 161 (suppl 18):97–102, 1992

Gould E, Glick ID: The effects of family presence and brief family intervention on global outcome for hospitalized schizophrenic patients. Fam Process 16:503–510, 1977

Greenley JR: The patient's family and length of psychiatric hospitalization, in The Psychiatric Hospital and the Family. Edited by Harbin HT. New York, SP Medical & Scientific Books, 1982, pp 213–237

Greenman DA, Gunderson JG, Canning D: Parents' attitudes and patients' behavior: a prospective study. Am J Psychiatry 146:226–230, 1989

Group for the Advancement of Psychiatry, Committee on the Family: The Family, the Patient, and the Psychiatric Hospital: Toward a New Model. New York, Brunner/Mazel, 1985

Haas GL, Glick ID, Clarkin JF, et al: Gender and schizophrenia outcome: a clinical trial of an inpatient family intervention. Schizophr Bull 16:277–292, 1990

Hahlweg K, Nuechterlein KH, Goldstein MJ, et al: Parental expressed emotion: attitudes and intrafamilial communication behavior, in Understanding Mental Disorder: The Contribution of Family Interaction Research. Edited by Hahlweg K, Goldstein MJ. New York, Family Process Press, 1987, pp 156–175

Haley J: Problem-Solving Therapy: New Strategies for Effective Family Therapy, 2nd Edition. San Francisco, CA, Jossey-Bass, 1987

Harbin HT: Families and hospitals: collusion or cooperation? Am J Psychiatry 135:1496–1499, 1978

Harbin HT: A family-oriented psychiatric inpatient unit. Fam Process 18:281–291, 1979

Harbin HT: Family treatment of the psychiatric inpatient, in The Psychiatric Hospital and the Family. Edited by Harbin HT. New York, SP Medical & Scientific Books, 1982, pp 3–25

Hatfield AB: Coping and adaptation: a conceptual framework for understanding families, in Families of the Mentally Ill: Coping and Adaptation. Edited by Hatfield AB, Lefley HP. New York, Guilford, 1987, pp 30–59

Haynes RB, Taylor DW, Sackett DL (eds): Compliance in Health Care. Baltimore, MD, Johns Hopkins University Press, 1979

Heinrichs DW: Recent developments in the psychosocial treatment of chronic psychotic illnesses, in The Chronic Mental Patient: Five Years Later. Edited by Talbott JA. New York, Grune & Stratton, 1984, pp 123–136

Herz MI: Recognizing and preventing relapse in patients with schizophrenia. Hospital and Community Psychiatry 35:344–349, 1984

Herz MI, Szymanski HV, Simon JC: Intermittent medication for stable schizophrenic outpatients: an alternative to maintenance medication. Am J Psychiatry 139:918–922, 1982

Hill R: Generic features of families under stress, in Crisis Intervention. Edited by Parad HJ. New York, Family Service Association, 1965, pp 32–52

Hoffman L: Foundations of Family Therapy: A Conceptual Framework for Systems Change. New York, Basic Books, 1981

Hogarty GE: Expressed emotion and schizophrenic relapse, in Controversies in Schizophrenia. Edited by Alpert M. New York, Guilford, 1985, pp 354–363

Hogarty GE, Goldberg SC, Schooler NR, et al: Drug and sociotherapy in the aftercare of schizophrenic patients, II: two-year relapse rates. Arch Gen Psychiatry 31:603–608, 1974

Hogarty GE, Schooler NR, Ulrich R, et al: Fluphenazine and social therapy in the aftercare of schizophrenic patients: relapse analyses of a two-year controlled study of fluphenazine decanoate and fluphenazine hydrochloride. Arch Gen Psychiatry 36:1283–1294, 1979

Hogarty GE, Anderson CM, Reiss DJ, et al: Family psychoeducation, social skills training, and maintenance chemotherapy in the aftercare treatment of schizophrenia, I: one-year effects of a controlled study on relapse and expressed emotion. Arch Gen Psychiatry 43:633–642, 1986

Hogarty GE, Anderson CM, Reiss DJ, et al: Family psychoeducation, social skills training, and maintenance chemotherapy in the aftercare treatment of schizophrenia, II: two-year effects of a controlled study on relapse and adjustment. Arch Gen Psychiatry 48:340–347, 1991

Hogarty GE, Reiss DJ, Kornblith SJ, et al: Social skills training for schizophrenia? (letter). Arch Gen Psychiatry 49:76–77, 1992

Hogarty GE, Greenwald D, Ulrich RF, et al: Three year trials of personal therapy among schizophrenic patients living with or independent of family, II: effects on adjustment of patients. Am J Psychiatry 154:1514–1524, 1997a

Hogarty GE, Kornblith SJ, Greenwald D, et al: Three year trials of personal therapy among schizophrenic patients living with or independent of family, I: description of study and effects on relapse rates. Am J Psychiatry 154:1504–1513, 1997b

Holden DF, Lewine RRJ: How families evaluate mental health professionals, resources and effects of illness. Schizophr Bull 8:626–633, 1982

Hooley JM: Expressed emotion: a review of the critical literature. Clin Psychol Rev 5:119–139, 1985

Horowitz MJ, Weisberg PS: Techniques for the group psychotherapy of acute psychosis. Int J Group Psychother 16:42–50, 1966

Johnson DL: The family's experience of living with mental illness, in Families as Allies in Treatment of the Mentally Ill. Edited by Lefley HP, Johnson DL. Washington, DC, American Psychiatric Press, 1990, pp 31–63

Kahn EM, Kahn EW: Group treatment assignment for outpatients with schizophrenia: integrating recent clinical and research findings. Community Ment Health J 28:539–550, 1992

Kanas N: Inpatient and outpatient group therapy for schizophrenic patients. Am J Psychother 39:431–439, 1985

Kanas N: Group therapy with schizophrenics: a review of controlled studies. Int J Group Psychother 36:339–360, 1986

Kanas N: Group therapy with schizophrenic patients: a short-term, homogeneous approach. Int J Group Psychother 41:33–48, 1991

Kanas N, Rogers M, Kreth E, et al: The effectiveness of group psychotherapy during the first three weeks of hospitalization: a controlled study. J Nerv Ment Dis 168:487–492, 1980

Kane JM: Treatment of schizophrenia. Schizophr Bull 13:133–156, 1987

Kane JM, Rifkin A, Woerner M, et al: Low-dose neuroleptic treatment of outpatient schizophrenics, I: preliminary results for relapse rates. Arch Gen Psychiatry 40:893–896, 1983

Katz HM, Frank A, Gunderson JG, et al: Psychotherapy of schizophrenia: what happens to treatment dropouts. J Nerv Ment Dis 172:326–331, 1984

Kavanagh DJ: Recent developments in expressed emotion and schizophrenia. Br J Psychiatry 160:601–620, 1992

Keith SJ, Matthews SM: Group, family and milieu therapies and psychosocial rehabilitation in the treatment of the schizophrenic disorders, in Psychiatry 1982: The American Psychiatric Association Annual Review. Edited by Grinspoon L. Washington, DC, American Psychiatric Press, 1982, pp 166–178

King S, Dixon MJ: The influence of expressed emotion, family dynamics, and symptom type on the social adjustment of schizophrenic young adults. Arch Gen Psychiatry 53:1098–1104, 1996

Krajewski T, Harbin HT: The family changes the hospital? in The Psychiatric Hospital and the Family. Edited by Harbin HT. New York, SP Medical & Scientific Books, 1982, pp 143–154

Kreisman DE, Joy VD: The family as reactor to the mental illness of a relative, in Handbook of Evaluation Research, Vol 2. Edited by Struening E, Guttentag M. Beverly Hills, CA, Sage, 1975, pp 483–518

Kuipers L, Bebbington PE: Expressed emotion research in schizophrenia: theoretical and clinical implications. Psychol Med 18:893–909, 1988

Kuipers L, Sturgeon D, Berkowitz R, et al: Characteristics of expressed emotion: its relationship to speech and looking in schizophrenic patients and their relatives. Br J Clin Psychol 22:257–264, 1983

Kuipers L, MacCarthy B, Hurry J, et al: Counseling the relatives of the long-term adult mentally ill, II: a low-cost supportive model. Br J Psychiatry 154:775–782, 1989

Langsley DG, Kaplan DM: The Treatment of Families in Crisis. New York, Grune & Stratton, 1968

Laqueur HP: Multiple family therapy, in Family Therapy and Major Psychopathology. Edited by Lansky MR. New York, Grune & Stratton, 1981, pp 57–69

Leff J: Stress reduction in the social environment of schizophrenic patients. Acta Psychiatr Scand Suppl 384:133–139, 1994

Leff J, Kuipers L, Berkowitz R, et al: A controlled trial of social intervention in the families of schizophrenic patients. Br J Psychiatry 141:121–134, 1982

Leff J, Kuipers L, Berkowitz R, et al: A controlled trial of social intervention in the families of schizophrenic patients: two-year follow-up. Br J Psychiatry 146:594–600, 1985

Leff J, Berkowitz R, Shavit N, et al: A trial of family therapy v a relatives group for schizophrenia. Br J Psychiatry 154:58–66, 1989

Lefley HP: Expressed emotion: conceptual, clinical and social policy issues. Hospital and Community Psychiatry 43:591–598, 1992

Lefley HP, Johnson DL (eds): Families as Allies in the Treatment of the Mentally Ill. Washington, DC, American Psychiatric Press, 1990

Lefley HP, Wasow M (eds): Helping Families Cope With Mental Illness. Baltimore, MD, Harwood Academic, 1994

Leszcz M, Yalom ID, Norden M: The value of inpatient group psychotherapy: patients' perceptions. Int J Group Psychother 35:411–433, 1985

Lewin K: Group decision and social change, in Readings in Social Psychology. Edited by Maccoby N, Newcomb TM. New York, Henry Holt, 1947, pp 330–344

Liberman RP: Social skills training, in Psychiatric Rehabilitation of Chronic Mental Patients. Edited by Liberman RP. Washington, DC, American Psychiatric Press, 1987, pp 147–198

Liberman RP, Wallace CJ, Vaughn CE, et al: Social and family factors in the course of schizophrenia: towards an interpersonal problem-solving therapy for schizophrenics and their families, in The Psychotherapy of Schizophrenia. Edited by Strauss JS, Bowers M, Downey TW, et al. New York, Plenum, 1980, pp 21–54

Linn MW: Partial hospitalization, in A Clinical Guide for the Treatment of Schizophrenia. Edited by Bellack AS. New York, Plenum, 1989, pp 163–185

Lukoff D, Wallace CJ, Liberman RP, et al: A holistic program for chronic schizophrenic patients. Schizophr Bull 12:274–282, 1986

MacCarthy B, Hemsley DR: Unpredictability as a correlate of expressed emotion in the relatives of schizophrenics. Br J Psychiatry 148:727–731, 1986

MacCarthy B, Kuipers L, Hurry J, et al: Counseling the relatives of the long-term mentally ill, I: evaluation of the impact on relatives and patients. Br J Psychiatry 154:768–775, 1989

Malm U: The influence of group therapy on schizophrenia. Acta Psychiatr Scand Suppl 297:5–65, 1982

Malm U: Group therapy, in Psychosocial Treatment in Schizophrenia. Edited by Herz MI, Keith SJ, Docherty JP. New York, Elsevier, 1990, pp 191–211

Marder SR, Wirshing WC, Mintz J, et al: Two-year outcome of social skills training and group psychotherapy for outpatients with schizophrenia. Am J Psychiatry 153:1585–1592, 1996

Markewich I: Multiple family group therapy for schizophrenic patients in a day treatment program: a comparison of patient-included and patient-excluded groups for families with different levels of expressed emotion. New York, New York University School of Education, Health, Nursing and Arts Professions, 1986

Maxmen JS: An educative model for inpatient group therapy. Int J Group Psychother 28:321–338, 1978

Maxmen JS: Helping patients survive theories: the practice of an educative model. Int J Group Psychother 34:355–368, 1984

McCreadie RG, Phillips K, Harvey JA, et al: The Nithsdale schizophrenia surveys, VIII: do relatives want family intervention—and does it help? Br J Psychiatry 158:110–113, 1991

McFarlane WR: Multiple family therapy in schizophrenia, in Family Therapy in Schizophrenia. Edited by McFarlane WR. New York, Guilford, 1983, pp 141–172

McFarlane WR: Multiple family groups and the treatment of schizophrenia, in Psychosocial Treatment of Schizophrenia. Edited by Herz MI, Keith SJ, Docherty JP. New York, Elsevier, 1990, pp 167–189

McFarlane WR, Dunne E: Family psychoeducation and multi-family groups in the treatment of schizophrenia. Directions in Psychiatry 11:2–8, 1991

McFarlane WR, Link B, Dushay R, et al. Psychoeducational multiple family groups: four-year relapse outcome in schizophrenia. Fam Process 34:127–144, 1995a

McFarlane WR, Lukens E, Link B, et al. Multiple family groups and psychoeducation and the treatment of schizophrenia. Arch Gen Psychiatry 52:679–687, 1995b

McGill CW, Falloon IRH, Boyd JL, et al: Family educational interventions in the treatment of schizophrenia. Hospital and Community Psychiatry 34:934–938, 1983

McGlashan TH, Hemsson RK, Fenton WS: Psychosocial treatment of negative symptoms in schizophrenia, in Modern Problems in Pharmacopsychiatry. Edited by Andreason NC. Basel, Switzerland. Karger, 1990, pp 175–200

Miklowitz DJ, Goldstein MJ, Falloon IRH: Premorbid and symptomatic characteristics of schizophrenics from families with high and low levels of expressed emotion. J Abnorm Psychol 92:359–367, 1983

Miklowitz DJ, Goldstein MJ, Falloon IRH, et al: Interactional correlates of expressed emotion in families of schizophrenics. Br J Psychiatry 144:482–487, 1984

Miklowitz DJ, Strachan AM, Goldstein MJ, et al: Expressed emotion and communication deviance in the families of schizophrenics. J Abnorm Psychol 95:60–66, 1986

Miklowitz DJ, Goldstein MJ, Doane JA, et al: Is expressed emotion an index of a transactional process? I: parents' affective style. Fam Process 28:153–167, 1989

Mintz LI, Nuechterlein KH, Goldstein MJ, et al: The initial onset of schizophrenia and family expressed emotion: some methodological considerations. Br J Psychiatry 154:212–217, 1989

Minuchin S: Families and Family Therapy. Cambridge, MA, Harvard University Press, 1974

Monti PM, Curran JP, Corriveau DP, et al: Effects of social skills training groups and sensitivity training groups with psychiatric patients. J Consult Clin Psychol 48:241–248, 1980

Mueser KT, Glynn SM: Behavioral Family Therapy for Psychiatric Disorders. Boston, MA, Allyn & Bacon, 1995

Mueser KT, Bellack AS, Douglas MS, et al: Prediction of social skill acquisition in schizophrenia and major affective disorder patients from memory and symptomatology. Psychiatry Res 37:281–296, 1991

Mueser KT, Bellack AS, Wade JH, et al: Expressed emotion, social skill and response to negative affect in schizophrenia. J Abnorm Psychol 102:339–351, 1993

Newmark M: A practical model for treating schizophrenia in the real world. Dulwich Centre Newsletter (Australia) 4:29–34, 1991

O'Brien CP: Group therapy for schizophrenia: a practical approach. Schizophr Bull 1:119–130, 1975

O'Brien CP: Group psychotherapy with schizophrenia and affective disorders, in Comprehensive Group Psychotherapy, 2nd Edition. Edited by Kaplan HI, Sadock BJ. Baltimore, MD, Williams & Wilkins, 1983, pp 242–249

Olarte SW, Masnik R: Enhancing medication compliance in coffee groups. Hospital and Community Psychiatry 32:417–419, 1981

O'Shea MD, Phelps R: Multiple family therapy: current status and critical appraisal. Fam Process 24:555–582, 1985

Otteson JP: Creative caring: the use of buddy groups with chronic schizophrenics. J Consult Clin Psychol 47:649–651, 1979

Parad HJ, Caplan G: A framework for studying families in crisis, in Crisis Intervention. Edited by Parad HJ. New York, Family Service Association, 1965, pp 53–72

Parker G, Johnston P, Hayward L: Parental "expressed emotion" as a predictor of schizophrenic relapse. Arch Gen Psychiatry 45:806–813, 1988

Pattison EM, Brissenden A, Wohl T, et al: Assessing the specific effects of inpatient group psychotherapy. Int J Group Psychother 17:283–297, 1967

Paul GL, Lentz RJ: Psychosocial Treatment of Chronic Mental Patients: Milieu Versus Social Learning Programs. Cambridge, MA, Harvard University Press, 1977

Powles WE: Varieties and uses of group psychotherapy. Canadian Psychiatric Association Journal 9:196–201, 1964

Rabkin R: Crisis intervention, in The Book of Family Therapy. Edited by Ferber A, Mendelsohn M. New York, Science House, 1972, pp 582–596

Randolph ET, Eth S, Glynn SM, et al: Behavioural family management in schizophrenia: outcome of a clinic-based intervention. Br J Psychiatry 164:501–506, 1994

Reiser GG, Schorske BJ: Relationships between family caregivers and mental health professionals: the American experience, in Helping Families Cope With Mental Illness. Edited by Lefley HP, Wasow M. Baltimore, MD, Harwood Academic, 1994, pp 3–26

Scharfstein B, Libbey M: Family orientation: initiating patients and their families to psychiatric hospitalization. Hospital and Community Psychiatry 33:560–563, 1982

Schooler C, Spohn HE: Social dysfunction and treatment failure in schizophrenia. Schizophr Bull 8:85–98, 1982

Schooler NR: Maintenance medication for schizophrenics: strategies for dose reduction. Schizophr Bull 17:311–324, 1991

Schooler NR, Keith SJ, Severe JB, et al: Relapse and rehospitalization during maintenance treatment of schizophrenia: the effects of dose reduction and family treatment. Arch Gen Psychiatry 54:453–463, 1997

Seaman M: Outpatient groups for schizophrenia—ensuring attendance. Can J Psychiatry 26:32–37, 1981

Selzer MA, Grimaldi JAR, Kulchycky S: The pre-alliance group: a new strategy for working with treatment-resistant schizophrenics. New Dir Ment Health Serv 55:35–45, 1992

Simon FB, Stierlin H, Wynne LC: The Language of Family Therapy: A Systemic Vocabulary and Sourcebook. New York, Family Process Press, 1985

Slavson SR: Group psychotherapy and the nature of schizophrenia. Int J Group Psychother 11:3–32, 1961

Solomon P, Draine J, Mannion E, et al: The impact of individualized consultation and group workshop family education interventions in ill relative outcomes. J Nerv Ment Dis 184:252–255, 1996

Solomon P, Draine J, Mannion E, et al: Effectiveness of two models of brief family education: retention of gains by family members of adults with serious mental illness. Am J Orthopsychiatry 67:177–186, 1997

Solomon P, Draine J, Mannion E, et al: Increased contact with community mental health resources as a potential benefit of family education. Psychiatr Serv 49:333–339, 1998

Stein LI, Test MA: Alternative to mental hospital treatment, I: conceptual model, treatment program, and clinical evaluation. Arch Gen Psychiatry 37:392–397, 1980

Steiner J: Holistic group therapy for schizophrenic patients. Int J Group Psychother 29:195–210, 1979

Steinglass P: Psychoeducational family therapy for schizophrenia: a review essay. Psychiatry 50:14–23, 1987

Stewart RP: Building an alliance between the families of patients and the hospital: model and process. National Association of Private Psychiatric Hospitals Journal 12:63–68, 1982

Stirling J, Tantum D, Thomas P, et al: Expressed emotion and early onset schizophrenia: a one year follow-up. Psychol Med 21:675–685, 1991

Strachan AM, Leff JP, Goldstein MJ, et al: Emotional attitudes and direct communication in the families of schizophrenics: a cross-national replication. Br J Psychiatry 149:279–287, 1986

Strachan AM, Feingold D, Goldstein MJ, et al: Is expressed emotion an index of a transactional process? II: patient's coping style. Fam Process 28:169–181, 1989

Strauss JS, Hafez H, Lieberman P, et al: The course of psychiatric disorder, III: longitudinal principles. Am J Psychiatry 142:289–296, 1985

Subotnik KL, Nuechterlein KH: Prodromal signs and symptoms of schizophrenic relapse. J Abnorm Psychol 97:405–412, 1988

Sullivan HS: Conceptions of Modern Psychiatry. New York, WW Norton, 1940

Tarrier N, Barrowclough C: Providing information to relatives about schizophrenia: some comments. Br J Psychiatry 149:458–463, 1986

Tarrier N, Barrowclough C, Vaughn C, et al: The community management of schizophrenia: a controlled trial of a behavioral intervention with families to reduce relapse. Br J Psychiatry 153:532–542, 1988

Terkelsen KG: Schizophrenia and the family, II: adverse effects of family therapy. Fam Process 22:191–200, 1983

Tharp RG, Otis GD: Toward a theory for therapeutic intervention in families. Journal of Counseling Psychology 30:426–434, 1966

Thompson KS, Griffith EEH, Leaf PJ: A historical review of the Madison model of community care. Hospital and Community Psychiatry 41:625–634, 1990

Torrey EF: Surviving Schizophrenia: A Family Manual. New York, Harper & Row, 1983

van den Bosch RJ, van Asma MJO, Rombouts R: Coping style and cognitive dysfunction in schizophrenic patients. Br J Psychiatry 161 (suppl 18):123–128, 1992

Vaughan K, Doyle M, McConaghy N, et al: The Sydney intervention trial: a controlled trial of relatives' counselling to reduce schizophrenic relapse. Soc Psychiatry Psychiatr Epidemiol 27:16–21, 1992

Vaughn CE: Patterns of emotional response in the families of schizophrenic patients, in Treatment of Schizophrenia: Family Assessment and Intervention. Edited by Goldstein MJ, Hand I, Hahlweg K. New York, Springer-Verlag, 1986, pp 97–106

Vaughn CE, Leff JP: The influence of family life and social factors on the course of psychiatric illness: a comparison of schizophrenic and depressed neurotic patients. Br J Psychiatry 129:125–137, 1976

Vine P, Beels CC: Support and advocacy groups for the mentally ill, in Psychosocial Treatment of Schizophrenia. Edited by Herz MI, Keith SJ, Docherty JP. New York, Elsevier, 1990, pp 387–405

Wallace CJ: Community and interpersonal functioning in the course of schizophrenic disorders. Schizophr Bull 19:233–257, 1984

Wallace CJ, Liberman RP: Social skills training for patients with schizophrenia: a controlled clinical trial. Psychiatry Res 15:239–247, 1985

Wallace CJ, Nelson CJ, Liberman RP, et al: A review and critique of social skills training with schizophrenic patients. Schizophr Bull 6:42–63, 1980

Walsh J: The family education and support group: a psychoeducational aftercare program. Psychosocial Rehabilitation Journal 10:51–61, 1987

Watzlawick P, Weakland J, Fisch R: Change: Principles of Problem Formation and Problem Resolution. New York, WW Norton, 1974

Withersty DJ: Family involvement on a psychiatric inpatient service. Am J Psychiatry 134:93–94, 1977

Wolman BB: Group psychotherapy with latent schizophrenics. Int J Group Psychother 10:301–312, 1960

Wynne LC: Current concepts about schizophrenia and family relationships. J Nerv Ment Dis 169:82–89, 1981

Wynne LC, McDaniel SH, Weber TT (eds): Systems Consultation: A New Perspective for Family Therapy. New York, Guilford, 1986

Wynne LC, McDaniel SH, Weber TT: Professional politics and the concepts of family therapy, family consultation and systems consultation. Fam Process 26:153–166, 1987

Zastowny TR, Lehman AF, Cole RE, et al: Family management of schizophrenia: a comparison of behavioral and supportive family treatment. Psychiatr Q 63:159–186, 1992

37

Psychiatric Rehabilitation

Charles J. Wallace, Ph.D.
Robert Paul Liberman, M.D.
Alex Kopelowicz, M.D.
Daniel Yaeger, B.A.

Treatment of individuals with serious and persistent mental illness (SPMI) is a challenging, long-term endeavor. SPMI, particularly schizophrenia, has adverse effects on almost every area of an individual's functioning, and reversing or attenuating these impairments and disabilities requires comprehensive, continuous, coordinated, and consumer-oriented services. Individuals with schizophrenia have "difficulties in interpersonal relationships and in achieving and maintaining competitive employment. They are often shy, awkward, passive, dependent, unmotivated, socially ill at ease, and occasionally aggressive in ways that are embarrassing or frightening to other people ... they tend to suffer from the negative effects of long-term psychotropic drug treatment, and they resist proper medical care. They also lack the basic survival skills necessary for coping in society" (Bachrach 1983, p. 165).

Improving this bleak picture has been a major aim of stakeholder groups in their efforts to establish a comprehensive standard of care for individuals with SPMI. The National Institute of Mental Health's *Caring for People With Severe Mental Disorders* (National Institute of Mental Health 1991) exemplifies this standard particularly well: "[F]our domains encompass the important areas to be [treated]: 1) clinical, reduction or elimination of symptoms; 2) rehabilitative, improvement or restoration of social and vocational functioning; 3) humanitarian, increase in a sense of well-being and personal fulfillment; and 4) public welfare, prevention of harm." The field of psychiatric rehabilitation has arisen specifically to help individuals restore and improve their social, instrumental, and vocational functioning. In this chapter we review the field's current procedures and summarize the evidence for their efficacy. Before beginning the review, however, we provide a general orientation by briefly discussing the rationale for psychiatric rehabilitation.

Rationale

Psychiatric rehabilitation is based on the assumption that adequate social and role functioning is the outcome of three factors: 1) the characteristics of the individual, 2) the community's requirements for adequate functioning, and 3) the supportiveness of the environment. The individual's characteristics—symptoms, cognitive functioning, past experiences, current role skills—limit his or her functioning; the community's requirements are the standards for evaluating that functioning, and the environment might be either responsive or indifferent to the individual's attempts to function.

The interaction among these three factors defines the process, form, and content of psychiatric rehabilitation's assessment and intervention procedures. The rehabilitation process begins with a comprehensive elicitation of the individual's personally relevant long-term goals for improved social and instrumental role functioning. These goals anchor the process and provide the specific foci for the next step: assessment of the three factors that influence functioning.

During the assessment, the clinician measures the individual's characteristics, particularly past and current functioning, and gathers information about the community's requirements for adequate role functioning and the environment's resources and support. The results are reviewed by the individual and the rehabilitation practitioner/team, and together they formulate the incremental short-term goals that are the steps to achieving the individual's personal long-term goals.

Next, the individual and the rehabilitation practitioner/team collaboratively design a rehabilitation plan that specifies the services needed for each incremental goal. Typically, the services include a flexible combination of teaching the individual the behavioral skills that comprise improved functioning, reducing the community's requirements for adequate functioning, and/or increasing environmental support. Once the services have been implemented, the individual's functioning is periodically assessed and compared with the incremental goals and the community requirements. These comparisons quantify the outcomes of rehabilitation and highlight potential areas for new or modified interventions.

In the remainder of this chapter, we review the field's assessment and intervention techniques, ending with summary conclusions and suggested directions for future research and clinical efforts.

Assessment

Rehabilitation Planning

Until recently, obtaining the comprehensive information needed to plan rehabilitation was a haphazard process. Practitioners typically administered either idiosyncratic measures or a battery of standardized tests, each of which assessed a relevant individual characteristic (e.g., symptoms, measures of functioning). Unfortunately, the psychometric soundness of practitioners' measures is usually unknown, and the different administrative and scoring procedures of standardized tests make it difficult to integrate the results. In the last several years, however, several tests, checklists, and computer programs have been developed to collect the comprehensive information needed to plan and evaluate psychiatric treatment (Diamond and Becker 1999; Kennedy 1992; Weaver 1994; Weiss and Chapman 1993). One of these, the Client's Assessment of Strengths, Interests, and Goals (CASIG; Wallace et al., in press), is specifically designed for psychiatric rehabilitation.

CASIG is administered as a structured interview that begins by eliciting the individual's medium-term goals in five areas of community living: housing, money/work, interpersonal relationships, health, and spiritual activities. Additional questions are asked to clarify these goals and obtain the individual's estimate of the services needed to achieve them. The interview continues with thoroughly specified questions that assess the individual's current and past community functioning, medication compliance and side effects, quality of life, quality of treatment, symptoms, and performance of intolerable community behaviors. The yes-no responses are summarized either manually or with the aid of a computer program that also produces a suggested rehabilitation plan. CASIG is sufficiently well structured that it can be administered accurately by SPMI inpatients and outpatients (Lecomte et al. 1999). CASIG's results can be supplemented with data from measures of individually relevant variables such as presence of comorbid disorders, physical health status, and performance on selected cognitive tests.

Functional Behaviors

A number of measures have been developed that focus specifically on assessing the individual's functional behaviors (see review articles by Dickerson 1997, Goldman et al. 1992, and Wallace 1986). Some are brief measures of the global outcomes of programs and providers (e.g., Role Functioning Scale; [McPheeters 1984]); others are thoroughly detailed measures that collect data from several sources (e.g., Independent Living Skills Survey [Wallace et al. 2000]). The cost for the greater detail is the time required to administer and score the data and interpret the results; the benefit is the greater precision of the information for pinpointing needed services and detecting changes in functioning.

Interventions

The core intervention of psychiatric rehabilitation is training the individual to perform the behavioral skills that comprise improved functioning. As necessary as it is, though, training is insufficient to guarantee that the individual will achieve his or her goals of improved functioning. The environment must provide the opportunities and encouragement to perform the skills and consistently deliver well-timed rewards. Hence, the rehabilitation plan includes services to train the individual and increase the environment's support.

Skills Training

Training closes the gap between the individual's current skills and those needed for improved functioning. Although its methods are straightforward (i.e., describe what will be trained, demonstrate it, practice it), its content is far from straightforward. Developing the curricula to teach skills such as managing one's money, maintaining employment, coping with SPMI symptoms, and participating in basic conversations is neither quick nor easy. Moreover, the instructional techniques must bypass or compensate for individuals' symptoms and cognitive dysfunctions that might interfere with learning.

Liberman and his colleagues have addressed this difficulty by producing modules that teach community living skills with thoroughly specified curricula and highly structured methodology (Liberman et al. 1993). Eight modules have been produced: medication self-management, symptom self-management, substance abuse management, recreation for leisure, basic conversation, workplace fundamentals, community reentry, and friendship and intimacy. All of them, as well as those under development, use the same methodology to train each skill in each module. Only the content varies from module to module, and the repetition of the methodology provides a predictable teaching/learning environment that helps trainers to conduct the modules and individuals to learn the skills.

For example, the workplace fundamentals module teaches nine skills: 1) knowing how work changes your life, 2) knowing your workplace, 3) knowing your workplace stressors, 4) solving problems, 5) solving health and substance abuse workplace problems, 6) solving mental health workplace problems, 7) coping with supervisors and improving task performance, 8) coping with peers and informal socializing, and 9) getting support and maintaining enthusiasm. Each skill is defined in terms of the specific behaviors required for successful performance. For example, coping with peers and informal socializing require identifying the workplace "rules" for social relationships, initiating and ending brief and friendly conversations, and solving relationship problems. These behaviors are the targets of training.

The training methodology consists of seven learning activities detailed in Figure 37–1. The introduction sets the stage for the learning; it tells the learners the "payoff" that they can expect from their investment of time and energy. The demonstration videotape provides a clear presentation of the skills that can be easily and consistently presented across diverse staff and settings. The videotape's periodic stops and the questions to assess viewers' comprehension are essential for ensuring that the training is achieving its instructional objectives. The role-play practice is similarly critical because learning is not just comprehension; it is ultimately the enactment of a skill. Furthermore, the more often that participants practice enacting the skill, the more polished their performances when the actual opportunities arise.

The problem-solving activities are the first steps in helping participants transfer their skills to their living environments. Two types of problems are considered: how to obtain the resources required to perform a skill and how to overcome obstacles in environments that do not respond as they should (Wallace and Boone 1984). The final two activities—exercises accompanied by a support person and homework assignments—extend training into the real world. Participants first complete real-life assignments accompanied by the trainer or case manager and then complete homework assignments on their own.

Each module is packaged with a trainer's manual, participant's workbook, and demonstration videotape. The manual specifies exactly what the trainer is to say and do to teach all of a module's skills; the videotape demonstrates the skills; and the workbook provides written material, forms, and exercises that help the individual learn the skills. A module can be easily conducted by one trainer with from one to eight participants. Having more than eight participants, however, reduces the opportunities for each to answer the questions and practice the skills and the problem-solving exercises.

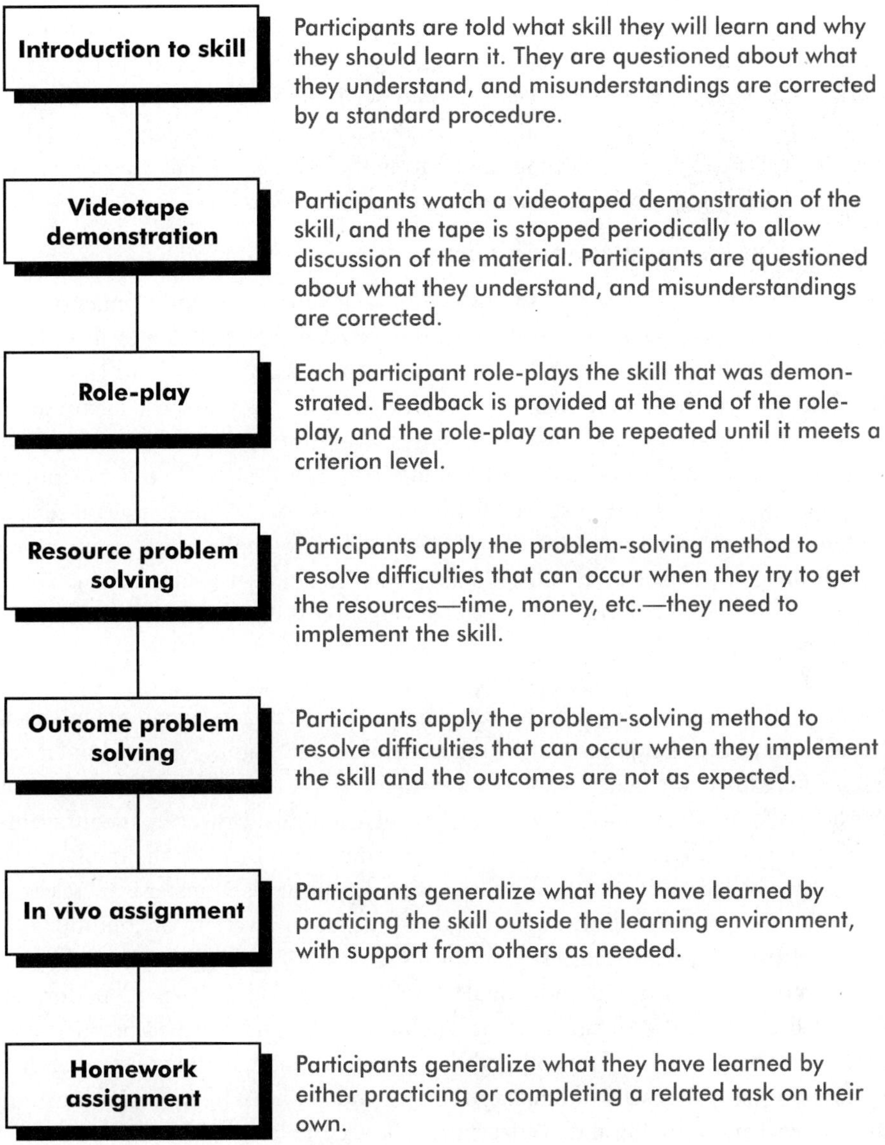
Introduction to skill
Participants are told what skill they will learn and why they should learn it. They are questioned about what they understand, and misunderstandings are corrected by a standard procedure.
Videotape demonstration
Participants watch a videotaped demonstration of the skill, and the tape is stopped periodically to allow discussion of the material. Participants are questioned about what they understand, and misunderstandings are corrected.
Role-play
Each participant role-plays the skill that was demonstrated. Feedback is provided at the end of the role-play, and the role-play can be repeated until it meets a criterion level.
Resource problem solving
Participants apply the problem-solving method to resolve difficulties that can occur when they try to get the resources—time, money, etc.—they need to implement the skill.
Outcome problem solving
Participants apply the problem-solving method to resolve difficulties that can occur when they implement the skill and the outcomes are not as expected.
In vivo assignment
Participants generalize what they have learned by practicing the skill outside the learning environment, with support from others as needed.
Homework assignment
Participants generalize what they have learned by either practicing or completing a related task on their own.

FIGURE 37–1. Seven learning activities.

Of course, the teaching must be modified to fit and compensate for the large variations in SPMI individuals' functioning, symptoms, and capabilities to benefit from training. Adaptations also should be made to fit the module into the particular characteristics of the clinical setting. The modules' repetitive, tight structure provides a completely reproducible starting point for these modifications. Experienced trainers can experiment with a variety of alterations, and inexperienced trainers can return to the structure should their modifications prove ineffective. The repetitive structure compensates for most symptomatic and cognitive limitations (Eckman et al. 1992) and forms a constant background of psychosocial treatment against which the effects of other treatments (e.g., medications) can be determined.

Empirical Evaluation of Skills Training

Over the past decade, a number of review articles have critically evaluated the evidence of the effects of skills training with SPMI individuals (e.g., Benton and Schroeder 1990; Dilk and Bond 1996; Heinssen et al. 2000; Penn and Mueser 1996; Scott and Dixon 1995). Their conclusions answer three key questions: 1) Do individuals learn and retain the skills? 2) If so, do individuals transfer their learning and perform the skills in the real world? and 3) Do the benefits of training generalize to improvements in other outcomes?

Learning the Skills and Retaining Them

Numerous studies have documented the significant and substantial improvements in participants' knowledge and behaviors as the result of training (e.g., Eckman et al. 1992; Kopelowicz et al. 1998; Liberman et al. 1998; Marder et al. 1996; Wallace et al. 1992, 1999). Furthermore, participants retain their improvements for up to 2 years, the maximum duration measured. These studies have been conducted in diverse treatment settings (inpatient, outpatient, partial/day hospitals, residential care of all types) by diverse practitioners (nursing staff, recreational therapists, mental health counselors, residential managers, and paraprofessional staff) covering a broad range of skills (steady employment, preparation for discharge from inpatient treatment, illness management, smoking cessation, human immunodeficiency virus (HIV) risk reduction, and conversation skills) (Heinssen et al. 2000).

Transfer of Training

The results are less conclusive for transferring skills to participants' environments. There is, of course, a transfer gradient, that is, the more alike the training and living environments, the more likely the behaviors will be transferred. But the gradient is steep, and the transfer falls off with even small differences between settings. However, encouragement and reinforcement evidence indicates that two procedures can increase the transfer. If opportunities are created in the living environment to use the skills, transfer is increased.

If the skills are automated through repeated practice in a variety of conditions, it is more likely that they will be transferred to diverse settings. Although this "overlearning" has not been directly tested with individuals with SPMI, studies of "expert" performance (Ericsson and Charness 1994) suggest that lengthy training and repeated practice are essential for producing stable, highly polished performances. These findings also suggest that infrequent training sessions are of limited value; too much time is spent reviewing and relearning rather than practicing and overlearning. The accumulated research and clinical experience indicates that skills training must be offered on at least a weekly basis for not less than 6 months to achieve substantial gains in persons with SPMI (Heinssen et al. 2000).

Generalization to Other Outcomes

Most, but not all, studies have reported few significant differences between participants in skills training and participants in control interventions in changes on measures of psychopathology, rehospitalization, and relapse (Dobson et al. 1995; Eckman et al. 1992; Liberman et al. 1998, 1999; Marder et al. 1996). The relative independence among the outcomes of treatment of persons with SPMI has been well documented (Carpenter et al. 1976), and outcomes tend to be specifically linked to particular treatments. For example, symptoms and relapse rates are more closely related to the quality and efficacy of psychopharmacotherapy, while psychosocial and community functioning are more responsive to behavioral treatments such as social skills training and supported employment (Heinssen et al. 2000; Marder et al. 1996).

Studies show one benefit unique to skills training: except for conceptual disorganization, skills training can be successfully conducted regardless of symptoms, even with inpatients with acute illness (Kopelowicz et al. 1998; Smith et al. 1996). The results also indicate that even during the acute phase of the illness individuals can profit from skills training. Indeed, the earlier one starts the rehabilitation process, the more opportunities become available to learn, practice, and adapt one's skills (Kopelowicz et al. 1998; MacKain et al. 1998; Smith et al. 1996).

Environmental Support

The individual's living environment is the ultimate test for his or her functional skills and provides both the opportunities to perform the skills and the rewards for doing so. The opportunities set the specific requirements for a successful performance; the regularity with which the success is actually rewarded depends on the recognition by people in the environment that a performance is successful and their willingness to then reward it.

A number of interventions have been developed to help an individual adapt his or her functional behaviors to the opportunities and/or to increase the environment's support. Most interventions have focused on increasing the family's general support; only a few have focused on improving residential care support or helping the individual adapt to the environment (DeRisi et al. 1975; Liberman et al. 2000).

Family Interventions

The family interventions—variously labeled family psychoeducation, behavioral family management/therapy, family-aided assertive community treatment, and multiple-family therapy—are designed to actively engage families in the rehabilitation process. All share several components, including educating about the nature of SPMI; assisting with using available community resources; and teaching better methods of managing stress, communicating, and problem solving (Mueser et al. 1994; Strachan 1992). Evaluations of these interventions have reported that adding them to a regimen of medication and customary case management produces substantially better outcomes than the latter two alone (Falloon et al. 1999; Hogarty et al. 1986; Leff et al. 1989; Liberman et al. 1984; MacFarlane et al. 1992; Randolph et al. 1994).

In contrast to the global nature of these family interventions, Kopelowicz and colleagues (1998) focused on improving families' support for the specific behaviors taught in two of the skills training modules, symptom management and medication management. The family intervention and skills training with patients in groups were conducted concurrently. Family members were taught how to provide opportunities for their SPMI relatives to implement the behaviors being taught in the modules, encourage their relatives to implement the behaviors, and reward them with positive feedback when they did so.

The effects of the intervention were evaluated in a rigorous experimental design with a total of 86 Latino families. The modules were translated into Spanish and culturally adapted, and half of the families were randomly assigned to the combined individual/family training and half were assigned to customary outpatient care. The results indicated that the participants with SPMI learned the skills, transferred them to their living environments, and maintained their use for at least 6 months after training, the duration of the follow-up in this study. Moreover, participants in skills training had lower rates of positive and negative symptoms at the end of training and at the 6-month follow-up as well as fewer hospitalizations during the 9 months of the study and 1 year later than did the individuals receiving customary care.

Community Reentry Module

The community reentry module (CRM) teaches individuals how to develop their own comprehensive community aftercare. The module is another of the Liberman et al. series, modified for use in the rapid-turnover operations of a typical, short-term-care, psychiatric inpatient facility. The module consists of sixteen 45-minute sessions divided into two 8-session sections: 1) planning for discharge and linking with service providers, and 2) understanding and managing mental illness. The CRM is formatted for continuous implementation, with participants "dropping in" and completing as many of the sessions as the cycling schedule and their schedules permit. An initial evaluation (Smith et al. 1996) found that participants not only learned the material, despite their acute illnesses, but their discharge level of knowledge and performance on the CRM skills was positively associated with their functioning 2 months after discharge.

Kopelowicz et al. (1998) conducted a rigorous evaluation of the CRM with 59 consecutive admissions to a short-term-care, psychiatric inpatient unit of a university-affiliated county hospital. The participants were randomly assigned either to the CRM or to equally intensive occupational therapy (OT) that used artistic and craft activities. Patients in both conditions received customary discharge planning services from social workers, including referrals to specific aftercare programs and housing.

The results again confirmed that the CRM participants with acute illness learned the material, improving from 54.5% correct on a pretest of knowledge and skills to 81.3% at discharge compared with a change from 50.4% to 54.8% for the OT group. Importantly, 85.2% of the CRM group attended their first aftercare appointments compared with 37% of the OT group. Because continuity of care is one of the key elements in successful long-term outcome, the results indicated that the CRM, with its well-focused and clear-cut outcome, had utility for participants, practitioners, and the system of care.

Nonfamilial Supporters

More common than training individuals to craft their own continuing care is increasing their nonfamilial environmental support. One approach is to teach patients to become their own advocates and case managers, using social skills training techniques that instigate and reinforce completion of assignments in the community that enable participants to attain their own personal goals (Hierholzer and Liberman 1986; Liberman et al. 1989). Another approach, described by Dobson (1996), is to create an ongoing support group of individuals who have participated in a common psychoeducational program. Periodic meetings provide opportunities for participants to refresh their skills, discuss problems, and encourage other participants' attempts to improve their lifestyle. Dobson conducted a randomized evaluation of this approach and reported that its costs were low, the participants were satisfied with its effects, and it may have reduced subsequent hospital use.

Alternatively, self-directed groups may be formed regardless of participants' common treatment experience. These groups create opportunities for social contact, recreation, and advocacy. Lane (1998), for example, described the establishment of a telephone peer counseling service staffed by individuals with SPMI. The service was a "win-win situation that resulted from an effective collaboration between clients, both as colleagues and consumers, and mental health professionals" (Lane 1998, p. 312).

Two other support procedures have been developed and evaluated, both explicitly designed to help participants in the skills training modules transfer their newly learned behaviors from training to their living environments. One, in vivo amplified skills training (IVAST), involves specialized case managers who routinely conduct additional training sessions in participants' environments. The sessions help participants adapt their behaviors to their environments and practice that adaptation. In addition, case managers "run interference" for individuals with SPMI so that opportunities and encouragement are provided for them to use their skills in everyday life. Evaluations of IVAST have reported that participants with the extra support achieved higher levels of interpersonal problem-solving skills, significantly greater social adjustment, and better quality of life over a 2-year period than did participants with the skills training alone (Liberman et al., in press).

The second procedure involves indigenous supporters—residential care staff, peers, and relatives—who similarly help participants in skills training adapt their newly learned behaviors to their living environments. Supporters are selected by participants based on the criteria of cooperativeness, accessibility, and familiarity with the specifics of their environments. Support consists of structured meetings between a participant and his or her supporter to review the participant's use of the newly learned behaviors, explore the causes of a less-than-satisfactory use, and generate a method to improve that use. No constraints are placed on the frequency or duration of a pair's meetings.

Tauber et al. (in press) evaluated the procedure with several process and outcome measures. Skills training participants chose primarily residential care staff and friends (89%) as supporters. The pairs had either established a long-term relationship (42% had known each other for more than 2 years) or met rather recently (40% had been acquainted for less than 6 months). The meetings between clients and supporters were frequent (average of 11 per month), lengthy (minimum of 30 minutes), and focused primarily on performance of the clients' newly learned behaviors. Both the supporters and the participants were highly satisfied with their relationship. Participants who received both the skills training and the added support improved their interpersonal and community functioning during training and continued to improve during the 18 months after training. In contrast, those without support lost some of their improvements during the follow-up.

Specialized Interventions

To address specialized problems, several psychiatric rehabilitation interventions have been developed: comorbid substance use disorder (SUD) and SPMI treatment, vocational rehabilitation, and cognitive rehabilitation.

Comorbid Substance Use Disorder Treatment

During the past two decades, the prevalence of dually diagnosed SPMI individuals—those with concurrent SPMI and SUD—has increased enormously. The combination of the two disorders greatly complicates individuals' treatment. SUD increases the risk of symptomatic relapse (Roberts et al. 1992; Sullivan et al. 1995; Swofford et al. 1996), interferes with the effects of antipsychotic medications, decreases compliance with treatment, increases the burden experienced by families and other caregivers (Clark et al. 1998), and multiplies the use of other services such as the legal system (Clark et al. 1999).

The reasons that dually diagnosed individuals use alcohol and drugs are the same as those of non-SPMI abusers (Bellack and DiClemente 1999; Carey et al. 1999; Cuffel et al. 1993). Dually diagnosed individuals report that alcohol and drug use makes them feel "euphoric, high, relaxed, or comfortable, and increases [their] ability to mix socially." They also report that it provides an opportunity to "be part of a crowd" and be with "others who were doing the same thing." Substance abuse also "fills [their] time and occupies [their] minds." Abstaining would "allow them to get more accomplished and be more productive..., go to educational programs," and be "attentive to [their] appearance and cleaning [their] home" (Carey et al. 1999, p. 291).

These responses suggest that psychiatric rehabilitation should be a major component of dually diagnosed individuals' treatment. Developing social networks, engaging in alternate activities, and participating in work or other productive pursuits are all part of psychiatric rehabilitation's goal of improving individuals' social and instrumental functioning. However, until recently, it has been difficult to introduce psychiatric rehabilitation even as a minor component in these individuals' care. The difficulty is that individuals have straddled two systems of care, one for SUD and one for SPMI. Each has its own personnel, funds, treatments, and mechanisms of authority and accountability, and dually diagnosed individuals have been shuffled between them.

Integration of SPMI and SUD services has now become the standard of care for dually diagnosed individuals (Center for Substance Abuse Treatment 1994). Drake and his colleagues define the standards of care as 1) treatment of both disorders by the "same clinicians who are trained in psychopathology, assessment, and treatment strategies for both"; 2) "emphasis on trust and learning rather than confrontation"; 3) "emphasis on reduction of harm from substance use rather than immediate abstinence"; 4) "slow pace and long-term perspective"; 5) "12-step groups available to those who choose and can benefit rather than being mandated for all"; 6) "neuroleptics and other pharmacotherapies indicated according to needs rather than being contraindicated for all"; 7) "some components specifically address substance use reduction"; and 8) "components focus on integrated treatment including substance abuse group interventions ... case management ... medications and medication management ... [and] psychosocial rehabilitation" (Drake et al. 1998).

Reviews and evaluations of integrated treatment have concluded that its effects are modest, with the most encouraging evidence coming from 10 studies "that included an array of components and followed participants for more than a year" (Drake et al. 1998, p. 601). One of these studies, Ridgely and Jerrell (1996), compared psychiatric rehabilitation services—specifically, training in social and instrumental role skills—with participation in either Alcoholics Anonymous groups or intensive case management. The training consisted of four of the Liberman and colleagues' (1993) skills training modules. The results indicated that the individuals who participated in the training "demonstrated substantially more positive outcomes across several indicators of client and system outcomes" (Ridgely and Jerrell 1996, p. 569) than did individuals who received either of the other two services. These indicators included symptoms, alcohol abuse, drug abuse, and community functioning.

To further increase the effectiveness of integrated treatment, a skills module has been produced to train the participants in the competencies needed to reduce current substance abuse and prevent it in the future. The module (Roberts et al. 1999) is based on a relapse prevention strategy that consists of seven tactics (e.g., practice damage control, avoid or escape high-risk situations, seek healthy alternatives) implemented with nine skills (e.g., quit before a slip becomes a full-blown relapse, report a slip, refuse drugs from a pushy dealer or friend, ask someone to join you in a healthy alternative). As with all other modules of the UCLA Social and Independent Living Skills Program, this module is available from its progenitors (Psychiatric Rehabilitation Consultants 2000).

The module is conducted as ongoing training that participants can join and exit at any point. The module has been in clinical use for approximately 4 years, and a pilot test of its efficacy was recently completed. A total of 56 individuals participated. All had extensive histories of SUD, and 75% had cocaine in their urine at the time of admission. Several outcome measures (e.g., Addiction Severity Index, urine toxicology, Brief Psychiatric Rating Scale) were administered pretest, posttest, and at a 3-month follow-up. Thirty-four individuals (61%) completed the study. The results indicated that days of complete abstinence in the past 30 days increased significantly from a mean of 12.76 to 24.26 and remained high at the 3-month follow-up (mean = 25.82). Moreover, there were significant and substantial reductions in all of the main drugs of abuse (cocaine, alcohol, and marijuana). Compliance with antipsychotic medication was significantly higher at the completion of treatment with the Substance Abuse Management Module and at follow-up, and psychiatric symptoms improved significantly at posttest and remained improved at the 3-month follow-up.

Vocational Rehabilitation

Helping physically disabled individuals find and keep competitive employment has long been the purview of a specialized system of care, the vocational rehabilitation system. Its services are generally time-limited, with a strong pressure on practitioners to successfully close cases as rapidly as possible with little, if any, follow-up. Unfortunately, such services are ill suited to the majority of SPMI individuals. A number of treatments, separate from the vocational rehabilitation system, have been developed to help SPMI individuals enter and stay in the workforce.

Transitional Employment

The first treatments were based on a train-place model that offered individuals time-limited work experiences and taught them vocational skills as they worked in these accommodating environments. Presumably, the workers would acquire the skills needed to get and keep competitive employment (Mastboom 1992).

Quasi-experimental evaluations of this model produced mixed results, and no well-controlled study found consistently higher rates of competitive employment than those under control conditions. A very different treatment, supported employment, had achieved superior rates of competitive employment with developmentally delayed individuals, and it was soon adapted for use with individuals with SPMI (Becker and Drake 1994).

Supported Employment

The supported employment (SE) model is based on a place-train sequence of services. Individuals are quickly placed in competitive employment and receive any and all services needed to keep them employed. Given the unpredictable course of SPMI and the changing nature of most jobs, the services are delivered as often as needed at the actual job site, consistent with employers' and individuals' preferences.

Evaluations of SE have confirmed its value when it is fully integrated into the care provided by a multidisciplinary psychiatric rehabilitation team. Drake and colleagues (1996) compared their integrated SE, individual placement and support (IPS), with traditional, brokered services conducted by a separate vocational rehabilitation agency. IPS was conducted by "employment specialists," each of whom served up to 25 individuals. The specialists collaborated with the individuals and their treatment teams to implement services that would achieve each individual's specific vocational goal.

Three findings of the Drake et al. (1996) study are applicable to the psychiatric rehabilitation procedures. First, IPS was significantly and substantially superior to the brokered services for helping individuals find jobs. Approximately one-half of the IPS participants obtained a competitive job; neither diagnosis nor symptoms were correlated with employment. Second, IPS and the brokered services did not differ on several measures of job retention. Both groups terminated their jobs at the same rates and for the same reasons: interpersonal problems, difficulty managing symptoms, dissatisfaction with the job, and poor work quality (Becker et al. 1998). Third, variations in the implementation of both IPS and the brokered services resulted in large differences in outcomes. As might be expected, the outcomes paralleled their accuracy or fidelity of utilization (Drake et al. 1999).

To help SPMI workers keep their jobs, Liberman and his colleagues (1993) produced another module in their series, the workplace fundamentals module, described previously. The skills it teaches explicitly address the reasons for job turnover by the SPMI, such as how to cope with stressors and how to socialize with co-workers. The thoroughly specified techniques it uses ensure its replication across a wide range of practitioners and treatment sites. Results from a quasi-experimental pilot implementation of the module were encouraging (Wallace et al. 1999), and a randomized clinical trial is now being conducted evaluating the effects of combining IPS and the module.

Cognitive Rehabilitation

A good deal of evidence indicates that individuals with SPMI, particularly those with schizophrenia, have enduring deficits in cognitive functions such as vigilance, working memory, secondary verbal memory, and executive functioning (Green and Nuechterlein 1999). A possible link between these deficits and social and instrumental role functioning seems obvious. Roles such as worker, spouse, and parent usually require processing complex information to make decisions and enact behaviors with uncertain and unknown outcomes. Hence, any deficiency in cognitive processing may lead to poor role functioning.

The treatment link seems just as obvious: improve cognitive functioning and role functioning will improve. These links, however, are not at all straightforward, and their thorny conceptual and methodological issues have been the subject of a decade's worth of reviews, opinions, and experiments (e.g., Bellack 1992; Bellack et al. 1999; Liberman and Green 1992; Spaulding et al. 1999).

Fueling the optimism that cognitive rehabilitation can be a valuable treatment strategy are two sets of findings: cognitive functioning is correlated with social and role functioning, and cognitive functioning can be modified. A number of studies have found that laboratory measures of cognitive functions such as vigilance, distractibility, and semantic memory are correlated with role-play and interview measures of social competence and social problem solving (e.g., Bellack et al. 1994, 1999; Bowen et al. 1994; Corrigan et al. 1994; Green 1996; Wykes et al. 1999). These cognitive measures are correlated with the outcomes of treatment designed to improve role functioning (Bowen et al. 1994; Corrigan et al. 1994; Kern et al. 1992; Mueser et al. 1991).

These results, however, must be interpreted cautiously. The measures of social competence and social problem solving are so narrowly operationalized that their results may not generalize to everyday social and role functioning. Performance in brief role-played interactions, for example, may have little relationship with performance in the ongoing complexities of spouse, parent, friend, and worker interactions.

A variation of this approach is to assess social and role functioning with broad measures and determine if these are related to cognitive functioning. Bellack et al. (1999) reported good vocational treatment outcomes (broadly defined as 1 year or more of full-time employment) that were associated with scores on two subtests of the Wechsler Adult Intelligence Scale–Revised (WAIS-R; Wechsler 1981), the Stroop Test (Stroop 1935), the Wisconsin Card Sorting Test (WCST; Heaton 1985), and the Trails B tests (Reitan and Wolfson 1993). Dickerson et al. (1996) found that spatial organization, aphasia, and visual spatial functioning were correlated with activities of daily living skills, social activities, and total social functioning. The functioning variables were assessed with a measure that was intermediate in breadth to the narrowness of the role-played interactions and the broad definition of vocational outcome used by Bellack et al. (1999). In a 2-year follow-up, Dickerson et al. (1999) reported that initial cognitive functioning predicted the 2-year changes on the three social functioning scales that did change (four did not change).

These results too must be interpreted cautiously. Functioning on broad measures may be affected by a host of variables that cannot be disentangled, and the findings cannot be unequivocally attributed to cognitive differences. Furthermore, the construct validity of the cognitive measures, which is typically difficult to establish, is the key to interpreting the results. What, for example, is (are) the construct(s) underlying the results reported in the study by Bellack et al. (1999)?

The evidence that cognitive functioning can be modified comes from studies of changing performance on specific cognitive tasks such as the WCST. Several much earlier studies changed performance with manipulations intended to explore the nature of the cognitive function and not treat it. For example, although individuals with SPMI recall information less accurately than individuals who are not mentally ill (e.g., Koh 1978), presenting the information in a manner that emphasizes its semantic organization substantially improves recall memory. Asking individuals to actively encode information into categories based on some characteristic, even a completely idiosyncratic one, improves memory (Koh et al. 1980, 1981; Larsen and Fromholt 1976). Rehearsal alone does not improve recall.

More recent studies have reported that cognitive functioning can be modified with manipulations relevant for treatment such as incentives and detailed instructions administered repeatedly. The cognitive tasks have included the Span of Apprehension Test and the WCST (Bellack et al. 1999; Green et al. 1992; Hellman et al. 1992; Kern et al. 1996). Changes on the WCST, at first so short-lived that their being labeled "learning" was questionable (Bellack et al. 1990), have been relatively durable when the manipulation involves detailed instructions (Bellack et al. 1999; Kern et al. 1996).

Again these results must be interpreted cautiously. Although the changes may be durable, only limited evidence exists showing that they generalize to other putative measures of the same cognitive function or to other functions. Bellack et al. (1999), for example, found no changes on the Vygotsky Category Test after WCST training, whereas Young and Freyslinger (1995) reported improvements on the Short Category Test after training on the WCST with scaffolded instruction. The construct validity of the cognitive measures is again the major problem in understanding these results. A lack of generalization can reflect insufficient shared common variance in the measures despite their purportedly measuring the same function, whereas generalization might reflect only shared method variance, not shared trait variance. A pattern of changes must be demonstrated that mirrors both convergent and discriminant validity.

Only a few clinical applications of cognitive rehabilitation techniques have been tried, and their results have been modest at best. One application (Spaulding et al. 1999) has carefully investigated the effects of Brenner's integrated psychological therapy (IPT) (Brenner et al. 1992, 1994). IPT is a series of training activities that systematically progress from visual and verbal memory to social and emotional perception to complex interpersonal problem solving. Brenner designed IPT based on somewhat arbitrary and theoretically derived conceptions of cognitive deficits in schizophrenia; thus, its tasks and measures are difficult to interpret.

Spaulding et al.'s (1999) positive results were limited to a subset of their outcome measures; their participants were long-term inpatients, and generalization of the findings to the larger population of community residents with less severe disorders is unknown. The durability of the results is similarly unknown. Hence, despite a decade of debate and research, efficacious and effective cognitive rehabilitation is still a promise waiting to be fulfilled.

Conclusions

The results of the numerous clinical trials and field tests summarized above reinforce the conclusions stated in this chapter in the second edition of the book (Wallace and Liberman 1995); individuals with SPMI can learn and "perform the…skills needed to live, learn, and work in the community" (Anthony 1979). Furthermore, these skills are retained without substantial degradation over a considerable period of time. Importantly, these results were produced with instructional tools whose thoroughly specified methodology makes them replicable across widely divergent practitioners and treatment settings.

Indeed, one of the conclusions drawn in this chapter in the previous edition was the desirability of producing standardized teaching methods "in a format that permits their wide-scale dissemination, adoption, and adaptation" (Wallace and Liberman 1995, p. 1037). The skills training modules provide these standardized teaching methods. Of course, no highly structured treatment fits perfectly the needs and characteristics of every individual with SPMI. The modules, however, fit a large proportion of individuals and offer accessible and well-defined starting points for building services adapted to each individual.

In addition to producing the modules, progress has been made toward fulfilling a number of other suggestions made in the second edition. Several assessment instruments have been developed that measure individuals' social and role functioning. The assessment instruments vary from a single item per major area of functioning to multiple items per basic area of independent living. Practitioners and managers can choose the instrument that balances the costs of collecting the data with the specificity of the results.

Methods of increasing the support of individuals' environments can offer solutions to the problem of generalizing individuals' functional behaviors from training to the real world. Considering that SPMI is a chronic condition, combining methods might make the most efficacious strategy for maintaining skills. Beginning generalization with a case manager who has competence in IVAST would place the process in the hands of a knowledgeable practitioner who could rapidly assess the environment and help individuals adapt their skills and/or alter the environment. Quickly shifting the process to indigenous supporters would add on-site assistants who could be routinely consulted by practitioners to assess generalization and modify the process accordingly. Enrolling individuals in a support group and/or a self-directed, self-help group would add peer social support and help with solving various problems. The practitioner's interventions at this later point would likely consist of periodic monitoring and occasional assistance. This flexible, multilevel approach to rehabilitation has been shown to have promise when tailored to severity of individuals' illnesses (Stein et al. 1999).

New Directions

As befits any area of mental health services with a growing base of empirical evidence and new techniques, numerous directions for future research and clinical efforts present themselves. Although psychometrically sound measures of social and role functioning have been developed, no methods have been developed for interpreting their results and integrating them into individualized treatment planning. A method based on practice guidelines, experts' rules, local norms, and individual resources and constraints could help practitioners implement more efficacious treatment. The interpretations and resulting treatment plans would document practitioners' standards of care; monitoring the treatment plans and observing the actual services would document the quality of that care.

The promise of cognitive rehabilitation has yet to be fully realized. Although the results of recent clinical trials are modestly encouraging, they are limited to a subset of outcome measures, and their durability and generalization to the much larger population of individuals with SPMI with less severe disorders are unknown. To improve cognitive functioning, innumerable methods could be used, such as thinking-skills programs developed for a wide range of children, self-help memory enhancement techniques, and computer-delivered exercises typically administered to individuals with traumatic brain injuries. It is entirely speculative as to which ones are more or less efficacious. Indeed, participation in skills training per se may improve general cognitive functioning, particularly if participation includes a regimen of overlearning mimicking the repeated trials of computer-delivered exercises for cognitive improvements in traumatic brain injuries. Even if participation did not generalize to improved cognitive functions, the repeated practice—conducted with planned variations that mirrored variations in participants' environments—could improve the skills' durability and generalizability and obviate the need for cognitive rehabilitation.

Integrated treatment of comorbid SUD and SPMI should be the standard of care and should be implemented in all treatment facilities. SUD sabotages rehabilitation, and its prevalence among individuals with SPMI is high enough that most individuals need treatment for both disorders.

Although the skills training modules are convenient and replicable, each encompasses a large block of material that is difficult to adapt to different settings and participants. Developing methods to assemble custom modules consisting of skills selected for particular sites or participants could increase the training's efficiency.

Furthermore, the modules' efficacy and effectiveness might be improved by adopting more sophisticated instructional methods such as Brown's (1997) flexible learning environment. Brown's method is based on reciprocal teaching: trainees systematically teach and quiz each other, summarizing the material as they present it, answering other trainees' questions, and clarifying the material as needed. The teaching and Socratic dialogues, always conducted cooperatively and never competitively, help trainees form a finely differentiated, conditional model of the causal connections among the elements of the subject matter. Trainees respond to test items and discussions with answers that extend beyond simple repetition to include complex analogies and multiply justified conclusions.

The potential value for psychiatric rehabilitation is participants' development of a differentiated, conditional causal model that guides their functioning and helps them generalize their skills. Each participant lives in a unique environment with its specific set of complex conditional connections that can vary considerably over time. Additionally, the social context of the technology might enhance the supportiveness of the training group during and after individuals' participation.

Participants' generalization might also be increased by bringing the living environment into training, the converse of IVAST and the use of indigenous supporters. Altering the modules' videotape to incorporate snapshots, sounds, and other aspects of participants' living environments would increase the reality of training. Of course, these alterations could profitably be combined with the other support procedures to diminish the differences between training and the real world.

Finally, dissemination of the methods of psychiatric rehabilitation and ongoing support of practitioners might be improved by using more advanced communication technologies such as the Internet. Although publications such as the American Psychiatric Association practice guidelines (e.g., American Psychiatric Association 1997) have contributed toward providing more favorable conditions for dissemination of psychiatric rehabilitation, the specific form, content, and value of psychiatric rehabilitation's assessment and treatment techniques are still not widely known or used. Making the information easily accessible to practitioners, managers, administrators, individuals with SPMI and their families, and advocacy groups could speed the adoption of psychiatric rehabilitation's techniques by the systems of care. Furthermore, the same communication technologies could be used to connect participants and practitioners across settings and times, offering support that is delivered when and where it is needed.

References

American Psychiatric Association: Practice guideline for the treatment of patients with schizophrenia. Am J Psychiatry 154 (4 suppl):1–63, 1997

Anthony WA: Principles of Psychiatric Rehabilitation. Baltimore, MD, University Park Press, 1979

Bachrach LL: Planning services for chronically mentally ill patients. Bull Menninger Clin 47:163–188, 1983

Becker DR, Drake RE: Individual placement and support: a community mental health center approach to vocational rehabilitation. Community Ment Health J 30:193–206, 1994

Becker DR, Drake RE, Bond GR, et al: Job terminations among persons with severe mental illness participating in supported employment. Community Ment Health J 34:71–82, 1998

Bellack AS: Cognitive rehabilitation for schizophrenia: is it possible? Is it necessary? Schizophr Bull 18:43–50, 1992

Bellack AS, DiClemente CC: Treating substance abuse among patients with schizophrenia. Psychiatr Serv 50:75–80, 1999

Bellack AS, Mueser KT, Morrison RL, et al: Remediation of cognitive deficits in schizophrenia. Am J Psychiatry 147:1650–1655, 1990

Bellack AS, Sayers M, Mueser KT, et al: An evaluation of social problem solving in schizophrenia. J Abnorm Psychol 103:371–378, 1994

Bellack AS, Gold JM, Buchannan RW: Cognitive rehabilitation for schizophrenia: problems, prospects, and strategies. Schizophr Bull 25:257–275, 1999

Benton MK, Schroeder HE: Social skills training with schizophrenics: a meta-analytic evaluation. J Consult Clin Psychol 58:741–747, 1990

Bowen L, Wallace CJ, Glynn SM, et al: Schizophrenics' cognitive functioning and performance in interpersonal interactions and skills training procedures. J Psychiatr Res 28:289–301, 1994

Brenner HD, Hodel B, Roder V, et al: Treatment of cognitive dysfunctions and behavioral deficits in schizophrenia. Schizophr Bull 18:21–26, 1992

Brenner HD, Roder V, Hodel B, et al: Integrated Psychological Therapy for Schizophrenic Patients. Toronto, ON, Hogrefe & Huber, 1994

Brown AL: Transforming schools into communities of thinking and learning about serious matters. Am Psychol 52:399–413, 1997

Carey KB, Purine DM, Maiso SA, et al: Decisional balance regarding substance use among persons with schizophrenia. Community Ment Health J 35:289–299, 1999

Carpenter WT, Bartko JJ, Carpenter CL, et al: Another view of schizophrenia subtypes: a report from the International Pilot Study of Schizophrenia. Arch Gen Psychiatry 33:508–516, 1976

Center for Substance Abuse Treatment: Assessment and Treatment of Patients With Coexisting Mental Illness and Alcohol and Other Drug Abuse (SAMHSA Publ No 94-2078). TIP series. Rockville, MD, U.S. Department of Health and Human Services, 1994

Clark RE, Teague GB, Ricketts SK, et al: Cost-effectiveness of assertive community treatment versus standard case management for persons with severe mental illness and substance use disorders. Health Serv Res 33:1283–1306, 1998

Clark RE, Ricketts SK, McHugo GJ: Legal system involvement and costs for persons in treatment for severe mental illness and substance use disorders. Psychiatr Serv 50:641–647, 1999

Corrigan PW, Wallace CJ, Schade ML, et al: Learning medication self-management skills in schizophrenia: relationships with cognitive deficits and psychiatric symptoms. Behaviour Therapy 25:5–15, 1994

Cuffel BJ, Heithoff KA, Lawson W: Correlates of patterns of substance abuse among patients with schizophrenia. Hospital and Community Psychiatry 44:247–251, 1993

DeRisi WJ, Myron M, Goding M: Building the behavioral bridge to continuity of care: training staff of community care facilities. Hospital and Community Psychiatry 26:472–475, 1975

Diamond RB, Becker M: The Wisconsin Quality of Life Index: a multidimensional model for measuring quality of life. J Clin Psychiatry 60 (suppl 3):29–31, 1999

Dickerson FB: Assessing clinical outcomes: the community functioning of persons with serious mental illness. Psychiatr Serv 48:897–902, 1997

Dickerson FB, Boronow JJ, Ringel N, et al: Neurocognitive deficits and social functioning in outpatients with schizophrenia. Schizophr Res 21:75–83, 1996

Dickerson FB, Boronow JJ, Ringel N, et al: Social functioning and neurocognitive deficits in outpatients with schizophrenia: a 2-year outcome. Schizophr Res 37:13–20, 1999

Dilk MN, Bond GR: Meta-analytic evaluation of skills training research for individuals with severe mental illness. J Consult Clin Psychol 64:1337–1346, 1996

Dobson D: Long-term support and social skills training for patients with schizophrenia. Psychiatr Serv 47:1195–1196, 1996

Dobson DJG, McDougall G, Busheikin J, et al: Effects of social skills training and social milieu treatment on symptoms of schizophrenia. Psychiatr Serv 46:376–380, 1995

Drake RE, McHugo GJ, Becker DR, et al: The New Hampshire study of supported employment for people with severe mental illness. J Consult Clin Psychol 64:391–399, 1996

Drake RE, Mercer-McFadden C, Mueser KT, et al: Review of integrated mental health and substance abuse disorders for patients with dual disorders. Schizophr Bull 24:589–608, 1998

Drake RE, Becker D, McHugo GJ, et al: A randomized clinical trial of supported employment for inner-city patients with severe mental disorders. Arch Gen Psychiatry 56:627–633, 1999

Eckman TA, Wirshing WC, Marder SR, et al: Techniques for training patients in illness self-management: a controlled trial. Am J Psychiatry 149:1549–1555, 1992

Ericsson KA, Charness N: Expert performance: its structure and acquisition. Am Psychol 49:725–748, 1994

Falloon IRH, Held T, Coverdale JH, et al: Family interventions for schizophrenia: a review of long-term benefits of international studies. Psychiatric Rehabilitation Skills 3:268–290, 1999

Goldman HH, Skodol AE, Lave TR: Revising Axis V for DSM-IV: a review of measures of social functioning. Am J Psychiatry 149:1148–1156, 1992

Green MF: What are the functional consequences of neurocognitive deficits in schizophrenia? Am J Psychiatry 153:321–330, 1996

Green MF, Nuechterlein KN: Should schizophrenia be treated as a neurocognitive disorder? Schizophr Bull 25:309–321, 1999

Green MF, Satz P, Ganzell S, et al: Wisconsin Card Sorting Test performance in schizophrenia: remediation of a stubborn deficit. Am J Psychiatry 149:62–67, 1992

Heaton R: Wisconsin Card Sorting Test. Odessa, FL, Psychological Assessment Resources, 1985

Heinssen RK, Liberman RP, Kopelowicz A: Psychosocial skills training for schizophrenia: lessons from the laboratory. Schizophr Bull 26:21–46, 2000

Hellman SH, Green MF, Kern RS, et al: The effects of instruction versus reinforcement on the Wisconsin Card Sorting Test. J Clin Exp Neuropsychol 14:63–67, 1992

Hierholzer RW, Liberman RP: Successful living: a social skills and problem-solving group for the chronic mentally ill. Hospital and Community Psychiatry 37:913–918, 1986

Hogarty GE, Anderson CM, Reiss DJ: Family education, social skills training and maintenance chemotherapy in aftercare treatment of schizophrenia. Arch Gen Psychiatry 43:633–642, 1986

Kennedy JA: Fundamentals of Psychiatric Treatment Planning. Washington, DC, American Psychiatric Press, 1992

Kern RS, Green MF, Satz P: Neuropsychological predictors of skills training for chronic psychiatric patients. Psychiatry Res 43:223–230, 1992

Kern RS, Wallace CJ, Hellman SG, et al: A training procedure for remediating WCST deficits in chronic psychotic patients: an adaptation of errorless learning principles. J Psychiatr Res 30:283–294, 1996

Koh SD: Remembering of verbal materials by schizophrenic young adults, in Language and Cognition in Schizophrenia. Edited by Schwartz S. Hillsdale, NJ, Erlbaum, 1978, pp 175–189

Koh SD, Marusarz TW, Rosen AJ: Remembering of sentences by schizophrenic young adults. J Abnorm Psychol 89:291–294, 1980

Koh SD, Grinker RR, Marusarz TW: Affective memory and schizophrenic anhedonia. Schizophr Bull 7:292–303, 1981

Kopelowicz A, Wallace CJ, Zarate R: Teaching psychiatric patients to re-enter the community: a brief method of improving continuity of care. Psychiatr Serv 49:1313–1316, 1998

Lane AB: Combining telephone peer counseling and professional services for clients in intensive psychiatric rehabilitation. Psychiatr Serv 49:312–314, 1998

Larsen SF, Fromholt P: Mnemonic organization and free recall in schizophrenia. J Abnorm Psychol 85:61–65, 1976

Lecomte TB, Wilde MS, Wallace CJ: Interviewing one's peers: mental health consumers as mental health workers. Psychiatr Serv 50:693–695, 1999

Leff J, Berkowitz R, Shavit N, et al: A trial of family therapy versus a relatives' group for schizophrenia. Br J Psychiatry 154:58–66, 1989

Liberman RP, Green MF: Whither cognitive therapy for schizophrenia? Schizophr Bull 18:27–35, 1992

Liberman RP, Falloon IRH, Aitchison RA: Multiple family therapy for schizophrenia: a behavioral, problem-solving approach. Psychosocial Rehabilitation Journal 7:60–77, 1984

Liberman RP, DeRisi WJ, Mueser KT: Social Skills Training for Psychiatric Patients. New York, Pergamon, 1989

Liberman RP, Wallace CJ, Blackwell GA, et al: Innovations in skills training for the seriously mentally ill: the UCLA Social and Independent Living Skills Modules. Innovations and Research 2:43–60, 1993

Liberman RP, Wallace CJ, Blackwell GA, et al: Skills training vs occupational therapy for persons with persistent schizophrenia. Am J Psychiatry 155:1087–1091, 1998

Liberman RP, Kopelowicz A, Smith TE: Psychiatric rehabilitation, in Comprehensive Textbook of Psychiatry, 7th Edition. Baltimore, MD, Lippincott Williams & Wilkins, 1999, pp 3218–3245

Liberman RP, Blair KE, Glynn SM, et al: Generalization of skills training to the natural environment, in Current Status of Schizophrenia Treatment. Edited by Brenner HD, Boker W, Genner R. Toronto, ON, Hogrefe & Huber, 2000, pp 175–192

Liberman RP, Glynn SM, Marder SR: In vivo amplified skills training for promoting social adjustment in schizophrenia. Psychiatry (in press)

MacKain SJ, Smith TH, Wallace CJ, et al: Evaluation of a community re-entry program. Int Rev Psychiatry 10:76–83, 1998

Marder SR, Wirshing WC, Mintz J, et al: Two-year outcome of social skills training and group psychotherapy for outpatients with schizophrenia. Am J Psychiatry 153:1585–1592, 1996

Mastboom J: Forty clubhouses: model and practices. Psychosocial Rehabilitation Journal 16:9–23, 1992

McFarlane WR, Stastny P, Deakins S: Family-aided assertive community treatment: a comprehensive rehabilitation and intensive case management approach for persons with schizophrenic disorders, in Effective Psychiatric Rehabilitation: New Directions for Mental Health Services (No 53). Edited by Liberman RP. San Francisco, CA, Jossey-Bass, 1992, pp 43–54

McPheeters HL: Statewide mental health outcome evaluation: a perspective of two southern states. Community Ment Health J 20:44–55, 1984

Mueser KT, Bellack AS, Douglas MS, et al: Predictions of social skill acquisition in schizophrenic and major affective disorder patients from memory and symptomatology. Psychiatry Res 37:281–296, 1991

Mueser KT, Glynn SM, Liberman RP: Behavior family management for serious psychiatric illness, in Family Interventions for the Mentally Ill Relatives: New Directions for Mental Health Services. Edited by Hatfield AB. San Francisco, CA, Jossey-Bass, 1994, pp 37–50

National Institute of Mental Health: Caring for people with severe mental disorders: a national plan of research to improve services (DHHS Publ No ADM 91-1762). Washington, DC, U.S. Government Printing Office, 1991

Penn DL, Mueser KT: Research update on the psychosocial treatment of schizophrenia. Am J Psychiatry 153:607–617, 1996

Psychiatric Rehabilitation Consultants: Modules of the UCLA Social and Independent Living Skills Program. Camarillo CA, Psychiatric Rehabilitation Consultants (P.O. Box 2867, Camarillo, CA 93011), 2000

Randolph E, Eth S, Glynn S, et al: Efficacy of behavioral family management in reducing relapse in veteran schizophrenics. Br J Psychiatry 164:501–506, 1994

Reitan RM, Wolfson D: The Halstead-Reitan Neuropsychological Test Battery: Theory and Clinical Interpretation, 2nd Edition. Tucson, AZ, Neuropsychology Press, 1993

Ridgley MS, Jerrell JM: Analysis of three interventions for substance abuse treatment of severely mentally ill people. Community Ment Health J 32:561–578, 1996

Roberts LJ, Shaner A, Eckman TA, et al: Effectively treating stimulant-abusing schizophrenics: mission impossible? In Effective Psychiatric Rehabilitation: New Directions for Mental Health Services (No 53). Edited by Liberman RP. San Francisco, CA, Jossey-Bass, 1992, pp 55–66

Roberts LJ, Shaner A, Eckman TA: Overcoming Addictions: Skills Training for Persons With Schizophrenia. New York, WW Norton, 1999

Scott JE, Dixon LB: Psychological interventions for schizophrenia. Schizophr Bull 21:621–630, 1995

Smith TE, Hull JW, MacKain SJ, et al: Training hospitalized patients with schizophrenia in community reintegration skills. Psychiatr Serv 47:1099–1103, 1996

Spaulding W, Flemming K, Reed D, et al: Cognitive functioning in schizophrenia: implications for psychiatric rehabilitation. Schizophr Bull 25:275–291, 1999

Stein LI, Barry KL, VanDien G, et al: Work and social support: a comparison of consumers who have achieved stability in ACT and clubhouse programs. Community Ment Health J 35:193–203, 1999

Strachan A: Family management, in Handbook of Psychiatric Rehabilitation. Edited by Liberman RP. New York, Macmillan, 1992, pp 183–212

Stroop JR: Studies of interference in serial verbal reactions. J Exp Psychol 18:643–662, 1935

Sullivan G, Wells KB, Morgenstern H, et al: Identifying modifiable risk factors for rehospitalization: a case-control study of 1995 seriously mentally ill persons in Mississippi. Am J Psychiatry 152: 1749–1756, 1995

Swofford CD, Kasckow JW, Scheller-Gilkey G, et al: Substance use: a powerful predictor of relapse in schizophrenia. Schizophr Res 20:145–151, 1996

Tauber R, Wallace CJ, Lecomte TB: Generalization of skills training for people with severe and persistent mental illness: enlisting indigenous community supporters. Psychiatr Serv (in press)

Wallace CJ: Functional assessment. Schizophr Bull 12:604–630, 1986

Wallace CJ, Boone SE: Cognitive factors in the social skills of schizophrenic patients: implications for treatment, in The Nebraska Symposium on Motivation: Theories of Schizophrenia and Psychosis, Vol 31. Edited by Spaulding W, Cole J. Lincoln, NE, University of Nebraska Press, 1984, pp 215–257

Wallace CJ, Liberman RP: Psychiatric rehabilitation, in Treatments of Psychiatric Disorders, 2nd Edition. Edited by Gabbard GO. Washington, DC, American Psychiatric Press, 1995, pp 1019–1038

Wallace CJ, Liberman RP, MacKain SJ: Effectiveness and replicability of modules to train social and instrumental skills in the severely mentally ill. Am J Psychiatry 149:654–658, 1992

Wallace CJ, Tauber R, Wilde MS: Teaching fundamental workplace skills to persons with serious mental illness. Psychiatr Serv 50:1147–1153, 1999

Wallace CJ, Liberman RP, Tauber R, et al: The Independent Living Skills Survey: a comprehensive measure of the community functioning of severely and persistently mentally ill individuals. Schizophr Bull 26:631–658, 2000

Wallace CJ, Lecomte TB, Wilde MS, et al: CASIG: a consumer-centered assessment for planning individualized treatment and evaluating program outcomes. Schizophr Res (in press)

Weaver RA: Computerized treatment planning. Psychiatr Serv 45:825–827, 1994

Weiss KM, Chapman HA: A computer-assisted inpatient psychiatric assessment and treatment planning system. Psychiatr Serv 44:1097–1100, 1993

Wechsler D: Wechsler Adult Intelligence Scale–Revised. San Antonio, TX, Psychological Corporation, 1981

Wykes T, Reeder JC, Williams C, et al: The effects of neurocognitive remediation on executive functioning in patients with schizophrenia. Schizophr Bull 25:291–309, 1999

Young DA, Freyslinger MG: Scaffolded instructions and the remediation of the WCST deficits in schizophrenia. Schizophr Res 16:199–207, 1995

38

Treatment Settings

Providing a Continuum of Care for Patients With Schizophrenia or Related Disorders

Richard L. Munich, M.D.
William H. Sledge, M.D.

It is clear from the preceding five chapters that our understanding of the treatment needs of the patient with schizophrenia or a related disorder has changed dramatically in a relatively few years. Similarly, major changes have taken place in the settings in which that treatment occurs. Rather than being oriented toward facilities, modern treatment organizations focus on integrated systems of care comprising a continuum of various locations and functional programs graded by degree of patient-staff contact, structure, and containment. In a system of care, the choice of setting of a particular patient's treatment depends on the phase of illness and on efforts to maximize contact with the patient's environment, to provide the least restrictive alternative, and to maintain continuity of treatment.

Less than 40 years ago, most treatment of patients with schizophrenia took place on locked units of mental hospitals. Hospital bed utilization was extensive and either of very long duration or custodial, with little or no continuity of care extending into the ambulatory setting. Over the next three decades, however, utilization of inpatient resources in psychiatry and medicine declined. Even for treatment of the most serious illnesses or disturbed mental states, modal lengths of stay have shifted from months to days, and powerful arguments are being made to reduce lengths of stay even further. Partial and day hospitalization, respite care, and supported living arrangements, such as outpatient surgery, have also been proven to be effective in the containment and management of complex treatment situations.

Dramatic reductions in inpatient length of stay as well as the development of alternatives to traditional care have also led to changes in milieu treatment. The centrality of the milieu in treatment has diminished. A more hierarchical structure has replaced the egalitarianism of the therapeutic community, and the medical model is regaining its hegemony over the multidisciplinary team. Regardless of the location, however, the social system or context in which the treatment takes place has an impact on the treatment itself. And even though it is difficult to conceptualize a therapeutic community in the midst of crisis intervention or in a system or continuum of care, well-established principles of social psychiatry and group and organizational theory continue to inform practice. When managed poorly, a system of care can lead to fragmentation and a diffusion of responsibility, thus fostering regression and loss of autonomy and identity; when managed well, a system can provide support and containment, lead to a continuous and coherent treatment, and enhance patient motivation and internalization of treatment values.

The role of the social system in treatment had its intellectual birth in the 18th-century debate between Rousseau and Diderot about the relative prominence of the individual and the social (Munich 1993). In his book *The Birth of the Clinic,* Michel Foucault (1973) noted that 18th-century economists and doctors in France felt that

> the only possible locus for recovering from disease was the natural environment of social life, the family. There the cost of sickness to the nation was reduced to a minimum, and the risk of the disease leading to artificial complications, spreading of its own accord, and assuming, as in hospitals, the aberrant form of the disease was avoided. (p. 39)

As we shall see, more than two centuries of changes in the location of treatment have more or less returned us remarkably close to some of these ideals.

The so-called moral treatment of the 19th century, based on the revolutionary work of William Tuke in England and Philippe Pinel in France, focused on the treatment situation itself and emphasized a humanitarian approach to patients and their environment (Mora 1980). The focus on the social system continued in both the work of Dorothea Dix and, extending into the 20th century, the mental hygiene movement (Grob 1983). The primacy of the social system in the treatment of patients came to fruition in England during and shortly after World War II in the work of Maxwell Jones, who used large-group methods to treat soldiers who were hospitalized with severe character disorders. Closely studied by M. Robert Rappaport and colleagues, Jones's Belmont Hospital unit attracted wide attention and generated various therapeutic principles such as democratization, permissiveness, communalism, and reality confrontation (Jones 1953; Rappaport 1960).

Ideas concerning the role of the social system in treatment quickly spread to traditional psychiatric hospitals, whose milieus were organized primarily around containment and custodial care, and to populations of patients with more complex diagnoses. For the next 30 years, until approximately the late 1970s, the theory and practice of milieu therapy for patients with schizophrenia and related disorders flourished amid great controversy (Almond 1974; Bettelheim 1950; Cumming and Cumming 1962; Edelson 1964; Stanton and

Schwartz 1954). At its height, milieu therapy was thought by some to be misfocused (Ayllon and Azrin 1968; Paul and Lentz 1977), by others to be overstimulating (Van Putten 1973; Van Putten and May 1976), by others to be essential (Edelson 1970a, 1970b; Rubinstein and Lasswell 1966), and by yet others, albeit a minority, to be curative by itself (Laing 1967; Mosher et al. 1975).

The decline of the therapeutic community movement followed the medicalization of psychiatry and reduced lengths of stay in the context of a paucity of research demonstrating the effectiveness of the milieu. This decline coincided with the reemergence of a community-oriented paradigm for the delivery of services, important clinical aspects of which were the development of alternatives to inpatient treatment and the philosophy of keeping patients closer to their natural environments and in the least restrictive settings. Rehabilitative and psychoeducational techniques with patients and their families also served, as suggested by the French physicians and economists more than two centuries ago, to make the alternative approaches to extended hospitalization much more effective and viable.

Schizophrenia presents as a heterogeneous and phasic illness, with defects and disabilities affecting thought, communication, adaptation, and social intercourse. Thus, modern treatment includes pharmacology to alter the neurochemical aspects of the vulnerability; flexible psychotherapy, assertive case management, and psychoeducation to mitigate the impact of stress; and rehabilitation to promote the development of adaptive, social, cognitive, and vocational skills and learning strategies to enhance the capacity to cope (Michels and Marzuk 1993; Mueser 1993; Mueser and Lieberman 1988; Munich and Lang 1993). Because of the fluctuating and phasic nature of the illness, including wide swings in levels of acuity, the ways these various treatments are integrated and the settings in which they are provided may be quite variable.

In this chapter, keeping the above historical and clinical perspective in mind, we outline the general and basic principles of short-term and extended hospital care for the severely mentally ill patient. We then elaborate on the specifics of various alternatives to hospital-based care, moving from the inpatient setting to continuous day and partial hospitalization, residential treatment, inns, and respite care in supportive living arrangements, and, finally, to a community setting to which the patient returns and undergoes outpatient follow-up. Rather than advocating a specific location for treatment, we describe a system, or continuum, of treatment options. We note that such a system requires flexibility of approach, accommodates adjustment to the various phases of psychotic illness, depends primarily on the needs of the patient, and provides different levels of intensity of care, management, continuity, and access.

Inpatient Treatments

> The decision to hospitalize is the single most important event in the career of a psychiatric patient. If taken too lightly, it can change a patient with a problem into a chronic user of psychiatric hospitals. If avoided at "all costs," it may lead to the patient's suicide.
> *Jerzy E. Henisz (1981), p. 11*

Indications for Hospitalization

The new practice environment, with its emphasis on cost-effectiveness and containment, has forced inpatient providers to become increasingly clear about the indications for hospitalization and the justifications for continuation. In medicine and surgery, the diagnosis-related groups provide the relevant guidelines, but such guidelines and consensus for psychiatric hospitalization have been slower to develop. However, psychiatric inpatient treatment is useful and at times absolutely essential, particularly for the patients described in this section of the present volume who are in the midst of florid psychotic decompensation. Although some patients with an acute psychosis can be managed outside the hospital, as is discussed, others, in whom the momentum of the psychopathological process is difficult to interrupt, will require hospitalization. In some of these decompensations, patients might erect barriers to treatment by viewing with fear those who might provide assistance and responding to them antagonistically. In other cases, patients experience internal commands that leave them on the edge of paralyzing, violent, or self-destructive behavior. Some patients are out of contact altogether.

When patients are gravely disabled and have a condition that requires secure structure, the obvious guidelines for hospital admission are providing asylum in the general sense of an inviolable refuge and ensuring safety in the specific sense of protection from danger to themselves or others. Dangerousness is most apparent in the midst of psychotic depression with suicidal ideation, mania, impulse-driven excitement, the loss of reality testing, command hallucinations, and bizarre and unpredictable behaviors associated with psychosis. Both biological vulnerabilities and psychosocial stressors that lead to the exacerbation of psychotic conditions require interventions that can be safely and efficiently achieved only in an inpatient setting. For example, although some medications are rapidly effective, they still take time for equilibration; in the meantime, psychosocial interventions can be introduced even while the affected patient is in a volatile state. Many patients with acute schizophrenia present with combinations of biologically, psychologically, and socially based conditions that require simultaneous use of several treatment approaches. For example, the patience and sensitivity associated with the treatment of a patient with a psychotic depression might be in conflict with the firmness and nonpunitive limit setting necessary in the treatment of a patient with difficulties controlling impulses. A patient with another type of psychotic decompensation and comorbid narcissistic personality disorder might experience profound humiliation because of having to take an antipsychotic. In both of these examples, the treatment requires a combination of containment, exploration, management, and education that is most efficiently and effectively provided in the hospital, where patient and staff can coordinate the appropriate approach to the multiple problems.

Many investigators have elaborated the indications for hospitalization (Gabbard 1992; Gruenberg 1970; Hanson and Babigian 1974; Henisz 1981; Maxmen and Tucker 1973; Rose et al. 1977; Sederer and Centorrino 1997). They have variously recommended hospitalization for the following purposes:

- Definitive and comprehensive medical and psychiatric diagnostic services
- Protection of the patient and others
- Crisis intervention, providing relief and safety
- Symptom stabilization involving changing or reestablishing a medication regimen
- Consultation or treatment planning in the face of resistance, deterioration, stalemate, or noncompliance in outpatient therapy

All of these reasons to hospitalize a patient can apply to the patient with schizophrenia, particularly in the midst of a decompensating phase of the illness.

Often the patient needs to be removed from the contextual stressors that have precipitated or are maintaining the decompensation. In the case of persistently ill patients with schizophrenia, significant changes, such as illness or infirmity in a reliable caregiver, in an otherwise stable environment can lead to the need for hospitalization. Although it is true that any location away from the original stressor might be beneficial, the milieu of the modern psychiatric hospital is designed to reduce stimulation and at the same time provide the right amount of support, structure, and containment. We have been impressed that some severely and persistently ill patients require inpatient stays not only to manage short-term episodes but also to obtain assistance with the awkwardness, humiliation, and anxiety associated with acknowledging, revealing, and beginning to rehabilitate their profound deficits in activities of daily living and social, vocational, and interpersonal skills. In an increasingly technological age, it may be more stigmatizing to be considered incompetent or a dropout than to have a mental illness.

Finally, the early stages of recovery from a severe mental illness may be the time when the patient is most vulnerable. Many suicides occur shortly after treatment has begun, when patients begin to feel they have enough energy to act. The readmission rates for recently hospitalized patients with psychotic disorders are generally high. The psychotic patient in recovery may be at risk from the suddenly increased expectations of family and friends. Again, the modern hospital milieu is particularly sensitive to the vicissitudes and clinical course of these illnesses.

Brief Hospitalization

As a result of economic restrictions instituted by third-party payers, availability of more effective somatic and focused psychosocial therapies, lack of findings from well-controlled research studies, and various alternatives to hospitalization that have been developed (as are discussed later in this chapter), brief hospitalization has become the modal form of inpatient practice (Glick and Hargreaves 1979; Sederer 1992). Although a brief hospitalization might be as short as 5–10 days, anything less than 1 month is still considered brief. Brief hospitalization has several simultaneous goals: rapid medical and psychological assessment, emotional support and symptom stabilization, identification of precipitating factors, consultation to a preexisting treatment, adjustment of the relevant environmental factors, and discharge planning. Usually the newly admitted patient is observed carefully in a highly structured milieu in which the focus is on behavioral control and functional adaptation. This structure is usually provided by stepwise privilege systems; regular schedules for meetings, meals, and medication; and clear boundaries between patients and staff. Seclusion rooms with one-to-one staff observation might be used to provide structure for the patient who is particularly agitated or disruptive.

Communication of staff expectations should be clear and commensurate with the patient's level of organization, and interventions should be directed toward gathering relevant information and problem solving rather than exploring intrapsychic processes. Unless the clinical course reverses, in brief hospitalization every effort should be made to provide the least restrictive setting as soon as it appears safe to do so. Contact with outside supports must be facilitated to inhibit regression and enhance reality testing, collect information, and prepare the patient for a return to ambulatory status. On many inpatient units with a brief length of stay, staff strive to have patients interact with each other to combat passivity and isolation, improve communication patterns, and help reinforce socially acceptable behaviors and treatment values. As the acute psychosis subsides, movement off the unit in the form of passes and home visits is encouraged. At about this time, active work with the patient's support system can begin in preparation for the patient's discharge.

Extended Hospitalization

A small number of patients might qualify for stays of intermediate (1–3 months) or extended (3 or more months) length. When this controversial option for a more extended length of stay exists, the population consists of a high percentage of persons whose current condition has been resistant to treatment or whose mental illness is chronic. Patients referred for extended hospitalization often are those who are unremittingly suicidal, who cycle in and out of brief hospitalizations, who cannot negotiate the discharge phase at the end of a brief inpatient stay, who demonstrate repeated medication noncompliance, or who need extra time to establish a therapeutic alliance. Often, the availability of appropriate ambulatory services will determine the length and goals of a particular hospitalization.

If the patient is younger, longer-term hospitalization might be indicated after fewer numbers of previous treatments and brief hospitalizations. For example, an 18-year-old student with no previous psychiatric contact who becomes acutely psychotic just before his or her first midterm examinations should have every opportunity to restore his or her previous level of functioning as quickly as possible, even if it means undergoing intensive outpatient treatment and taking some time off from school. Because with such a patient the stressors might be playing a greater role than the vulnerabilities, the clinician might try two brief hospitalizations before recommending a longer hospital stay. A 32-year-old mother of two who decompensates after the delivery of her third child might have three brief hospitalizations before such a recommendation, whereas a 15-year-old boy or girl who begins hallucinating with no obvious precipitant might undergo only one brief hospitalization before the clinician recommends long-term inpatient treatment.

Diagnostically, any severe illness potentially qualifies a patient for a longer inpatient stay, but a reliable criterion for extended hospitalization is the comorbidity of Axis I and Axis II psychopathology. In addition to the standard measures of dangerousness and inability to care for self, treatment resistance, treatment stalemate, ego-dystonic symptoms, and conflict with (rather than acquiescence to) the illness are also indicators for a longer stay. A psychodynamic criterion in patient selection is that extended inpatient treatment may be indicated when interventions needed to keep the patient alive, such as hands-on help to control impulsive or grossly inappropriate behaviors or regular and active limit setting, would compromise the psychiatrist's or psychotherapist's capacity to form a treatment alliance. Severe antisocial behavior, substance abuse, organically based psychopathology, significantly below-average intelligence, and a previous long-term hospital stay argue against long-term inpatient treatment just as they usually argue against intensive psychotherapy. For milieu integrity, staff morale, and utilization review, it is extremely important to differentiate between those severely ill patients who can engage in a useful treatment process and those patients who cannot and who, therefore, would benefit from a less active treatment approach or custodial care. These latter patients include those with difficult-to-control violence, persistent florid psychotic states, and/or treatment resistance and extreme denial of illness.

The essential rationale for a long-term hospital stay is to provide an opportunity to deal with extremely complex issues such as 1) finding the proper medication and dosage; 2) dealing with persistent suicidal and other severe self-destructive behaviors; 3) treating comorbid conditions such as mental retardation, substance abuse, dyscontrol, or severe characterological problems; or 4) establishing a therapeutic alliance to enhance motivation, treatment compliance, and insight. A long-term inpatient treatment staff is organized and trained to assist patients to learn more about themselves and their illnesses. These discoveries are brought about through the vicissitudes of establishing a treatment alliance, by learning opportunities in the therapeutic milieu, and by a carefully graded provision of assessment and implementation of psychiatric rehabilitation. In theory this discovery or insight will strengthen the patient's coping capacity by giving the patient a greater perspective on vulnerabilities and relevant stressors and by assisting the clinician in determining those psychosocial factors contributing to treatment resistance, medication noncompliance, and disrupted community integration and tenure. A longer stay also provides the opportunity for the clinician to more carefully stabilize the appropriate psychopharmacological regimen and institute timely rehabilitation interventions while protecting and supporting the patient's self-esteem.

Like brief hospitalization, extended hospitalization also provides asylum, support, structure, and containment. Because the goals of extended hospitalization are somewhat more ambitious, however, the techniques may be less directed toward symptom stabilization and more toward symptom significance, that is, understanding of the symptom's psychodynamics and its relationship to underlying personality features (Smith et al. 1993). Anxiety associated with psychosis is medicated according to the principles outlined in Chapter 34, but the patient is not sedated to the extent that he or she cannot identify the anxiety. Under these circumstances the treatment plan might not call for the least restrictive setting, and the patient might have to be reassured that discharge is not imminent and that protection from environmental factors will be maintained. The treating physician must always be mindful that regression is not promoted and that adaptive behavior is supported.

Custodial treatment must be considered when longer hospitalization as described above is not available or has been unsuccessful or when active treatment is overstimulating or conveys too high a level of expectation for the severely impaired and unmotivated patient. Custodial treatment provides asylum and containment for the patient with unmanageable impulses, self- and other destructive behaviors, and severely limited capacity for self-care. Schizophrenic patients in custodial treatment should have their status, especially their psychopharmacological usage, evaluated no less than annually. In evaluating the status, the clinician may discover that a patient is more prepared or motivated for an active treatment.

Residential Treatment

Residential treatment provides much of what the longer-term hospital provides. With lower staff-to-patient ratios (compared with inpatient facilities), variable length of stay, and levels of intensity, residential treatment represents the final inpatient alternative. Residential treatment facilities might exist in a large, institution-like setting or in a regular house in a residential neighborhood. Not necessarily run by physicians, the program typically has a combination of professionals and paraprofessionals (e.g., a program director with at least a master's degree, a consulting psychologist, and residential counselors). Beyond a careful monitoring of mental status, medication compliance, and possible relapse, most residential programs provide a curriculum of psychiatric rehabilitation activities directed toward improving the resident's adaptive skills: capacity to cope in the activities of daily living, social skills, use and enjoyment of leisure time, and early vocational adjustment. The emphasis is on providing the least restrictive setting and a postdischarge support system, developing a family-like environment, avoiding rehospitalization, and facilitating the patient's transition to community living. Much more than in the traditional inpatient setting, patients are involved in the development of their treatment plans with an interdisciplinary team, and additionally they might be responsible for room care, meal plans and preparation, and laundry (Carpenter 1978; Fenton et al. 1998; Hawthorne et al. 1994; Wherley and Bisgaard 1987). Some issues in the conceptualization of residential services are discussed later in this chapter.

Alternatives to Hospitalization

Clinical experience and published reports over the last 30 years have demonstrated repeatedly that a variety of programmatic services can function as effective and safe alternatives to psychiatric hospitalization for patients with acute disturbance, particularly schizophrenia in the acute stages. These programs function as alternatives to hospitalization by reducing the need for hospitalization. This reduction is effected by engaging patients more effectively in treatment services and thereby preventing or modulating the crises that precipitate the need for hospitalization, by responding effectively to crises when they occur (e.g., crisis response services), and by offering alternatives to full hospitalization through the provision of services that are different from and in lieu of psychiatric hospitalization (e.g., partial hospital and respite programs). The function, structure, and goals of these strategies are different, but these strategies share the philosophy of providing treatment services in the least restrictive environment, emphasizing rehabilitation and adaptation to "normal" (i.e., noninstitutional) environments rather than treatment or custodial services provided in institutional settings.

Engagement Services

The well-known Program for Assertive Community Treatment (PACT) and Assertive Continuous Treatment (ACT) (Stein and Test 1980; Stein et al. 1975; Test and Stein 1976) are the most articulated and investigated examples of services that vigorously attempt to engage patients through aggressive outreach and active management of daily living problems and opportunities. The hallmark of the PACT and ACT models is the conceptualization of the service delivery system as a small, multidisciplinary team that provides all of the services (e.g., clinical, supportive, rehabilitative, and social services) regardless of the intensity of the services needed (e.g., inpatient, outpatient). The result of this approach to organizing and delivering services is that accountability, continuity, and staff mutual support are maximized. At times the techniques are coercive, but they are always aimed toward ensuring that the patient is able to stay out of the hospital. Essential services such as psychopharmacological treatment are provided in a manner that makes it difficult for the patient not to utilize them (Thompson et al. 1990).

Assertive treatment of this sort is clearly effective in keeping patients with serious mental illness out of hospital settings, but it is not at all clear if it is effective in improving these patients' quality of life (Olfson 1990), nor are the cost benefits clear (Olfson 1990; Weisbrod et al. 1980). Weisbrod and colleagues (1980) found that the costs of ACT and those of hospital care were about the same, but this work has come under criticism for underestimating the cost of ACT. Future studies that compare the cost-effectiveness of ACT models with other case management models of intensive community-oriented treatment will help clarify this very important policy matter.

Crisis Response Services

It has been hypothesized that timely recognition and intervention with intensive crisis services will avert the need for short-term hospitalization in many patients with schizophrenia or other forms of psychosis (Fisher et al. 1990; Geller 1991). Indeed, such intervention seems to be effective and is probably more usefully deployed in the context of a system of care for persons with severe mental illness (Langsley 1980). It is generally believed that any such system of care should have substantial capacity for mobility and outreach and should be available to be accessed by patients at all hours every day. In addition, other elements of a complete crisis response service should include a telephone service, the opportunity for face-to-face evaluations, and a crisis residential component (Stroul 1993).

Other Treatment Settings in Lieu of Hospital Services

The most thoroughly investigated alternative to hospitalization has been day hospital, or partial hospital, programs. Day hospitals, functioning as alternatives to full hospitalization, are not to be confused with day care or continuous day treatment programs that provide maintenance and supportive care for patients with severe, persistent mental illness (Creed et al. 1990; Hoge et al. 1992; Wilder et al. 1966). Other models have included the rearrangement of existing services in order to divert patients from conventional hospitalization (Gudeman et al. 1983), special settings for recovery (Mosher et al. 1975), and crisis residential programs (Kresky-Wolff et al. 1984; Lamb and Lamb 1984).

Investigators at the Massachusetts Mental Health Center have reorganized their system of care to include an inn, day hospital, and intensive inpatient care. All patients except those who are dangerous to self or others are admitted to the day hospital program for psychiatric care; those patients who require some residential service are boarded in the inn, a lightly staffed dormitory-type program on the grounds of the hospital. For those patients who require 24-hour hospitalization, the intensive care of the inpatient service, which is well staffed with nursing personnel, is provided (Gudeman et al. 1983). This program has been shown to be effective in reducing the number of patients who require hospital care.

The Soteria Project (Mosher 1991; Mosher et al. 1975) was designed to be an effective alternative to hospital-based treatment for young, first-episode psychotic persons. The project took place in the Soteria House, a six-bed facility staffed by nonprofessionals, and emphasized adaptation through one-to-one therapeutic contact with staff. Medications were used only sparingly.

For the past two decades, short-term residential alternatives to psychiatric hospitalization have grown steadily in both the United States and the United Kingdom despite the lack of a coherent definition, purpose, or conceptualization for their use. These services have frequently been referred to as "respite" or "crisis respite" services. With the use of the term *crisis respite care* we do not include the use of mental health service sleepover settings to provide respite for family members of severely mentally ill adults (Geiser et al. 1988) or the placement of such patients with carefully selected families in the community to provide respite to the families or to residential service providers (Britton and Mattson-Melcher 1985). These programs exist and serve a purpose in a system of care. Although "crisis hostels"

(Brook 1973) may have represented an early form of acute crisis respite care, crisis respite services are distinct from "hostel" services because the latter usually function as an alternative to hospital-based institutionalization for patients who require extended hospitalization (Gibbons 1986; Hyde et al. 1987; Simpson et al. 1989).

The literature contains considerable evidence of the value and potential importance of acute crisis respite care. Studies of family members of deinstitutionalized mental patients consistently indicate a need for respite care among family members (Zirul et al. 1989), including families with members living in board-and-care homes (Segal and Kotler 1989). Evidence for this need is also provided by the requests from community providers of care for severely mentally ill patients (Ghaziuddian 1988).

Thus far, acute crisis respite care has been found to be appropriate for a wide range of adults with psychiatric difficulties. Although services are most commonly designed for persistently mentally ill adults who experience an acute exacerbation of their illness, acute crisis respite care also has been found to be appropriate for young adults experiencing a first acute episode of major mental illness (Brunton and Howthorne 1989), long-stay users of day hospitals (MacCarthy et al. 1989), adolescents with psychiatric difficulties (Schwartz 1989), and persons in acute psychiatric emergency resulting from a life crisis (Brunton and Howthorne 1989).

A number of authors (Fields 1990; Shadoan 1985) have argued that acute crisis respite care should be part of a full range of residential treatment programs that function to maintain severe mentally ill adults in the community. The emphasis in such models is on the integration of various levels of residential care within a service system. In such a conceptualization, residential care should not be regarded as merely "housing" but rather as "treatment in a residential setting" in the community, regardless of its focus or length (Fields 1990). Levels of care are conceptualized in terms of the staff-patient ratio and the degree of structure required: high intensity (crisis housing and lodge programs), moderate intensity (board-and-care homes), low intensity (cooperative living arrangements), and psychiatric outreach for patients living independently (Shadoan 1985). In all instances, treatment services for patients in acute crisis are provided on-site or through an outpatient setting.

Until relatively recently, systematic evaluation of the effectiveness of acute crisis respite care and its impact on the service system has been only limited. In the only known published comparative outcome study, Brook (1973) compared patients in a 7-day crisis respite alternative with a nonequivalent comparison group of patients who received hospital services. The crisis respite patients were found to have a lower readmission rate than the control patients and to have better outcomes on 11 of 12 measures of functioning. Descriptive accounts of crisis respite care services have also reported the effectiveness of these services, under specific circumstances. Walsh (1986) suggested that medication compliance and substance use problems do not predict favorable outcomes in acute crisis respite care, and Brunton and Howthorne (1989) noted that crisis respite care programs work best when located in or near residential neighborhoods and staffed by a multidisciplinary clinical team.

Our own work (Sledge et al. 1996a, 1996b) examined the effectiveness, impact, and costs of acute crisis respite care in a randomized comparative trial with short-term psychiatric hospitalization. The program is a combined day hospital and crisis respite living arrangement that is structured to serve as an alternative to conventional inpatient treatment for most voluntary patients. Results indicate that the program, compared with conventional hospitalization, is equally effective clinically and significantly less costly.

Popular and widely used in Europe for some time, home visits by psychiatrists and related mental health professionals are gaining acceptance in the United States. This modality requires flexibility, creativity, responsiveness, and sensitivity on the part of the practitioner (Terkelsen and McCarthy 1994).

Supported Living

Housing, like work, is an important dimension to the recovery of and support of recovery for those persons with schizophrenia or other psychotic conditions. In the last 50 years, there has been a movement from maintaining residence in the hospital, to aggregate living in the community (in the form of halfway houses and group homes), and now to scattered-site living supported by flexible, wraparound services (Carling 1993). This movement toward noncongregate living arrangements is not without controversy and disagreement, particularly between providers and patients (Carling 1993; Tanzman 1993).

In the scattered-site model, in which a continuum of care is not provided, halfway and quarterway houses (Dickey et al. 1986), with their resident staff, congregate living, and treatment programs, give way to individual living arrangements and the provision of substantial material support and human services support for persons with persistent mental illness. Group homes and nursing homes (except when special nursing/medical needs are present) have a diminished role in such a vision of the posthospital care phase of treatment. This move toward scattered-site dwellings in part reflects patient and family preferences but is probably more a function of the separation of housing from treatment in the conceptualization of these services. It has become clear that the mandatory coupling of treatment services with housing has been a subtle, although unintended, form of discrimination against severely mentally ill persons. The services that are required to support such an arrangement must be comprehensive as well as flexible. Continuity of care should be provided as well as care planning so that the patients in such a program have the benefit of familiar and trusted staff. The services should emphasize problem solving in their approach so that the staff assists without actually doing the work of adaptation. Budget maintenance, transportation, food preparation, leisure time, family relationships, and work adjustment (when appropriate) are skills and activities that should be supported.

One of the substantial difficulties with this means of providing services is that no clear mechanism exists for the financing of affordable, safe housing. Consequently, the solutions to the provision of housing services tend to be dependent on local conditions and services.

Systemic Considerations

A modern approach to the treatment of schizophrenia emphasizes a systemic approach to the organization of services rather than one based on setting or institution. Indeed, this approach to the treatment of schizophrenia offers several advantages, including the clear provision of access to needed care, a variety of services in a coordinated and integrated system, and continuity of care, all delivered in an accountable and cost-effective manner that is efficient and of high quality. The creation of a system of care begins with a careful specification of the goals of such a program, the target population of patients to be served, and the clinical service context in which the program is to exist. Once these considerations are resolved, subsequent decisions concerning funding, location, staffing, program features, policies and procedures, and other matters follow logically.

Persons are hospitalized because they are perceived to require inpatient-level care or because no suitable alternative, community-based services are available (Oldham et al. 1990). Patients can be diverted from hospitalization by the mental health professional's intervening at the earliest signs of an exacerbation of the disorder and assigning them to a viable alternative to hospitalization. Because many mental health professionals are unfamiliar with the growing literature indicating that alternatives are cost-effective and safe, they are inclined to seek to hospitalize patients who are very ill. Thus, for a system of care to function effectively and to be well managed, it is essential that a strong admissions function exist that will allow for patients to be triaged appropriately. The triage function and hospitalization decision are best accomplished at a single point of entry managed by staff who are not part of the treatment staff of the unit that is referring the patient or receiving the patient.

Program Design Features

A system of care for patients with schizophrenia and other psychotic conditions must have several design features:

1. *A single point of entry for all services, allowing for ease of access, coordination of care, tracking of potential referrals, evaluation and triage, and centralization of tracking of resources.*
2. *Effective crisis response.* By crisis response, we refer to the rapid availability and deployment of clinical resources for patients who require an intense level of services and who are in a rapid state of change and at risk for hospitalization. Crisis response differs from access in that access defines who becomes a patient, whereas crisis response is a particular reaction to a specific clinical state. Crisis response can refer to changes in treatment plans for patients presently in active treatment as well as to the deployment of clinical resources for patients who are not in treatment at the moment but who are at risk for hospitalization.
3. *Medical and psychiatric evaluation.* Such evaluation is essential in making a proper diagnosis and in guiding a proper medical treatment approach. Such an approach depends on a careful diagnosis of psychopathology as well as a functional assessment of social and rehabilitative needs. Diagnosis and evaluation should be ongoing activities, but these functions also need to be organized to occur rapidly during the admission and early-treatment phase. A psychiatrist who can adequately evaluate, judge medication need, and prescribe accordingly must be a part of this program approach.
4. *Multiple levels of care.* Level of care is a key to the particular needs of the patient. The levels of care range in intensity from brief (once every 2 months) dyadic contact and relatively unstructured supportive drop-in experiences to highly organized structures and controlled inpatient services.
5. *Flexible structures of care that allow the engagement of patients in nontraditional settings.* For many patients, flexible structures for engagement are primarily embodied in case management services (Sledge et al. 1995) but can also include other programs such as supported living arrangements and crisis residences. Although case management might have been oversold as a solution to the fragmentation of the mental health service system, it is an essential and cost-effective way to coordinate and integrate ongoing care for patients with schizophrenia. Case managers are not only brokers and

advocates for services (Intagliata 1982) but are also clinicians who must be skilled in the provision of direct clinical care services for their patients (Lamb 1980).

6. *Coordination and liaison with other providers.* Clinical services must be integrated and coordinated with other types of services, such as vocational and psychosocial rehabilitation efforts, in order to ensure continuity of treatment planning and maximization of efforts. Usually, this coordination service is provided by case management personnel.
7. *Continuity of care.* A major principle or goal of any system of care for persons with psychotic disorders is continuity of care. Embodied in this concept is both continuity of caregiver and continuity of treatment planning. Learning to trust and collaborating are difficult processes for many persons with schizophrenia or other psychotic disorders, and consequently the establishment of an effective therapeutic alliance and patient involvement in treatment planning are major undertakings and substantial achievements when they occur. Continuity of care should be ensured in the program design whenever possible (Bachrach 1993). When treatment is viewed from a longitudinal perspective, a myriad of details arise, which must be considered for the proper care of the psychotic patient. For example, when a patient with schizophrenia requires hospitalization or when another group of caregivers becomes involved in the patient's care, the tendency arises to duplicate previous efforts or to redo the work of other caregivers. This process is usually wasteful and can be destructive for the patient, enhancing rather than reducing resistances. The presence of a caregiver who follows the patient through a variety of different settings will minimize this kind of inefficiency of care.
8. *Exit functions from high-intensity services.* An exit function that includes discharge planning should be in place to ensure that the appropriate housing, case management, and clinical services are available when the patient is ready to leave the inpatient program. Another exit function that must be a part of the design is ready and easy access to a higher level of care (e.g., hospitalization) for those patients for whom alternatives to inpatient care are not structured enough or are otherwise inappropriate. It is important for the staff to have immediate and quick access to security, clinical backup, and a high level of intensity of care should any one of these become necessary in the evolution of a clinical presentation that may rapidly require more care.

Treatment Functions

Treatment functions in the system of care include medical evaluation and treatment addressing clinical conditions and medication requirements, as well as assessment of patients' rehabilitation readiness and special needs for psychosocial and vocational rehabilitation. Rehabilitation functions must emphasize aspects of self-care and autonomy and act as bulwarks against the compelling pull toward regression that is a feature of many psychotic states. The rehabilitative goals that can be usefully addressed include, but are not limited to, sustaining symptomatic improvement, establishing or reestablishing interpersonal supports and full independent living skills, and helping the person access resources and opportunities (Munich and Lang 1993).

A system of care must have a clearly defined mission and must be appropriately managed and led to provide the structures and resources to carry out that mission. Administrative, fiscal, and other resource issues such as staff credentials, education, and morale must be addressed continually and integrated with the provision of clinical services. In closing, however, a caveat seems to be in order. In the United States now, the trend is clearly a move away from conceptualizing the hospital as the primary locus of care for persons with schizophrenia. The hospital is increasingly viewed as a place for the limited functions of rapid assessment and initiation of a treatment plan. Except for special cases, the community is becoming the locus of care, and the system of care is the treatment instrument. Although these developments seem to be reasonable and progressive in terms of offering patients with schizophrenia a better chance at a meaningful life, we must not submit to the tendency to erect idealized conceptualizations that become subscribed to in a faddish way. We must not lose sight of the fact that treatment is delivered by persons with expertise and experience to persons who are disabled and vulnerable and greatly in need of assistance. It is through the quality of this interaction and the subsequent relationship that the person with a mental disorder and his or her caregiver establish an alliance that will determine the outcome of care.

References

Almond R: The Healing Community: Dynamics of the Therapeutic Milieu. New York, Jason Aronson, 1974

Ayllon T, Azrin N: The Token Economy: A Motivational System for Therapy and Rehabilitation. New York, Appleton-Century-Crofts, 1968

Bachrach LL: Continuity of care and approaches to case management for long-term mentally ill patients. Hospital and Community Psychiatry 44:465–468, 1993

Bettelheim B: Love Is Not Enough: The Treatment of Emotionally Disturbed Children. Glencoe, IL, Free Press, 1950

Britton JG, Mattson-Melcher DM: The crisis home: sheltering patients in emotional crisis. J Psychosoc Nurs Ment Health Serv 23:18–23, 1985

Brook BD: Crisis hostel: an alternative to psychiatric hospitalization for emergency patients. Hospital and Community Psychiatry 24:621–624, 1973

Brunton J, Howthorne H: The acute non-hospital: a California model. Psychiatric Hospital 20:95–99, 1989

Carling PJ: Housing and supports for persons with mental illness: emerging approaches to research and practice. Hospital and Community Psychiatry 44:439–449, 1993

Carpenter MP: Residential placement for the chronic psychiatric patient: a review and evaluation of the literature. Schizophr Bull 4:384–398, 1978

Creed F, Black D, Anthony P, et al: Randomised controlled trial of day patient versus inpatient psychiatric treatment. BMJ 300:1033–1037, 1990

Cumming J, Cumming E: Ego & Milieu: Theory and Practice of Environmental Therapy. New York, Atherton Press, 1962

Dickey B, Cannon NL, McGuire TG, et al: The Quarterway House: a two-year cost study of an experimental residential program. Hospital and Community Psychiatry 37:1136–1143, 1986

Edelson M: Ego Psychology, Group Dynamics and the Therapeutic Community. New York, Grune & Stratton, 1964

Edelson M: The Practice of Sociotherapy: A Case Study. New Haven, CT, Yale University Press, 1970a

Edelson M: Sociotherapy and Psychotherapy. Chicago, IL, University of Chicago Press, 1970b

Fenton WS, Mosher LR, Herrell JM, et al: Randomized trial of general hospital and residential alternative care for patients with severe and persistent mental illness. Am J Psychiatry 155:516–522, 1998

Fields S: The relationship between residential treatment and supported housing in a community system of services. Psychosocial Rehabilitation Journal 13:105–113, 1990

Fisher WH, Geller JL, Wirth-Cauchon J: Empirically assessing the impact of mobile crisis capacity on state hospital admissions. Community Ment Health J 26:245–253, 1990

Foucault M: The Birth of the Clinic: An Archaeology of Medical Perception. New York, Pantheon, 1973

Gabbard GO: Comparative indications for brief and extended hospitalizations, in American Psychiatric Press Review of Psychiatry, Vol 11. Edited by Tasman A, Riba MB. Washington, DC, American Psychiatric Press, 1992, pp 503–517

Geiser R, Hoche L, King J: Respite care for mentally ill patients and their families. Hospital and Community Psychiatry 39:291–295, 1988

Geller JL: "Anyplace but the state hospital": examining assumptions about the benefits of admission diversion. Hospital and Community Psychiatry 42:145–152, 1991

Ghaziuddian M: Referral of mentally handicapped patients to the psychiatrist: a community study. Journal of Mental Deficiency Research 32:491–495, 1988

Gibbons JS: Care of "new" long-stay patients in a district general hospital psychiatric unit: the first two years of a hospital-hostel. Acta Psychiatr Scand 73:582–588, 1986

Glick ID, Hargreaves WA: Psychiatric Hospital Treatment for the 1980's: A Controlled Study of Short Versus Long Hospitalization. Lexington, MA, DC Heath, 1979

Grob GN: Mental Illness and American Society: 1875–1940. Princeton, NJ, Princeton University Press, 1983

Gruenberg EM: Hospital treatment in schizophrenia: the indications for and the value of hospital treatment, in The Schizophrenic Reactions: A Critique of the Concept, Hospital Treatment, and Current Research. Edited by Cancro R. New York, Brunner/Mazel, 1970, pp 121–136

Gudeman JE, Shore MF, Dickey B: Day hospitalization and an inn instead of inpatient care for psychiatric patients. N Engl J Med 308:749–753, 1983

Hanson GD, Babigian HM: Reasons for hospitalization from a psychiatric emergency service. Psychiatr Q 48:336–351, 1974

Hawthorne WB, Fals-Stewart W, Lohr JB: A treatment outcome study of community-based residential care. Hospital and Community Psychiatry 45:152–155, 1994

Henisz JE: Psychotherapeutic Management on the Short-Term Unit: Glimpses at Inpatient Psychiatry. Springfield, IL, Charles C Thomas, 1981

Hoge MA, Davidson L, Hill WL, et al: The promise of partial hospitalization: a reassessment. Hospital and Community Psychiatry 43:345–354, 1992

Hyde C, Bridges K, Goldberg D, et al: The evaluation of a hostel ward: a controlled study using modified cost-benefit analysis. Br J Psychiatry 151:805–812, 1987

Intagliata J: Improving the quality of community care for the chronically mentally disabled: the role of case management. Schizophr Bull 8:655–674, 1982

Jones M: The Therapeutic Community. New York, Basic Books, 1953

Klutier G, Giel R, Nienhusis EF, et al: Predicting feasibility of day treatment for unselected patients referred for inpatient psychiatric treatment: results of a randomized trial. Am J Psychiatry 149:1199–1205, 1992

Kresky-Wolff M, Matthews S, Kalibat F, et al: Crossing Place: a residential model for crisis intervention. Hospital and Community Psychiatry 35:72–74, 1984

Laing RD: The Politics of Experience. New York, Pantheon, 1967

Lamb HR: Therapist–case managers: more than brokers of services. Hospital and Community Psychiatry 31:762–764, 1980

Lamb HR, Lamb DM: A nonhospital alternative to acute hospitalization. Hospital and Community Psychiatry 35:728–730, 1984

Langsley DG: Crisis intervention and the avoidance of hospitalization. New Dir Ment Health Serv 6:81–90, 1980

MacCarthy B, Lesage E, Brewin CR, et al: Needs for care among the relatives of long-term users of day care: a report from the Camberwell High Contact Survey. Psychol Med 19:725–736, 1989

Maxmen JS, Tucker GJ: The admission process. J Nerv Ment Dis 156:327–340, 1973

Michels R, Marzuk PM: Progress in psychiatry. N Engl J Med 329:552–560, 1993

Mora G: Historical and theoretical trends in psychiatry, in Comprehensive Textbook of Psychiatry/III, 3rd Edition, Vol 1. Edited by Kaplan HI, Freedman AM, Sadock BJ. Baltimore, MD, Williams & Wilkins, 1980, pp 4–98

Mosher LR: Soteria: a therapeutic community for psychotic persons. International Journal of Therapeutic Communities 12:53–67, 1991

Mosher LR: Soteria and other alternatives to acute hospitalization, a personal and professional review. J Nerv Ment Dis 187:142–149, 1999

Mosher LR, Menn A, Matthews SM: Soteria: evaluation of a home-based treatment for schizophrenia. Am J Orthopsychiatry 45:455–467, 1975

Mueser KT: Commentary on Liberman and Corrigan. Psychiatry 56:250–253, 1993

Mueser KT, Lieberman RP: Skills training in vocational rehabilitation, in Vocational Rehabilitation of Persons With Prolonged Psychiatric Disorders. Edited by Ciardiello JA, Bell MD. Baltimore, MD, Johns Hopkins University Press, 1988, pp 81–103

Munich RL: Group dynamics, in Comprehensive Group Psychotherapy, 3rd Edition. Edited by Kaplan HI, Sadock BJ. Baltimore, MD, Williams & Wilkins, 1993, pp 21–32

Munich RL, Lang E: The boundaries of psychiatric rehabilitation. Hospital and Community Psychiatry 44:661–665, 1993

Oldham JM, Lin A, Breslin L: Comprehensive psychiatric emergency services. Psychiatr Q 61:57–67, 1990

Olfson M: Assertive community treatment: an evaluation of the experimental evidence. Hospital and Community Psychiatry 41:634–641, 1990

Paul GL, Lentz RJ: Psychosocial Treatment of Chronic Mental Patients: Milieu Versus Social Learning Programs. Cambridge, MA, Harvard University Press, 1977

Rappaport RN: Community as Doctor: New Perspectives on a Therapeutic Community. Springfield, IL, Charles C Thomas, 1960

Rose SO, Hawkins J, Apodaca L: Decision to admit: criteria for admission and readmission to a Veterans Administration hospital. Arch Gen Psychiatry 34:418–421, 1977

Rubinstein R, Lasswell H: Sharing of Power in a Psychiatric Hospital. New Haven, CT, Yale University Press, 1966

Schwartz IM: Hospitalization of adolescents for psychiatric and substance abuse treatment: legal and ethical issues. Journal of Adolescent Health Care 10:473–478, 1989

Sederer LI: Brief hospitalization, in American Psychiatric Press Review of Psychiatry, Vol 11. Edited by Tasman A, Riba MB. Washington, DC, American Psychiatric Press, 1992, pp 518–534

Sederer L, Centorrino F: Schizophrenia, in Acute Care Psychiatry: Diagnosis and Treatment. Edited by Sederer LI, Rothschild AJ. Baltimore, MD, Williams & Wilkins, 1997, pp 167–193

Segal SP, Kotler PL: Do we need board and care homes? Adult Respite Care Journal 3:24–32, 1989

Shadoan RA: Levels of care for residential treatment in an urban setting. Psychiatric Annals 15:639–641, 1985

Simpson CJ, Hyde CE, Faragher EB: The chronically mentally ill in community facilities: a study of quality of life. Br J Psychiatry 154:77–82, 1989

Sledge W, Astrachan B, Thompson K, et al: Case management in psychiatry: an analysis of tasks. Am J Psychiatry 152:1259–1263, 1995

Sledge W, Tebes J, Rakfeldt J, et al: Day hospital/crisis respite care vs inpatient care, I: clinical outcomes. Am J Psychiatry 153:1067–1073, 1996a

Sledge WH, Tebes J, Wolff N, et al: Day hospital/crisis respite care vs inpatient care, II: service utilization and costs. Am J Psychiatry 153:1074–1083, 1996b

Smith TE, Deutsch A, Schwartz F, et al: The role of personality in treatment of schizophrenic and schizoaffective disorder inpatients: a pilot study. Bull Menninger Clin 57:88–99, 1993

Stanton AH, Schwartz MS: The Mental Hospital: A Study of Institutional Participation in Psychiatric Illness and Treatment. New York, Basic Books, 1954

Stein LI, Test MA: Alternative to mental hospital treatment, I: conceptual model, treatment program, and clinical evaluation. Arch Gen Psychiatry 37:392–397, 1980

Stein LI, Test MA, Marx AJ: Alternative to the hospital: a controlled study. Am J Psychiatry 132:517–522, 1975

Stroul B: Psychiatric Crisis Response Systems: A Descriptive Study (Publ No CS 00-0055). Rockville, MD, Community Support Program, Center for Mental Health Studies, Substance Abuse and Mental Health Services Administration, 1993

Tanzman B: An overview of surveys of mental health consumers' preferences for housing and support services. Hospital and Community Psychiatry 44:450–455, 1993

Terkelsen KG, McCarthy RH: Home visits in the era of cost containment: comments on Reding, Raphelson & Montgomery's paper. Community Ment Health J 30:297–301, 1994

Test MA, Stein LI: Training in community living: a follow-up look at a gold-award program. Hospital and Community Psychiatry 27:193–194, 1976

Thompson KS, Griffith EEH, Leaf PJ: A historical review of the Madison model of community care. Hospital and Community Psychiatry 41:625–634, 1990

Van Putten T: Milieu therapy: contraindications? Arch Gen Psychiatry 29:640–643, 1973

Van Putten T, May PRA: Milieu therapy of the schizophrenias, in Treatment of Schizophrenia: Progress and Prospects. Edited by West LJ, Flinn DE. New York, Grune & Stratton, 1976, pp 217–243

Walsh SF: Characteristics of failures in an emergency residential alternative to psychiatric hospitalization. Soc Work Health Care 11:53–64, 1986

Weisbrod BA, Test MA, Stein LI: Alternative to mental hospital treatment, II: economic benefit-cost analysis. Arch Gen Psychiatry 37:400–405, 1980

Wherley M, Bisgaard S: Beyond model programs: evaluation of a countywide system of residential treatment programs. Hospital and Community Psychiatry 38:852–857, 1987

Wilder JF, Levin G, Zwerling I: A two-year follow-up evaluation of acute psychotic patients treated in a day hospital. Am J Psychiatry 122:1095–1101, 1966

Zirul DW, Lieberman AA, Rapp CA: Respite care for the chronically mentally ill: focus for the 1990s. Community Ment Health J 25:171–184, 1989

Index

Page numbers printed in ***boldface*** type refer to tables or figures.

Acetylcholinesterase inhibitors *(continued)*
physostigmine, 484
rivastigmine, 487
tacrine, 484–485, 554–555
ACOA (Adult Children of Alcoholics), 901
Acquired immunodeficiency syndrome (AIDS). *See* Human immunodeficiency virus infection
Acrylamide, 590
ACT. *See* Assertive Community Treatment
ACTH (adrenocorticotropic hormone), 8, 1237
Action potentials, seizures and, 449–451
Acupuncture
for chronic pain, 1794
for male erectile disorder, 1881
for opioid detoxification, 629, 794
Acute crisis respite care, 1121–1122
Acute stress disorder, 1567–1570
diagnostic criteria for, **1568**
as predictor of posttraumatic stress disorder, 1567, 1569–1570
prevalence of, 1567–1569
role of social support in, 1570
types of trauma associated with, 1568–1569
Acute stress disorder treatment, 1570–1580
models for, 1573–1577
cognitive-behavioral therapies, 1575–1576
eye movement desensitization and reprocessing, 1577
frontline combat treatment, 1577
hypnosis, 1576–1577
psychodynamic psychotherapies, 1574–1575
psychological debriefing, 1573–1574
pharmacotherapy, 1577–1580
antidepressants, 1579
antipsychotics, 1580
noradrenergic blockers, 1578–1579
principles of, 1570–1573
considering context of trauma, 1572
establishing safety, 1571
establishing therapeutic alliance, 1570–1571
facilitating social support, 1572–1573
focusing on trauma, 1571–1572
providing patient information/education, 1571
recognizing need for self-care, 1573
timing, 1571
AD. *See* Alzheimer's disease
"Adam." *See* Methylenedioxymethamphetamine
Adaptive functioning
dissociative symptoms and, 1629–1630, 1632
mental retardation and, 76, 77
Tourette's disorder and, 197
ADAS (Alzheimer's Disease Assessment Scale), 485, 487, 524
Adderall®, for persons with tic disorders, **203**
Addiction Severity Index (ASI), 649, 660, 1103
ADDTC (Alzheimer's Disease Diagnostic and Treatment Centers), 518
Adenosine reuptake inhibitors, for anxiety, 1610
S-Adenosyl-L-methionine (SAMe), 547
for treatment-resistant depression, **1336**, 1339
Adenotonsillectomy, for sleep apnea in children, 372
Adenylate cyclase, **1146**
ADHD. *See* Attention-deficit/hyperactivity disorder
ADHD Rating Scale, 196
ADI (Adolescent Drinking Inventory), 659
Adjustment disorders, 1446, 1715–1725
comorbidity with, 1718
transvestism, 2014
diagnostic criteria for, 1716, **1717**
stress as precipitant of, 1716, 1719
treatment of, 1717–1725
course and prognosis in plan for, 1723–1725
literature review of randomized controlled trials, 1717–1718
outcome studies, 1718–1719
pharmacotherapy, 1721–1722
in primary care, 1722
psychotherapy, 1719–1721
support groups, 1720–1721
uncertainty regarding diagnosis of, 1715–1717
Adolescent Drinking Inventory (ADI), 659
Adolescents. *See also* Childhood-adolescent disorders
choice of therapist for, 26
conflicts around body image and reproduction, 34
marijuana use by, 704, **704**, **705**
mental retardation in, 82
self-esteem of girls, 33

suicidal behavior of, 283–286
culture and, 56
treating gender identity disorder in, 2085–2086
Adoption studies, of oppositional defiant disorder, 180
ADRDA (Alzheimer's Disease and Related Disorders Association), 506
Adrenal insufficiency, 546
α-Adrenergic agonists
for alcohol withdrawal, 667
for attention-deficit/hyperactivity disorder, 151, 162–163, **163**
interaction with methylphenidate, 162–163
in persons with tic disorders, **203**, 203–204
for autism, 138
for conduct disorder, 185–186
effect on γ-aminobutyric acid, 186
for opioid detoxification, 790–792, **791**
for posttraumatic stress disorder in alcoholic patients, 673
for self-injurious behaviors, 204
side effects of, **163**, **201**, **203**
sleep disorders, **2418**
for tic disorders, 200, **201**
β-Adrenergic blockers
for alcohol withdrawal, 667
for Alzheimer's disease, **498**, 501–502
for anxiety disorders
in children/adolescents, 237–238, 299
generalized anxiety disorder, 1609–1610
panic disorder, 1456
posttraumatic stress disorder, 238, 299, 1545
social phobia, 1492–1493, 1498
specific phobias, 1503
for attention-deficit/hyperactivity disorder, 151, **163**
for behavioral problems in patients with dementia, 554–555
contraindications to, 555
effects on growth, 238
for elderly persons, 502
for esophageal varices in alcoholic patients, 675
penetration of blood-brain barrier by, 1609, 1610
for self-injurious behaviors, 204
side effects of, **163**, 238, 555, 1610
sleep disorders, 377, **2418**
Adrenocorticotropic hormone (ACTH), 8, 1237
Adrenoleukodystrophy, 545
Adult Children of Alcoholics (ACOA), 901
Adult protective service interventions, for substance abuse, 954
Affect bridge technique, for dissociative amnesia, 1641
Affective disorders. *See* Mood disorders
African-Americans
cultural experience and development of, 54
cultural variability of, 53
pharmacotherapy for, 64
psychotherapy for, 61
racial stereotypes and diagnosis in, 57
validity of psychometric assessment instruments for, 57
African traditional healing practices, 59–60
Aftercare
inpatient substance abuse treatment and, 946–947
therapeutic community treatment and, 975
Age regression, for dissociative amnesia, 1641–1642
Aggressive behavior
in Alzheimer's disease, 497
in antisocial personality disorder, **2252**, 2255–2256
affective vs. predatory aggression, 2263
pharmacotherapy for, **2262**, 2262–2263
biological factors and, 179–180
conduct disorder, 177–186
in Huntington's disease, 539, 540
intergenerational stability of, 180
intermittent explosive disorder, 2439–2442
mental retardation and, 84
lithium for, 99
paroxetine for, 100
sexual, 1951–1970 (*See also* Paraphilias and paraphilia-related disorders)
treatment in patients with dementia, 554–555
toward women, 33, 1541, 1547
Aging
Alzheimer's disease and, 481–507
delirium and, 387, 389–391, **390**
drug-induced, 421–422
dementia and, 390, 535–536
drug metabolism and, 421
effect on elimination of neurotoxins, 422
male erectile disorder and, 1875

Amitriptyline *(continued)*
for borderline personality disorder, 2283
for chronic pain, 1788, 1789
combined with phenelzine, 1331, **1334**
combined with psychotherapy for depression, 1252–1255
behavior therapy, 1253–1254
cognitive therapy, 1255
marital and family therapy, 1252
compared with interpersonal therapy for depression, **1195**, 1196
depersonalization induced by, 1697
interaction with levodopa, 420
for maintenance treatment of depression, 1163–1164
for mentally retarded persons, 101
neuroleptic malignant syndrome and, **436**
for posttraumatic stress disorder, 1543
for premature ejaculation, 1922
for progressive supranuclear palsy, 543
for sleep disorders, **2381**, 2386, 2408
switching to mirtazapine from, **1335**, 1338
therapeutic plasma levels of, 1171
for trichotillomania, 2452
use in patients with alcoholism, 672
for vulvar vestibulitis syndrome, 1938
Ammonia aversion
for paraphilias and paraphilia-related disorders, 1963–1964
for pedophilia, 1986–1987
Ammonium chloride, for urine acidification, 739
Amnestic disorder. *See also* Memory impairment
brain areas affected in, 612–614, **614**
dissociative amnesia, 610, 1623–1647
due to general medical condition or not otherwise specified, 609–622
assessment and differential diagnosis of, 615–617
definition of, 610
diagnostic criteria for, 610, **611**
epidemiology of, 610
prevention of, 617
transient vs. chronic, 610
treatment of, 617–622
etiology of, 611–615
memory rehabilitation for, 617–621
pharmacotherapy for, 621–622
psychogenic, 582
substance-induced persisting, 575–599, 610
transient global amnesia, 613–614
Amobarbital, withdrawal from, **687**
Amobarbital-assisted interviews, 1547, 1680
for conversion disorder, 1765–1766
for dissociative amnesia and fugue, 1634, 1645–1646
indications for, 1645
Amotivation, in schizophrenia, 1013
Amoxapine
for depression, 1155
psychotic, 1421
for panic disorder, 1453
for premature ejaculation, 1922
side effects of, 1155
for sleep disorders, **2381**
Amphetamine, **1147**, 1153
abuse of, 723 (*See also* Stimulant abuse)
for attention-deficit/hyperactivity disorder, 147, 153, **154**
deliriogenic effects of, **415**
excitotoxic effects of, **450**
"ice," 724
psychosis induced by, 724
routes of administration of, 724
use in dual diagnosis patients, **983**
withdrawal from, 635, 724–725
β-Amyloid, in Alzheimerís disease, 490–491, 494
Amyloid precursor protein (APP), 490–491
Amyotrophic lateral sclerosis dementia syndrome, 539
Amytal. *See* Amobarbital
Anal stimulation, for male orgasmic disorder, 1927, 1929
Analgesics. *See also* Pain management for chronic pain
for chronic pain, 1784–1791
acetaminophen, 1786
anticonvulsants, 1790
antidepressants, 1787–1789
benzodiazepines, 1789–1790
nonsteroidal anti-inflammatory drugs, 1786
opioid analgesics, 1784–1786
other agents, 1790–1791
dementia induced by, 587
for patients on methadone maintenance, 806
for patients on naltrexone maintenance, 820–821
Anandamide, 709

Anaracetam, 597
Androgens. *See also* Antiandrogens
  Alzheimer's disease and, 493–494
  effect on women's sexual response, 1902
  for hypoactive sexual desire, 1862
  for male erectile disorder, 1889
Anesthesia
  dissociative anesthetics, 735, 753
  for electroconvulsive therapy, 1281–1283
  for patients on methadone maintenance, 805–806
  ultrarapid opioid detoxification under, 792–793
"Angel Dust." *See* Phencyclidine
Anger attacks, 2440. *See also* Aggressive behavior
  depression with, 1316
  intermittent explosive disorder, 2439–2442
Anger management training
  for conduct disorder, 183
  for intermittent explosive disorder, 2440–2441
Aniracetam, for Alzheimer's disease, 495
Anorexia nervosa. *See also* Eating disorders
  assessment of, 2103–2108, **2104–2105**
  case examples of, 2175–2185
  diagnostic criteria for, 2099–2100, **2101**, 2144–2145
  epidemiology of, 2100
  genetics and, 2171, 2188–2189
  personality and, 2179
  psychodynamics of, 2169–2171
  symptoms and psychological structure of, 2185–2187
    starvation-related symptoms, 2100–2102
Anorexia nervosa treatment
  approaches to, 2100–2103
  choice of provider for, 2108–2109
  cognitive-behavioral therapy, 2145
    compared with behavioral family therapy, 2145
    in day hospital program, 2132–2133, **2133**
    future directions for, 2151–2152
    during hospitalization, 2121–2122
  components of, 2109–2111
  comprehensive program for, **2112**
  day hospital treatment, 2127–2136
    advantages and disadvantages of, 2128
    cognitive-behavioral therapy, 2132–2133, **2133**
    contraindications to, 2129
    effectiveness of, 2136
    goals of, 2130–2131
    group therapy, 2128–2129, 2134–2135
    medical and psychopharmacological management, 2131–2132
    patient selection for, 2129
    setting behavioral expectations for, 2130
    staff issues, 2135
    structure of, 2130
  establishing working alliance for, 2103
  family therapy, 2110, 2193–2202
    behavioral, 2145
    compared with individual psychodynamic psychotherapy, 2171–2173, 2190
    contraindications to, 2199
    guidelines for, 2199
    during hospitalization, 2122
    opinions of laypeople and patients about, 2195–2196
    outcome studies of, 2196–2198
    practices and opinions of therapists about, 2194–2195
    pragmatic and constructive approach to, 2199–2200
    separation-individuation of adolescent and, 2200
    sibling therapy, 2200–2202
    special issues in, 2200
    theoretical considerations for, 2194
    varieties of, 2198
  group therapy, 2110
    in day hospital program, 2128–2129, 2134–2135
  inpatient treatment, 2119–2122
    brief hospitalization, 2120
    discharge criteria, 2120, 2121
    extended hospitalization, 2120–2122
    specialized units for, 2121
  lack of patient cooperation with, 2103, 2112–2113
  legal and ethical issues in compulsory treatment, 2111–2114
  marital therapy, 2202–2205
    guidelines for, 2204–2205
    marital interaction, 2202–2203
    role of spouse in therapy, 2203–2204
  multifactorial approach to, 2171
  nutritional counseling, 2110

Anorexia nervosa treatment *(continued)*
pharmacotherapy, 2159, 2163–2165
antidepressants, 1138, 2164
antipsychotics, 2163–2164
in day hospital program, 2132
during hospitalization, 2122, 2163
other agents, 2164
"Practice Guideline for the Treatment of Patients with Eating Disorders," 2127–2128
principles of, **2111**
psychodynamic psychotherapy, 2169–2190
compared with family therapy, 2171–2173, 2190
costs and benefits of, 2189
countertransference responses in, 2173–2174, 2179
for less "typical" cases, 2179–2185
therapeutic alliance for, 2177–2178
transference reactions and, 2176, 2178
for "typical" cases, 2175–2179
Antabuse. *See* Disulfiram
Anti-inflammatory agents, for Alzheimer's disease, 492–493
Antiamyloid strategies, for Alzheimer's disease, 490–491
Antiandrogens
for intermittent explosive disorder, 2442
for male-to-female transsexuals, **2042**, 2043
for paraphilias and paraphilia-related disorders, 1964–1967
for pedophilia, 1989–1990
for transvestism, 2024–2025
Antibiotics
deliriogenic effects of, **415**
dementia induced by, **549**, 587
Anticholinergic agents, premedication for electroconvulsive therapy, 1281–1282
Anticholinergic effects of drugs, **426**
antipsychotics, 404
monoamine oxidase inhibitors, 1461
tricyclic antidepressants, 586, 1395, 1461
Anticholinergic toxicity, 426–427
clinical features of, 426
diagnosis of, 426
pathophysiology of, 427
location and function of muscarinic cholinergic receptor subtypes, **428–429**
treatment of, 401, 427, 502
Anticoagulants, after cardioembolic stroke, 523
Anticonvulsants
for aggressive behavior, **2262**, 2263
for Alzheimer's disease, **498**, 501
for bipolar depression, 1354, **1355**
carbamazepine, 1158–1159
for conduct disorder, 186
dementia induced by, **549**, 587
dose titration for, **1170**
gabapentin, 1162
hypersomnia induced by, **2419**
for intermittent explosive disorder, 2441–2442
lamotrigine, 1161–1162
management before and during course of electroconvulsive therapy, 1279
for mania, 1158–1162
for mentally retarded persons, 100
for neuropathic pain, 1790
for panic disorder, 1456
topiramate, 1162
for treatment-resistant depression, 1324–1325, **1328**, **1336**, 1339
valproic acid, 1160
Antidepressants, 13, 1144–1156
for acute-phase treatment of depression, 1144–1162, 1167–1171, **1168**, 1310, 1420–1429
comorbidity and, 1421–1423
declaring initial treatment failure, 1423
adjunctive medications used with, 1426–1427
for anxiety disorders
acute stress disorder, 1579
in children/adolescents, 156, 235–239
generalized anxiety disorder, 1605–1608
panic disorder, 1138, 1443, 1444, 1450–1453, 1461
for attention-deficit/hyperactivity disorder, 148–151, 156–162, **157–160**
to augment effects of electroconvulsive therapy, 1279
for autism, 138–139
for body dysmorphic disorder, 1816–1817
for chronic pain, 1787–1789
classification of, 156, 1144–1145, **1147**
drugs with mixed pharmacological properties, 1154–1156
monoamine oxidase inhibitors, 1151–1153
monoamine-releasing agents, 1153

Attention-deficit/hyperactivity disorder (ADHD), 145–168
in adults, 147
comorbidity with, 147, 148
anxiety disorders, 227
bipolar disorder, 1346
conduct disorder, 177, 178
depression, 261, 1322
learning disorders, 110, 112–113
mental retardation, 84
paraphilias, 1957
substance abuse, 155, 729, 992–993
Tourette's disorder, 194
course of, 147
definition of, 145
etiology of, 146–147
nicotine hypothesis of, 151–152
prevalence of, 146
Attention-deficit/hyperactivity disorder (ADHD) treatment, 147–168
in dual diagnosis patients, 992–993
pharmacotherapy, **146**, 147–163
antidepressants, 148–151, 156–162, **157–160**, 261
antihypertensives, 151, 162–163, **163**
antipsychotics, 151
anxiolytics, 151
carbamazepine, 151
nicotinic drugs, 151–152
other agents, 152
in persons with Tourette's disorder, 202–204, **203**
stimulants, 147–148, 153–156, **154**
psychosocial treatment, 163–168
cognitive-behavioral therapy, 165
combinations of medical and nonmedical therapy, 165–166
goodness-of-fit model for, 164
Multimodal Treatment Study for ADHD, 164–168
operant procedures, 164
theoretical basis for, 164
Attention deficits
delirium and, 393
progressive supranuclear palsy and, 543
AUDIT (Alcohol Use Disorders Identification Test), 649, 659
Autistic disorder, 125–128
autistic learning disability model, 127–128
autistic learning disabilities, 128, **129**
nomenclature-based literature, 127–128
"primary deficits" research, 127
symptom- vs. diagnosis-specific treatment, 126, 128, 130
intelligence testing in, 140
mental retardation and, 86
Autistic disorder treatment, 128–140
early intervention, 125–126
future research on, 140
methodological problems in research on, 126–127
omnibus approaches, 128–135
applied behavioral analysis, 130–133
comparison of, **131**
inclusive education, 134–135
TEACCH, 133–134
pharmacotherapy, 137–140
antidepressants, 138–139
antipsychotics, 139
clonidine, 138
effectiveness of, 139–140
naltrexone, 137–138
stimulants, 137
vitamin B_6 and magnesium, 139
specific nonpharmacological treatments, 135–137
behaviorally focused treatments, 137
floor time, 135–136
picture exchange communication system, 136
pivotal response training, 135
social stories, 136–137
state of the art, 125–126
Autoerotic asphyxia, **1952**
Autonomic dysfunction
in depression, 1390
in generalized anxiety disorder, 1588
in neuroleptic malignant syndrome, 443–444
Autonomy, interdependence, and culture, 50–51
Aversive techniques
for kleptomania, 2444
for mentally retarded persons, 96–97
for paraphilias and paraphilia-related disorders, 1963–1964
for pathological gambling, 2448
for pedophilia, 1986–1987
for transvestism, 2019–2021
Avoidant personality disorder, 2327–2337
cognitive distortions in, 2334–2335

for cocaine abuse, 727–728
opiate agonist action of, 821
for opioid detoxification, 629, 794, 806
Bupropion, 156, **1147**, 1150–1151
for anxiety disorders
panic disorder, 1453
social phobia, 1493
for attention-deficit/hyperactivity disorder, 148, 150, **159**, 162
for bulimia nervosa, **2162**
for cocaine abuse, 727
combined with selective serotonin reuptake inhibitors, 1332
for compulsive buying, 2454
for depression, 1151, 1172–1173
associated with traumatic brain injury, 553
atypical depression, 1312, 1421
bipolar depression, 1352, **1353**, **1354**
in children/adolescents, **258–259**, 261
for depressive dementia, 553
dosage of, 162, 1151
dose-response relationship, 1309
titration of, **1170**
mechanism of action of, 1151, 1394
for Parkinson's disease, 542
for sexual disorders
male orgasmic disorder, 1927
paraphilias and paraphilia-related disorders, 1969
side effects of, **159**, 162, **258**, 261, 1394
seizures, 162, 1151, 1394
for sleep disorders, 2387, 2409
for smoking cessation, **767–768**, 769
sustained-release, 261, 1151
switching from another antidepressant to, **1335**, 1337
use in medically ill patients, 1394
cardiovascular disease, 1400–1401
use in persons with tic disorders, 162
Burn encephalopathy, 391
BuSpar. *See* Buspirone
Buspirone, **687**
for Alzheimer's disease, **498**, 501, 503
for anxiety disorders
in alcoholic patients, 673, 990
in children/adolescents, 234–235
generalized anxiety disorder, 1608
obsessive-compulsive disorder, **202**, 1524, 1529
panic disorder, 1456
social phobia, 1492, 1498
for attention-deficit/hyperactivity disorder, 151
for behavioral problems in patients with dementia, 555
for body dysmorphic disorder, 1817
for delirium, 404
for male orgasmic disorder, 1927
mechanism of action of, 1394
for mood disorders, 1138
treatment-resistant depression, 1323, **1327**
for sedative-hypnotic withdrawal, 585
side effects of, 235, 1608
for transvestism, 2021–2022
for trichotillomania, 2453
use in medically ill patients, 1394
Butabarbital, withdrawal from, **687**
Butalbital, withdrawal from, **687**
Butisol. *See* Butabarbital
Butyrylcholinesterases, 484
Buying mania. *See* Compulsive buying
BZs. *See* Benzodiazepines

CA. *See* Cocaine Anonymous
CAD. *See* Coronary artery disease
CADASIL (cerebral autosomal dominant arteriopathy with subcortical infarcts and leukoencephalopathy), 517
Cadmium exposure, 591
Caffeine, 644
eating disorders and, 2107
side effects of, 2388
delirium, **415**
excitotoxicity, **450**
sleep disorders and, 2378, 2388, **2418**
CAGE questionnaire, 649, 659, 713
Calcium acetyl homotaurinate, for alcoholism, 640, 671
Calcium channel blockers
for Alzheimer's disease, 491, 494
for cognitive impairments, 557–558
for conduct disorder, 186
for mood disorders associated with traumatic brain injury, 553
for treatment-resistant bipolar disorder, 1360
CAM (Confusion Assessment Method), 397

eye movement desensitization and reprocessing for, 1551–1552
frontline combat treatment for acute stress reactions, 1577
group therapy for, 1549
posttraumatic stress disorder among, 1541, 1546–1547
feigned, 1833, 1838
relaxation training for, 1554
Communication
conversion as, 1759
mental retardation and, 87–89
picture exchange communication system for autism, 136
schizophrenia and, 1014
sexual functioning and, 1850, 1900–1901
Community-based treatment of substance abuse, 951–959
brief intervention in colleges, 952
brief intervention in primary care settings, 951–952
in children/adolescents, 333–334
criminal justice system intervention, 954–955
drug courts, 954–955, **955**
drunk driving, 955
non-hospital-based services, 955–959
case management, 958–959
community residential facilities, 957
day hospital and intensive outpatient treatment, 956–957
detoxification centers, 957–958
outpatient detoxification, 958
social service agency intervention, 952–954
adult protective services, 954
child protective services, 952–953
disability and public support, 953–954
therapeutic communities, 963–977
Community reentry training, 1100
Community resources, for Alzheimer's disease, 506–507
Compression ring, for male erectile disorder, 1882
Compulsions. *See also* Obsessive-compulsive disorder
definition of, 1516, **1517**
in impulse-control disorder, 2436–2438
Compulsive buying, 2437, 2453–2455
comorbidity with, 2454
definition of, 2453
preliminary diagnostic criteria for, **2454**
prevalence of, 2453–2454
treatment of, 2454–2455
pharmacotherapy, 2454–2455
psychological treatments, 2454
Computed tomography (CT)
in dementias, 538, 580
in depersonalization, 1697
hydrocephalus on, 552
lacunar infarcts on, 516
in substance-induced persisting dementia and amnestic disorder, 594
in Tourette's disorder, 197
in vascular dementia, 518
Computer use, problematic, 1846, 2437, 2460
Conceptual disorganization, in schizophrenia, **1011**, 1014
Concrete thinking, in schizophrenia, 1014
Conduct disorder (CD), 177–181
childhood-onset, 177
comorbidity with, 178–179
attention-deficit/hyperactivity disorder, 177, 178
learning disorders, 112
mental retardation, 84, 85
paraphilias, 1957
substance abuse, 179, 327
definition of, 177
diagnostic criteria for, 177, **178**
differential diagnosis of, 178–179
etiological factors in, 179–181
biological, 179–180
psychological, 180–181
gender distribution of, 179
outcome of, 179
prevalence of, 179
severity of, 177
Conduct disorder (CD) treatment, 181–186
assessment and planning for, 181–182
cognitive-behavioral techniques, 184
functional family therapy, 184
long-term effectiveness of, 184
parent management training, 184, 2263
group homes/residential treatment, 182
group therapy, 182
at home, 182
inpatient programs, 182
multisystemic therapy, 182
pharmacotherapy, **146**, 152–153, 184–186
anticonvulsants, 186
antidepressants, 185
antipsychotics, 186

goal of full remission, 1308, 1310
monitoring response to, 1170–1171, **1171**
no or inadequate response to, 1308–1311
residual symptoms after, 1307–1308
for specific subtypes of depression, **1169**
therapeutic plasma levels of, 1171, 1308
for chronic depression, 1249
combined medication and psychotherapy, 13–14, 1247–1262
for acute-phase treatment, 1250–1257, 1430–1432
AHCPR recommendations against use of, 1248
applications and procedures for, 1260
behavior therapy, 1253–1254
case examples of, 1260–1261
cognitive therapy and related cognitive-behavioral approaches, 1254–1257
for continuation/maintenance-phase treatment, 1258–1259
contraindications to, 1250
dynamic psychotherapy, 1251
effect on acceptability of treatment, 1248–1249, 1259–1260
effect on breadth of treatment response, 1248, 1257–1258, 1262
effect on magnitude of treatment response, 1248, 1262
effect on probability of treatment response, 1248
indications for, 1249–1250
interpersonal psychotherapy, 1252–1253
marital and family therapy, 1251–1252
for patients with comorbid conditions, 1249–1250
potential benefits of, 1248–1249
side effects of, 1259–1260
continuation/maintenance-phase treatment, **1143**, 1144, 1163–1165, 1172, 1419, 1432–1434
antidepressants, 1163–1165, 1310, 1432–1434
cognitive therapy, 1207–1208, **1208**, 1432
combined medications and psychotherapy, 1258–1259, 1432
duration of, 1432–1434
electroconvulsive therapy, 1271–1273, 1286–1287, 1419
goals of, 1418
interpersonal psychotherapy, 1198–1199, **1199**, **1200**, 1258–1259
light therapy, 1299–1300
in medically ill patients, 1433
in pregnancy, 1433
psychodynamic psychotherapy, 1231
symptom breakthrough during, 1433
definition of response to, 1307
depression-focused psychotherapies, 1181–1215, 1429–1430
behavior therapy, 1187–1188, 1199–1204
cognitive therapy, 1188–1191, 1204–1209
definition of, 1181
efficacy of, 1191–1209, **1192–1196**, **1201**
guidelines for use of, 1212–1215
history of, 1182–1183
interpersonal psychotherapy, 1185–1187, 1191–1199
pharmacotherapy and, 1252–1257
predictors of response to, 1211–1212, **1213**, **1214**
for severe depression, 1209–1211, **1210**
shared features of, 1183–1185, **1184**
in dual diagnosis patients, 986–988, 1421
alcoholism, 672–673
electroconvulsive therapy, 1267–1289
for acute-phase treatment, 1270–1271
case examples of, 1287–1289
for continuation/maintenance-phase treatment, 1271–1272, 1286–1287
gender and outcome of, 38–39
light therapy, 1295–1303
for acute-phase treatment, 1299
for continuation/maintenance-phase treatment, 1299–1300
contraindications to, 1297–1298
formal aspects of, 1300–1301
indications for, 1295–1297, **1297**
novel treatment devices for administration of, 1301
practical aspects of, 1301–1302
in medically ill patients, 1389–1407, 1422–1423
cancer, 1406–1407
cardiovascular disease, 1399–1401
diabetes mellitus, 1402–1404

Electroencephalography (EEG)
  for child with initial episode of psychosis, 342
  in delirium, 388, **396**, 396–397, 416, 582
  in depersonalization, 1697
  effect of sensory deprivation on, 392
  in generalized anxiety disorder, 1588
  in idiopathic recurring stupor, 427
  in mercury poisoning, 592
  monitoring of electroconvulsive therapy-induced EEG response, 1285
  in schizophrenia, 1015–1016
  sleep stages on, 359
  in substance-induced persisting dementia and amnestic disorder, 594
Elimination disorders, 211–219
  encopresis, 216–219
  enuresis, 211–216
EMDR. *See* Eye movement desensitization and reprocessing
Emotional states, 7
  antisocial personality disorder and, 2257–2258
  binge eating triggered by negative affect, 2209–2210, 2213–2214
  in dissociative amnesia and fugue, 1629, 1633, 1636
  family expressed emotion and schizophrenia relapse, 349–351, 1073–1074, **1075**, 1078
  lability in delirium, 395
  substance abuse relapse and, 867
Employment
  back problems and return to work, 1781
  individual placement and support for, 1104
  learning disorders and, 111
  skills training for, 1104
  somatization disorder and, 1748
  substance abuse and, 636–637
  supported, 1103–1104
  transitional, 1103
Encephalitis
  AIDS-related, 550
  delirium and, 399
  herpes simplex, 614, 621
  sleep disorders and, **2411**
Encephalopathy
  gold-induced, 593
  hepatic, 401
  HIV, 550
  hypertensive, 399, 401
  lead, 591–592
  subcortical arteriosclerotic, 517
  substance-induced, 424–460
    anticholinergic toxicity, 426–427
    inhibitotoxicity, 427–433
    neuroleptic malignant syndrome, 433–447
    seizures, 447–453
    serotonin syndrome, 453–460
    varieties of, 425–426
  Wernicke's, 399, 401, 584–585, 668, 674
Encopresis, 216–219
  assessment of, 217
  conditions associated with, 217
    constipation, 216, 217
    enuresis, 217
  diagnostic criteria for, 216, **216**
  epidemiology of, 217
  etiology of, 217
  natural history of, 217
  treatment of, 218–219
    behavioral-educational therapy, 218
    biofeedback therapy, 218–219
    medical, 218
Encounters, in therapeutic communities, 971
Endocrine factors. *See also* Hormonal therapies
  dementia and, **537**, 545–547
  depression and, 1390
    stress responses of depressed women with history of childhood abuse, 1236–1237
  hormonal effects of psychotherapeutic interventions, 13
  hypoactive sexual desire and, 1857, 1862
  posttraumatic stress disorder and, 1542
  sleep disorders and endocrinological disease, **2414**
Endozepine-4, 427–429
Engel, G. L., 3
English as a second language, 56
Enuresis, 211–214
  assessment of, 213
  conditions associated with, 213
    encopresis, 217
  diagnostic criteria for, 211, **212**
  epidemiology of, 212
  etiology of, 212–213
    detrusor instability, 213
    genetic factors, 212–213
    psychological factors, 213
  natural history of, 212

Group therapy *(continued)*
for substance abuse, 891–898
in children/adolescents, 333
gender and, 24–25
marijuana, 715
for transvestism, 2018
Growth, drug effects on
β-blockers, 238
stimulants, 155–156
Guanabenz, for alcohol withdrawal, 667
Guanfacine
for attention-deficit/hyperactivity disorder, 151, 163, **163**
in persons with tic disorders, 203, **203**
for posttraumatic stress disorder in alcoholic patients, 673
side effects of, **163**, **203**
for tic disorders, 200
Guidelines for Clinical Practice: From Development to Use, 1718
Guidelines for Treating Dissociative Identity Disorder (Multiple Personality Disorder) in Adults, 1674
Guilty ruminations, 85
Gut function, serotonin in, 453–454

Habit reversal training
for onychophagia, 2459–2460
for trichotillomania, 2451
Hachinski Ischemia Score (HIS), 518
Hair pulling. *See* Trichotillomania
Hair toxicology screening. *See* Toxicology testing for substance abuse
Halazepam, withdrawal from, **685**
Halcion. *See* Triazolam
Haldol. *See* Haloperidol
Halfway houses
for bulimic patients, 2125
for patients with borderline personality disorder, 2286
for schizophrenic persons, 1123
for substance-abusing persons, 957
Hallervorden-Spatz syndrome, 543
Hallucinations
in alcohol-induced psychotic disorder, 673
in Alzheimer's disease, 497
in children/adolescents, 341
in delirium, 393
hallucinogen-induced, 693, 694
hypnagogic and hypnopompic, 373
mental retardation and, 85
in narcolepsy, 2372
in psychotic depression, 1313
in schizophrenia, 1010, 1012–1013
Hallucinogens, 693–700
absorption of, 694
definition of, 693
differential diagnosis of exposure to, 695–696
dose-response curve for, 694, 697
drug interactions with, 698
drugs classified as, 693
incidence of use of, 627, 628
intervention for acute adverse reactions to, 696–698
intervention for chronic adverse reactions to, 698–700
anxiety and depressive states, 699
flashbacks, 699–700
personality changes induced by, 695, 698–699
psychological effects of, 694–695
terminology for, 693–694
Haloperidol
for acute adverse reactions to hallucinogens, 698
for Alzheimer's disease, **498**, 499
for anxiety disorders in children/adolescents, 238
for autism, 139
for childhood-onset schizophrenia, 344–347
for conduct disorder, 186
for delirium, **402**, 403–404, **405**, 423–424, **424**
effect on regional cerebral blood flow/metabolism, 1019
for Huntington's disease, 540
for insomnia, 2408
interaction with lithium, 549
for intermittent explosive disorder, 2441
intravenous, 403–404
for ketamine intoxication, 745
for mentally retarded persons, 98, 99
neuroleptic malignant syndrome and, **436**
for obsessive-compulsive disorder, 1529
in children/adolescents, 318
in Tourette's disorder, 202, **202**
for personality disorders
paranoid personality disorder, 2234
schizotypal personality disorder, 2247
for phencyclidine delirium, 741
for rapid tranquilization, 1029

Lecithin, for Alzheimer's disease, 483
Legal issues
  Alzheimer's disease and, 507
  criminal behavior and conduct disorder, 177–186
  gender transition, 2040
  implications of hypnosis, 1639
  informed consent
    for electroconvulsive therapy, 1277–1278
    for estrogen therapy for transvestism, 2024
    for treatment of dissociative identity disorder, 1673–1674
  lawsuits related to "false" memories of childhood abuse, 1625–1626
  malingering, 1836–1839
  pain management for patients involved in litigation or workers' compensation claims, 1794–1795
  responsibility for illegal acts during fugue state, 1634–1635
  sex crimes, 1955–1957
    pedophilia, 1981–2000
  in treatment of eating disorders, 2111–2114
Leiter International Performance Scale, 140
Length of stay
  brief hospitalization, 1117–1118
  custodial treatment, 1119
  extended hospitalization, 1118–1119
  reductions in, 1114
  for treatment of substance use disorders, 947
Leritine, withdrawal from, **788**
Lesch-Nyhan syndrome, 86
Leukoariosis, 517
Leuprolide acetate (LPA)
  for gender-dysphoric adolescents, 2086
  for inappropriate sexual behaviors in Huntington's disease, 540
  for paraphilias and paraphilia-related disorders, 1967
  for pedophilia, 1990
Levodopa
  for attention-deficit/hyperactivity disorder, 152
  for cognitive effects of traumatic brain injury, 553
  interaction with amitriptyline, 420
  neuroleptic malignant syndrome and, **435**
  for Parkinson's disease, 541
  for progressive supranuclear palsy, 543
  psychosis induced by, 542
  for REM sleep behavior disorder, 2404
  sexual effects of, 1961
  for Wilson's disease, 544
Levodopa-carbidopa
  neuroleptic malignant syndrome and, **435**
  for restless legs syndrome and periodic limb movements, **2385**, 2399–2400
Levomethadyl acetate (LAAM), 806, 858
Levonorgestrel, for trichotillomania, 2453
Levorphanol, withdrawal from, **788**
Levothyroxine, for treatment-resistant bipolar disorder, 1359
Lewy bodies, 540, 543
Lewy body disorders with dementia, 540
LHRH (luteinizing hormone-releasing hormone) agonists, for paraphilias and paraphilia-related disorders, 1966–1967
Librium. *See* Chlordiazepoxide
Liddle's multidimensional family therapy, for substance abuse in children/adolescents, 333
Lidocaine
  antidepressant interactions with, 1401
  deliriogenic effects of, **418**
Liebowitz Social Anxiety Scale, 1491, 1493
Life experiences
  adjustment disorders and, 1715–1725
  childhood/adolescent events and female sexual dysfunction, 1898–1899
  early stressors
    conduct disorder and, 180
    enuresis and, 213
  gender, choice of therapist and, 30–31
  hypoactive sexual desire and, 1857
  life-cycle events, 29
    gender differences in, 34–35
  mental retardation and, 89
  stressful (*See* Stress)
  traumatic
    acute stress disorder and, 1567–1580
    conversion as response to, 1760
    delayed recall of, 1625–1626, 1645
    depersonalization and, 1697–1700
    dissociative amnesia, dissociative fugue and, 1623–1647
    dissociative identity disorder and, 1653–1687
    posttraumatic stress disorder and, 1539–1559

Methyprylon
sleep disorders and, 2387, **2417**
withdrawal from, **687**
Methysergide, for progressive supranuclear palsy, 543
Metoclopramide
for migraine, 1791
neuroleptic malignant syndrome and, **435**, **436**
Metaidoioplasty, 2046–2047
Metrifonate, for Alzheimer's disease, 487, **488**
Metyrapone, for treatment-resistant depression, **1336**, 1339
Mexiletine, for neuropathic pain, 1790
MFT (multiple-family treatment), of schizophrenia, 1081–1082
Mianserin
combined with isocarboxazid, 1331, **1334**
neuroleptic malignant syndrome and, **436**
for trichotillomania, 2452
Michigan Alcohol Screening Test (MAST), 649, 659
"Midas touch syndrome," 2261
Midazolam
neuroleptic malignant syndrome and, **436**
withdrawal from, **685**
Migraine headache
antidepressants for, 1788
intermittent explosive disorder and, 2440
"triptans" for, 1791
Migration and mental health, 60–61
Milieu therapy
for antisocial personality disorder, 2264–2265
for schizophrenia, 1114–1115
Millon, T.
characterization of avoidant personality disorder, 2328–2330
characterization of dependent personality disorder, 2356
Millon Clinical Multiaxial Inventory-III, 2252
Miltown. *See* Meprobamate
Mind and brain, 3–16
diathesis-stress model of disease, 9–10
chronic pain, 1782
schizophrenia, 349, 1005, 1048–1049
etiology and pathogenesis of psychiatric disorders, 6–9
gender and, 21–40
mind-body problem, 4–6
biological naturalism, 5
dualistic thinking, 4, 383
materialism theories, 4–5
role of meaning, 10–12
treatment considerations and, 12–15
biological effects of psychotherapy, 5–6, 12–13, 22
combined psychotherapy-medication regimens, 13–14
personality and, 14–15
therapeutic alliance, 15
windows in human development for major brain structural changes, 8
Mini-Mental State Exam (MMSE), 392, 397, 486, 525, **525**, 527, 528
Minnesota Model of substance abuse treatment, 942, 956
Minnesota Multiphasic Personality Inventory (MMPI), 967
"Conversion V" configuration on, 1780
to differentiate genuine vs. feigned posttraumatic stress disorder, 1838
for patients with antisocial personality inventory, 2252
for sex offenders, 1957
for transvestites, 2015
utility in African-American population, 57
Minoxidil gel, for male erectile disorder, 1883
Mirtazapine, 156, 1155–1156
active metabolite of, 1156
for attention-deficit/hyperactivity disorder, **160**
dose-response relationship for, 1309
dose titration for, **1170**
mechanism of action of, 1155–1156, 1324
for melancholic depression, 1312
for mood disorders in children/adolescents, 261
for panic disorder, 1453
pharmacokinetics of, 1156
for posttraumatic stress disorder, 1545
side effects of, **160**, **2383**
for sleep disorders, **2383**
switching from another antidepressant to, **1335**, 1338
for treatment-resistant depression, 1324, **1327**
use in medically ill patients, 1394
Mivacurium, for electroconvulsive therapy, 1282
Mizoribine, for multiple sclerosis, 551

Monoamine reuptake inhibitors *(continued)*
selective serotonin reuptake inhibitors, 1148–1149, **1149**
Monomanias, 2435. *See also* Impulse-control disorders
Montgomery-Asberg Depression Rating Scale (MADRS), 1324
Mood disorders. *See also* Bipolar disorder; Depression; Mania
chronicity of, 1141
impulse-control disorders and, 2437, 2438
intermittent explosive disorder and, 2440
in medically ill patients
bipolar disorder, 1346
depression, 1314–1315
prevalence of, 1390
psychodynamic themes in, 1233–1235
recovery from, 1141
recurrence of, 1141
sleep disorders and, 2404, **2405**
substance use disorders and, 985–988
diagnosis of, 986
prevalence of, 985–986
treatment of, 986–988
Mood disorders of childhood/adolescence, 253–287
age-specific symptoms of, 254, **254**
assessment of, 253–255
comorbidity with, 254
anxiety disorders, 227
attention-deficit/hyperactivity disorder, 261
conduct disorder, 178, 179
learning disorders, 112
mental retardation, 84, 85
education for patients/families about, 255, **255**
preventive interventions for children at risk for, 281–283
relapse rate for, 255, 257, 281
Mood disorders treatment, 1133–1135
acute-phase treatment of depression, 1419–1432
antidepressants, 1144–1162, 1167–1171, **1168**, 1310, 1420–1421
declaring unsatisfactory response to, 1423, 1428–1429
determining need for, 1419
electroconvulsive therapy, 1270–1271, 1340
evaluating outcome of, 1420, 1428
light therapy, 1299
making diagnosis and choosing treatment, 1420–1423
medications combined with psychotherapy, 1250–1257, 1430–1432
objectives of, 1418, 1419
patient adherence to, 1418
psychotherapy, 1229–1230, 1429–1430
selecting initial treatment, 1420
selecting second treatment options, 1424–1425
settings for, 1418
antidepressant and antimanic agents, 1137–1173
for acute-phase treatment, 1144–1162, 1167–1171, **1168**, 1310, 1420–1429
case examples of, 1172–1173
combined with psychotherapy, 13–14, 1247–1262
for continuation/maintenance-phase treatment, 1162–1165, 1171–1172, 1310, 1432–1434
contraindications to, 1141
for depression, 1167–1172
discontinuation of, 1310
guidelines for treatment with, 1141–1144
indications for, 1138–1141
monitoring response to, 1170–1171, **1171**
no or inadequate response to, 1308–1311, 1423, 1428–1429
pharmacological properties of antidepressants, 1144–1156
pharmacological properties of antimanic agents, **1156**, 1156–1162
side effects of, 1165–1167
for chronic depression, 1249
combined medication and psychotherapy, 13–14, 1247–1262
for acute-phase treatment, 1250–1257, 1430–1432
AHCPR recommendations against use of, 1248
applications and procedures for, 1260
behavior therapy, 1253–1254
case examples of, 1260–1261
cognitive therapy and related cognitive-behavioral approaches, 1254–1257

Opiate antagonists *(continued)*
naltrexone for impulse-control disorders
compulsive buying, 2455
kleptomania, 2445
pathological gambling, 2450
psychogenic excoriation, 2459
repetitive self-mutilation, 555, 2456–2457
trichotillomania, 2453
naltrexone for opioid-detoxified patients, 809–823
benefits of, 812–814
compared with methadone, 813
dose and administration schedules for, 812, 818–819
for health care professionals, 812–815
pain management and, 820–821
as part of comprehensive treatment program, 813
for patients in heroin addiction programs, 817–818
for probationers in work-release programs, 816–817, **817**
side effects of, 813
for white-collar populations, 815–816
for obsessive-compulsive disorder, 1530
Opiate dependence
antagonist treatment for, 809–823
antisocial personality disorder and, 995
buprenorphine for, 794, 806, 821–822
deliriogenic effects of, **415**
dementia induced by, 588–589
detoxification for, 783–796
evaluation and diagnosis of, 785–787
interview, 786–787
laboratory testing, 787
methadone maintenance for, 799–806
new drugs for legal substitution treatment for, 806
treating mood disorders comorbid with, 987
Opiate detoxification, 783–796
acupuncture for, 794
buprenorphine for, 794
clonidine for, 790–792, **791**
clonidine-naltrexone ultrarapid withdrawal, 792, **793**
factors influencing severity of withdrawal symptoms, 784
medical conditions and, 795
for mixed addictions, 794
before naltrexone treatment, 811
onset and duration of withdrawal symptoms, 785, **785**
in pregnancy, 795
protracted abstinence syndrome, 785
seizures induced by, 794
setting for, 783
symptoms and signs of withdrawal, **784**, 784–785
ultrarapid withdrawal under anesthesia/sedation, 792–793
vomiting induced by, 795
withdrawal technique, 787–790
length of withdrawal, 789
methadone substitution, 787–789, **788**
for patients taking prescribed opioid analgesics for chronic pain, 1785–1786
short-term and long-term, 787
supportive measures and medications, 790
withdrawal from methadone maintenance, 789
Opiate receptors
agonist, antagonist, and partial agonist interactions with, 809–811
phencyclidine effects on, 736
Opiates
for chronic pain, 1784–1785
sleep disorders and, **2385**, **2418**
for terminally ill patients, 1795–1796
Opium tincture, withdrawal from, **788**
Oppositional defiant disorder, 152–153
genetic factors and, 180
mental retardation and, 85
pharmacotherapy for, **146**, 152–153
Orality and eating disorders, 2187–2189
Organic mental disorders, 383. *See also* Neuropsychiatry
phencyclidine-induced, 741
substance-related, 644, 646
Organic solvents, 589–590
Orgasmic disorder
female, 1895–1908 (*See also* Female sexual arousal disorder and female orgasmic disorder)
hypoactive sexual desire and, 1853
male, 1924–1929
Osheroff v. Chestnut Lodge, 1182
Ouabain, 451
Outcomes of treatment
for adjustment disorders, 1718

imaginal desensitization, 1988–1989
olfactory aversion, 1986–1987
satiation, 1987–1988
selective serotonin reuptake inhibitors, 1990–1991
surgical interventions, 1989
to resolve intrapsychic conflicts, 1995–1996
family systems therapy, 1996
psychodynamic psychotherapy, 1996
sexual addiction treatment, 1996–1997
steps in, 1983
trauma model treatment, 1997
Peer interventions
for conduct disorder, 183
in therapeutic communities, 972
Pellagra, 585
D-Penicillamine
for lead poisoning, 592
for Wilson's disease, 544
Penicillin, **450**, 453
Penile prostheses, 1882–1883
Pentamidine, **418**
Pentobarbital
for drug-facilitated interview, 1680
mechanism of action of, 451
withdrawal from, 679, **687**
Pentoxifylline, for vascular dementia, 524
Perceptual distortions
in delirium, 393
in schizophrenia, 1012
Pergolide
for restless legs syndrome and periodic limb movements, **2385**, 2400
for treatment-resistant depression, 1321, 1322, **1326**
Periodic limb movements (PLM) during sleep, 2399–2400
definition of, 2399
treatment of, 2399–2400
behavioral/psychotherapeutic treatment, 2399
pharmacotherapy, **2380**, **2385**, 2399–2400
Perphenazine, for Huntington's disease, 540
Persistence, 14
Personal therapy (PT), for schizophrenia, 1047
Personality disorders, 2223–2225
antisocial personality disorder, 2251–2267
avoidant personality disorder, 2327–2337
borderline personality disorder, 2273–2287
comorbidity with
bipolar disorder, 1345–1346
conversion disorder, 1757–1758
mental retardation, 82, 84
mood disorders, 1316, 1421–1422
Munchausen syndrome, 1827
other personality disorders, 2223
repetitive self-mutilation, 2455–2456
somatization disorder, 1743
substance use disorders, 995–996
dependent personality disorder, 2353–2365
early trauma and, 31–32
gender and, 33
histrionic personality disorder, 2293–2306
long-term stability of, 2225
narcissistic personality disorder, 2309–2325
obsessive-compulsive personality disorder, 2341–2349
paranoid personality disorder, 2227–2235
recent literature on, 2225
schizoid and schizotypal personality disorders, 2237–2247
temperament, character and, 14–15
theories of, 2224
treatment of, 2223–2225 (*See also* specific personality disorders)
with concurrent depression, 1228–1229
cost-effectiveness of, 2225
in dual diagnosis patients, 996
history of, 2224
pharmacotherapy, 2224–2225
psychotherapy, 2223–2224
recent trends in, 2224–2225
Personality Inventory for Children, **229**
Personality traits
anorexia nervosa and, 2179
bulimia nervosa and, 2124
cultural influences on, 54
delirium and, 392
dependency, 2354, 2356–2357
development of, 31
mental retardation and, 81–82
dissociative identity disorder and, 1655 (*See also* Alters in dissociative identity disorder)
generalized anxiety disorder and, 1588
hallucinogen effects on, 695, 698–699
paranoid, 2229
substance abuse and, 640
persons entering therapeutic communities, 967
transvestism and, 2015

circadian rhythm sleep disorder, 2398–2399
due to general medical condition, 2415
hypersomnia, 2393
insomnia, 2392–2393
narcolepsy, 2394–2395
nightmare disorder, 2401
REM sleep behavior disorder, 2404
restless legs syndrome and periodic limb movements, 2399–2400
sleep terror disorder and sleepwalking disorder, 2403
substance-induced sleep disorder, 2420
for somatoform disorders
body dysmorphic disorder, 1816–1817
chronic pain, 1784–1791
conversion disorder, 1767
hypochondriasis, 1810–1811
for substance use disorders, 629, 781–823
alcoholism, 628, 669–675, 841–842
antagonist treatment, 809–823
in children/adolescents, 334
detoxification, 783–796
in dual diagnosis patients, 982–983, **983**
inappropriate uses of, 639–640
methadone maintenance, 799–806
nicotine dependence, 766–769, **767–768**
stimulant abuse, 725–728
for Tourette's disorder, 199–204, **200–203**
for vulvar vestibulitis syndrome, 1938
Phenacetin, 587
Phenazepam, for depersonalization, 1709
Phencyclidine (PCP), 628, 735–743
abuse of and dependence on, 741–743
clinical features and diagnosis of, 741–742
management of, 742–743
central nervous system effects of, 736
as contaminant in other drugs, 735
craving for, 742
delirium caused by, 740–741
dementia induced by, 589
epidemiology of use of, 736
excitotoxic effects of, **450**
history of, 735
incidence of use of, 627, 628
intoxication with, 737–740
complications of, 739–740
diagnosis of, 737
differential diagnosis of, 737
laboratory testing for, 737
management of, 737–739
stages of, 737, **738**
manufacture of, 735
organic mental disorder caused by, 741
patterns of abuse of, 736
pharmacokinetics of, 736
prenatal exposure to, 740
psychological effects of, 736–737
routes of administration for, 736
street names for, 737
withdrawal from, 742
Phenelzine, 161, **1147**, 1152
for anxiety disorders
in children/adolescents, 238–239
obsessive-compulsive disorder, 1525
panic disorder, 1452, 1458, 1461
posttraumatic stress disorder, 1544
social phobia, 238, 1488, 1490–1491, 1498, 2333
for attention-deficit/hyperactivity disorder, **158**
for bulimia nervosa, **2162**
for depression
atypical depression, 1312, 1421
combined with amitriptyline, 1331, **1334**
compared with cognitive therapy, 1204, **1205**
with concurrent borderline personality disorder, 1316
maintenance treatment, 1164
with panic attacks, 1315
dosage of, 1152
for personality disorders
avoidant personality disorder, 2333
avoidant personality disorders, 2333
borderline personality disorder, 2283
for premature ejaculation, 1922
side effects of, 1498
for sleep disorders, 2386
switching from tricyclic antidepressant to, **1335**, 1338
Phenobarbital
substitution equivalents for sedative-hypnotic withdrawal, **687**
high-dose benzodiazepine withdrawal, **685**, 685–686
low-dose benzodiazepine withdrawal, 687–688
withdrawal from, 680
Phenoxybenzamine intracavernous injections, for male erectile disorder, 1884

Phentolamine, for male erectile disorder, 1889
  intracavernous injections, 1884–1885
DL-Phenylalanine, for attention-deficit/hyperactivity disorder, 152
Phenylketonuria, 85, 99
Phenytoin
  for aggressive behavior, **2262**, 2263
  for alcohol withdrawal seizures, 668
  for bulimia nervosa, 2160
  hypersomnia induced by, **2419**
  for intermittent explosive disorder, 2441–2442
  for neuropathic pain, 1790
Phobias, 1485–1506
  comorbidity with
    mental retardation, 84, 85
    panic disorder, **1449**
  gender and, **37**
  social phobia, 1486–1499
  specific, 1499–1506
Phoenix House, 892
Phosphatidylcholine, for Alzheimer's disease, 483
Photosensitivity, as contraindication to light therapy, 1298
Phototherapy. *See* Light therapy
Physical Self-Maintenance Scale (PSMS), 485
Physical therapy
  for chronic pain, 1792–1794
  for conversion disorder, 1767
Physician-assisted suicide, 1795–1796
Physostigmine
  for Alzheimer's disease, 484, **488**, 502, 554
  for anticholinergic toxicity, 401, 427, 502
  contraindications to, 401
  for Friedreich's ataxia, 544
Piaget, Jean, 52
Pica, 592
Pick bodies, 539
Pick complex, 539
Pick's disease, 538–539
  clinical features of, 539
  differentiation from Alzheimer's disease, 539
  genetics of, 538–539
  neuropathology of, 539
Picture exchange communication system, 136
Pills Anonymous, 883
Pilocarpine
  for Alzheimer's disease, 489
  excitotoxic effects of, **450**
Pimozide
  for anorexia nervosa, 2163–2164
  for anxiety disorders in children/adolescents, 238
  for factitious disorder, 1829
  neuroleptic malignant syndrome and, **435**
  side effects of, **201**, **202**
  for tic disorders, 200, **201**, **202**, **202**
  for trichotillomania, 2452
PIMRA (Psychopathology Instrument for Mentally Retarded Adults), 84
Pindolol
  for attention-deficit/hyperactivity disorder, 151
  for behavioral problems in patients with dementia, 554
  for obsessive-compulsive disorder, 1530
  for treatment-resistant depression, 1323–1324, **1327**
Piperidines, 486
Piracetam, 597
  for Alzheimer's disease, 495
Piribedil, for treatment-resistant depression, 1321, 1322
Pivotal response training, for autism, 135
Placidyl. *See* Ethchlorvynol
Plasma exchange, for obsessive-compulsive disorder, 1530
Platelet aggregation inhibitors, for vascular dementia, 524–525
Play therapy, for posttraumatic stress disorder in children/adolescents, 295–298
Poisoning
  aluminum, 590–591
  arsenic, 593
  cadmium, 591
  delirium and, 400
  dementia and, **549**, 549–550, 590–593
  lead, 591–592
  manganese, 592–593
  mercury, 592
  thallium, 593
  tin, 593
Polycystic ovary disease, divalproex-induced, 269
Polysomnography, 2374
  for children, 366, 372
    for sleep apnea, 372
  indications for, 2374
Pornography dependence, **1954**

Side effects, of drugs *(continued)*
gamma-hydroxybutyrate, 754
guanfacine, **163, 203**
haloperidol, **201, 202**, 403–404
lamotrigine, 1161–1162
lithium, 185, 1158
magnesium pemoline, 1322, 2388
N-Methyl-D-aspartate receptor antagonists, 598
mirtazapine, **160, 2383**
moclobemide, 1153
modafinil, 2388
monoamine oxidase inhibitors, 150, **158**, 161, 239, 263, 1152, 1165–1167, 1396, 1452, 1498
naltrexone, 813, 842
nefazodone, **159, 258,** 1155
olanzapine, 347–348, 1034
paroxetine, **258**
phenelzine, 1498
pimozide, **201, 202**
propranolol, **163**
risperidone, 200–201, **201, 202**
selective serotonin reuptake inhibitors, **158, 202,** 237, 257, 260, 457–458, **458,** 1148–1149, 1165–1167, 1166, 1391, 1459–1460, 1526, 1607, 1887, 1927, 1960, **2382**
sertraline, **258**
stimulants, **154,** 154–155, **203,** 1153, 1323, 1396–1397, **2384,** 2388
tacrine, 485
topiramate, 1162
trazodone, 263, 1154, 1607, **2383**
tricyclic antidepressants, 156, **157,** 185, **203,** 215, 235–236, 261–263, 1150, 1165–1167, 1426, 1461, 1607, **2381**
valproic acid, 269, 1160
venlafaxine, **159, 258,** 1150
yohimbine, 1886
of electroconvulsive therapy, 1275–1277
of light therapy, 1302, 2389
Sildenafil, 1873, 1886–1889
for antidepressant-induced sexual dysfunction, 1886–1887
case example of, 1887
cardiovascular effects of, 1888
cost of, 1888
deaths after use of, 1888
dosage and timing of administration of, 1887, 1888
drug interactions with, 1888
for erectile dysfunction of various etiologies, 1886
for male orgasmic disorder, 1927
mechanism of action of, 1886
patient counseling before initiation of, 1888
pharmacokinetics of, 1886
psychosocial factors and use of, 1888–1889
Simple phobias. *See* Specific phobias
Single photon emission computed tomography (SPECT), 12
in degenerative dementias, 581
in substance-induced persisting dementia and amnestic disorder, 594
SIPAD. *See* Substance-induced persisting amnestic disorder
SIPD. *See* Substance-induced persisting dementia
SIT. *See* Stress inoculation training
β-Site APP cleaving enzyme (BACE), 491
Skills training, 1095–1099. *See also* Problem-solving skills training; Social skills training
curriculum modules for, 1096, 1106
empirical evaluation of, 1098
generalization to other outcomes, 1098
in vivo amplified, 1101
instructional methods for, 1097, 1107–1108
learning activities for, 1096, **1097**
learning skills and retaining them, 1098
symptomatology and, 1099
transfer of, 1098
Skin cancer
group therapy for melanoma patients, 13
light therapy for persons with history of, 1297
Skin picking. *See* Psychogenic excoriation
Sleep apnea. *See* Breathing-related sleep disorder
Sleep deprivation
sleep restriction for patients with for sleep disorders, 2377
for treatment-resistant depression, 1339–1340
Sleep disorders, 2371–2374
in Alzheimer's disease, **498,** 503–504
classification of, 360–361, 2372
dyssomnias, 360, **361–363,** 2372, **2373**
parasomnias, 360, **364, 365, 2373**